Imaging in Neurology

OSBORN | DIGRE

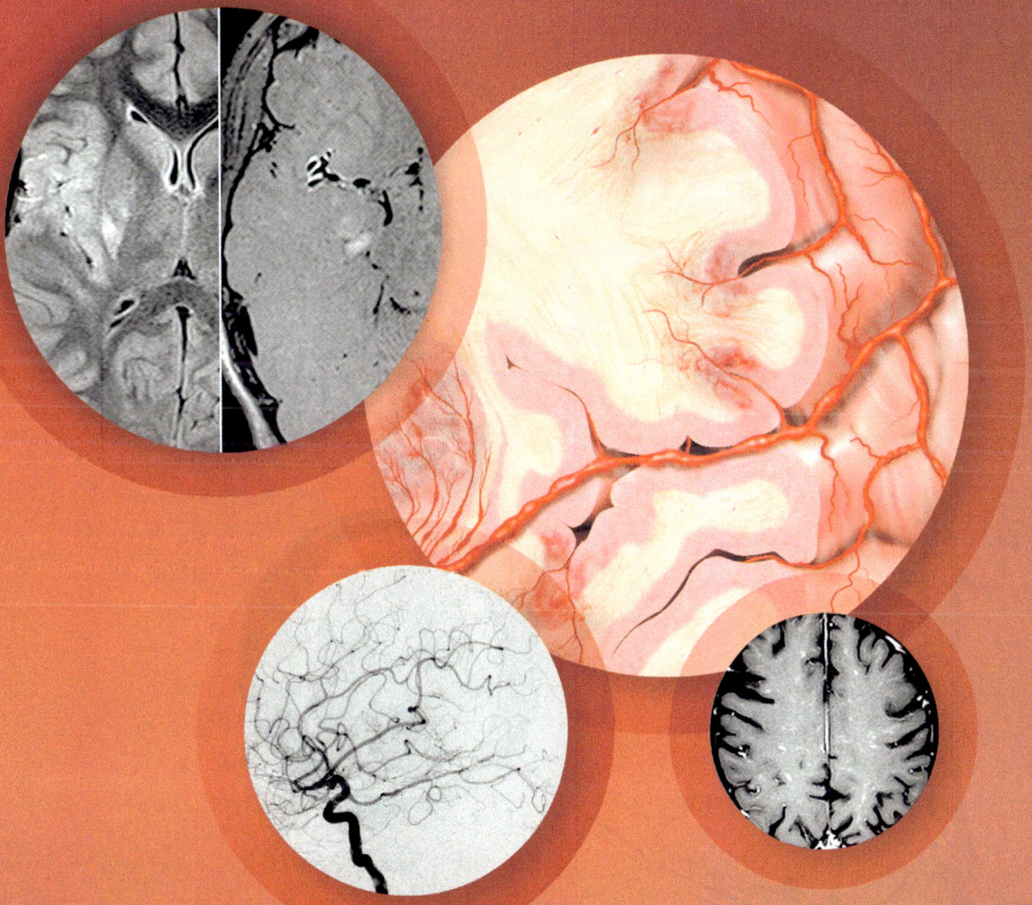

ELSEVIER

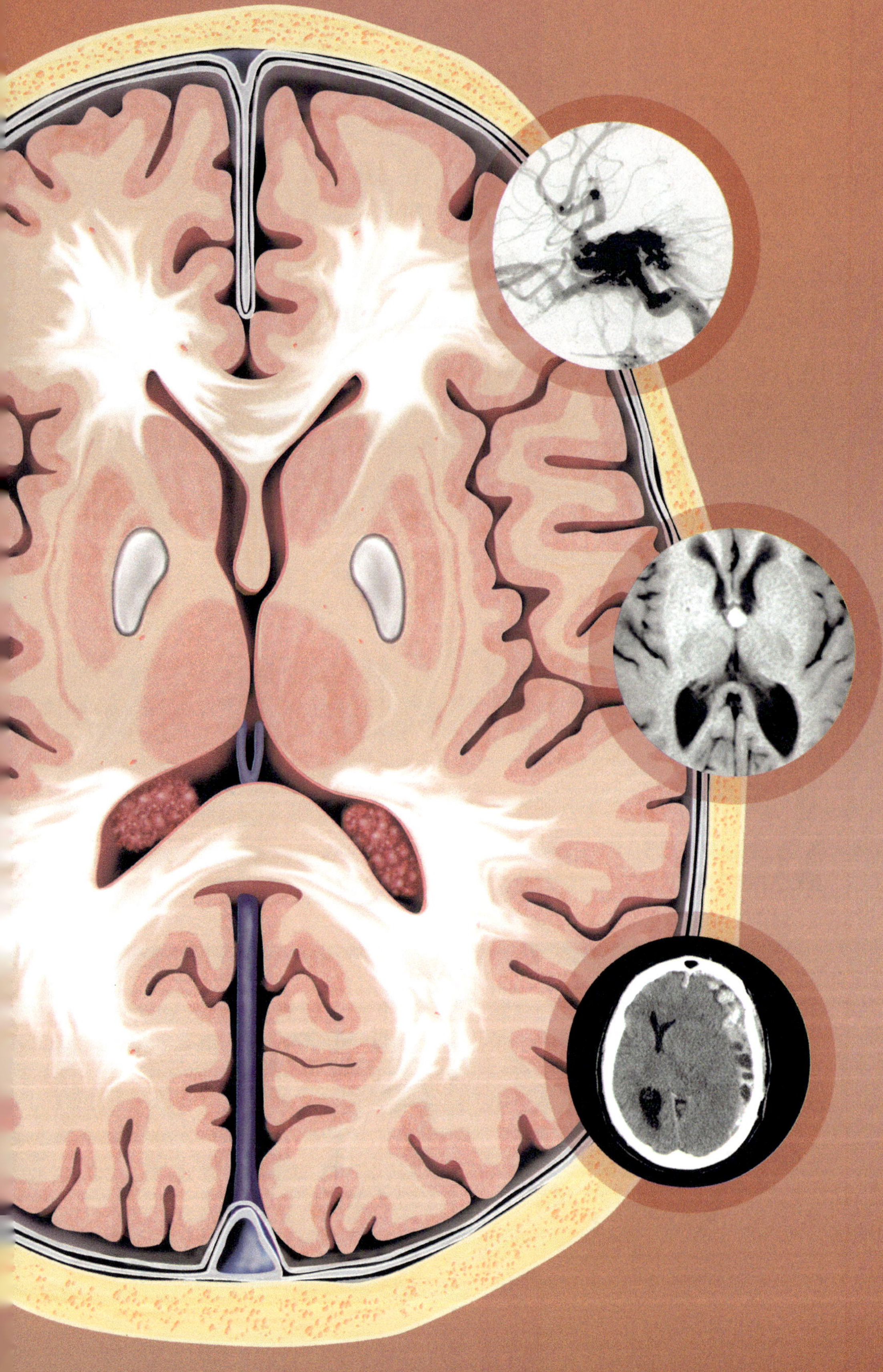

Imaging in Neurology

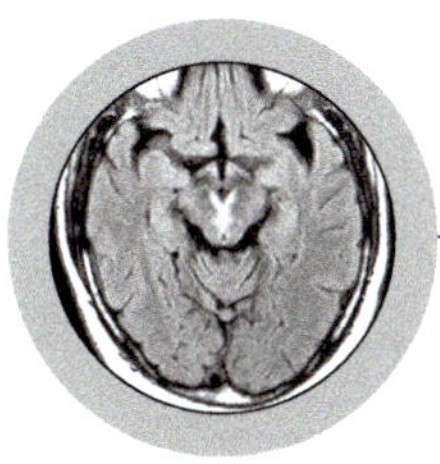

Anne G. Osborn, MD, FACR

University Distinguished Professor
William H. and Patricia W. Child Presidential Endowed Chair
University of Utah School of Medicine
Salt Lake City, Utah

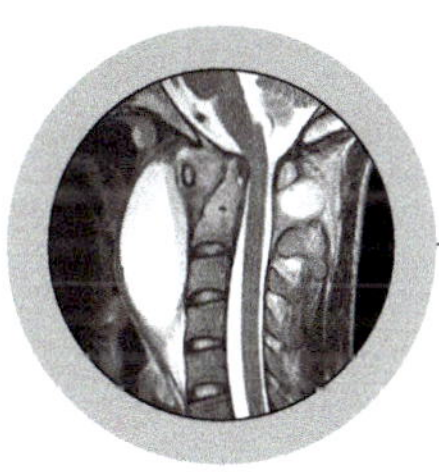

Kathleen B. Digre, MD

Professor of Neurology, University of Utah School of Medicine
Chief, Division of Headache and Neuro-Ophthalmology
John A. Moran Eye Center
Salt Lake City, Utah

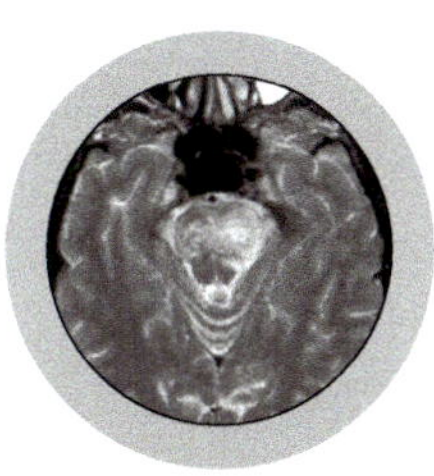

ELSEVIER

1600 John F. Kennedy Blvd.
Ste 1800
Philadelphia, PA 19103-2899

IMAGING IN NEUROLOGY

ISBN: 978-0-323-44781-2

Notices

Knowledge and best practice in this field are constantly changing. As new research and experience broaden our understanding, changes in research methods, professional practices, or medical treatment may become necessary.

Practitioners and researchers must always rely on their own experience and knowledge in evaluating and using any information, methods, compounds, or experiments described herein. In using such information or methods they should be mindful of their own safety and the safety of others, including parties for whom they have a professional responsibility.

With respect to any drug or pharmaceutical products identified, readers are advised to check the most current information provided (i) on procedures featured or (ii) by the manufacturer of each product to be administered, to verify the recommended dose or formula, the method and duration of administration, and contraindications. It is the responsibility of practitioners, relying on their own experience and knowledge of their patients, to make diagnoses, to determine dosages and the best treatment for each individual patient, and to take all appropriate safety precautions.

To the fullest extent of the law, neither the Publisher nor the authors, contributors, or editors, assume any liability for any injury and/or damage to persons or property as a matter of products liability, negligence or otherwise, or from any use or operation of any methods, products, instructions, or ideas contained in the material herein.

Publisher Cataloging-in-Publication Data

Names: Osborn, Anne G., 1943- | Digre, Kathleen B.
Title: Imaging in neurology / [edited by] Anne G. Osborn and Kathleen B. Digre.
Description: First edition. | Salt Lake City, UT : Elsevier, Inc., [2016] | Includes bibliographical references and index.
Identifiers: ISBN 978-0-323-44781-2
Subjects: LCSH: Neurology--Handbooks, manuals, etc. | Nervous system--Imaging----Handbooks, manuals, etc. | MESH: Neurology--Atlases. | Nervous System--Atlases. | Functional Neuroimaging--Atlases.
Classification: LCC RC349.D52 O83 2016 | NLM WL 141 | DDC 616.804754--dc23

International Standard Book Number: 978-0-323-44781-2

Cover Designer: Tom M. Olson, BA

Printed in the United States of America

Last digit is the print number: 9 8 7 6 5 4 3

Dedication

To my husband, Michael Varner, for his neverending love and encouragement.

KBD

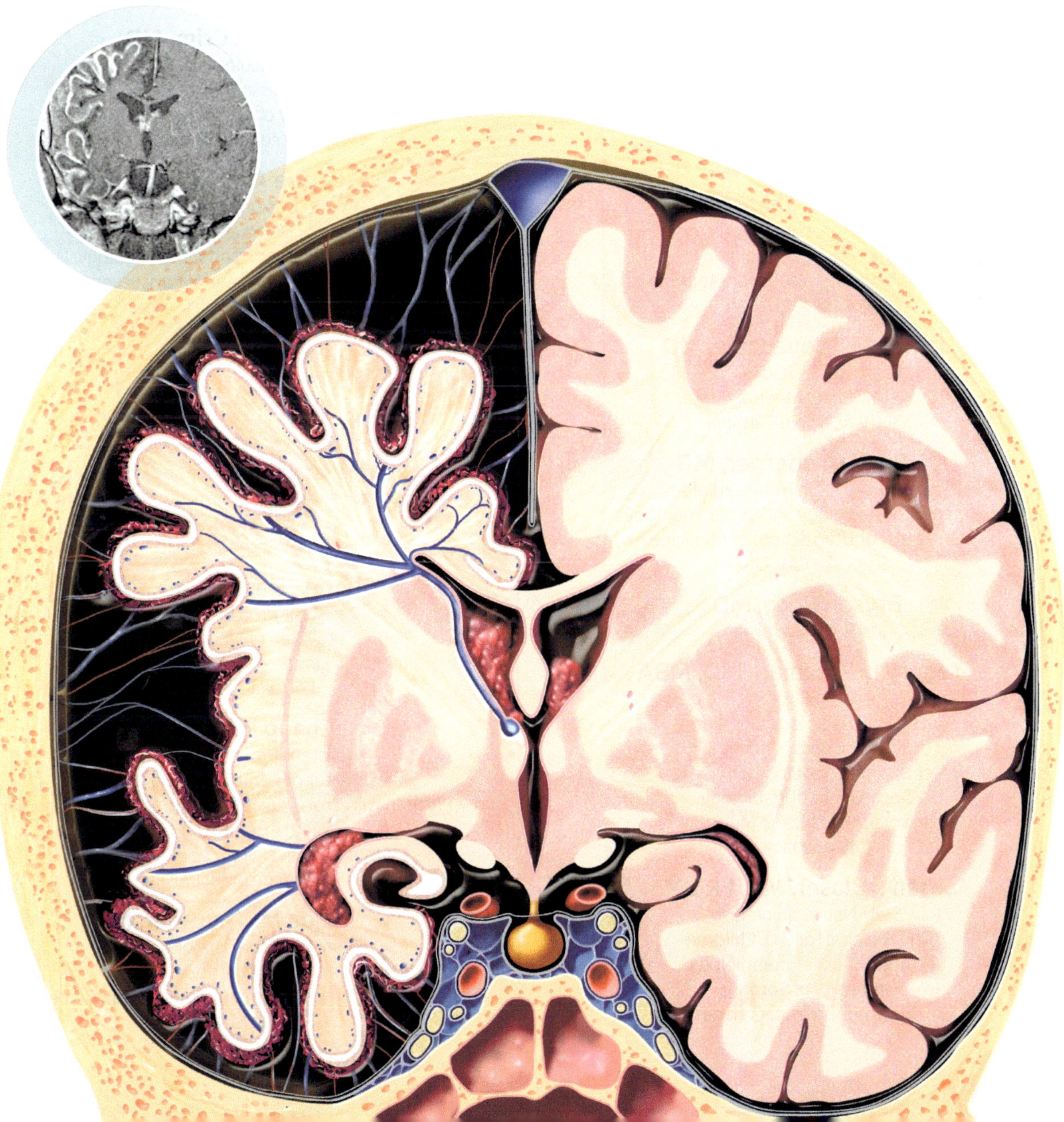

Contributing Authors

Miral D. Jhaveri, MD
Associate Professor
Director of Neuroradiology
Department of Diagnostic Radiology & Nuclear Medicine
Rush University Medical Center
Chicago, Illinois

Karen L. Salzman, MD
Professor of Radiology
Leslie W. Davis Endowed Chair in Neuroradiology
University of Utah School of Medicine
Salt Lake City, Utah

Jeffrey S. Ross, MD
Senior Associate Consultant
Neuroradiology Division
Department of Radiology
Mayo Clinic Arizona
Professor of Radiology
Mayo Clinic College of Medicine
Phoenix, Arizona

Kevin R. Moore, MD
Pediatric Neuroradiologist
Primary Children's Hospital
Salt Lake City, Utah

Lubdha M. Shah, MD
Associate Professor of Radiology
Division of Neuroradiology
University of Utah School of Medicine
Salt Lake City, Utah

James M. Provenzale, MD
Professor of Radiology
Duke University Medical Center
Durham, North Carolina

H. Ric Harnsberger, MD
R.C. Willey Chair in Neuroradiology
Professor of Radiology and Otolaryngology
University of Utah School of Medicine
Salt Lake City, Utah

Bryson Borg, MD
Fairfield, California

Gregory L. Katzman, MD, MBA
Professor, Neuroradiology
Vice Chair, Radiology Operations
Chief Quality Officer
Chief Business Development Officer
Department of Radiology
University of Chicago Medicine
Chicago, Illinois

Susan I. Blaser, MD, FRCPC
Staff Neuroradiologist
The Hospital for Sick Children
Professor of Neuroradiology
University of Toronto
Toronto, Ontario, Canada

Bronwyn E. Hamilton, MD
Professor of Radiology
Oregon Health & Science University
Portland, Oregon

Perry P. Ng, MBBS (Hons), FRANZCR
Adjunct Associate Professor, Department of Radiology
University of Utah School of Medicine
Salt Lake City, Utah
Interventional Neuroradiologist
Centura Health Physician Group
Denver, Colorado

A. James Barkovich, MD
Professor of Radiology and Biomedical Imaging, Neurology, Pediatrics and Neurological Surgery
UCSF-Benioff Children's Hospital
University of California, San Francisco
San Francisco, California

Julia R. Crim, MD
Chief of Musculoskeletal Radiology
Professor of Radiology
University of Missouri at Columbia
Columbia, Missouri

Laurie A. Loevner, MD
Chief, Division of Neuroradiology
Director, Head and Neck Radiology
Professor of Radiology, Otorhinolaryngology: Head and Neck Surgery, and Neurosurgery
University of Pennsylvania Health System Perelman School of Medicine at the University of Pennsylvania
Philadelphia, Pennsylvania

Gilbert Vézina, MD
Director, Program in Neuroradiology
Children's National Medical Center
Professor of Radiology and Pediatrics
The George Washington University School of Medicine and Health Sciences
Washington, DC

Sheri L. Harder, MD, FRCPC
Assistant Professor of Radiology
Division of Neuroradiology
Loma Linda University Medical Center
Loma Linda, California

Chang Yueh Ho, MD
Assistant Professor of Radiology
Director of Pediatric Neuroradiology
Program Director, Pediatric Neuroradiology Fellowship
Riley Hospital for Children
Indiana University School of Medicine
Indianapolis, Indiana

Majda M. Thurnher, MD
Associate Professor of Radiology
Medical University of Vienna
Department of Biomedical Imaging and Image-Guided Therapy
Vienna, Austria

H. Christian Davidson, MD
Professor of Radiology
University of Utah School of Medicine
Salt Lake City, Utah

Yoshimi Anzai, MD, MPH
Professor of Radiology
Associate Chief Medical Quality Officer
University of Utah
Salt Lake City, Utah

Anna Illner, MD
Pediatric Neuroradiologist
Texas Children's Hospital
Assistant Professor of Radiology
Baylor College of Medicine
Houston, Texas

Ulrich Rassner, MD
Associate Professor of Radiology
Division of Neuroradiology
University of Utah School of Medicine
Salt Lake City, Utah

Charles Raybaud, MD, FRCPC
Derek Harwood-Nash Chair in Medical Imaging
Division Head of Neuroradiology
The Hospital for Sick Children
Professor of Radiology
University of Toronto
Toronto, Ontario, Canada

John H. Rees, MD
Chief of Neuroradiology: Partners Imaging
Sarasota, Florida
Assistant Professor of Radiology
Georgetown University
Previously: Visiting Scientist
Armed Forces Institute of Pathology
Washington, DC

Jeffrey S. Anderson, MD, PhD
Associate Professor of Radiology and Bioengineering
University of Utah School of Medicine
Salt Lake City, Utah

P. Ellen Grant, MD
Associate Professor in Radiology, Harvard Medical School
Founding Director, Center for Fetal-Neonatal Neuroimaging
and Developmental Science
Director of Fetal and Neonatal Neuroimaging Research
Boston Children's Hospital Endowed Chair in Neonatology
Boston Children's Hospital
Boston, Massachusetts

Gary L. Hedlund, DO
Adjunct Professor of Radiology
University of Utah School of Medicine
Pediatric Neuroradiologist
Department of Medical Imaging
Primary Children's Hospital
Salt Lake City, Utah

Blaise V. Jones, MD
Associate Director of Radiology
Neuroradiology Section Chief
Cincinnati Children's Hospital Medical Center
Professor of Clinical Radiology and Pediatrics
University of Cincinnati College of Medicine
Cincinnati, Ohio

Luke N. Ledbetter, MD
Assistant Professor of Radiology
Division of Neuroradiology
University of Kansas Medical Center
Kansas City, Kansas

Deborah R. Shatzkes, MD
Professor of Radiology
Hofstra North Shore-LIJ School of Medicine
Chief, Head & Neck Radiology
Lenox Hill Hospital and
The New York Head & Neck Institute
North Shore-LIJ Health System
New York, New York

Rebecca S. Cornelius, MD, FACR
Professor of Radiology and Otolaryngology-
Head and Neck Surgery
University of Cincinnati College of Medicine
University of Cincinnati Medical Center
Cincinnati, Ohio

Patricia A. Hudgins, MD, FACR
Professor of Radiology/Otolaryngology
Director of Head & Neck Radiology
Department of Radiology and Imaging Sciences
Emory University School of Medicine
Atlanta, Georgia

Nicholas A. Koontz, MD
Assistant Professor of Clinical Radiology
Department of Radiology and Imaging Sciences
Indiana University School of Medicine
Indianapolis, Indiana

Gary M. Nesbit, MD
Professor of Radiology, Neurology, Neurological Surgery
and the Dotter Interventional Institute
Oregon Health & Science University
Portland, Oregon

Edward P. Quigley, III, MD, PhD
Assistant Professor of Radiology
Division of Neuroradiology
University of Utah School of Medicine
Salt Lake City, Utah

Palmi Shah, MD
Assistant Professor
Rush University Medical Center
Chicago, Illinois

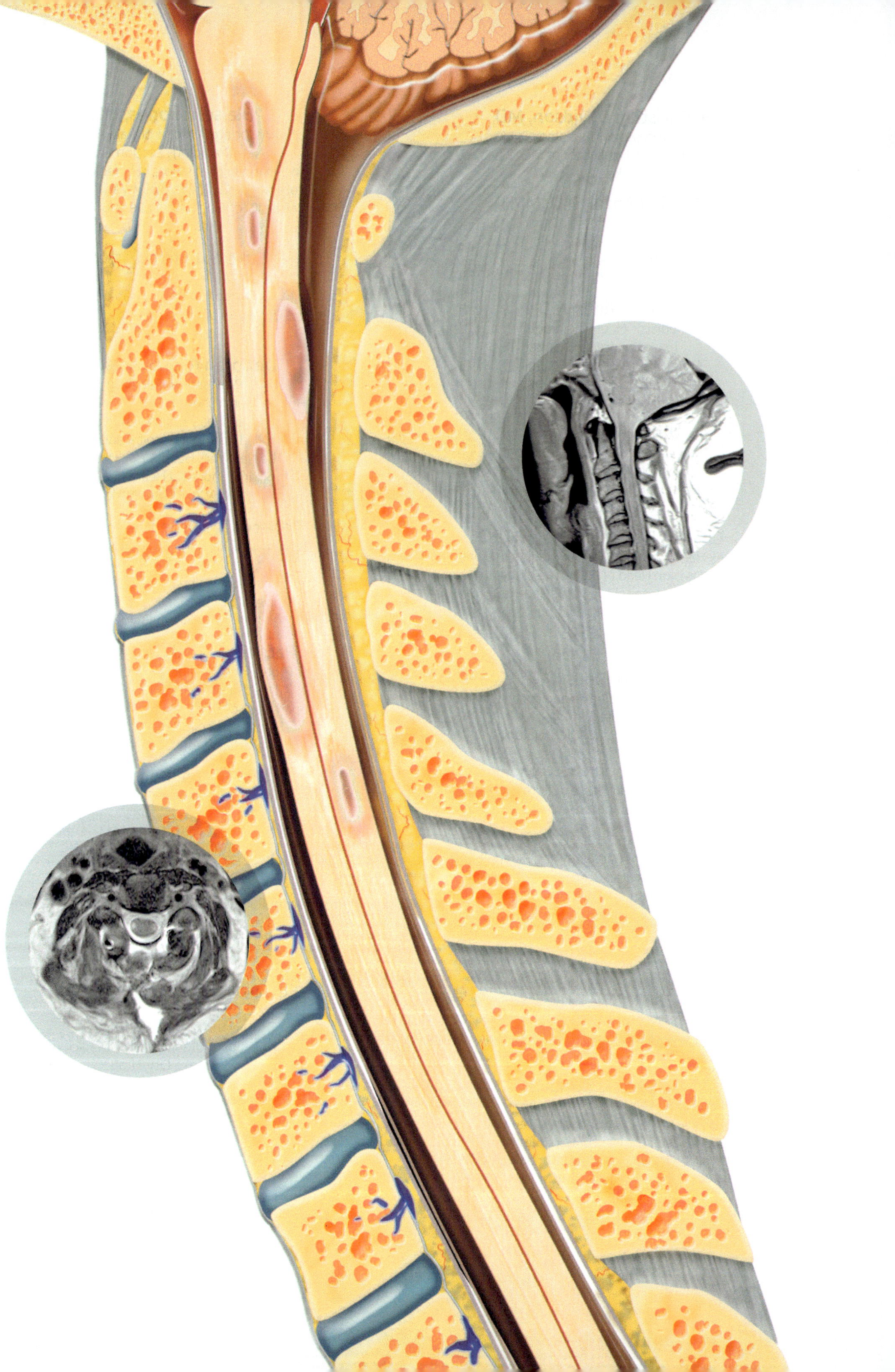

Preface

Anne Osborn and I have been colleagues for almost our entire careers. When she approached me about joining her to edit a book for neurologists on imaging, I didn't have to think twice. Neurologists use imaging every day as an extension of the neurological examination. In fact, imaging is critical to making the correct diagnosis and following patients. Yet, the best imaging books are all in neuroradiology. Here was a chance to partner with one of the premier neuroradiologists to produce a book that would be practical and useful to my neurological colleagues around the world. What wasn't to like?!

The book's purpose is to provide key imaging findings to the most common and important neurological disorders in an easy-to-understand format, using typical imaging examples, pathological examples when appropriate, and gorgeous drawings that illustrate key findings. We have also included clinical photos where indicated.

The book is divided into three parts—an introduction to imaging in general, imaging of the brain from pathology-based and anatomic-based diagnoses, and spine imaging. There are overview chapters to difficult subjects like congenital malformations, trauma, vascular anatomy, neoplasms, infectious diseases, and metabolic disorders. There are anatomic overviews of the ventricles, the pituitary, cerebellar pontine angle, and the orbit. The spine section also has a wonderful review of normal anatomy and then develops a complex subject made simple.

Each chapter is written by outstanding neuroradiologists who point out the main imaging findings for each disorder or anatomic area. We then addressed key clinical features. The organization of each chapter makes it really easy for a neurologist to quickly know the key terminology, imaging findings, pathologic underpinnings, and important clinical details. Images were specifically chosen to be classic examples, and Anne Osborn labored for many hours putting arrows on every structure that is described so that all of us neurologists know exactly what the key findings are.

We see this book being of value to every practicing neurologist or physician who sees general neurology patients. In addition, we see residents using this book to study for in-service and board exams.

We have many people to thank in producing this book. First, we relied on two fellows from the University of Utah who completed neurological residencies and are currently in fellowship—Dr. Kelsey Juster-Switlyk and Dr. Reuben Valenzuela. These two highlighted areas that were not clear or key points that were missing. Our fabulous senior editor, Dr. Karen E. Concannon, kept us on schedule.

Finally, we thank our families and colleagues for giving us the time and space to finish the project.

Kathleen B. Digre, MD

Professor of Neurology, University of Utah School of Medicine
Chief, Division of Headache and Neuro-Ophthalmology
John A. Moran Eye Center
Salt Lake City, Utah

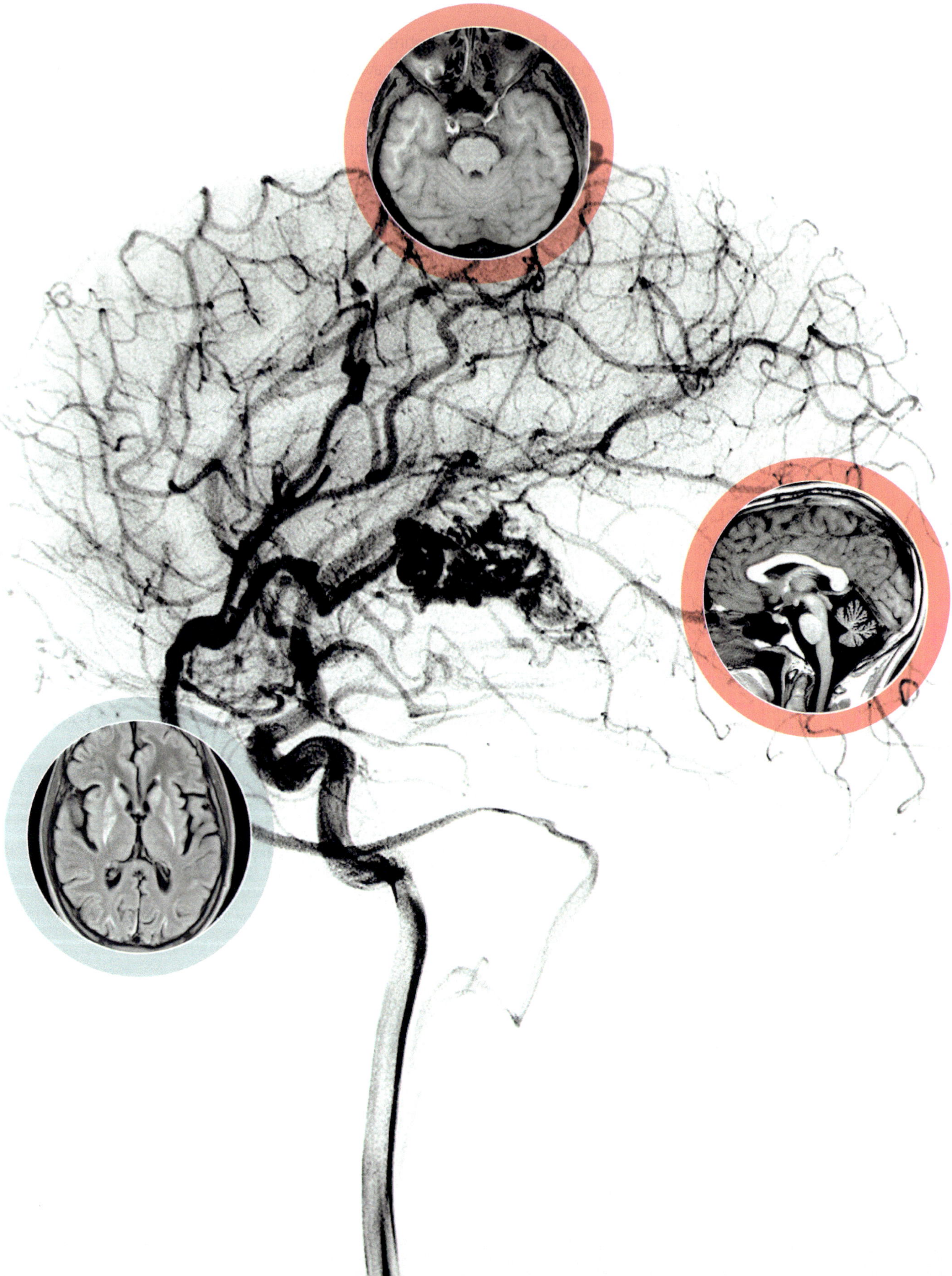

Acknowledgments

Text Editors

Arthur G. Gelsinger, MA
Nina I. Bennett, BA
Tricia L. Cannon, BA
Terry W. Ferrell, MS
Lisa A. Gervais, BS
Emily C. Fassett, BA

Image Editors

Jeffrey J. Marmorstone, BS
Lisa A. M. Steadman, BS

Medical Editors

Kelsey Juster-Switlyk, MD
Reuben Mari Valenzuela, MD

Illustrations

Laura C. Sesto, MA
Lane R. Bennion, MS
Richard Coombs, MS

Art Direction and Design

Tom M. Olson, BA
Laura C. Sesto, MA

Lead Editor

Karen E. Concannon, MA, PhD

Production Coordinators

Angela M. Terry, BA
Rebecca L. Hutchinson, BA

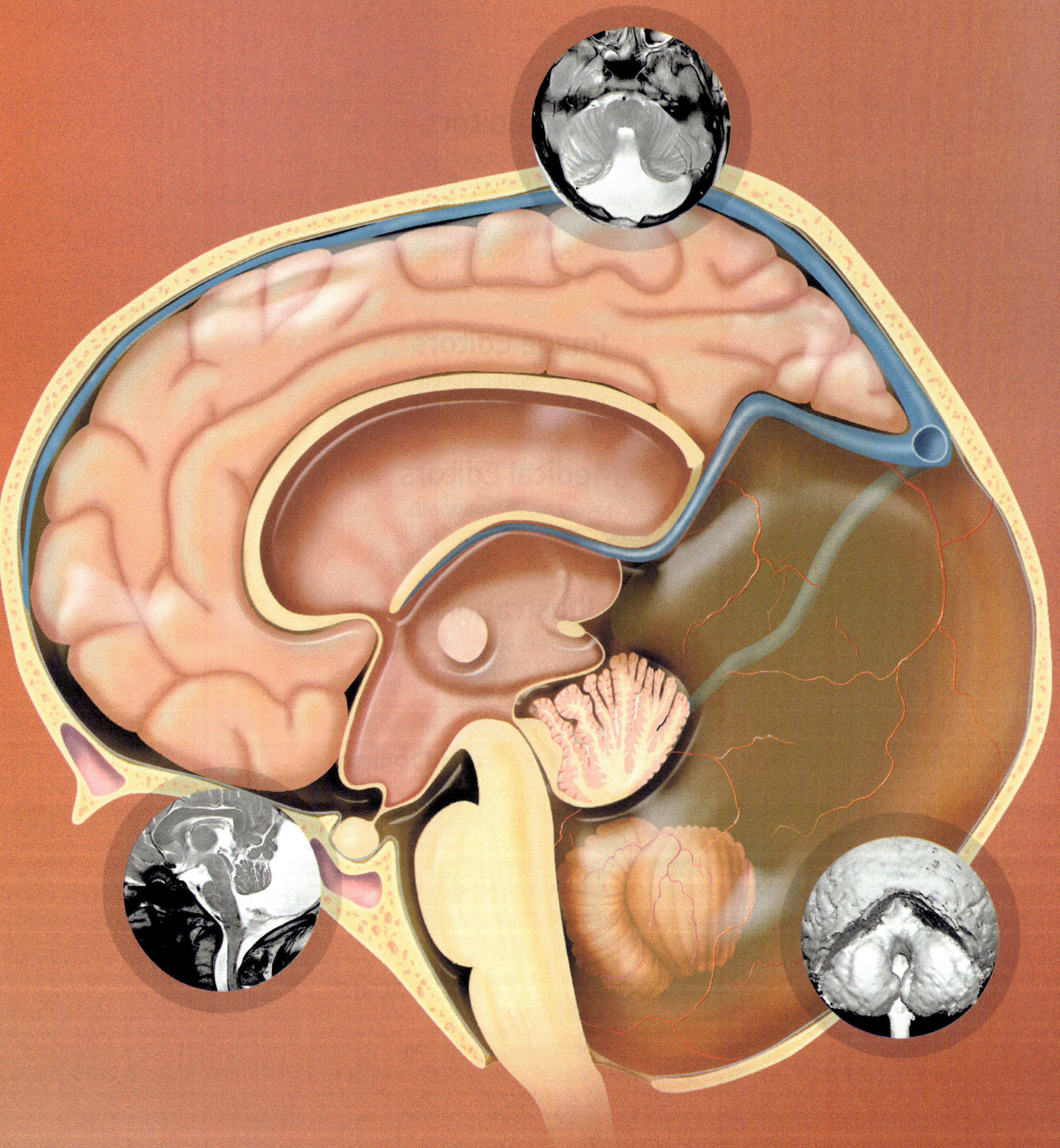

Sections

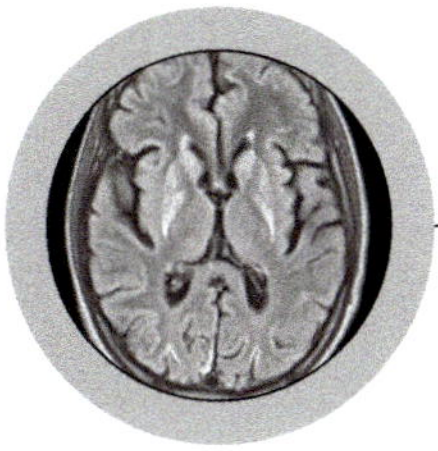

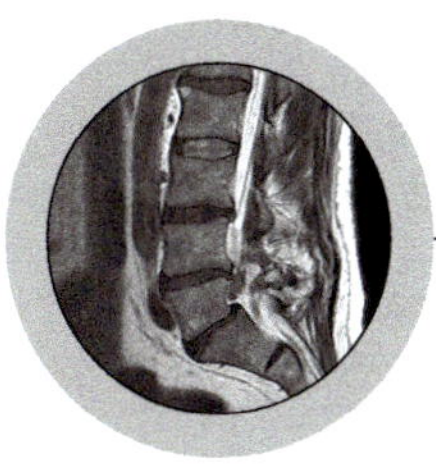

TABLE OF CONTENTS

Part I: Brain

SECTION 1: PATHOLOGY-BASED DIAGNOSES: MALFORMATIONS, TRAUMA, AND STROKE

CONGENITAL MALFORMATIONS

TRAUMA

TABLE OF CONTENTS

TABLE OF CONTENTS

TABLE OF CONTENTS

TABLE OF CONTENTS

TABLE OF CONTENTS

TABLE OF CONTENTS

TABLE OF CONTENTS

Imaging in Neurology

OSBORN | DIGRE

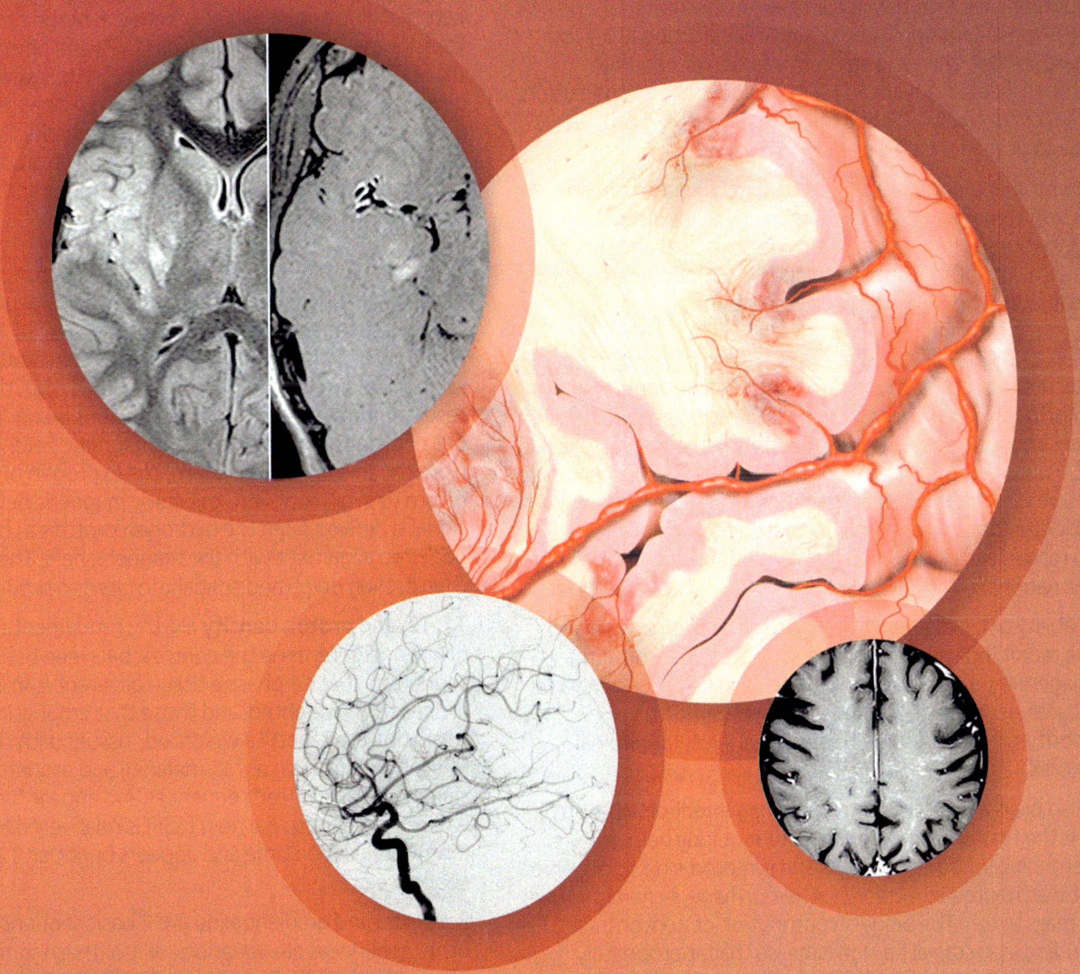

ELSEVIER

Introduction

Rapid advancement of medical imaging in the last couple of decades has significantly enhanced the role of imaging in medicine. Imaging plays an integral role in the evaluation of neurological disorders. It is performed for diagnosis, assessing efficacy of therapy, follow-up, and guidance for procedures.

Benign neurological disorders and life-threatening neoplasms may present with similar overlapping symptomatology, which could be relatively nonspecific. Clinical history combined with a good neurological evaluation is often followed by lab investigations, electroencephalography, lumbar puncture, and other investigations. Computed tomography (CT) and magnetic resonance (MR) form the backbone of the imaging work-up of these patients. Neurological disorders tend to be complex, and arriving at a diagnosis involves knowledge of neuroanatomy, pathology, physiology, and diagnostic tools such as neuroimaging.

Imaging Modalities

In the past, radiography ("plain films" and more recently digital radiography) played a significant role in imaging. With the advent of advanced imaging like CT and MR, the role of radiography has significantly diminished. Currently CT and MR are the most commonly performed imaging modalities for diseases of the brain and spine. In addition to exquisite anatomical detail, advanced MR techniques like MR perfusion, MR spectroscopy (MRS) and functional MR (fMRI) provide physiological information.

Likewise single-photon emission CT (SPECT) and positron emission tomography (PET)-CT imaging have a distinct contribution, as they can also provide structural and functional images of the brain. Ultrasound and color Doppler are useful in evaluating the head and neck vasculature.

CT

CT technology relies on the same physical principles as x-rays do. The differential absorption of the x-ray beam by different tissues produces varied levels of density in the image, which on CT scans are measured in Hounsfield units (HU). This can be displayed in cross-sectional format or in multiple planes. Multidetector CT (MDCT) has increased the capability of CT with faster scans, greater spatial resolution, and multiplanar reformations.

The ability of CT to image traumatic conditions of brain and spine rapidly has made it invaluable in acute neurotrauma management. Lesions commonly seen on CT include calvarial fractures, acute intraaxial and extraaxial hemorrhage, hemorrhagic contusions, diffuse axonal injury, and spinal fractures.

CT also plays a pivotal role in the management of acute stroke and is the first-line imaging modality. It quickly helps in determining whether the signs and symptoms being observed can be attributed to intracranial hemorrhage, ischemic stroke, or a mass lesion. The biggest contribution of noncontrast CT is excluding intracranial hemorrhage, so that appropriately selected patients can be started on tissue plasminogen activator (tPA). Although CT is less sensitive than MR in detecting acute cerebral ischemia-infarction, detectable changes are present on 50-60% of noncontrast CT (NECT) scans in patients with major territorial (not lacunar) infarcts.

Noncontrast CT is relatively insensitive for detection of neoplastic disease, especially when the tumor burden is small. A postcontrast CT should always be obtained when evaluating neoplastic conditions using CT.

CT Angiogram (CTA)

CTA is the study of choice for all emergent and nonemergent neurovascular conditions, including acute stroke. It is fast and less prone to artifact than MR angiography (MRA). A combined CTA of the head and neck, from the aortic arch to the cranial vertex, can be obtained with as little as 70 ml of IV contrast in < 15 seconds. Given the high prevalence of cardiogenic acute strokes, it now is possible to extend the field of coverage of CTA to include the heart in the evaluation.

CT Venogram (CTV)

CTV is similar to CTA except for an added delay for optimal visualization of the venous system. It is a fast, reliable modality to exclude dural sinus thrombosis in an emergent setting.

CT Perfusion (CTP)

CTP imaging uses the dynamics of first-pass bolus through the brain parenchyma to derive perfusion maps. Repeated CT scans through a limited region of the brain yield a time-attenuation curve for each pixel that documents the changes in tissue contrast during the bolus contrast passage. CTP software is used to process these images and generate cerebral blood volume (CBV), cerebral blood flow (CBF) , mean transit time (MTT), time to peak (TTP), and permeability (kPS) maps. CTP aims to detect the mismatch between the brain already infarcted (ischemic "core") and that at risk of infarction ("penumbra" or potentially salvageable brain). Permeability maps (kPS) are helpful in tumor imaging to grade gliomas and to differentiate between tumor recurrence and radiation necrosis.

MR

The primary origin of the MR signal used to generate almost all clinical images comes from hydrogen nuclei. Hydrogen nuclei consist of a single proton that is constantly spinning. A radio frequency pulse (RF pulse) emitted from the scanner results in some of the hydrogen protons being "knocked" 180° out of alignment with the static magnetic field. As the energy from the RF pulse is dissipated, the hydrogen protons will return to alignment with the static magnetic field. The MR signal is derived from the hydrogen protons as they move back into alignment with the magnetic field. The MR signal is then broken down and spatially located to produce images.

T1, T2, and proton density are the fundamental parameters of MR and determine the contrast between tissues. MR sequences that emphasize tissue differences in T1 relaxation are called T1 weighted, and those that emphasize T2 relaxation are called T2 weighted. Tissues with short T1 relaxation time such as fat, melanin, and protein produce high signal on T1-weighted sequences and appear "bright," whereas cerebrospinal fluid (CSF) is relatively dark. CSF has a long T2 relaxation time and appears bright on T2-weighted sequences.

Spin echo and gradient echo are 2 basic sequences in MR. All other sequences are variations of 1 of these sequences and are used to better characterize specific tissue types. MPRAGE is a 3-dimensional, thin-section T1-weighted volumetric acquisition that is increasingly utilized for evaluating a broad spectrum of brain disorders.

Fluid-attenuation inversion recovery (FLAIR) sequence is used to eliminate the signal from CSF, which thus appears dark. It is useful for highlighting parenchymal lesions that lie close to ventricles or sulci like multiple sclerosis plaques or small cortical infarcts, which are not as conspicuous on T2-weighted sequences. "Bright" CSF sulcal signal on FLAIR could suggest leptomeningeal disease with replacement of the normal CSF by pus (meningitis), blood (subarachnoid hemorrhage), or tumor cells (leptomeningeal carcinomatosis).

Short tau inversion recovery (STIR) sequence is used to eliminate signal from fat. This is useful in diagnosing fat-containing lesions like lipoma and dermoid cyst.

Diffusion-weighted imaging (DWI) is a way to display the molecular motion or diffusion of water protons within tissue. DWI generates diffusion and apparent diffusion coefficient (ADC) maps. ADC is a measure of the rate of diffusion. True restricted diffusion will be bright on diffusion and low (dark) on ADC maps. Acute cerebral infarction with cytotoxic edema is the most commonly encountered pathologic process to restrict diffusion and can be seen as early as 30 minutes after ictus. Restricted diffusion can also be seen in other processes like pyogenic abscess, highly cellular tumor, epidermoid cyst, and Creutzfeldt-Jakob disease. Pathologies with vasogenic edema (most cases of PRES) typically do not cause restricted diffusion.

Diffusion tensor imaging (DTI) is an interesting application of diffusion imaging, which assesses diffusion in at least 6 different directions and yields a more complete diffusivity information compared with standard DWI. This information can be used to deduce axonal fiber orientation and create 3D color-encoded maps of white matter tracts in the brain. Red indicates right to left, green encodes anterior to posterior, and blue denotes superior to inferior tract orientation.

Gradient echo sequence (GRE) is sensitive to small amounts of blood breakdown products as well as calcium and metallic deposits, fat, and air.

Susceptibility weighted imaging (SWI) is a very sensitive type of gradient echo MR sequence. The most common use of SWI is for the identification of small amounts of hemorrhage/blood product or calcium, both of which may be inapparent on other MR sequences. Compounds that have paramagnetic, diamagnetic, and ferromagnetic properties all interact with the local magnetic field and result in loss of signal. Paramagnetic compounds include deoxyhemoglobin, ferritin, and hemosiderin. Diamagnetic compounds include bone minerals and dystrophic calcifications. SWI is more sensitive than GRE for cerebral microbleeds.

MRA

Time-of-flight (TOF) imaging is most commonly used for MRA. Signal in intracranial arteries is related to flow phenomenon, and thus no IV gadolinium is needed. TOF MRA can be performed by both 2D and 3D techniques.

Contrast-enhanced MRA is often used to evaluate the neck vasculature. Contrast-enhanced intracranial MRA is useful in patients with stent and/or coils.

MR Venogram (MRV)

MRV can be performed with 2D/3D TOF techniques, which do not need administration of IV gadolinium. Contrast-enhanced MRV is, however, more robust and is less susceptible to artifacts compared with the TOF techniques.

MR Perfusion

Perfusion MR (with contrast) can be performed using 2 major techniques: Dynamic susceptibility contrast MR perfusion (DSC) and dynamic contrast-enhanced perfusion (DCE). DSC perfusion gives information on relative CBV, relative CBF, MTT, and TTP, useful in stroke patients. DCE perfusion examines the leakiness of blood vessels to generate permeability maps. Both DSC and DCE techniques can be used in evaluation of brain tumors.

Arterial spin labeling (ASL) is an MR perfusion method for quantitatively measuring CBF by taking advantage of arterial water as a freely diffusible tracer. ASL is completely noninvasive, repeatable, and is performed without gadolinium.

MRS

MRS provides metabolite/biochemical information about tissues noninvasively in vivo. The basic metabolite changes common to brain pathology include elevation in choline (Cho), lactate, and lipid and decrease in *N*-acetylaspartate (NAA) and creatine (Cr). MRS is useful in the clinical setting of focally enhancing lesions, metabolic disorders, dementia, epilepsy, and brain infections.

fMRI

fMRI is a technique used to obtain functional information by visualizing cortical activity. fMRI detects subtle alteration in blood flow in response to stimuli or actions. It is used in clinical practice typically for presurgical mapping of eloquent areas (e.g., speech and motor skills) and in research aimed at elucidating novel neural networks.

SPECT

SPECT provides structural and functional images of the brain with perfusion agents or with neuroreceptor imaging radiopharmaceuticals.

Brain perfusion imaging agents 99mTc-HMPAO and 99mTc-ECD are sensitive indicators of regional CBF changes and can be used in acute ischemia, transient ischemic attacks, stroke, and assessment of CBF reserve (e.g.,in arterial stenosis, moyamoya disease). Classification of perfusion defects into several perfusion patterns is useful in dementias.

Brain SPECT with thallium-201 and 99mTc-sestamibi have been useful in distinguishing radiation effects from residual or recurrent tumor. Thallium-201 SPECT can help differentiate lymphoma from toxoplasmosis in patients with HIV/AIDS.

Dopamine-transporter SPECT (DaT-SPECT) is used to differentiate a true parkinsonian syndrome from vascular parkinsonism, drug-induced changes, or essential tremor.

PET

PET involves injection of a radioactive tracer. A tracer is essentially a biological compound of interest labeled with a positron-emitting isotope, such as 11C, 18F, and 15O. PET enables in vivo examination of brain functions and quantification of CBF, metabolism, and receptor binding.

PET tracers used to study neurological disorders include 18F-2-deoxyglucose (F-18 FDG) for glucose metabolism, 11C-raclopride for dopamine D2 receptors, 11C-methionine for cellular amino acid uptake, and 11C-flumazenil for central benzodiazepine binding.

18F-6-fluorodopa (18F-dopa) is 1 of the most commonly used ligands for studying the dopaminergic system in movement disorders. Differentiating various types of parkinsonian syndromes clinically, especially in the early stages of the disease, can be difficult, and PET may be employed as an adjunct to clinical diagnosis in equivocal cases.

CT Hounsfield Units

Tissue	Hounsfield Unit
Air	-1000
Fat	-120
Water/cerebrospinal fluid	0
White matter	22-32
Gray matter	36-46
Hemorrhage	70-80
Calcification	80-100
Bone	+400

Comparison of CT and MR in Neurology

CT	MR
Few contraindications	Multiple contraindications (implantable devices)
Fast, readily available	Slower, less available
Radiation exposure	No radiation exposure
Very good for acute hemorrhage	Excellent for different phases of hemorrhage
Poor soft tissue contrast	Excellent soft tissue contrast
Nephrotoxic contrast	Nephrogenic systemic fibrosis
Higher incidence of contrast reaction	Lower incidence of contrast reaction
Need contrast for CTA	Noncontrast MRA (flow related)

MR Signal Characteristic of Different Tissues

	T1	T2
Dense bone	Low signal	Low signal
Fat	High signal	Loses signal compared with T1
Water (cerebrospinal fluid)	Low signal	High signal
Hemorrhage	Variable (depends on stage of hemoglobin breakdown)	Variable (depends on stage of hemoglobin breakdown)
Gray/white matter	White matter higher signal than gray matter	White matter lower signal than gray matter

Main clinical use of PET in epilepsy is localization of epileptogenic foci in potential surgical candidates with partial seizures.

F-18 FDG PET can provide important prognostic information, as increased glucose metabolism of gliomas correlates with higher histological grades (III and IV) and shorter survival period. Similarly, increased uptake of 11C-methionine, which reflects cellular amino acid uptake, is indicative of high-grade glioma and poorer survival.

F-18 FDG PET has been used extensively to study dementia, and it may be an effective tool for early diagnosis and differentiation of various types of dementia. Amyloid PET imaging using 11C-Pittsburg compound (PiB) and 18F-AV-45 (florbetapir) have high sensitivity in detecting amyloid plaques.

Ultrasound and Doppler

Grayscale is used to for extracranial atherosclerotic disease and plaque morphology. Color Doppler detects turbulent blood flow. Doppler spectral analysis measures blood flow velocity, which correlates with the degree of vascular stenosis.

Digital Subtraction Angiography (DSA)

Digital subtraction angiography (DSA) is still considered the "gold standard" in vascular imaging. However, DSA is an invasive procedure associated with risk of complications, 1% overall incidence of neurologic deficit and 0.5% incidence of persistent deficit.

Diagnostic indications for DSA include assessing for aneurysms in subarachnoid hemorrhage when CTA/MR are negative, accurate assessment of arteriovenous malformations, and intracerebral hemorrhage of unknown etiology.

Selected References

1. Audebert HJ et al: Brain imaging in acute ischemic stroke—MRI or CT? Curr Neurol Neurosci Rep. 15(3):6, 2015
2. Brinjikji W et al: Contemporary carotid imaging: from degree of stenosis to plaque vulnerability. J Neurosurg. 1-16, 2015
3. Naqvi J et al: Transcranial Doppler ultrasound: a review of the physical principles and major applications in critical care. Int J Vasc Med. 2013:629378, 2013
4. Tai YF et al: Applications of positron emission tomography (PET) in neurology. J Neurol Neurosurg Psychiatry. 75(5):669-76, 2004

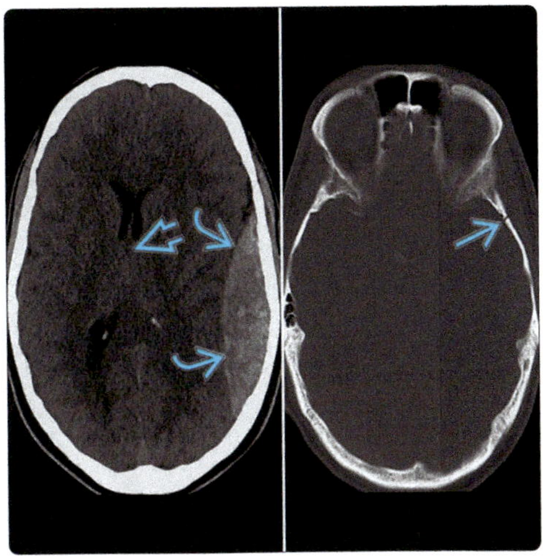

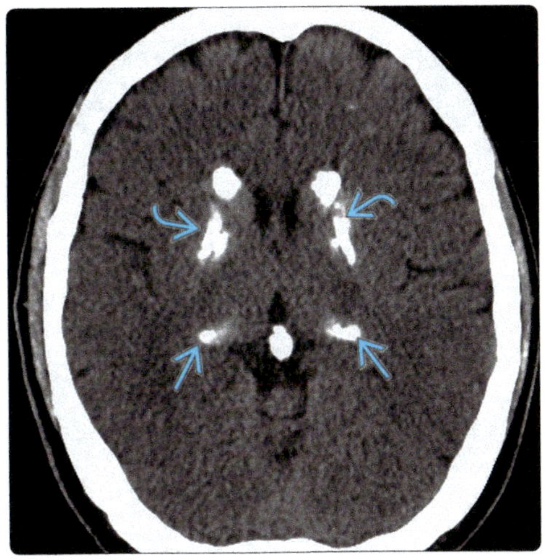

(Left) *Axial NECT images in soft tissue windows (L) and bone windows (R) in a patient with head trauma demonstrates an acute epidural hematoma* → *along the left cerebral convexity with mass effect and midline shift* →*. Bone windows demonstrate an undisplaced skull fracture* →*.* **(Right)** *Axial NECT in a patient with Fahr syndrome demonstrates extensive calcifications in the basal ganglia* → *and pulvinar nucleus* → *of the thalamus. CT is very sensitive in depicting acute hemorrhage, calcification, and fat.*

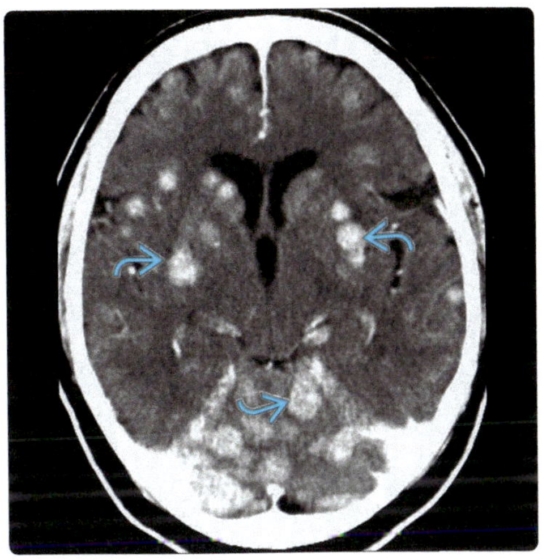

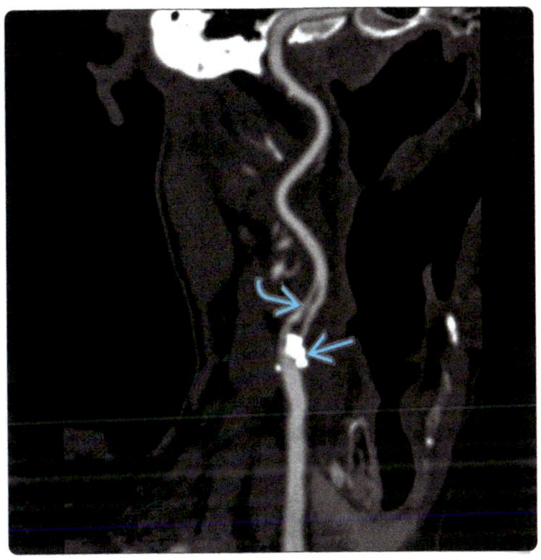

(Left) *Axial CECT in a patient with lung carcinoma demonstrates numerous enhancing lesions* → *in the brain parenchyma consistent with metastases. IV contrast is always needed when evaluating neoplastic conditions with CT.* **(Right)** *CTA with curved sagittal oblique multiplanar reconstruction (MPR) shows a calcified plaque* → *at the origin of the left internal carotid artery with a floating hypodense intraluminal thrombus* →*. CTA is fast, reliable, and accurate for evaluating vascular disorders.*

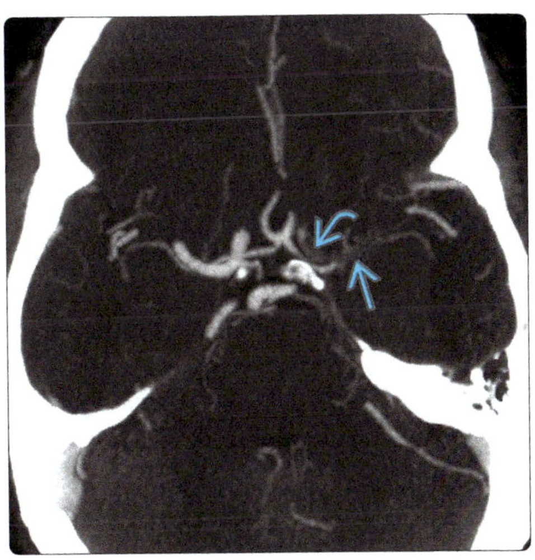

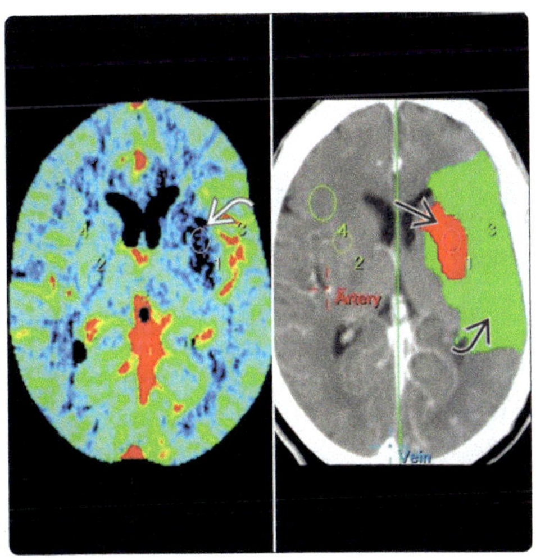

(Left) *Axial CTA maximum intensity projection (MIP) image in a patient with acute right hemiparesis shows a filling defect due to a thrombus in the terminal left ICA* → *and proximal MCA* →*. There is resultant occlusion and nonvisualization of the distal MCA.* **(Right)** *CT perfusion cerebral blood flow map (L) in the same patient shows an infarct core* → *with very low CBF. A color-coded map (R) derived from the CT perfusion data of CBV and MTT mismatch shows the infarct core (red)* → *and the ischemic penumbra (green)* →*.*

(Left) *Sagittal FLAIR MR in a patient with multiple sclerosis demonstrates classic demyelinating plaques oriented perpendicular to the ventricular margin. The lesions are more conspicuous on FLAIR due to the CSF signal suppression in the ventricles and sulci.* **(Right)** *Axial T1 MR in a patient with malignant melanoma shows multiple T1 hyperintense metastatic lesions. Melanin, methemoglobin, fat, and protein are hyperintense on T1 MR.*

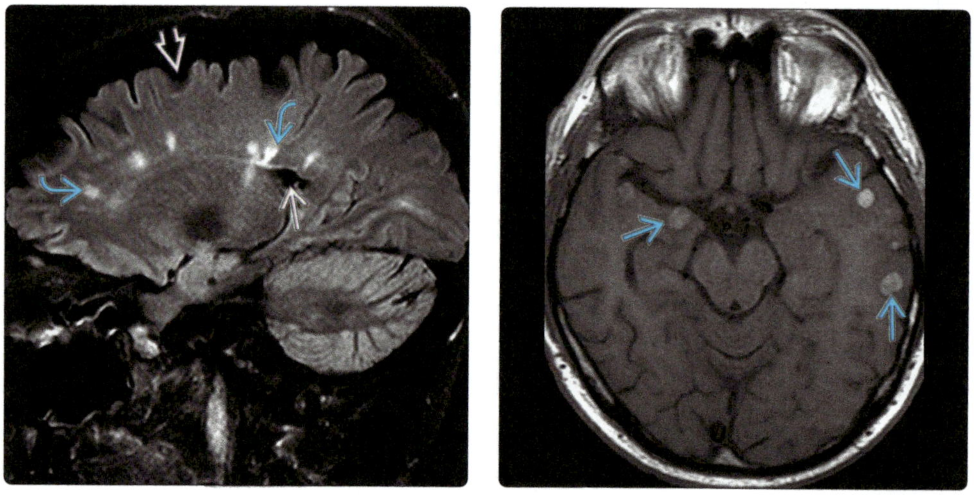

(Left) *Axial DWI (L) and corresponding ADC map (R) demonstrate a large acute infarct in the distribution of the left middle cerebral artery. The acute infarct is bright on DWI and dark on ADC map. DWI is very sensitive for acute infarcts.* **(Right)** *3D-TOF MIP image in the same patient shows nonvisualization of the left internal carotid and left middle cerebral arteries due to proximal occlusion of the left internal carotid artery in the neck. Note normal right-sided circulation.*

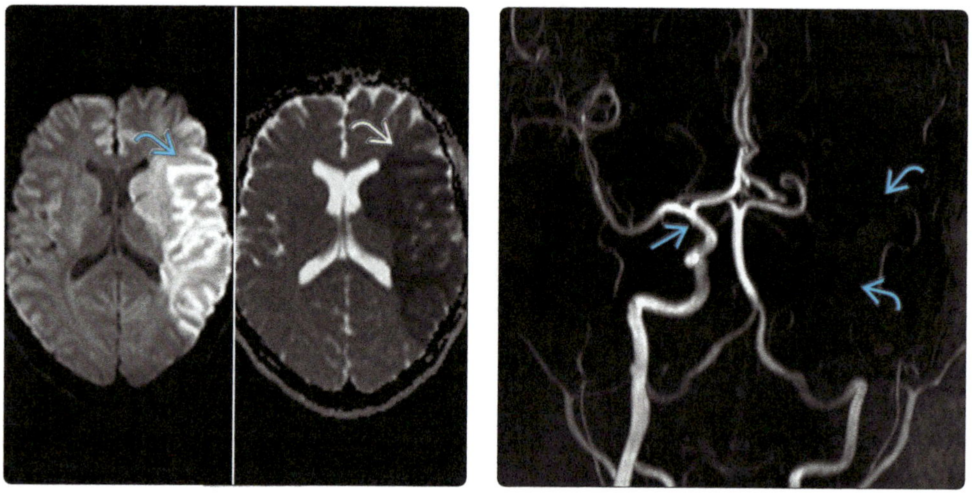

(Left) *Axial SWI MIP image in a 75-year-old man shows a large area of signal void in the left frontal lobe due an intracranial hemorrhage. Remote microbleeds are also noted predominantly in a cortical/subcortical distribution. Findings are typical of cerebral amyloid disease.* **(Right)** *MIP image of a contrast-enhanced MR venogram study demonstrates normal dural venous sinuses and cortical veins. Superior sagittal sinus, transverse sinus, sigmoid sinus, straight sinus, and cortical veins are shown.*

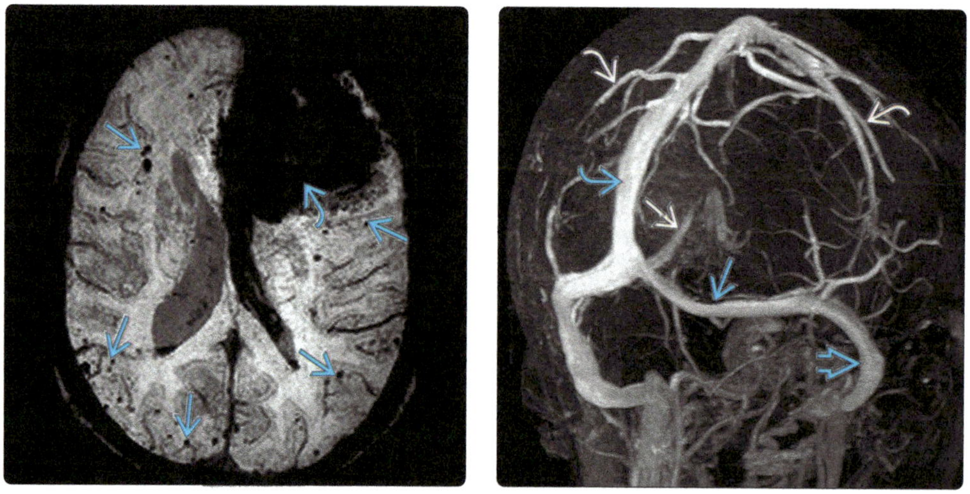

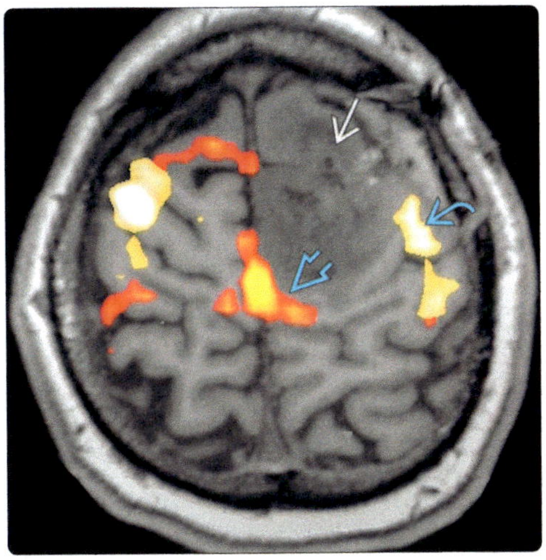

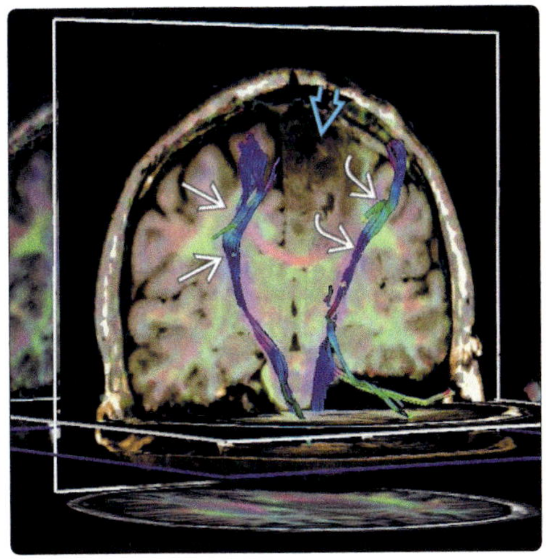

(Left) *Axial fMRI performed with motor paradigm demonstrates activation of the left hand motor area at the lateral margin of the left frontal tumor. There is posterior displacement of the left lower extremity motor area by the tumor. fMRI is helpful in preoperative localization of eloquent areas of the brain.* **(Right)** *DTI tractography in the same patient shows lateral displacement of the left corticospinal tract by the frontal lobe mass. Note normal course of the right corticospinal tract.*

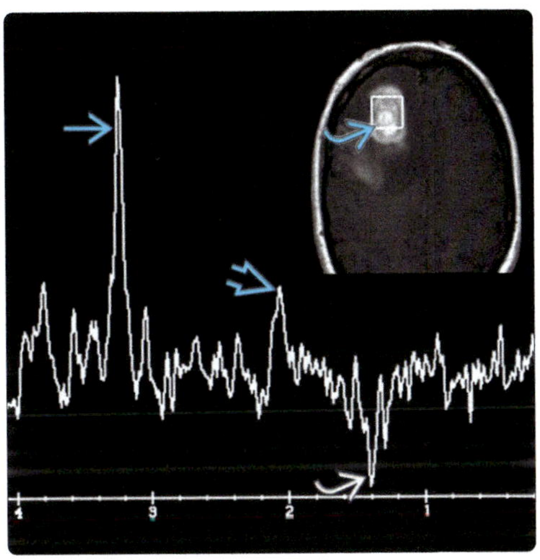

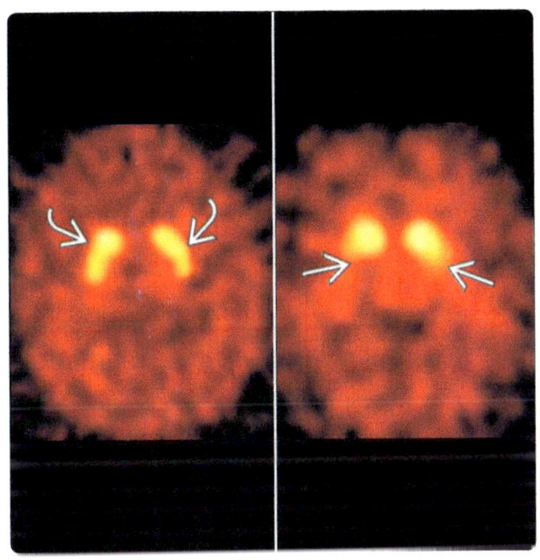

(Left) *MRS in this patient with a proven glioblastoma shows elevated choline, decreased NAA, and an inverted lactate peak, which can be seen in a high-grade neoplasm.* **(Right)** *Axial DaT-SPECT in a healthy control (L) demonstrates normal symmetric "comma-shaped" uptake in the caudate nuclei and putamina. In a patient with idiopathic Parkinson disease (R), there is asymmetric reduction in putaminal uptake, right greater than left. The uptake looks more like "dots" than "commas."*

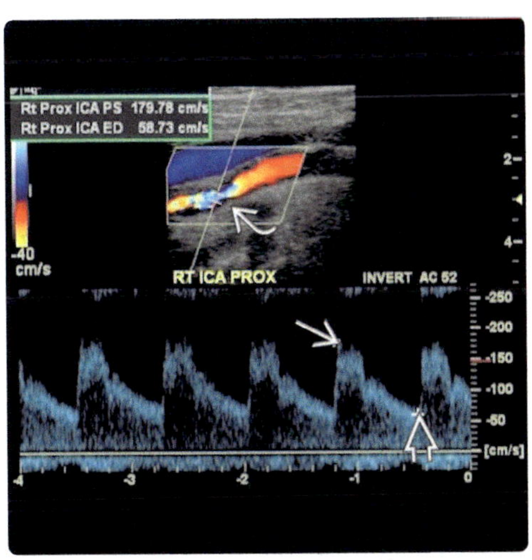

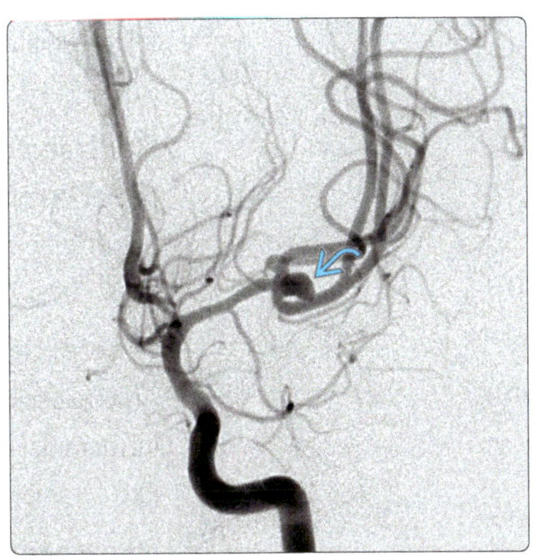

(Left) *Color and spectral Doppler of the origin of the right internal carotid artery shows high velocity jet at the site of carotid stenosis. The peak systolic velocity measured up to 237 cm/s and end-diastolic velocity 85 cm/s. This was a > 70% stenosis.* **(Right)** *AP view of a DSA performed with selective left internal carotid injection demonstrates a saccular aneurysm at the left middle cerebral artery bifurcation projecting laterally.*

PART I: BRAIN
SECTION 1

Pathology-Based Diagnoses: Malformations, Trauma, and Stroke

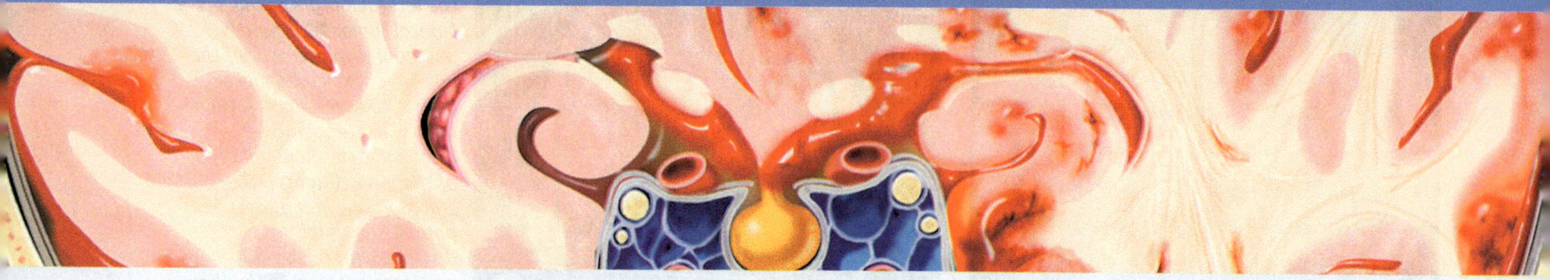

Congenital Malformations

Trauma

Vascular Anatomy and Stroke

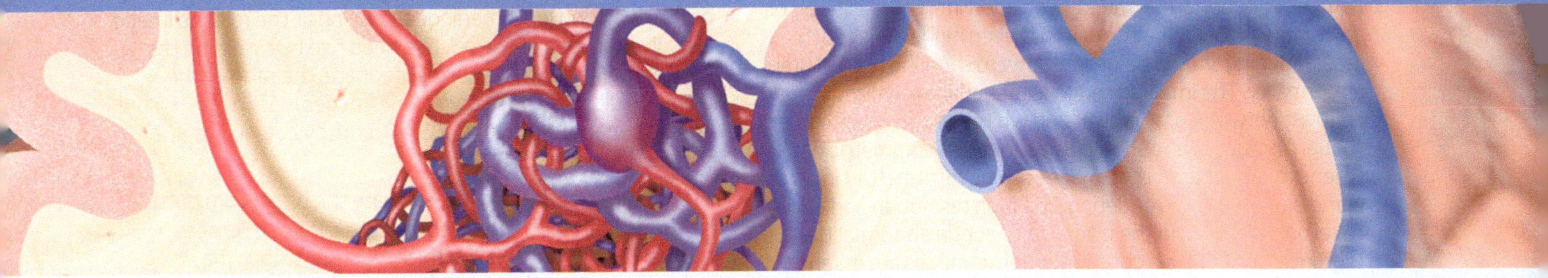

Cerebral Ischemia and Infarction

Subarachnoid Hemorrhage and Aneurysms

Vascular Malformations

General Imaging Approach to Brain Malformations

Whenever an infant or child is referred for imaging because of either seizures or delayed development, a brain malformation is a possible cause. If the child appears dysmorphic in any way (low-set ears, abnormal facies, hypotelorism), the likelihood of an underlying brain malformation is even higher. In all such cases, imaging should be geared toward showing a structural abnormality. The imaging sequences should maximize contrast between gray matter and white matter, have high spatial resolution, and should be acquired as volumetric data whenever possible so that images can be reformatted in any plane or as a surface rendering. The high resolution and ability to reformat will aid in the diagnosis of subtle abnormalities. High-resolution T1-weighted volumetric images are essential for this purpose. If possible, volumetric T2-weighted images can be acquired, but the images must have excellent spatial resolution and sharp contrast between gray matter and white matter, which is not currently easy to achieve with volumetric T2-weighted sequences. If contrast between gray and white matter is poor with volumetric acquisition, acquire two-dimensional sequences (2D) in at least two planes and with relatively thin (3-4 mm) section size. FLAIR images are not particularly useful in looking for malformations, as the contrast between gray matter and white matter is often poor. Diffusion-weighted images are not currently of diagnostic utility, although the use of DTI to acquire color fractional anisotropy maps and perform tractography is useful to better understand the connectivity of the malformed brain and may become clinically useful in the near future.

After acquisition of appropriate images, image analysis must take place in an orderly manner. The midline structures (including cerebral commissures, septum pellucidum, nose and rhinencephalon, pituitary gland, and hypothalamus), the cerebral cortex (cortical thickness, gyral pattern, and cortical-white matter junction), cerebral white matter (myelination, presence of nodules or clefts), the basal ganglia, the ventricular system (are all ventricles completely present and normally shaped), the interhemispheric fissure, and the midbrain hindbrain structures (brainstem and cerebellum) should all be scrutinized in every patient.

Evaluate the midline structures first, as many disease processes of children take place in the midline, including anomalies of the cerebral commissures (corpus callosum, anterior commissure, and hippocampal commissure), midline tumors (suprasellar, pineal, brainstem, and 4th ventricle), anomalies of the cerebellar vermis, and anomalies of the craniocervical junction. Anomalies of the cerebral commissures are the most common of brain malformations; more than 130 syndromes involving them have been described. Many of these are associated with anomalies of the hypothalamus, so remember to always look at the hypothalamus and pituitary gland to ensure that the posterior pituitary gland is in the sella turcica and not in the median eminence of the hypothalamus. The midline leptomeninges are important in commisural development, so make sure to look for other anomalies associated with abnormal midline leptomeninges, such as interhemispheric lipomas and interhemispheric cysts when the commissures are absent or dysmorphic. Remember that large cerebrospinal fluid (CSF) spaces in the posterior fossa (mega cisterna magna) are often associated with anomalies of the cerebellum. The reason for this has only recently been discovered. Several cerebellar growth factors derive from the overlying leptomeninges. Therefore, abnormalities of the cerebellar leptomeninges may result in anomalies of the cerebellum itself, as well as abnormalities of the surrounding CSF spaces. This is the basis of development of the Dandy-Walker malformation; it requires abnormal development of the cerebellum itself and of the overlying leptomeninges. Looking at the midline image also gives an idea of the relative head size by assessing the craniofacial ratio. In the normal neonate, the ratio of the cranial vault to the face on midline images is 5:1 or 6:1. By the age of 2 years, it should be 2.5:1.0, and, by age 10 years, it should be about 1.5:1.0.

After looking at the midline, evaluate the brain from outside to inside. Start with the cerebral cortex. Is the thickness normal (2-3 mm)? If it is too thick, think of pachygyria or polymicrogyria. Is the cortical-white matter junction smooth or irregular? If it is irregular, think of polymicrogyria or the cobblestone cortex seen associated with congenital muscular dystrophies such as muscle-eye-brain disease. The location of these abnormalities is important as well. Pachygyria more severe in the parietal and occipital lobes suggests a mutation of *TUBA1A*, whereas pachygyria worst in the frontal lobes suggests a mutation of *DCX*. Similarly, there are many different polymicrogyria syndromes that depend on the location of the polymicrogyria: Bilateral frontal polymicrogyria is a different entity than bilateral perisylvian polymicrogyria or bilateral parasagittal parietooccipital polymicrogyria; it is important to be specific in reporting the location of the abnormality. If the cortex is abnormally thin, one should think of a prenatal injury (infectious or ischemic), particularly if the thinning is focal or multifocal.

After the cortex, look at the cerebral white matter. Make sure myelination is appropriate for age (there are many sources of normal myelination charts). Then look for areas of abnormal myelination within the deep white matter. Diffuse layers of hypomyelination or amyelination associated with overlying polymicrogyria should raise suspicion for congenital cytomegalovirus infection. More localized foci of delayed or absent myelination are often seen in deep white matter of patients with congenital muscular dystrophy and in the subcortical white matter of those with focal cortical dysplasias (FCDs). With FCDs, the absent myelination may be localized to a gyrus or may extend centrally as a curvilinear cone-shaped abnormality coursing from the cortex to the superolateral margin of a lateral ventricle (this is known as the "transmantle" sign). Also, look for nodules of heterotopic gray matter in the periventricular or deep white matter. Subcortical heterotopia typically extend from the cortex all the way to the lateral ventricular wall, whereas periventricular nodular heterotopia are more localized to the immediate subependymal/periventricular region.

The basal ganglia are sometimes abnormal in disorders of neuronal migration, as they are formed from neurons generated in the medial and lateral ganglionic eminences, the same germinal zones that produce GABAergic neurons that migrate to the cerebral cortex. In particular, the basal ganglia tend to be dysmorphic in appearance in patients with subcortical heterotopia. In addition, the hippocampi are often abnormal in malformations of cortical development. In patients with lissencephaly, in particular, the hippocampi are incompletely folded. Sometimes, the only structural abnormalities in children with developmental delay are

Brain Anomaly Imaging Checklist

Anomaly	Findings
Anomalies of Cerebral Cortex	
Agyria/pachygyria	Thick cortex, smooth inner margin, few shallow sulci
Polymicrogyria	Thin undulating cortex, irregular inner margin
Cobblestone cortex	Thick cortex, irregular inner margin, abnormal myelin
Focal cortical dysplasia	Blurred gray-white junction, ± abnormal myelination
White Matter Abnormalities With Cortical Malformation	
Polymicrogyria	Enlarged perivascular spaces
Cobblestone cortex	Delayed myelination, patchy hypomyelination
Congenital cytomegalovirus	Deep layers of hypomyelination/gliosis
Focal cortical dysplasia	Focal subcortical hypomyelination
Malformations Associated With Absent Septi Pellucidi	
Septooptic dysplasia	
Holoprosencephaly	
Bilateral schizencephaly	
Bilateral polymicrogyria	
Rhombencephalosynapsis	
Malformations with prolonged severe hydrocephalus	

Classification for Malformation of Cortical Development

Mechanism	Examples
Abnormal cellular proliferation	Polymicrogyria; focal cortical dysplasia
Abnormal neuronal migration	Lissencephaly I; lissencephaly II; heterotopia
Abnormal cortical organization	Schizencephaly; cortical dysplasia (balloon cells)

hippocampal; always look to make sure that they are fully folded and not too round.

Always look at the entire interhemispheric fissure (IHF); if the cerebral hemispheres are continuous across the midline, holoprosencephaly should be diagnosed. In severe holoprosencephalies, the interhemispheric fissure is completely absent, whereas in milder forms of holoprosencephaly certain areas of the IHF will be absent (anterior IHF in semilobar holoprosencephaly, central IHF in syntelencephaly). Look at the septum pellucidum; absence of the septum is seen in corpus callosum dysgenesis/agenesis, septooptic dysplasia, and in some cases of schizencephaly or bilateral polymicrogyria. While checking the septum, look at the lateral ventricles to ensure that they are normal in size and shape. Abnormally enlarged trigones and temporal horns are often associated with callosal anomalies and pachygyria. Enlarged frontal horns are often seen in bilateral frontal polymicrogyria.

Don't forget to look carefully at the posterior fossa; anomalies of the brainstem and cerebellum are commonly overlooked. Make sure that the 4th ventricle and cerebellar vermis are normally sized. In newborns, the vermis should extend from the inferior colliculi to the obex, whereas infants and older children should have a vermis that extends from the intercollicular sulcus to the obex. Also, make sure you see normal vermian fissures. If the fissuration of the vermis looks abnormal, look at an axial or coronal image to make sure the vermis is present; if the cerebellar hemispheres are continuous without a vermis between them, make a diagnosis of rhombencephalosynapsis. If the 4th ventricle has an abnormal rectangular shape (with a horizontal superior margin) with a narrow isthmus and small vermis, think about a molar tooth malformation. To confirm this diagnosis, look for the molar tooth sign of the lower midbrain, consisting of large, horizontal superior cerebellar peduncles extending posteriorly toward the cerebellum and a longitudinal cleft in the superior vermis. Make sure that the components of the brainstem are of normal size; in a child, the height of the pons should be double that of the midbrain on the midline sagittal image. An important clue can be provided by looking at the size of the pons compared with that of the cerebellar vermis. Because much of the anterior pons is composed of the decussation of the middle cerebellar peduncles, development hypoplasia of the cerebellum is nearly always associated with hypoplasia of the ventral pons. If the pons is normal in the setting of a small cerebellum, it is most likely that the cerebellum lost volume near the end of gestation or after birth. Remember that a small posterior fossa, intracranial **hypo**tension, **or** intracranial **hyper**tension can result in descent of the cerebellum below the foramen magnum. Look for causes of a small posterior fossa (clival anomaly, anomaly of the craniovertebral junction), intracranial hypertension (space-occupying mass, hydrocephalus), or evidence of intracranial hypotension (large dural venous sinuses, large pituitary gland, "slumping" brainstem) before making a diagnosis of Chiari 1 malformation.

(Left) *Midline analysis using sagittal T1WI MR shows classic findings of Dandy Walker spectrum with a large posterior fossa cyst ➔, high torcular ➔, and a small, upwardly rotated vermis ➔. There is also a significant commissural anomaly with only a small corpus callosum remnant present ➔. The rostrum and splenium are absent. The anterior commissure ➔ is present and appears normal.* **(Right)** *T2WI in the same case shows that the 4th ventricle is open dorsally ➔, contiguous with the huge posterior fossa cyst.*

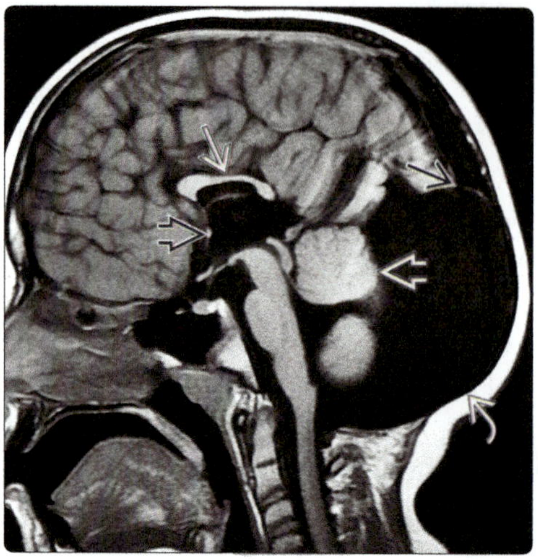

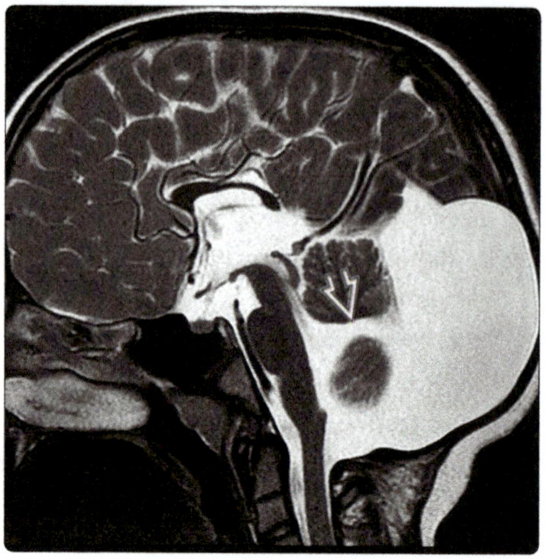

(Left) *Sagittal T1WI shows a hypoplastic callosum rostrum and splenium, plus a small interhemispheric lipoma ➔.* **(Right)** *Sagittal T2WI shows a very small posterior fossa with a low-lying torcular ➔ and an elongated 4th ventricle ➔ that lacks a fastigium. This patient has a classic Chiari 2 malformation.*

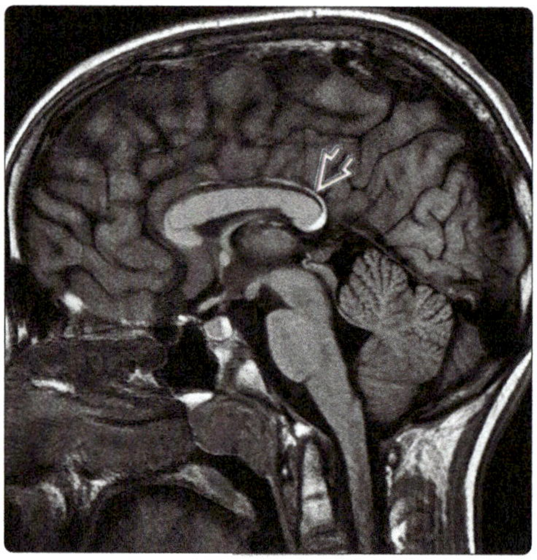

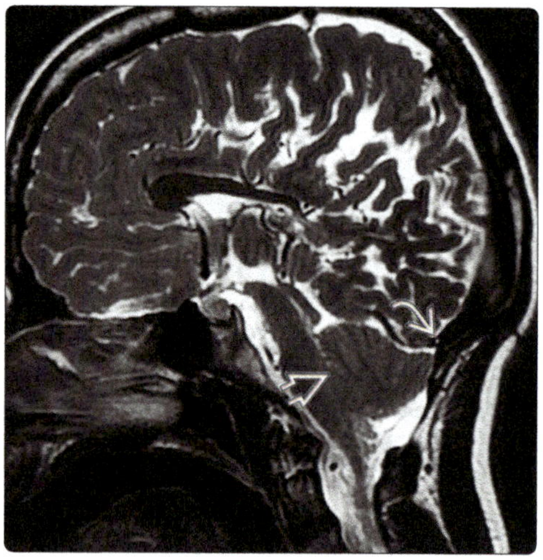

(Left) *Midline analysis of a sagittal T2WI shows a normal-sized posterior fossa. The cerebellar tonsils are pointed ➔ and displaced inferiorly 1 cm below the foramen magnum. Note cord hyperintensity ➔, suggesting a "presyrinx" state in this case of Chiari 1 malformation.* **(Right)** *Axial T2WI in the same case shows the mass-like thickening of the right medial parietal gray matter and distorted sulcal-gyral pattern of cortical dysplasia.*

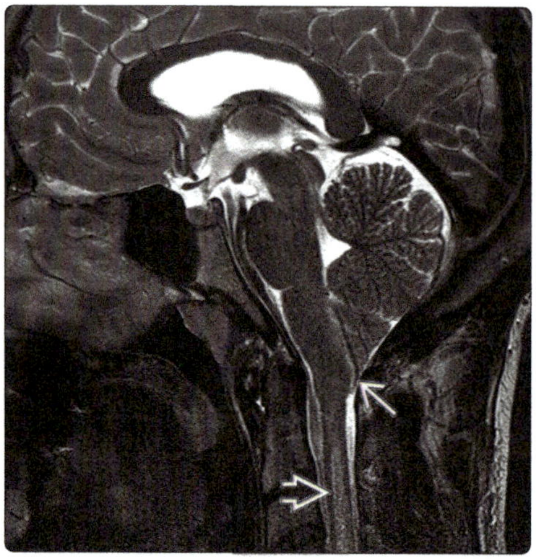

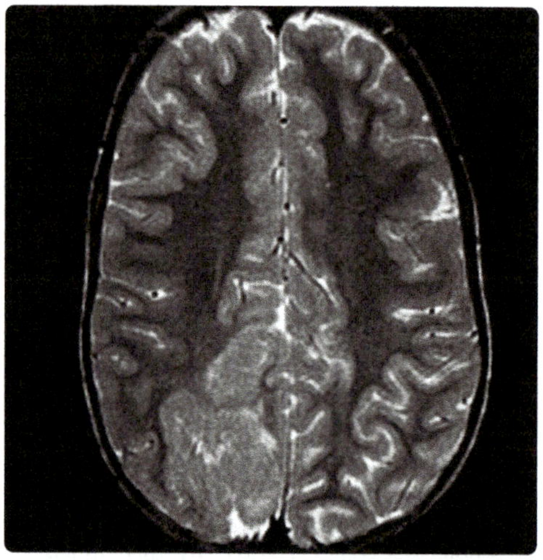

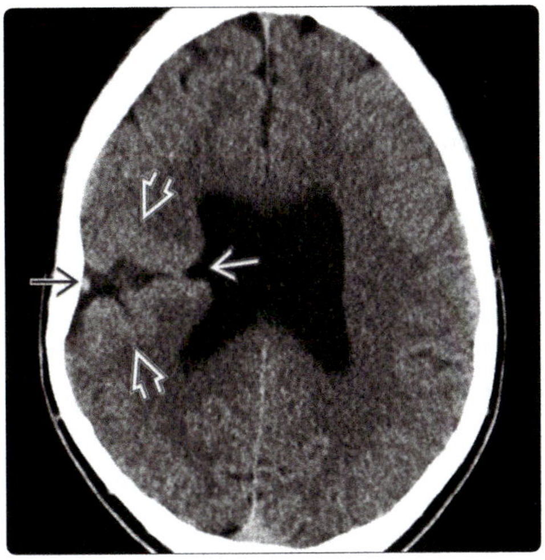

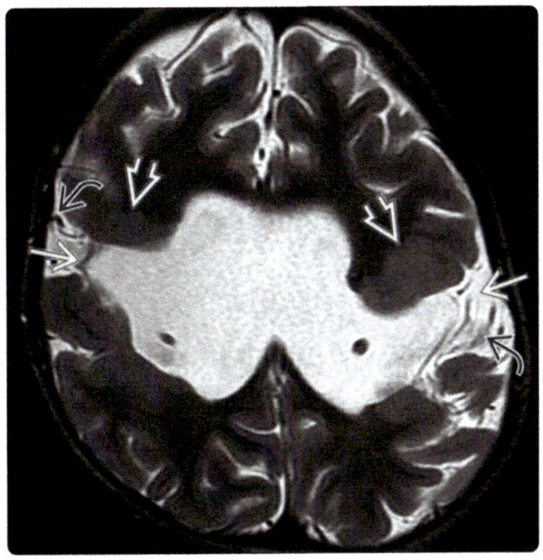

(Left) *Axial NECT scan in an 18-year-old man with seizures shows a unilateral schizencephalic cleft extending from the pial surface of the brain to the ventricle. Note the characteristic cerebrospinal fluid "nipple" at the ventricular margin. The cleft is lined by thickened, dysplastic gray matter.* **(Right)** *Axial T2WI shows bilateral schizencephalic clefts lined by dysplastic gray matter. Note the abnormal cortical veins associated with the clefts.*

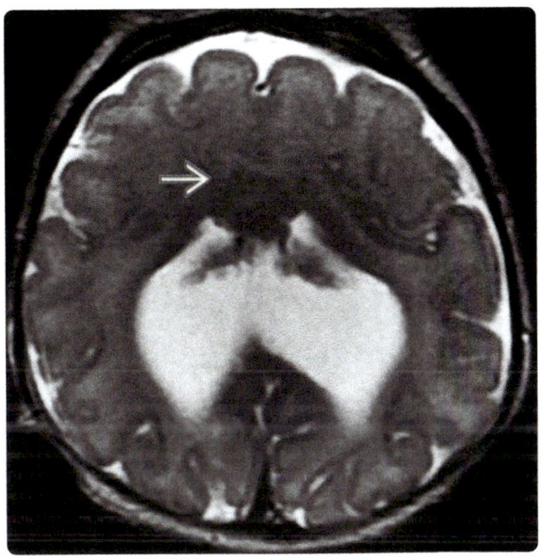

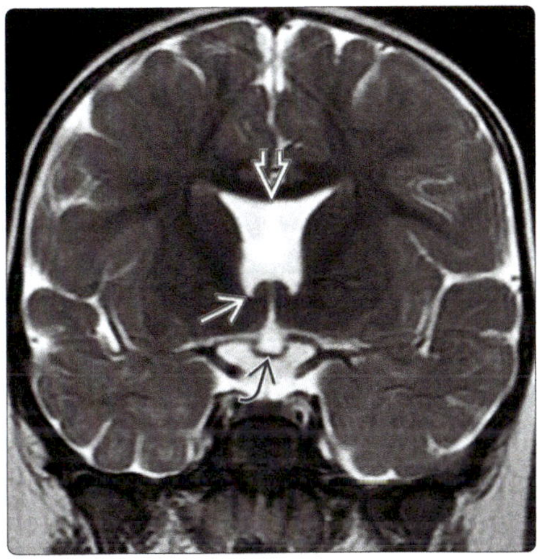

(Left) *Axial T2WI MR allows analysis of midline and shows absent interhemispheric fissure in frontal lobes (white matter continuous across midline). This finding, plus the absence of frontal horns, gives the diagnosis of holoprosencephaly.* **(Right)** *Analysis of coronal images shows a squared-off appearance to the lateral ventricles with inferiorly pointed frontal horns, absent septum pellucidum, and hypoplastic optic chiasm characteristic of septooptic dysplasia.*

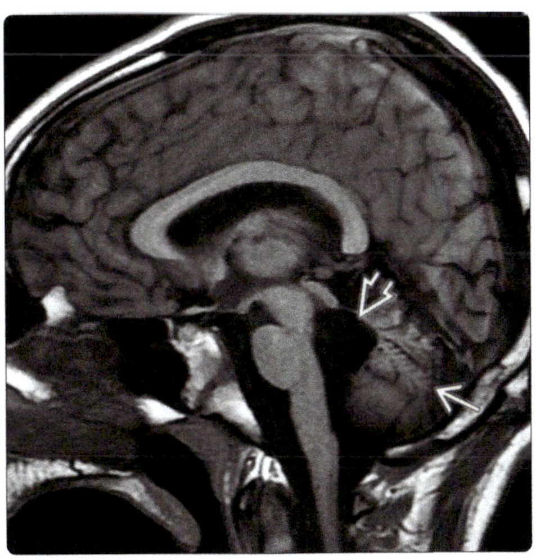

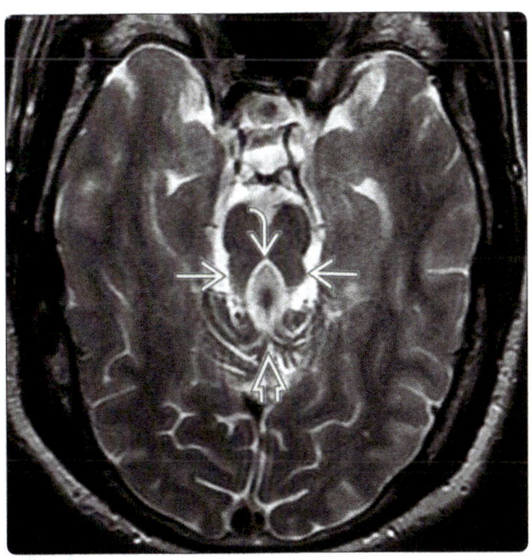

(Left) *Midline analysis of posterior fossa structures shows an upwardly convex superior 4th ventricle and a dysplastic-appearing vermis.* **(Right)** *Axial T2WI in the same case shows the elongated 4th ventricle, cleft vermis, and thickened, horizontally oriented superior cerebellar peduncles forming the classic molar tooth sign of Joubert syndrome.*

Chiari 1

KEY FACTS

TERMINOLOGY

- Chiari 1 malformation (CM1): Constellation of findings (not disease, not simply measurement)
- No clear consensus definition of what constitutes CM1
  - Traditional: Elongated, peg-shaped cerebellar tonsils extend below foramen magnum (FM) into upper cervical spinal canal
  - 5-mm criterion for tonsillar position (TP) below FM is flawed criterion
    - TP is morphometric distribution, also changes with time
    - TP **plus** shape/configuration (elongated, pointed)
    - TP also risk factor for syrinx (lower the tonsils, higher the risk)
  - "Crowded" posterior fossa + compressed CSF spaces
    - +/- obex displaced below FM
  - Evaluate skull base, upper cervical spine
    - Posterior fossa may be small, shallow (especially children)
    - Short clivus, craniovertebral junction assimilation anomalies common

TOP DIFFERENTIAL DIAGNOSES

- Normal variant (normal-shaped tonsils below FM)
- Intracranial hypotension
  - Critical not to mistake this for CM1
- Acquired tonsillar herniation (don't call "acquired Chiari 1")
- "Complex Chiari malformation" (neurosurgery: "Chiari 1.5")
  - Tonsillar herniation complicated by other abnormalities (caudal descent of brainstem with low-lying obex, bony anomalies, such as "retroflexed" odontoid)

CLINICAL ISSUES

- Up to 50% of CM1 is asymptomatic
  - Headache, ataxia, downbeat nystagmus, progressive spastic quadriparesis
- Caution: Look for findings of intracranial hypotension before making diagnosis of CM1

(Left) *Sagittal graphic demonstrates pointed peg-like tonsils extending below foramen magnum, elongating the normally positioned 4th ventricle. Note low position of obex.* **(Right)** *Sagittal T2WI in a 23-year-old man with classic Chiari 1 malformation shows low-lying pointed tonsils, obex below the foramen magnum, and hyperintensity in the upper cervical cord that may represent "presyrinx" state, nucleus gracilis.*

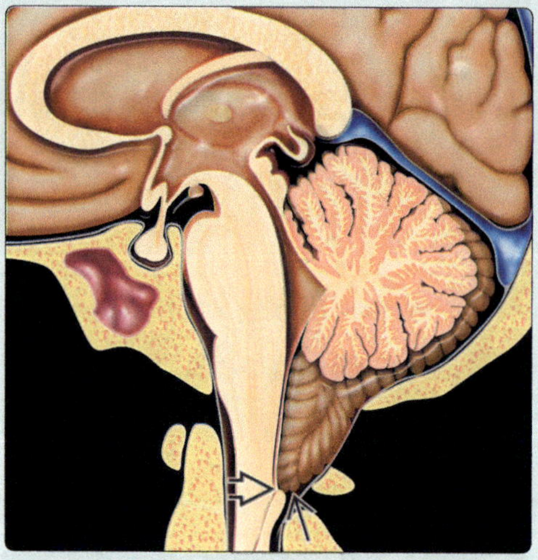

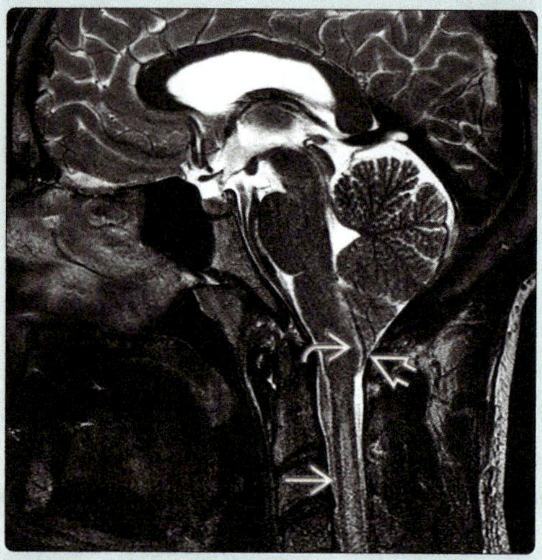

(Left) *Sagittal T1WI MR shows normal 4th ventricle position and appearance. The fastigium is in normal position, helping to distinguish from Chiari 2 malformation. There is inferior displacement of the ectopic cerebellar tonsils through the foramen magnum with odontoid process retroflexion and clivus foreshortening.* **(Right)** *Axial T2WI MR confirms inferior displacement of ectopic cerebellar tonsils through the foramen magnum, producing foramen magnum crowding.*

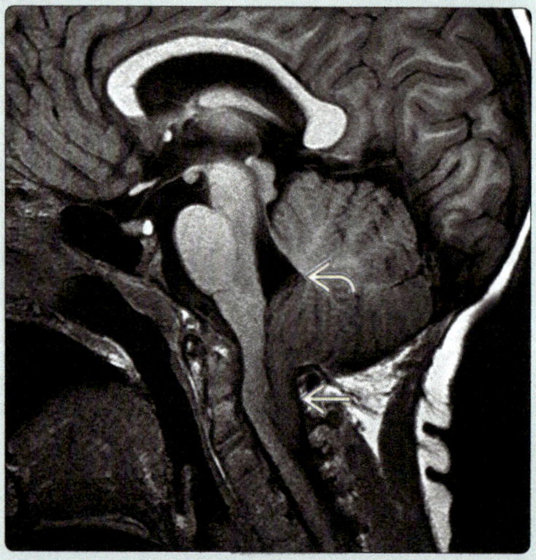

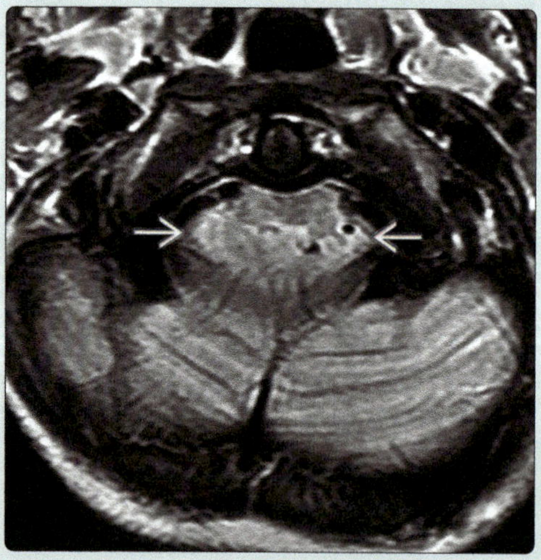

KEY FACTS

TERMINOLOGY

- Complex hindbrain malformation
- Virtually 100% associated with neural tube closure defect, usually lumbar myelomeningocele (MMC)

IMAGING

- Crowded posterior fossa, widened tentorial incisura, tectal beaking, inferior vermian displacement
- Cascade or waterfall of cerebellum/brainstem downward
  - Uvula/nodulus/pyramid of vermis → sclerotic peg
  - Cervicomedullary kink (70%)
  - Towering cerebellum → compresses midbrain, associated beaked tectum
  - 4th ventricle elongated with no posterior point (fastigium)
- Lacunar skull: Focal calvarial thinning with scooped-out appearance

TOP DIFFERENTIAL DIAGNOSES

- Chiari 1 malformation
- Chiari 3 malformation
- Intracranial cerebral spinal fluid (CSF) hypotension
- Severe, chronic shunted hydrocephalus (congenital)

PATHOLOGY

- Secondary to sequelae of CSF leakage through open spinal dysraphism during gestation (4th fetal week)
- Methylenetetrahydrofolate reductase (*MTHFR*) mutations → abnormal folate metabolism
- Spine- and brain/skull-associated anomalies common (myelomeningocele ~ 100%)

CLINICAL ISSUES

- Progressive hydrocephalus
  - Most common cause of death in myelomeningocele patients

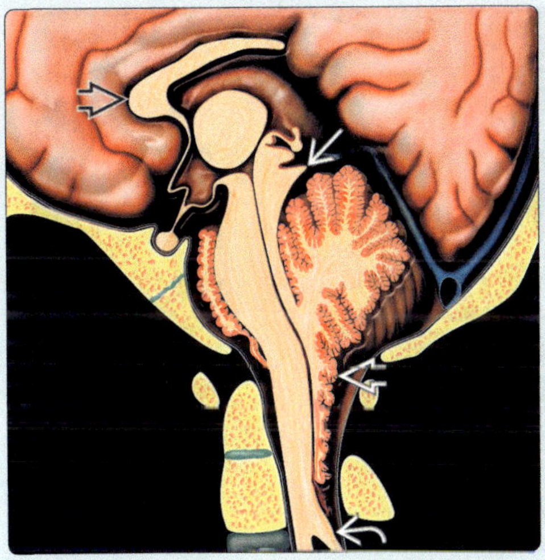

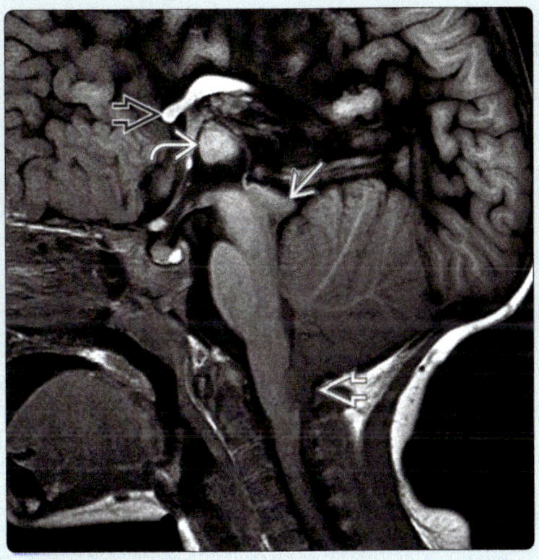

(Left) *Sagittal graphic of the posterior fossa and upper cervical spine demonstrates characteristic findings of Chiari 2 malformation, including callosal dysgenesis ➔, tectal beaking ➔, small posterior fossa, vermian ectopia ➔, and medullary kinking ➔.* **(Right)** *Sagittal T1WI MR reveals characteristic Chiari 2 malformation findings. Note the tectal beaking ➔, vermian displacement ➔ through the foramen magnum, large massa intermedia ➔, and dysplastic corpus callosum ➔.*

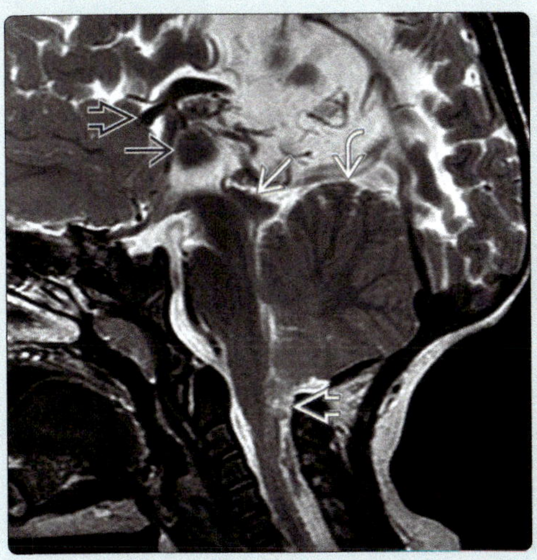

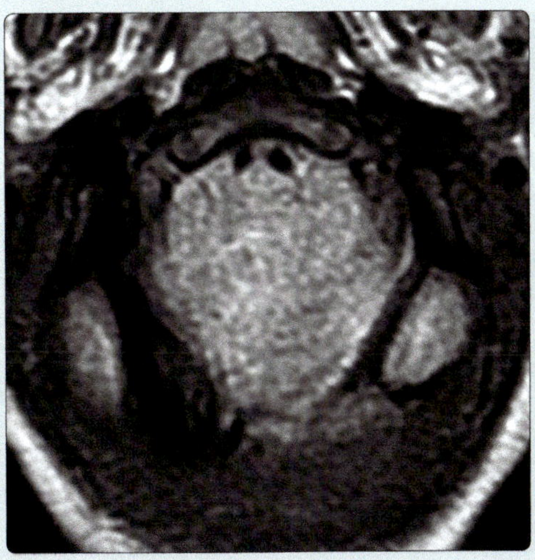

(Left) *Sagittal T2WI MR confirms characteristic findings of Chiari 2 malformation, including tectal beaking ➔, vermian displacement through the foramen magnum ➔, "towering" cerebellum ➔, large massa intermedia ➔, and dysplastic corpus callosum ➔.* **(Right)** *Axial T2WI MR shows characteristic posterior fossa crowding at the foramen magnum, reflecting small dimensions of the posterior fossa combined with cerebellar ectopia and vermian displacement through the foramen magnum.*

KEY FACTS

TERMINOLOGY

- Partial or complete absence of corpus callosum (CC), hippocampal commissure, or anterior commissure (AC); can be isolated or associated with additional cerebral malformations
- Spectrum of congenital CC structural abnormalities
  - Total agenesis (absence from birth of all anatomically defined regions of CC)
  - Partial agenesis (absence from birth of at least 1, but not all, regions of CC)
  - Hypoplasia (thinner CC with normal anteroposterior extent)
  - Hyperplasia (thick CC resulting from decreased postnatal axonal pruning)
  - Dysgenesis (CC present but malformed in some way, including partial AC and hypoplasia of CC)

IMAGING

- Absent corpus callosum on sagittal, coronal views
- Atrium/occipital horns often dilated (colpocephaly)
- DTI: Callosal fiber tracts form Probst bundles instead of crossing, where corpus callosum is absent
- Vertical/posterior course of anterior cerebral artery

CLINICAL ISSUES

- Any age; classically identified in early childhood, most common malformation found in fetuses
- Seizures, developmental delay, cranial deformity/hypertelorism
- Sporadic/isolated agenesis/dysgenesis corpus callosum: Normal/near normal at 3 years (75%), but subtle cognitive defects apparent with increasing complexity of school tasks
- Agenesis/dysgenesis CC with associated/syndromic anomalies = worst

DIAGNOSTIC CHECKLIST

- Look for absent/incomplete CC rather than indirect signs
- Fully assess for associated lesions

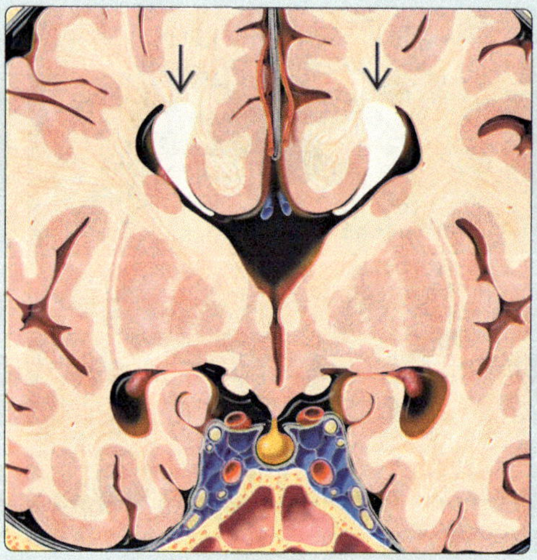

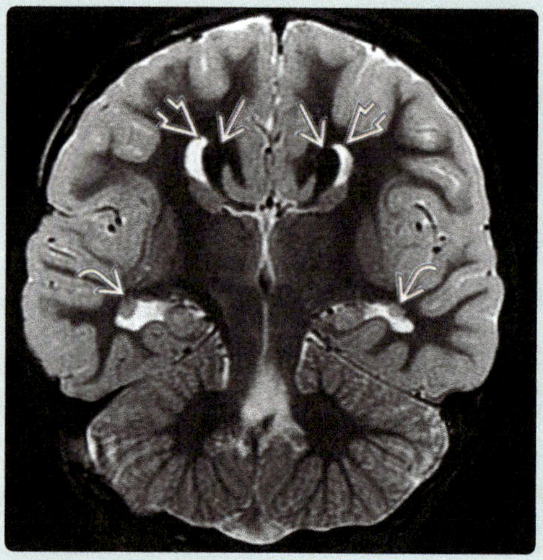

(Left) *Coronal graphic shows a lack of transverse corpus callosum and separate lateral ventricles. The interhemispheric fissure extends to the 3rd ventricle. The bundles of Probst* ➾ *contain the parasagittally rerouted callosal fibers.* **(Right)** *Coronal T2WI with callosal dysgenesis shows Viking helmet or moose head appearance of widely separated lateral ventricles* ➡. *The very hypointense white matter tracts medial to the lateral ventricles are the Probst bundles* ➡. *Note the heterotopic GM* ➡.

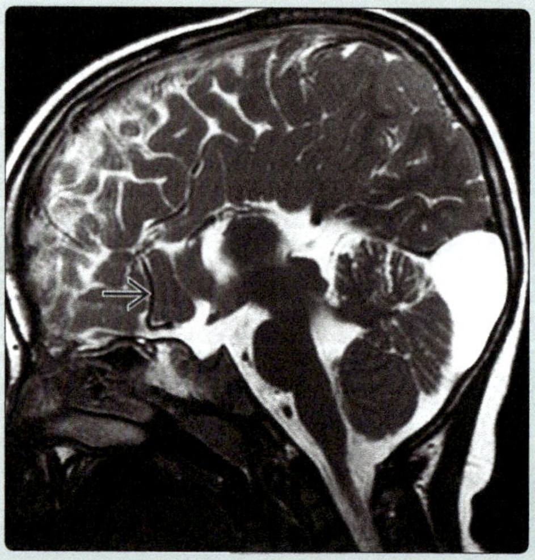

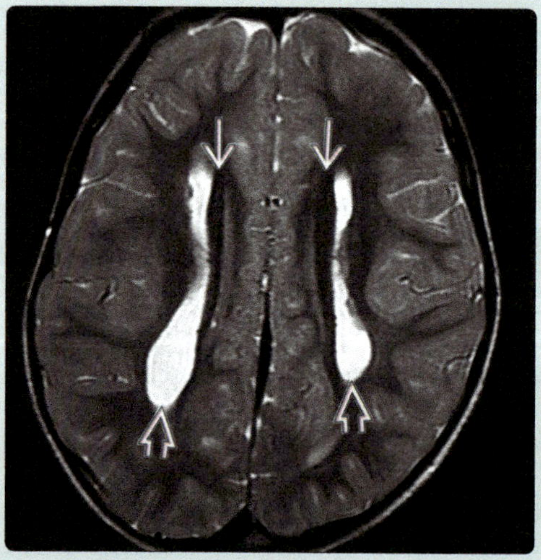

(Left) *Sagittal T2WI in the same patient shows absence of the corpus callosum, radially oriented gyri converging on a high-riding 3rd ventricle. Note the azygous anterior cerebral artery* ➾. *The anterior commissure is also absent.* **(Right)** *Axial T2WI in the same case shows the characteristic parallel, nonconverging lateral ventricles* ➡ *seen in corpus callosum agenesis. Heavily myelinated Probst bundles* ➡ *are seen just medial to the lateral ventricles.*

KEY FACTS

TERMINOLOGY

- Intracranial lipoma (ICL)
- Mass of mature adipose tissue (congenital malformation, not true neoplasm)

IMAGING

- Well-delineated lobulated extraaxial mass with fat attenuation/intensity
  - CT: -50 to -100 Hounsfield units (HU) (fat density); Ca++ varies from none to extensive
  - MR: Hyperintense on T1WI (becomes hypointense with fat suppression); may encase vessels and cranial nerves; often occurs with corpus callosum dysgenesis
- 80% supratentorial
  - 40-50% interhemispheric fissure (over corpus callosum; may extend into lateral ventricles, choroid plexus)
  - 15-20% suprasellar (attached to infundibulum, hypothalamus)
  - 10-15% tectal region (usually inferior colliculus/superior vermis)
- 20% infratentorial
  - Cerebellopontine angle (may extend into internal auditory canal, vestibule)

TOP DIFFERENTIAL DIAGNOSES

- Teratoma: Locations similar to lipoma; tissue from all 3 embryonic germ layers

CLINICAL ISSUES

- Most are asymptomatic; some present with seizures or headaches mainly affecting interhemispheric fissure

DIAGNOSTIC CHECKLIST

- When in doubt, use fat-saturation sequence
- Could high signal on T1WI be due to other substances with short T1 (e.g., subacute hemorrhage)
- Beware: Lipoma can mimic intracranial air on nonenhanced CT (use bone windows to distinguish)

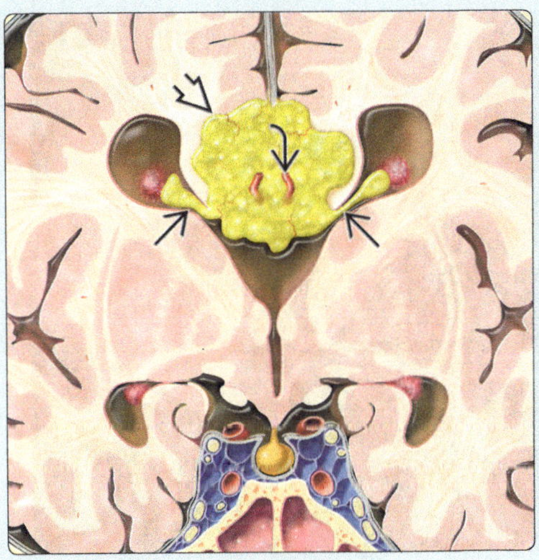

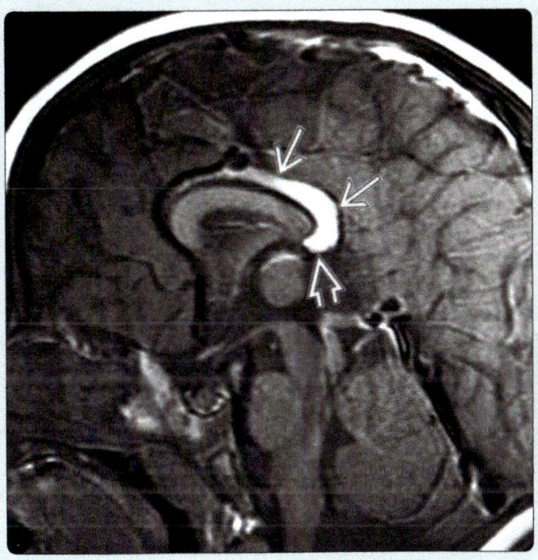

(Left) *Coronal graphic shows callosal agenesis with a bulky tubulonodular interhemispheric lipoma that encases the arteries and extends into the lateral ventricles.* **(Right)** *Sagittal T1WI MR shows a rather thin curvilinear interhemispheric lipoma in a 9-month-old infant. Note that the hyperintense lipoma is thicker posteriorly than anteriorly. It wraps around the back of the corpus callosum and extends beneath the corpus into the velum interpositum.*

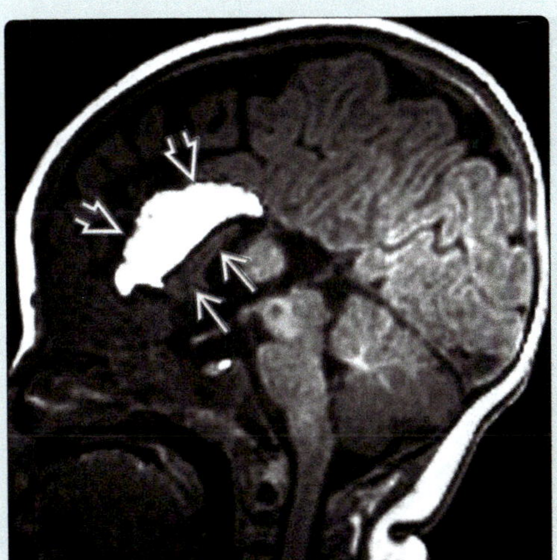

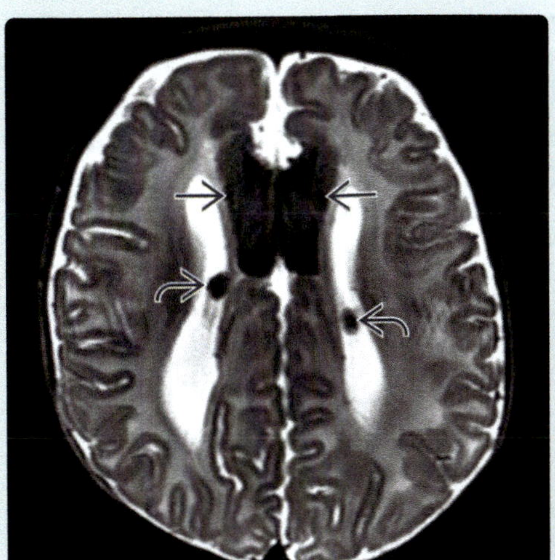

(Left) *Sagittal T1WI MR in a neonate shows a large, tubulonodular, interhemispheric lipoma dorsal to a wedge-shaped callosal remnant (absent body, splenium).* **(Right)** *Axial T2WI FS MR in the same patient shows the lipoma as hypointense and lying between the 2 cerebral hemispheres. The lipoma extends through the choroidal fissures into the lateral ventricles, where it is in the stroma of the choroid plexuses.*

KEY FACTS

TERMINOLOGY

- Dandy-Walker spectrum (DWS) represents broad spectrum of cystic posterior fossa (PF) malformations
  - DWS/complex
  - "Classic" DW malformation (DWM)
  - Hypoplastic vermis with rotation (HVR)
  - Persistent embryonic Blake pouch cyst (BPC)
  - Mega cisterna magna (MCM)

IMAGING

- "Classic" DWM
  - Cystic dilatation of 4th ventricle → enlarged PF
  - Vermis hypoplastic, rotated superiorly
- HVR
  - Variable vermian hypoplasia
  - PF/brainstem normal-sized
  - No or small cyst, keyhole-shaped 4th ventricle
- BPC
  - "Open" 4th ventricle communicates with cyst
  - Fastigial recess, primary fissure, PF/brainstem normal
- MCM
  - Enlarged pericerebellar cisterns communicate with basal subarachnoid spaces
- Occipital bone may appear scalloped/remodeled with **all** DWS types (including MCM)
- Routine MR (thin sagittal views crucial)

PATHOLOGY

- Most severe to mildest: DWM with 4th ventriculocele → classic DWM → HVR → BPC → MCM
- Numerous syndromes associated with DWS

CLINICAL ISSUES

- Marked heterogeneity in genetic, clinical findings
- DWM: 80% diagnosed by 1 year

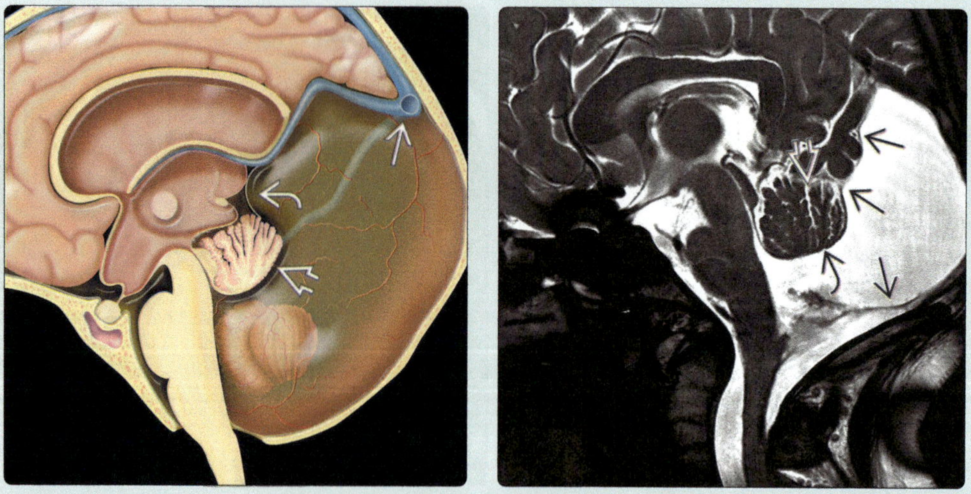

(Left) *Sagittal graphic of classic Dandy-Walker malformation shows an enlarged posterior fossa, elevated torcular herophili, superior rotation of hypoplastic cerebellar vermis, an overexpanded 4th ventricle with a thin wall, and a dilated ventricle (hydrocephalus).* **(Right)** *Sagittal T2WI MR DWS shows a hypoplastic, rotated vermis, lack of fastigial crease, and incomplete vermian lobulation of the posterior lobules beyond the primary fissure. The cyst wall is faintly seen.*

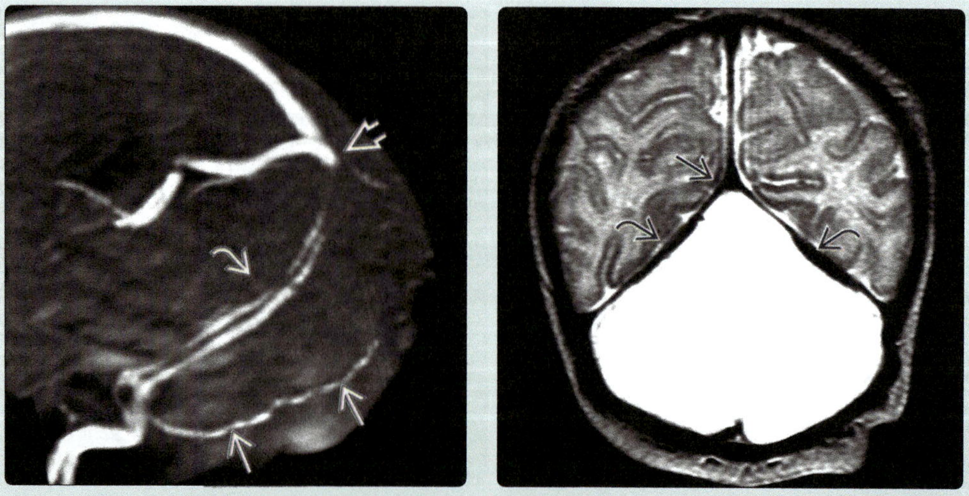

(Left) *Sagittal MRV demonstrates torcular-lambdoid inversion. The transverse sinuses angle upward toward the torcular, as the cyst has prevented normal fetal torcular descent. Note the persistent fetal occipital sinus.* **(Right)** *Coronal T2WI MR demonstrates a huge, fluid-filled posterior fossa. Again, notice that the transverse sinuses are angled upward toward the torcular herophili.*

KEY FACTS

TERMINOLOGY

- Septooptic dysplasia (SOD)
- De Morsier syndrome

IMAGING

- Absent septum pellucidum, small optic chiasm
- Optic nerves, pituitary gland, septum pellucidum
- Coronal imaging shows
  - Flat-roofed ventricles
  - Downward-pointing anterior horns
- 3 orthogonal planes crucial to identify all findings
  - Absent septum pellucidum, flat roof of frontal horns, small optic chiasm

CLINICAL ISSUES

- Newborns: Hypoglycemic seizures, apnea, cyanosis, hypotonia, prolonged conjugated jaundice, and (in boys) microphallus
- Abnormal endocrine function (60%): Look for multiple pituitary deficiencies
- Normal endocrine function (40%): Often have schizencephaly, seizures
- Child with short stature, endocrine dysfunction
- Normal or color blindness, visual loss, nystagmus, strabismus
- ± mental retardation, spasticity, microcephaly, anosmia
- 75-90% have brain abnormalities; 45% have pituitary insufficiency
- Bilateral optic nerve hypoplasia (70%)

DIAGNOSTIC CHECKLIST

- SOD in small-stature pediatric patient with absent septum pellucidum
- Small optic nerves, with ectopic posterior pituitary lobe, with absent septum pellucidum

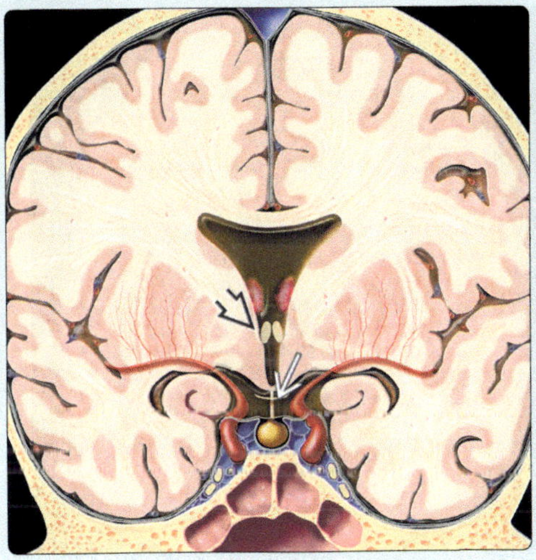

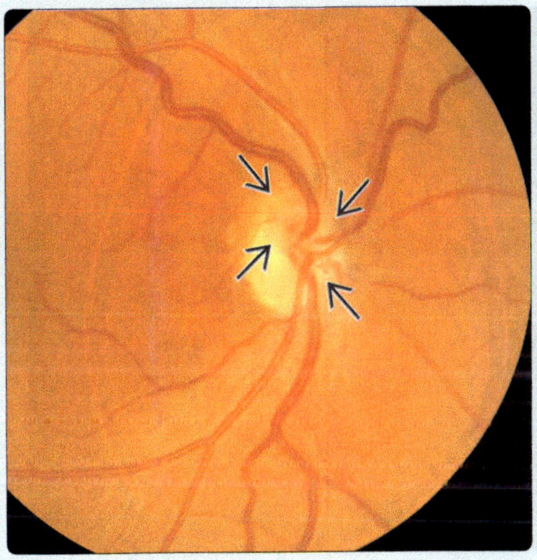

(Left) *Coronal graphic depicts flat-roofed anterior horns and the absence of a midline septum pellucidum. The anterior horns are draped inferiorly around the fornices* ⇨*, and the optic chiasm* ➡ *is small.* **(Right)** *Funduscopic photograph in a patient with absent septum pellucidum, bilateral optic nerve hypoplasia, and ectopic posterior pituitary gland shows a hypoplastic optic disc* →*.*

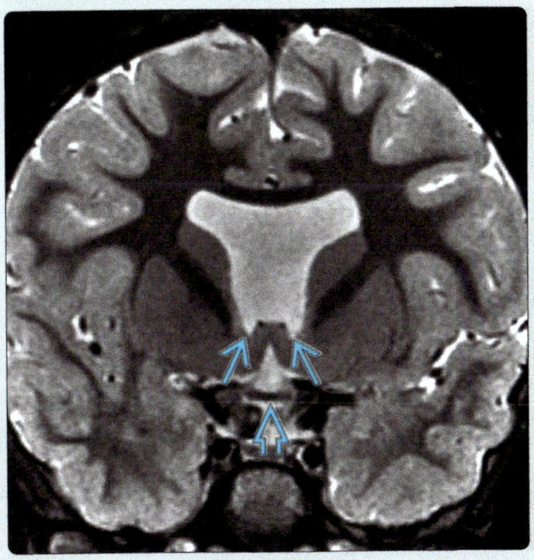

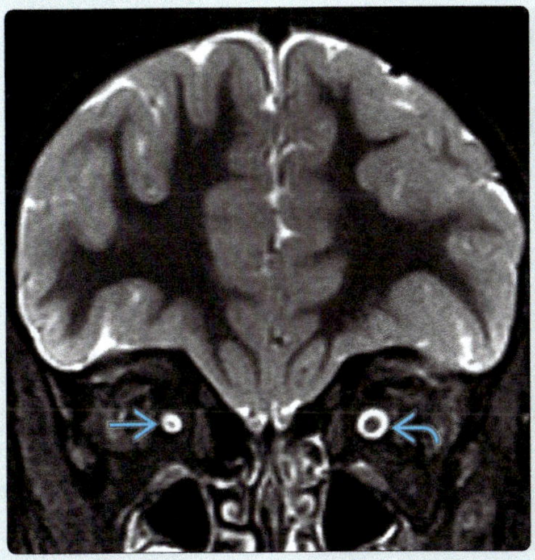

(Left) *Coronal T2WI FSE MR shows the absence of septum pellucidum and pointing* → *of the inferior margins of the frontal horns draped over fornices. Note that the optic chiasm* ⇨ *is normal in size, as is often the case in septooptic dysplasia.* **(Right)** *Coronal T2WI FSE MR in the same patient at the level of the intraorbital optic nerves shows unilateral optic nerve hypoplasia. The right optic nerve* → *is tiny, running through a small optic nerve sheath. The left optic nerve* ↩ *is normal.*

Heterotopic Gray Matter

KEY FACTS

TERMINOLOGY

- Heterotopia (HTP)
- Arrested/disrupted migration of groups of neurons from periventricular germinal zone (GZ) to cortex

IMAGING

- Ectopic nodule or ribbon, isointense with gray matter on every MR sequence
- Periventricular, subcortical/transcerebral, molecular layer
- Periventricular HTP located next to periventricular white matter (GZ of cerebral mantle) but not in corpus callosum (fiber tract) or next to basal ganglia (GZ of ganglionic eminence)
- Variable: From tiny to huge, isolated to diffuse
- Thin-slice, high-definition 3D acquisition, heavily weighted T1 provides optimal contrast and definition
- Large nodular HTP: Often thinned, polymicrogyric-looking overlying cortex

TOP DIFFERENTIAL DIAGNOSES

- Tuberous sclerosis
- "Closed-lip" schizencephaly
- Tumors

PATHOLOGY

- Periventricular nodular HTP often genetic when diffuse
  - *FLNA* gene commonly involved (required for cell migration to cortex) on Xq28
- Band HTP: Mild form of type 1 (classic) lissencephaly (agyria/pachygyria/double cortex)
  - Predominantly posterior lissencephaly/band HTP: Deletion LIS1 located on 17p13.3
  - Predominantly anterior lissencephaly/band HTP: Deletion *DCX* = double cortin on Xq22.3-q23

(Left) *Axial T2WI MR in a 6-year-old girl with refractory epilepsy shows massive right posterior subcortical heterotopia (HTP) containing cortex-like GM, WM, cerebrospinal fluid spaces, and blood vessels. The mass may suggest a tumor, but the hemisphere is small. Note the thin overlying cortex.* **(Right)** *Axial DTI color FA map (same patient) depicts the complete disorganization of WM in and around nodular subcortical HTP. Red, R-L; green, A-P; blue, S-I fiber orientation. Other hues imply intermediate directions.*

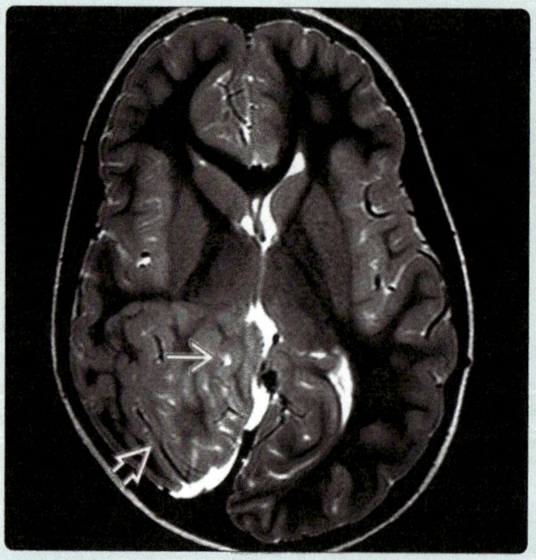

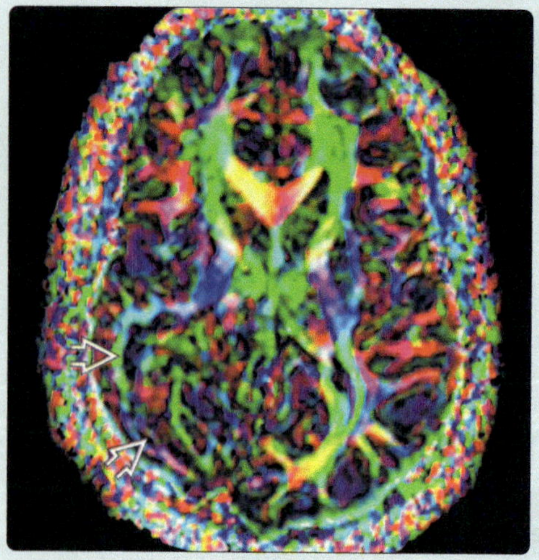

(Left) *Axial 3D T2WI MR shows subcortical band heterotopia in a 12-year-old boy. The symmetric HTP lies below an intermediate layer of WM. It is thicker posteriorly, in keeping with LIS1 mutation (autosomal recessive). The overlying cortex looks essentially normal.* **(Right)** *Axial T1WI MR in the same patient coregistered with magnetoencephalography (MEG) shows that the MEG spikes (triangles) originate from HTP, yet both the HTP and overlying cortex participate in the epileptogenic loop.*

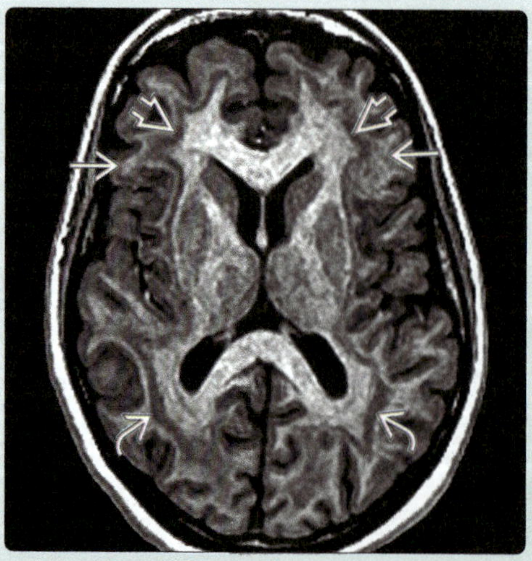

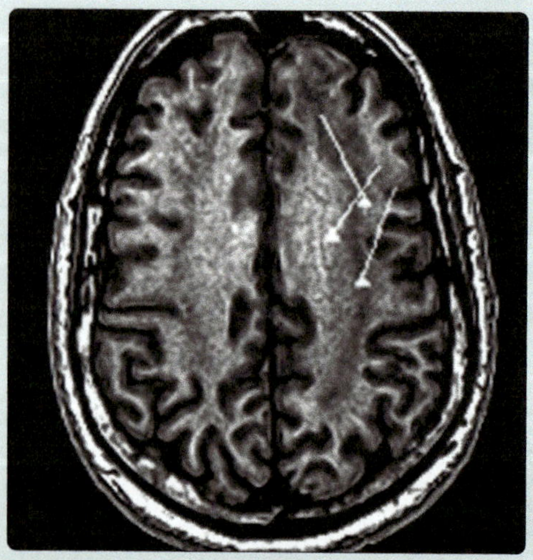

KEY FACTS

TERMINOLOGY

- Malformation due to abnormality in late neuronal migration and cortical organization
  - Neurons reach cortex but distribute abnormally, forming multiple small, undulating gyri
  - Result is cortex containing multiple small sulci that often appear fused on gross pathology and imaging

IMAGING

- Excessively small and prominent convolutions
- Predilection for perisylvian regions; when bilateral, often syndromic
- Small irregular gyri, but cortex appears normal or thick on MR
- May appear as deep infolding of thick cortex
- MR comprehensively assesses malformation; NECT for suspected Ca++ (TORCH)

TOP DIFFERENTIAL DIAGNOSES

- Microcephaly with simplified gyral pattern
- Hemimegalencephaly
- Congenital cytomegalovirus
- Pachygyria
- "Cobblestone" malformations

CLINICAL ISSUES

- Polymicrogyria most commonly → developmental delay, seizure
- Onset and severity of seizures, neurological deficits relate to extent of malformation, presence of associated anomalies

DIAGNOSTIC CHECKLIST

- Remember that polymicrogyria can result from injury, infection, or metabolic or destructive causes
- If visual or auditory symptoms, rule out congenital infection

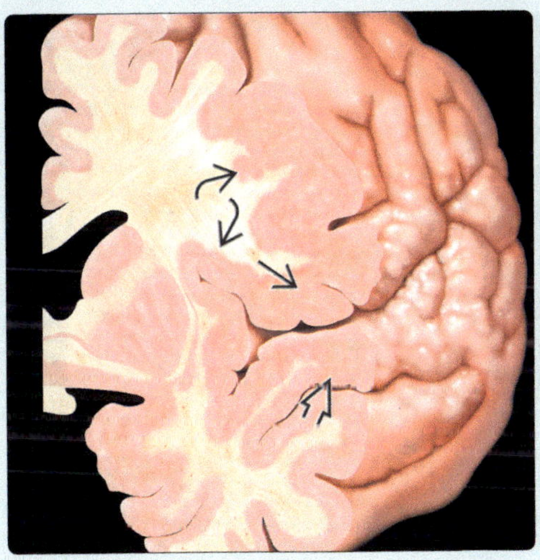

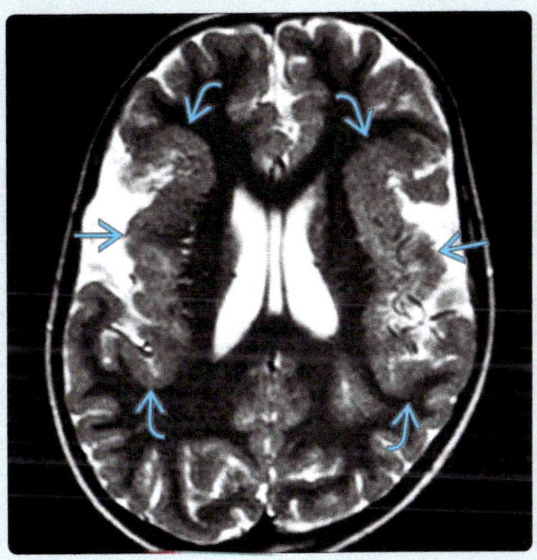

(Left) *Coronal oblique graphic shows the thickened pebbly gyri of polymicrogyria involving the frontal → and temporal → opercula. Note the abnormal sulcation and the irregular cortical-white matter junction → in the affected regions.* **(Right)** *Axial T2WI MR of a patient with bilateral perisylvian polymicrogyria shows a thickened, irregular cortex in the insulae →, as well as frontal and parietal opercula →. Incidental cavum septi pellucidi is also seen.*

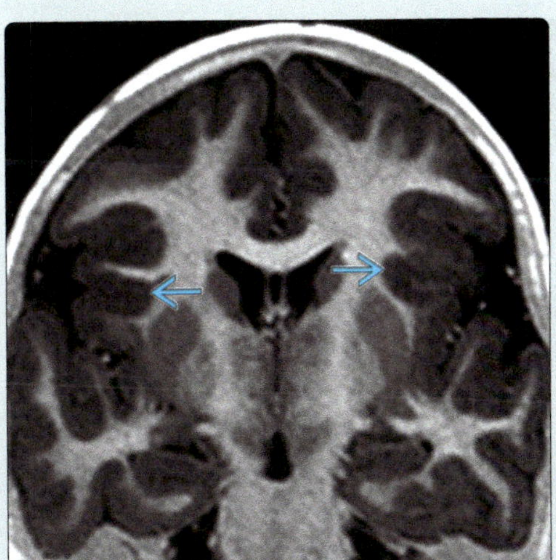

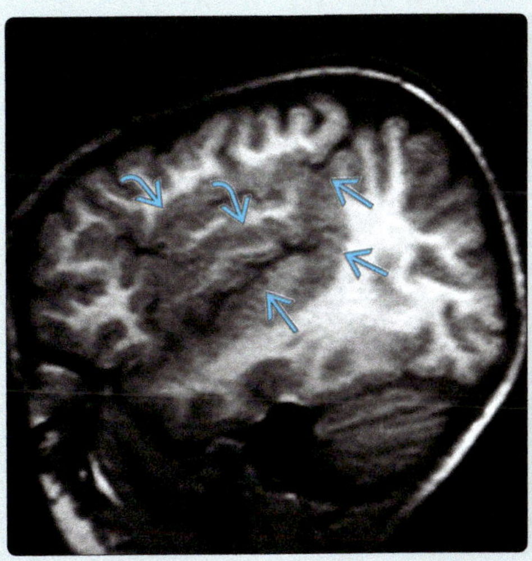

(Left) *Coronal T1WI MR of the same patient shows thickened, deeply undulating insulae → and opercula around the abnormal sylvian fissures. Polymicrogyria is often more poorly characterized in the coronal plane. The microgyri are not as well seen.* **(Right)** *Sagittal T1WI MR shows the characteristic continuation of the perisylvian polymicrogyria posteriorly into the superior parietal lobule →, which establishes the diagnosis. Other abnormal horizontal sulci with thick, irregular cortex → are present.*

KEY FACTS

IMAGING

- Transmantle gray matter (GM) lining clefts
  - Look for dimple in wall of ventricle if cleft is narrow/closed
- Up to 1/2 of schizencephalies are bilateral
  - When bilateral, 60% are open-lipped on both sides
- GM lining clefts may appear hyperdense
- Ca++ when associated with CMV or *COL4A1* mutations
- Prior to myelination, T2WI more clearly defines lesion

TOP DIFFERENTIAL DIAGNOSES

- Encephaloclastic porencephaly
  - Lined by gliotic white matter, not dysplastic GM
- Hydranencephaly
  - Residual tissue is supplied by posterior circulation
- Semilobar holoprosencephaly
  - Can mimic bilateral open-lip schizencephaly

PATHOLOGY

- Can be result of acquired in utero insult affecting neuronal migration
- 1/3 of children with schizencephaly have non-CNS abnormalities
- Infection (CMV), vascular insult, maternal trauma, toxin

CLINICAL ISSUES

- Unilateral: Seizures or mild motor deficit
- Bilateral: Developmental delay, paresis, microcephaly, spasticity
- Seizure more common with unilateral clefts
- Size of clefts and presence of associated malformative lesions govern severity of impairment

(Left) *Coronal graphic shows right closed-lip ➔ and left open-lip ➔ schizencephaly, both lined by gray matter. Note absence of septum pellucidum ➔.* **(Right)** *Coronal T2FS MR shows bilateral schizencephaly. A closed-lip defect is seen on the right ➔, extending from the pial surface to the ventricular outpouching ➔, while a mildly open-lip defect lined with dysplastic gray matter is present on the left ➔. Note the abnormal vessels in the left-sided schizencephalic cleft ➔.*

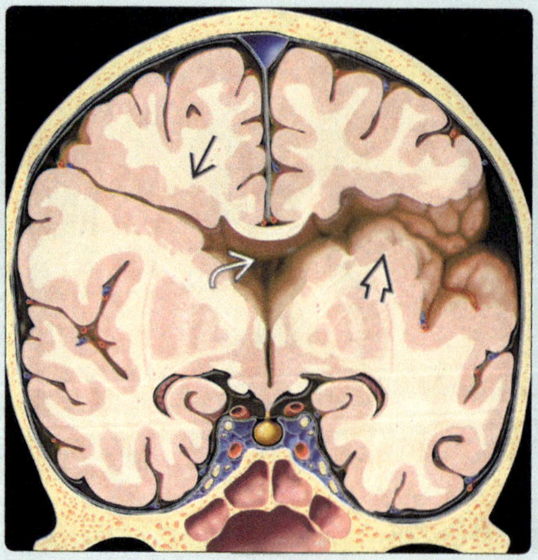

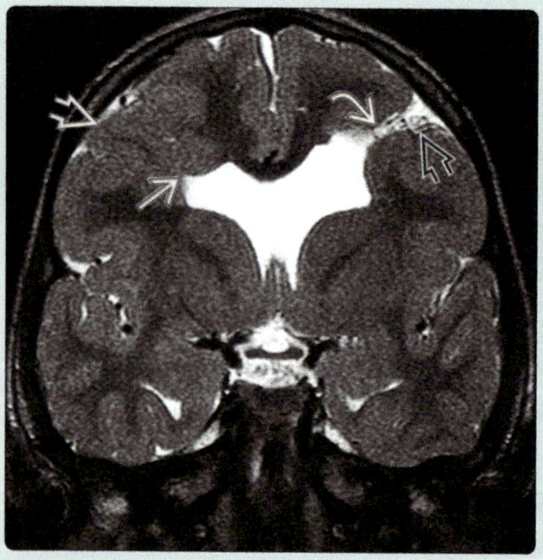

(Left) *Axial NECT in a 19-year-old man in the ER for trauma shows a "nipple" or outpouching of the left lateral ventricle ➔ that extends into a full-thickness cerebrospinal fluid cleft ➔. The cleft is lined with heterotopic gray matter ➔. This is a classic unilateral schizencephaly.* **(Right)** *Coronal T2WI shows large bilateral open-lip schizencephalic clefts ➔.*

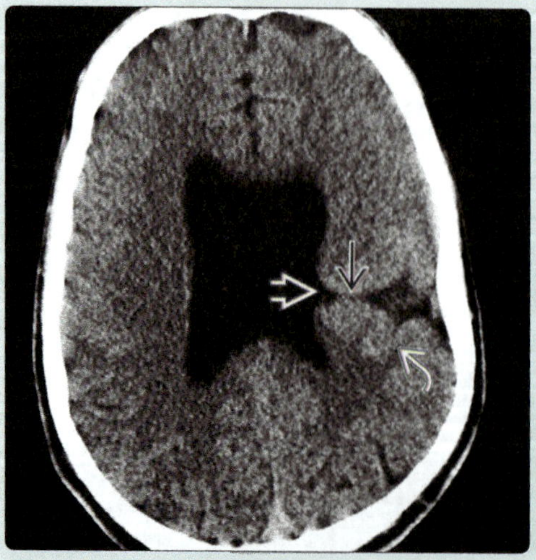

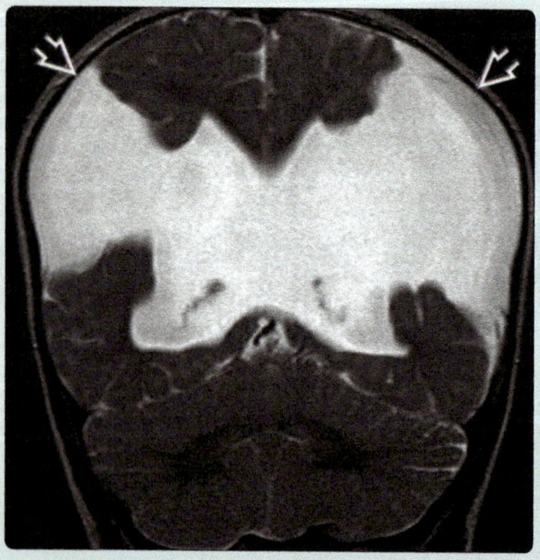

KEY FACTS

TERMINOLOGY

- Autosomal-dominant familial syndrome with hemangioblastomas (HGBLs), clear cell renal carcinoma, cystadenomas, pheochromocytomas

IMAGING

- 2 or more CNS HGBLs or 1 HGBL plus visceral lesion or retinal hemorrhage
- HGBLs vary from tiny mass to very large with even larger associated cysts

TOP DIFFERENTIAL DIAGNOSES

- Vascular metastasis
- Solitary HGBL
- Pilocytic astrocytoma
- Hemispheric medulloblastoma in teenager or young adult
- Multiple arteriovenous malformations in vascular neurocutaneous syndrome

PATHOLOGY

- von Hippel-Lindau (VHL) phenotypes, subtypes based on absence or presence of pheochromocytoma
  - Type 1: Low risk of pheochromocytoma
  - Type 2: High risk of pheochromocytoma
    - Type 2A (low risk of renal cell carcinoma)
    - Type 2B (high risk of renal cell carcinoma)
    - Type 2C (familial pheochromocytoma without either HGBL or Rathke cleft cyst)

CLINICAL ISSUES

- Earliest symptom in VHL often visual
  - Retinal HGBL, peak in teenage years
- HGBLs → multiple periods of tumor growth (usually associated with increasing cyst size) separated by periods of arrested growth

DIAGNOSTIC CHECKLIST

- Check retina, cerebellum

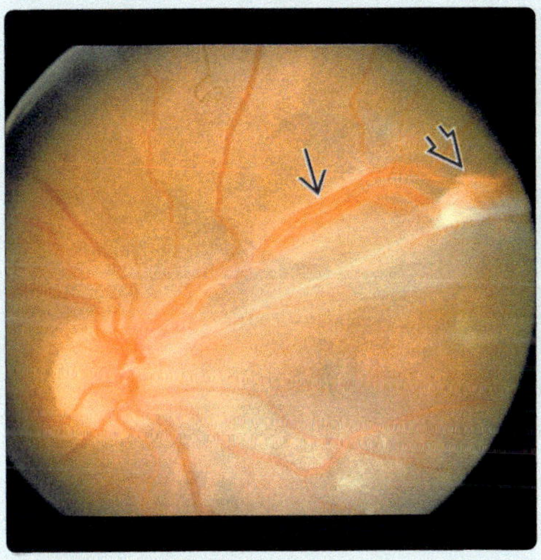

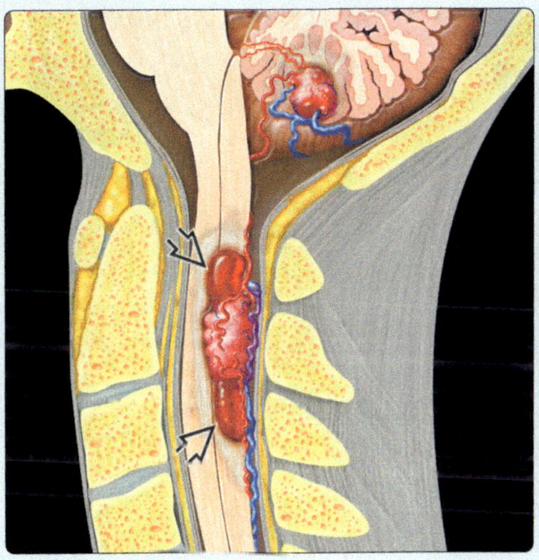

(Left) *Funduscopic examination in a patient with von Hippel-Lindau syndrome (VHL) shows a peripheral retinal angioma supplied by prominent arteries.* **(Right)** *Sagittal graphic shows 2 hemangioblastomas (HGBLs) in VHL. In this patient, the spinal cord tumor has an associated cyst and would cause myelopathy. The small cerebellar HGBL would be asymptomatic.*

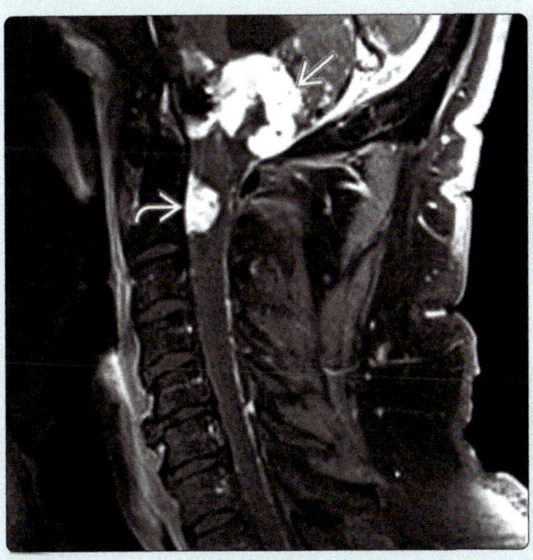

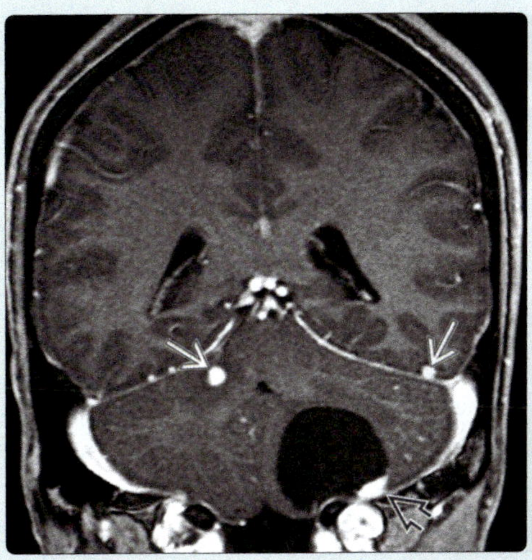

(Left) *Sagittal T1C+FS MR in a patient with VHL shows multiple cerebellar, spinal HGBLs.* **(Right)** *Coronal T1 C+ FS in an asymptomatic 26-year-old man with pancreatic cysts and a family history of VHL shows 2 solid and 1 cystic HGBL with a mural nodule.*

KEY FACTS

TERMINOLOGY

- Neurofibromatosis type 1 (NF1), von Recklinghausen disease, peripheral neurofibromatosis

IMAGING

- Benign hyperintense white matter (WM) lesions on T2WI in 70-90% of preteen children
  - Lesions are poorly defined, no mass effect/enhancement
  - May also involve cerebellar WM, globus pallidus, thalamus, brainstem
  - Wax, then wane; disappear by 20 years of age
- Neoplasms
  - Plexiform neurofibromas
    - Sphenoid wing and occipital bone dysplasia found in association with plexiform tumors
  - Optic pathway gliomas (OPGs)
  - Parenchymal gliomas
- Vascular dysplasias → stenosis, moyamoya, aneurysm

PATHOLOGY

- Autosomal dominant; gene locus is chromosome 17q12
- Gene product is neurofibromin (negative regulator of RAS protooncogene)
  - Neurofibromin also regulates neuroglial progenitor function
  - Required for normal glial and neuronal development
  - Inactivated in NF1 → tissue proliferation, tumor development
- Focal areas of signal intensity related to (transient) intramyelinic edema

CLINICAL ISSUES

- ~ 50% have macrocephaly; in part secondary to ↑ WM volume
- OPG can cause progressive vision loss
- Café au lait spots are earliest finding
- Most common neurocutaneous and inherited tumor syndrome

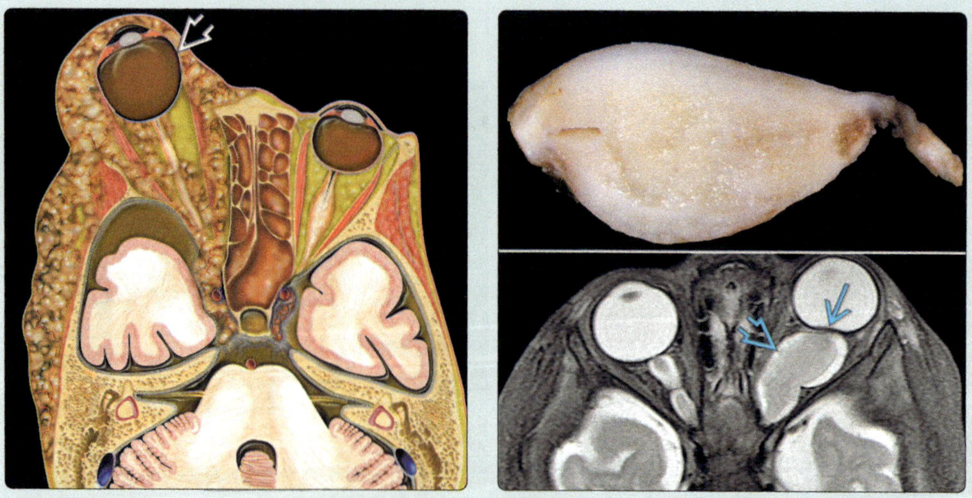

(Left) *Axial graphic shows enlarged right middle cranial fossa, dysplastic sphenoid wing, and a large orbital/periorbital plexiform neurofibroma. Note the exophthalmos and buphthalmos of the involved globe.* **(Right)** *Gross pathology of optic pathway glioma (top) shows classic well-delineated fusiform enlargement of the optic nerve. Axial T2WI (bottom) shows optic nerve glioma enlarging the left optic nerve. Note anterior displacement and posterior deformity of the globe.*

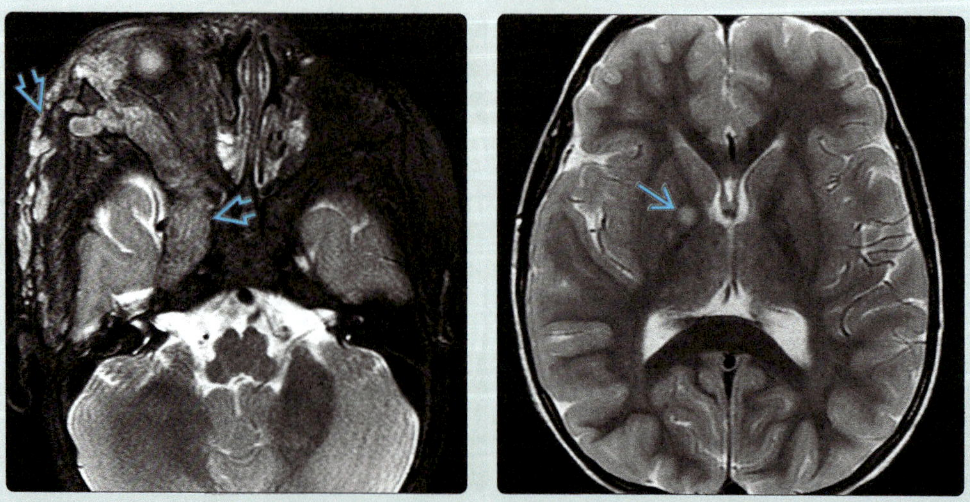

(Left) *Axial T2FS MR in an 18-month-old child shows an extensive plexiform neurofibroma infiltrating the scalp and orbit and extending into the cavernous sinus through the superior orbital fissure. Note the bag of worms appearance.* **(Right)** *Axial T2WI in a 4-year-old child with neurofibromatosis type 1 shows 2 prominent hyperintense foci in the right internal capsule. The lesions disappeared by age of 15 years.*

Neurofibromatosis Type 2

KEY FACTS

TERMINOLOGY

- Familial cancer syndrome
  - Multiple cranial nerve (CN) schwannomas, meningiomas, and spinal tumors

IMAGING

- Best diagnostic clue: Bilateral vestibular schwannomas
- Multiple extraaxial tumors
  - Schwannomas of CNs and spinal nerve roots
  - Meningiomas on dural surfaces (up to 50%)
- Intraaxial tumors
  - Ependymomas in spinal cord and brainstem (6%)
- Recommendation: Use high-resolution T1 C+ FS MR through basal cisterns to evaluate cranial nerves

TOP DIFFERENTIAL DIAGNOSES

- Schwannomatosis
- Multiple meningiomas
- Metastases

PATHOLOGY

- All neurofibromatosis type 2 (NF2) families have chromosome 22q12 abnormalities
- *NF2* gene encodes for merlin protein

CLINICAL ISSUES

- Usually presents between 2nd and 4th decades with hearing loss, ± vertigo
- Incidence: 1:25,000-30,000
- Life span substantially shortened by presence of meningiomas and by complications related to lower cranial neuropathies (i.e., aspiration)

DIAGNOSTIC CHECKLIST

- Carefully evaluate other cranial nerves in any new diagnosis of schwannoma or meningioma in child/adolescent/young adult

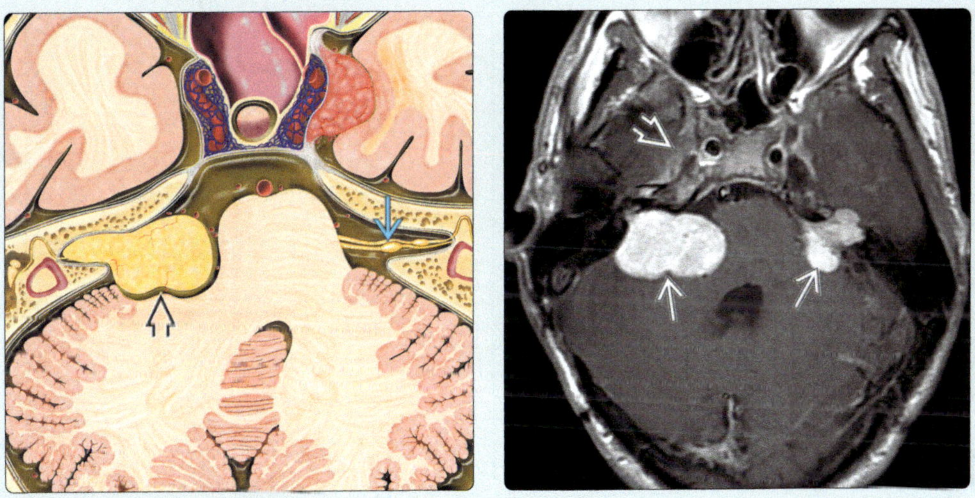

(Left) *Axial graphic shows bilateral cerebellopontine angle schwannomas pathognomonic of neurofibromatosis type 2 (NF2). The tumor ⇨ on the right is large, and several small schwannomas → are seen on the left vestibulocochlear nerves.* **(Right)** *Axial T1 C+ MR in a patient with typical NF2 shows bilateral vestibular schwannomas ➡ and a right cavernous sinus meningioma ⇨.*

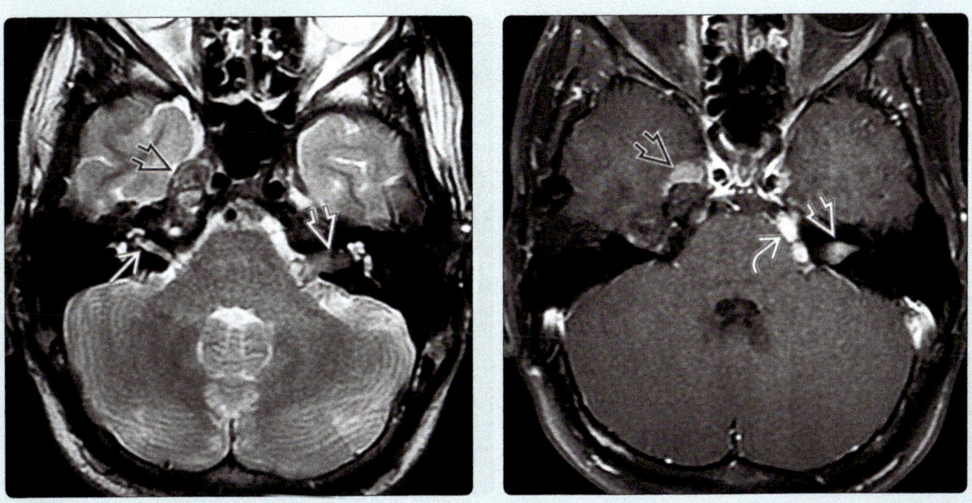

(Left) *Axial T2WI in a 14-year-old boy with left sensorineural hearing loss shows a mass in the left internal auditory canal ➡ and another lesion in the right cavernous sinus ⇨. Note the small nodules ➡ along the right vestibular nerve.* **(Right)** *T1 C+ FS in the same patient shows the left internal auditory canal mass enhances ➡, as does the right cavernous sinus lesion ⇨. In addition, 2 enhancing nodules are seen along the cisternal left trigeminal nerve ➡. The patient was subsequently diagnosed with NF2.*

KEY FACTS

TERMINOLOGY

- Tuberous sclerosis complex (TSC)
- Multisystem genetic disorder with epilepsy, multiorgan tumors, and hamartomas
  - Spectrum of CNS hamartomas; all contain dysplastic neurons and giant (balloon) cells
  - Caused by mutation in *TSC1* or *TSC2* gene
  - Now considered an infantile (developmental) tauopathy
    - Tau abnormally expressed in many dysmorphic neurons and glial cells of TSC
    - Similar to focal cortical dysplasia (FCD) 2

IMAGING

- FLAIR and T1 MR most sensitive sequences for diagnosis
- Calcified subependymal nodules (SENs)
  - < 1.3 cm, often enhance (more on MR than CT)
- Subependymal giant cell astrocytoma (SEGA) (15% of TSC)
  - Most located at foramen of Monro
    - > 1.3 cm; enhance strongly, enlarge over time
- Cortical/subcortical tubers (95%)
  - Early T1 ↑ but variable after myelin maturation
- Other findings
  - White matter (WM) radial migration lines
  - Cyst-like WM lesions (cystoid brain degeneration)

TOP DIFFERENTIAL DIAGNOSES

- Taylor-type cortical dysplasia (FCD type 2)
- X-linked subependymal heterotopia

PATHOLOGY

- Mutations in TSC tumor suppressor genes → abnormal germinal matrix proliferation, differentiation

CLINICAL ISSUES

- Classic clinical triad = facial angiofibromas (90%), mental retardation (50-80%), seizures (80-90%) (all 3 = 30%)

DIAGNOSTIC CHECKLIST

- SEN (< 1.3 cm) vs. SEGA (> 1.3 cm, enlarging)

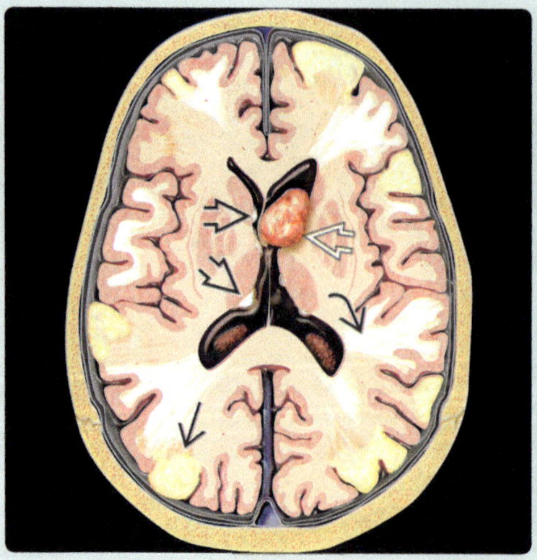

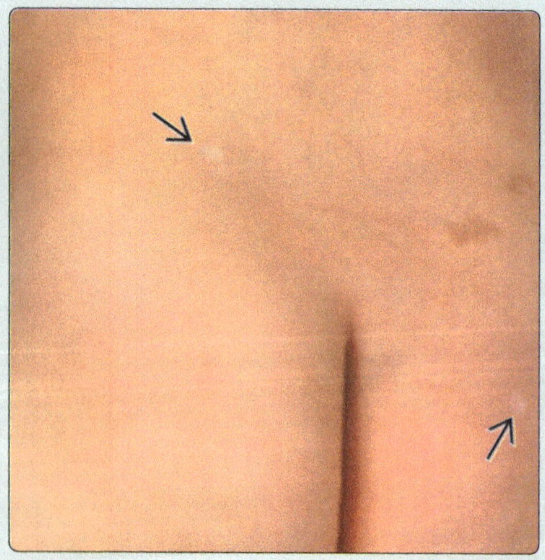

(Left) *Axial graphic of typical brain involvement in tuberous sclerosis complex (TSC) shows a giant cell astrocytoma ➔ in the left foramen of Monro, subependymal nodules ➔, radial migration lines ➔, and cortical/subcortical tubers ➔.* **(Right)** *Clinical photograph of a patient with TSC shows the hypopigmented "ash leaf" spots ➔ characteristic of TSC.*

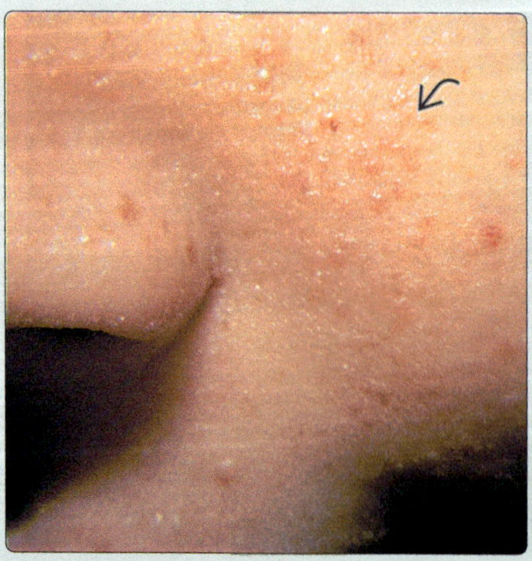

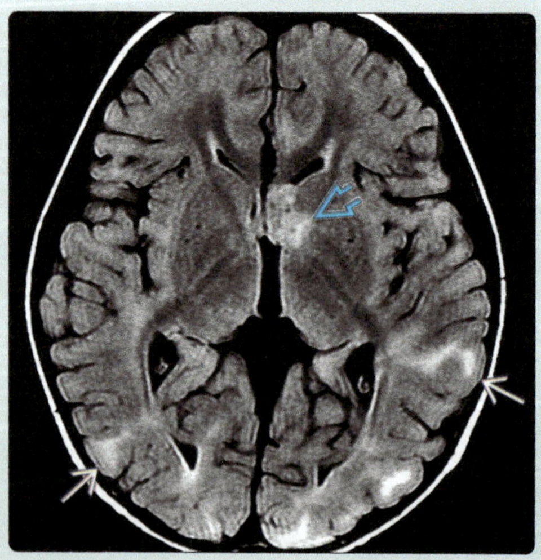

(Left) *Clinical photograph of a patient with TSC shows numerous facial angiofibromas ➔ characteristic of the disorder. (Courtesy B. Krafchik, MD.)* **(Right)** *Axial FLAIR surveillance scan in a 14-year-old boy with known TSC shows a well-demarcated lobulated mass in the left frontal horn ➔, a subependymal giant cell astrocytoma. Note multiple expanded gyri with poor gray-white differentiation (tubers ➔), subcortical WM hyperintensities.*

KEY FACTS

TERMINOLOGY

- Synonyms: Sturge-Weber-Dimitri, encephalotrigeminal angiomatosis

IMAGING

- Imaging features are pial angioma with sequelae of chronic venous ischemia
  - Pial angiomatosis unilateral (80%), bilateral (20%)
  - Cortical Ca++, atrophy, and enlarged ipsilateral choroid plexus
  - "Tram-track" calcification in cortex (not angioma)
- Early: Transient hyperperfusion → "accelerated" myelin maturation
- Late: Increased signal in region of gliosis and decreased cortical signal in regions of calcification
- Early: Serpentine leptomeningeal enhancement, pial angiomatosis of subarachnoid space
- SWI delineates enlarged, tortuous medullary white matter veins providing collateral drainage to deep veins

PATHOLOGY

- Somatic mutation of *GNAQ* causes Sturge-Weber syndrome and nonsyndromic "port-wine" stains

CLINICAL ISSUES

- "Port-wine" stain, seizures, hemiparesis
- Rare: 1:20,000-50,000
- ↑ extent of lobar involvement and atrophy leading to increased likelihood of seizures
- Seizures cause further brain injury

DIAGNOSTIC CHECKLIST

- FLAIR C+ most sensitive sequence to detect pial angioma (especially in infancy)
- T2 hypointensity of white matter underlying angioma is clue to early diagnosis
- Identification of retinal angioma critical in subtle/early cases

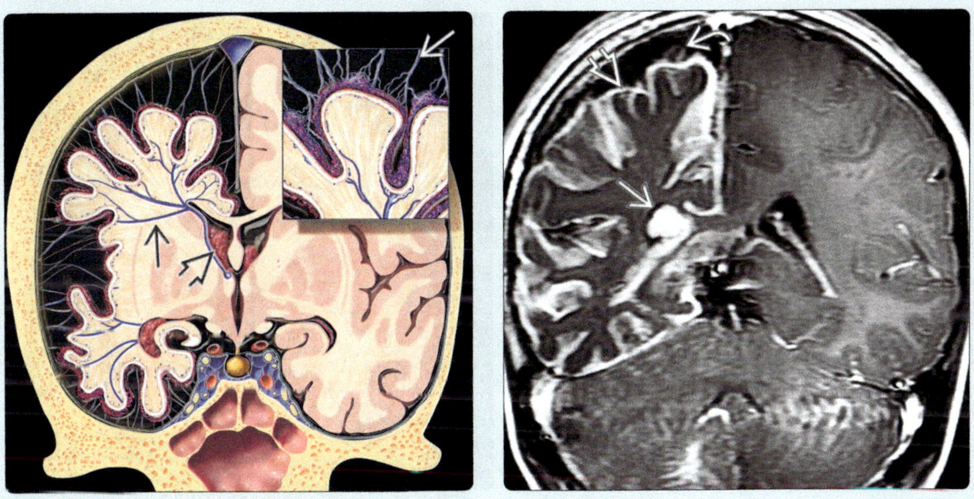

(Left) *Coronal graphic shows extensive pial angiomatosis ➔ surrounding affected gyri, prominent deep medullary collaterals ⇨, shunt venous blood to deep system, enlarged ipsilateral choroid plexus ⇨, and atrophy of the right cerebral hemisphere.* **(Right)** *Coronal T1C+ MR in an 8 year old with Sturge-Weber syndrome (SWS) shows atrophy of the right hemisphere with vessels ➔ crossing the prominent subarachnoid space from the pial angioma ➔. Note enlarged ipsilateral choroid plexus ➔.*

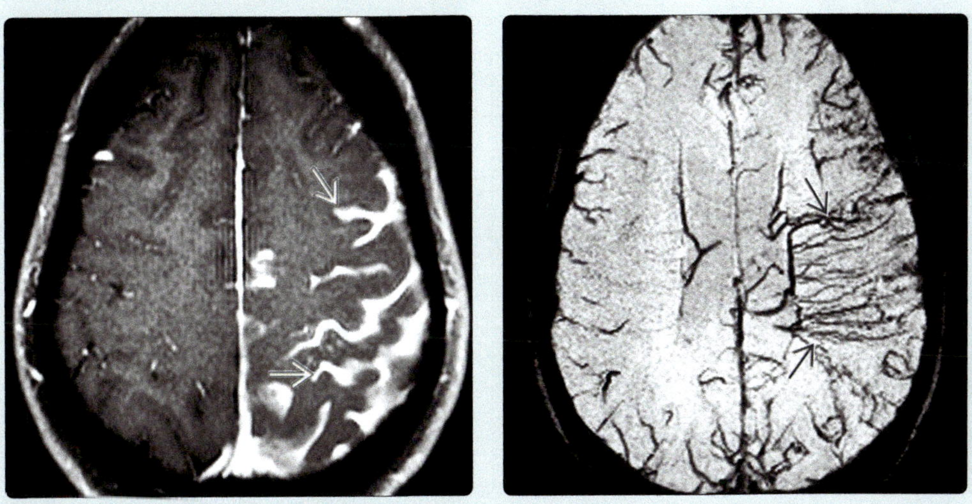

(Left) *T1 C+ FS scan in another patient with SWS shows enlarged convexity sulci that are entirely filled with an intensely enhancing pial angioma ➔.* **(Right)** *T2* SWI in the same case shows multiple enlarged, tortuous medullary veins ⇨ draining the left hemisphere into the deep venous system. There is a paucity of normal cortical veins in SWS, so the enhancing pial angioma must drain into the ipsilateral subependymal veins and choroid plexus.*

KEY FACTS

TERMINOLOGY

- Hereditary hemorrhagic telangiectasia (HHT)
  - Rendu-Osler-Weber, Osler-Weber-Rendu syndrome
- Autosomal dominant disorder with widely distributed, multisystem angiodysplastic lesions
  - Mucocutaneous telangiectasias with arteriovenous malformations (AVMs) in visceral organs (primarily lungs, brain, liver)

IMAGING

- Best diagnostic clue
  - Multiple pulmonary or cerebral malformations (pAVM/cAVM) in patient with recurrent epistaxis
- MR
  - "Blooming" of capillary telangiectasias (SWI > GRE)
    - "Fluffy" enhancement on T1 C+
  - cAVM: Nest ("tangle") of flow voids, gliosis
- Useful: Multislice CT/CTA of lungs and liver

PATHOLOGY

- Genetically heterogeneous disorder caused by mutations in TGF-β/BMP signaling pathway
  - Endoglin (*ENG*) mutations cause HHT1
  - Activin A receptor type II-like 1 (*ACVRL1/ALK1*) mutations cause HHT2
  - *SMAD4* mutations cause the combined Juvenile Polyposis/HHT syndrome
- 3 types of vascular malformations in HHT
  - Most common: Capillary vascular malformation (61%)
    - Tangle of abnormal vessels
    - No shunt, no dilated feeding artery or draining vein
  - Nidus-type AVM: 43%
    - Dilated network of abnormal vessels
    - AV shunting (early draining vein)
  - Direct high-flow arteriovenous fistula: 12%
    - Shunt with absence of intervening nidus between feeding artery, draining vein

(Left) *Photograph of a patient with hereditary hemorrhagic telangiectasia (HHT), multiple episodes of severe epistaxis shows numerous cutaneous telangiectasias ⇨, with visible lesions on mucosa of the mouth → and nose ↷.* **(Right)** *Axial FLAIR MR in an 18-year-old man with family history of HHT was obtained as part of routine screening. A small left medial frontal hyperintensity ⇨ with associated flow voids → is present.*

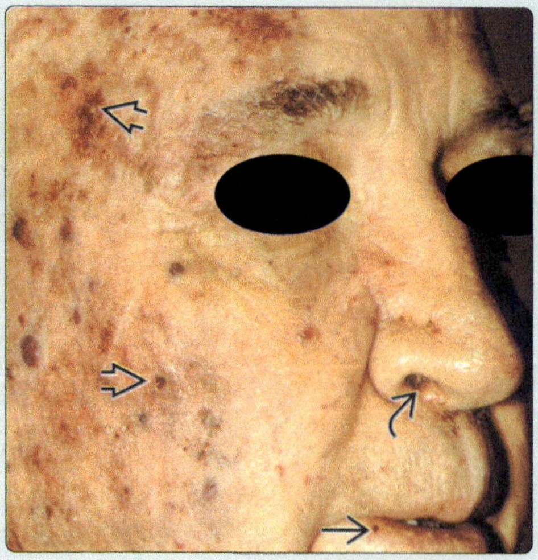

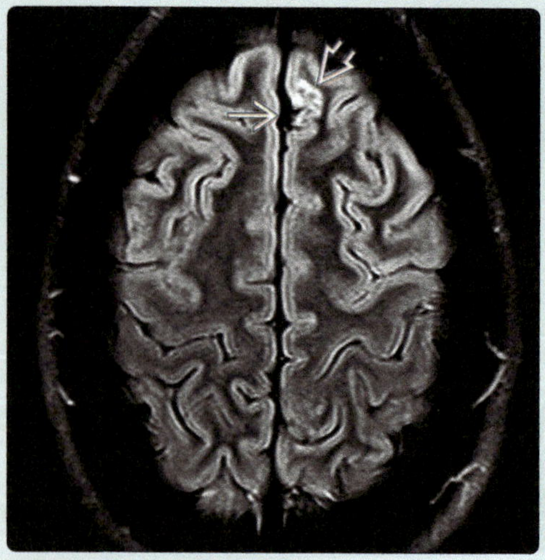

(Left) *Axial T1 C+ MR in the same patient shows that the lesion ⇨ enhances intensely.* **(Right)** *Lateral view of the left internal carotid DSA obtained in the same patient shows a small arteriovenous malformation (AVM) nidus ⇨ ("micro-AVM") with an early draining vein →. Genetic profiling showed ENG mutation.*

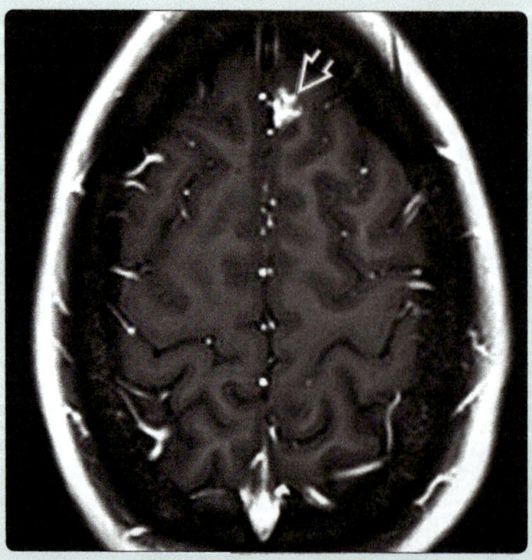

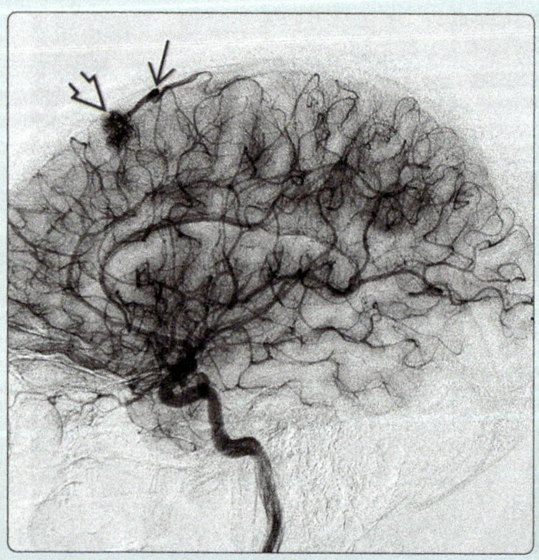

KEY FACTS

TERMINOLOGY

- Lhermitte-Duclos disease (LDD)
  - Benign cerebellar lesion; unclear if neoplastic, malformative, or hamartomatous
- Multiple hamartoma syndrome (MHAM) → autosomal dominant, mutation in *PTEN* gene, associated with increased incidence of malignancy
  - MHAM = Cowden syndrome (CS); Cowden plus Lhermitte-Duclos = MHAM with LDD
    - CS is most common phenotype of PTEN hamartoma tumor syndrome
  - LDD now considered manifestation of MHAM and neurocutaneous syndrome

IMAGING

- Relatively well-defined cerebellar mass with striated/corduroy/tigroid/gyriform pattern
- LDD always in cerebellum and may be large → mass effect, tonsillar herniation, hydrocephalus

TOP DIFFERENTIAL DIAGNOSES

- Subacute cerebellar infarction
- Cerebellitis
- Unclassified cerebellar dysplasias
- Ganglioglioma
- Medulloblastoma

CLINICAL ISSUES

- Most common presentation: Headache, nausea and vomiting, ataxia, blurred vision
  - Can present in coma
- Shunting or surgical debulking for symptomatic patients with hydrocephalus

DIAGNOSTIC CHECKLIST

- If LDD, screen for MHAM; if MHAM, screen for LDD
- Long-term cancer screening needed, especially thyroid and breast (↑ malignancy in MHAM)

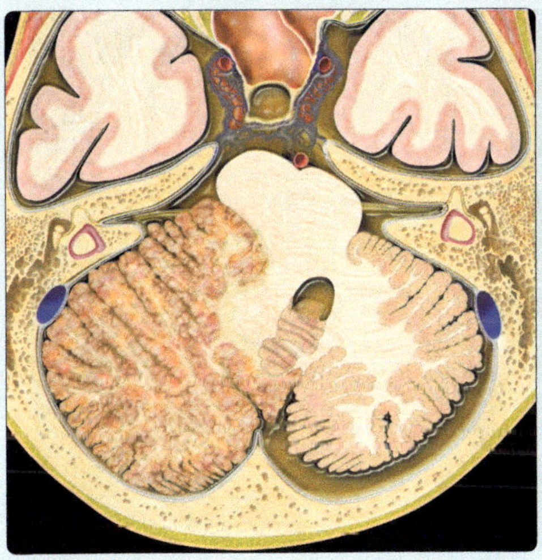

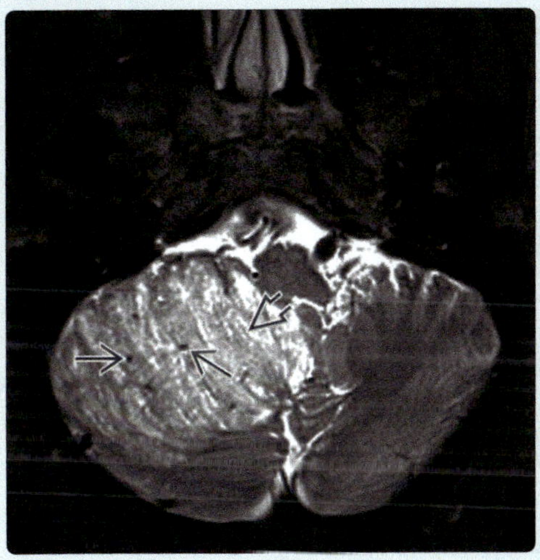

(Left) *Axial graphic shows thickened and irregular cerebellar folia in the right cerebellar hemisphere. This results in the enlargement of the hemisphere & mass effect upon the brainstem that are typical of Lhermitte-Duclos disease (LDD).* **(Right)** *Axial T2WI in a 76-year-old man with nonspecific headaches shows a hyperintense right cerebellar hemispheric mass. The widened "gyriform" folia ⇨ give the mass a distinctive striated appearance. Several dot-like flow voids ⇨ are present in between the enlarged folia.*

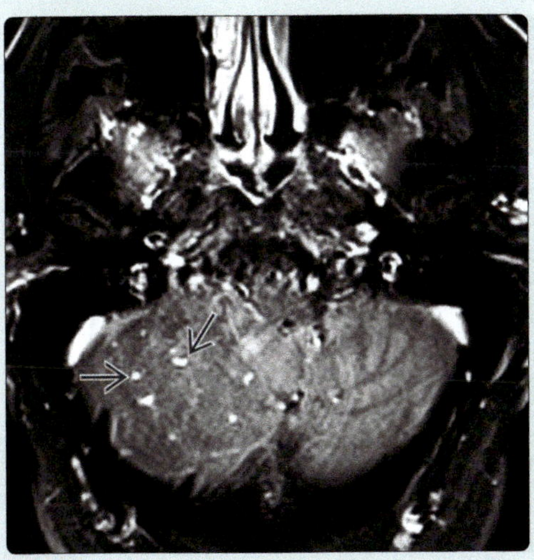

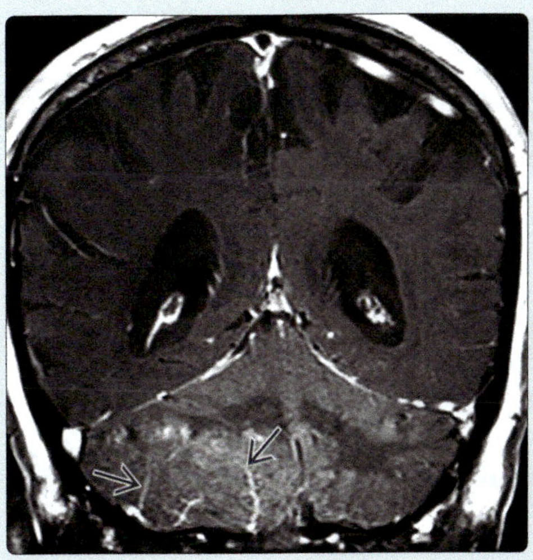

(Left) *Axial T1 C+ FS in the same patient shows that the thickened folia do not enhance, but the prominent flow voids seen on the T2WI show strong, uniform enhancement ⇨, suggesting that they are vascular structures.* **(Right)** *Coronal T1 C+ scan in the same case shows the enhancing vessels ⇨ nicely. The findings were pathognomonic of LDD, so the mass was not biopsied.*

KEY FACTS

TERMINOLOGY

- Li-Fraumeni syndrome (LFS)
- Autosomal-dominant familial cancer syndrome
  - 75% of LFS cases have loss of function mutations in *TP53* tumor suppressor gene
  - Lifelong ↑ risk of osteosarcoma, soft tissue sarcoma, leukemia, breast cancer, brain tumors, melanoma, adrenal cortical tumors

IMAGING

- Astrocytoma: Cerebrum > cerebellum > spine
- Choroid plexus carcinoma: Lateral ventricle > > 4th ventricle

TOP DIFFERENTIAL DIAGNOSES

- Hereditary syndromes causing familial cancers, including brain tumors
- Tuberous sclerosis
- von Hippel-Lindau
- Medulloblastoma
- Basal cell nevus syndrome
- Turcot
- Neurofibromatosis type 1
- Carney complex
- Melanoma-astrocytoma syndrome

PATHOLOGY

- p53: Transcription factor important in apoptosis, cell cycle control; frequently mutated in tumors
- Breast cancer (24-30%), soft tissue sarcoma (12-18%), brain tumors (12-14%), bone sarcoma (12-13%), adrenocortical carcinoma (6%)

CLINICAL ISSUES

- Propensity to develop additional primary neoplasms
- Brain tumors: High prevalence below 10 years of age

(Left) *A 38-year-old woman with a history of breast cancer presented to the ER with several months of increasingly severe headache and visual difficulties. NECT scan shows a large hyperdense mass ➡ in the right occipital region.* **(Right)** *Axial T1 C+ FS in the same patient shows a large, intensely enhancing right occipital mass ⇨.*

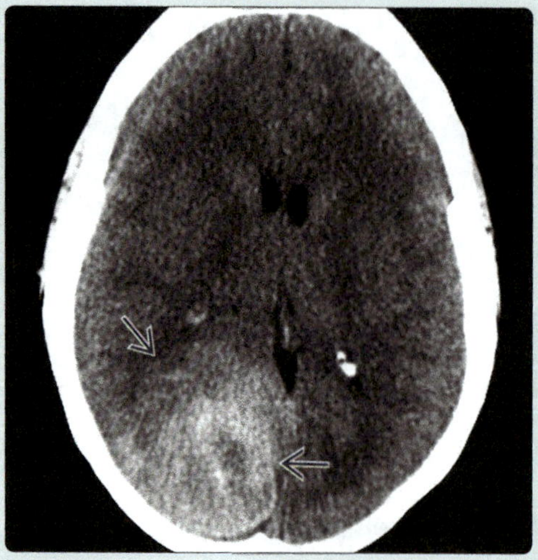

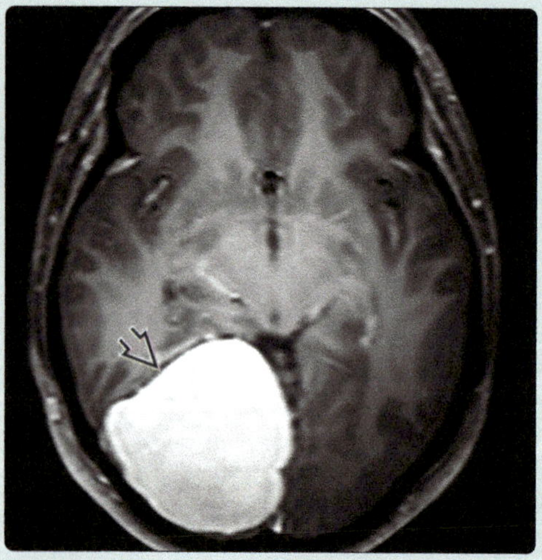

(Left) *Sagittal T1 C+ FS MR shows that the well-demarcated, intensely enhancing mass ⇨ abuts the dura.* **(Right)** *Axial presurgical contrast-enhanced SPGR shows a subtle dural "tail" along the tentorium cerebelli ➡. Preoperative diagnosis of meningioma was confirmed at surgery. Further evaluation disclosed TP53 germline mutation, and Li-Fraumeni syndrome was diagnosed.*

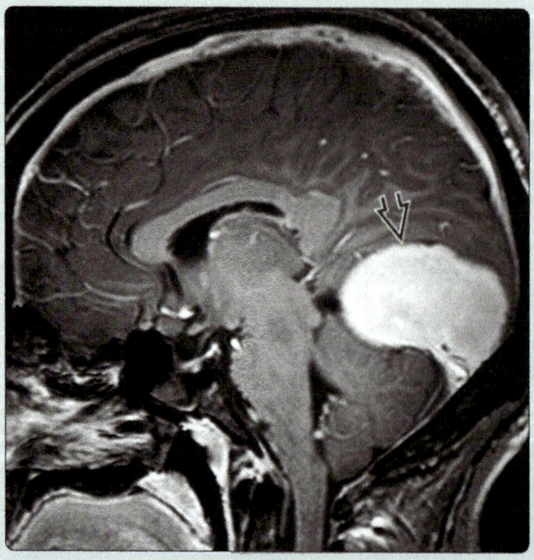

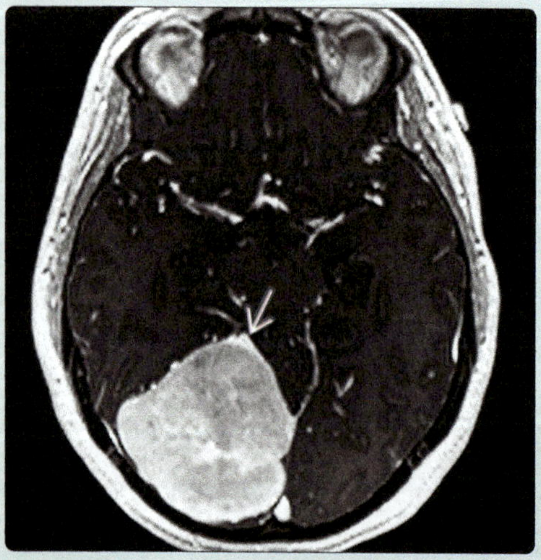

Approach to Head Trauma

General Considerations

Epidemiology: Trauma is the most common worldwide cause of death and disability in children and young adults. In these patients, neurotrauma is responsible for the vast majority of cases. In the USA and Canada, emergency departments (ED) treat more than 8 million patients with head injuries annually, representing 6-7% of all ED visits.

The vast majority of patients with head trauma are classified as having minimal or minor injury. Minimal head injury is defined as no neurologic alteration or loss of consciousness (LOC). Minor head injury or concussion is epitomized by a walking, talking patient with a Glasgow Coma Score (GCS) of 13-15, who has experienced LOC, amnesia, or disorientation.

Of all head-injured patients, ~ 10% sustain fatal brain injury, whereas another 5-10% of neurotrauma survivors have permanent serious neurologic deficits. A number have more subtle deficits ("minimal brain trauma"), whereas 20-40% of patients have moderate disability.

Etiology and Mechanisms of Injury

The etiology of traumatic brain injury (TBI) varies according to patient age. Falls are the leading cause of TBI in children younger than 4 years and in elderly patients older than 75 years. Gunshot wounds are most common in adolescent and young adult male patients but relatively rare in other groups. Motor vehicle and auto-pedestrian collisions occur at all ages without gender predilection.

TBI can be a missile or nonmissile injury. Missile injury results from penetration of the skull, meninges, &/or brain by an external object (such as a bullet).

Nonmissile closed head injury (CHI) can be caused by direct blows, blasts, or penetrating injuries. However, nonmissile CHI is a more common cause of neurotrauma. High-speed accidents exert significant acceleration/deceleration forces, causing the brain to move suddenly within the skull. Forcible impaction of the brain against the unyielding calvaria and hard, knife-like dura results in gyral contusion. Rotation and abrupt changes in angular momentum may deform, stretch, and damage long vulnerable axons, resulting in axonal injury.

Classification of Head Trauma

The most widely used **clinical** classification of brain trauma, the GCS, depends on the assessment of 3 features: Best eye, verbal, and motor responses. With the use of the GCS, TBI can be designated as mild (13-15), moderate (9-12), or severe (≤ 8).

TBI can also be divided pathoetiologically into primary and secondary injuries. Primary injuries occur at the time of initial trauma. Skull fractures, epi- and subdural hematomas, contusion, and axonal injuries are examples of primary traumatic injuries.

Secondary injuries occur later and include cerebral edema, perfusions, and brain herniations. Large arteries, such as the internal carotid, vertebral, and middle meningeal arteries, can be injured either directly at the time of initial trauma or indirectly as a complication of brain herniations.

How to Image Acute Head Trauma

Imaging is absolutely critical to the diagnosis and management of the patient with acute TBI. The goal of emergent imaging is 2-fold: (1) identify treatable injuries and (2) detect and delineate the presence of secondary injuries, such as herniation syndromes.

MDCT: Multidetector row CT (MDCT) is the "workhorse" of brain trauma imaging and is also used as a screening procedure in a wide variety of clinical settings. Whenever possible, helically acquired, thin-section, nonenhanced CT scans from the foramen magnum to the vertex with both soft tissue and bone algorithm should be obtained. Coronal and sagittal images reformatted from the axial source data are extremely helpful, especially in detecting thin peritentorial subdural hematomas. Subdural windowing (e.g., window width of 150-200 HU) of the soft tissue images on PACS (or film, if PACS is not available) is also highly recommended. The scout view should always be displayed and evaluated as part of the study.

Whole-body, CT-based studies for patients with multiple traumas are becoming increasingly more common. Soft tissue and bone algorithm reconstructions with multiplanar (usually coronal and sagittal) reformatted images of the spine are often included as part of the initial trauma evaluation.

CTA: CTA is an appropriate modality in the setting of penetrating neck injury, cervical fracture/subluxation, skull base fractures that traverse the carotid canal or a dural venous sinus, and suspected vascular dissections.

MR: MR is generally a secondary modality most often used in the late acute or subacute stages of brain injury. It is helpful in detecting focal/regional/global perfusion alterations, assessing the extent of hemorrhagic and nonhemorrhagic injuries, and assisting in long-term prognosis. MR should also be considered if nonaccidental trauma is suspected either clinically or on the basis of initial CT scan findings.

Who and When to Image?

Liberal use of head CT scans even in minor trauma (normal neurologic examination, no loss of consciousness) is increasingly common. Many clinical studies have attempted to determine whom to image and when. Three major clinically based appropriateness criteria for imaging acute head trauma are currently in widespread use. These are: (1) The American College of Radiology (ACR) Appropriateness Criteria, (2) the New Orleans Criteria (NOC), and (3) the Canadian Head CT Rule (CHCR).

The American College of Radiology has delineated and published updated appropriateness criteria for imaging head trauma. Emergent NECT in mild/minor CHI with the presence of a focal neurologic deficit &/or other risk factors is deemed very appropriate, as is imaging all traumatized children under 2 years of age.

Between 6-7% of patients with minor head injury have positive findings on head CT scans; most also have headache, vomiting, drug or alcohol intoxication, seizure, short-term memory deficits, or physical evidence of trauma above the clavicles. CT should be used liberally in these cases as well as in patients over 60 years of age and in children under the age of 2.

Repeat CT of patients with head injury should be obtained if there is sudden clinical deterioration, regardless of initial imaging findings. Delayed development or enlargement of both extra- and intraaxial hemorrhages typically occurs within 36 hours following the initial traumatic event.

Approach to Skull Base and Facial Trauma

Fractures involving the base of the skull (BOS) range from a solitary linear fracture to complex injuries involving the craniofacial bones. BOS fractures are often associated with intracranial injuries, such as cerebral contusion, intra- and extraaxial hemorrhages, and vascular or cranial nerve injuries. The objective of imaging patients with BOS &/or facial trauma is to depict the location and extent of the fractures and identify associated injuries to vital structures. Accurate imaging interpretation also aids in surgical planning and in the prevention of complications, such as cerebrospinal fluid leak.

Skull Base Trauma

Anterior skull base (ASB) fractures: ASB trauma is frequently associated with sinonasal cavity &/or orbital injuries. The majority of these patients have facial fractures. Imaging should determine whether the fractures cross the cribriform plate, traverse the frontal sinuses, and involve the orbital apex or optic canals.

Central skull base (CSB) fractures: Imaging patients with CSB trauma may involve the sphenoid bone, clivus, cavernous sinuses, and carotid canal. Injury to the internal carotid artery and CN 3, 4, 6, &/or the trigeminal nerve divisions can be present.

Temporal bone (T-bone) fractures: T-bone fractures can be oriented parallel (longitudinal) or perpendicular (transverse) to the petrous ridge. Longitudinal fractures are more common and traverse the mastoid and middle ear cavity, often disrupting the ossicles and extending into the squamous portion of the T-bone. Transverse fractures often cross the inner ear and extend into the occipital bone.

Imaging evaluation should include the determination of ossicular chain integrity, inner ear &/or facial nerve canal involvement, and whether the T-bone tegmen (roof) is transgressed.

Posterior skull base (PSB) fractures: Fractures of the occipital bones may be isolated or associated with transverse petrous T-bone fractures. PSB fractures may extend into the transverse or sigmoid sinuses, jugular foramen, or hypoglossal canal. Craniocervical junction injuries are also common in patients with trauma to the PSB.

Facial Trauma

Orbit fractures: There are 2 types of orbit fractures: (1) those that involve the orbital walls/rim and (2) so-called blowout fractures. Blowout fractures may involve the orbital floor (inferior blowout) or ethmoid (medial blowout), but the rim is intact. Imaging should determine whether (1) there are other orbital or facial fractures and (2) whether there is entrapment of the inferior ± medial rectus muscles and fat.

Facial bone (Le Fort) fractures: There are 3 types of Le Fort fractures. Le Fort I is a horizontal fracture through the maxilla that involves the piriform aperture. Le Fort II is a pyramidal fracture that involves the nasofrontal junction, infraorbital rims, medial orbital walls, orbital floors, and the zygomaticomaxillary suture lines.

Le Fort III, a.k.a. craniofacial separation, consists of nasofrontal junction fractures that extend laterally through the orbital walls and zygomatic arches.

All 3 Le Fort fractures involve the pterygoid plates and often exhibit elements of > 1 type of facial bone fracture.

Zygomaticomaxillary fractures: The prominent position of the zygomatic arch renders it susceptible to trauma. A zygomaticomaxillary complex (ZMC) fracture, formerly referred to as a "tripod fracture," has 4 involved articulations and 5 distinct fractures.

Imaging in ZMC fractures should determine how displaced/comminuted the fracture is, whether there is involvement of the orbital floor/apex &/or lamina papyracea, and how the lateral orbital wall is displaced.

Complex midfacial fracture: Complex midfacial fracture, or "facial smash injury," consists of multiple facial fractures that cannot be classified as 1 of the named patterns. It is important to determine the posterior displacement of the midface, as this is a highly cosmetically deforming injury. Associated injuries to the orbit &/or skull face must be delineated in detail.

Nasoorbitoethmoid (NOE) fracture: NOE fractures may disrupt the medial canthal tendon and extend into the lacrimal apparatus. Displacement or comminution of the bony fragments posteriorly into the ethmoid or superiorly into the anterior fossa should be identified.

Mandible fracture: Mandibular fractures can occur within or posterior to the teeth. The mandible essentially functions as a "ring of bone" and multiple, often bilateral, fractures are common. The fractures should be located, the degree/direction of fragment displacement identified, and the condyles evaluated for subluxation or dislocation. Involvement of the inferior alveolar canal and teeth should be determined.

Approach to Spine and Cord Trauma

Imaging Acute Spine Injuries

Although radiographs are still used for evaluating the spine, MDCT has become the procedure of choice in rapidly assessing patients with possible spine injuries. In patients with moderate to severe injuries, obtaining large datasets that are subsequently parsed into C-, T-, and L-spine studies together with chest, abdomen, and pelvis is increasingly common.

Thin-section axial images are easily reformatted into sagittal and coronal views. Both bone algorithm and soft tissue reconstructions are typically performed. CTA is a helpful adjunct if vascular injury is a risk (BOS fractures that cross carotid canal or dural venous sinus, cervical spine fractures that traverse foramen transversarium, posterior element subluxation, etc.). Emergent MR is especially helpful in patients with suspected ligamentous complex damage, traumatic disc herniation, or cord injury.

Spine Fracture Classification

Craniovertebral junction (CVJ): Initial evaluation in patients with suspected CVJ injury should begin with a focus on identification of craniocervical malalignment followed by delineation of specific fractures. These are classified by level and type of injury as well as potential for instability. Although an exhaustive description is beyond the scope of this text, a few selected fractures are briefly delineated here.

C1 fractures often involve the posterior arch. A Jefferson fracture is a vertical compression fracture in which both the anterior and posterior rings are disrupted and displaced radially. A combined lateral mass displacement (relative to C2 lateral masses) of ~ 7 mm indicates disruption of the transverse ligament and potential instability.

Odontoid fractures are classified anatomically into 3 types: Type I = avulsed tip, type II = transverse dens fracture above the C2 body, and type III fractures involve the superior portion

New Orleans Criteria in Minor Head Injury

CT Indicated If GCS = 15 Plus Any of Following
Headache
Vomiting
Patient > 60 years
Intoxication (drugs, alcohol)
Short-term memory deficits (anterograde amnesia)
Visible trauma above clavicles
Seizure

Thoracolumbar Injury Severity Score

	Description	Qualifier	Points
Injury Mechanism			
	Compression		
		Simple	1
		Lateral angulation > 15°	1
		Burst	1
	Translation/rotational		3
	Distraction		4
Posterior Ligamentous Complex			
	Intact		0
	Suspected/indeterminate for disruption		2
	Injured		3
Neuro Status			
	Nerve root involvement		2
	Cord, conus involvement (incomplete)		3
	Cord, conus involvement (complete)		2
	Cauda equina involvement		3

Score is a total of 3 components. Score ≤ 3 suggests nonoperative treatment, whereas score of 4 is indeterminate. Score ≥ 5 suggests operative treatment. For injury mechanism, the worst level is used, and the injury is additive. An example is a distraction injury with burst without angulation is 1 (simple compression) + 1 (burst) + 4 (distraction) = 6 points. Modified from Vaccaro AR et al: Reliability of a novel classification system for thoracolumbar injuries: the Thoracolumbar Injury Severity Score. Spine (Phila Pa 1976). 31(11 Suppl):S62-9; discussion S104, 2006.

of the C2 body. Odontoid fractures are especially common in elderly osteoporotic patients who experience falls.

Cervical spine fracture classification: Cervical spine fractures are classified functionally, according to presumed mechanism of injury. Cervical hyperflexion injuries range from simple compression fractures and "clay shoveler fracture" (C7-T1 spinous process avulsion) to unstable injuries, such as posterior ligament disruption with anterior subluxation, bilateral interfacetal dislocation, and flexion teardrop fracture.

In cervical hyperflexion and rotation injury, unilateral facet dislocation (± fracture) is common. Forward displacement of a vertebra < 50% of the AP diameter of the body is typical. The articular pillars are fractured in hyperextension with rotation injury.

Cervical vertical compression injury can cause a Jefferson fracture. In cervical "burst" fractures, there is middle column involvement with bony retropulsion.

Thoracolumbar fracture classification: Multiple systems for classifying thoracolumbar fractures have been developed. In the increasingly popular thoracolumbar injury classification and severity score (TLICS), injury mechanism, integrity of the posterior ligamentous complex, and neurologic status are each scored. The total number of TLICS points is then used to guide treatment.

Selected References

1. Gordic S et al: Whole-body CT-based imaging algorithm for multiple trauma patients: radiation dose and time to diagnosis. Br J Radiol. 88(1047):20140616, 2015
2. Mietto BS et al: Neurotrauma and inflammation: CNS and PNS responses. Mediators Inflamm. 2015:251204, 2015
3. Readdy WJ et al: A review and update on the guidelines for the acute non-operative management of cervical spinal cord injury. J Neurosurg Sci. 59(2):119-28, 2015
4. Furlow B: Computed tomography imaging of traumatic brain injury. Radiol Technol. 84(3):273CT-94CT, 2013

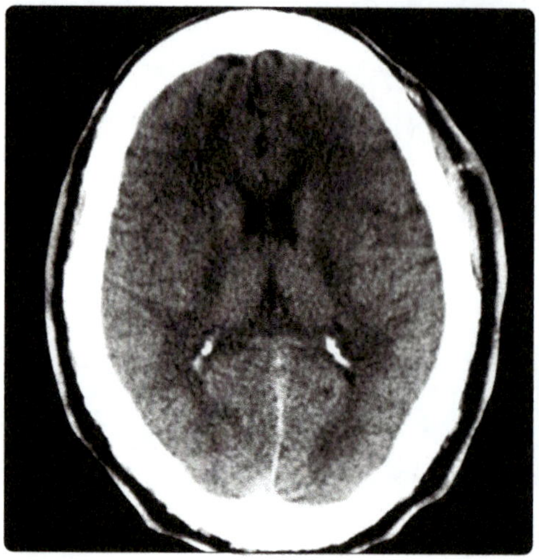

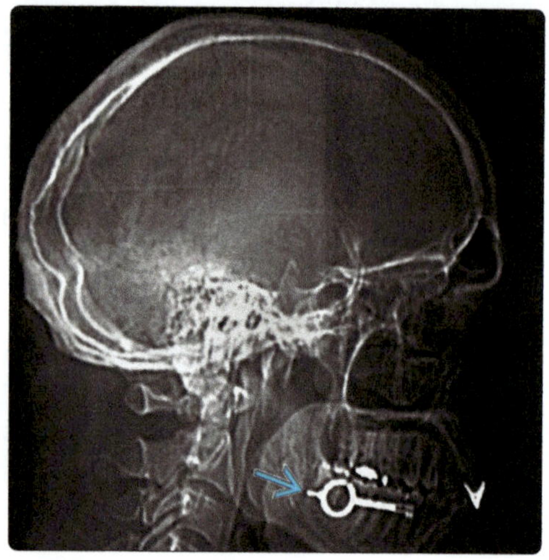

(Left) *NECT scan of a prisoner imaged for head trauma shows no gross abnormality.* **(Right)** *Scout view in the same patient shows a foreign object* → *(a handcuff key) in the prisoner's mouth. He faked the injury and was planning to escape, but the radiologist alerted the guards and thwarted the plan. This case illustrates the importance of looking at the scout view in every patient, especially those being imaged for trauma. (Courtesy J. A. Junker, MD.)*

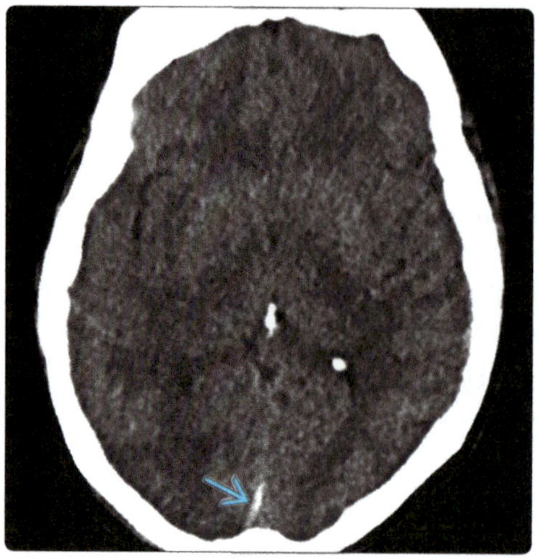

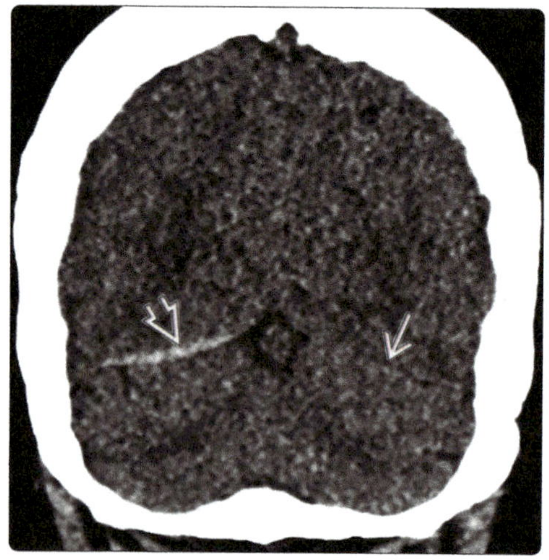

(Left) *Axial NECT scan in a 64-year-old woman with a ground-level fall shows only a small linear hyperdensity* → *adjacent to the falx cerebri and torcular Herophili. The scan was initially considered normal.* **(Right)** *Coronal NECT in the same patient was reformatted from the axial source data. Note thin peritentorial acute subdural hematoma* →*, nicely contrasted with the nearly invisible, normal left side of the tentorium* →*.*

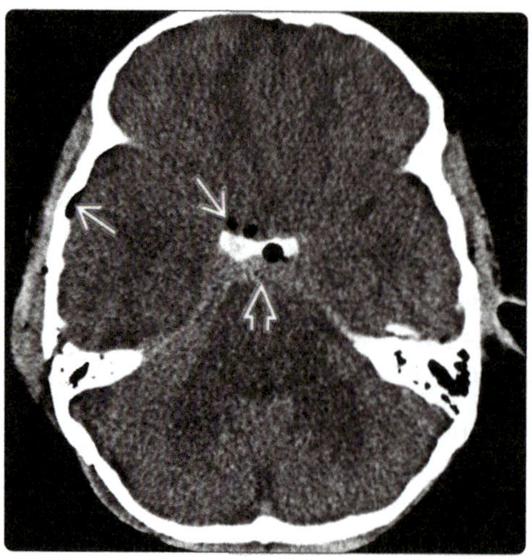

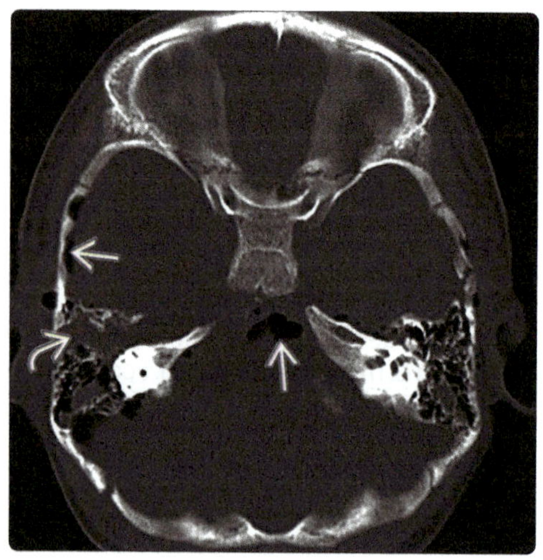

(Left) *NECT scan in a 3-year-old boy with severe head trauma shows brain swelling with obliteration of all sulci and subarachnoid cisterns, intracranial air ("pneumocephalus")* →*, and subarachnoid hemorrhage* →*.* **(Right)** *Bone CT in the same patient shows the importance of determining why intracranial air* → *is present. Multiple skull fractures are present, including a longitudinal fracture through the aerated right temporal bone* →*.*

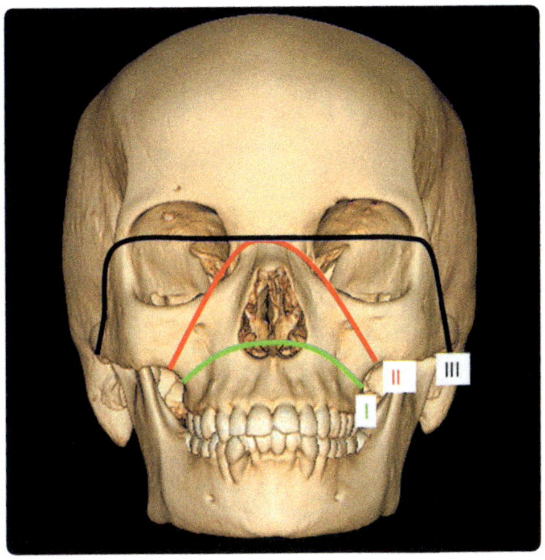

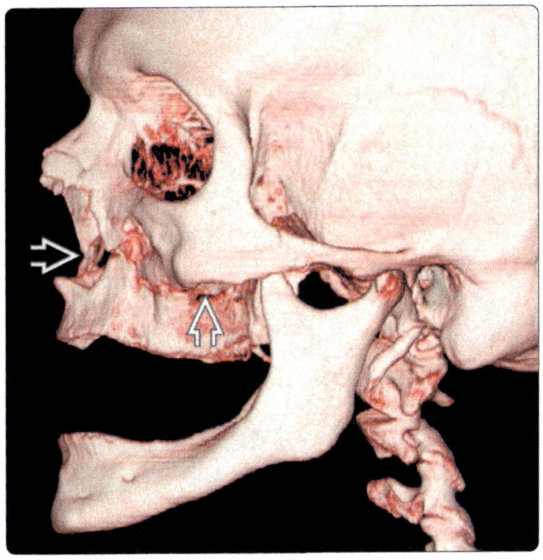

(Left) *Coronal graphic shows 3 lines defining the 3 classic types of Le Fort fractures. Le Fort I (green) involves the maxilla and nasal aperture. Le Fort II (red), a.k.a. pyramidal fracture, extends upward across the maxilla and across the inferior orbital rim and nose. Le Fort III (black), a.k.a. craniofacial separation, extends through the orbits and zygomatic arches.* **(Right)** *3D CT shows a Le Fort I fracture ➔ through the maxillary alveolus and nose.*

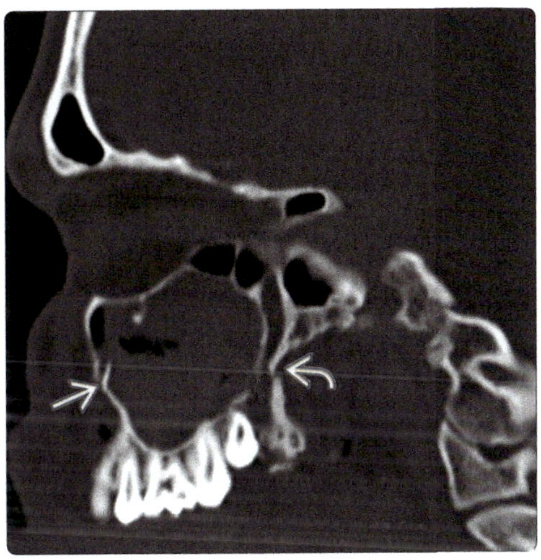

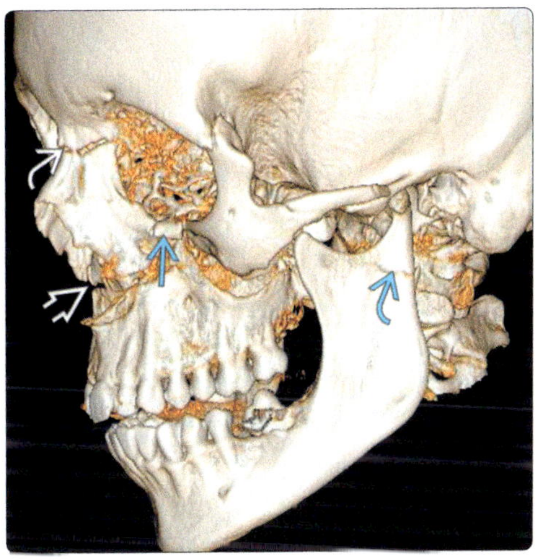

(Left) *Sagittal reformatted bone CT shows a Le Fort I fracture extending from maxillary alveolus ➔ into the posterior sinus wall and pterygoid plate ➔.* **(Right)** *3D CT shows a Le Fort II fracture through the nasofrontal junction ➔ that descends obliquely through the inferior orbital rim ➔. A Le Fort I fracture ➔ is also present through the maxillary alveolus and nose. A nondisplaced mandibular fracture ➔ is also present. It is common to have multiple types of facial fractures in the same patient.*

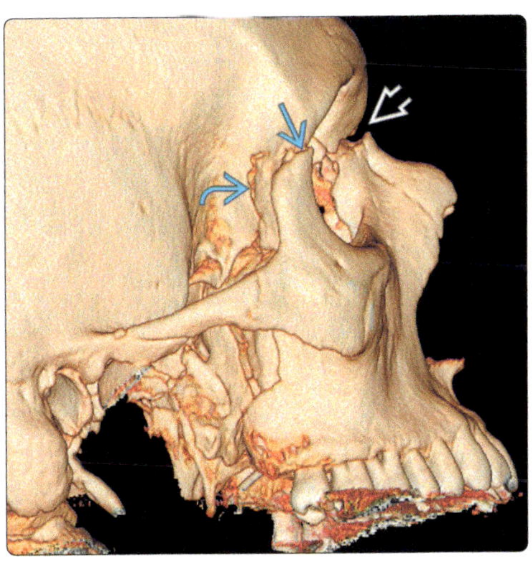

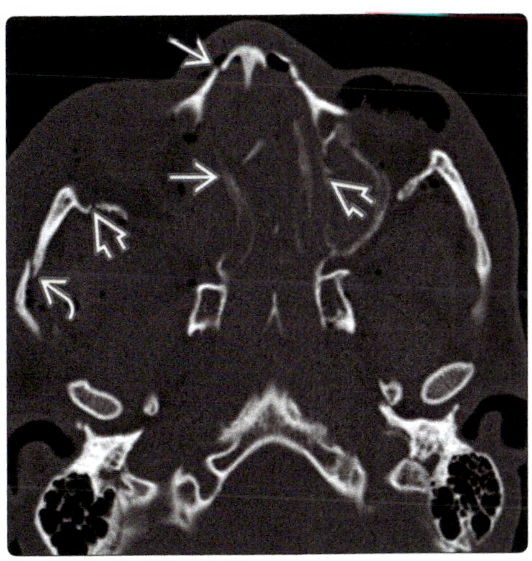

(Left) *3D CT shows a Le Fort III fracture with frontonasal diastasis ➔, orbital wall fracture ➔, and diastasis of the zygomaticofrontal suture ➔.* **(Right)** *Axial bone CT in a complex midface "smash" injury shows comminuted, depressed nasal bone and ethmoid fractures ➔, maxillary sinus fractures ➔, and zygoma fractures ➔.*

(Left) *Bone CT with sagittal reformatting shows that the anteroposterior alignment of the cervical spine appears normal. However, there is increased distance between the occipital condyle and C1 lateral mass as well as widening of the C1-C2 articulation.* **(Right)** *Sagittal STIR scan in the same patient shows how MR better depicts soft tissue injuries. Widened occipital condyle-C1 and C1-C2 articulations with hyperintensity in both joints and posterior ligamentous C2-C4 injury are present.*

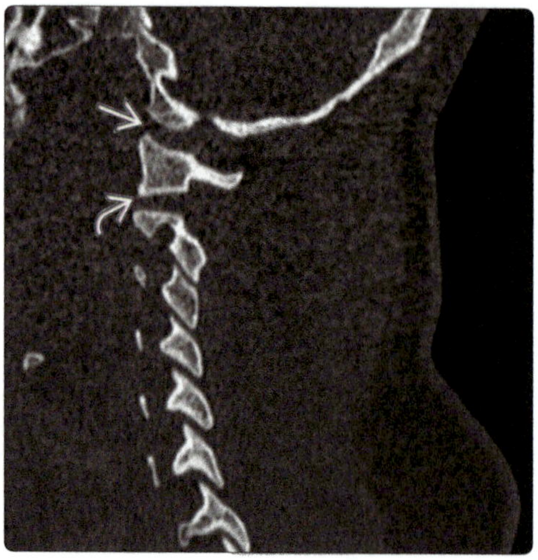

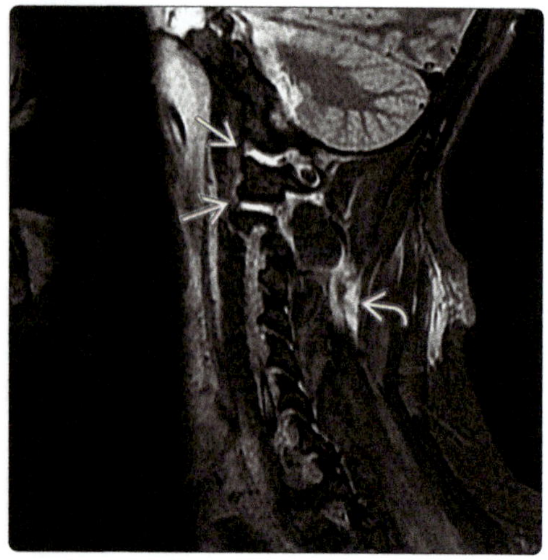

(Left) *Lateral radiograph of the upper cervical spine shows malalignment with the spinolaminar line of C1 in front of C2 and C3. Lucencies through the posterior C1 ring are fractures.* **(Right)** *Coronal reformatted bone CT shows coronal displacement of both C1 lateral masses. Also seen is a bony fragment due to transverse ligament tubercle avulsion.*

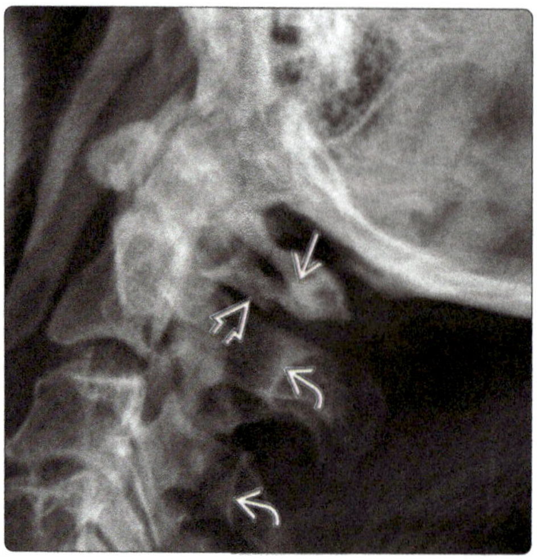

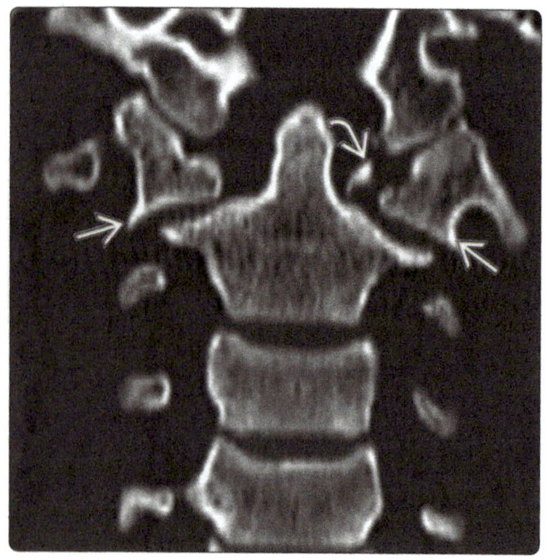

(Left) *Sagittal graphic shows an unstable cervical hyperflexion injury with disruption of the anterior and posterior longitudinal ligaments as well as the interspinous ligament, traumatic disc herniation, epidural hemorrhage, and cord injury.* **(Right)** *Sagittal reformatted bone CT of a cervical spine fracture in a patient with ankylosing spondylitis nicely shows the bone injuries but does not depict the extent of soft tissue damage. MR is complementary to multiplanar CT.*

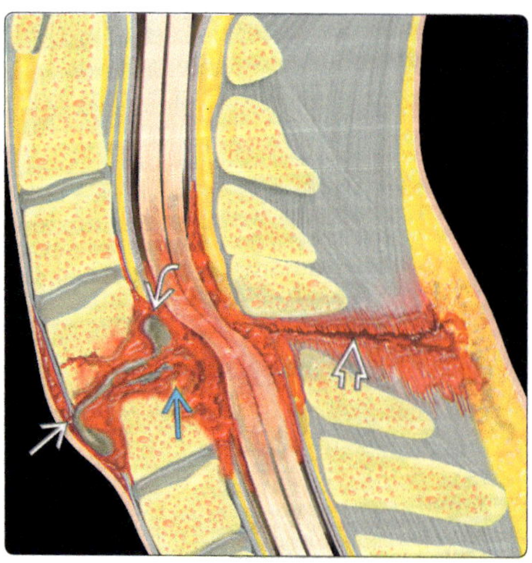

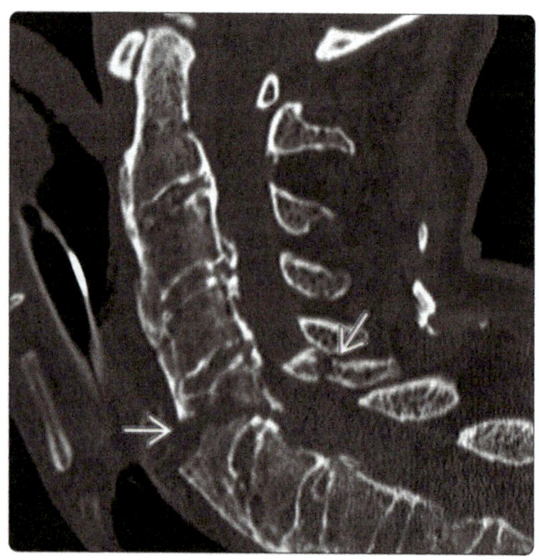

Acute Subdural Hematoma

KEY FACTS

TERMINOLOGY

- Acute blood between inner border cell layer of dura, arachnoid

IMAGING

- NECT as initial screening study
  - Use both bone, soft tissue algorithms
  - Use both standard brain, wide windows (150 HU)
  - Coronal, sagittal reformatted scans best for detecting small subdural hematomas (SDHs)
- Crescentic hyperdense extraaxial collection
  - Spreads diffusely over cerebral convexity
  - Often extends along falx, tentorium
- Inward displacement of cortical veins, sulci
- May cross sutures, not dural attachments

TOP DIFFERENTIAL DIAGNOSES

- Other subdural fluid collections
  - Mixed SDH (acute on chronic/subacute SDH): Hyperdense foci in pockets of iso-, hypodense fluid
  - Subdural hygroma: Clear CSF, no encapsulating membranes
  - Subdural effusion: Near CSF density
  - Subdural empyema: Peripheral enhancement, hyperintensity on FLAIR; restricted diffusion on DWI
- Acute epidural hematoma (typically crescentic)

PATHOLOGY

- Common: Tear of bridging cortical veins
- Nontrauma (spontaneous) more common in elderly

CLINICAL ISSUES

- Mental status & focal neurological changes can have rapid deterioration

DIAGNOSTIC CHECKLIST

- Multiplanar reconstructions, wide windows best for subtle acute SDHs; inform clinician if unsuspected finding

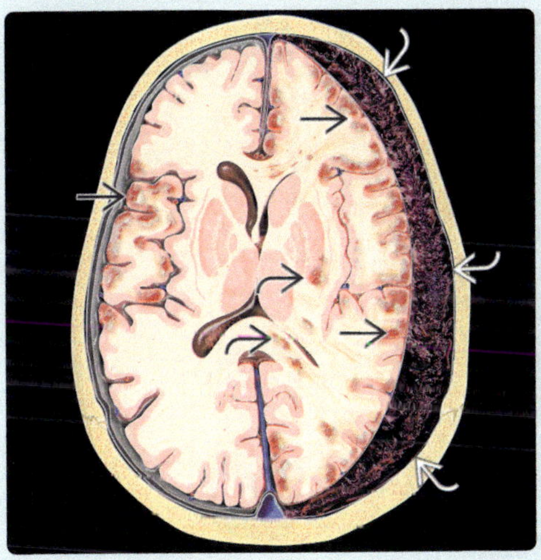

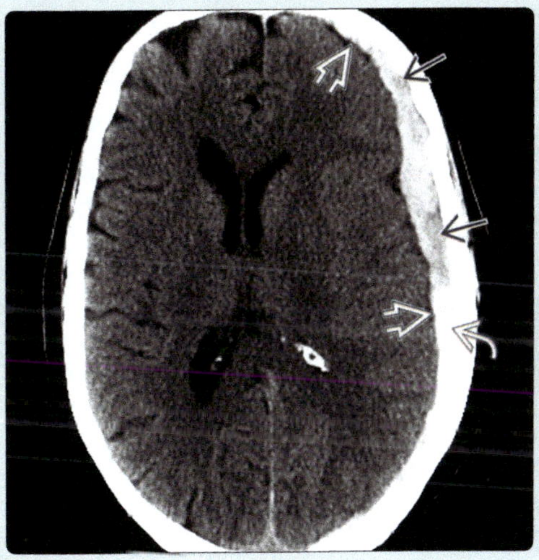

(Left) *Graphic shows acute subdural hematoma (aSDH) ➡ compressing the left hemisphere and lateral ventricle, resulting in midline shift. Coexisting cortical contusions ➡ and axonal injuries ➡ are common in aSDHs.* **(Right)** *Axial NECT in a 58-year-old woman with head trauma shows a classic aSDH ➡ extending over the left convexity and compressing the underlying subarachnoid space ➡. The subtle hypodense foci ➡ within the hyperdense aSDH represent unclotted blood and risk for rapid hematoma expansion.*

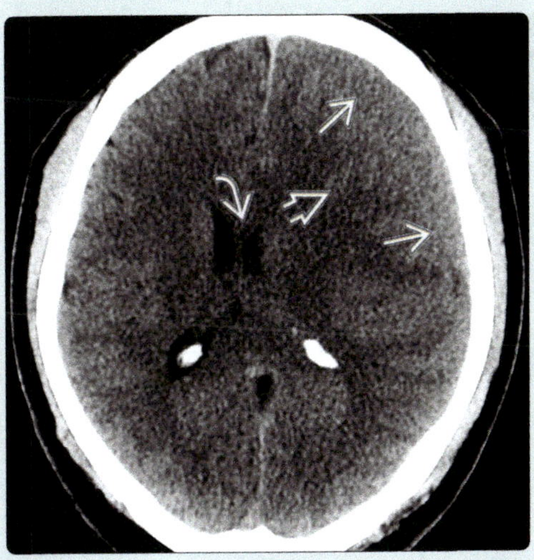

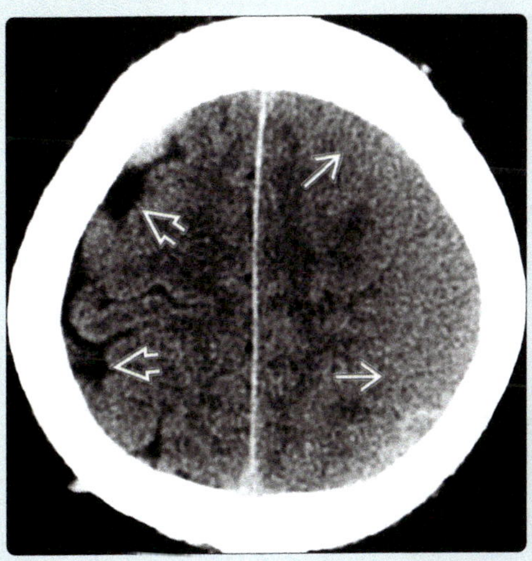

(Left) *Occasionally, aSDHs are isodense to the underlying brain. Note the aSDH ➡ with mass effect, inward displacement of the underlying gray-white interface ➡, and left-to-right subfalcine herniation of the lateral ventricles ➡.* **(Right)** *More cephalad NECT scan in the same patient again shows the isodense aSDH ➡. The underlying sulci are completely effaced. Compare this appearance of "absent sulci" with the normal-appearing cerebrospinal fluid-filled sulci ➡ over the right hemisphere.*

Subacute Subdural Hematoma

KEY FACTS

TERMINOLOGY

- Subacute (~ 3 days to 3 weeks) collection
  - In subdural space (between arachnoid and dura or within inner border cell layer)
  - Partially liquefied clot, resorbing blood products
  - Surrounded by granulation tissue ("membrane")

IMAGING

- Crescent-shaped, iso- to hypodense extraaxial collection
  - Spreads diffusely over hemisphere
  - May cross sutures, not dural attachments
  - May be of same density as underlying cortex
  - Look for inwardly displaced "dots" of cerebrospinal fluid
- MR
  - T1 iso- to hyperintense
  - T2/FLAIR hyperintense (does not suppress)
  - DWI may show double-layer appearance
  - Enhancing membranes may be seen on postcontrast imaging
- General imaging recommendations
  - NECT initial screen; consider CECT for membranes/loculations; MR is more sensitive for subdural hematoma, detecting additional traumatic brain injuries

TOP DIFFERENTIAL DIAGNOSES

- Other subdural collections: Effusion, hygroma; empyema
- Pachymeningopathies, thickened dura (look for other signs of intracranial hypotension)
- Chronic dural sinus thrombosis

PATHOLOGY

- Traumatic stretching/tearing of bridging cortical veins as they cross subdural space
- Trauma may be minor (particularly in elderly patients)

CLINICAL ISSUES

- Can present with headache, seizures, gait abnormalities in elderly & present weeks after initial minor trauma

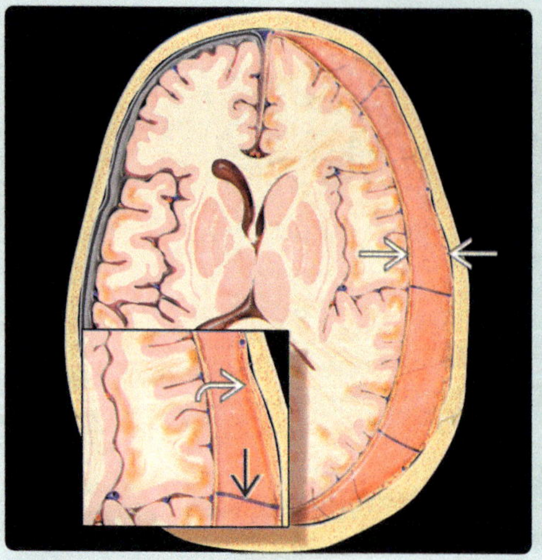

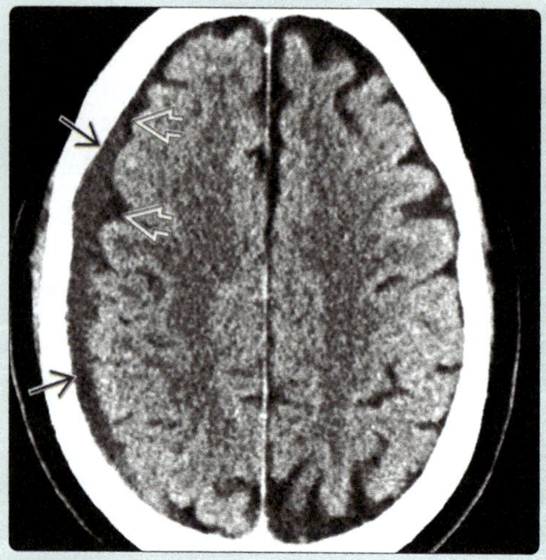

(Left) *Axial graphic shows a typical subacute subdural hematoma (sSDH) →. Inset shows the traversing "bridging" vein → and developing membranes →. These are often related to relatively minor trauma in the elderly.* **(Right)** *Axial NECT scan shows a right sSDH as a crescentic extraaxial fluid collection → that appears slightly hyperdense compared with the "dots" of cerebrospinal fluid (CSF) in the underlying sulci →.*

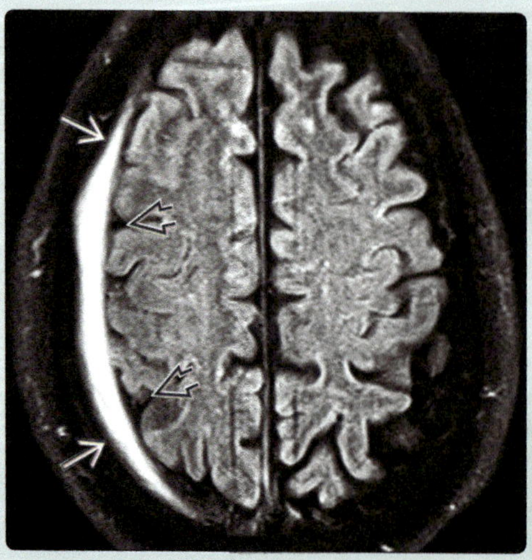

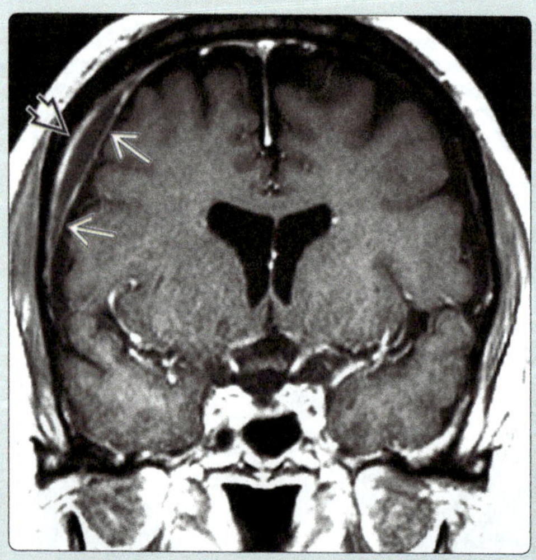

(Left) *FLAIR MR in the same case shows that the sSDH is hyperintense → and does not suppress (compared with the normal "dark" CSF in the underlying subarachnoid spaces →).* **(Right)** *Coronal T1 C+ MR in the same case shows enhancing membranes surrounding the sSDH. The outer membrane → is generally thicker, more prominent than the inner membrane →.*

KEY FACTS

TERMINOLOGY

- Chronic subdural hematoma (cSDH)
- Chronic (> 3 weeks to months) subdural blood products
  - Mixed chronic and acute hemorrhage is common

IMAGING

- Crescent-shaped extraaxial collection
  - Spreads diffusely over affected hemisphere
  - Surrounded by enhancing membranes
  - Often septated, loculated, with fluid-fluid levels
  - Recurrent, mixed-age hemorrhage is common and raises suspicion of nonaccidental trauma in children
- Imaging recommendations
  - NECT is good initial screen
  - Use wide window settings (150-200 HU)
  - MR better demonstrates cSDH

TOP DIFFERENTIAL DIAGNOSES

- Subdural hygroma
- Subdural effusion
- Subdural empyema

PATHOLOGY

- Serosanguineous fluid
- Encapsulated by granulation tissue: "Neomembranes" with fragile capillaries
- 5% multiloculated with fluid-blood density levels

CLINICAL ISSUES

- Treatment
  - Surgical drainage with resection of membranes
- Older age, brain atrophy are contributory factors in conversion of traumatic SDH into cSDH
- Recurrence risk varies with type
  - Separated SDH has highest risk
  - Large > small preoperative collections
  - Residual postoperative volume > 80 mL

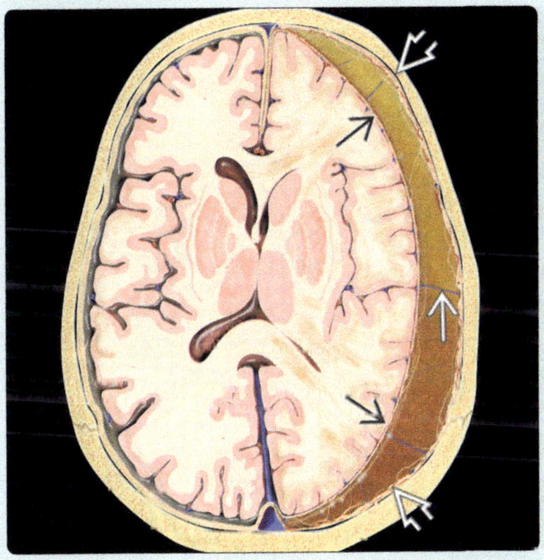

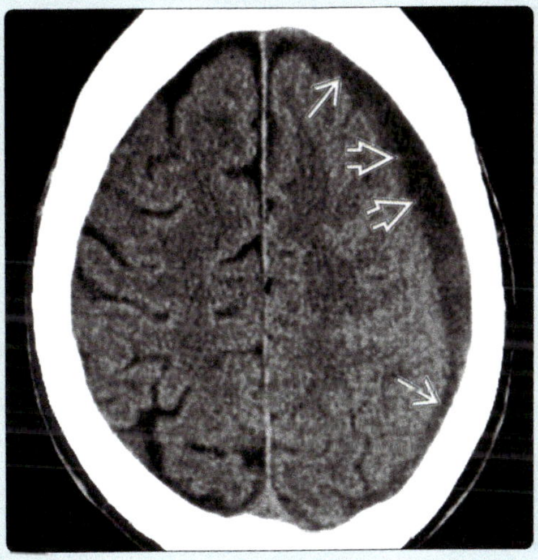

(Left) *Axial graphic depicts pathology of classic chronic subdural hematoma (SDH) with the formation of thin internal ➡, thicker external ➡ membranes. Note the stretched bridging veins ➡ crossing the SDH, top-to-bottom gradation of fluid from serosanguinous to more proteinaceous contents.* **(Right)** *Axial NECT depicts chronic SDH (cSDH) as crescentic hypodense extraaxial fluid collection ➡ over the left hemisphere. Stretched cortical veins ➡ are faintly visible as they cross the SDH.*

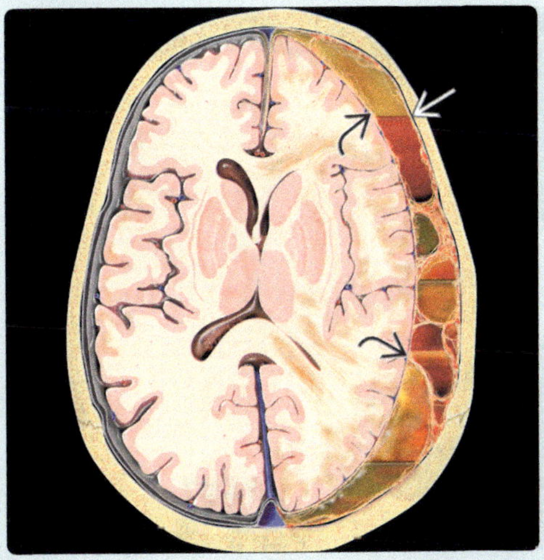

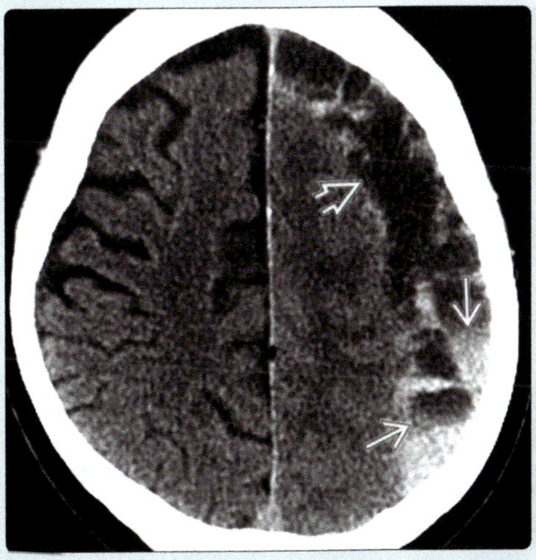

(Left) *Axial graphic depicts "mixed" subdural hematoma. Numerous loculations ➡ that contain hemorrhages of multiple ages are present. Note the fluid-fluid levels with mixed acute, subacute blood ➡. Rehemorrhage into preexisting subacute &/or cSDH is common.* **(Right)** *Axial NECT shows classic left-sided "mixed" SDH ➡. Note the multiple loculations and fluid-fluid levels ➡ formed by acute rehemorrhage into preexisting loculated cSDH.*

KEY FACTS

TERMINOLOGY

- Blood collection between skull and dura

IMAGING

- NECT
  - Hyperdense, biconvex, extraaxial collection
  - > 95% unilateral, supratentorial
  - Does not cross sutures unless venous or sutural diastasis/fracture is present
  - Compresses/displaces underlying brain, subarachnoid space
  - Low-density swirl sign: Active/rapid bleeding with unretracted clot
  - 1/3-1/2 have other significant lesions
- Bone CT
  - Skull fracture in 90-95%

TOP DIFFERENTIAL DIAGNOSES

- Subdural hematoma
- Neoplasm
- Infection/inflammation
- Extramedullary hematopoiesis

PATHOLOGY

- Arterial (90-95%)
  - Arterial epidural hematoma (EDH) is most often near middle meningeal artery groove fracture
- Venous EDH (5-10%)
  - Fracture is adjacent to dural sinus
  - Common sites: Vertex, anterior middle cranial fossa

CLINICAL ISSUES

- Classic "lucid interval"
  - ~ 50% of cases
- Good outcome if promptly recognized and treated
- Some EDHs < 1 cm may be managed nonoperatively
  - Anterior middle fossa epidural hematoma is usually venous, benign

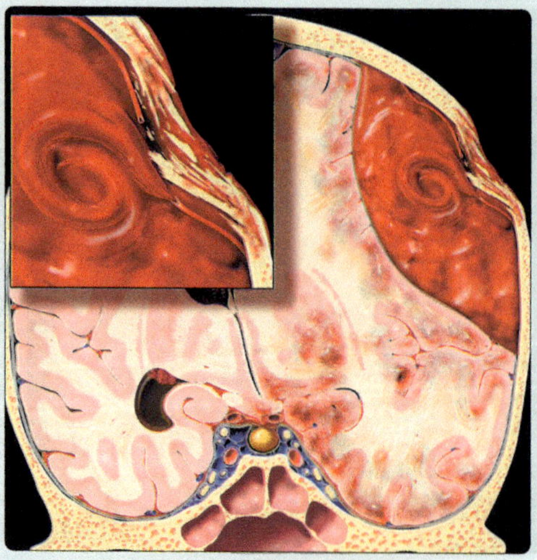

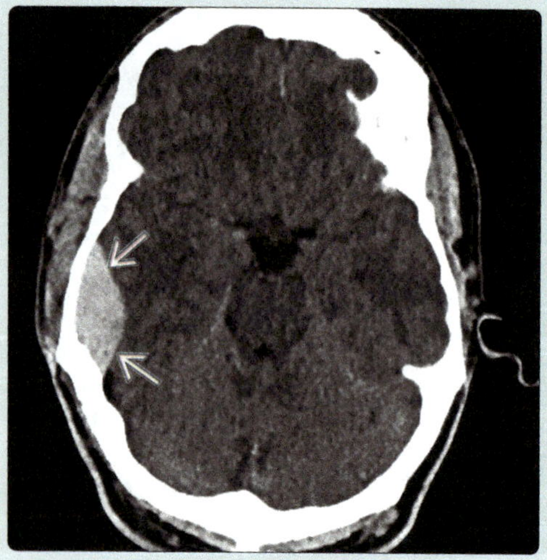

(Left) *Coronal graphic illustrates swirling acute hemorrhage from a laceration of the middle meningeal artery by an overlying skull fracture. The epidural hematoma displaces the dura inward as it expands.* **(Right)** *Axial NECT scan in a 47-year-old man with head trauma shows a classic biconvex (lentiform) uniformly hyperdense epidural hematoma (EDH)* ➔ *in the right middle fossa. Bone CT (not shown) disclosed a nondisplaced skull fracture underlying the hematoma.*

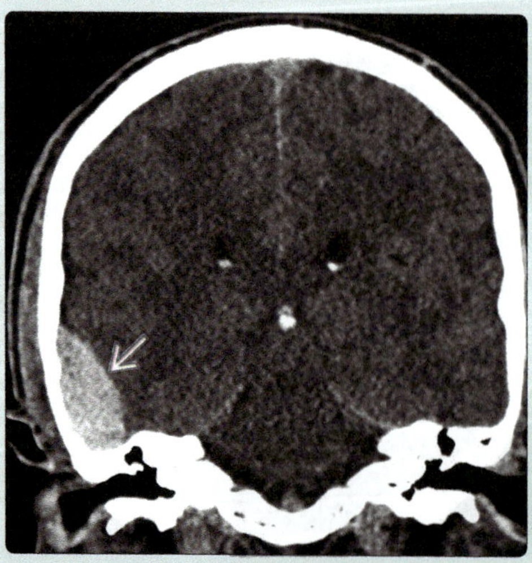

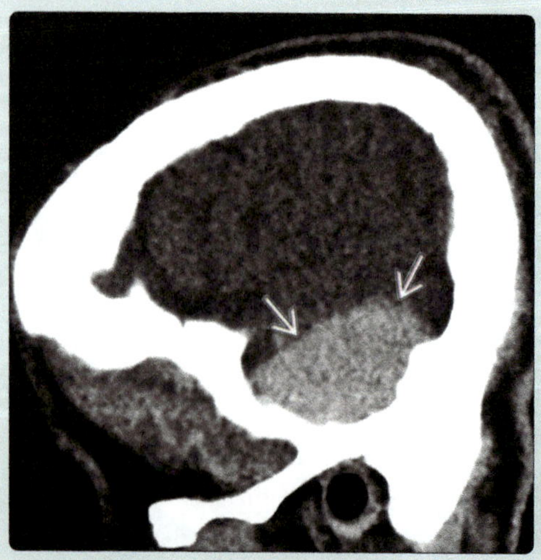

(Left) *Coronal scan reformatted from the axial date nicely demonstrates the classic middle cranial fossa acute EDH* ➔. **(Right)** *Sagittal NECT scan reformatted from the axial source date in the same patient shows that the classic biconvex configuration of the acute middle fossa EDH* ➔ *is present in all 3 major imaging planes.*

KEY FACTS

TERMINOLOGY

- "Typical" epidural hematoma (EDH)
  - Arterial laceration
  - 90-95% supratentorial (temporoparietal most common)
  - Biconvex, unilateral
- Atypical EDH
  - Unusual etiology
  - Unusual location
  - Unusual shape or density

IMAGING

- Venous EDH (10% of EDHs)
  - Fracture (linear, diastatic) crosses dural venous sinus
  - Skull base, vertex
  - Easily overlooked
  - Coronal, sagittal reformats key to diagnosis
- Anterior temporal EDH (10% of EDHs)
  - Middle cranial fossa
    - In front of, not lateral to, temporal lobe
  - Fracture crosses sphenoparietal sinus
  - Generally asymptomatic (1-2 cm, stable size)
  - No reported cases requiring surgery
- Vertex EDH (1-2% of EDHs)
  - Fracture crosses, lacerates superior sagittal sinus
  - Accumulates slowly
  - Symptoms often delayed
  - Easily overlooked, size underestimated on axial CT
  - Coronal, sagittal reformatted images key
- Clival EDH (< 1% of EDHs)
  - Lacerates clival venous plexus
  - Self-limited; dura tightly attached, so rarely large
  - Asymptomatic unless associated vascular, cranial nerve injury
  - Biconvex hyperdensity immediately posterior to clivus
  - Sagittal reformatted images key to diagnosis

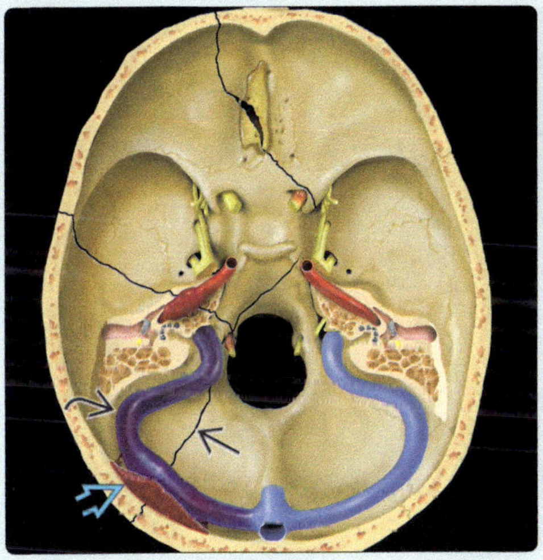

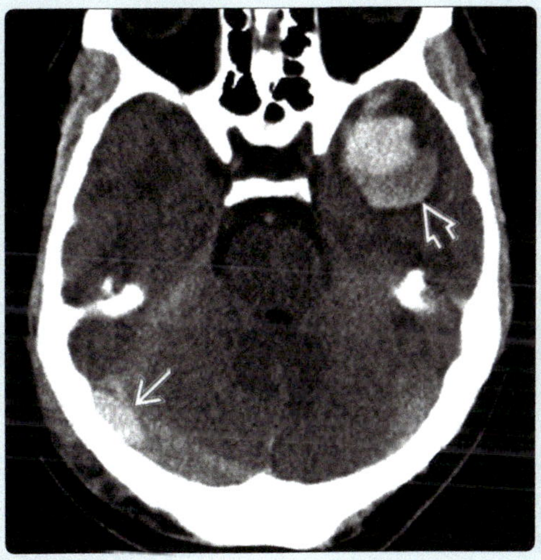

(Left) *Axial graphic depicts different basilar skull fractures that cross, and may injure, important vascular structures. Linear skull fracture crosses the right transverse sinus. The lacerated sinus causes a venous epidermal hematoma (EDH) to accumulate. The injured sinus often thromboses.* **(Right)** *Axial NECT scan in a 26-year-old man who fell 10 meters onto his head shows a large left temporal lobe contusion. A small biconvex hyperdense fluid collection is seen adjacent to the right transverse sinus.*

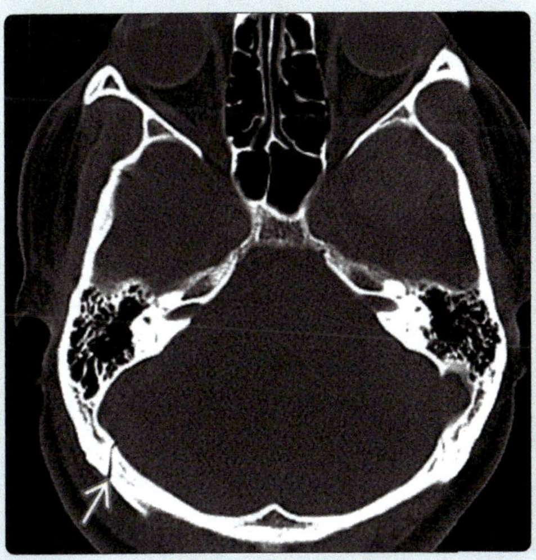

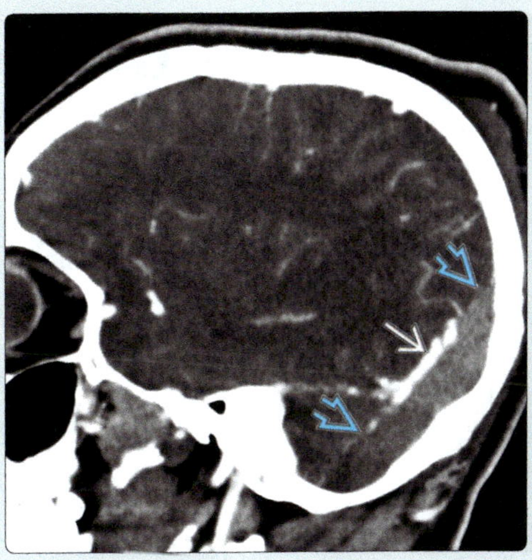

(Left) *Bone CT in the same patient shows a diastatic fracture through the right lambdoid suture.* **(Right)** *Sagittal CT venogram shows that the transverse sinus is elevated and displaced anteriorly by a hyperdense venous EDH. Note that the venous EDH lies both above and below the site of dural attachment. Venous EDHs commonly cross dural attachments, whereas classic arterial EDHs rarely do.*

KEY FACTS

TERMINOLOGY

- Intentionally inflicted injury; abusive head trauma, inflicted head injury, nonaccidental head injury

IMAGING

- Plays key role in early diagnosis
  - Disparate brain injuries relative to proffered history
- Skeletal survey, NECT as initial primary imaging tools
  - Detection/characterization of intracranial hemorrhage
  - Detection/characterization of fractures
- MR
  - Delayed (24-72 hours) for detection of parenchymal injuries, demonstration of unexplained, different-aged subdural hemorrhages (SDHs)
    - Use T1WI, T2WI, T2*/SWI (best sequence varies with SDH age)
    - DWI key for identification of parenchymal insult
    - Use T1W1 C+ to detect subdural membranes of chronic SDH
    - Sagittal/coronal best for small peritentorial SDHs

PATHOLOGY

- Direct impact injury
  - Skull fractures
  - Underlying brain injury
- Violent "to and fro" shaking
  - Diffusely distributed subdural hematomas
  - Cortical contusions, axonal injury, parenchymal lacerations
- Ischemic injury
  - Global hypoxic brain injury
  - Territorial infarcts
  - Excitotoxic edema

CLINICAL ISSUES

- Most common cause of traumatic death in infants
- Signs of trauma (e.g., Battle sign, raccoon eyes) may be present but often are not

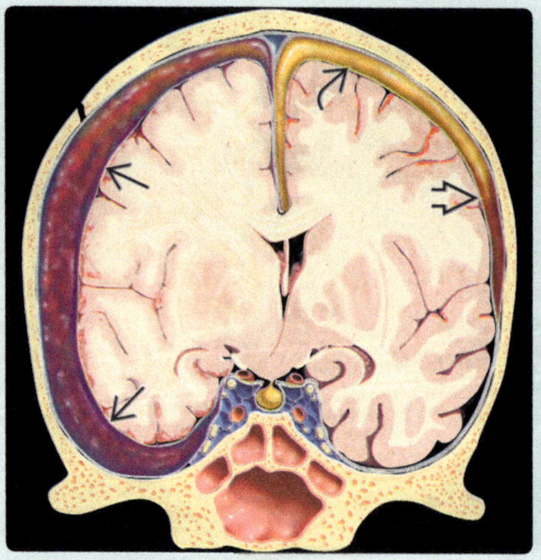

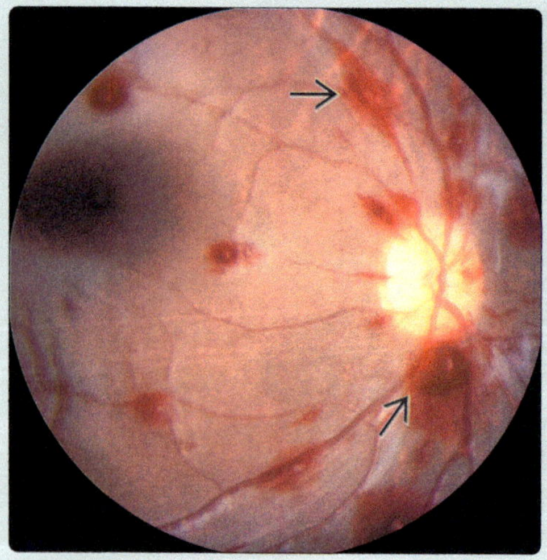

(Left) *Coronal graphic of abusive head trauma (AHT) shows an acute subdural hemorrhage (SDH) over the right hemisphere ➔ and a smaller left SDH ➔ with hematocrit effect producing layering of blood products ➔. Other injuries (traumatic SAH, cortical contusions) are illustrated and are common in AHT.* **(Right)** *Funduscopic examination in an infant with suspected AHT shows multiple retinal hemorrhages ➔. Retinal hemorrhages are present in up to 95% of AHT cases.*

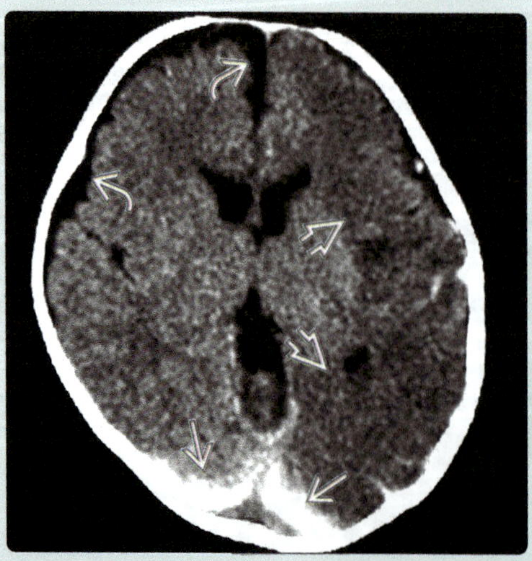

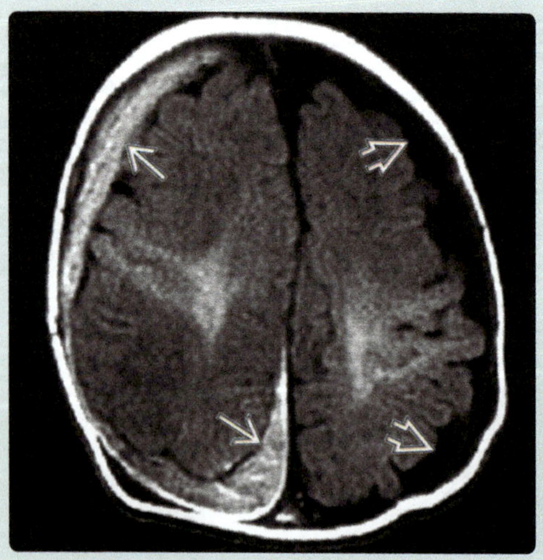

(Left) *Axial NECT in suspected AHT shows varied attenuation SDHs with right low attenuation ➔, bilateral high attenuation ➔ SDHs. The diffuse edema involves almost the entire left hemisphere ➔.* **(Right)** *Axial T1WI MR in an infant with AHT shows subacute right SDH ➔ extending into the interhemispheric fissure and a more chronic-appearing left subdural collection (chronic SDH vs. hygroma) ➔.*

KEY FACTS

TERMINOLOGY

- Blood within subarachnoid spaces
  - Contained between pia and arachnoid membranes

IMAGING

- High density on CT, hyperintensity on FLAIR

TOP DIFFERENTIAL DIAGNOSES

- Nontraumatic SAH
- Meningitis: Cellular and proteinaceous debris
- Carcinomatosis meningitis
- Pseudosubarachnoid hemorrhage
- Gadolinium administration
- High inspired oxygen

PATHOLOGY

- Associated with contusions, subdural or epidural hematoma, diffuse axonal injury

CLINICAL ISSUES

- Headache, emesis, decreased consciousness
- Trauma is most common cause of subarachnoid hemorrhage (SAH)
- Outcome is related in logistic regression analysis to
  - Admission Glasgow Coma Scale score
  - Amount of subarachnoid blood
- Isolated traumatic SAH, no other injuries usually benign
- Poor prognosis if associated with other intracranial injuries
- Vasospasm develops earlier than with aneurysmal SAH
- Associated with ↓ neuropsychologic profiles, worse vocational outcomes in 1 year follow-up

DIAGNOSTIC CHECKLIST

- Isolated supratentorial sulcal blood common
- Hyperdense blood in interpeduncular cistern may be only manifestation of subtle SAH

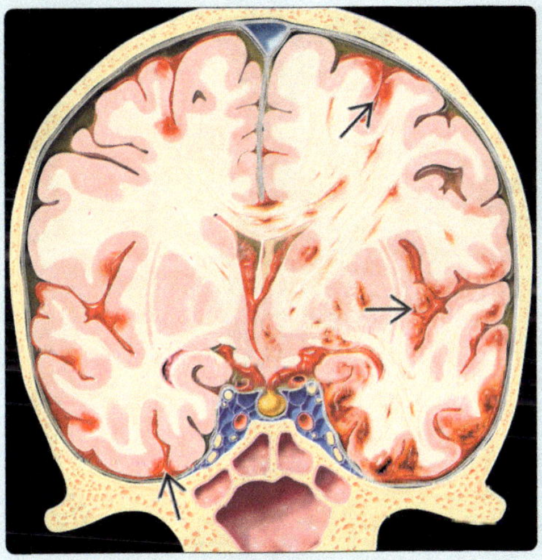

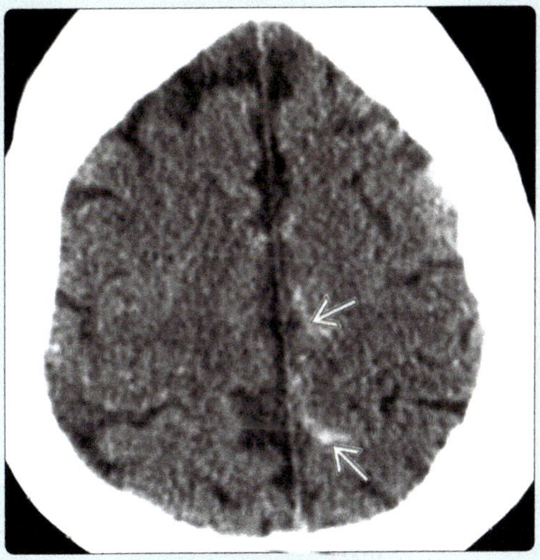

(Left) *Coronal graphic depicts findings in a severe traumatic brain injury. Closed head trauma has resulted in multiple gyral contusions and subarachnoid hemorrhage (SAH). Most traumatic SAHs (tSAHs) ➡ occur adjacent to parenchymal brain injuries and are found centered around the sylvian fissures, inferior frontotemporal, and convexity sulci.* **(Right)** *Axial NECT in a patient with head trauma and tSAH demonstrates focal hyperdense collections in a few left posterior frontal sulci bordering the interhemispheric fissure ➡.*

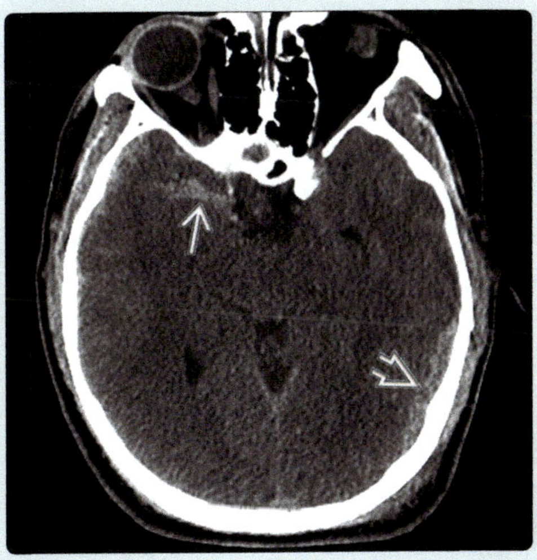

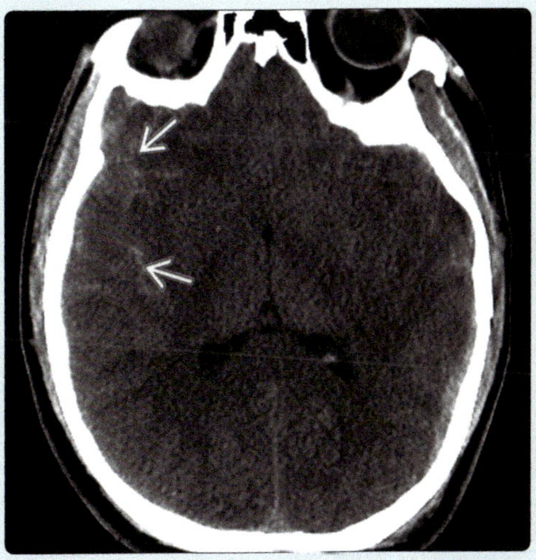

(Left) *Axial NECT scan in a 28-year-old man with closed head injury shows tSAH in the right sylvian fissure ➡. Note the absence of blood in the adjacent suprasellar cistern, a more common site for aneurysmal SAH. A left parietal epidural hematoma ➡ is also present. tSAH often occurs in combination with other injuries.* **(Right)** *Axial NECT scan in the same patient shows the typical curvilinear configuration of tSAH ➡ in the sulci of the right temporal lobe.*

KEY FACTS

TERMINOLOGY

- Brain surface injuries involving gray matter and contiguous subcortical white matter

IMAGING

- Best diagnostic clue: Patchy hemorrhages within edematous background
- Characteristic locations: Adjacent to irregular bony protuberance or dural fold
- Anterior inferior frontal lobes and anterior inferior temporal lobes most common
- FLAIR: Best for hyperintense cortical edema and subarachnoid hemorrhage
- GRE: Hypointense hemorrhagic foci "bloom"
- Best imaging tool
  - CT to detect acute hemorrhagic contusions, other intracranial lesions, and herniations
  - MR to detect presence and delineate extent of lesions
- Coup: Direct injury to brain beneath impact site
- Contrecoup: Injury opposite impact site; usually more severe than coup

TOP DIFFERENTIAL DIAGNOSES

- Infarct
- Venous sinus thrombosis
- Cerebritis
- Low-grade neoplasm
- Transient postictal changes

PATHOLOGY

- Inflammation → worsening/enlarging lesions

CLINICAL ISSUES

- Initial symptom: Confusion → obtundation
- Central goal: Prevent and treat secondary injury
- Mass effect and herniation may require evacuation

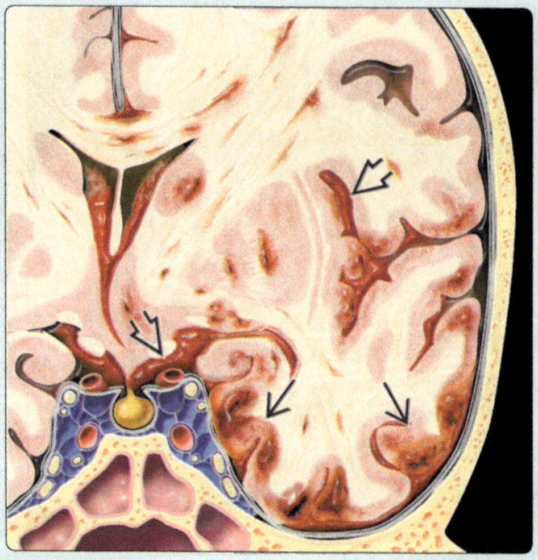

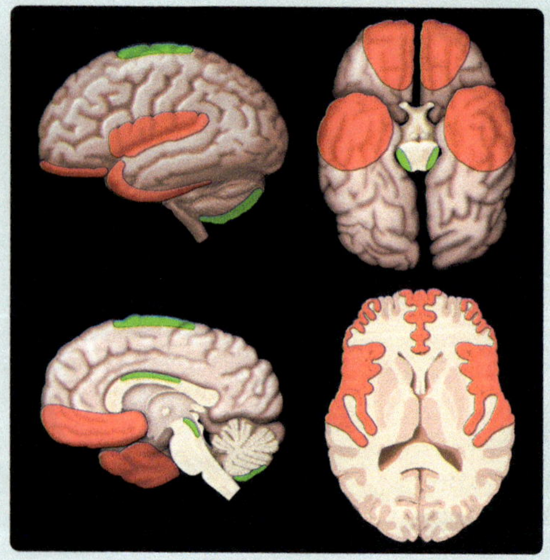

(Left) *Coronal graphic illustrates the pathology of closed head injury. Note the hemorrhagic foci involving gray matter of several contused gyri ⇨, axonal and deep gray injuries, and traumatic subarachnoid hemorrhage ⇨ in the basal cisterns and sylvian fissure.* **(Right)** *Graphics depict the most common sites of cerebral contusions in red. Less common sites are shown in green. The most common locations of all are the anteroinferior frontal and temporal lobes.*

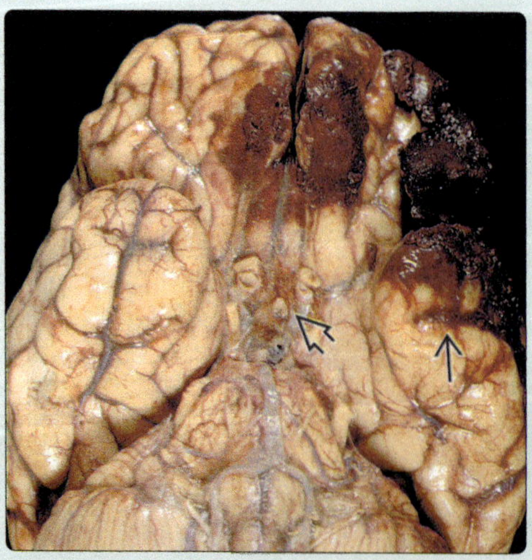

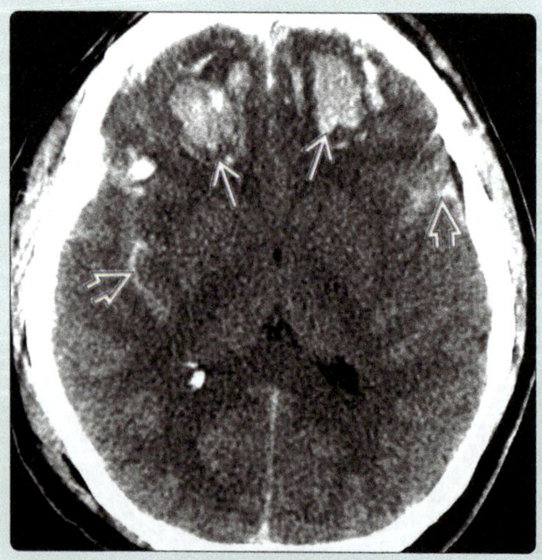

(Left) *Gross pathology of the brain from a patient who died from a severe closed head injury shows bifrontal, temporal hemorrhagic contusions ⇨, as well as traumatic subarachnoid hemorrhage in the suprasellar cistern ⇨. (Courtesy R. Hewlett, MD.)* **(Right)** *NECT scan shows extensive frontotemporal contusions ➡ and traumatic subarachnoid hemorrhage ➡ in a patient with severe brain injury.*

KEY FACTS

TERMINOLOGY

- Traumatic axonal stretch injury

IMAGING

- General features
  - Can be hemorrhagic or nonhemorrhagic
    - Microbleeds important imaging marker for diffuse axonal injury (DAI)
    - Intraventricular hemorrhage correlates with DAI
  - Location
    - Subcortical/deep white matter (WM), corpus callosum
    - Deeper brain involvement = ↑ severity, poor prognosis
- NECT often normal (50-80%)
- MR
  - FLAIR: Hyperintense foci
  - T2* GRE: Hypointense "blooming" foci (hemorrhage)
  - SWI: Depicts significantly more DAI foci than GRE
  - DWI: May show restricted diffusion

PATHOLOGY

- Closed head injury (CHI)
  - Sudden deceleration, abrupt changes in angular momentum
- Cortex, WM have different densities, rotate at different speeds in CHI
  - Axons stretched (rarely disconnected or "sheared")
  - Occurs at interfaces between tissues of differing density
- 80% of lesions are microscopic, nonhemorrhagic

DIAGNOSTIC CHECKLIST

- Consider DAI if
  - Low GCS, minimal findings on NECT
- Remember
  - Deeper the abnormalities, more severe the brain injury
  - Remember: Visible lesions are "tip of iceberg"

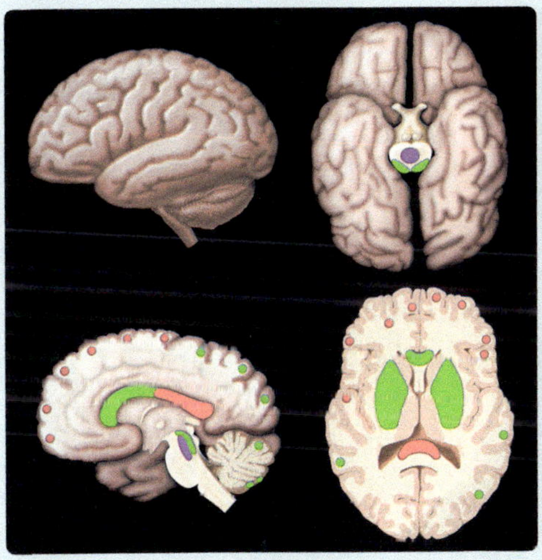

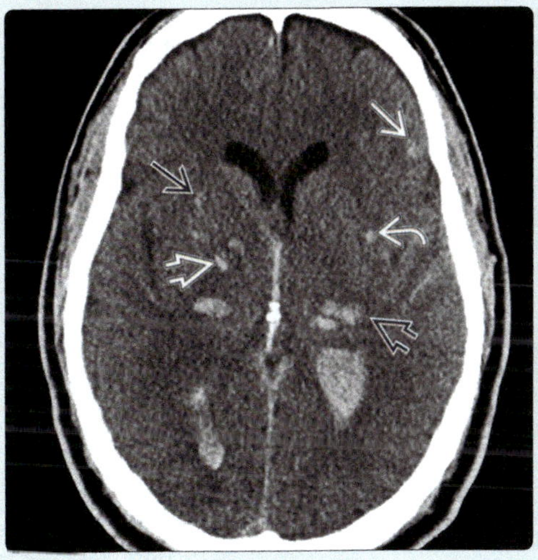

(Left) *Most common sites of axonal injury are shown in red; frequent but less common locations are in green. Injury to the midbrain/upper pons (purple) is uncommon but often lethal; generally, the deeper the abnormalities, the more severe the injury.* **(Right)** *Axial NECT scan in a 25-year-old man involved in a high-impact motor vehicle accident (MVA) shows multiple hemorrhagic foci in the subcortical WM →, external → and internal → capsules, basal ganglia →, and thalami →. Blood is also present in 3rd & lateral ventricles.*

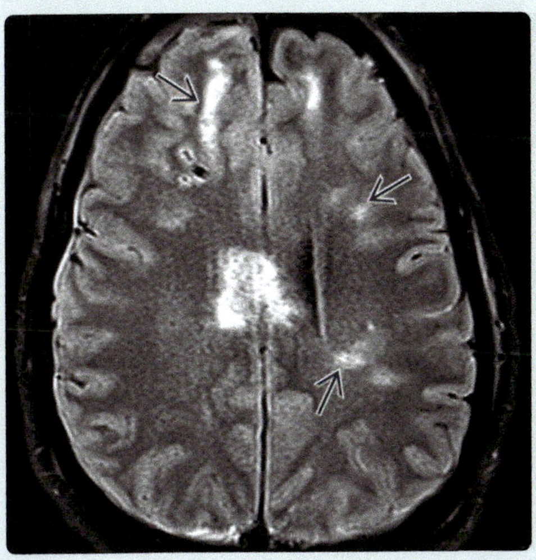

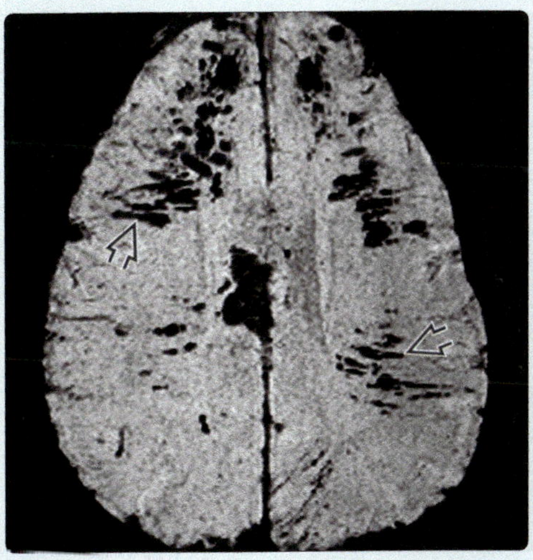

(Left) *FLAIR MR in a 26-year-old man involved in a high-speed roll-over MVA shows scattered hyperintense foci → in the subcortical and deep WM consistent with diffuse axonal injury.* **(Right)** *Axial SWI in the same case shows innumerable punctate and linear hypointense foci → that follow the course of the axons within the corona radiata. T2* scans (GRE, SWI) are very sensitive to susceptibility artifact from hemorrhage.*

KEY FACTS

TERMINOLOGY

- Subcortical injury (SCI): Deep diffuse axonal injury lesions of brainstem, basal ganglia, thalamus, and regions around 3rd ventricle
- Intraventricular hemorrhage (IVH): Hemorrhage within ventricular system
- Choroid hemorrhage (CH): Hemorrhage localized to choroidal plexus

IMAGING

- SCI: FLAIR most sensitive → hyperintense foci
- IVH: Hyperdense intraventricular blood; fluid-heme level common
- CH: Localized hyperdense choroidal hemorrhage

TOP DIFFERENTIAL DIAGNOSES

- SCI: Cavernous malformation, lacunar infarcts, small-vessel ischemia
- IVH: None
- CH: Normal calcification may mask small hemorrhages

PATHOLOGY

- SCI: Most commonly induced by shear-strain forces that disrupt penetrating &/or choroidal vessels
- IVH: Disruption of subependymal veins
- CH: Traumatic shear forces damage to choroid tissue

CLINICAL ISSUES

- SCI: Profound neurologic deficits
- IVH: Obtundation, seizures
- CH: Can lead to IVH

DIAGNOSTIC CHECKLIST

- Delayed development of deep lesions common
  - Initial scan may show only diffuse brain swelling
  - Focal lesions often appear 24-48 hours later
- Remember: The deeper the lesion, the more severe the injury

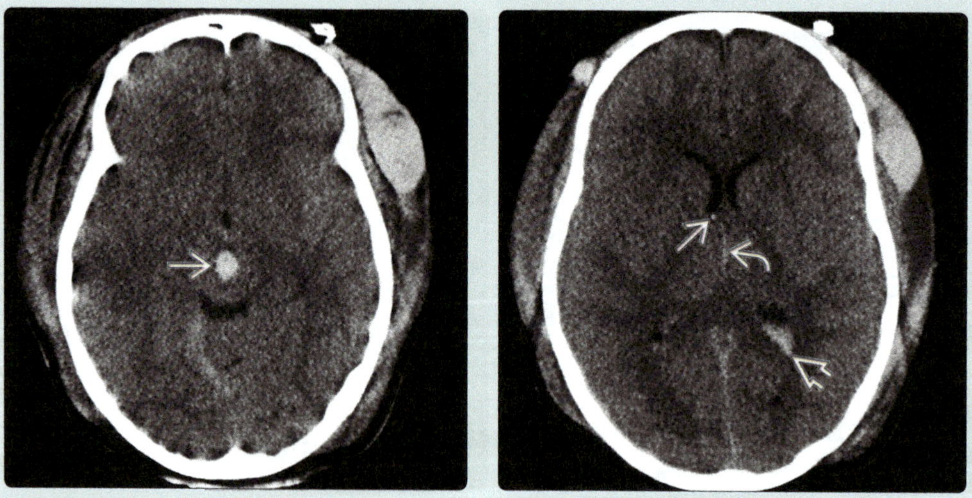

(Left) *Initial axial NECT in a 17-year-old girl involved in a high-speed MVA demonstrated only diffuse brain swelling (not shown). Because of persisting low GCS, repeat scan was obtained 24 hours later, showing a focal midbrain hemorrhage ➔.* **(Right)** *More cephalad scan shows a punctate hemorrhage in the right fornix ➔ and in the 3rd ➔ and lateral ventricles ➔. The patient expired 1 week later. The presence of deep lesions and intraventricular hemorrhage indicate severe subcortical injury.*

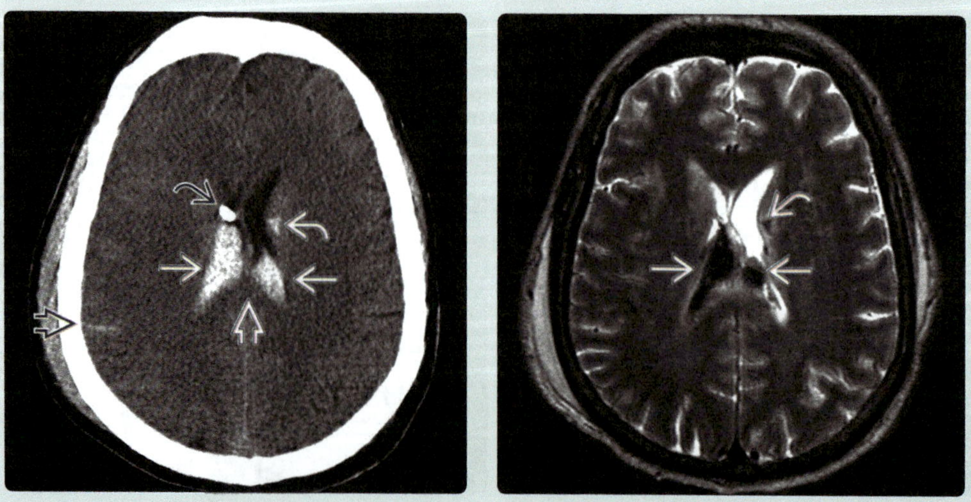

(Left) *Axial NECT in a patient with subcortical injury shows a hyperdense choroidal hemorrhage within choroid plexus substance of both ventricles ➔. Note the subarachnoid hemorrhage ➔, corpus callosum diffuse axonal injury (DAI) ➔, left caudate hemorrhagic DAI ➔, and a ventriculostomy tube tip ➔.* **(Right)** *Axial T2WI MR in the same patient shows hypointense hemorrhages distending the choroid plexi ➔. A left caudate hemorrhagic DAI ➔ is again seen.*

KEY FACTS

TERMINOLOGY

- Brain displaced from 1 compartment into another

IMAGING

- Subfalcine herniation
  - Cingulate gyrus displaced under falx
  - Lateral ventricle compressed/displaced across midline
  - Contralateral ventricle dilated
- Unilateral descending transtentorial herniation (DTH)
  - Temporal lobe displaced medially into incisura
  - Encroaches on, then effaces suprasellar cistern
- Bilateral DTH ("central herniation")
  - Both temporal lobes herniated into tentorial hiatus
  - Diencephalon crushed against skull base
  - Suprasellar cistern, cerebrospinal fluid spaces obliterated
  - Midbrain/pons displaced inferiorly
- Ascending transtentorial herniation
  - Cerebellum displaced up through incisura
  - Quadrigeminal cistern, tectum flattened
- Tonsillar herniation
  - Tonsils impacted into foramen magnum
  - Cisterna magna obliterated
- Transalar herniation
  - Ascending (middle fossa mass) or descending (frontal mass)
  - Brain, middle cranial artery herniated up/over sphenoid
- Transdural/transcranial herniation
  - Brain extruded through dural/skull defect

TOP DIFFERENTIAL DIAGNOSES

- Intracranial hypotension

CLINICAL ISSUES

- Uncal herniation: Ipsilateral pupil-involving CN3 palsy, contralateral hemiparesis
- Progressive bilateral ("central") herniation: Decorticate → decerebrate → death

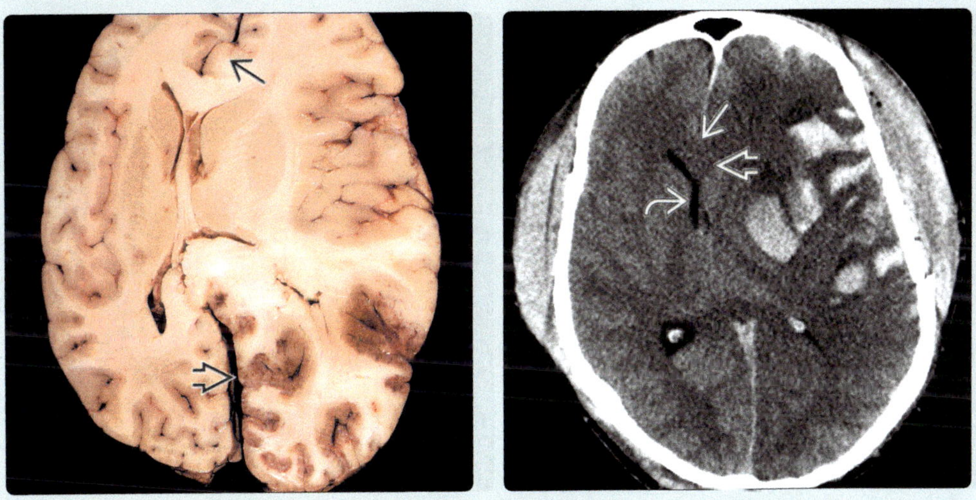

(Left) *Axial gross pathology section through the ventricles in a patient who died of multiple traumatic injuries shows findings of severe subfalcine herniation. Ventricles are displaced across the midline, and the cingulate gyrus is herniated under the falx. Left PCA infarct occurred secondary to descending transtentorial herniation. (Courtesy R. Hewlett, MD.)* **(Right)** *Axial NECT in severe trauma shows subfalcine herniation with severely compressed left and slightly dilated right lateral ventricle.*

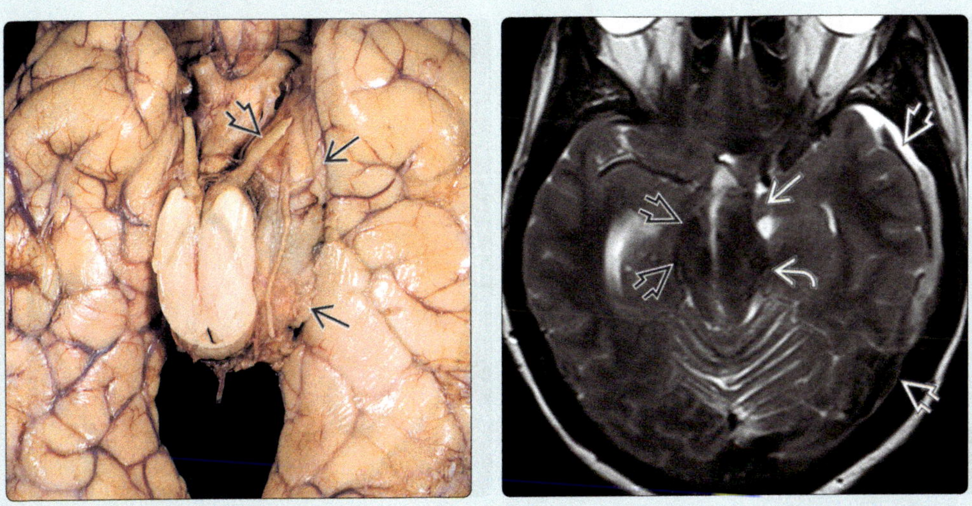

(Left) *Submentovertex gross pathology shows unilateral descending transtentorial herniation. Undersurface of herniated temporal lobe shows "grooving" from impaction against the tentorium. Note the 3rd nerve compression and midbrain displacement. (Courtesy R. Hewlett, MD.)* **(Right)** *Axial T2WI shows mixed-age subdural hematomas causing typical uncal herniation. The herniating uncus, hippocampus compress, displace the midbrain against the opposite edge of the tentorium.*

KEY FACTS

TERMINOLOGY

- Posttraumatic cerebral ischemia (PTCI)
- Hemodynamic alterations induced by traumatic brain injury (TBI)
  - Can be local, regional, generalized perfusion alteration(s)

IMAGING

- Best diagnostic clue: Restricted diffusion
- Most commonly occurs in PCA vascular distribution
  - MCA and ACA, vertebrobasilar relatively common
  - Less common: Perforating, cerebellar arteries
- Best imaging tool: MR + DWI/ADC
  - Diffusion most sensitive sequence
  - Midsagittal imaging to evaluate for herniation

TOP DIFFERENTIAL DIAGNOSES

- Nontraumatic ischemia/infarction; vascular (multiinfarct) dementia
- Atherosclerotic occlusion
- Subarachnoid-induced vasospasm

PATHOLOGY

- Primary TBI = direct damage at time of trauma
- Secondary brain injury occurs after initial trauma
  - Due to systemic responses to initial injuries
  - PTCI may be most common cause of secondary brain injury in setting of severe TBI
  - Secondary injuries often more devastating than primary TBI
  - Secondary injury can occur after negative initial imaging
- Mechanical shift of brain with herniation across falx &/or tentorium → 80-90% of PTCI

CLINICAL ISSUES

- Most common sign: GCS ≤ 8
- Symptoms often delayed 12-24 hours to several weeks
- PTCI occurs in 1.9-10.4% of craniocerebral trauma
- Ischemic damage present in 90% of TBI deaths

(Left) *Submentovertex view of autopsied brain in a patient with uncal herniation and occlusion of the adjacent posterior cerebral artery (PCA) against the tentorium shows a secondary hemorrhagic infarct in the ipsilateral occipital lobe. (Courtesy R. Hewlett, MD.)* **(Right)** *Axial NECT in a patient with a large mixed-age subdural hematoma shows herniation of the right uncus and compression of the ipsilateral PCA.*

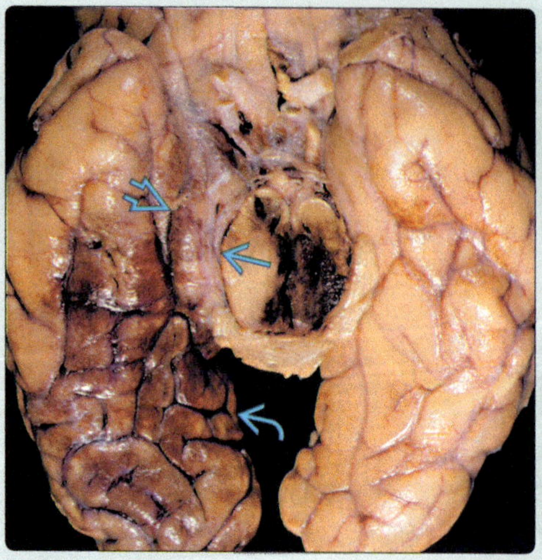

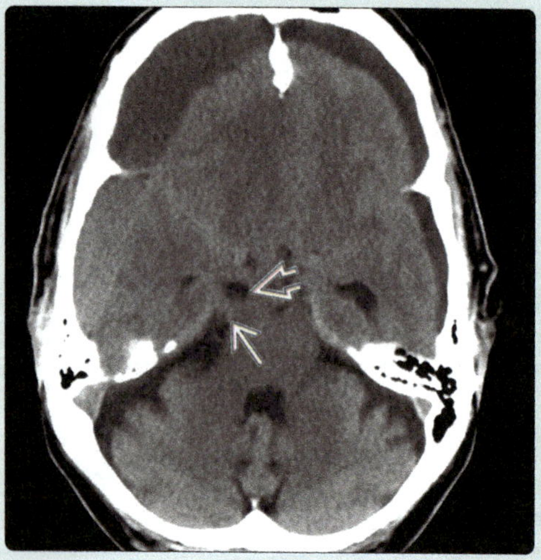

(Left) *Lateral DSA shows an inferiorly displaced PCA secondary to descending transtentorial herniation of the adjacent temporal lobe. Note the points at which the herniated PCA passes over the edge of the tentorium. The distal PCA is severely kinked and narrowed. Worsening herniation will occlude the PCA and result in secondary infarction.* **(Right)** *Axial NECT scan in a patient with severe bifrontal traumatic contusions shows a right PCA infarct.*

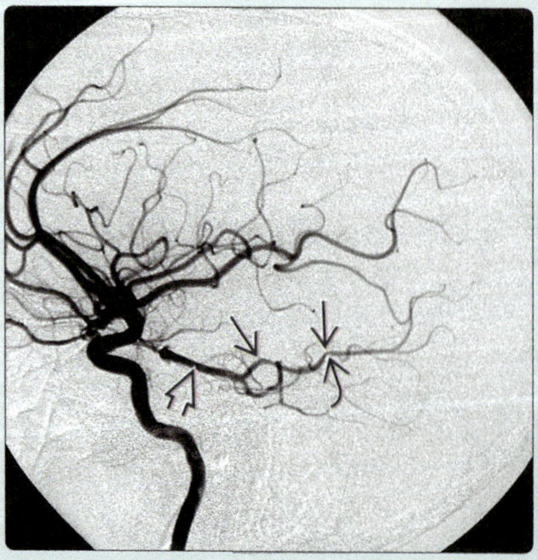

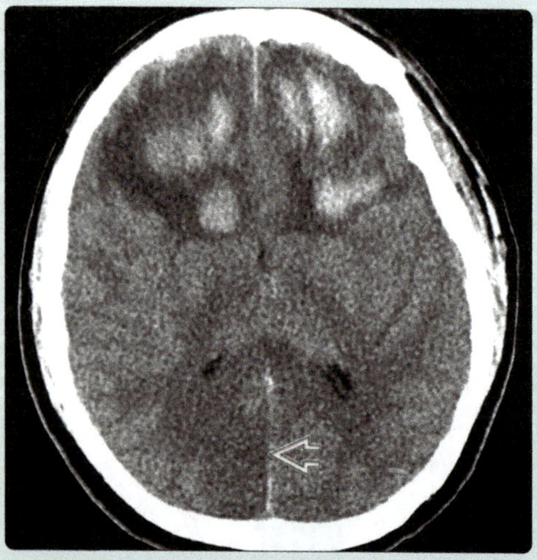

Brain Death

KEY FACTS

TERMINOLOGY

- Brain death (BD); death by neurological criteria (DNC)
- Complete, irreversible cessation of brain function

IMAGING

- No flow in intracranial arteries or venous sinuses
  - No intravascular enhancement on CT or MR
  - Light-bulb sign on radionuclide study
- Diffuse cerebral edema
  - Gyri swollen, ventricles/cisterns compressed
  - Gray-white matter borders effaced

TOP DIFFERENTIAL DIAGNOSES

- Reversible diffuse cerebral edema
  - Drug overdose
  - Status epilepticus (clinically can mimic BD)
  - Acute metabolic dysfunction (e.g., fulminant hepatic failure)
- Technical difficulty
  - Missed bolus (nuclear study, CTA)
  - Dissection (catheter angiography)
  - Vasospasm (catheter angiography)
- Massive cerebral infarction/edema

PATHOLOGY

- Severe cell swelling, ↑ intracranial pressure

CLINICAL ISSUES

- Complex assessment, often misunderstood by nonspecialists and families
  - DNC highly reliable with
    - Experienced examiners
    - Using established criteria
- Imaging may confirm but does not substitute for clinical criteria
- Reversible causes of coma must be excluded
- Remember: BD is primarily clinical diagnosis, legal criteria vary

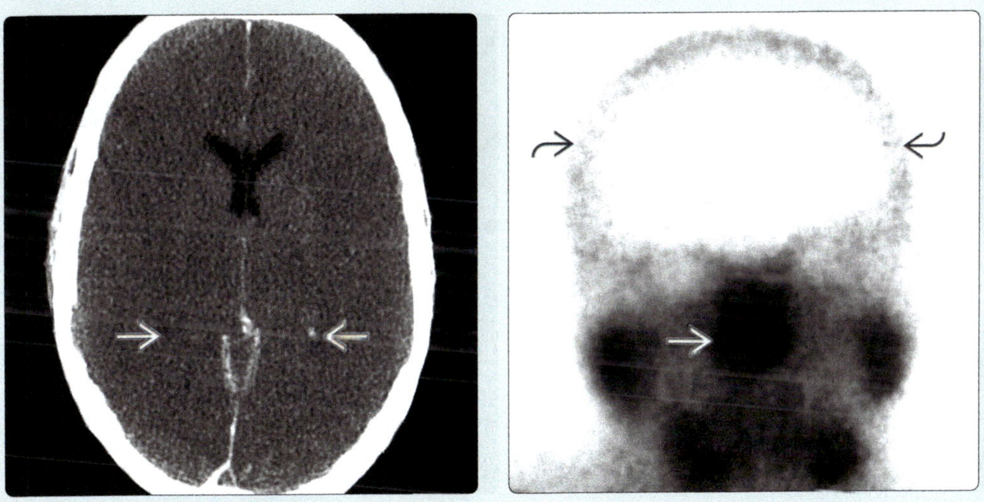

(Left) *Axial NECT shows complete loss of gray-white matter differentiation and diffuse sulcal and gyral effacement in this patient with diffuse cerebral edema and clinical brain death. The lateral ventricles are also effaced posteriorly ➡.* **(Right)** *Anteroposterior Tc-99m HMPAO scan shows the classic light-bulb ⤻ and hot-nose signs ➡ related to lack of intracerebral blood flow in brain death. No radionuclide is seen in the intracranial arteries or veins. (Courtesy B. Vomocil, MD.)*

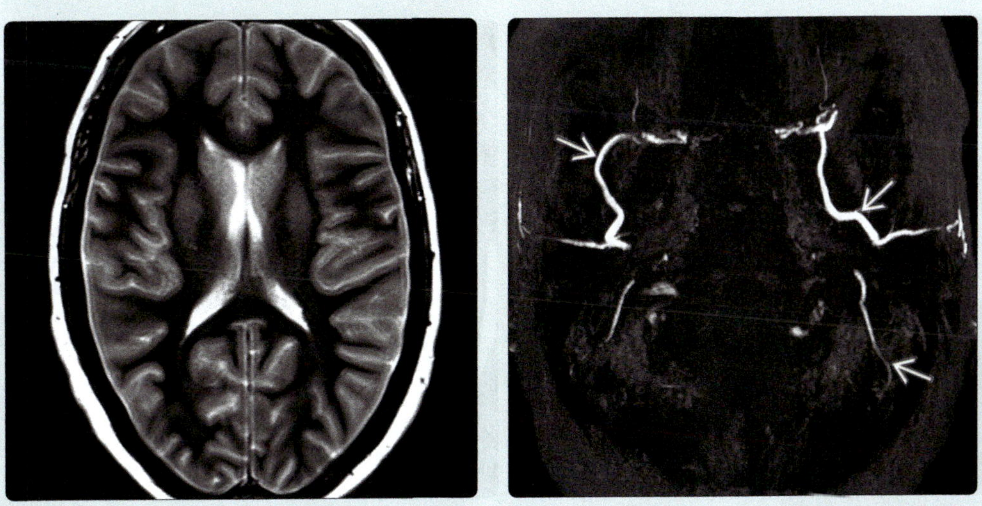

(Left) *Antemortem axial T2WI in a 50-year-old woman with clinical brain death obtained just before death shows small ventricles and swollen gyri with near-complete obliteration of the surface sulci.* **(Right)** *Submentovertex maximum intensity projection (MIP) view of MRA in the same patient shows flow only in extracranial branches of the external carotid arteries ➡. No flow is present in the intracranial vasculature.*

KEY FACTS

TERMINOLOGY

- Dysautoregulation/second impact syndrome
- Repeated head trauma within "window of vulnerability" before brain recovers from initial concussive injury
- May cause catastrophic brain swelling

IMAGING

- Thin, acute subdural hematoma (aSDH)
  - Disproportionate mass effect
    - Midline (subfalcine) shift more than accounted for by thickness of aSDH
- Swollen, hypodense cerebral hemisphere under aSDH
  - Underlying sulci compressed, then obliterated
- Best imaging tools
  - NECT (initial screening) ± MR with T2*, DWI

TOP DIFFERENTIAL DIAGNOSES

- aSDH (without underlying dysautoregulation)
- Nonaccidental trauma (child abuse)

PATHOLOGY

- Thin subdural hematoma
- Underlying brain swollen, hyperemic
  - May represent excitotoxic injury
  - ± secondary infarcts
  - ± uncal, central, tonsillar herniations

CLINICAL ISSUES

- Severe headache
- Vomiting
- May have dramatic, sudden collapse, coma
- Most common in
  - Adolescent male patients involved in high-impact sports
  - Abused infants
  - Elderly patients with repeated falls, head impacts

(Left) *Axial NECT in an abused infant with repeated inflicted head trauma shows a mixed-density right subdural hematoma (SDH) ⇨. The underlying right hemisphere is diffusely swollen and hypodense. Note disproportionate mass effect, subfalcine herniation ➡ compared with relatively thin SDH.* **(Right)** *Axial NECT in an elderly patient with repeated falls and head trauma shows a thin acute SDH ⇨. Underlying cortex is swollen ➡ with disproportionate mass effect on left lateral ventricle.*

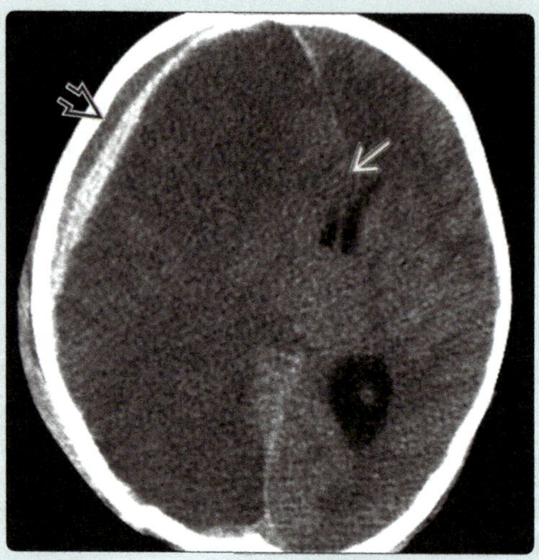

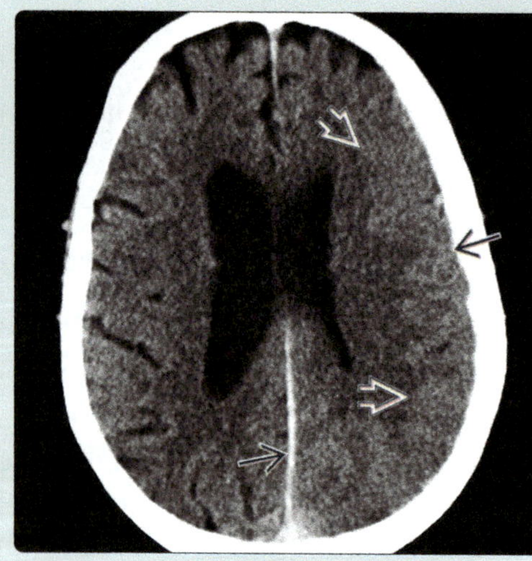

(Left) *Axial NECT in an abused infant shows mixed acute, subacute/chronic SDH overlying a swollen, hypodense hemisphere.* **(Right)** *Axial fat-suppressed T2WI in the same case 2 days later, after evacuation of the SDH, shows swollen hyperintense cortex ➡ underlying bilateral SDHs. Note hyperintensity in the corpus callosum splenium ➡. Findings are consistent with excitotoxic injury.*

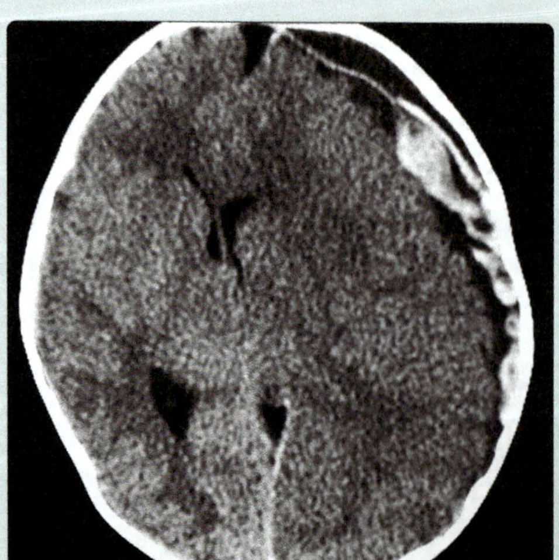

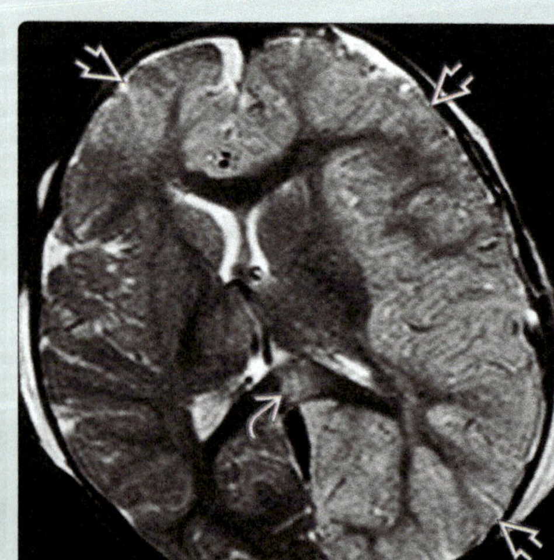

KEY FACTS

TERMINOLOGY

- Dissection
  - Intramural hematoma extends along vessel wall
- Dissecting aneurysm
  - Dissection + aneurysmal dilation contained by adventitia
- Pseudoaneurysm
  - Lumen contained by thrombus outside vessel wall

IMAGING

- Location
  - Often adjacent to falx, skull, tentorium, or region of significant motion
  - Posterior circulation most common
    - Vertebral arteries most common site (72%)
    - Extension into basilar artery rare
  - Anterior circulation uncommon
    - Supraclinoid internal carotid artery
    - Distal, more peripheral (A2, M2, P2, and beyond) where vessel contacts dura or skull
- NECT: Basal subarachnoid hemorrhage (SAH)
  - Looks like aneurysmal SAH
  - In unusual locations, more extensive than traumatic SAH
- MR: Hyperintense hematoma + central "flow void"
  - Target or crescent sign
- CTA/MRA/DSA
  - "Fat" vessel (dissecting aneurysm or mural thrombus)
  - Long segment narrowing or tapered occlusion
  - Intraluminal flap (± on DSA/MRA; best seen on DSA)
  - ± dissecting aneurysm (irregular, wide neck; at side wall, usually not at vessel bifurcations)

TOP DIFFERENTIAL DIAGNOSES

- Intracranial artery narrowing/occlusion
  - Atherosclerosis
  - Vasospasm
  - Vasculitis
- Traumatic SAH
  - Aneurysmal, perimesencephalic nonaneurysmal SAH

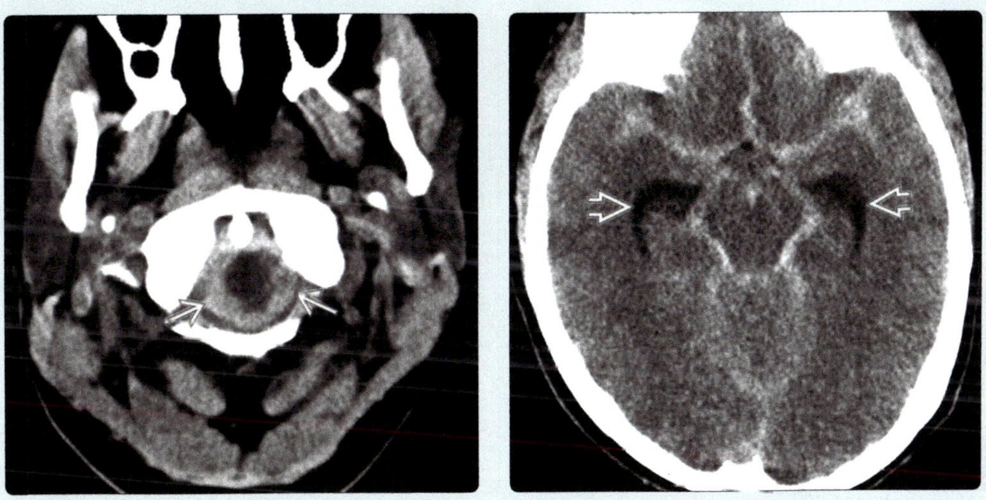

(Left) *Axial NECT scan in a 29-year-old woman involved in a high-speed MVA shows subarachnoid hemorrhage (SAH) ➡ surrounding the lower medulla.* **(Right)** *More cephalad NECT scan in the same patient shows extensive SAH filling the basal cisterns, outlining the midbrain. Note the enlargement of the temporal horns ➡, indicating early extraventricular obstructive hydrocephalus.*

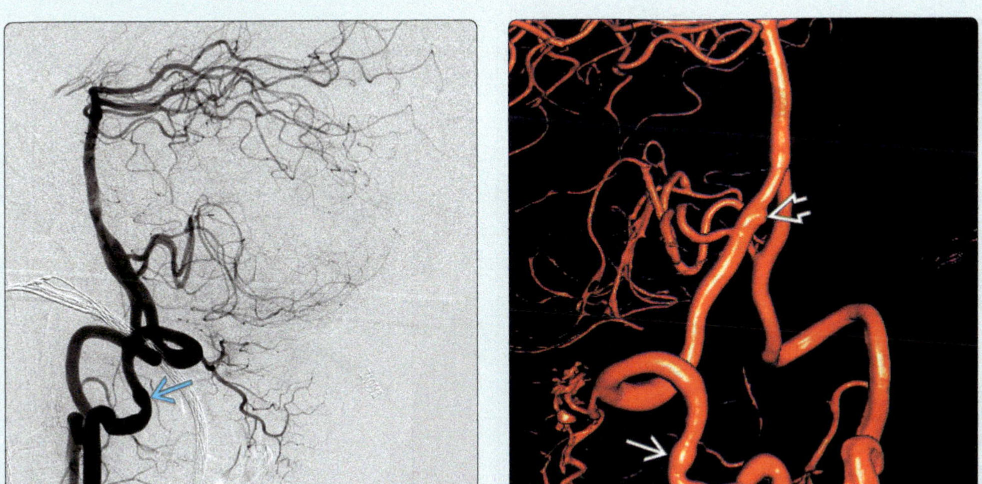

(Left) *Slightly oblique lateral DSA in the same patient shows focal fusiform enlargement of the left vertebral artery ➡, suggesting a dissecting pseudoaneurysm may be the etiology for the SAH.* **(Right)** *Oblique 3D color-shaded surface display in the same patient shows the focal right dissecting aneurysm ➡ as well as a 2nd dissecting aneurysm along the distal right vertebral artery ➡. The patient had a cardiac arrest after the DSA and expired.*

KEY FACTS

TERMINOLOGY

- Direct carotid cavernous fistula (CCF), high-flow CCF
- Single-hole tear/transection of cavernous internal carotid artery (ICA) with arteriovenous shunt into cavernous sinus (CS)

IMAGING

- General features
  - Proptosis, dilated superior ophthalmic vein (SOV) and CS, extraocular muscle enlargement
  - Skull base fracture involving sphenoid bone/carotid canal ↑ likelihood of ICA injury
- MRA: ↑ flow-related signal in CS and SOV
- CT/CTA may be suggestive; should proceed to DSA to confirm and treat
- DSA is definitive
  - Early filling of CS + outflow pathways including retrograde filling of SOV, angular + facial veins
  - Reduced or absent antegrade flow in ICA beyond fistula, depending on size of ICA tear

TOP DIFFERENTIAL DIAGNOSES

- Indirect CCF
  - Low-flow CCF
  - CS dural arteriovenous fistula
  - Often older patient without history of trauma

CLINICAL ISSUES

- Bruit, pulsating exophthalmos, orbital edema/erythema, ↓ vision, glaucoma, headache
- Hemispheric ischemia if ↓ flow in ICA beyond CCF
- Focal deficits → cranial nerves 3-6 (ptosis)
- Endovascular treatment options include
  - Transarterial-transfistula balloon embolization
  - Transvenous embolization
  - Pipeline/covered stent placement
  - ICA sacrifice

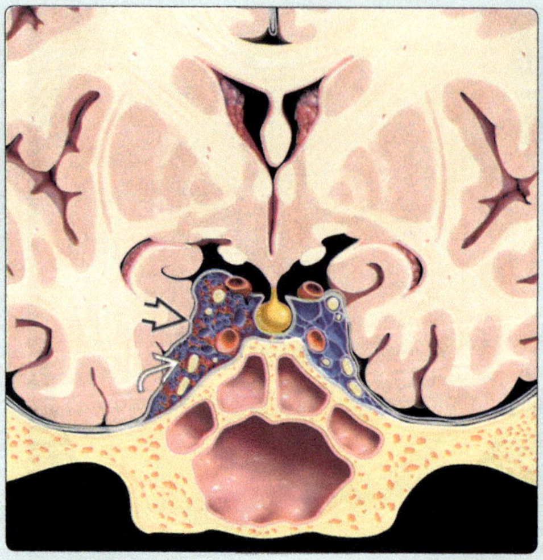

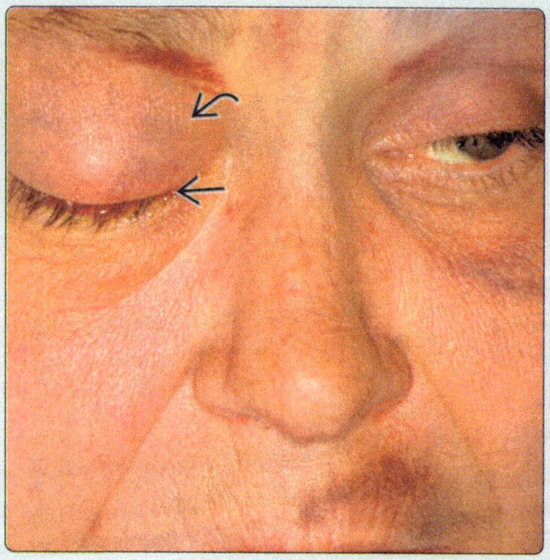

(Left) *Coronal graphic depicts a carotid cavernous fistula (CCF). The right cavernous sinus → is enlarged. Note numerous dilated arterial and venous channels → within the laterally bulging cavernous sinus.* **(Right)** *Clinical photograph depicts findings in posttraumatic right carotid cavernous fistula. Pulsatile exophthalmos → with 3, 4, and 6 nerve palsies including ptosis → was present.*

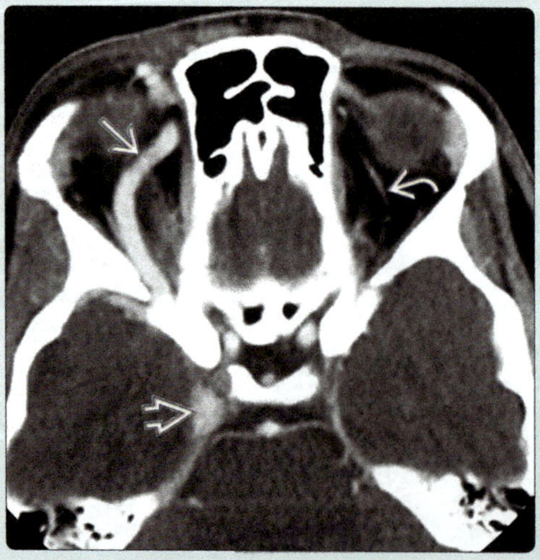

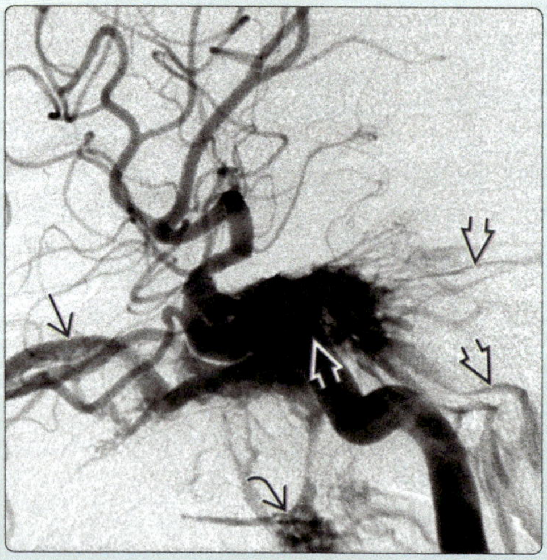

(Left) *CECT scan in a patient with posttraumatic pulsatile exophthalmos shows that the right cavernous sinus → is enlarged. The ipsilateral superior ophthalmic vein → is more than 4x the size of the left superior ophthalmic vein →.* **(Right)** *DSA in the same case shows opacification of the cavernous sinus → in the arterial phase. Also outlined are many of the venous outflow pathways of the cavernous sinus, including the superior ophthalmic vein →, superior and inferior petrosal sinuses →, and pterygoid and pharyngeal venous plexi →.*

KEY FACTS

TERMINOLOGY

- Definition
  - Neurodegenerative disease secondary to repetitive concussive/subconcussive head injuries
- Synonyms
  - Dementia pugilistica ("punch-drunk")
  - Postconcussion syndrome

IMAGING

- MR
  - Age-inappropriate volume loss
    - Voxel-based morphometry shows disproportionate involvement of medial temporal lobes
  - Nonspecific T2/FLAIR punctate, confluent hyperintensities in deep, periventricular white matter (WM)
  - DTI shows loss of WM integrity
    - Uncinate and superior/inferior longitudinal fasciculi
  - T2* shows microbleeds in ~ 10%
- PET
  - Temporoparietal hypometabolism on FDG-PET
  - PET imaging ligands for phosphorylated tau may be in vivo biomarker

PATHOLOGY

- Etiology
  - Repetitive head trauma
  - Contact sports (football, soccer, hockey, boxing, wrestling, mixed martial arts, etc.)
  - Battlefield exposure to blast waves generated by improvised explosive devices
- Gross: Likened to octogenarian Alzheimer patient
- Microscopic: Neurofibrillary tangles, Aβ plaques

CLINICAL ISSUES

- Cognitive dysfunction, memory loss
- Variable mood, personality, behavior disorders

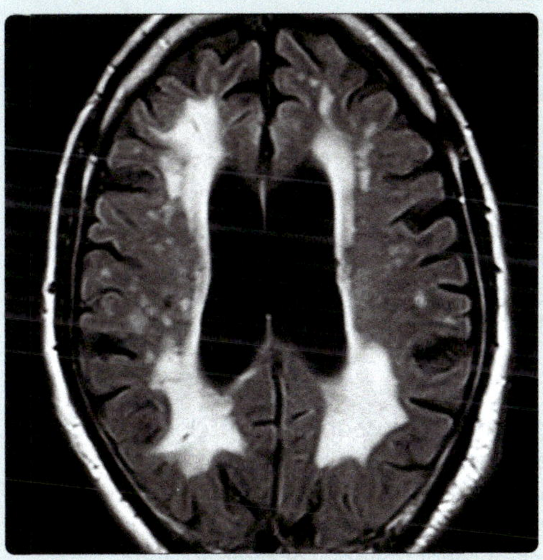

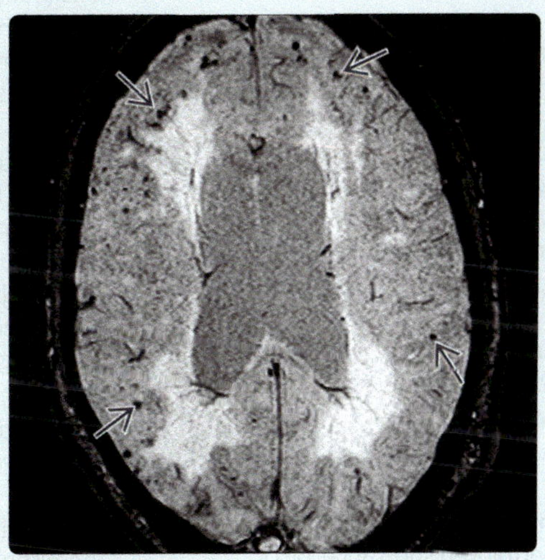

(Left) *Axial FLAIR scan in a middle-aged former professional athlete with early-onset dementia shows diffuse bihemispheric volume loss with extensive confluent and punctate hyperintensities in the subcortical and deep cerebral white matter (WM).* **(Right)** *Axial T2* SWI scan in the same patient shows numerous punctate "blooming" foci in the subcortical and deep WM ➙, consistent with microbleeds in this case of clinically diagnosed chronic traumatic encephalopathy.*

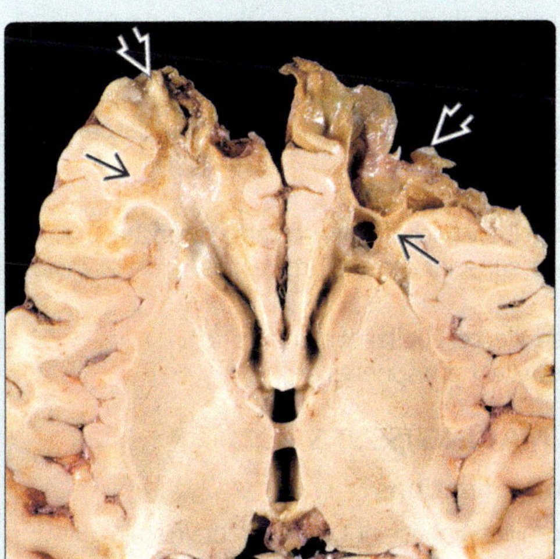

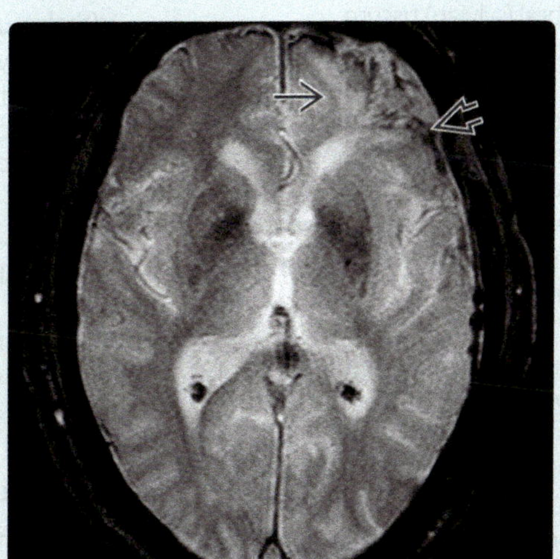

(Left) *Autopsy in a patient who survived a single episode of severe head injury shows remote effects of head trauma. Note the bifrontal encephalomalacia ➡ and extensive gliosis in the subcortical WM ➙. Note absence of microbleeds.* **(Right)** *Axial T2* GRE in an elderly patient with a single episode of moderate head trauma shows left frontal encephalomalacia and gliosis ➙ with superficial siderosis of the adjacent cortex ⇨. Note the absence of microbleeds in this case.*

TERMINOLOGY

Abbreviations

- Anterior, middle, posterior cerebral arteries (ACA, MCA, PCA)
- Anterior, posterior communicating arteries (ACoA, PCoA)
- Basilar artery (BA)
- Vertebral artery (VA)
- Anterior, posterior inferior cerebellar arteries (AICA, PICA)
- Anterior choroidal artery (AChoA)
- Recurrent artery of Heubner (RAH)

GROSS ANATOMY

Anterior Circulation

- ICA and its branches + ACoA, PCoA

Posterior Circulation

- BA and its branches

IMAGING ANATOMY

Overview

- **Internal carotid artery**
  - Proximal to termination gives off ophthalmic artery, AChoA, PCoA
  - Terminal bifurcation into ACA (smaller, medial), MCA (larger, lateral)
  - **ACA** has 4 segments
    - Horizontal or precommunicating (A1) segment courses medially above optic chiasm, joined by ACoA to contralateral A1
    - Vertical or postcommunicating (A2) segment courses superiorly in interhemispheric fissure, around corpus callosum genu
    - Distal (A3) segment courses posteriorly under inferior free margin of falx cerebri, gives off cortical branches
    - Perforating arteries arise from A1, ACoA
    - RAH arises from distal A1 or proximal A2
  - **MCA** has 4 segments
    - Horizontal (M1) segment courses laterally to sylvian fissure below anterior perforated substance, bi- or trifurcates
    - "Genu" or "knee" of MCA is gentle posterosuperior turn toward lateral cerebral (sylvian) fissure
    - Insular (M2) segments course within lateral cerebral fissure, over insula
    - Opercular (M3) segments begin at top of insula, turn laterally in sylvian fissure to reach overhanging frontal/parietal/temporal opercula
    - Cortical (M4) branches emerge from lateral cerebral fissure, course over hemispheric surface
    - Perforating arteries arise from M1
- **Basilar artery**
  - Courses cephalad in prepontine cistern to terminal bifurcation ventral to midbrain
    - Gives off **AICA**, superior cerebellar arteries (**SCAs**), pontine, midbrain perforating arteries
  - Bifurcates into **PCAs**, each of which has 4 segments
    - Mesencephalic or precommunicating (P1) segment lies within interpeduncular cistern, curves posterolaterally from BA to PCoA junction
    - Ambient (P2) segment extends from PCA-PCoA junction, curving around cerebral peduncles just above tentorium, above oculomotor nerve
    - Quadrigeminal (P3) segment extends posteromedially from level of quadrigeminal plate
    - Cortical (P4) branches arise from distal PCA at or just before reaching calcarine fissure
    - Multiple perforating branches arise from BA bifurcation, proximal P1s
      - Important variant = Artery of Percheron (thalamic, midbrain perforators all arise from single trunk)
  - **Vertebral arteries**
    - Intracranial (V4) segments enter dura near foramen magnum
    - Give off anterior/posterior spinal arteries, perforating arteries to medulla, PICA

Vascular Territory

- Vascular distributions of ACA, MCA, PCA vary from individual to individual, have typical as well as maximum, minimum territories
- **2 vascular "watershed" zones** exist at confluence of territorial supply, are vulnerable to hypoperfusion
  - Cortical watershed = subpial confluence of cortical ACA/MCA/PCA branches
  - Deep white matter watershed zone = confluence of deep cortical penetrating branches, perforating branches from circle of Willis
- **ACA**
  - Perforating branches: Corpus callosum rostrum, heads of caudate nuclei, anterior commissure, anteromedial putamen/globus pallidus/anterior limb internal capsule (if RAH present)
  - Cortical branches: Inferomedial frontal lobes, anterior 2/3 of medial hemisphere surface, 1-2 cm over brain convexity
- **MCA**
  - Perforating branches: Most of putamen, globus pallidus, superior half of internal capsule, most of caudate nucleus, some deep white matter
  - Cortical branches: Most of lateral surface of cerebral hemispheres, anterior tip (pole) of temporal lobe
- **PCA**
  - Perforating branches: Much of central brain base (thalamus, hypothalamus), midbrain, choroid plexus
    - Artery of Percheron = thalami, midbrain
  - Cortical branches: Most of inferior surface of temporal lobe, occipital pole, variable amount of posterolateral surface of hemisphere
- **BA**
  - All of PCA territory (including perforating branches), most of pons, superior cerebellum/vermis
- **VA**
  - Most of medulla, cerebellar tonsils, inferior vermis/cerebellar hemispheres

ANATOMY IMAGING ISSUES

Imaging Recommendations

- Late arterial (capillary) phase of DSA with "brain stain" shows vascular territory

GRAPHIC & MRA

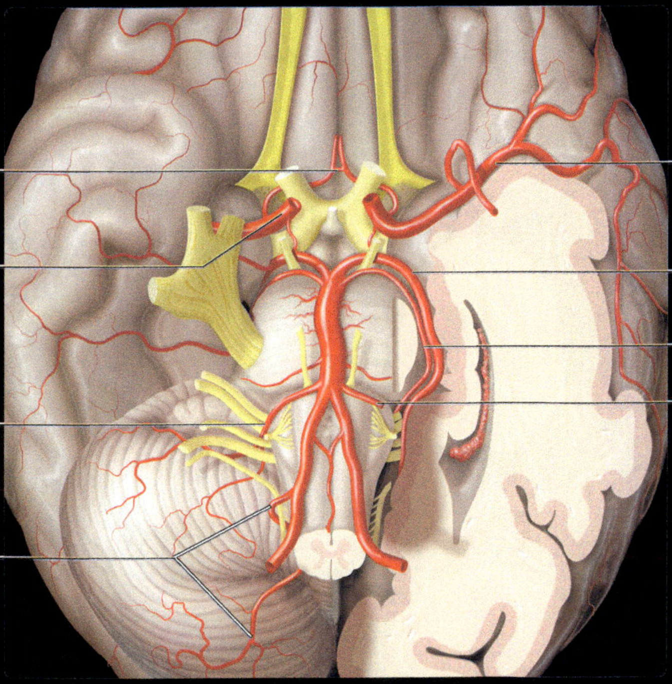

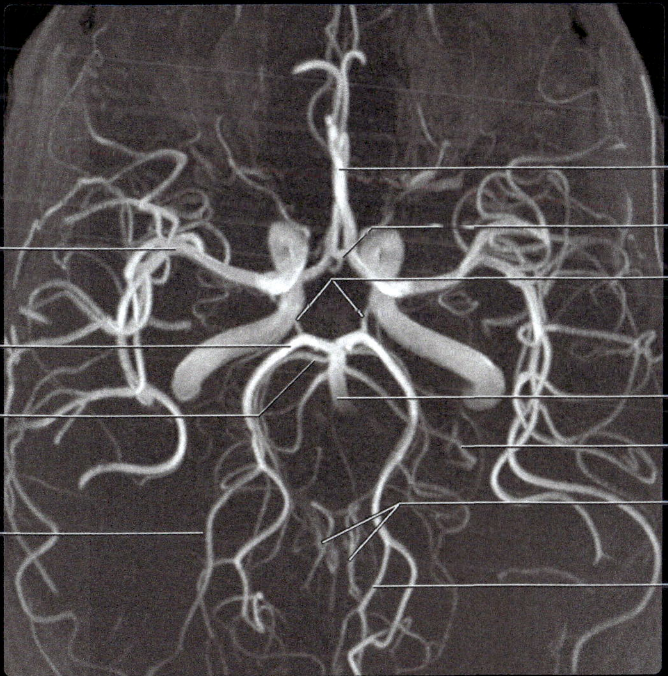

(Top) *Graphic depicts the brain vascular system and its relationship to the base of the brain. The anterior cerebral arteries course cephalad in the interhemispheric fissure from their junction at the anterior communicating artery. They supply most of the medial brain surface except for the posterior 3rd, which is supplied by the middle cerebral artery (MCA). The MCA supplies most of the lateral surface of the hemispheres. The posterior cerebral artery (PCA) supplies most of the undersurface of the temporal lobe except for its most anterior tip. The right anterior and posterior inferior cerebellar arteries (AICA and PICA) are shown on the right. On the left, a common AICA-PICA trunk is present, a frequent normal variant.* **(Bottom)** *Submentovertex view of a 3T MRA depicts normal intracranial circulation. Compare with graphic above.*

GRAPHICS

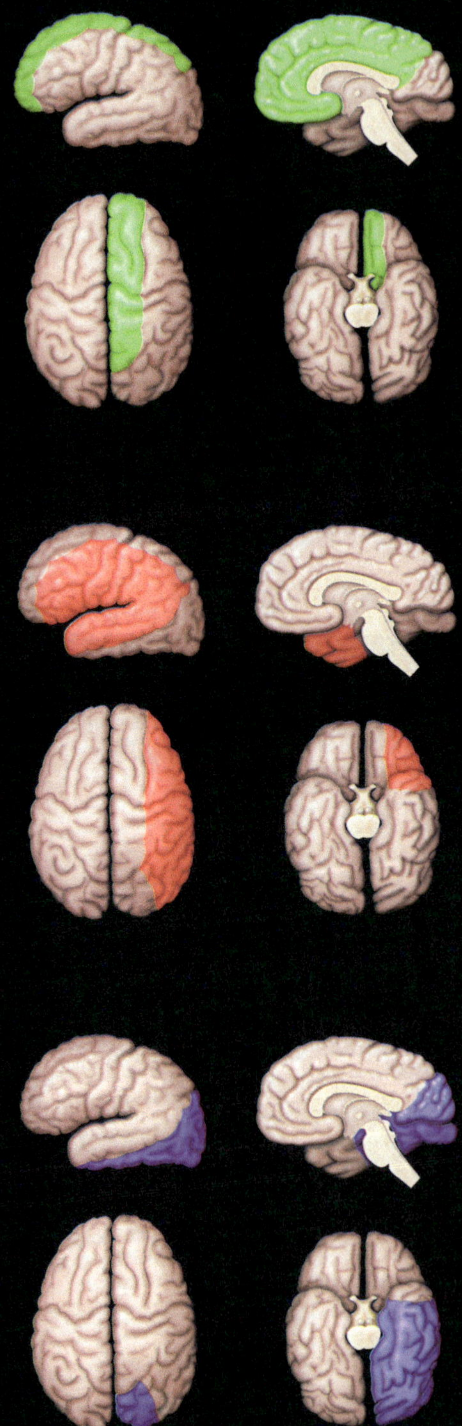

(Top) *Typical vascular territories of the 3 major cerebral arteries are depicted. The most common distribution of the anterior cerebral artery (ACA) is shown in green, as seen from lateral (upper left), medial (upper right), from top down (lower left) and from the submentovertex perspective (lower right). The ACA supplies most of the medial hemispheric surface except for the occipital lobe.* **(Middle)** *Usual vascular territory of the MCA is shown in red. MCA typically supplies most of the lateral and superior surface of the hemisphere except for a small strip over the vertex (ACA), occipital pole, and inferolateral temporal lobe (PCA).* **(Bottom)** *Usual vascular territory of the PCA is depicted in purple. The PCA supplies the occipital poles and most of the undersurface of the temporal lobe except for its tip, which is usually supplied by the MCA.*

GRAPHICS

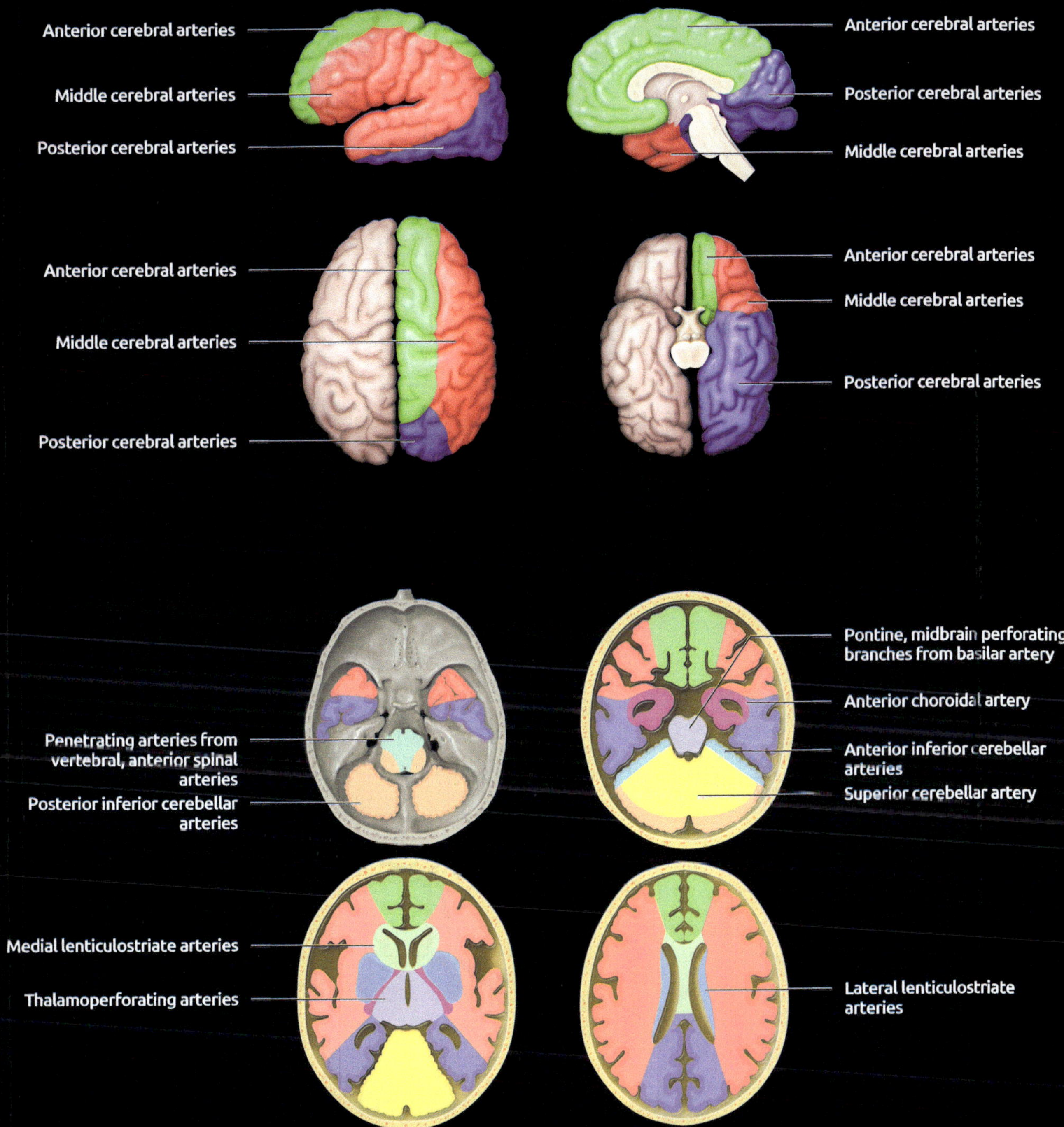

(Top) *The 3 major cerebral artery territories fit together like a jigsaw puzzle as they supply the hemispheres. ACA is depicted in green. MCA is shown in red. The PCA is colored purple. The junction of territories forms the cortical watershed zone. The posterior confluence where all 3 vascular distributions meet together, seen on the lower left at the vertex, is especially vulnerable to cerebral hypoperfusion.* **(Bottom)** *Penetrating artery territories are shown in axial plane. PICA (tan) supplies inferior cerebellum, lateral medulla. Superior cerebellar artery is shown in yellow, AICA in light blue. Medullary (aqua), pontine, and thalamic perforating arteries (light purple) are derived from the vertebrobasilar territory. Anterior choroidal (magenta), lateral (medium blue), and medial (light green) lenticulostriate arteries supply basal ganglia, caudate, much of corpus callosum.*

GRAPHICS

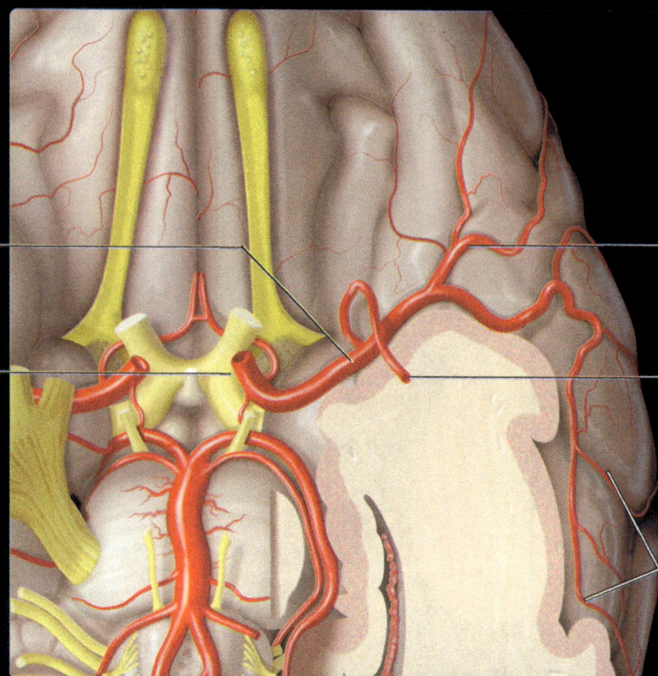

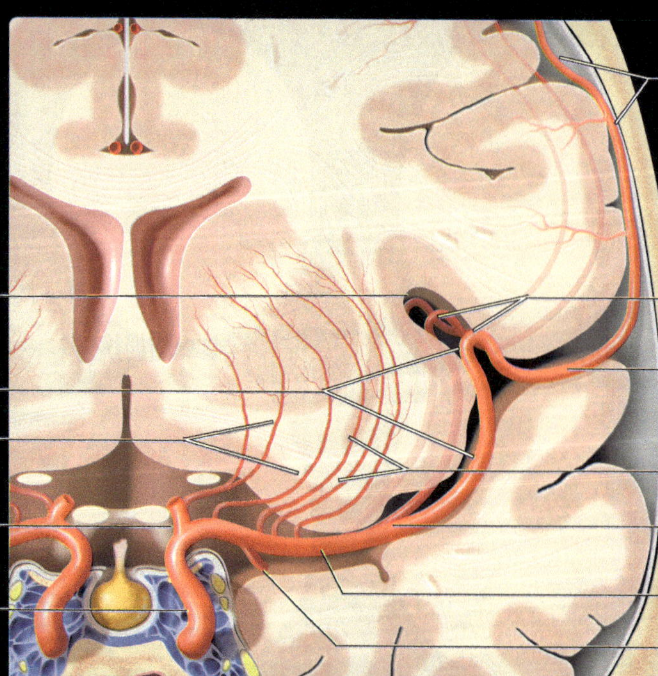

(Top) *The MCA and its relationship to adjacent structures is depicted on these graphics. Submentovertex view with the left temporal lobe sectioned through the temporal horn of the lateral ventricle is illustrated. The MCA supplies much of the lateral surface of the brain and is the larger of the 2 terminal branches of the internal carotid artery.* **(Bottom)** *AP view shows the MCA and its relationship to the adjacent brain. The MCA courses through the sylvian fissure, and the M1-M4 segments are well delineated. A few medial and numerous lateral lenticulostriate arteries arise from the top of the horizontal (M1) MCA segment, course superiorly through the anterior perforated substance, and supply the lateral basal ganglia + external capsule.*

GRAPHICS

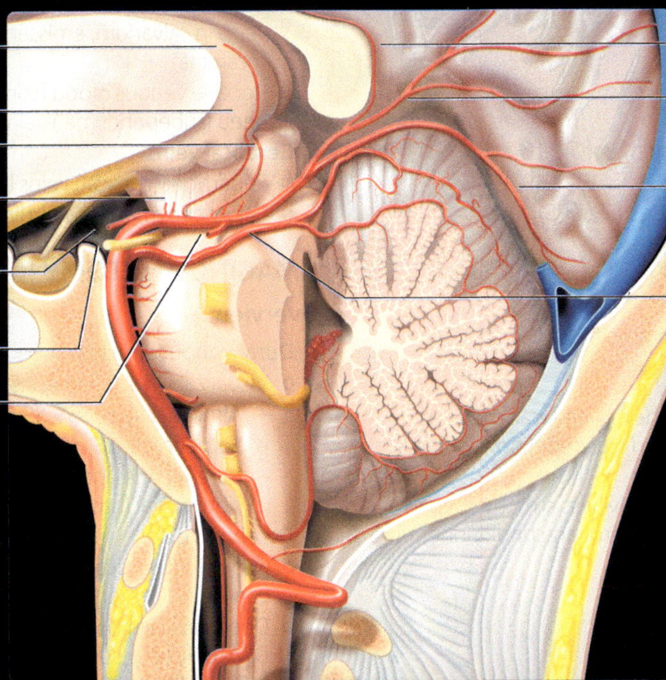

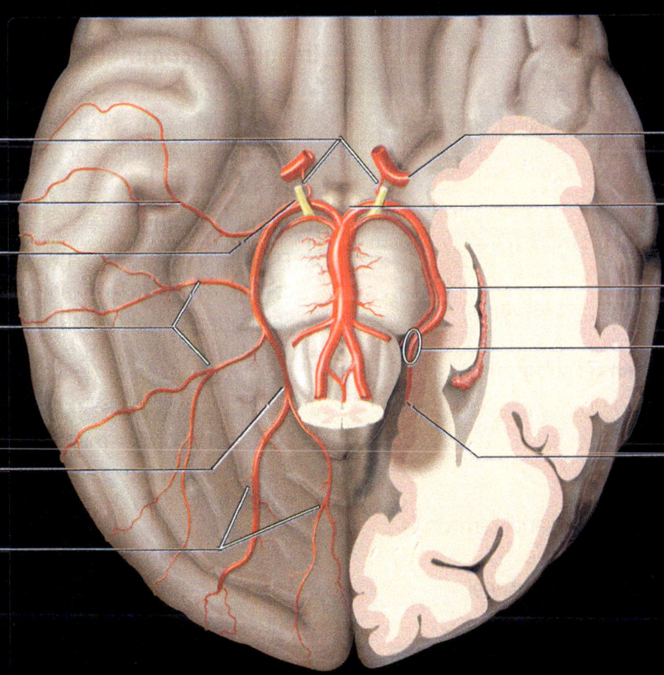

(Top) *Lateral graphic depicts the PCA and its branches. The tentorium and CN3 lie between the PCA above and the superior cerebellar artery below. The PCA has central (perforating), choroidal, and cortical branches as well as a small branch to the corpus callosum splenium.* **(Bottom)** *Submentovertex graphic shows the PCA and the relationship of its segments to the midbrain. The PCA supplies the occipital lobe and almost all of the inferior surface of the temporal lobe (except for its tip). The precommunicating (P1) PCA segment extends from the basilar bifurcation to the posterior communicating artery junction. The ambient (P2) segment swings posterolaterally around the midbrain. The quadrigeminal segment (P3) lies behind the midbrain. The PCA terminal segment is the calcarine (P4) segment.*

TERMINOLOGY

Abbreviations

- Superior sagittal sinus (SSS)
- Inferior sagittal sinus (ISS)
- Internal cerebral vein (ICV)
- Straight sinus (SS)
- Great cerebral vein (vein of Galen, VofG)
- Transverse sinus (TS)
- Superior/inferior petrosal sinuses (SPS/IPS)
- Cavernous sinus (CS)
- Internal jugular vein (IJV)
- Basal vein of Rosenthal (BVR)
- Superficial, deep middle cerebral veins (SMCV; DMCV)

Definitions

- **Dural sinuses** are large, endothelial-lined trabeculated venous channels encased within folds/reflections of dura that define, form their walls
- **Cerebral veins** are thin-walled, valveless structures that cross subarachnoid space (SAS), pierce arachnoid/inner dura to enter dural venous sinus

GROSS ANATOMY

Overview

- **Dural venous sinuses** (divided into 2 groups)
  - **Anteroinferior group** (CS, SPS/IPS, clival, sphenoparietal)
  - **Posterosuperior group** (SSS, ISS, SS, TS, sigmoid, occipital)
- **Cerebral veins** (divided into 3 groups)
  - **Superficial ("external") veins** (3 subgroups)
    - Superior: 8-12 smaller cortical veins over hemispheres, vein of Trolard
    - Middle: SMCV, vein of Labbé
    - Inferior: DMCV, BVR
  - **Deep ("internal") veins**
    - Subependymal veins
    - ICVs (formed by thalamostriate, septal veins)
    - Great cerebral vein (VofG)
  - **Brainstem/posterior fossa veins** (3 subgroups)
    - Superior (galenic) group
    - Anterior (petrosal) group
    - Posterior (tentorial) group
- **Venous vascular territories**
  - More variable, less well-known than arterial territories
  - General concepts
    - Venous drainage generally radial, centrifugal (exception = deep cerebral structures)
    - Much of middle/superior brain surfaces (cortex, subcortical white matter) drained by cortical veins to SSS
    - Posterior/inferior temporal lobe, adjacent parietal lobe drained by vein of Labbé to TS
    - Insular cortex, parenchyma around sylvian (middle cerebral) fissure drained by sphenoparietal sinus to CS
    - Deep cerebral structures (central/deep white matter, basal ganglia) drained by medullary/subependymal veins to ICVs, VofG, SS; medial temporal lobe via DMCV/BVR to VofG

Anatomy Relationships

- **Dural venous sinuses**
  - Communicate with extracranial veins directly (via diploic veins in calvarium, emissary veins through basilar foramina)
  - Receive venous blood from superficial (cortical) veins, deep (subependymal) veins
- **Cerebral veins**
  - Superficial (cortical) veins lie in SAS, mainly follow sulci
  - Subependymal veins outline ventricles

IMAGING ANATOMY

Overview

- **Dural venous sinuses**
  - Visualization at DSA varies widely
    - Almost always: SSS, SS, TS, sigmoid sinus, IJVs
    - Sometimes: ISS, SPS/IPS
    - Rare/inconstant: CS, sphenoparietal sinus, occipital sinus, clival (basal) venous plexus
- **Cerebral veins**
  - Superficial cortical veins almost always seen (number, configuration vary)
  - Deep veins almost always seen on late venous phase of DSA, only largest (e.g., thalamostriate veins) seen on MR/MRV
  - ICVs, VofG almost always seen on DSA, CTV, MRV

ANATOMY IMAGING ISSUES

Imaging Recommendations

- Obtain source images for MR venogram perpendicular to main axis of dural sinus (e.g., coronal for SSS)
- MRV, CTV excellent for general overview of dural sinuses, cerebral veins but DSA best for detailed delineation

Imaging Pitfalls

- TSs often asymmetric, hypoplastic/atretic segment common (do not misdiagnose as occlusion)
- Saturation bands on MR disguise flow
- Jugular bulb flow often very asymmetric, turbulent (pseudolesion)
- Unopacified venous blood streaming into dural sinus on DSA should not be mistaken for filling defect (thrombus)
- "Giant" arachnoid granulations appear as round/ovoid CSF-equivalent filling defects in dural sinuses (especially TS), are normal variant, should not be mistaken for thrombus
- Acute dural sinus, cortical vein thrombi isointense with brain on T1WI, so T2* (GRE) or T1 C+ imaging very helpful
- Subacute clot is hyperintense on T1WI (do not mistake for enhancement)

GRAPHICS

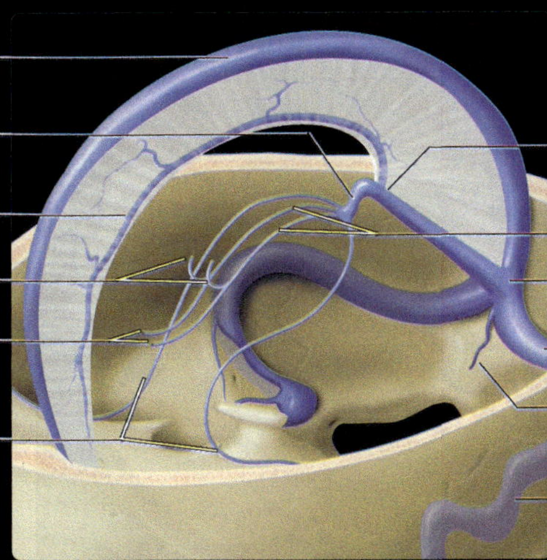

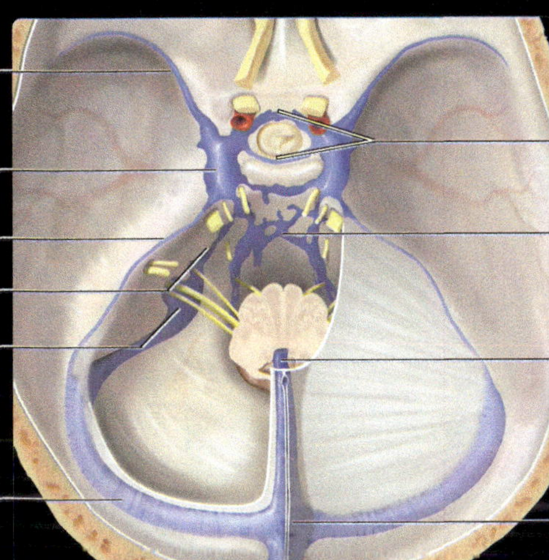

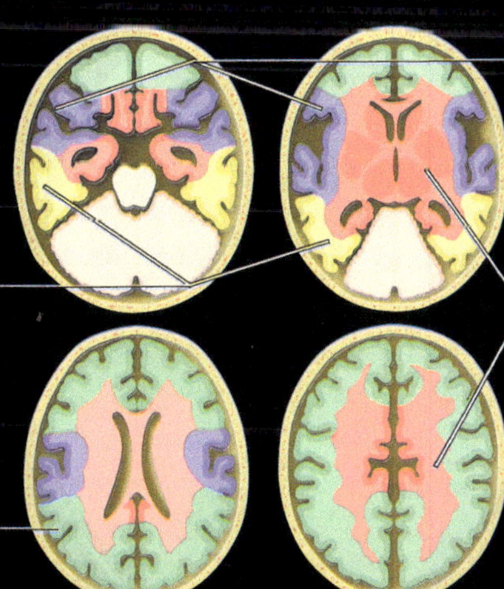

(Top) *A series of 3 graphics provides an overview of the intracranial veins and their drainage territories. The first of these, a 3D rendering of falx cerebri with major dural sinuses and deep veins, shows the interconnections between these 2 venous systems.* **(Middle)** *Intracranial view depicts the major dural venous sinuses as seen from top down. The cerebral hemispheres, midbrain, and pons as well as the left half of the tentorium cerebelli have been removed. Note the numerous interconnections between both halves of the cavernous sinus, the clival venous plexus, and the petrosal sinuses.* **(Bottom)** *A series of 4 axial sections depicts typical venous drainage patterns of the cerebral hemispheres. In general, the deep white matter and basal ganglia are drained by the internal cerebral vein and its tributaries (such as medullary veins).*

AXIAL CECT

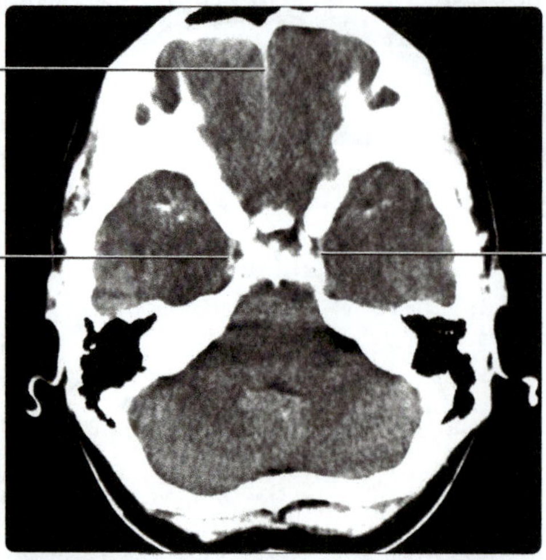

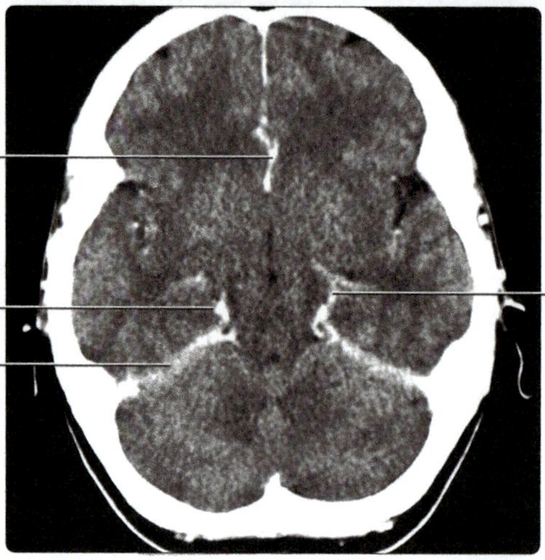

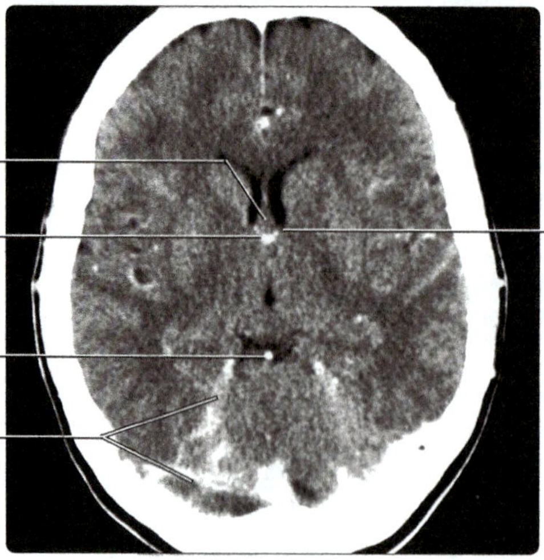

(Top) *Series of 6 selected axial CECT images through the brain from inferior to superior are shown. Contrast in the lateral dural wall of the cavernous sinus is seen on this section.* **(Middle)** *Section through the midbrain shows dura of the tentorium cerebelli with adjacent basal veins of Rosenthal and lateral mesencephalic veins.* **(Bottom)** *Section through the foramen of Monro shows septal veins as they curve around the pillars of the fornix behind the frontal horns of both lateral ventricles. The larger, midline enhancing area represents choroid plexus as it is passing inferiorly from the lateral ventricles and forming the posterior border of the foramen of Monro. The anterior border is formed by the pillars of the fornix.*

AXIAL CECT

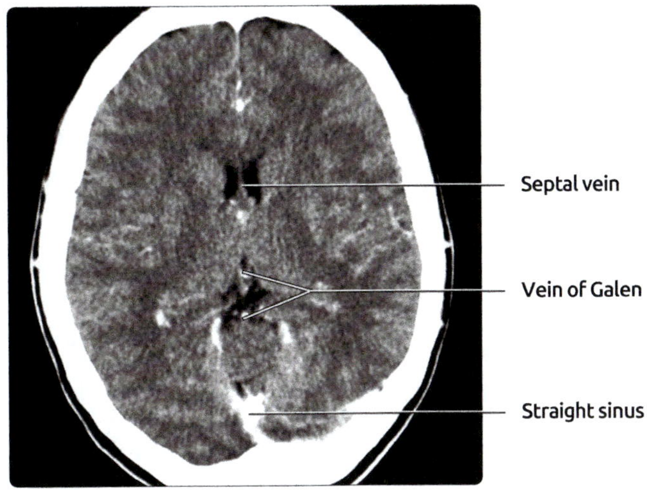

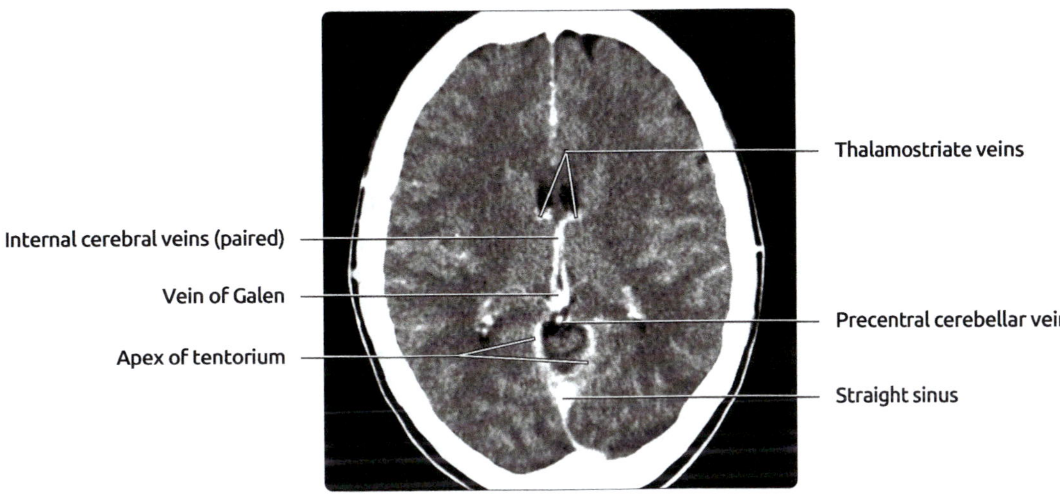

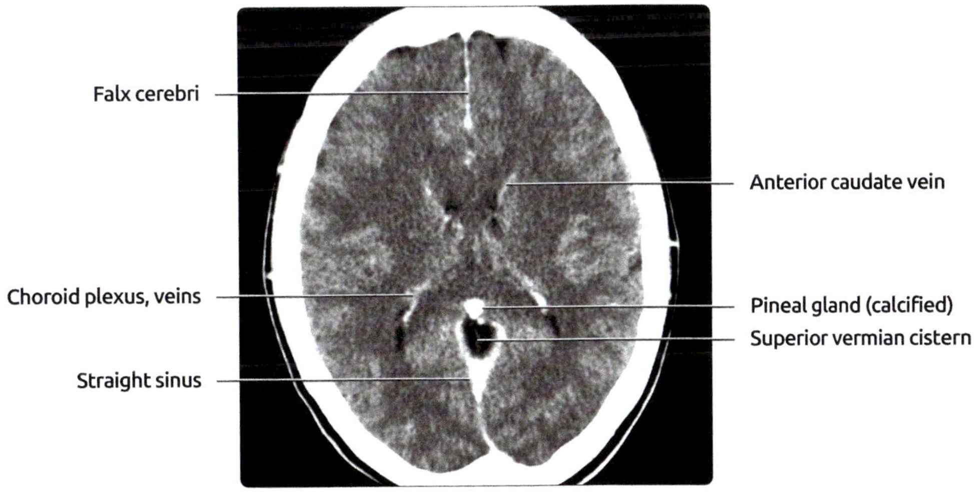

(Top) *Scan at the level of the upper foramen of Monro. The vein of Galen, a U-shaped structure, is seen here with its anterior and posterior segments seen as 2 contrast-filled "dots" that curve above the pineal gland and under the corpus callosum splenium.* **(Middle)** *Section through the internal cerebral veins, paired paramedian structures, shows their extent from the thalamostriate tributaries anteriorly to the vein of Galen posteriorly.* **(Bottom)** *Scan through the upper ventricles and tentorial apex is depicted. Anterior caudate veins are subependymal tributaries of the thalamostriate veins. The septal and thalamostriate veins join to form the internal cerebral veins.*

AXIAL T1 C+ MR

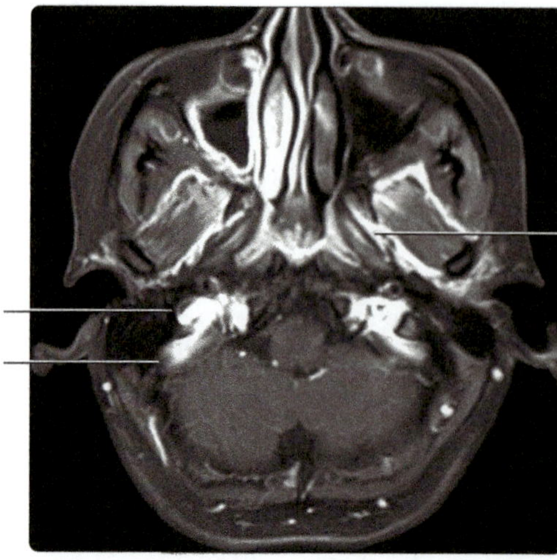

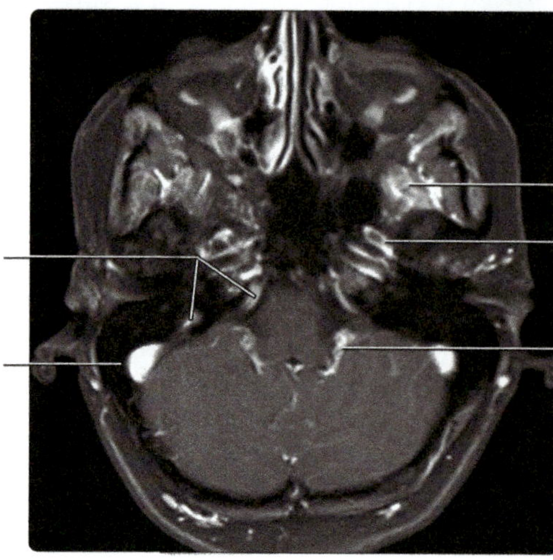

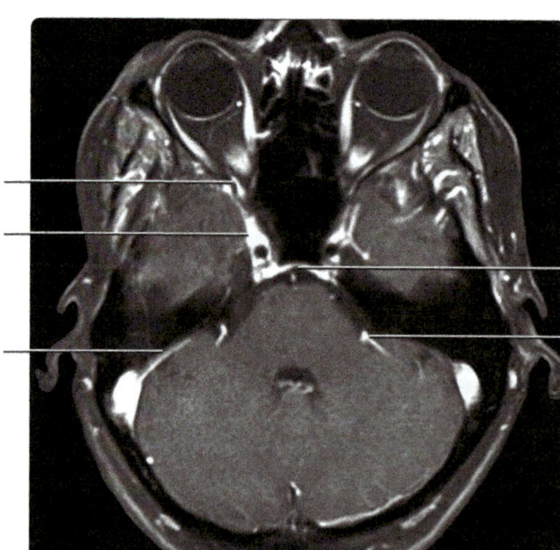

(Top) *Series of axial T1 C+ MR scans from inferior to superior are depicted. Note inhomogeneous flow in the jugular bulb. This is normal and should not be mistaken for a mass or thrombus (jugular "pseudolesion").* **(Middle)** *Section through the lateral recesses of the 4th ventricle shows the inferior petrosal sinuses, tributaries of the jugular bulb. The pterygoid venous plexus and the venous plexus in the foramen ovale are connected through the skull base to the cavernous sinus. These intra- to extracranial connections may provide an important source of collateral venous drainage if the cavernous sinus becomes occluded.* **(Bottom)** *Section through the cavernous sinus shows connections with the clival plexus and the orbit (inferior ophthalmic vein). Petrosal veins in the cerebellopontine angle cistern are prominent but normal in this case.*

AXIAL T1 C+ MR

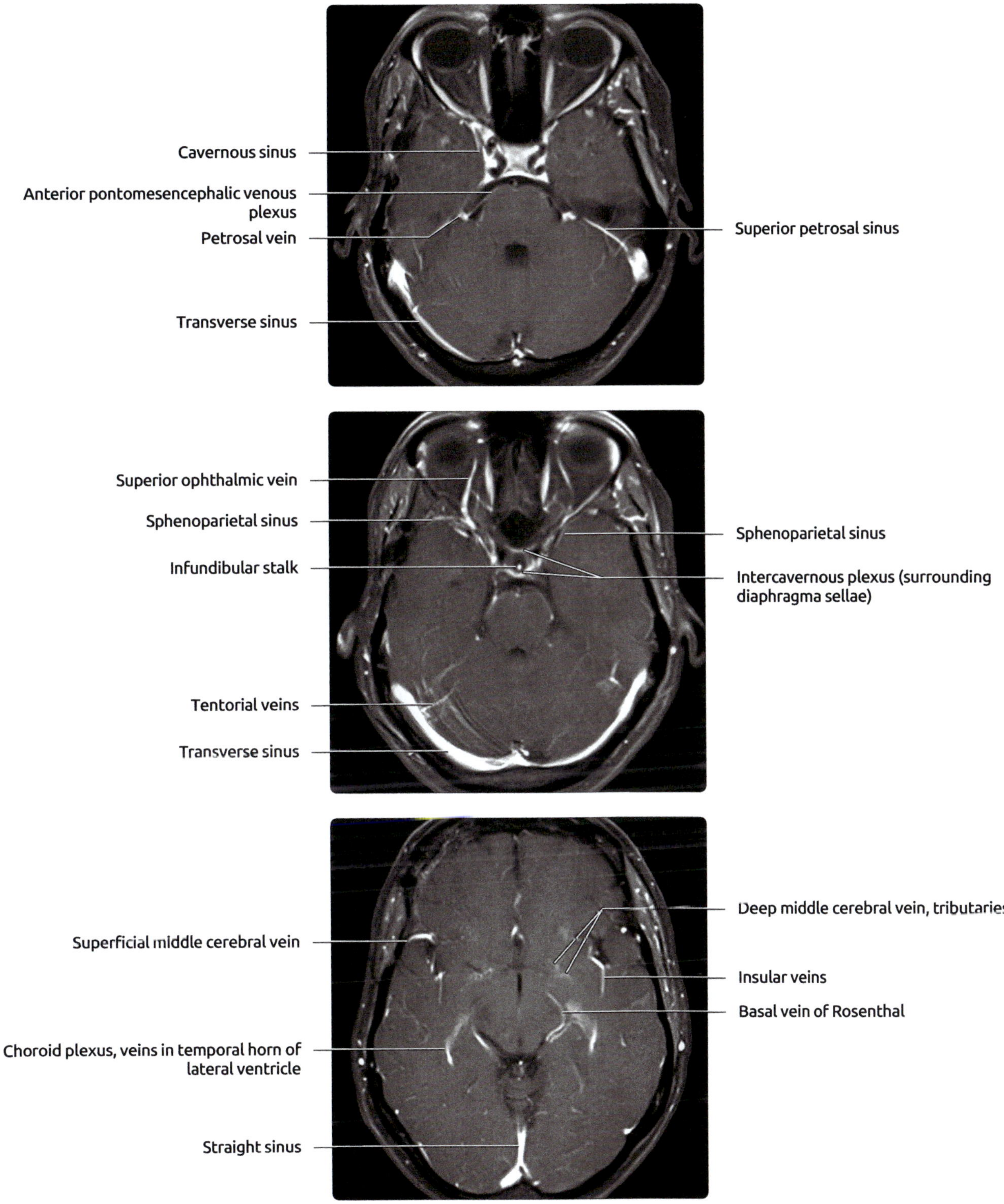

(Top) *The cavernous sinus is especially well seen on this scan. Again note prominent petrosal veins in the upper cerebellopontine angle cisterns. The faint enhancement seen along the anterior belly of the pons is the anterior pontomesencephalic venous plexus and is normal, should not be mistaken for meningitis or leptomeningeal carcinomatosis.* **(Middle)** *Section through the upper cavernous sinus shows the intercavernous plexus surrounding the opening of the diaphragma sellae, which contains the infundibular stalk. Superior ophthalmic vein drains posteriorly into the cavernous sinus.* **(Bottom)** *Section through upper vermis shows the left basal vein of Rosenthal curving around midbrain, coursing posteriorly toward its confluence with the inner cerebral veins at the vein of Galen. The superficial middle cerebral vein drains into the sphenoparietal sinus (shown on the lower section, above). Deep middle cerebral vein drains into basal vein of Rosenthal and vein of Galen.*

AXIAL T1 C+ MR

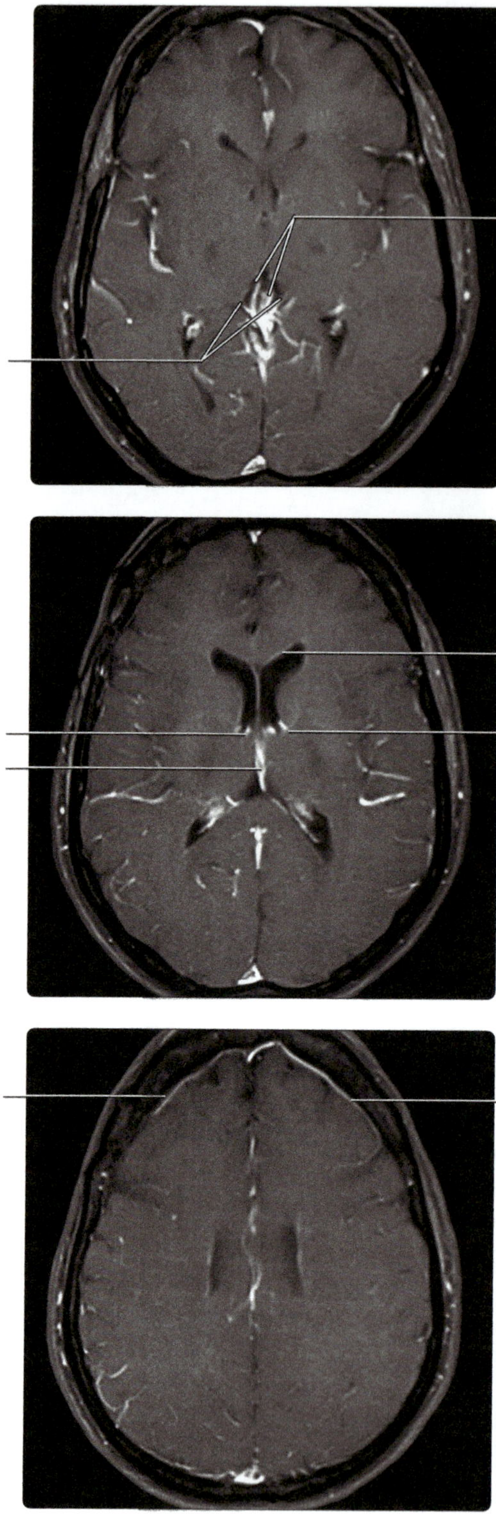

(Top) *The paired internal cerebral veins as they terminate in the vein of Galen are shown. Note the basal veins of Rosenthal terminating with the internal cerebral veins to form the great cerebral vein (of Galen).* **(Middle)** *Section through the foramen of Monro shows the septal, anterior caudate vein and thalamostriate tributaries of the internal cerebral veins.* **(Bottom)** *Most cephalad sections show prominent frontal superficial cortical veins, tributaries of the superior sagittal sinus.*

LAT, OBL, & AP MRV

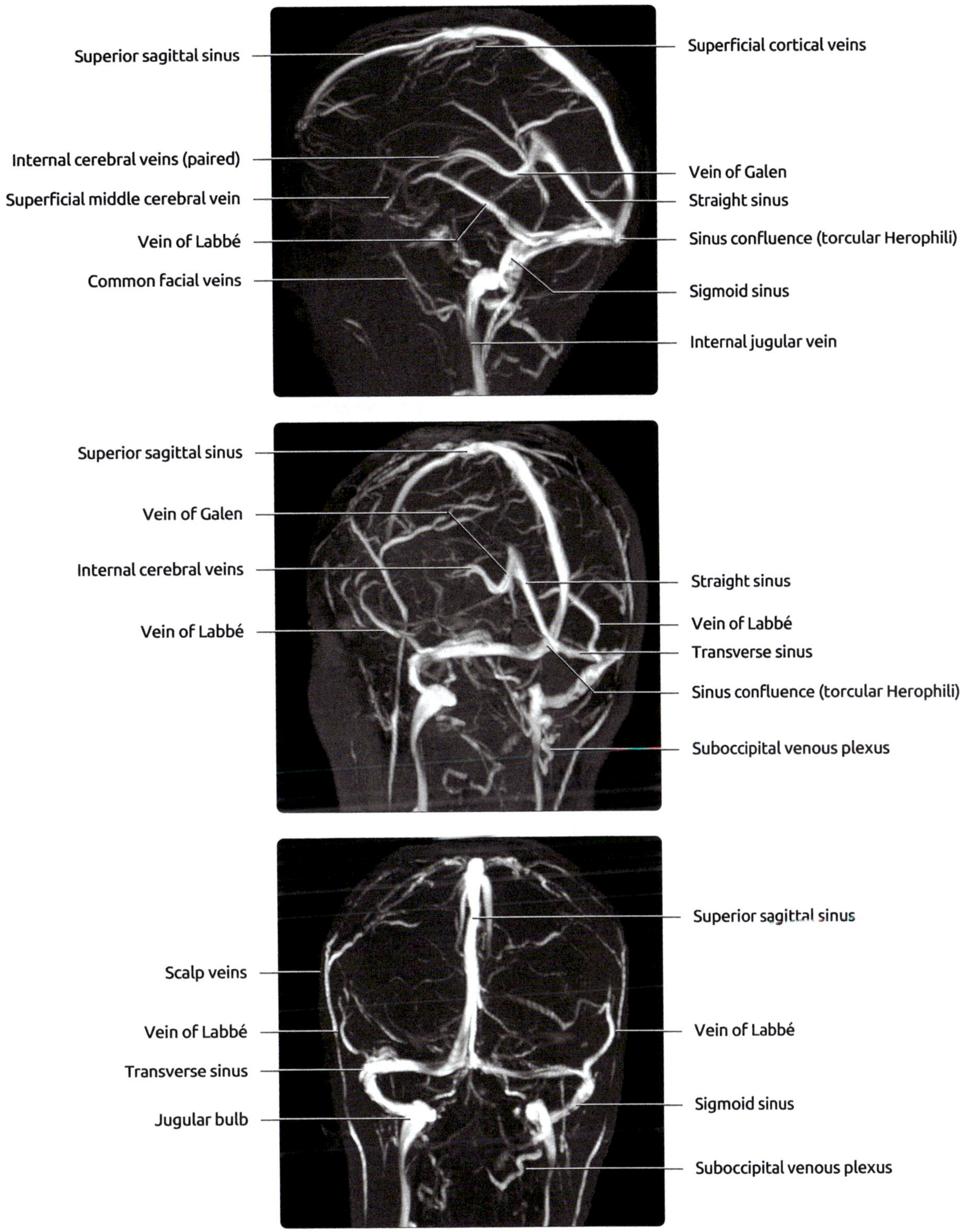

(Top) *Lateral view from an MRV demonstrates cerebral venous drainage. Dural venous sinuses and superficial cortical veins are well depicted on this lateral view.* **(Middle)** *Oblique view of the MRV shows dural sinuses draining posteroinferiorly to torcular Herophili, which splits into 2 nearly symmetric transverse sinuses.* **(Bottom)** *AP view shows superimposed superior sagittal and straight sinuses, which demonstrates slight but normal asymmetry of transverse sinuses. Larger (left) and smaller (right) veins of Labbé are seen here as they drain into the transverse sinus. The vein of Labbé can be quite large and drain a significant territory over the inferolateral cerebral hemisphere. If the transverse sinus becomes occluded, the vein of Labbé may also thrombose and cause a large venous infarct.*

Introduction

Stroke is a generic term that describes the clinical event of a sudden onset of neurologic deficit secondary to cerebrovascular disease. Stroke has 4 main etiologies, including cerebral infarction (80%), intraparenchymal hemorrhage (15%), nontraumatic subarachnoid hemorrhage (5%), and venous infarction (~ 1%). Clinically, ischemic infarction is the most common etiology and will be the main topic of this introduction. The principal cause of cerebral infarction is atherosclerosis and its sequelae.

Ischemic Infarction

There are 3 major clinical ischemic stroke subtypes based on the classification from a multicenter clinical trial [trial of drug ORG 10172 in acute stoke treatment (TOAST)]. These 3 subtypes include large artery/atherosclerotic infarctions, cardioembolic infarctions, and small vessel occlusion (lacunar) infarctions.

Large artery/atherosclerotic strokes represent ~ 40% of strokes and can arise from thrombosis at the site of a plaque or from emboli produced at the plaque that lodge downstream. The most common site of atherosclerotic plaque is at the carotid bifurcation with involvement of the distal common carotid artery and the 1st 2 cm of the internal carotid artery. The most frequently occluded intracranial vessel is the middle cerebral artery (MCA). Other common locations for atherosclerotic plaque include the carotid siphon and proximal anterior artery and MCA. The vertebral and basilar arteries are also commonly involved by atherosclerosis.

Cardioembolic disease accounts for 15-25% of ischemic strokes. Risk factors include myocardial infarction, ventricular aneurysm, atrial fibrillation or flutter, cardiomyopathy, and valvular heart disease.

Lacunar infarcts are small in size (< 15 mm), typically in the basal ganglia and thalamus, and account for 15-30% of all strokes. They are often multiple and are due to embolic, atheromatous, or thrombotic lesions in the single penetrating end arterioles that supply the deep gray nuclei, including the lenticulostriate and thalamoperforating arteries. Other common locations for lacunar infarcts include the internal capsule, pons, and corona radiata.

Intraparenchymal Hemorrhage

Intraparenchymal hemorrhage represents ~ 15% of all strokes and includes multiple etiologies. Hypertensive hemorrhage is the most common etiology, representing ~ 40-60% of all primarily intracranial hemorrhages. Other etiologies include amyloid angiopathy in elderly patients, as well as vascular malformations, vasculitis, drugs, and bleeding diathesis.

Risk factors for hemorrhagic stroke include increasing age, hypertension, smoking, excessive alcohol consumption, prior ischemic stroke, abnormal cholesterol, and anticoagulant medications.

Although the MR physics related to hemorrhage are complex, the stages are generally accepted as hyperacute, acute, early subacute, late subacute, and chronic.

Nontraumatic Subarachnoid Hemorrhage

Nontraumatic subarachnoid hemorrhage is typically related to an aneurysm (75%) or a vascular malformation, such as an arteriovenous malformation or cavernous angioma. Nonaneurysmal "perimesencephalic" subarachnoid hemorrhage is uncommon.

Venous Infarction

Dural sinus or cerebral vein occlusion is rare, representing < 1% of strokes. Venous thrombosis risk factors include pregnancy, trauma, dehydration, infection, oral contraceptives, coagulopathies, malignancies, collagen vascular diseases, and protein C and S deficiencies. Venous infarcts occur in only ~ 50% of venous thrombosis cases and can be differentiated from arterial infarcts by the location of the ischemia. Superior sagittal sinus thrombosis typically results in T2/FLAIR hyperintense parasagittal lesions, whereas thrombosis of the transverse sinus often results in T2/FLAIR hyperintensities in the posterior temporal lobe. Additionally, venous infarcts more commonly present with associated hemorrhage. CECT is useful to identify the "empty delta" sign representing nonenhancing thrombus within a major dural sinus, typically the superior sagittal or transverse sinus.

Approach to Stroke Imaging

Cerebral ischemia results from significantly decreased blood flow to selected areas or the entire brain. Stroke progresses in stages from ischemia to actual infarction. In the most common situation, MCA occlusion, there is a densely ischemic central core and a less densely ischemic "penumbra." The central core is usually irreversibly damaged unless reperfusion is quickly established, whereas the cells within the penumbra may remain viable but at risk for several hours. Current stroke therapies attempt to rescue the "at-risk" cells.

Currently, acute stroke protocols vary among different institutions. The exact protocol is often based on the availability of CT vs. MR, technology/software, time of stroke, physician expertise, and the possibility of neurointervention. Typically, stroke neurologists work with neuroradiologists to devise a plan that best serves the patient's needs.

Most stroke protocols begin with a noncontrast head CT to evaluate for hemorrhage or mass, which directly affects treatment decisions. Additionally, > 1/3 of MCA territory hypodensity at presentation is considered by most to be a contraindication to thrombolysis, as it is associated with a greater risk of fatal hemorrhage. CTA is useful to evaluate for large-vessel occlusion. When available, CT perfusion is an excellent way to evaluate for large=vessel ischemia.

MR with DWI is particularly useful for acute ischemia when CT perfusion is negative and the clinical suspicion for stroke remains. MR is also the primary imaging tool when the clinical question includes a posterior fossa or brainstem lesion. MR with PWI has been found extremely helpful in guiding therapy when available.

Most stroke protocols use 3-hour and 6-hour windows for treatment of nonhemorrhagic ischemic stroke. If the patient presents within 6 hours after the initial onset of symptoms, an unenhanced CT is typically the initial study of choice to exclude a mass or hemorrhage. If there is a hemorrhage or mass, no thrombolytic therapy is initiated. If there is no hemorrhage or mass and the patient is within 3 hours after onset of symptoms, the patient is eligible for intravenous (IV) thrombolysis. If the patient is between 3 and 6 hours of onset, either a CTA with CT perfusion or an MR with DWI and PWI is performed to determine whether they are eligible for treatment. If the patient has an intracranial thrombus with a penumbra, intraarterial (IA) thrombolysis or IA thrombectomy is recommended. If there is no penumbra, IA therapy may not benefit the patient, so each case is evaluated individually.

5 Stages of Intraparenchymal Hemorrhage

Stage	Time (Range)	Blood Products	T1	T2
Hyperacute	< 24 hours	Oxyhemoglobin	Isointense	Bright
Acute	1-3 days (hours to days)	Deoxyhemoglobin	Isointense	Dark
Early subacute	> 3 days (days to 1 week)	Intracellular methemoglobin	Bright	Dark
Late subacute	> 7 days (1 week to months)	Extracellular methemoglobin	Bright	Bright
Chronic	> 14 days (≥ months)	Hemosiderin	Dark	Dark

The effective therapeutic window for the posterior circulation is thought to be longer than the 3-6-hour window, but the exact time is variable and depends on collateral circulation. Therefore, patients with vertebrobasilar thrombosis are evaluated individually for risk vs. benefit of IA thrombolysis or thrombectomy.

Ischemic Penumbra

Ischemic stroke results in a core of tissue that has undergone irreversible injury. The ischemic penumbra is the area of brain that may be salvageable with appropriate therapy. The penumbra typically surrounds the ischemic core and is supported by collateral circulation.

The ischemic penumbra can be identified by a combination of MR diffusion (DWI) and perfusion (PWI). DWI is the most reliable estimate of the ischemic core and generally correlates with irreversible injury. However, with early reperfusion following thrombolysis, some reversal of DWI can be observed. PWI evaluates the presence of a penumbra. With MR, the mismatch between the DWI and PWI defines the penumbra. This model provides a practical means to estimate the ischemic penumbra. In general, if there is no diffusion/perfusion mismatch, therapy may be ineffective.

With the newer CT perfusion techniques, an ischemic penumbra may also be measured with CT.

With the urgency of acute stroke, MR may be impractical. However, with new faster MR protocols and the superiority of MR to CT in detecting small vessel ischemia and brainstem ischemia, MR may be a preferred technique.

CT Perfusion

Cerebral perfusion refers to the tissue-level blood flow in the brain. This flow is evaluated by 3 main parameters at CT perfusion (pCT): Cerebral blood flow (CBF), cerebral blood volume (CBV), and mean transit time (MTT).

CBF is defined as the volume of blood moving through a given unit of volume of brain per unit time. CBF uses units of milliliters of blood per 100 g of brain tissue per minute. Studies suggest that CBF is a reasonable marker for the ischemic penumbra.

CBV is defined as the total volume of blood in a given unit of volume of brain. This includes blood in the tissues as well as blood in the large-capacitance vessels, such as arteries, arterioles, capillaries, venules, and veins. CBV uses units of milliliters of blood per 100 g of brain tissue. Some studies suggest that pCT-acquired CBV is a reasonably reliable marker of the ischemic core.

MTT is defined as the average of the transit time of blood through a given brain region. The transit time of blood through the brain parenchyma varies depending on the distance traveled between arterial inflow and venous outflow. MTT equals CBV/CBF.

CBF/CBV mismatch correlates with stroke enlargement in untreated or unsuccessfully treated patients. Those patients with a CBF/CBV match or those with early complete recanalization do not exhibit progression of the ischemic stroke.

The general treatment guidelines for pCT are as follows. If there is a CBF/CBV mismatch, with a larger CBF suggesting an ischemic penumbra, the patient is likely a good candidate for therapy. Many treatment guidelines suggest that a ≥ 20% CBF/CBV mismatch should be present to consider thrombolysis. Some authors propose that, if there is no mismatch between CBV and CBF, treatment is unlikely to benefit the patient.

CT Perfusion Interpretation Pearls

The MTT is the most sensitive parameter for perfusion deficits. Although it is generally elevated due to a thromboembolic process, it may be elevated in a patient with significant arterial atherosclerotic narrowing. In early ischemia, MTT is elevated, and CBF is decreased. However, the CBV can be preserved or even elevated due to capillary bed dilatation in very early ischemia. Once a CBF threshold is reached, CBV starts to decline. This results in the ischemic core, which has a matched decrease in CBF and CBV, whereas a mismatch between CBF and CBV suggests a penumbra.

Differential Diagnosis

When considering **stroke** in a **child** or **young adult**, several possible etiologies should be addressed, including arterial dissection, vascular malformation with hemorrhage, drug abuse, or clotting disorder. In **young children**, other possibilities include congenital heart disease with emboli and idiopathic progressive arteriopathy of childhood (moyamoya disease).

In a middle-aged or older **adult**, the typical stroke etiologies include arterial thromboembolism, hypertensive hemorrhage, and cerebral amyloid angiopathy.

When evaluating a **hemorrhagic stroke**, etiologies in **children** include vascular lesions, hematologic disorder, vasculopathy, and venous infarct. In a **young adult**, considerations include vascular malformations, drug abuse, and less commonly venous occlusions or vasculitis. In **older adults**, common considerations for intracranial hemorrhage include hypertensive hemorrhage, neoplasm, cerebral amyloid angiopathy, and, less commonly, dural sinus/cerebral venous occlusion and coagulopathy.

(Left) *Axial NECT scan shows a hyperattenuating left middle cerebral artery (MCA) (hyperdense MCA sign) in this patient with acute onset of right hemiparesis. Compare to the normal right MCA.* **(Right)** *More cephalad NECT in the same case shows the disappearing basal ganglia sign caused by the occluded MCA. The basal ganglia should normally be hyperdense compared with white matter. In this case, they are hypodense and thus "disappear" (compare to the normal right side).*

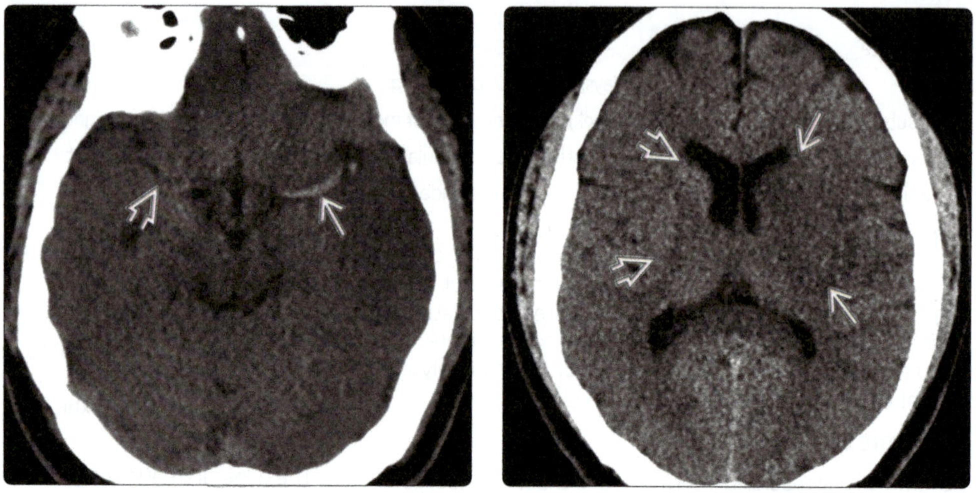

(Left) *Axial DWI MR shows diffusion restriction in the left anterior cerebral artery (ACA) distribution within the medial parafalcine frontal lobe.* **(Right)** *Axial ADC map in the same case shows hypointensity in the distribution of the left ACA, confirming the presence of an acute infarct in this territorial distribution.*

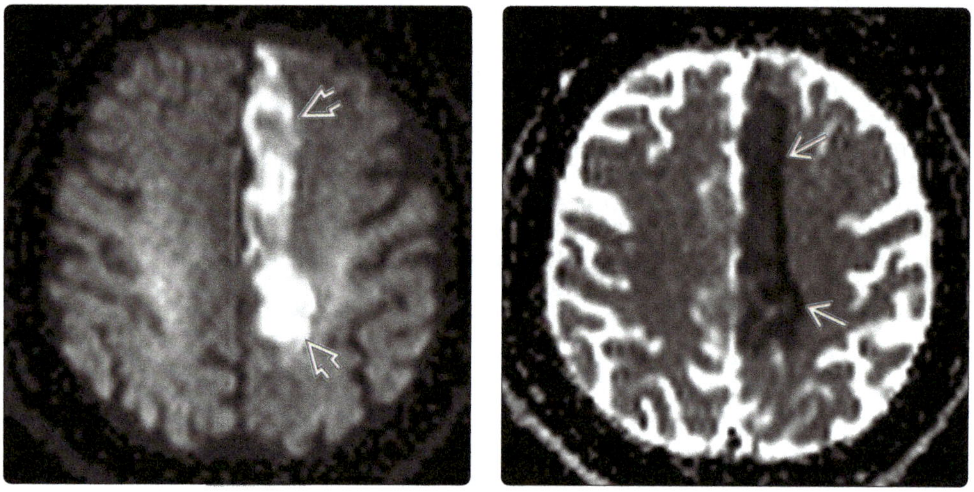

(Left) *Axial DWI MR shows diffusion restriction in the occipital lobe related to posterior cerebral artery (PCA) ischemia. DWI is the most sensitive MR sequence for acute ischemia.* **(Right)** *Axial NECT scan shows a hyperattenuating basilar artery in this patient with acute onset of ataxia and multiple cranial nerve palsies. Note bilateral cerebellar infarcts.*

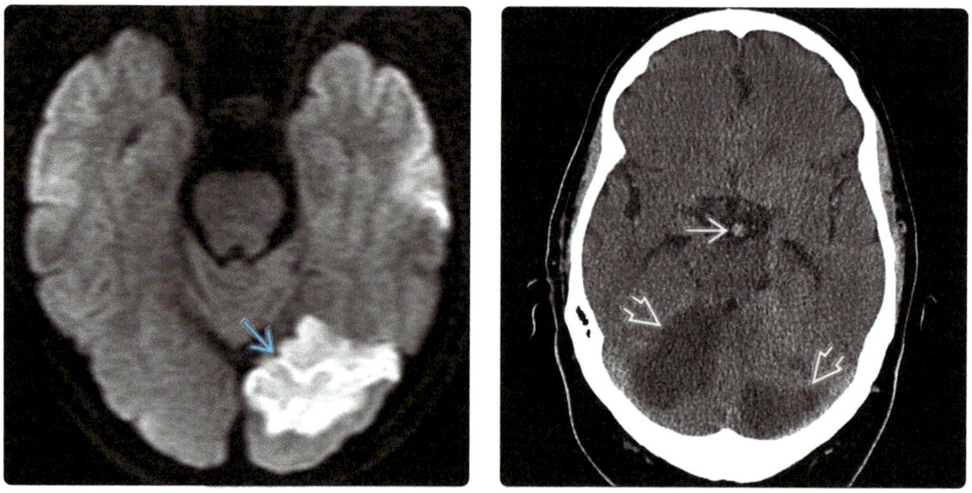

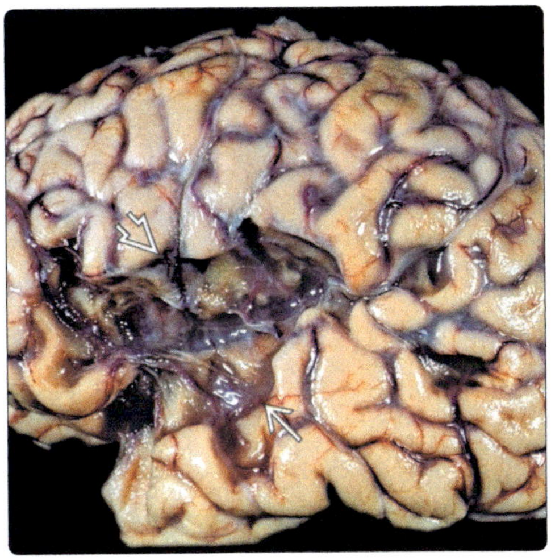

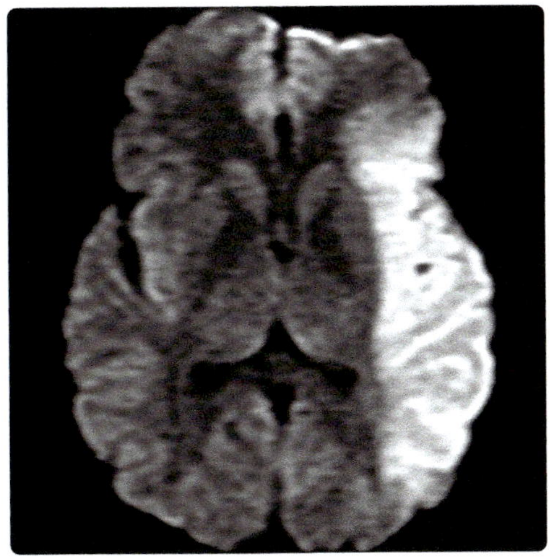

(Left) *Lateral gross pathology shows a chronic MCA infarct with hemorrhage and encephalomalacia in the frontal operculum* ➡ *and temporal lobe* ➡. **(Right)** *Axial DWI MR shows restriction in left MCA territory with preservation of the basal ganglia. The MCA territory is the most common location for ischemic stroke.*

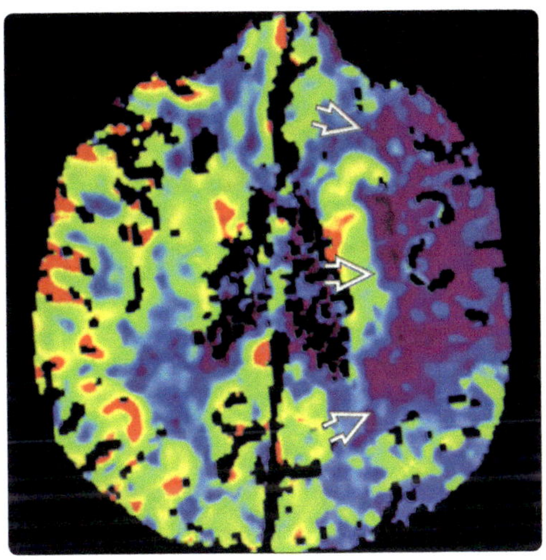

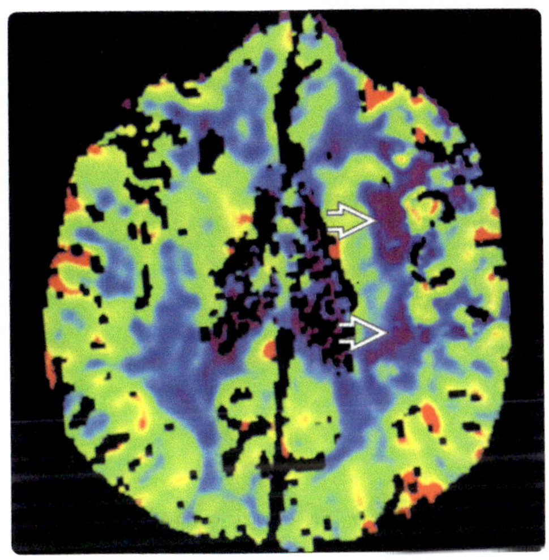

(Left) *Axial CT perfusion cerebral blood flow (CBF) color map shows a large area of decreased blood flow* ➡ *in the left hemisphere related to hyperacute MCA ischemia.* **(Right)** *Axial CT perfusion cerebral blood volume (CBV) color map in the same patient shows a much smaller area of decreased blood volume* ➡. *The CBV is a marker for the ischemic core. This CBF/CBV mismatch correlates with the presence of a large ischemic penumbra, which suggests the patient would benefit from intraarterial thrombolytic therapy or clot retrieval.*

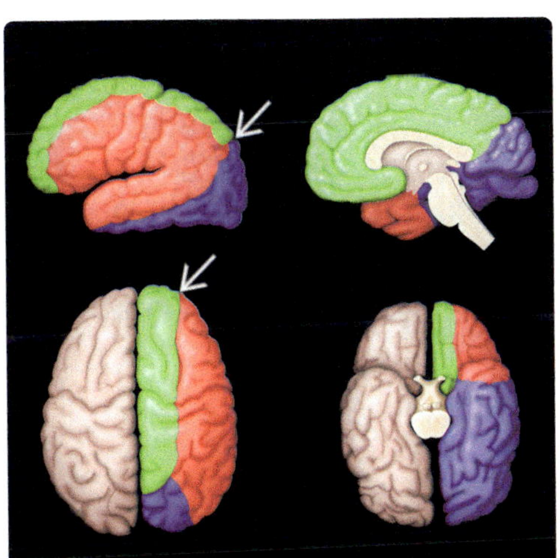

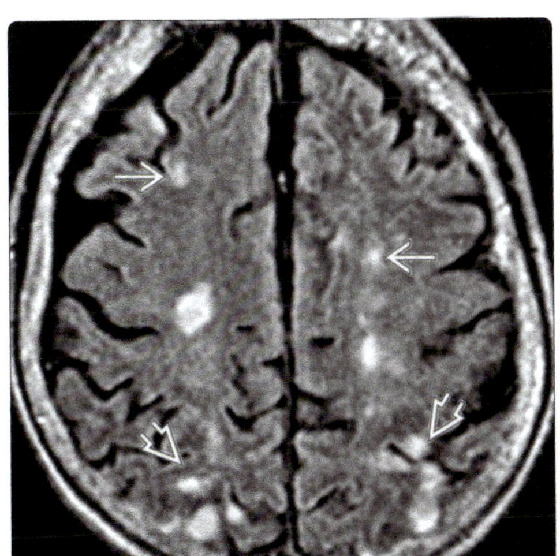

(Left) *The MCA (red) supplies the lateral aspects of the frontal/temporal lobes; ACA (green), the medial hemispheres; PCA (purple) the occipital & inferior temporal lobes. Watershed zone* ➡ *is the border between the major vascular territories.* **(Right)** *Axial FLAIR MR shows multiple hyperintense foci* ➡ *in the watershed zones between the major areas (MCA, PCA, ACA) related to acute ischemia from hypoperfusion; posterior confluence where all 3 vascular distributions meet at the vertex* ➡ *is vulnerable to cerebral hypoperfusion.*

(Left) *Axial DWI MR shows hyperintensity related to acute ischemia in the lateral midbrain, posterior hippocampus. This represents penetrating artery infarction (thalamoperforating, thalamogeniculate arteries).* **(Right)** *Axial DWI MR shows diffusion restriction related to acute ischemia in a pontine-perforating artery distribution.*

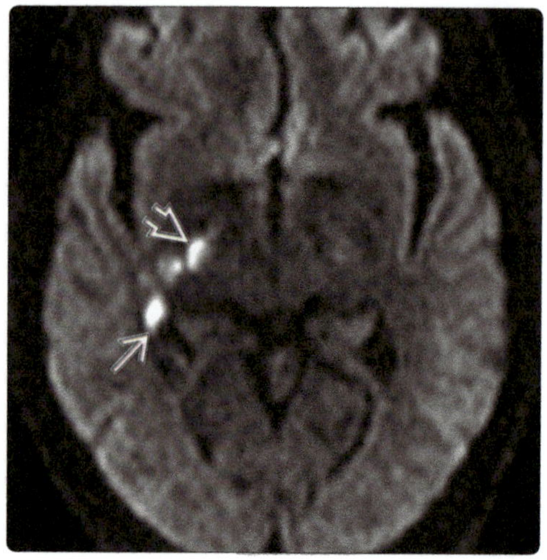

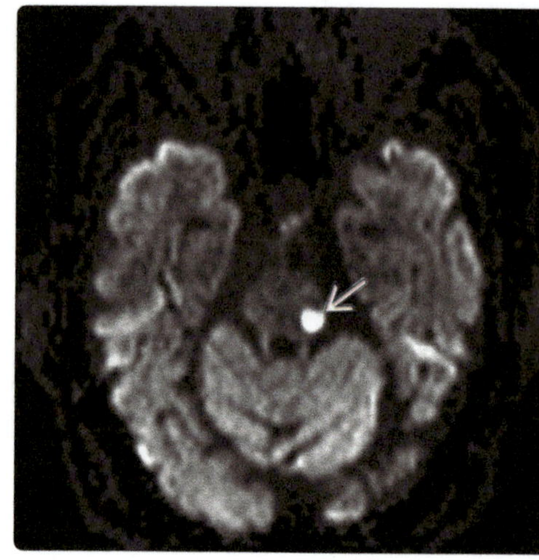

(Left) *Axial graphic shows the cerebellar artery distributions. The superior cerebellar artery (SCA) (green) supplies the superior cerebellum. The posterior inferior cerebellar artery (PICA) (peach) supplies the majority of the inferior cerebellum and lateral medulla. The anterior inferior cerebellar artery (AICA) (yellow) supplies the petrosal surface of the cerebellum.* **(Right)** *Axial T2WI MR shows hyperintensity in the right inferior cerebellum and lateral medulla related to a PICA infarct from a vertebral artery embolus.*

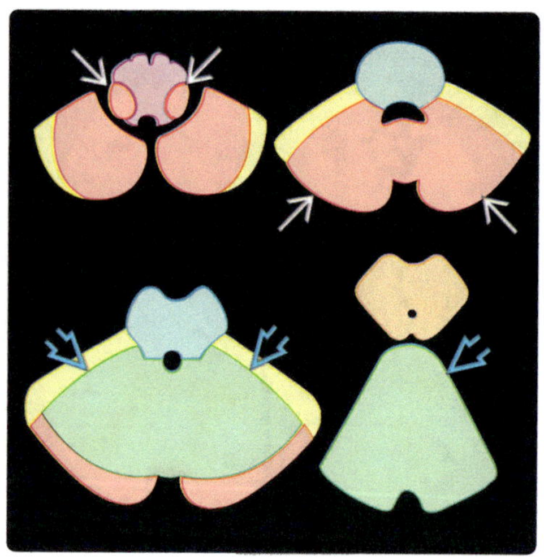

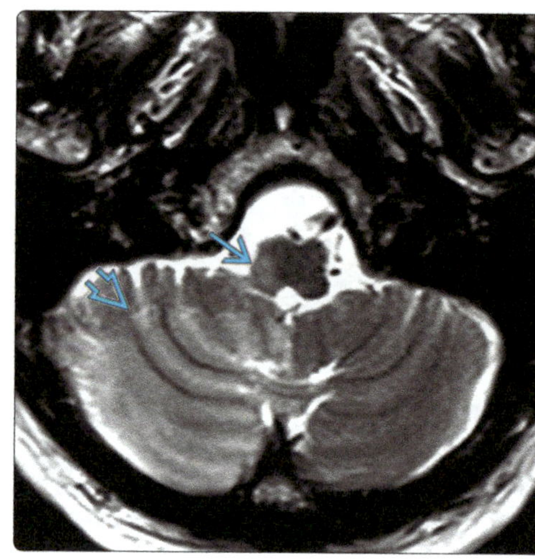

(Left) *Axial T2WI MR shows hyperintensity and local mass effect in the right superior cerebellum related to an acute SCA infarct. SCA infarcts may involve the superior cerebellum and the upper lateral pons.* **(Right)** *Axial DWI MR shows acute diffusion restriction in the anterior, inferior cerebellum laterally in an AICA distribution. AICA primarily supplies the ventral pons and petrosal surface of the cerebellar hemispheres, the brachium pontis, flocculus, and inner ear as well as CN7 and CN8.*

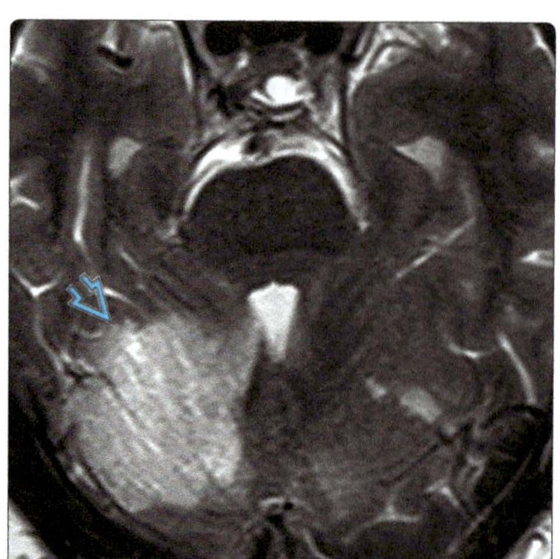

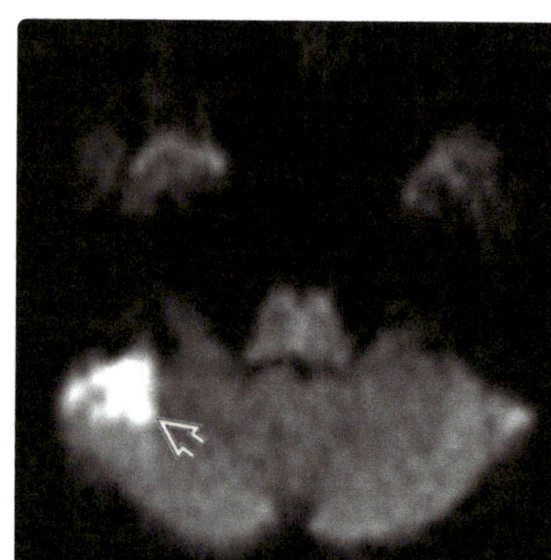

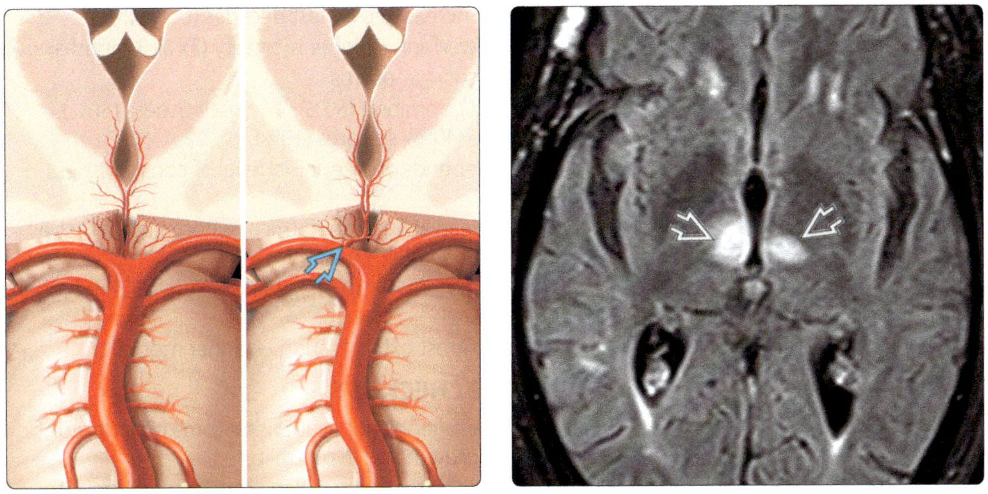

(Left) *Coronal oblique graphic of the rostral basilar artery shows (L) the typical arterial supply to the medial thalami by multiple PCA and basilar tip perforators. The anatomic variant, artery of Percheron* ➩*, is shown (R), in which a single large perforating artery from P1 supplies bilateral thalami and the medial midbrain.* **(Right)** *Axial FLAIR MR shows hyperintensity in the bilateral medial thalami* ➩ *related to an acute artery of Percheron infarct. Extension to the medial midbrain is often present.*

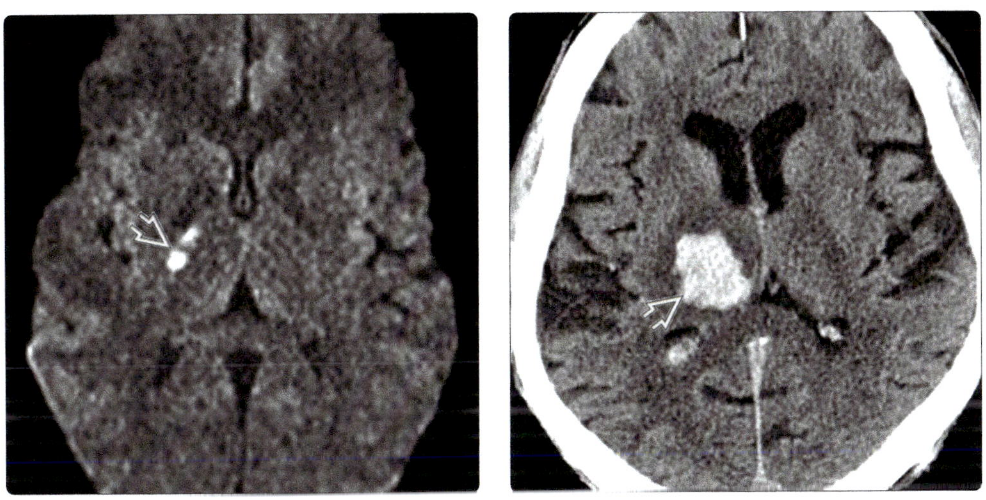

(Left) *Axial DWI MR shows hyperintensity related to acute ischemia in the posterior limb of the internal capsule* ➩ *in an anterior choroidal artery distribution. The anterior choroidal artery typically supplies the lateral midbrain, uncus, thalamus, posterior limb of internal capsule, and the optic tract. The posterior choroidal artery typically supplies the pulvinar, thalamus, medial temporal lobe, splenium, and choroid plexus.* **(Right)** *Axial CT shows a classic thalamic hypertensive hemorrhage* ➩*, the 2nd most common cause of stroke.*

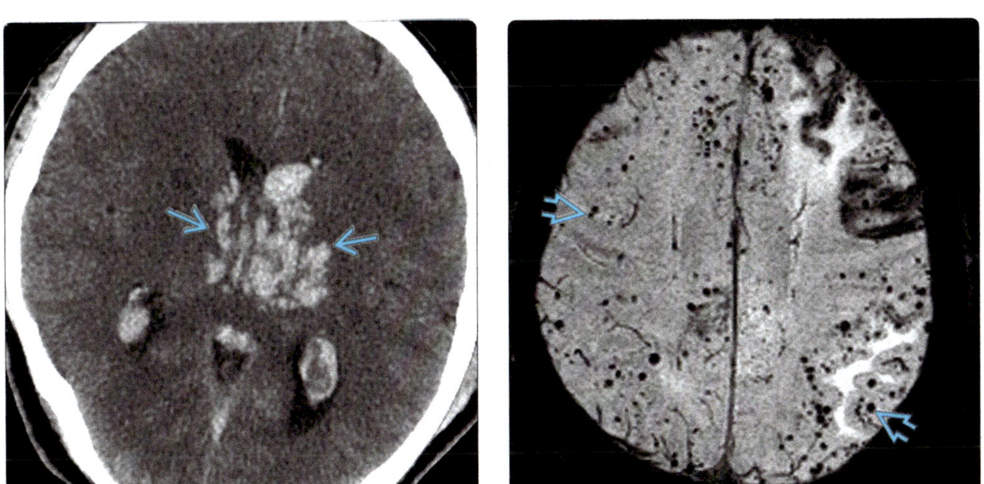

(Left) *Axial CT shows bilateral thalamic hemorrhage* → *related to deep venous thrombosis. Venous thrombosis risk factors include pregnancy, trauma, dehydration, infection, oral contraceptives, coagulopathies, malignancies, collagen vascular diseases, and protein C and S deficiencies.* **(Right)** *Axial SWI MR in an elderly patient shows extensive susceptibility artifact-related microhemorrhages* ➩ *in the bilateral hemispheres. Pattern is typical of cerebral amyloid angiopathy.*

KEY FACTS

IMAGING

- CT: Hemorrhage appearance based on density
  - Hyperdense mass (50-70 Hounsfield units) on NECT
  - Peripheral edema develops over 1st few days
- MR: Intracranial hemorrhage staging based on T1 and T2 signal characteristics
  - Hematoma matures more slowly in center (core) than in periphery
    - Therefore MR signal change proceeds peripherally to centrally

PATHOLOGY

- Very common: Hypertension (HTN), cerebral amyloid angiopathy, trauma, hemorrhagic vascular malformations
- Common: Infarct with reperfusion, coagulopathy, blood dyscrasia, drug abuse, tumor (glioma, metastases)

CLINICAL ISSUES

- HTN, ↑ age most important risk factor
  - Rate of anticoagulant-related intracerebral hematoma (ICH) has increased over last decades (up to 20%)
  - ICH with warfarin = higher mortality (2x at 3 months)
- Common signs, symptoms
  - HTN (90%), vomiting (50%), ↓ consciousness (50%), headache (40%), seizures (10%)
- Prognosis depends on size, initial level of consciousness, location
  - 35-52% dead at 1 month (50% of whom died in first 2 days); 59% dead at 1 year
  - Large hematoma (> 30 mL), swirl sign on NECT → higher mortality
  - Active contrast extravasation → higher mortality

DIAGNOSTIC CHECKLIST

- Marked heterogeneity of acute hematoma on CT predicts hematoma growth and ↑ mortality
- Swirl sign, contrast extravasation enhancement indicate hematoma growth and ↑ mortality

(Left) *Axial graphic shows the evolution of parenchymal hemorrhage from hyperacute → (intracellular oxy-Hgb) to acute → (intracellular deoxy-Hgb with surrounding edema). Early → and late subacute (intra- and extracellular met-Hgb, respectively) are followed by a chronic cystic cavity → with a hemosiderin stain.* **(Right)** *Axial NECT shows a hyperdense mass related to an acute left cerebellar hemorrhage → with minimal surrounding edema in a patient with hypertension.*

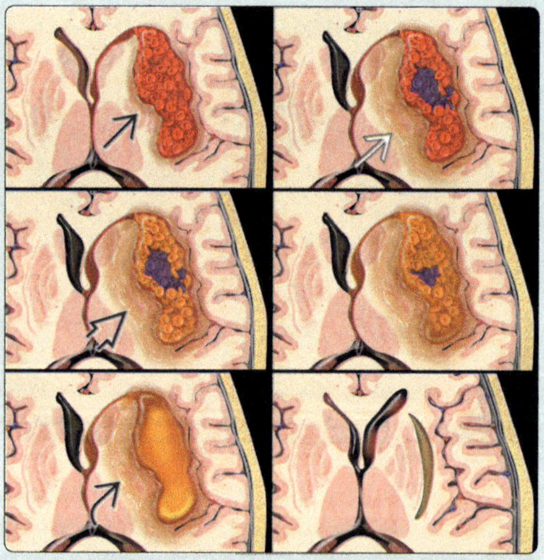

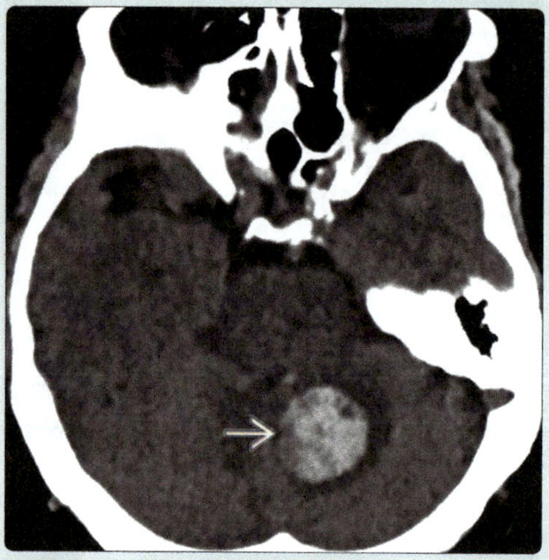

(Left) *Axial T1WI MR in the same patient shows that the cerebellar hemorrhage → is predominantly isointense and mildly hypointense to the surrounding brain parenchyma, indicating hyperacute blood products.* **(Right)** *Axial T2WI MR in the same patient shows the hyperacute hemorrhage to be hyperintense to the surrounding brain parenchyma with a peripheral hypointense rim →. Intraparenchymal hemorrhage evolves from peripheral to central with the central core maturing more slowly.*

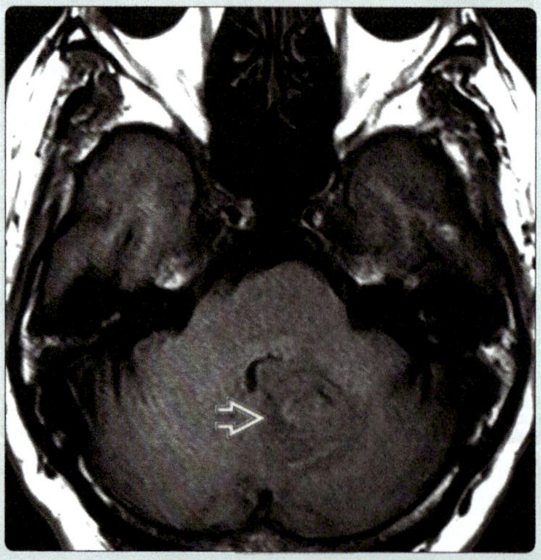

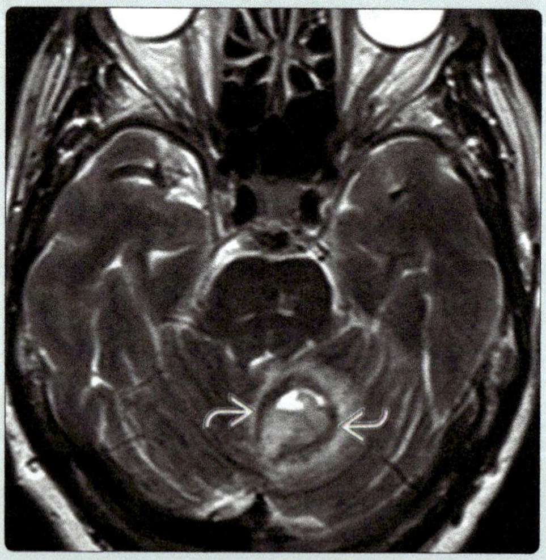

KEY FACTS

TERMINOLOGY

- Primary intraparenchymal hemorrhage (pICH)
- Acute nontraumatic intracranial hemorrhage (ICH)

IMAGING

- Acute round or oval intracerebral hematoma
- Subcentimeter "microbleeds" to massive ICH
- Hematoma location for common causes of pICH
  - HTN: Basal ganglia > thalamus > pons > cerebellum
  - Amyloid angiopathy: Lobar
  - Arteriovenous malformation: Any location
  - Cavernous malformation: Any location
  - Venous sinus thrombosis: Subcortical white matter
  - Neoplasm: Any location
- Recommended imaging: Begin with NECT
  - If HTN with striatocapsular hematoma → stop
  - If atypical hematoma → CTA or MR/MRA
  - Atypical hematoma or unclear history: MR (T2*, DWI, C+)
  - If standard study suggests vascular etiology → CTA/MRA
  - If concern for venous infarct → CTV/MRV

PATHOLOGY

- Pediatric patients, < 18 years old: Vascular malformation (~ 50%) > hematologic disorders, vasculopathy, venous infarct, neoplasm
- Young adults, < 45 years old: Vascular malformation, drug abuse, venous thrombosis, PRES, vasculitis, neoplasm
- Adults > 45 years old: HTN, amyloid > neoplasm (primary or metastatic), venous infarct, coagulopathy

CLINICAL ISSUES

- ICH causes ~ 15% of acute strokes
- Treatment: Control of intracranial pressure, hydrocephalus
- Surgical evacuation when clinically indicated
- If positive spot sign indicates active bleeding, predicts hematoma expansion and poor outcome
- 1-year mortality approaches 60%

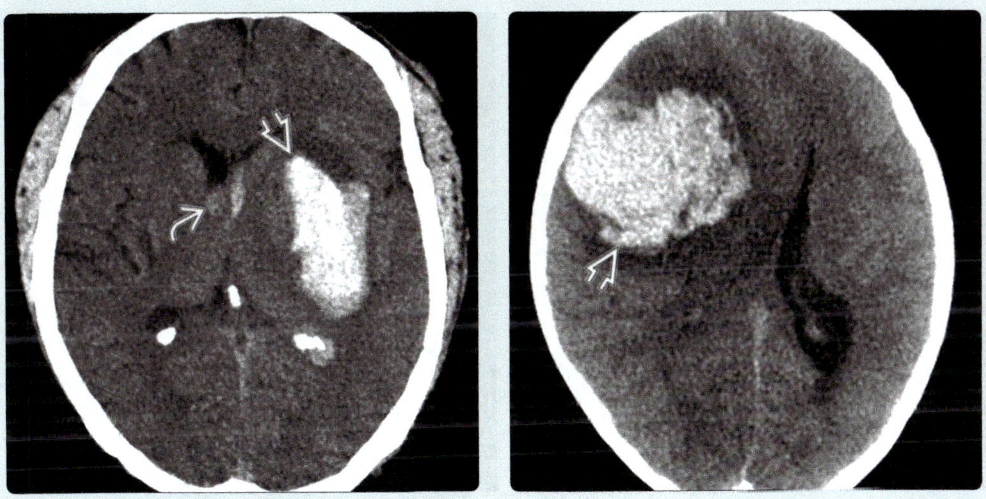

(Left) *Axial NECT in an elderly hypertensive patient shows a hyperdense hematoma centered in the left external capsule and putamen ➡ with intraventricular extension of hemorrhage ➡. This is the most common location for a hypertensive hemorrhage.* **(Right)** *Axial CT in this 5 year old shows a large frontal lobe hemorrhage ➡ with surrounding edema and mass effect. Additional imaging revealed an underlying cavernous malformation. In children, vascular lesions represent ~ 50% of all intracranial hemorrhages.*

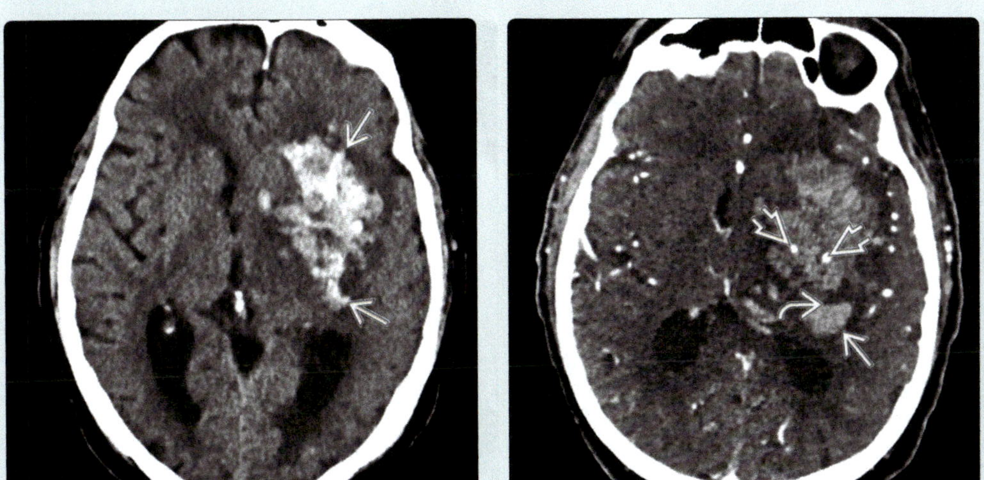

(Left) *Axial NECT in a 73-year-old hypertensive anticoagulated man with sudden onset of right hemiparesis shows a mixed-density hematoma centered in the lateral putamen/external capsule ➡.* **(Right)** *CTA in the same case shows 2 enhancing foci (spot sign) ➡ within the clot, which also is expanding ➡ and demonstrates a fluid-fluid level ➡. All are dire prognostic indicators. The patient expired shortly after the scan was obtained.*

KEY FACTS

TERMINOLOGY

- Hypertensive intracranial hemorrhage (hICH)
- Acute nontraumatic intracerebral hemorrhage (ICH) secondary to systemic hypertension
- 2nd most common cause of stroke

IMAGING

- Initial screen = NECT in patients with HTN
- CT: Acute round or oval hyperdense mass
  - Striatocapsular: Putamen/external capsule (60-65%)
  - Thalamus (15-25%)
  - Pons, cerebellum (10%)
- Multifocal "microbleeds" (1-5%)
- Heterogeneous density (coagulopathy, active bleed)
- Other findings: Intraventricular extension, mass effect, hydrocephalus, herniation
- MR signal intensity (varies with age of clot)
  - Hyperacute (< 24 hours): T1WI iso-hypo/T2WI hyper
  - Acute (~ 1-3 days): T1WI iso-hypo/T2WI hypo
  - Subacute (days): T1WI hyper/T2WI hypo-hyper
  - Chronic (weeks-months): T1WI hyper/T2WI hypo

TOP DIFFERENTIAL DIAGNOSES

- Cerebral amyloid angiopathy
- Hemorrhagic neoplasm
- Coagulopathy
- Deep cerebral venous thrombosis
- Drug abuse (especially in young patient)
- Vascular malformation (rare in elderly)

CLINICAL ISSUES

- HTN single most important risk factor for **all** types of stroke
- 10-15% of stroke patients have hICH
- 40-50% of nontraumatic ICHs caused by hICH
- HTN most common cause of spontaneous ICH in patients 45-70 years old
- 10-15% of hypertensive patients with spontaneous ICH have underlying aneurysm or arteriovenous malformation

(Left) *Axial CT in a 61-year-old hypertensive woman shows the classic appearance of a left basal ganglia hemorrhage involving the putamen and external capsule (striatocapsular). Note areas of periventricular hypodensity likely related to chronic small vessel ischemia.* **(Right)** *Axial SWI shows a large hypertensive basal ganglia hemorrhage, as well as multiple foci of susceptibility artifact from hemosiderin deposition related to microhemorrhages from chronic hypertension.*

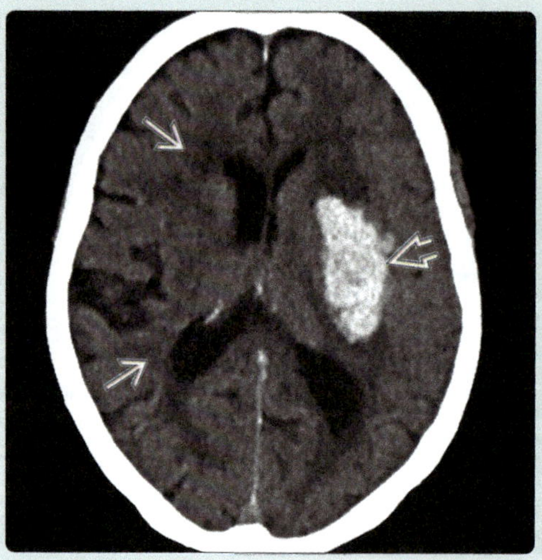

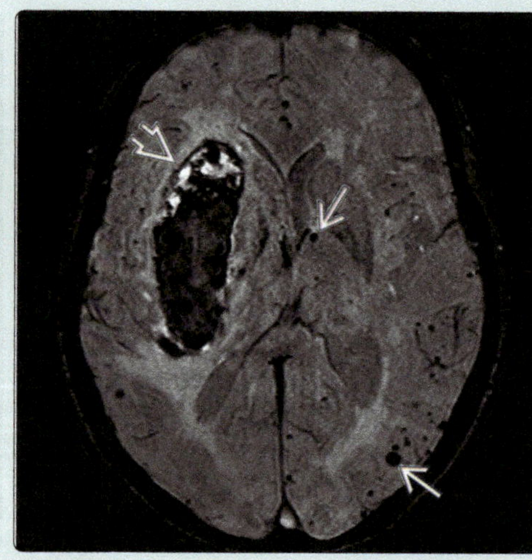

(Left) *Axial graphic shows a classic acute hypertensive basal ganglia/external capsule hemorrhage with dissection into the lateral ventricle. Hemorrhage extends through the foramen of Monro into the 3rd ventricle.* **(Right)** *A coronal CTA in a young patient with a right basal ganglia hemorrhage shows displacement of the lenticulostriate arteries medially, compared with the normal left side by the hematoma. There is no spot sign that would indicate active bleeding. No underlying vascular lesion is present.*

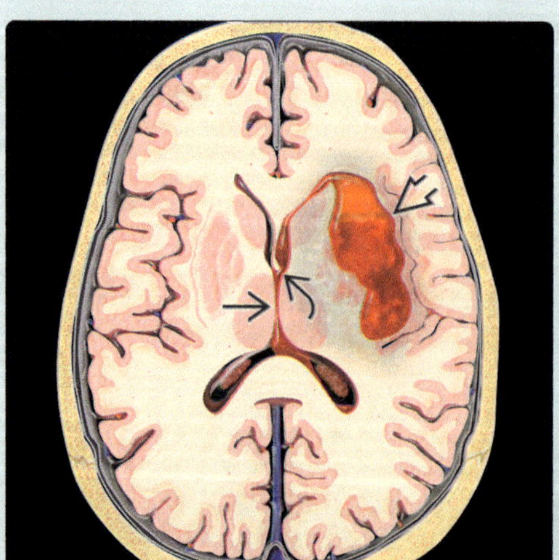

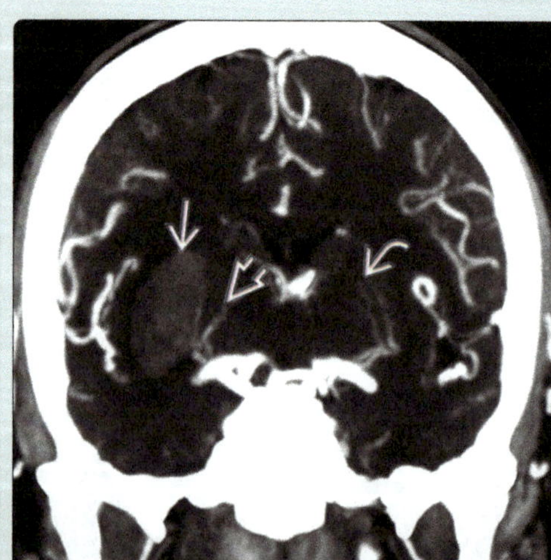

Arteriolosclerosis

KEY FACTS

TERMINOLOGY

- Sclerosis of small-sized arteries (arterioles)
  - Common with chronic hypertension (HTN) &/or diabetes
  - May lead to vascular dementia (VaD)

IMAGING

- Multifocal white matter (WM) hypodensity on CT
- Patchy/confluent ↑ T2/FLAIR hyperintensities
  - Broad or confluent base with ventricles
  - Periventricular > deep > juxtacortical involvement
- Findings nonspecific
  - Large number of causes other than arteriopathy
  - Demyelination, infection, inflammatory, drug related, metabolic, age related
- Caused by several types of arteriopathy
  - Arteriolosclerosis
  - Chronic hypertension (more basal ganglia, periventricular WM involvement)
  - Diabetes mellitus (more peripheral involvement)

TOP DIFFERENTIAL DIAGNOSES

- Age-related WM changes
- Perivascular (Virchow-Robin) spaces
- Demyelinating disease
- VaD
- Cerebral autosomal dominant arteriopathy with subcortical infarcts and leukoencephalopathy (CADASIL)
- Cerebral amyloid angiopathy (CAA)

CLINICAL ISSUES

- Clinical and radiographic picture overlaps
  - Multi-infarct (vascular) dementia: Caused by arteriolosclerosis &/or multiple infarcts
  - Subcortical arteriosclerotic encephalopathy (Binswanger disease)

DIAGNOSTIC CHECKLIST

- Use FLAIR, T2* (GRE, SWI) sequences in all elderly patients
  - Look for microbleeds (HTN, CAA)

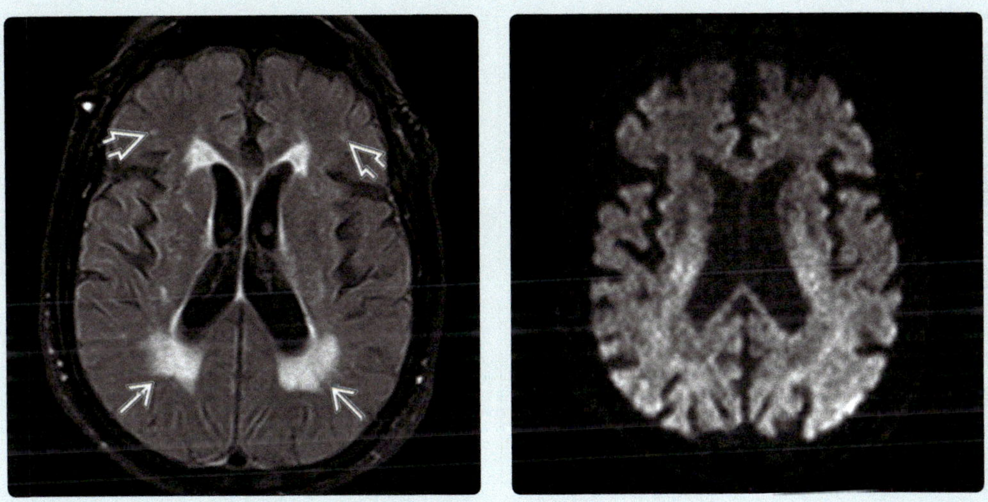

(Left) *Axial FLAIR MR shows mild atrophy and confluent periventricular ➡ and punctate subcortical ➡ white matter hyperintensity typical for arteriolosclerosis (chronic small vessel disease) in this elderly patient with mild cognitive impairment.* **(Right)** *Axial DTI trace shows no areas of diffusion restriction to suggest acute ischemia in this elderly patient. Arteriolosclerosis may mask an acute ischemic event, so DWI or DTI sequences are helpful to exclude acute ischemia in this patient population.*

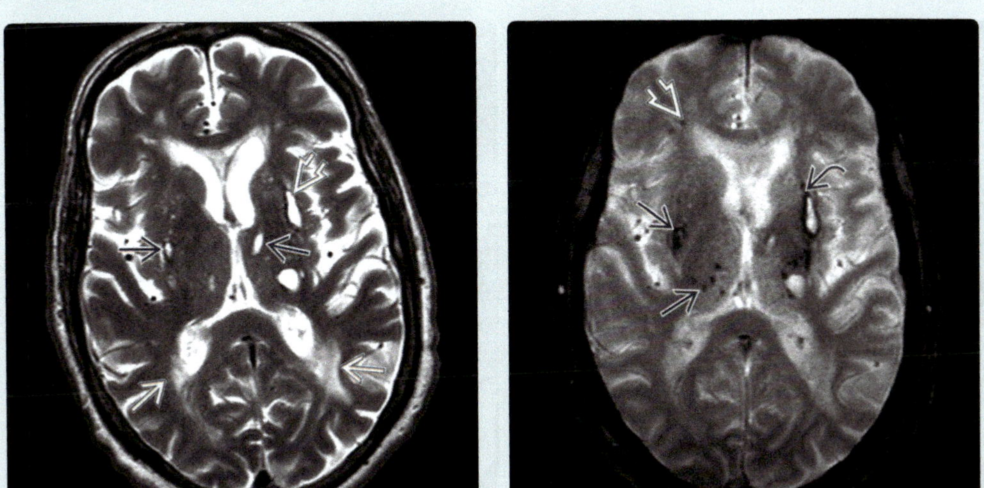

(Left) *Axial T2 MR in a patient with chronic hypertension shows confluent regions of periventricular hyperintensity ➡ related to arteriolosclerosis. There are chronic lacunar infarcts ➡ and a chronic hypertensive basal ganglia hemorrhage ➡.* **(Right)** *GRE in the same case shows blooming hypointensity ➡ around the chronic hypertensive hemorrhage. Multiple foci of susceptibility artifact or "blooming" are seen in the deep gray nuclei ➡ and white matter ➡ related to microhemorrhages from chronic hypertension.*

KEY FACTS

TERMINOLOGY

- Intracranial atherosclerotic vascular disease (ASVD)
- Intracranial atherosclerotic stenosis (ICAS)

IMAGING

- Gold standard is now high-resolution MR (HRMR) with direct vessel wall imaging
  - HRMR vessel wall imaging > > depicting lumen (DSA, CTA, MRA)
- Imaging findings (HRMR)
  - Crescent-shaped or eccentric thickening
  - May show asymmetric hyperintensity of intraplaque hemorrhage on T1WI
  - Noncircumferential, short segment, irregular enhancement
- CTA/MRA/DSA
  - Visualizes lumen, not wall
  - Warfarin-aspirin symptomatic intracranial disease method for calculating ICAS
    - % stenosis = [1- (diameter stenosis/diameter normal)] x 100
  - Focal stenosis, luminal irregularities in cortical vessels can mimic vasculitis
    - Most common cause of vasculitic-like appearance at angiography in middle-aged/older patient is intracranial ASVD

TOP DIFFERENTIAL DIAGNOSES

- Vasculitis/arteritis
- Vasospasm
- Dissection
- Nonocclusive thrombus or embolus

CLINICAL ISSUES

- Disease burden of intracranial ASVD greatly underestimated
- Most common cause of intracranial vascular stenosis in adults
- Independent correlation with T2/FLAIR hyperintensities

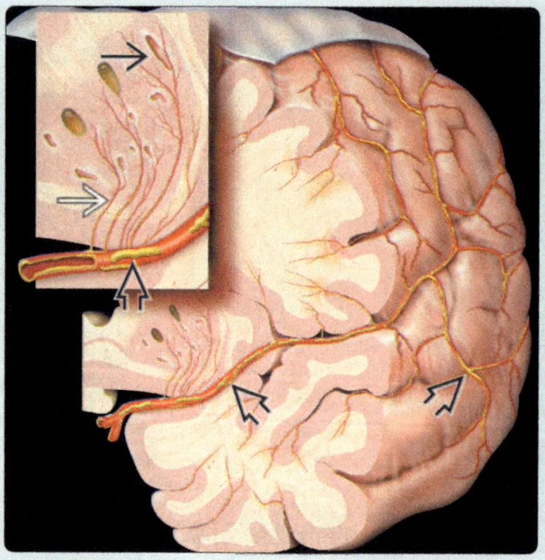

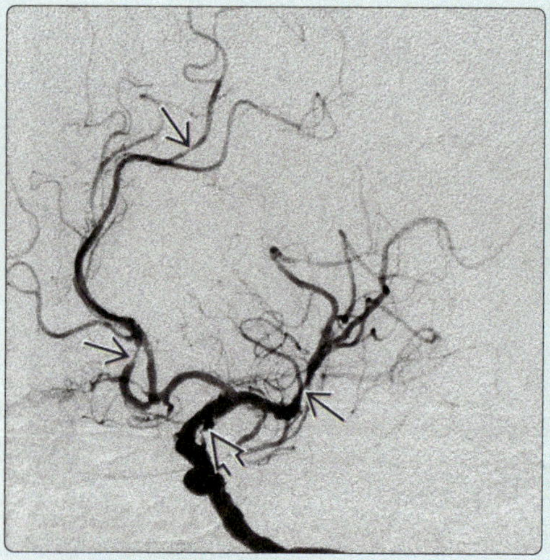

(Left) *Coronal graphic shows atherosclerotic plaques (ASVD) → involving the major intracranial arteries and their branches. Inset shows penetrating (lenticulostriate) arteries → and lacunar infarcts →. ASVD plaques are typically short segment, irregular, noncircumferential, and may enhance.* **(Right)** *DSA in a 68-year-old man in the ER with an acute stroke shows extensive intracranial ASVD. Note multiple areas of stenosis →. An ulcerating plaque → is also present in the supraclinoid internal carotid artery.*

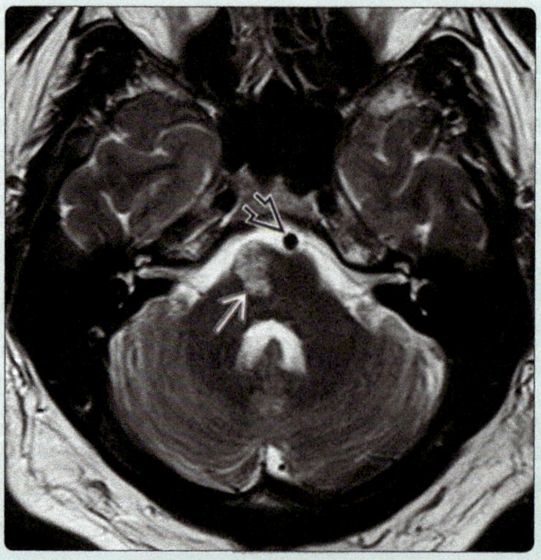

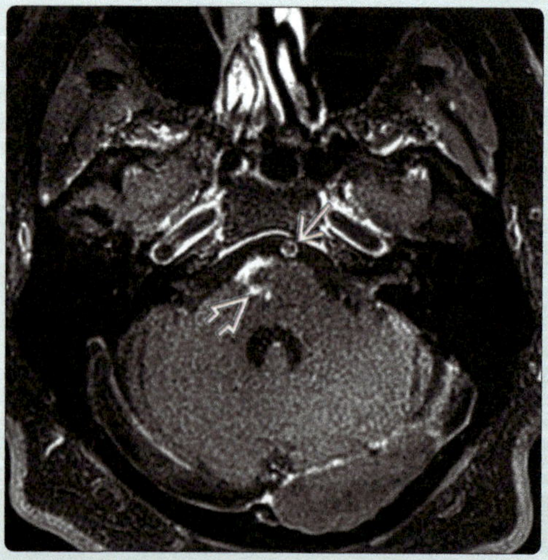

(Left) *Axial T2WI shows a typical pontine perforating artery infarct →. The basilar artery "flow void" → appears normal.* **(Right)** *Vessel wall imaging with thin-section 3T T1 C+ FS MR in the same patient shows enhancement of the subacute infarct →. A partial rim of crescentic enhancement in the basilar artery wall is also present →, consistent with chronic inflammation within an ASVD plaque.*

KEY FACTS

TERMINOLOGY

- Degenerative process resulting from plasma lipid deposition in arterial walls

IMAGING

- Smooth/irregular narrowing of proximal ICA
- Ca++ in arterial walls
- ICA, vertebrobasilar arteries most common sites
- Single diameter thresholds for CTA: 2.2 mm (50% stenosis), 1.3 mm (70% stenosis)
- Protocol advice: Color Doppler US as initial screen; CTA/MRA or contrast MRA; consider DSA before carotid endarterectomy, in equivocal cases or if CTA/MRA shows "occlusion"

PATHOLOGY

- NASCET method: % stenosis = (normal lumen - minimal residual lumen)/normal lumen x 100
- Mild (< 50%), moderate (50-70%), severe (70-99%)
- Intraplaque hemorrhage is independent stroke risk factor

CLINICAL ISSUES

- Carotid endarterectomy (CEA) if symptomatic carotid stenosis ≥ 70% (NASCET)
- Symptomatic moderate stenosis (50-69%) also benefits from CEA (NASCET)
- Asymptomatic patients benefit even with stenosis of 60% (ACAS)
- Carotid stenting depends on preop risk factors
- Signs/symptoms (can be asymptomatic)
  - Carotid bruit, TIA, stroke (may be silent)

DIAGNOSTIC CHECKLIST

- DSA remains gold standard, but acceptable noninvasive preoperative imaging includes any 2: US, CTA, TOF, or enhanced MRA
- Late-phase DSA important to rule out pseudocollusion
  - High-grade stenosis with string sign

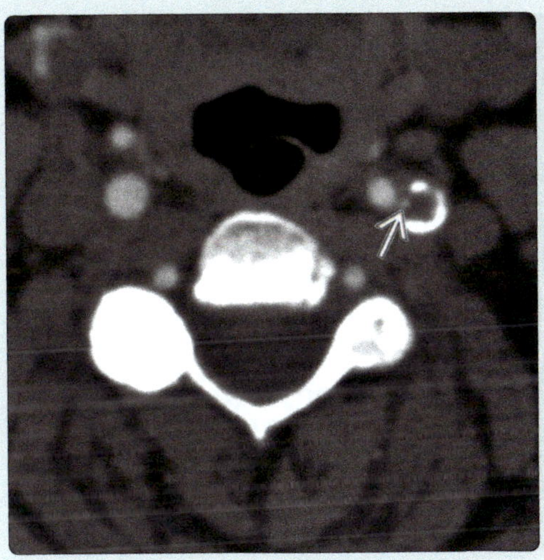

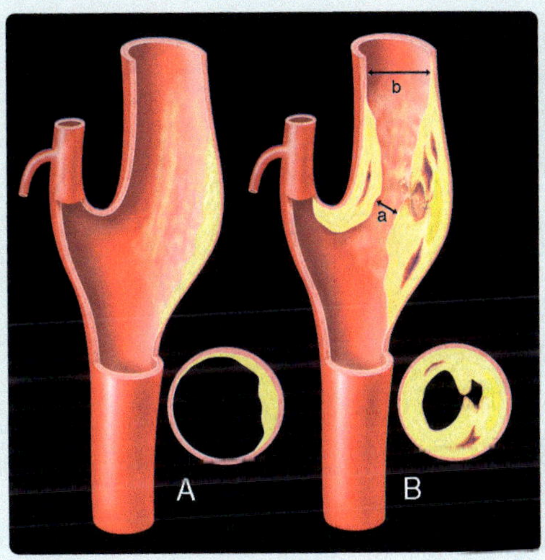

(Left) *Axial CTA shows severe stenosis of the proximal left internal carotid artery (ICA) with small residual lumen ➡. Peripheral mural calcification and the lower density lipid-rich core of the more central soft plaque in the left ICA are typical.* **(Right)** *Graphic shows the mild form of ASVD (A) with "fatty streaks" & slight intimal thickening. The severe form (B) is characterized by intraplaque hemorrhage, ulceration, & platelet thrombi. NASCET calculation for % of stenosis = (b-a)/b x 100, where b = normal ICA lumen & a = minimal residual ICA lumen.*

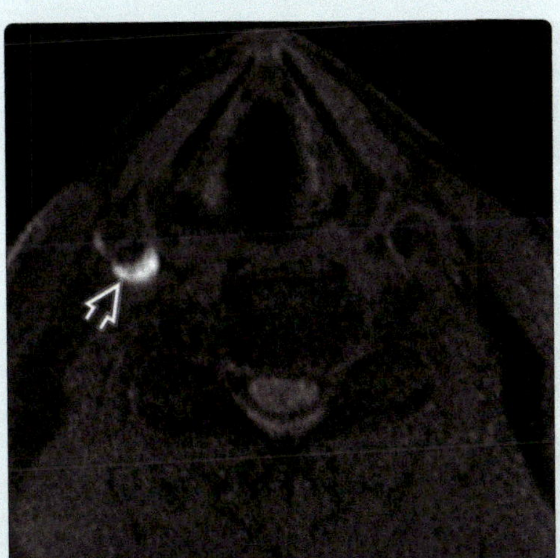

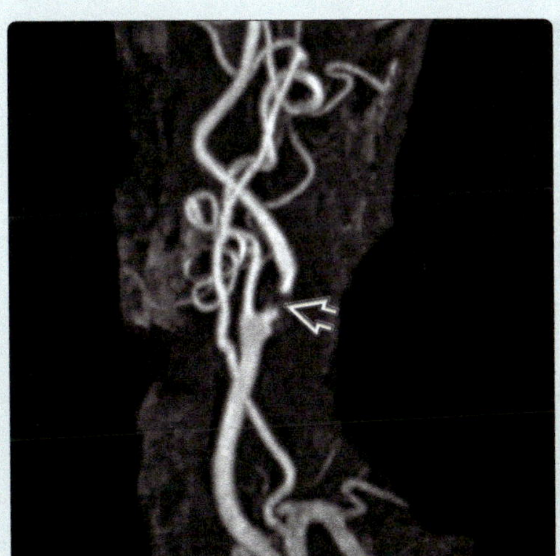

(Left) *Axial MP-RAGE sequence shows intraplaque hemorrhage ➡ in the right ICA as a hyperintense crescent. Intraplaque hemorrhage is an independent stroke risk factor, regardless of ICA percent stenosis. (Courtesy JS McNally, MD, PhD.)* **(Right)** *Coronal oblique MRA shows signal loss as a "flow gap" in the left internal carotid artery ➡, indicating severely restricted flow, typically > 95% stenosis. The patient underwent an emergency left carotid endarterectomy.*

KEY FACTS

TERMINOLOGY

- Progressive narrowing of distal internal carotid artery/proximal circle of Willis (COW) vessels with secondary collateralization
  - Collateral vessels → cloud-like "puff of smoke" (moyamoya) at angiography
- Moyamoya disease (MMD) = primary (idiopathic) moyamoya
  - Marked East-West gradient (more common in Japan, Korea)
- Moyamoya pattern of collaterals = secondary to many etiologies

IMAGING

- Best diagnostic clue: Attenuated COW with multiple tiny basal ganglia "flow voids" on MR
- Best imaging tool: T1 MR C+/MRA; DSA for delineating vascular details

PATHOLOGY

- Moyamoya disease
  - RNF213 polymorphism (95% of familial, 79% of sporadic)
    - Correlated with early onset, severe form of MMD
- Secondary "moyamoya"
  - Moyamoya pattern of collaterals in other conditions
    - Syndromic (e.g., neurofibromatosis type 1)
    - Sickle cell disease
    - Inflammatory or prothrombotic states
    - Suprasellar irradiation in childhood

CLINICAL ISSUES

- Bimodal age peaks (5-10 years and 2nd peak during 4th decade)
- Most frequent cause of stroke in Asian children
- Presentation
  - Children: Recurrent TIAs; hemorrhage rare
  - Adults: TIAs, infarcts, hemorrhage (20%), migraines

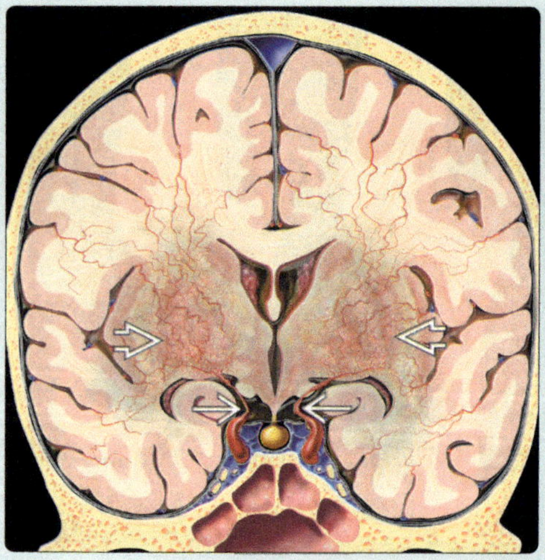
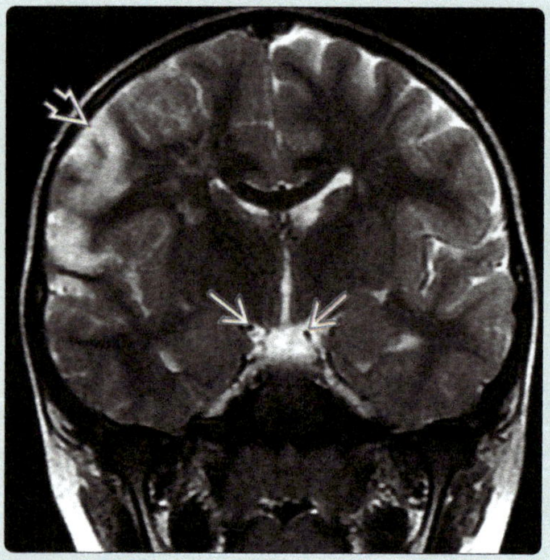

(Left) *Coronal graphic shows severe tapering of both distal internal carotid arteries* ➡ *and strikingly enlarged lenticulostriate arteries* ➡ *coursing through basal ganglia. This is the "puff of smoke" (moyamoya).* **(Right)** *Coronal T2WI in a 3-year-old girl with moyamoya disease shows severely attenuated supraclinoid internal carotid arteries* ➡*. An acute cortical infarct is present in the right middle carotid artery (MCA) distribution* ➡*.*

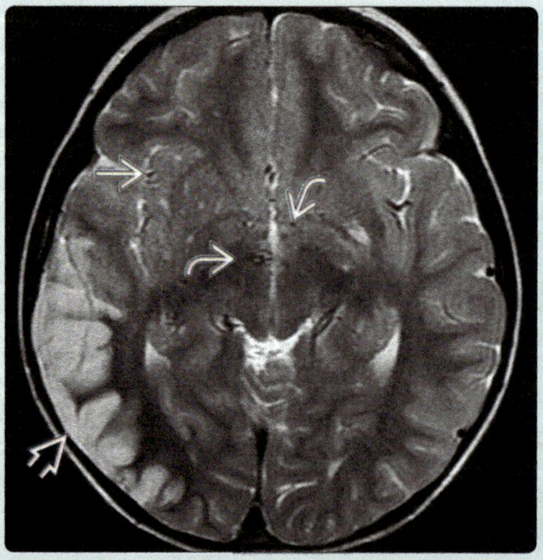
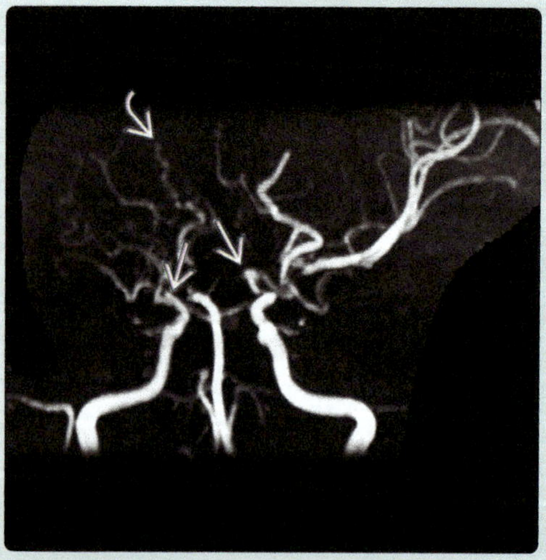

(Left) *Axial T2WI in the same patient shows tiny, almost inapparent "flow voids" of the right MCA branches in the sylvian fissure* ➡*. The acute cortical infarct has produced marked gyral edema, swelling* ➡*. Note the tiny "squiggly" flow voids* ➡ *from the basal collateral vessels.* **(Right)** *Coronal MIP of the time-of-flight MRA in the same patient shows the severely attenuated supraclinoid internal carotid arteries* ➡ *and the puff of smoke appearance of the basal collateral vessels* ➡*.*

KEY FACTS

TERMINOLOGY

- Primary arteritis of CNS (PACNS)
  - No evidence of secondary (systemic) vasculitis
  - May involve intracranial arteries of any size
- 2 features essential for histopathologic diagnosis
  - Inflammation and necrosis of blood vessel wall

IMAGING

- CT
  - Look for secondary signs of vasculitis (ischemia, infarction)
  - Hypodensities on CT
  - Especially basal ganglia, subcortical white matter
- MR (high resolution)
  - Multifocal punctate, linear hyperintensities on T2/FLAIR
  - Vessel wall imaging with thin-section, high-resolution (3T) T1 C+
    - Circumferential, smooth, long segment
  - ± patchy parenchymal enhancement, restricted diffusion
  - DWI variable (may restrict)
- DSA
  - Once considered imaging gold standard
  - "Beaded" arteries (irregular stenoses, dilatations) on DSA
    - Peripheral branches > proximal (circle of Willis)
  - Less common: Long-segment stenoses, pseudoaneurysms, occlusions

PATHOLOGY

- Brain biopsy may be required to confirm diagnosis
  - 75-80% sensitive
  - Negative biopsy does not exclude PACNS

CLINICAL ISSUES

- Wide age range (mean: 42 years)

DIAGNOSTIC CHECKLIST

- Atherosclerosis is by far most common cause of vasculitis-like DSA pattern in older adults, not PACNS

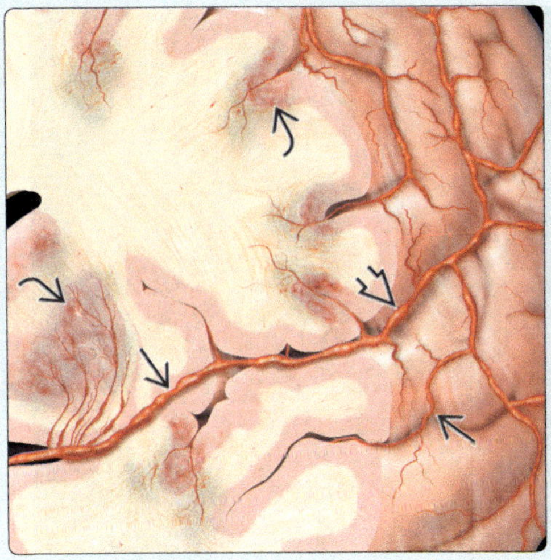

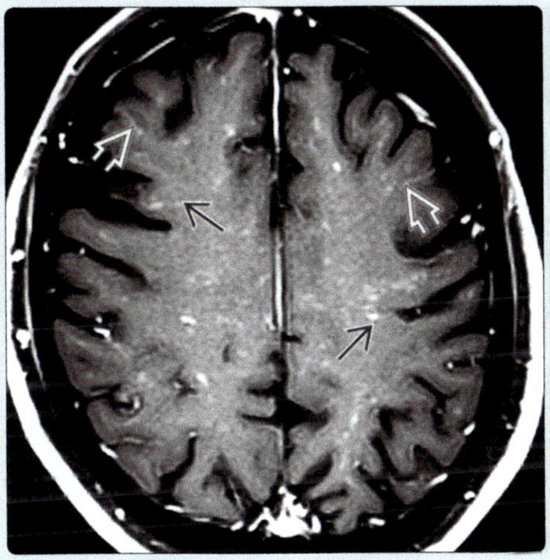

(Left) *Graphic depicts primary arteritis of the CNS with areas of narrowing and dilatation of the middle cerebral artery branches, as well as foci of patchy ischemia and microbleeds in the basal ganglia, cortex, and subcortical white matter.* **(Right)** *T1 C+ FS scan in a 62-year-old man with ataxia, diplopia, and confusion shows innumerable abnormal linear and dot-like areas of enhancement in the subcortical and deep white matter of both hemispheres. This is biopsy-proven primary arteritis of the CNS (PACNS).*

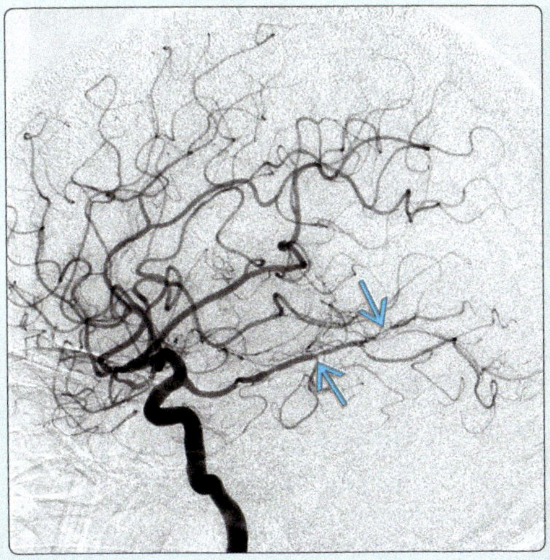

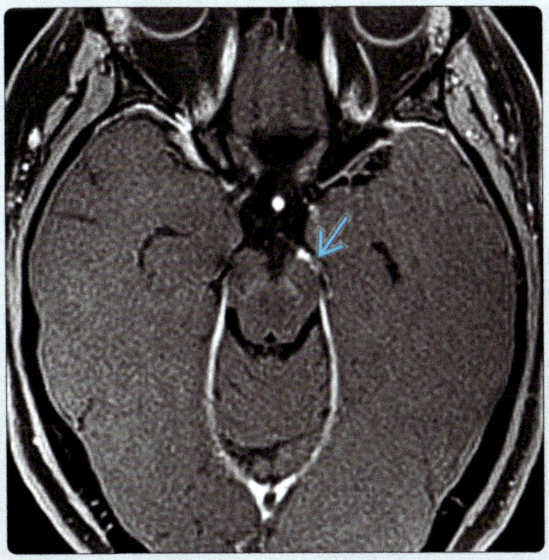

(Left) *Lateral DSA in a 34-year-old woman with multiple strokes shows markedly irregular posterior cerebral artery with alternating areas of stenosis and dilatation.* **(Right)** *Thin-section T1 C+ FS in the same patient shows enhancement in the wall of the left posterior cerebral artery. Wall enhancement can occur in both vasculitis and atherosclerosis with chronic inflammation. Patient was a smoker with cardiovascular risk factors, but young age and clinical features were most consistent with PACNS.*

KEY FACTS

TERMINOLOGY

- Heterogeneous group of CNS disorders
    - Characterized by nonatheromatous inflammation and necrosis of blood vessel walls
    - Both arteries, veins may be affected

IMAGING

- CTA/MRA useful screening; spatial resolution usually insufficient for subtle disease
- MR
    - Basal ganglia, cortex, subcortical white matter
        - Multifocal hypodensities/T2 hyperintensities
        - Look for secondary signs (ischemia/infarction)
    - High-resolution (3T, thin-section) T1 C+ may demonstrate wall enhancement
        - Smooth, concentric
        - Long segment
        - Distal involvement (e.g., M2, M3, M4 branches > intracranial internal carotid artery and basilar artery)
        - Multiple vessels usually affected
- DSA
    - Findings nonspecific (visualizes lumen, not vessel wall)
        - Multifocal areas of smooth or slightly irregular-shaped stenoses alternating with dilated segments
        - May occur in intracranial vessels of any size
        - Major differential diagnosis = intracranial atherosclerosis

TOP DIFFERENTIAL DIAGNOSES

- Intracranial atherosclerotic vascular disease
- Arterial vasospasm
- Reversible cerebral vasoconstriction syndrome

PATHOLOGY

- Vessel wall inflammation, necrosis common to all vasculitides

(Left) *Axial FLAIR scan in a case of secondary CNS vasculitis shows multiple hyperintense foci in the basal ganglia, thalami, and cortex* ➡. **(Right)** *Axial DWI MR in the same case shows multiple small foci of restricted diffusion in the basal ganglia, thalami, and cortex* ➡.

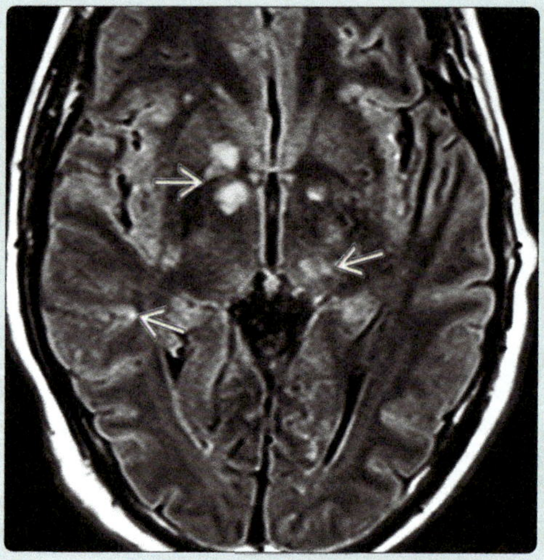

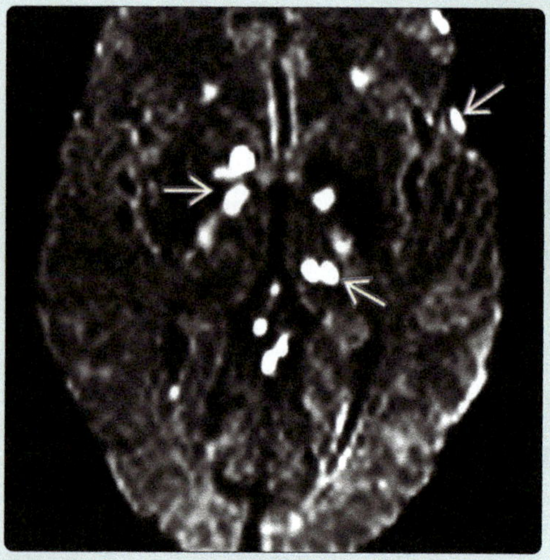

(Left) *Lateral view of the internal carotid angiogram obtained in the same case shows multiple cortical vessels* ➡ *with alternating areas of stenosis and dilatation ("beading"). The findings are consistent with multiple infarcts secondary to infectious (streptococcal) vasculitis.* **(Right)** *3T high-resolution axial T1 C+ FS in a 59-year-old woman with proven ANCA vasculitis shows intense enhancement of the distal internal carotid and proximal middle cerebral arteries* ➡.

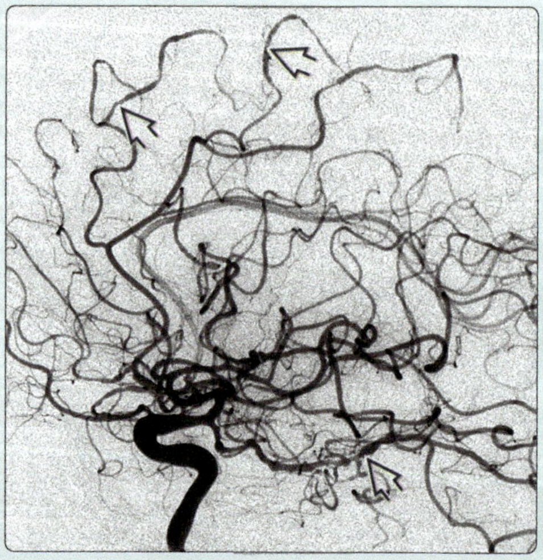

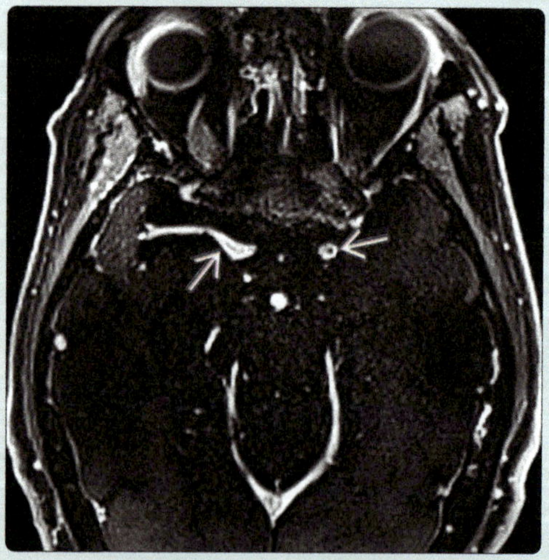

KEY FACTS

TERMINOLOGY

- Reversible cerebral vasoconstriction syndrome, a.k.a. Call-Fleming syndrome
- Group of disorders characterized by
  - Reversible, multifocal cerebral artery vasoconstrictions
  - Severe headaches ± focal neurological deficits

IMAGING

- Acute/recurrent headaches with vasculitic pattern (DSA)
- DSA = crucial for diagnosis (100% sensitive)
  - Involves large, medium-sized arteries
  - Diffuse, multifocal, segmental narrowing
  - Sometimes "string of beads" or "sausage strings"
- NECT often negative
  - Small cortical subarachnoid hemorrhages (20%) ± parenchymal hemorrhage
- CTA/MRA: May be normal if subtle changes (10%)
  - Diffuse segmental arterial constriction in 90%
- Transcranial Doppler: ↑ arterial velocities in MCA, ICA, & ACA

PATHOLOGY

- Thought to represent transient disturbance in control of cerebral vascular tone → vasoconstriction → ischemia, stroke, death
- Spontaneous (1/3 of cases) or precipitated by
  - Postpartum state
  - Exposure to vasoactive substances
- Can be associated with posterior reversible encephalopathy syndrome (PRES)

CLINICAL ISSUES

- Symptoms: Severe, acute "thunderclap" headache
  - Often recurrent (95%)
  - Ischemia/stroke (visual disturbance, aphasia, hemiparesis)
- Treatment: Discontinuation of vasoactive medications; vasodilators (e.g., Ca++ channel blockers)

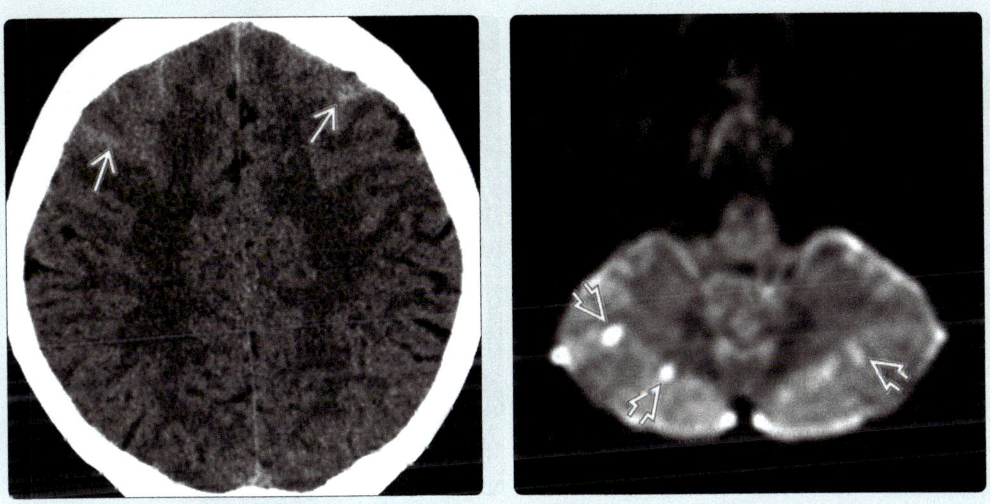

(Left) *Axial NECT in a female patient with acute onset of severe headache shows limited cortical subarachnoid hemorrhage (SAH) in the sulci of the frontal lobes ➡. DSA was performed to exclude a vascular lesion and showed multifocal arterial narrowings (not shown) related to RCVS.* **(Right)** *Axial DWI trace shows multiple foci of hyperintensity ➡ related to acute ischemia in this patient with RCVS who presented with an acute onset of a "thunderclap" headache. Ischemia is a common complication of RCVS.*

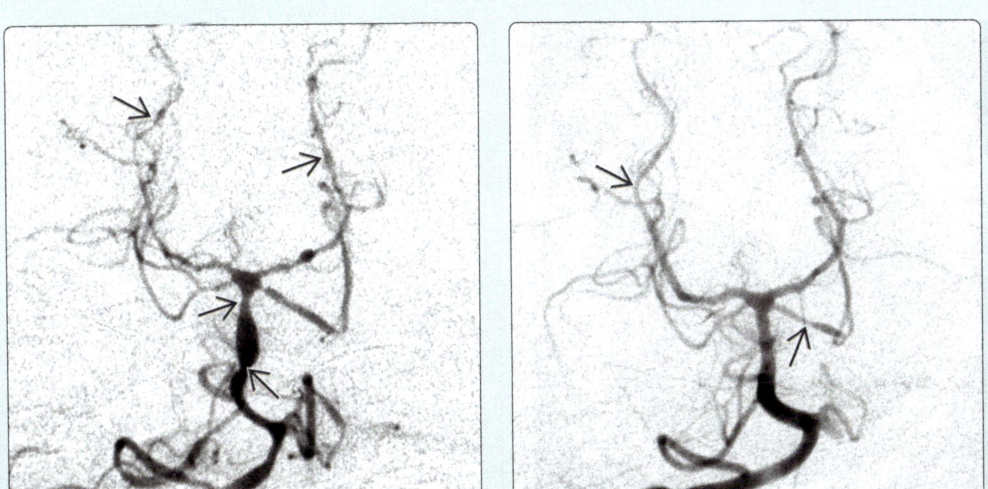

(Left) *Anteroposterior right vertebral artery DSA shows diffuse luminal irregularity and focal stenoses involving the basilar artery and posterior cerebral and superior cerebellar arteries ⇨. Similar changes were seen in the anterior circulation (not shown). The patient was treated with IA verapamil over the next 10 days.* **(Right)** *DSA repeated 2 weeks later shows significant interval resolution of the posterior circulation vasospasm. There are a few foci ⇨ of mild residual stenoses still evident.*

KEY FACTS

TERMINOLOGY

- Reversible stenosis of intracranial arteries
- Common with aneurysmal subarachnoid hemorrhage (SAH)
- Caused by exposure to blood breakdown products
  - Contraction of vascular smooth muscle
  - Histological changes in vessel wall

IMAGING

- General features (CTA/MRA/DSA)
  - Typically occurs 4-14 days after SAH
  - Smooth, relatively long segmental stenoses
  - Seen as arterial luminal irregularity/undulations
  - Multiple arteries, usually > 1 vascular territory
- CT perfusion
  - ↑ time to peak, ↑ mean transit time
  - ↓ cerebral blood flow in areas of hypoperfusion
- Transcranial Doppler shows ↑ mean flow velocity

TOP DIFFERENTIAL DIAGNOSES

- Non-SAH causes of vasospasm
  - Meningitis
  - Acute hypertensive encephalopathy (PRES)
  - Reversible cerebral vasoconstriction syndrome
  - Migraine headache
- Vasculitis
- Atherosclerosis

CLINICAL ISSUES

- Delayed ischemic neurological deficit
  - ~ 1 week after SAH is typical
- Management
  - "Triple H" therapy to prevent/treat vasospasm after SAH
    - Induced hypertension
    - Hypervolemia
    - Hemodilution
  - Endovascular (chemical or balloon angioplasty)

(Left) *Autopsied case of ruptured middle cerebral artery (MCA) aneurysm ➯ with subarachnoid hemorrhage (SAH) in a patient who survived several days shows severe vasospasm of the parent MCA →.* **(Right)** *Axial NECT in a 43-year-old man in the ER with "worst headache of life" shows diffuse SAH ➔ in the basal cisterns, especially in the left sylvian fissure.*

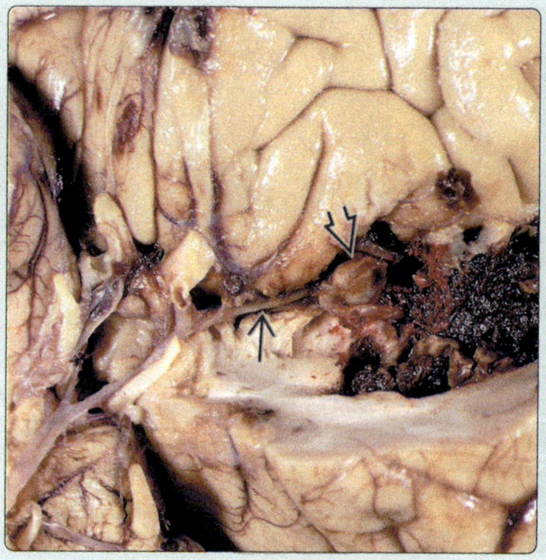

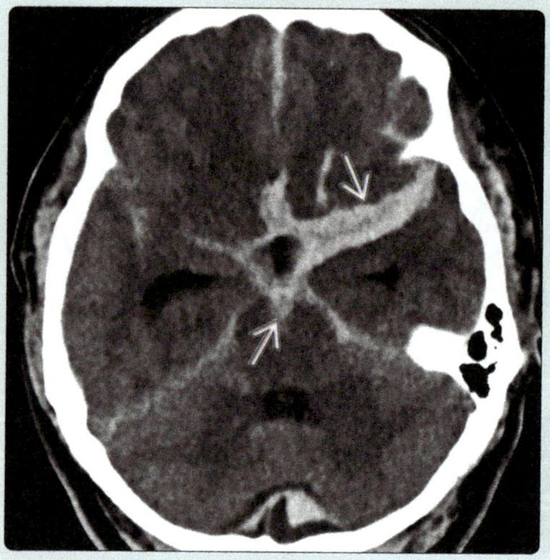

(Left) *CTA in the same patient shows a lobulated aneurysm ➔ at the left distal internal carotid artery bifurcation.* **(Right)** *Four days after emergency clipping of the aneurysm, the patient became drowsy and developed right-sided weakness. AP DSA of the left internal carotid artery shows mass effect, vasospasm →, seen here as narrowing of the proximal anterior cerebral artery and MCA. The patient responded well to intraarterial infusion of verapamil.*

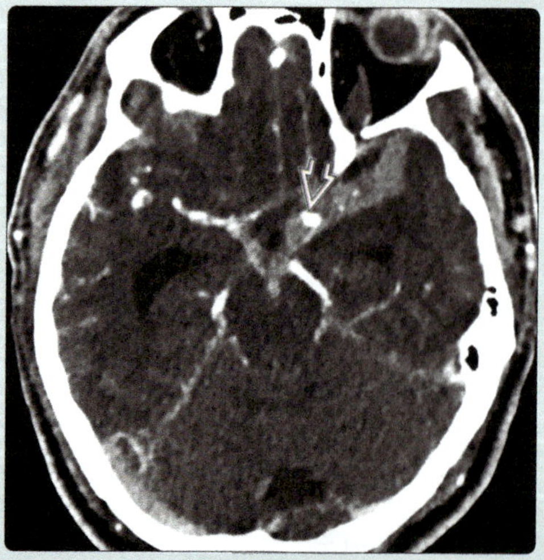

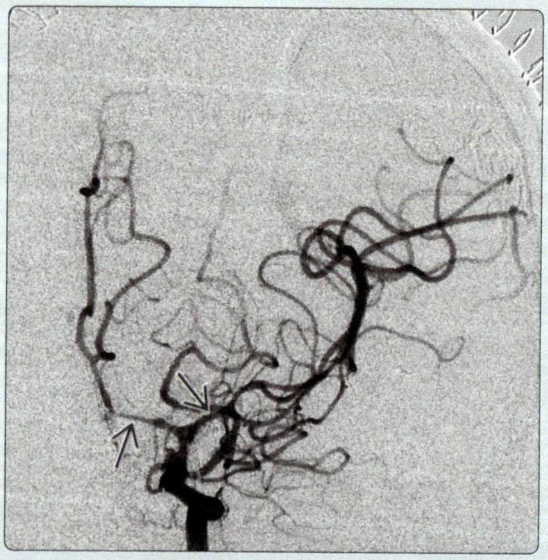

KEY FACTS

TERMINOLOGY

- Systemic lupus erythematosus (SLE), neuropsychiatric (NPSLE), CNS lupus
- Multisystem autoimmune disorder that affects respiratory, cardiovascular, GI, GU, musculoskeletal systems, and CNS
  - CNS involved in up to 75%

IMAGING

- 4 general patterns
  - New infarcts (associated with ↑ anticardiolipin, ↑ lupus anticoagulant antibodies)
  - Focal areas of hyperintensity, primarily in gray matter
  - Multiple T2WI hyperintensities (microinfarctions)
  - Extensive, reversible white matter (WM) changes (cerebral edema)
- Multifocal WM microinfarcts, cerebral atrophy common
- Mild SLE: PET/SPECT more sensitive than MR
- Restricted diffusion (cytotoxic edema) in ischemia/infarct
- Increased diffusion (vasogenic edema) in vasculopathy
- Acute/active CNS lesions may enhance

TOP DIFFERENTIAL DIAGNOSES

- Multiple sclerosis (MS), Susac syndrome
- Lyme encephalopathy
- Arteriolosclerosis (microvascular disease)
- Other vasculitides (e.g., primary angiitis of CNS)

CLINICAL ISSUES

- Cerebral involvement may precede full-blown SLE picture or may develop during course of disease
- SLE associated with antiphospholipid syndrome, posterior reversible encephalopathy syndrome (PRES), Lupus-related myelitis, Libman-Sacks endocarditis, emboli

DIAGNOSTIC CHECKLIST

- Look for elevated cerebrospinal fluid protein
- Role of imaging in SLE: Assess acute neurologic deficits
- Keep in mind: Negative brain MR does not exclude cerebral lupus

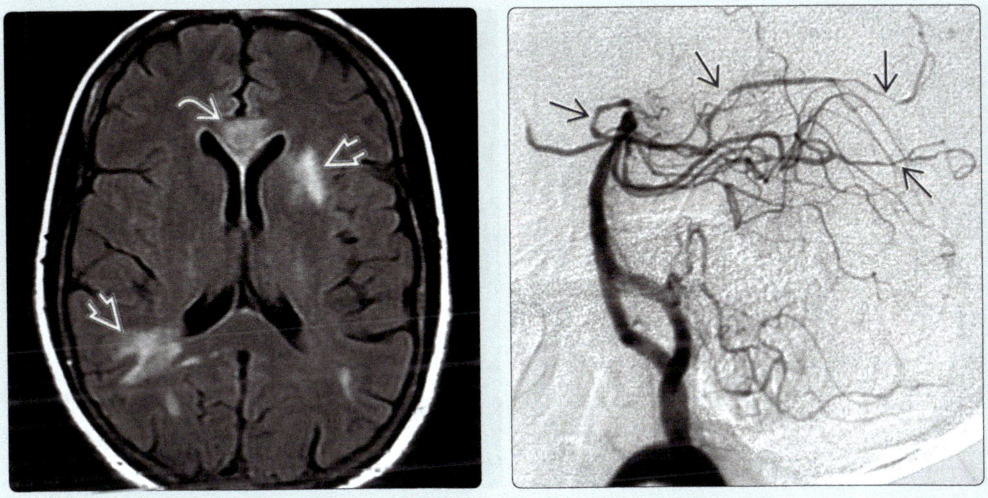

(Left) *Axial FLAIR MR in an SLE patient with new neurologic symptoms. Note the multiple foci of FLAIR hyperintensity in the white matter and the corpus callosum. This patient also had antiphospholipid syndrome, which is common in SLE patients.* **(Right)** *Lateral vertebrobasilar DSA shows multifocal stenoses typical of a nonspecific vasculitis. This is uncommonly seen with lupus, which is more of a small-vessel vasculitis than other inflammatory vasculitides. DSA is often normal in SLE patients.*

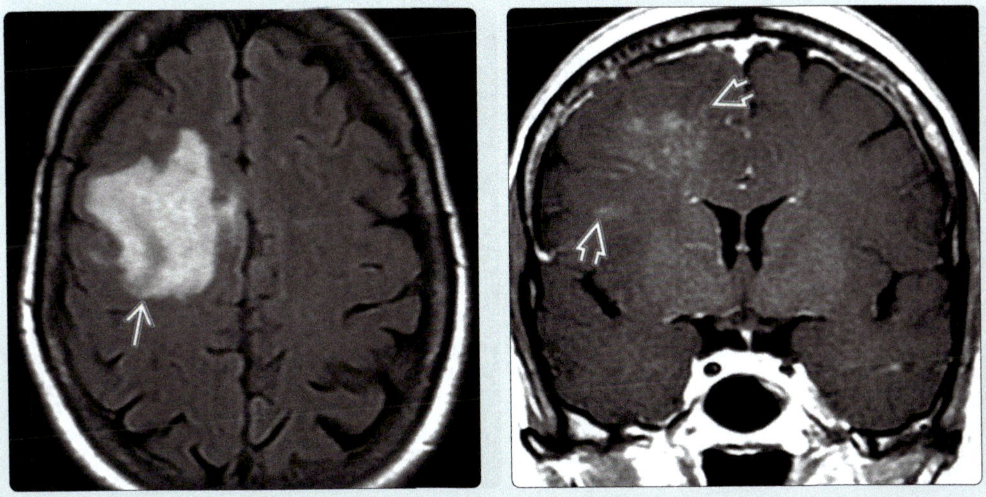

(Left) *Axial FLAIR MR in a 52-year-old woman with neuropsychiatric symptoms shows a large hyperintense frontal lobe lesion.* **(Right)** *Coronal T1 C+ MR in the same patient shows linear enhancement throughout the frontal lobe. Biopsy disclosed CNS lupus vasculitis. Although imaging of SLE is nonspecific, there are often multiple white matter hyperintensities as well as multifocal infarcts. Migratory edematous regions are also often seen.*

Cerebral Amyloid Angiopathy (CAA)

KEY FACTS

TERMINOLOGY

- Cerebral amyloid deposition occurs in 3 morphologic varieties
  - Common: Cerebral amyloid angiopathy (CAA)
  - Uncommon: Mass-like lesion (amyloidoma)
  - Rare: Inflammatory; diffuse (encephalopathic) white matter involvement

IMAGING

- General findings
  - Normotensive demented patient
  - Lobar hemorrhage(s) of different ages
  - Multifocal "black dots" on T2* or SWI MR
- Protocol advice
  - Best initial screening (for acute hemorrhage) = CT
  - MR with T2* &/or SWI

TOP DIFFERENTIAL DIAGNOSES

- Multifocal "black dots" on T2/T2* MR
  - Hypertensive microhemorrhages
  - Multiple cavernous malformations (type 4)
  - Ischemic stroke with microhemorrhage
  - Diffuse axonal injury
  - Hemorrhagic metastases
  - Posterior reversible encephalopathy syndrome

CLINICAL ISSUES

- CAA: Common cause of "spontaneous" lobar hemorrhage in elderly patients
  - Causes up to 15-20% of primary intracranial hemorrhage (ICH) in patients > 60 years old
  - Stroke-like clinical presentation with "spontaneous" lobar ICH
  - Chronic: Can cause vascular dementia
- CAA common in elderly patients with dementia
  - 2/3 normotensive, 1/3 hypertensive
  - 40% with subacute dementia/overt Alzheimer (overlap common)

(Left) *Axial graphic shows an acute hematoma ➡ with a blood-fluid level ➡. Multiple microbleeds ➡ and old lobar hemorrhages ⇨ are also typical findings in cerebral amyloid disease.* **(Right)** *Axial SWI MR in a 70-year-old man with cognitive impairment and acute visual changes shows multiple lobar hemorrhages ⇨ and microhemorrhages ➡ related to cerebral amyloid angiopathy (CAA). SWI and T2* sequences are the most sensitive sequences for identifying microhemorrhages characteristic of CAA.*

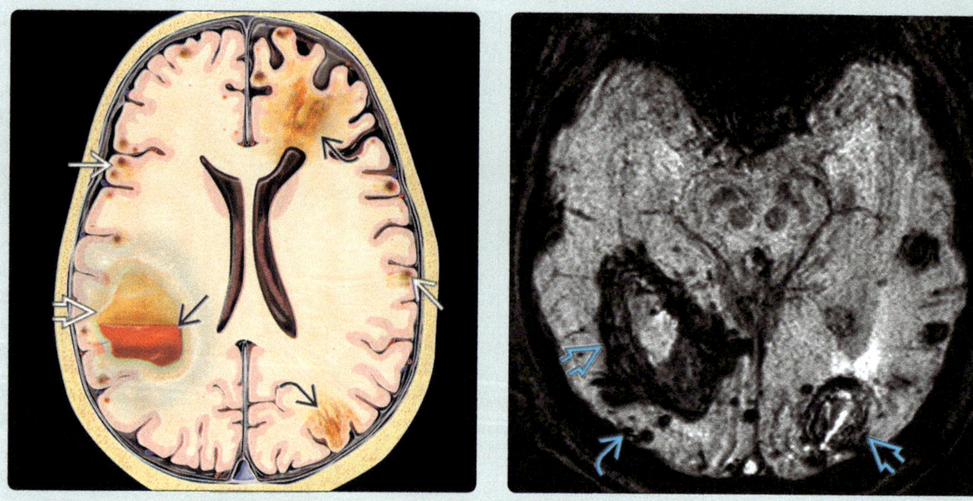

(Left) *Axial CT in a 72-year-old woman with no history of hypertension shows an acute right occipital lobe hemorrhage ➡.* **(Right)** *Axial GRE MR in the same patient shows multiple foci of susceptibility artifact ➡ "blooming" related to microhemorrhages in a typical location for CAA. CAA patients most often present with acute focal neurologic deficits related to the lobar hemorrhage. Patients also present with cognitive impairment related to the microhemorrhages.*

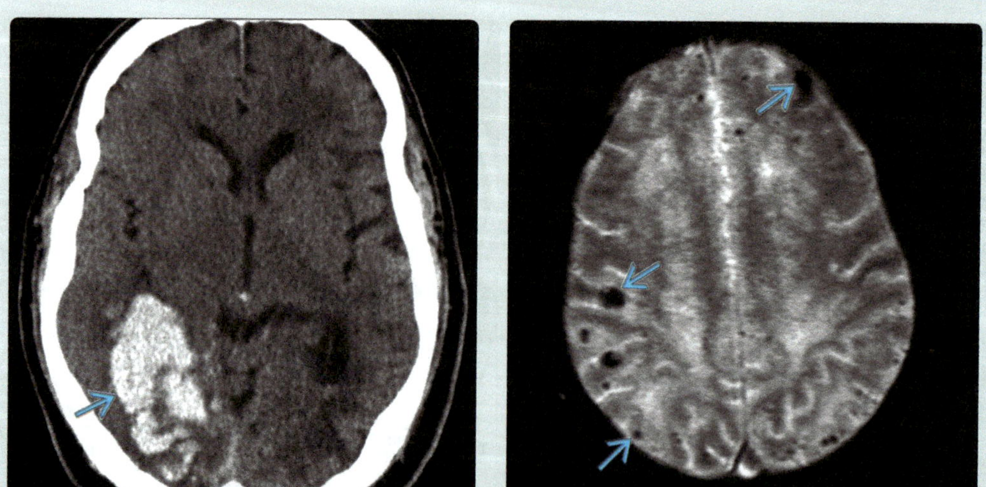

KEY FACTS

TERMINOLOGY

- **C**erebral **A**utosomal **D**ominant **A**rteriopathy with **S**ubcortical **I**nfarcts and **L**eukoencephalopathy (**CADASIL**)
- Hereditary small-vessel disease due to mutations in *NOTCH3* gene on chromosome 19, which causes stroke in young to middle-aged adults

IMAGING

- Diffuse white matter (WM) hyperintensities = leukoaraiosis, early finding
- Multiple lacunar infarcts
- Anterior temporal pole, external capsule, and paramedian superior frontal lobe highly sensitive and specific locations
- Diffusion restriction in acute lacunar infarcts
- Protocol advice: MR with T2, FLAIR, and DWI

TOP DIFFERENTIAL DIAGNOSES

- Arteriolosclerosis ("Binswanger"), MELAS, subcortical arteriosclerotic encephalopathy, primary angiitis of CNS

PATHOLOGY

- Autosomal dominant disease with mutation in *NOTCH3* results in arteriopathy affecting penetrating cerebral and leptomeningeal arteries

CLINICAL ISSUES

- Most frequent hereditary small-vessel disease of brain
- TIA/stroke or migraine with aura often initial presentation
- TIA or stroke most common manifestation of disease (60-85% of all patients)
    - Often absence of traditional risk factors
- Migraines, if present, often precede other findings
- Average onset of stroke slightly earlier for men, but not significantly different (M = 50.7, F = 52.5 yr)
- Clinical differential diagnosis includes multiple sclerosis, dementia, and CNS vasculitis
- No specific therapy, supportive therapy to reduce stroke and myocardial infarct risk

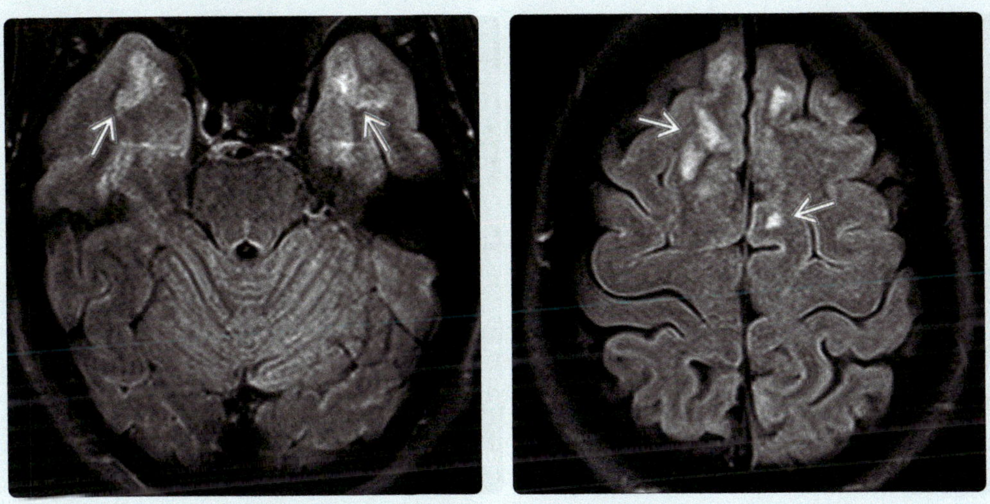

(Left) *Axial FLAIR MR of a young patient with migraines shows focal hyperintensity ➡ in the anterior temporal lobes highly suggestive of CADASIL. NOTCH3 mutation confirmed CADASIL.* **(Right)** *Axial FLAIR MR in the same patient shows additional subcortical hyperintense foci in the paramedian superior frontal lobes ➡, which is a highly sensitive and specific location for lesions in patients with CADASIL, in addition to the anterior temporal lobes and external capsule.*

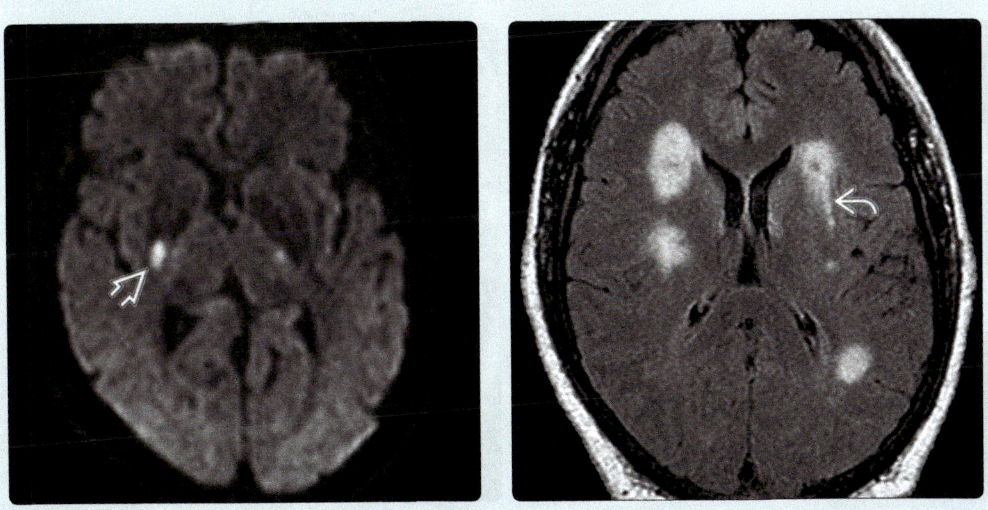

(Left) *Axial DWI trace in a young woman with no vascular risk factors shows an acute lacunar ➡ infarct in the right basal ganglia. CADASIL was diagnosed by the presence of a NOTCH3 mutation.* **(Right)** *Axial FLAIR MR shows multiple hyperintense white matter lesions with involvement of the external capsule ➡. External capsule disease location is characteristic for CADASIL and rarely seen with the more common arteriolosclerosis.*

Behçet Disease

KEY FACTS

TERMINOLOGY

- Chronic, idiopathic relapsing-remitting multisystem vascular-inflammatory disease characterized by recurrent orogenital ulcerations and uveitis
  - CNS involved in up to 20-25% of patients

IMAGING

- Best diagnostic clue: T2 hyperintense brainstem lesion in patient with oral and genital ulcers
  - Midbrain > pons > basal ganglia > thalami > white matter
  - Focal or multifocal lesions
  - May see expansion of involved structures acutely
- T2WI: Hyperintense lesions
- T1WI C+: Patchy enhancement typical
- ↓ *N*-acetylaspartate (NAA) in acute lesions
  - NAA may normalize when lesions resolve
- May see atrophy of involved structures chronically

TOP DIFFERENTIAL DIAGNOSES

- Gliomatosis cerebri
- Acute disseminated encephalitis
- Primary CNS lymphoma
- Vasculitis
- Multiple sclerosis

CLINICAL ISSUES

- Neurologic deficit (hemiparesis), headache, seizure common presenting features
  - Other: Recurrent meningoencephalitis
- Young adults, median age: 40 years

DIAGNOSTIC CHECKLIST

- Consider Behçet disease in young adult with brainstem or deep gray nucleus lesion
- Enhancement pattern may help differentiate Behçet disease from other etiologies

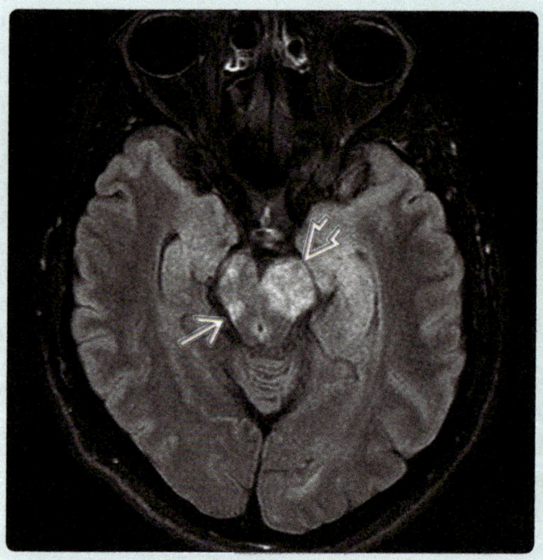
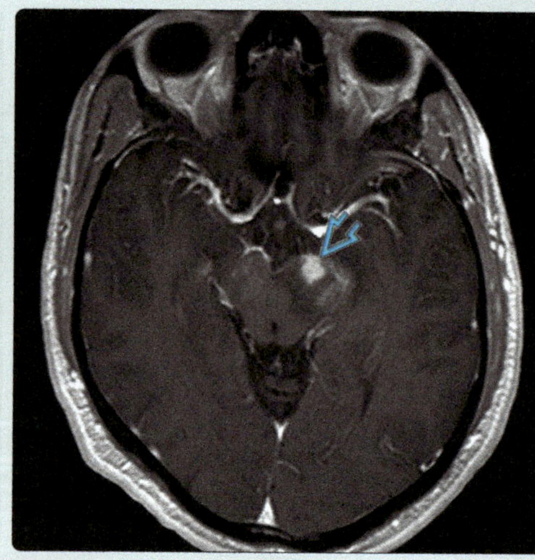

(Left) *Axial FLAIR MR shows abnormal hyperintensity and mild expansion of the left ventral midbrain ➡ and patchy hyperintensity in the right midbrain ➡ in this 35-year-old man with neuro-Behçet disease. This chronic, relapsing idiopathic multisystem vascular inflammatory disease is also characterized by oral and genital ulcers.* **(Right)** *Axial T1 C+ MR in the same patient shows enhancement of the large midbrain lesion ➡. Imaging typically mimics neoplasm, vasculitis, and demyelination.*

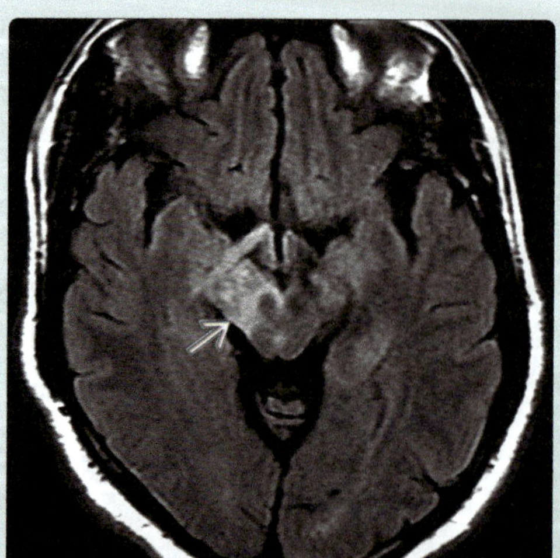
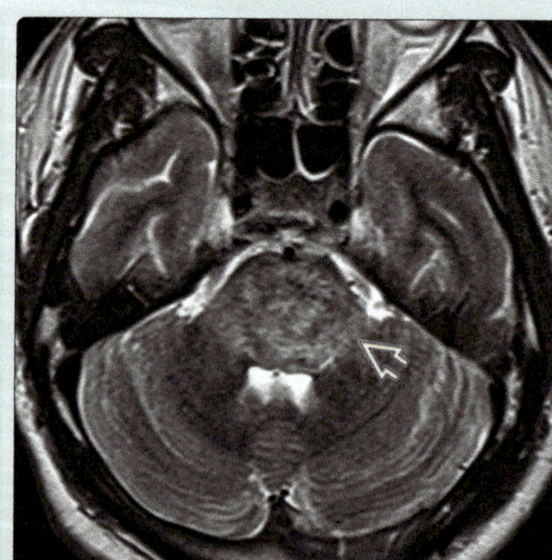

(Left) *Axial FLAIR MR in the same patient 2 years later shows resolution of the left midbrain lesion and development of a large right midbrain lesion ➡ involving the cerebral peduncle. A relapsing-remitting clinical course is typical.* **(Right)** *Axial T2WI MR shows hyperintensity in the pons with mild expansion ➡ in a young man with oral ulcers and a clinical diagnosis of Behçet disease. Other lesions were present in the midbrain and basal ganglia. Thalamic and white matter involvement is less common in this disease.*

KEY FACTS

TERMINOLOGY

- Microangiopathy of brain, retina, and cochlea

IMAGING

- T2 hyperintense corpus callosum lesions in patient with clinical triad
  - Encephalopathy, bilateral hearing loss, and branch retinal artery occlusions
- Multifocal T2 hyperintensities similar to MS
  - More often round, midcallosal rather than callososeptal location
- May involve brainstem, basal ganglia, thalamus, subcortical white matter, centrum semiovale
- Lesions may show acute diffusion restriction
- Variable enhancement of lesions and leptomeninges

TOP DIFFERENTIAL DIAGNOSES

- Multiple sclerosis
- Acute disseminated encephalomyelitis (ADEM)
- Systemic lupus erythematosus
- Vasculitis

PATHOLOGY

- Microinfarctions in cerebral cortex that are generally not seen on imaging
- No demyelination seen on pathology

CLINICAL ISSUES

- 20-40 year old (F > > M)
- Sudden visual loss, deafness; headache, variable encephalopathy
- Usually self-limited (2-4 years), but may lead to permanent deafness or blindness

DIAGNOSTIC CHECKLIST

- Most patients do not exhibit entire triad (up to 97% at time of presentation)
- Complete triad seen after 2 weeks or after 2 years

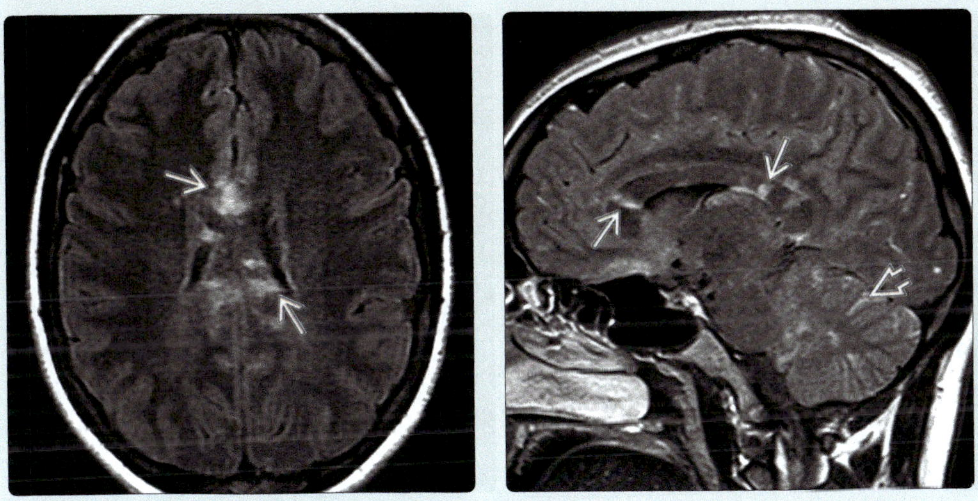

(Left) *Axial FLAIR MR shows multiple hyperintensities ➡ in corpus callosum of this 27-year-old woman with Susac syndrome who presented with headache and confusion. The classic clinical triad includes encephalopathy, bilateral hearing loss, and branch retinal artery occlusions.* **(Right)** *Postcontrast sagittal FLAIR in the same patient shows classic involvement ➡ of corpus callosum body with hyperintense lesions. Note leptomeningeal enhancement ➡, which may be seen in up to 50% of patients.*

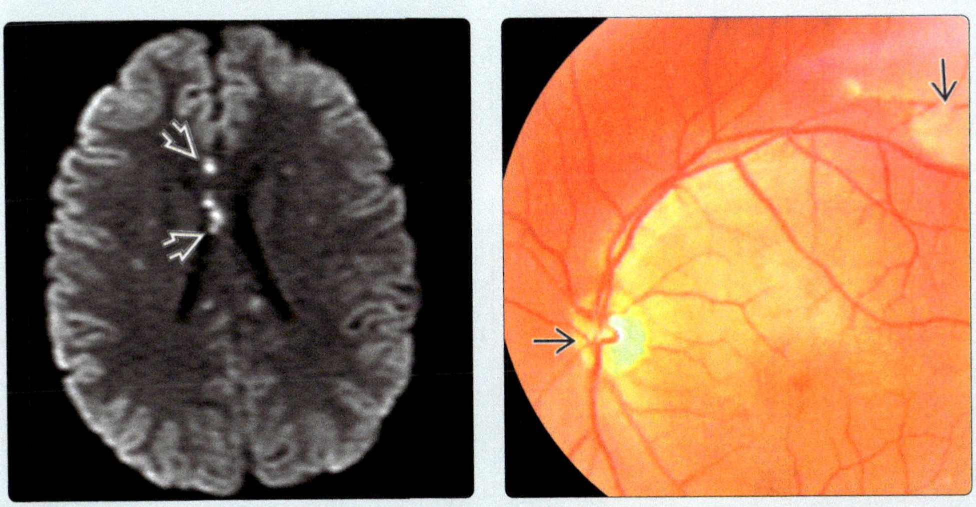

(Left) *Axial DWI trace shows multiple hyperintense lesions ➡, many of which had corresponding low ADC values representing true diffusion restriction. Acute lesions may mimic vasculitis.* **(Right)** *Funduscopic examination shows multiple retinal artery branch occlusions and irregularities ➡, classic for Susac syndrome. Susac syndrome is often mistaken for multiple sclerosis on imaging studies. Its etiology is uncertain but most likely represents an autoimmune microangiopathy, not a demyelinating disorder.*

KEY FACTS

TERMINOLOGY

- Fibromuscular dysplasia (FMD)
  - Arterial disease of unknown etiology
  - Overgrowth of smooth muscle, fibrous tissue
  - Affects medium/large arteries

IMAGING

- Renal artery is most common overall site (~ 75%)
- Cervicocranial FMD (~ 70%)
  - Internal carotid artery (ICA) (30-50%) > external carotid artery > vertebral arteries (10-20%)
  - Carotid bifurcation is typically spared
  - > 50% of cases are bilateral
  - Intracranial rare (supraclinoid ICA, middle carotid artery)
- CTA
  - Arterial luminal irregularity or "beading" ± stenosis or aneurysm (rare)
- DWI-MR
  - Most sensitive for ischemic sequela of FMD
- DSA
  - Type 1 (85%): Classic "string of beads" = medial fibroplasia
  - Type 2 (10%): Long, tubular stenosis = intimal fibroplasia
  - Type 3 (5%): Asymmetric outpouching from 1 side of artery = periadventitial fibroplasia

TOP DIFFERENTIAL DIAGNOSES

- Atherosclerosis
- Standing waves
- Nonatherosclerotic vasculopathies

CLINICAL ISSUES

- Symptoms: hypertension, stroke, dissection
- Treatment
  - Antiplatelet ± anticoagulant Rx to reduce risk of thromboembolic sequela (stroke)
  - Balloon angioplasty
  - Covered stent, arterial reconstruction for aneurysm

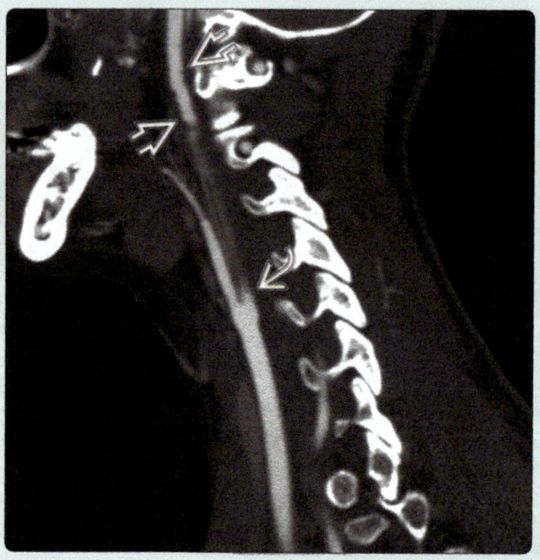

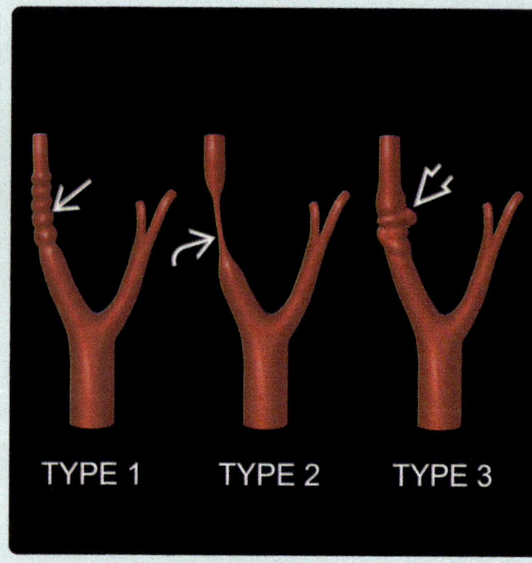

(Left) *Sagittal CTA shows classic fibromuscular dysplasia (FMD) in a 40-year-old woman following trauma. There is type I FMD in the cervical carotid artery with alternating areas of constriction and dilatation. C1-C2 is the most common location. Note the typical sparing of the carotid bulb.* **(Right)** *Carotid bifurcation shows principal subtypes of FMD. Type 1 appears as alternating areas of constriction and dilatation, type 2 as tubular stenosis, and type 3 as focal corrugations ± diverticulum.*

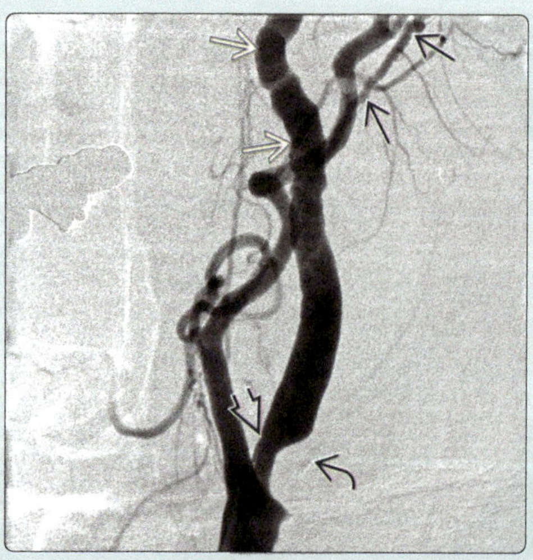

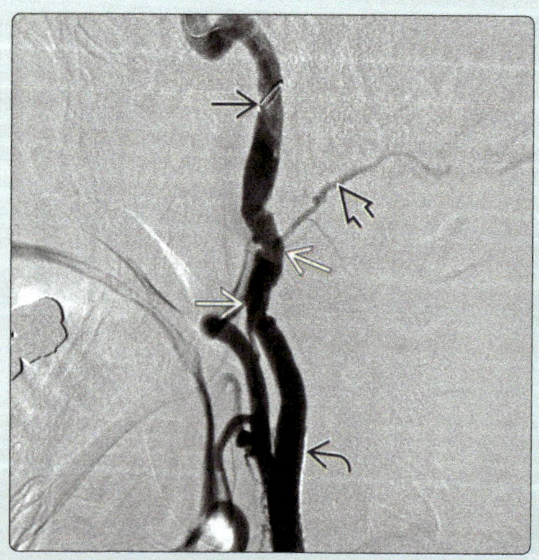

(Left) *Oblique DSA of the left carotid artery shows ASVD stenosis of the carotid bulb. Mural calcification is faint subtraction artifact. Superiorly, the internal carotid artery (ICA) shows luminal irregularity and beading, consistent with FMD. Additional FMD involvement of an external carotid artery branch is evident.* **(Right)** *Lateral DSA after carotid stenting across the ASVD stenosis shows a distal protection device in situ. Note the irregularity of the ICA and occipital artery due to FMD.*

KEY FACTS

TERMINOLOGY

- Internal carotid artery (ICA) dissection (ICAD)
- ICAD: Tear in ICA wall allows blood to enter & delaminate wall layers

IMAGING

- Pathognomonic findings of dissection: **Intimal flap** or **double lumen** (seen in < 10%)
- Aneurysmal dilatation seen in 30%
  - Commonly in distal subcranial segment of ICA
  - Focal pseudoaneurysm unusual
- Flame-shaped ICA occlusion (acute phase)
- ICAD most commonly originates in ICA 2-3 cm distal to carotid bulb & variably involves distal ICA
- Stops before petrous ICA
- MR T1 with fat suppression best sequence for **hyperintense mural hematomas**

TOP DIFFERENTIAL DIAGNOSES

- Fibromuscular dysplasia
- Carotid artery fenestration
- Traumatic ICA pseudoaneurysm
- Atheromatous plaque
- Glomus vagale paraganglioma
- Carotid space schwannoma

CLINICAL ISSUES

- Ipsilateral pain in face, jaw, head, or neck
- Oculosympathetic palsy (miosis and ptosis, partial Horner syndrome)
- Ischemic symptoms (cerebral or retinal TIA or stroke)
- Bruit (40%)
- Lower cranial nerve palsies (especially CN10)
- Pulsatile tinnitus

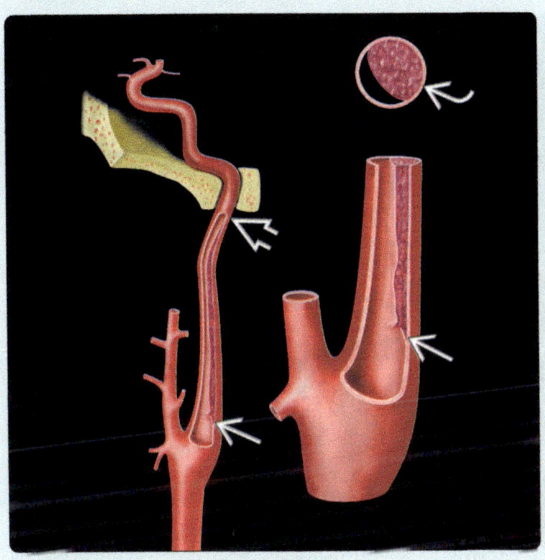
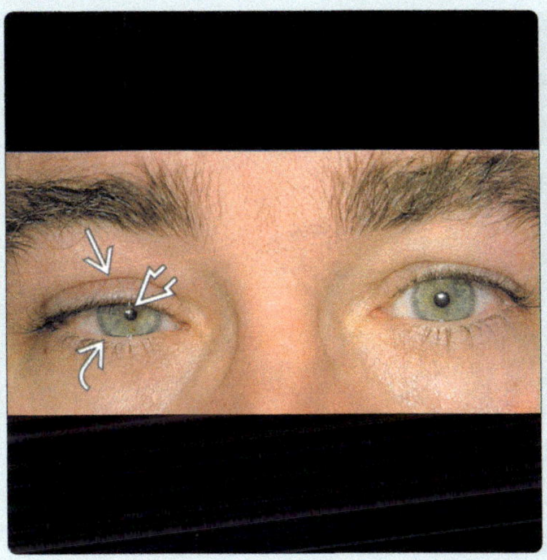

(Left) *Lateral graphic depicts typical internal carotid artery (ICA) dissection. Note dissection begins above bifurcation ➡ & ends at skull base ➡. Cross section of subintimal hematoma ➡ is also shown.* **(Right)** *Clinical photograph of a patient with an acute postganglionic Horner syndrome shows ptosis ➡, "upside-down" ptosis (lower lid is up ➡), and meiosis (constricted pupil ➡).*

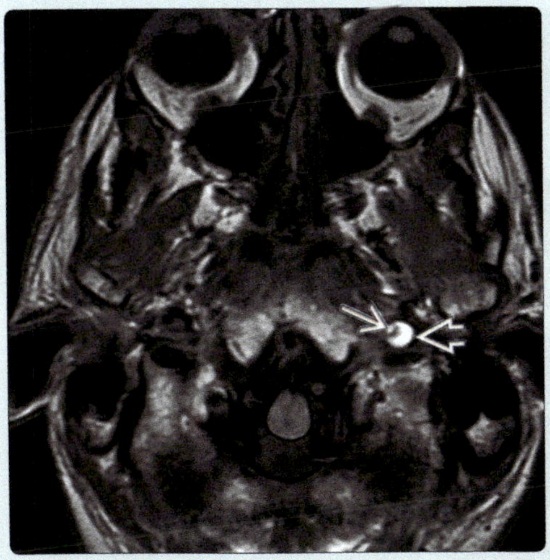
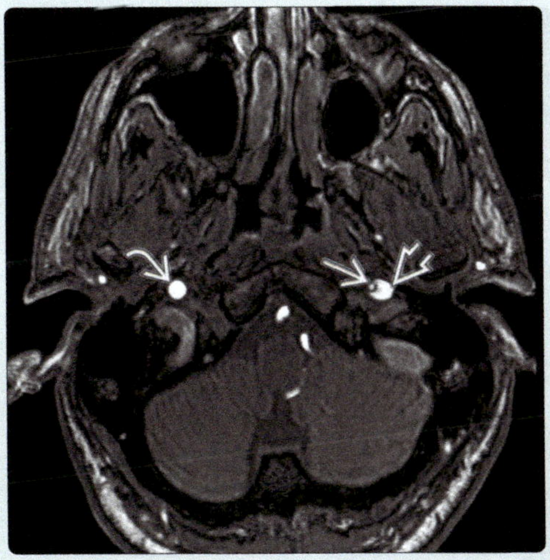

(Left) *Axial T1WI MR in a 47-year-old man who fell skiing 3 weeks prior to developing left frontotemporal headache shows T1 shortening within the crescentic subacute clot ➡ in the false lumen of the dissected left ICA. Note the high signal thrombus ➡ within the true lumen of the vessel, which was occluded.* **(Right)** *Axial MRA source image in the same patient shows the high signal thrombus in the false lumen ➡ as well as the thrombosed true lumen ➡. Compare to normal flow signal of the right ICA ➡.*

KEY FACTS

TERMINOLOGY

- Vertebral artery (VA) dissection
- Irregularity of VA contour from intimal tear or subadventitial hematoma

IMAGING

- **Stenoocclusive dissection**
  - Dissection to subintimal plane with vessel luminal narrowing or occlusion
- **Dissecting aneurysm**
  - Dissection into subadventitial plane with dilatation of outer wall
- Intramural hematoma is pathognomonic
  - Best seen as **bright crescent** on T1 FS MR
- CTA source images show contour changes of lumen
- Conventional angiography is gold standard

TOP DIFFERENTIAL DIAGNOSES

- Extracranial atherosclerosis
- Fibromuscular dysplasia
- Miscellaneous vasculitis
- Congenital VA hypoplasia

PATHOLOGY

- **Traumatic** VA dissection
  - Direct or indirect arterial injury
- **Spontaneous** VA dissection
  - Many associations and predisposing factors

CLINICAL ISSUES

- Age: Adults < 45 years

DIAGNOSTIC CHECKLIST

- Check other vessels carefully for 2nd dissection
- Subadvential/intramural hematoma can sometimes occur without narrowing vessel lumen
- Cerebellar infarction in young to middle-aged adults; need to exclude posterior inferior cerebellar artery infarction due to VA dissection

(Left) *Axial CECT in a patient with idiopathic vertebral artery dissection demonstrates normal caliber of left vertebral artery and narrowed, eccentric lumen of right vertebral artery. Note normal and symmetric foramina transversarium.* **(Right)** *Axial T1 FS MR in the same patient reveals a hyperintense crescent of mural hematoma with small hypointense patent lumen. Contralateral vertebral artery shows no methemoglobin hyperintensity. This is unilateral vertebral artery dissection.*

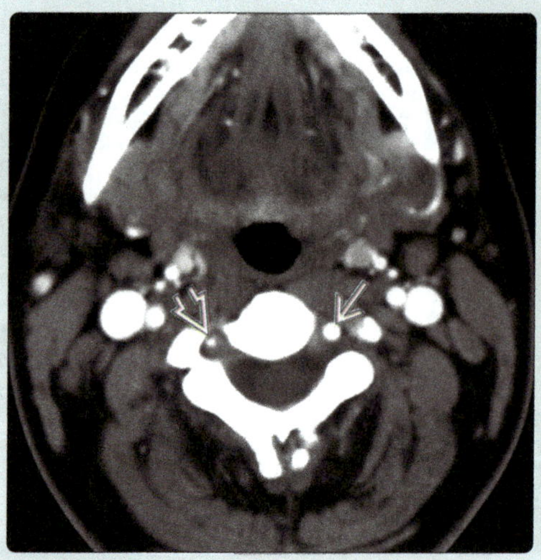

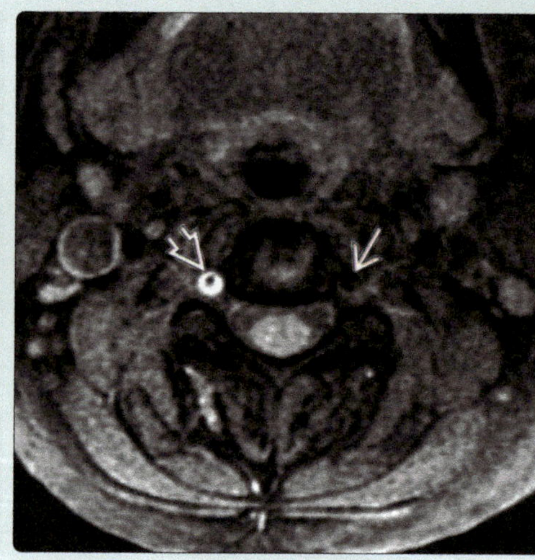

(Left) *Axial CTA shows rim enhancement of the left vertebral artery with low-density mural hematoma and contrast filling the narrowed lumen. Subtle linear lucency in the right vertebral artery proved not to be a dissection flap.* **(Right)** *Axial T2 MR in a patient with neck trauma and cervical fractures reveals traumatic vertebral artery dissection as loss of right vertebral flow void, compared with the normal left side. Note right cervical hemicord hyperintensity from cord ischemia.*

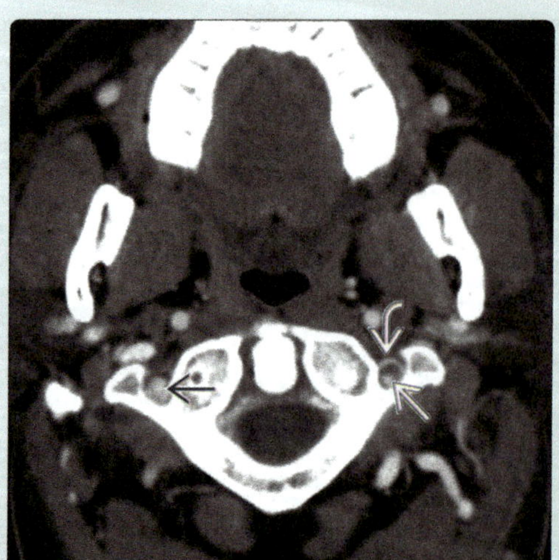

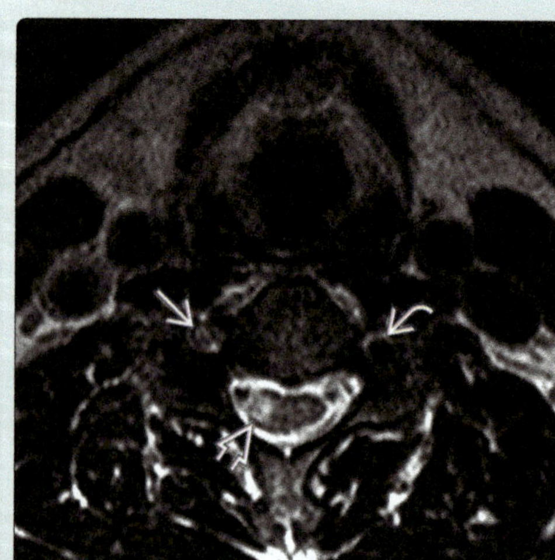

KEY FACTS

TERMINOLOGY

- Hypoxic ischemic injury (HII): Global hypoxic ischemic injury, global anoxic injury, cerebral hypoperfusion injury
  - Etiologies: Cardiac arrest, cerebrovascular disease, drowning, asphyxiation

IMAGING

- Injury patterns highly variable depending on brain maturity, severity, and length of insult
  - Mild to moderate: Watershed zone infarcts
  - Severe: Gray matter structures (basal ganglia, thalami, cortex, cerebellum, hippocampi)
- MR best to assess overall extent of injury within hours after HII event
  - DWI: 1st modality to be positive (within hours)
  - DWI: Restriction in deep nuclei ± cortex
  - T2/FLAIR: ↑ signal in cerebellum, basal ganglia, cortex
  - Acute changes not reliably identified with T2
- MRS: More sensitive and indicative of severity of injury in first 24 hours after HII
  - ↑ lactate, ↑ glutamine-glutamate

TOP DIFFERENTIAL DIAGNOSES

- Ischemic territorial infarction
- Traumatic cerebral edema
- Toxic/metabolic disorder
- Acute hypertensive encephalopathy, posterior reversible encephalopathy syndrome (PRES)
- Creutzfeldt-Jakob disease
- MELAS

PATHOLOGY

- Common underlying process regardless of cause
  - ↓ cerebral blood flow and ↓ blood oxygenation
  - Switch from oxidative phosphorylation to anaerobic metabolism
  - Glutamate-related cytotoxic processes

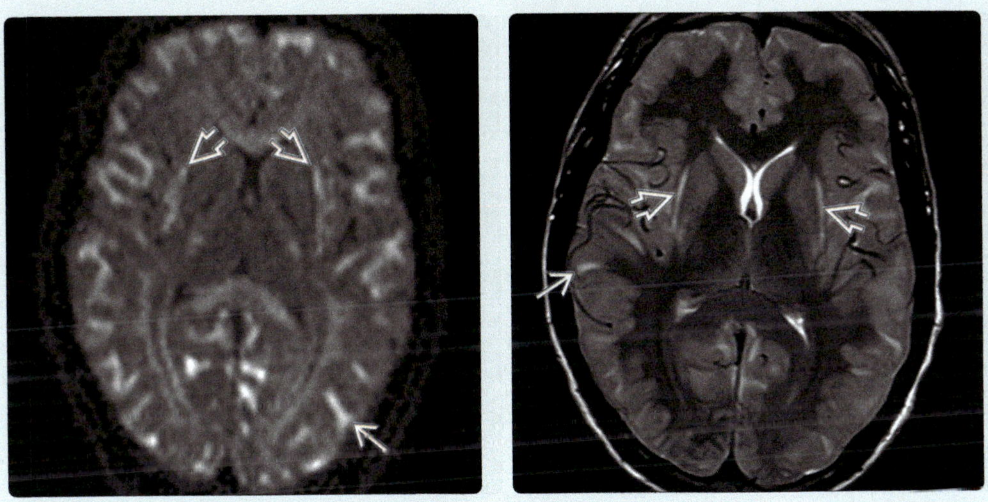

(Left) *Axial DTI trace image in a 21-year-old unresponsive man shows extensive hyperintensity related to cytotoxic edema throughout the cortex and subcortical WM ➡ as well as the external capsules ➡ in this patient with severe hypoxic ischemic injury (HII).* **(Right)** *Axial T2 MR in the same patient shows hyperintensity throughout the cortex, subcortical WM ➡ and the external capsules ➡. Complete effacement of the sulci is related to gyral swelling. Involvement of the visual and sensorimotor cortex is common in severe HII.*

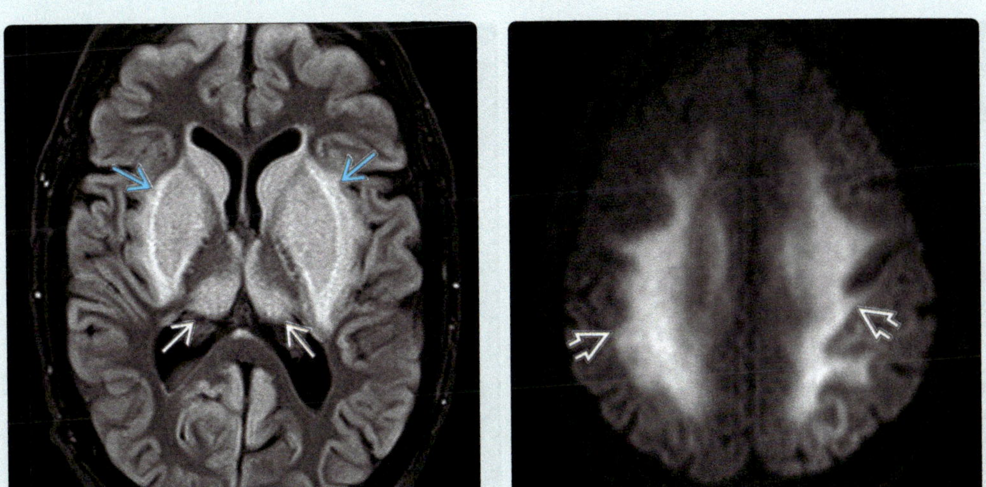

(Left) *Axial FLAIR MR shows symmetric hyperintensity of the basal ganglia → and thalami ➡ in this patient status post cardiac arrest. T2 and FLAIR images typically become positive in the early subacute period (> 24 hours to 2 weeks) with increased signal and swelling of the injured GM structures.* **(Right)** *Axial DTI trace shows extensive WM hyperintensity ➡ related to cytotoxic edema in this 43-year-old woman with mild to moderate HII. DWI signal abnormalities may pseudonormalize by the end of the 1st week.*

Hypotensive Cerebral Infarction

KEY FACTS

TERMINOLOGY

- Hypotensive cerebral infarction (HCI)
  - Infarction resulting from insufficient cerebral blood flow (CBF) to meet metabolic demands (low-flow state)
  - 2 types of border zone or watershed infarcts
    - Border zone between major arterial territories
      - Typically at cortex, gray matter (GM)-white matter (WM) junctions
    - Border zone between perforating arteries
      - Typically in deep WM

IMAGING

- Best imaging tool
  - MR with DWI/ADC ± MR perfusion
- Cortical border zone
  - Between major arterial territories
  - Typically at GM-WM matter junctions
  - Hypodensity between vascular territories
- WM matter border zone
  - Between perforating arteries
  - Typically in deep WM (centrum semiovale)
  - ≥ 3 lesions
  - Linear AP orientation → string of pearls appearance
  - If unilateral, look for stenosis of major vessel
- Imaging recommendations
  - MR + GRE, DWI, MRA (both cervical, intracranial)
  - ± pMR (may show ↓ CBF to affected areas)
  - NECT, pCT, CTA if MR not available
  - CTA/DSA > MRA for determining total vs. near occlusion of internal carotid artery

TOP DIFFERENTIAL DIAGNOSES

- Acute embolic cerebral infarction(s)
- Arteriosclerosis ("small vessel disease")
- Posterior reversible encephalopathy (PRES)
- Vasculitis
- Pseudolaminar necrosis (other causes, e.g., Reye, lupus, etc.)

(Left) *T1WI show 2 watershed (WS) zones. External WS zones are depicted in turquoise. Yellow lines indicate internal (deep white matter) watershed zones between perforating arteries and major territorial vessels.* **(Right)** *Axial gross pathology shows classic external (cortical) watershed infarcts ➡ from cerebral hypoperfusion. The patient survived several days, allowing for petechial hemorrhagic transformation to occur.*

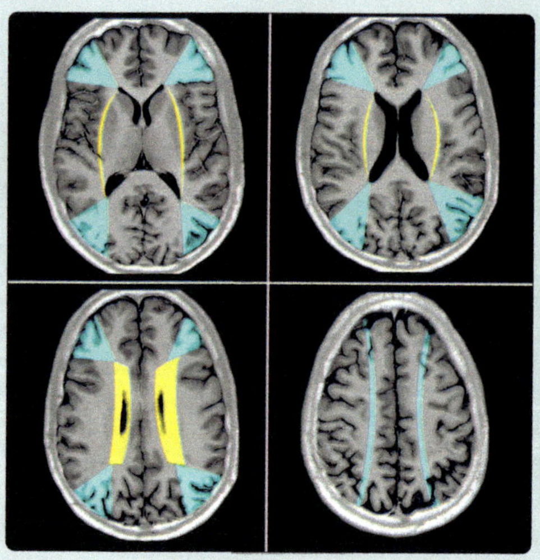

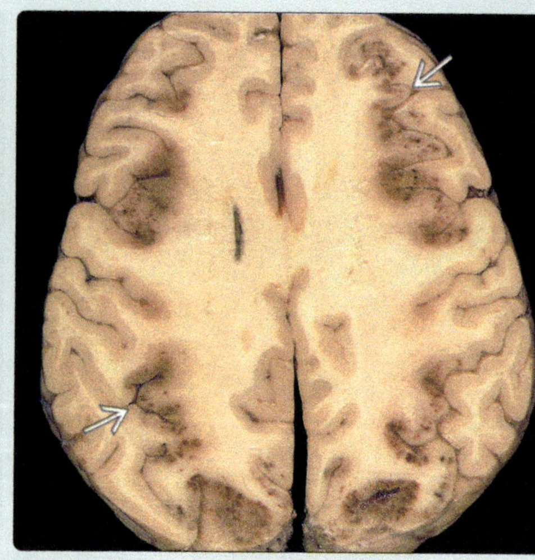

(Left) *Axial FLAIR MR in a patient with transient global hypoperfusion secondary to a hypotensive episode shows multifocal hyperintensities along the cortical WS zone ➡. Changes are most severe at the confluence of the anterior cerebral, posterior cerebral, and middle cerebral artery cortical vascular territories ➡.* **(Right)** *DWI in the same patient shows corresponding areas of restricted diffusion in the cortical WS zones bilaterally ➡, most severe at the trivascular confluence ➡. The diagnosis was hypotensive WS cerebral infarctions.*

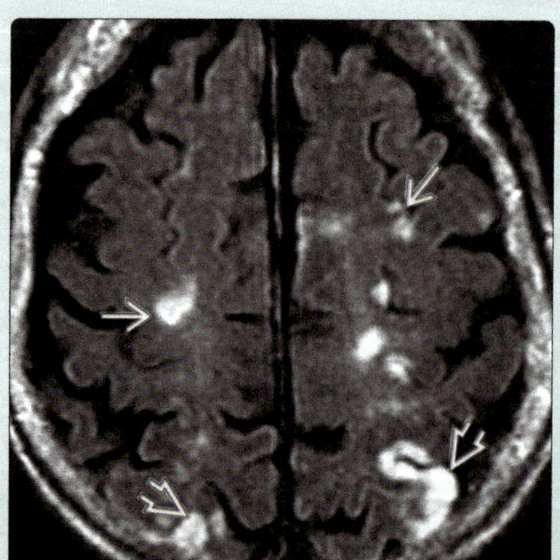

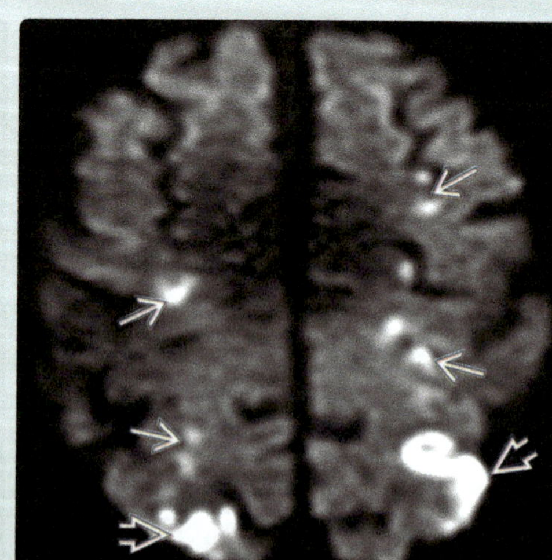

KEY FACTS

TERMINOLOGY

- Acute alteration of neurologic function due to loss of vascular integrity

IMAGING

- Best imaging
  - MR with diffusion, perfusion, MRA
  - MRV if MRA negative and DWI positive
  - Can do emergent "limited" MR (FLAIR, DWI, SWI)
- Imaging findings
  - CT
    - Insular-ribbon sign = loss of distinction of insular cortex
    - Hyperdense MCA sign = increased density of thrombosed MCA
    - Look for calcified emboli (suggests heart disease)
    - ± CTA
  - MR
    - DWI is most sensitive imaging sequence for ischemic injury
    - Perfusion studies can identify ischemic penumbra
    - FLAIR may show intravascular signal
    - Arterial wall imaging may identify vasculopathy

PATHOLOGY

- Etiology
  - Most common: Cardiac disease (25-50%)
  - Other: Sickle cell (200-400x increased risk), trauma
  - No underlying cause discovered in > 33% of cases

CLINICAL ISSUES

- Under-recognized as significant source of morbidity in pediatric population
  - Can be mistaken for seizure (postictal), migraine
  - Children with stroke often have delayed presentation
  - High risk of recurrence (20-40%), especially with calcified emboli

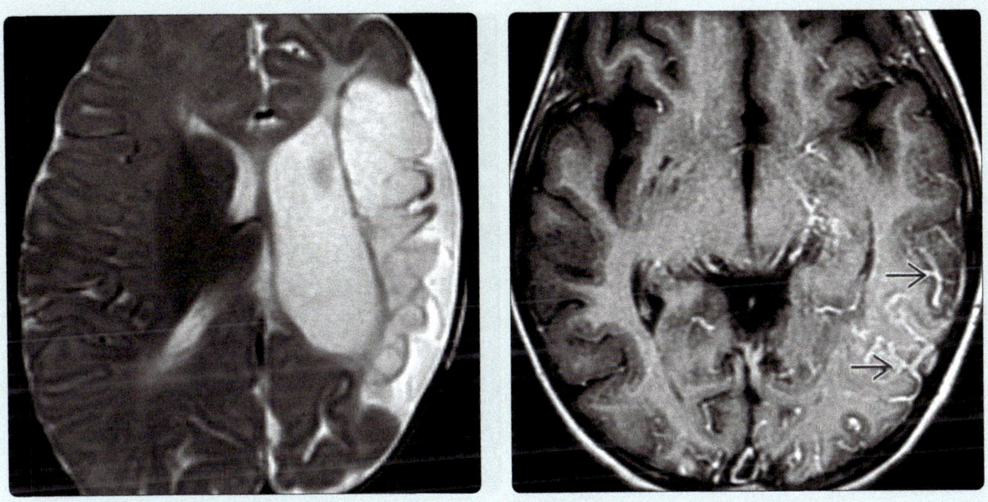

(Left) *Axial T2WI MR shows mature encephalomalacia in the vascular territory of the left MCA in this 4-month-old infant with left hand preference. Handedness should not be apparent before 12-18 months.* **(Right)** *Axial T1WI C+ MR shows the characteristic climbing-ivy sign of enhancing sulcal arteries ➡ in a child with moyamoya vasculopathy secondary to sickle cell disease. Slow flow in MCA branches distal to the stenosis allows T1 shortening from contrast to overcome flow void effects.*

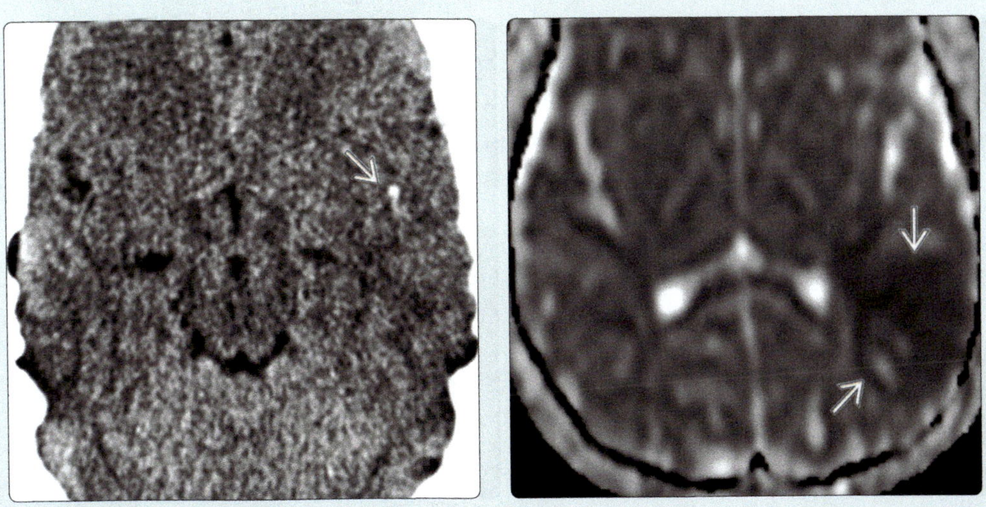

(Left) *Axial NECT in 15 year old with difficulty speaking and right hand weakness shows a hyperdense MCA ➡. The patient presented 12 hours after symptom onset and was treated with aspirin only.* **(Right)** *Axial ADC in the same teenager shows reduced diffusion ➡ in the distal left middle carotid artery territory. Encephalomalacia developed, but the patient had a normal neurologic exam 6 months later. Children often have a much greater capacity for neurologic recovery than adults, even with similar imaging findings.*

KEY FACTS

TERMINOLOGY

- Interrupted blood flow to brain resulting in cerebral ischemia/infarction with variable neurologic deficit

IMAGING

- Major artery (territorial) infarct
  - Generally wedge-shaped; both GM and WM involved
- Embolic infarcts
  - Often focal/small, at GM-WM interface
- NECT
  - Hyperdense vessel = clot (dense middle cerebral artery sign)
  - Loss of GM-WM distinction in first 3 hours (50-70%)
    - Insular-ribbon sign: GM-WM interface lost
    - Disappearing basal ganglia sign
  - Calcified embolus
    - Do not miss this (high risk of recurrent stroke)
- CTA: Excellent for major vessel occlusions
- pCT: CBF/CBV "mismatch" estimates penumbra
- MR
  - Parenchymal ± intraarterial FLAIR hyperintensity
  - ↑ intensity on DWI with corresponding ↓ on apparent diffusion coefficient
  - ↓ cerebral blood flow (CBF), cerebral blood volume on perfusion MR

TOP DIFFERENTIAL DIAGNOSES

- Normal vessel (MCA normally slightly hyperdense to brain)
- Nonvascular causes of hypodense brain (neoplasm, cerebritis, etc.)

PATHOLOGY

- Severely ischemic core; CBF < (6-8 cm^3)/(100 g/min)
- Peripheral penumbra; CBF between (10-20 cm^3)/(100 g/min)

CLINICAL ISSUES

- 2nd most common cause of death worldwide
- Rx: IV thrombolysis (< 3 hours of onset), clot retrieval

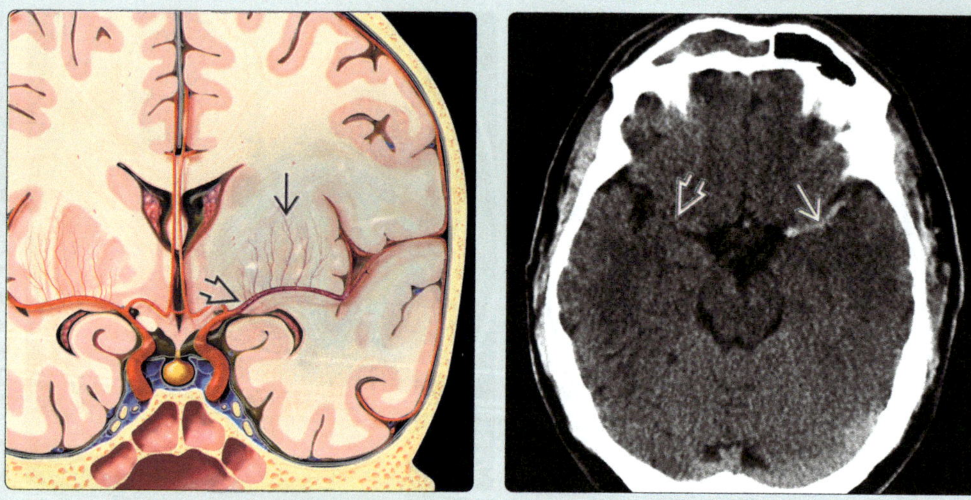

(Left) *Coronal graphic illustrates left M1 occlusion. Proximal occlusion ⇨ affects the entire middle cerebral artery (MCA) territory, including the basal ganglia (perfused by lenticulostriate arteries →). Acute ischemia is often identified by subtle loss of the gray-white interfaces with blurring of the basal ganglia and an insular-ribbon sign on the initial CT.* **(Right)** *NECT scan in a 46-year-old man shows a very dense left MCA → compared with the normal minimally hyperdense right MCA ⇨.*

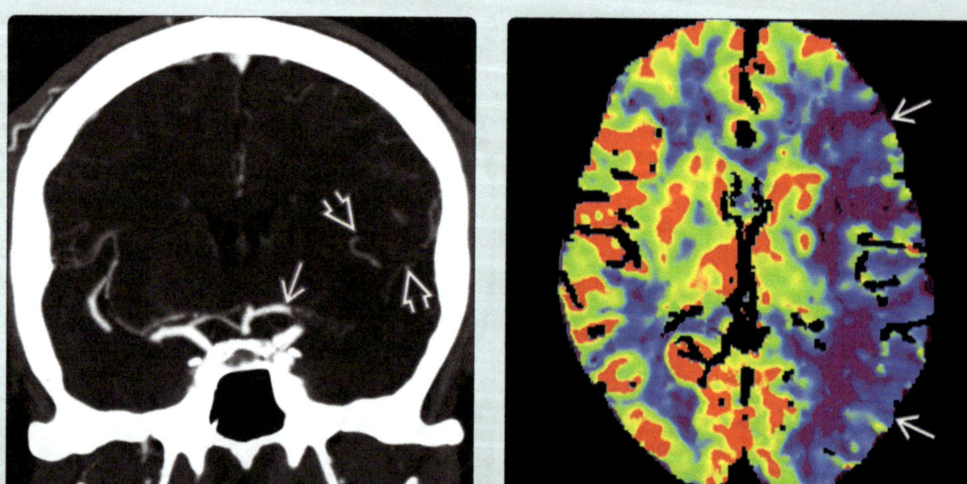

(Left) *Coronal maximal intensity projection view of the CTA in the same patient shows a proximal left MCA occlusion →. Minimal filling of the distal MCA branches ⇨ is occurring via collaterals from the anterior cerebral artery and posterior cerebral artery.* **(Right)** *Axial CT perfusion shows decreased cerebral blood flow in the left MCA distribution →.*

KEY FACTS

TERMINOLOGY

- Subacute infarction ~ 2-14 days following initial ischemic event

IMAGING

- Best diagnostic clue: Gyral edema and enhancement within basal ganglia and cortex
- Typically wedge-shaped abnormality involving gray and white matter within vascular distribution
- Hemorrhagic transformation of initially ischemic infarction occurs in 20-25% of middle cerebral artery occlusions, usually by 48-72 h
- "2-2-2" rule = enhancement begins at 2 days, peaks at 2 weeks, disappears by 2 months
- MRS: ↑ lactate, ↓ NAA within infarcted tissue
- DWI: ↑ diffusion restriction, ↓ ADC initially, reversing as it proceeds into/through subacute stage
- "Fogging" effect = normal T2WI with striking enhancement on T1WI C+ 1-2 weeks following ictus

TOP DIFFERENTIAL DIAGNOSES

- Neoplasm
- Venous infarction
- Encephalitis/cerebritis

CLINICAL ISSUES

- Acute-onset focal neurologic deficit
- Elderly patient with typical risk factors: Hypertension, diabetes, smoking history, obesity, hypercholesterolemia
- 1st month after infarction, mortality predominantly from neurologic complications; 1:4 die of recurrent stroke event
- Acute anticoagulation after 1st infarction reduces mortality

DIAGNOSTIC CHECKLIST

- Enhancement is key to defining subacute stage of cerebral infarction
- Subacute ischemia often mimics neoplasm
    - Recommend short-term follow-up to ensure expected course of evolution

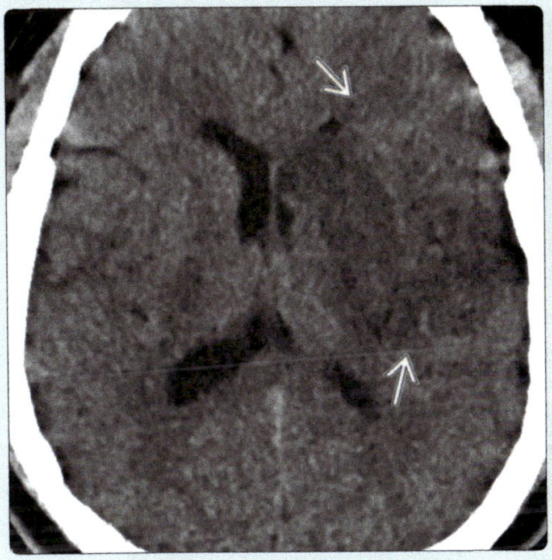

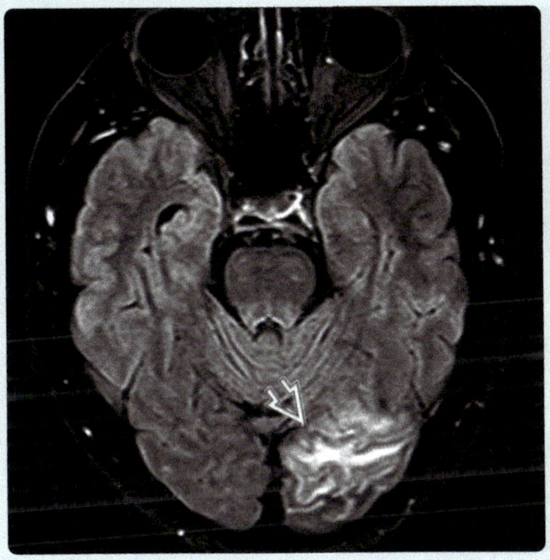

(Left) *Axial CT obtained 48 h after initial onset of weakness and speech difficulties shows the classic appearance of an early subacute cerebral infarct. Note the wedge-shaped, low-density area ➡ involving both the gray and white matter in the left middle cerebral artery distribution.* **(Right)** *Axial FLAIR MR in a 58-year-old man 1 week after onset of visual changes shows classic imaging of a subacute infarct with hyperintensity in the cortex and subcortical WM of the occipital lobe ➡ in a posterior cerebral artery (PCA) distribution.*

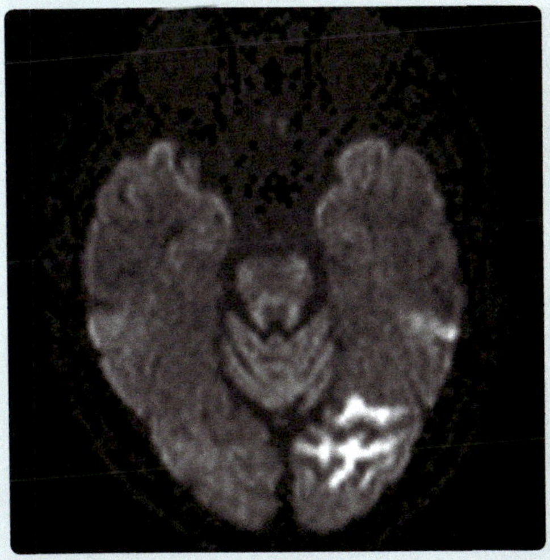

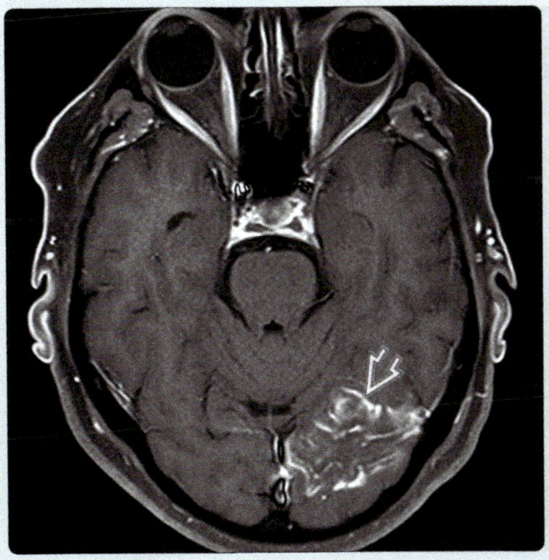

(Left) *Axial DWI in the same patient shows hyperintensity within the left PCA distribution. The hyperintensity represents a combination of true diffusion restriction and T2 shine through.* **(Right)** *Axial T1 C+ MR in the same patient shows gyriform enhancement along the cortex of the occipital lobe ➡. This enhancement may be seen as early as 2 days and may last up to 2 months after the patient's initial ischemic event. Without clinical history, imaging may mimic a tumor, venous infarct, or cerebritis.*

Chronic Cerebral Infarction

KEY FACTS

IMAGING

- Volume loss with gliosis along affected margins
- Classic: Wedge-shaped area of encephalomalacia
- Territorial infarction
  - Involves brain supplied by major cerebral artery
- Watershed infarction
  - Involves brain **between** main vascular territories
- Lacunar infarction(s)
  - Most common in basal ganglia/thalami, deep white matter

TOP DIFFERENTIAL DIAGNOSES

- Porencephalic cyst
- Arachnoid cyst
- Postsurgical/posttraumatic encephalomalacia
- Low-attenuating tumors

PATHOLOGY

- Volume loss, gliosis are pathological hallmarks

CLINICAL ISSUES

- Elderly patient with typical risk factors
- Focal neurologic deficit
  - Varies depending on size, location of cerebral infarction
- Stroke severity most consistent predictor of 30-day mortality after stroke
- Lacunar stroke most common stroke subtype associated with vascular dementia

DIAGNOSTIC CHECKLIST

- Evaluate for associated acute infarcts in same or different vascular territory
- Evaluate for underlying cause
  - CTA/MRA of extra-/intracranial vasculature
  - If negative, consider cardiac source
- Evaluate for risk factors

(Left) *Axial graphic shows chronic infarct involving the posterior left middle cerebral artery (MCA) territory. Infarct is lined with gliotic WM. Small lacunar infarctions and atrophy also depicted.* **(Right)** *Axial gross pathology, sectioned through the midventricular level, shows a chronic left MCA infarct with encephalomalacia in the classic MCA vascular distribution →. Note the adjacent WM gliosis ⇨ and the mild compensatory enlargement of the left lateral ventricle ↷. (Courtesy R. Hewlett, MD.)*

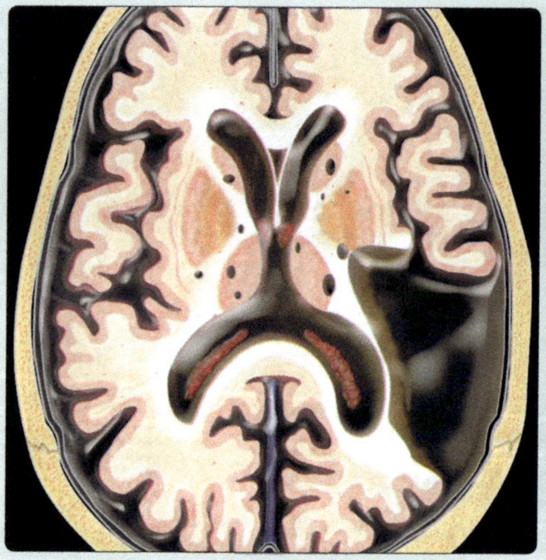

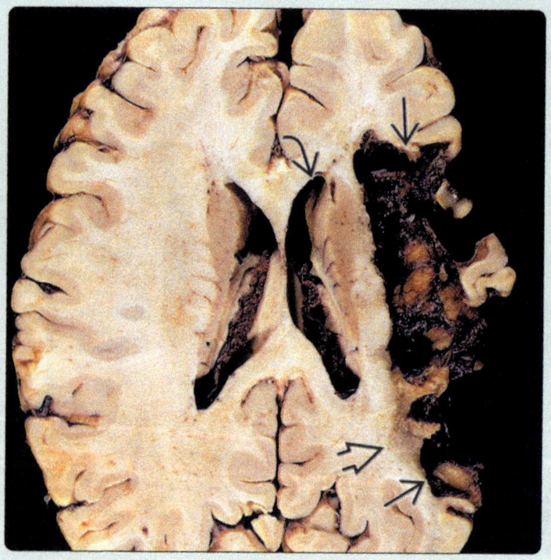

(Left) *Axial NECT scan 2 days after large territorial infarction in the left MCA territory shows wedge-shaped hypodensity → involving both cortex, WM, and basal ganglia. Moderate mass effect is present, with subfalcine herniation of the lateral ventricles.* **(Right)** *Follow-up scan 2 months later shows findings of chronic infarct. The mass effect has resolved completely, and there is frank encephalomalacia in the left MCA territory →. The left lateral ventricle shows compensatory enlargement ⇨.*

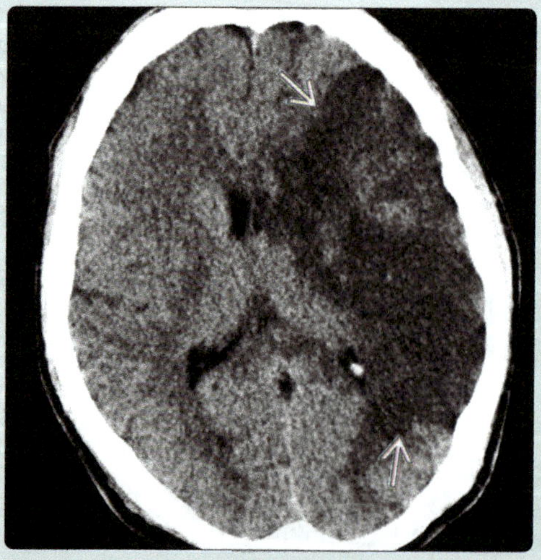

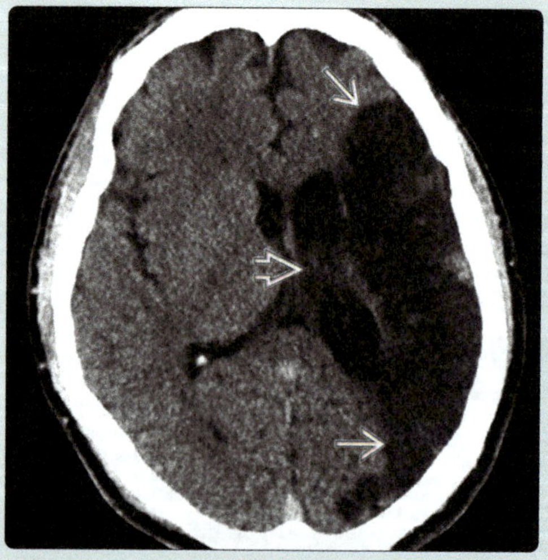

Multiple Embolic Cerebral Infarctions

KEY FACTS

TERMINOLOGY

- Infarcts in multiple arterial distributions from embolic source, often cardiac origin

IMAGING

- Best imaging clue: DWI restriction in multiple vascular distributions
- NECT: Multiple regions of low attenuation, loss of gray-white differentiation
- T2/FLAIR: Multiple supratentorial and infratentorial regions of hyperintensity, often in vascular distribution
  - May be of different ages
- Embolic infarcts tend to involve terminal cortical branches, producing wedge-shaped infarcts
- Cardiac echocardiography may show valve vegetations, intracardiac filling defect, or atrial or ventricular septal defect
- Best imaging tool: MR with DWI, FLAIR, T1WI C+

TOP DIFFERENTIAL DIAGNOSES

- Hypotensive cerebral infarction
- Multiple sclerosis
- Parenchymal metastases
- Vasculitis

CLINICAL ISSUES

- Multiple focal neurologic complaints not conforming to singular vascular distribution
- Peripheral signs of emboli, such as splinter hemorrhages or paradoxical emboli
- Cardiac source most common etiology of multiple embolic infarcts
  - May be septic or benign
- Carotid artery disease may cause multiple embolic infarct, if associated with variant posterior cerebral artery origin
- Cardiac and vascular evaluation → treat underlying disease

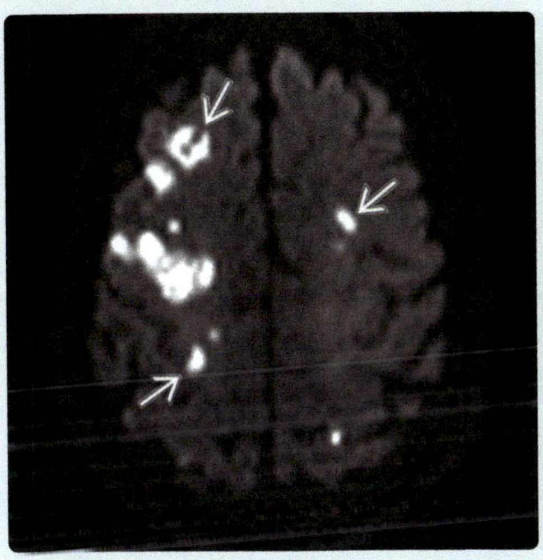

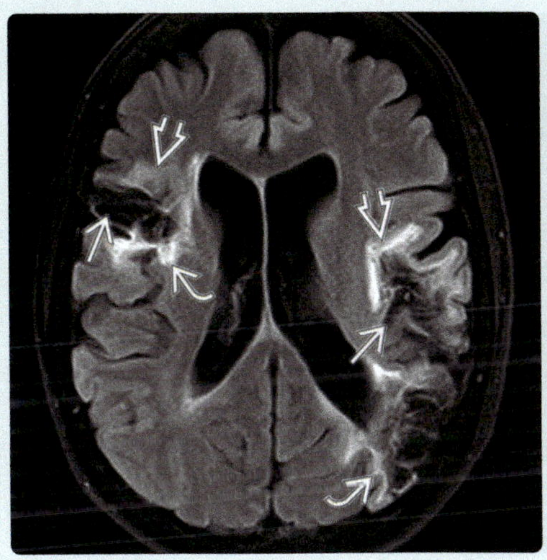

(Left) *Axial DTI trace image shows multiple regions of diffusion hyperintensity ➡ related to acute middle cerebral artery (MCA) distribution ischemia in bilateral hemispheres in a patient with embolic disease from a cardiac source.* **(Right)** *Axial FLAIR MR shows bilateral chronic MCA distribution ischemia ➡ related to untreated atrial fibrillation. Note the areas of encephalomalacia ➡ with surrounding gliosis ➡, typical of chronic ischemia.*

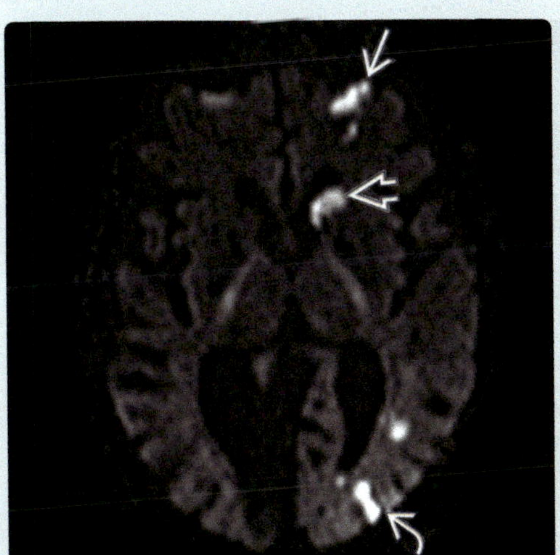

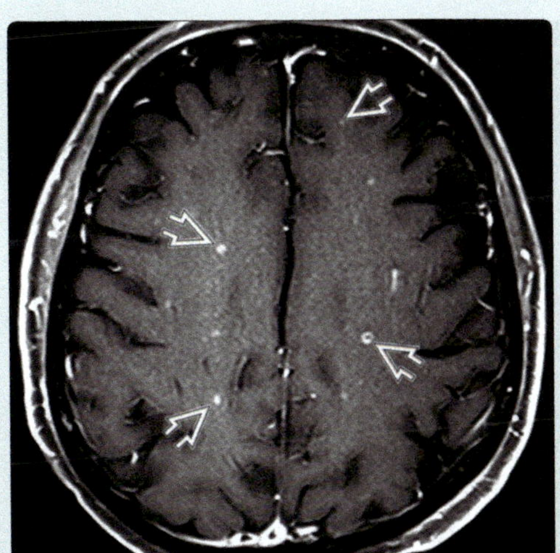

(Left) *Axial DTI trace shows acute ischemia in the left hemisphere in multiple vascular distributions. Note the involvement of the recurrent artery of Heubner from the ACA distribution (head of caudate) ➡, as well as the MCA ➡ and PCA ➡ territories, in this patient with severe internal carotid artery atherosclerotic disease and a fetal origin PCA.* **(Right)** *Axial T1 C+ FS MR shows multiple foci of enhancement ➡ in bilateral hemispheres related to septic emboli in a patient with cardiac valve vegetations.*

KEY FACTS

TERMINOLOGY

- Acute stroke related to fat emboli

IMAGING

- Acute ischemia with appropriate clinical history
  - Long bone or pelvic fractures, cardiac surgery, joint replacement surgery
- Often mimics thromboembolic stroke
- Commonly affects both gray and white matter
  - May affect deep and periventricular white matter
  - May affect deep gray nuclei
- May involve typical vascular territory
- May mimic "watershed" infarct
- NECT: Typically negative acutely
  - Hypodense MCA sign related to fat within MCA
- T2WI: Multiple small, scattered hyperintense foci
- DWI: Acute diffusion restriction

TOP DIFFERENTIAL DIAGNOSES

- Acute cerebral ischemia-infarction
- Acute hypertensive encephalopathy, PRES
- Vasculitis

PATHOLOGY

- Fat emboli can pass through pulmonary capillaries without shunting lesions and result in systemic embolization (brain, kidneys most commonly)

CLINICAL ISSUES

- Fat embolism syndrome: Pulmonary, CNS, and cutaneous manifestations
  - Hypoxia, deteriorating mental status, petechiae
- Neurological dysfunction varies from confusion to encephalopathy with coma and seizures
- Uncommon but potentially life threatening
- Fat embolism syndrome after fractures: Up to 2.2%

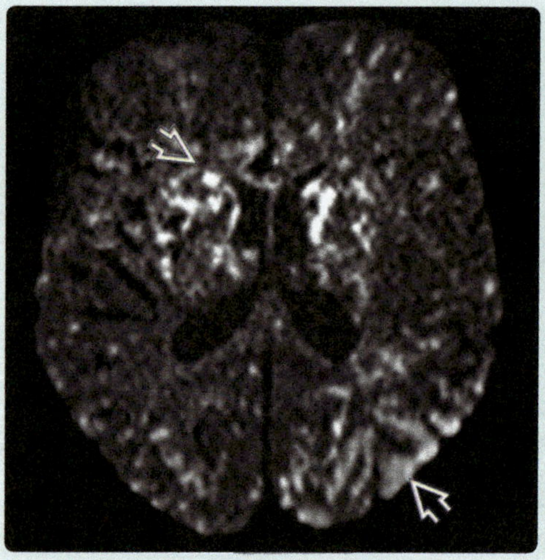
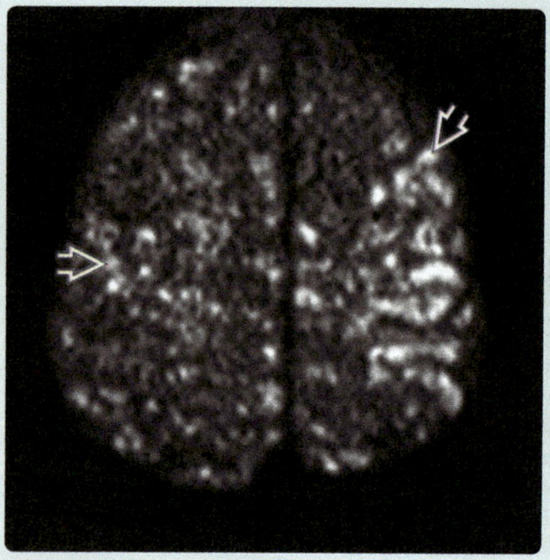

(Left) *Axial DWI MR shows innumerable punctate foci of restriction ➡ throughout the white matter and gray matter of this 68-year-old patient with mental status changes post hip surgery. Note the extensive involvement of the basal ganglia and thalami.* **(Right)** *Axial DWI in the same patient shows the extensive foci of restriction ➡ related to acute ischemia from the patient's fat emboli. Note the more focal involvement of the left middle carotid artery territory with frontal and temporal lobe involvement.*

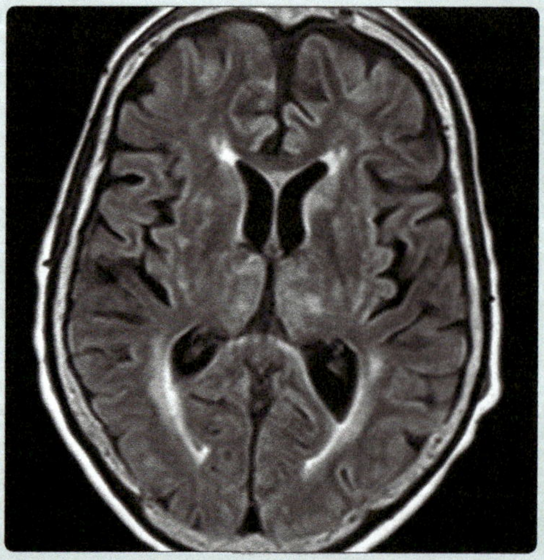
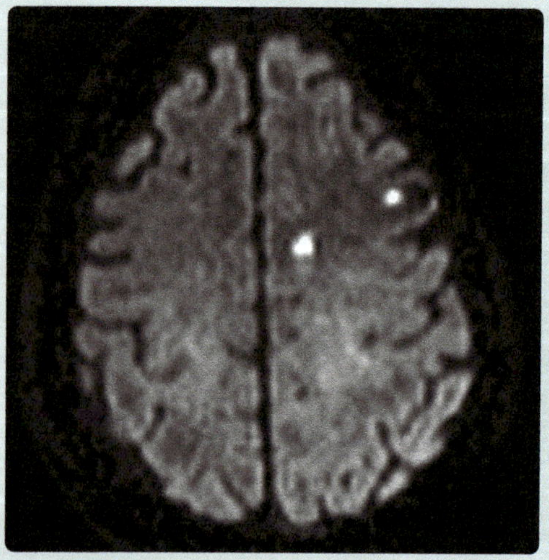

(Left) *Axial FLAIR MR in the same patient shows minimal abnormal hyperintensities in the deep gray nuclei and periventricular white matter. Diffusion imaging is the most sensitive sequence for acute stroke imaging.* **(Right)** *Axial DTI trace shows 2 punctate foci of restriction related to fat emboli in this 39-year-old trauma patient with bilateral acetabular fractures. DTI may be more sensitive than DWI in acute ischemia. Imaging of fat emboli often mimics a typical thromboembolic stroke.*

Lacunar Infarction

KEY FACTS

TERMINOLOGY

- Small, deep cerebral infarcts located in basal ganglia and thalamus, pons, or cerebral white matter (WM), ≤ 15 mm

IMAGING

- Commonly deep gray nuclei, especially putamen, thalamus, caudate nuclei; internal capsule, pons
    - Other locations include deep and periventricular WM
- Range in size from microscopic to 15 mm
- Because of small size, most acute lacunar infarcts are not seen on CTs
- Acute: T2/FLAIR increased signal
- Chronic: FLAIR central low signal with increased peripheral signal (gliosis)
- DWI: Restricted diffusion (hyperintense) if acute/subacute
    - May show small lesions otherwise undetectable
- Prominent perivascular spaces are main imaging differential diagnosis

PATHOLOGY

- Embolic, atheromatous, or thrombotic lesions in long, single-penetrating-end arterioles supplying deep cerebral gray matter
- Size of lacunar infarct depends on level of occlusion and anatomy of affected vessel

CLINICAL ISSUES

- Many different presentations, depending on size, location, number
- Most lacunar infarctions are clinically "silent," often subtle neurological deficits that may go unnoticed by patient and physician
- Typical risk factors for cerebrovascular disease: Hypertension, diabetes, smoking history, obesity, hypercholesterolemia, etc.
- Lacunar infarcts account for up to 25% of all strokes
- Lacunar stroke is most common stroke subtype associated with vascular dementia

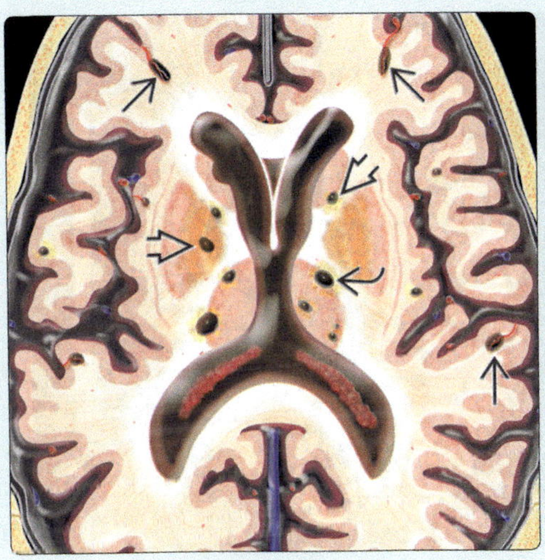

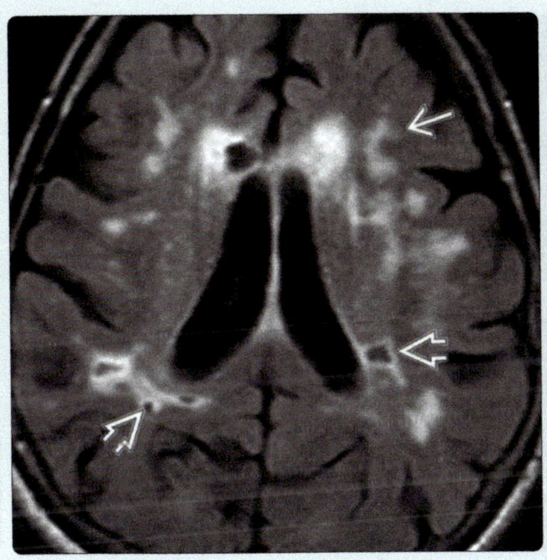

(Left) *Axial graphic illustrates numerous bilateral lacunar infarcts within the thalami ⇨ and basal ganglia ⇨, the most common locations. Also shown are prominent perivascular (Virchow-Robin) spaces ⇨, a common normal variant.* **(Right)** *Axial FLAIR MR shows multiple chronic lacunar infarcts in the periventricular white matter ➡ with central hypointense encephalomalacia and mild peripheral hyperintense gliosis in a patient with chronic hypertension. Note the hyperintensity ➡ related to chronic small vessel ischemia.*

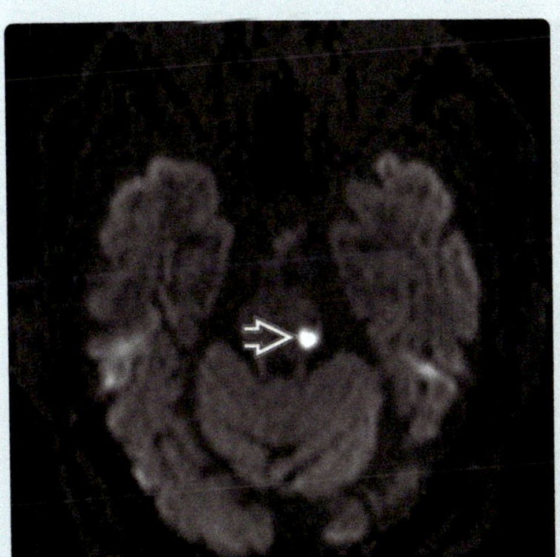

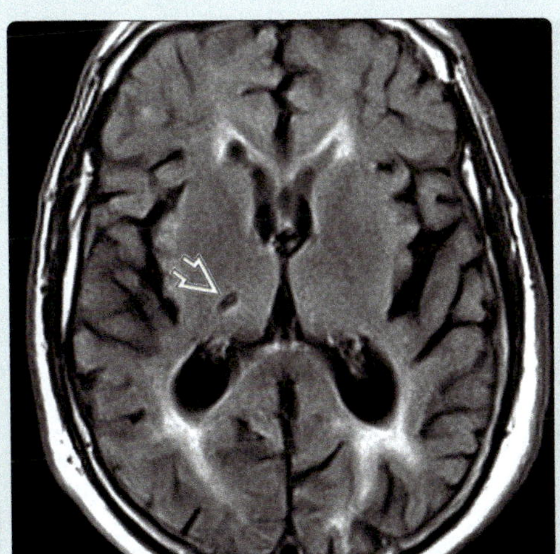

(Left) *Axial DWI MR shows focal diffusion hyperintensity ➡ related to an acute lacunar infarct in the pons, a common location for lacunar infarcts. Risk factors for lacunar infarcts include hypertension, diabetes, smoking history, obesity, and hypercholesterolemia.* **(Right)** *Axial FLAIR MR shows a chronic lacunar infarct in the right thalamus ➡ with central encephalomalacia and mild peripheral gliosis. The surrounding gliosis and typical location can help differentiate a chronic lacunar infarct from a perivascular space.*

KEY FACTS

TERMINOLOGY

- Rare (1-3%) disorder most commonly occurring as complication of cerebral revascularization
  - Other etiologies less common
    - Status epilepticus
    - MELAS
- Major increase in ipsilateral cerebral blood flow (CBF) well above normal metabolic demands

IMAGING

- Ipsilateral gyral swelling, sulcal effacement in post-carotid endarterectomy (CEA) patient
- ↑ CBF, CBV on perfusion MR, perfusion CT

TOP DIFFERENTIAL DIAGNOSES

- Acute cerebral ischemia-infarction
- Status epilepticus
- MELAS
- Acute hypertensive encephalopathy, PRES
- Hypercapnia

PATHOLOGY

- Cerebral hyperperfusion syndrome (CHS) probably caused by maladaptive autoregulatory mechanisms, altered cerebral hemodynamics
  - Normal perfusion pressure breakthrough
  - Rapid restoration of normal perfusion following revascularization → hyperperfusion in previously underperfused brain

CLINICAL ISSUES

- ~ 3% of post-CEA patients develop CHS
- Classic: Triad of unilateral headache, neurologic deficit, & seizures
  - Variable cognitive impairment; ipsilateral face, eye pain

DIAGNOSTIC CHECKLIST

- Need to distinguish stroke/TIA from CHS

(Left) *A 56-year-old man with > 70% stenosis of proximal left cervical ICA underwent carotid endarterectomy. A few hours after surgery, he became acutely confused and developed right-sided weakness; perfusion source image shows markedly increased vasculature in the left hemisphere* ⇨. **(Right)** *CT perfusion obtained in the same patient appears relatively normal, but cerebral blood flow on the left (as measured by circled regions of interest 2a, 2b) increased compared to the right side (1a, 1b).*

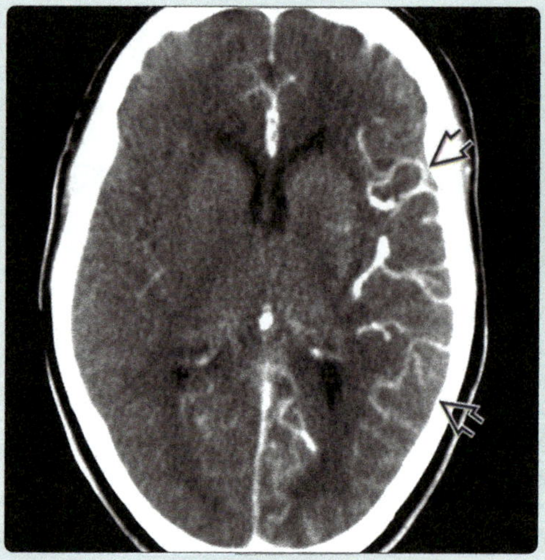

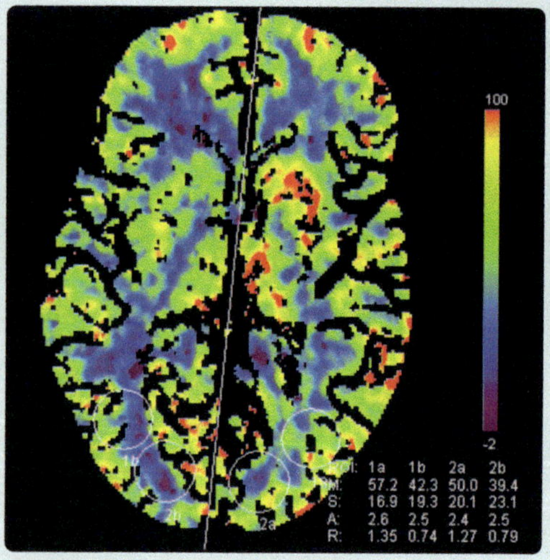

(Left) *Time to peak (TTP) in the same patient is even more striking. The abnormal side is not the right middle carotid artery distribution (green) but is the left side* ➡ *(blue), where the TTP is markedly shortened.* **(Right)** *Axial T2WI in the same patient shows gyral swelling, sulcal effacement, and hyperintensity in the left temporal and parietooccipital cortex/subcortical white matter* ➡, *basal ganglia* ⇨. *DWI (not shown) was normal. This is a classic example of postcarotid endarterectomy hyperperfusion syndrome.*

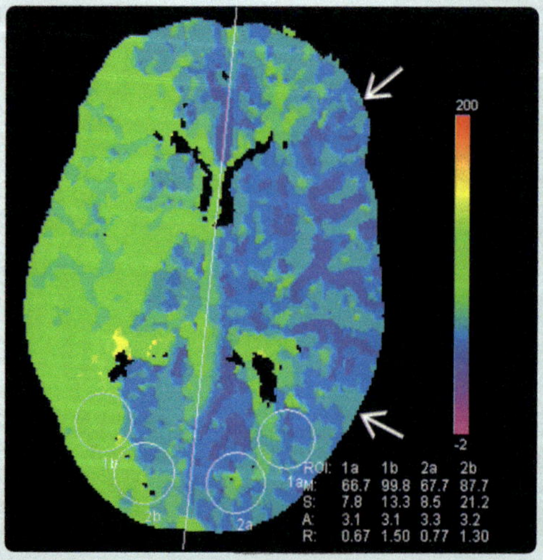

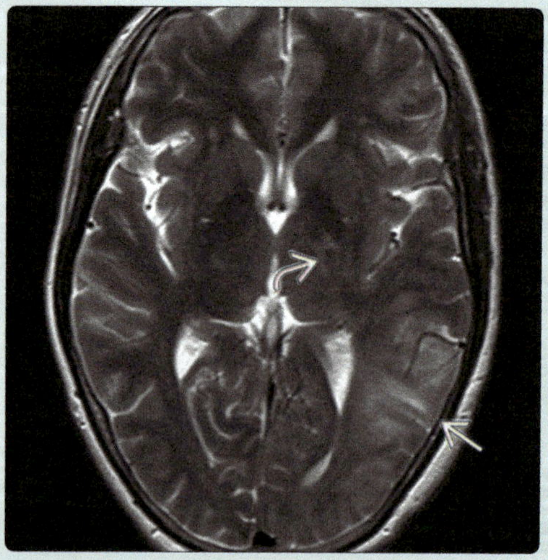

KEY FACTS

IMAGING

- General features
  - Empty-delta sign on CECT, T1WI C+ MR
- CT
  - Hyperdense sinus on NECT (usually > 70 Hounsfield units)
  - ± hyperdense cortical veins (cord sign)
  - CTV: Filling defect (thrombus) in dural sinus
- MR
  - Hypointense thrombus "blooms" on T2* GRE
  - Absence of flow in occluded sinus on 2D TOF MRV
- Protocol recommendations
  - NECT, CECT scans ± CTV as initial screening
  - If CTs negative, MR + MRV (T2*, DWI, T1WI C+)
  - If MRV equivocal, DSA is gold standard

TOP DIFFERENTIAL DIAGNOSES

- Normal (arteries, veins normally slightly hyperdense)
- High hematocrit (newborns, polycythemia)
- Dural sinus hypoplasia/aplasia: No "blooming"; collaterals/venous infarcts absent
- "Giant" arachnoid granulations: Round/ovoid, not elongated like thrombus
- Acute subdural hematoma: Blood layered on tentorium can mimic transverse sinus (TS) thrombosis

CLINICAL ISSUES

- May present with headache and papilledema

DIAGNOSTIC CHECKLIST

- Review MRV source images; exclude pseudocollusions (e.g., hypoplastic TS)
- Review T1 images to exclude false-negative MRV
- Review NECT to exclude dense thrombus as false-negative CECT or CTV
- Brain looks normal; does not exclude CVT
- DSA helpful if noninvasive imaging inconclusive
- Chronic thrombosis may enhance; recanalization or granulation tissue enhances

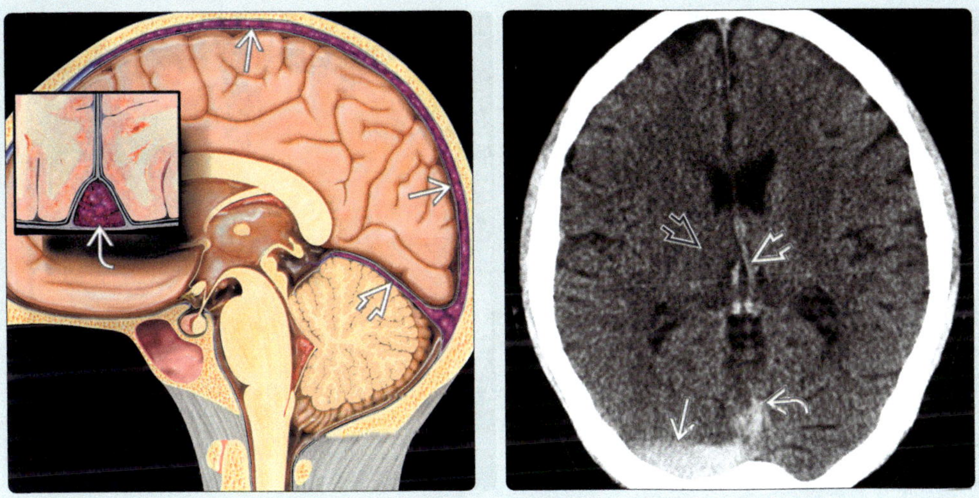

(Left) *Sagittal graphic shows thrombosis of the superior sagittal sinus and straight sinus. Inset in the upper left reveals a thrombus in the superior sagittal sinus in cross section (empty = delta sign) seen on contrast-enhanced imaging.* **(Right)** *NECT scan in a 25-year-old man with progressively increasing headaches shows hyperdensity in the right transverse and straight sinuses. Both internal cerebral veins are hyperdense, and the right thalamus is hypodense and edematous.*

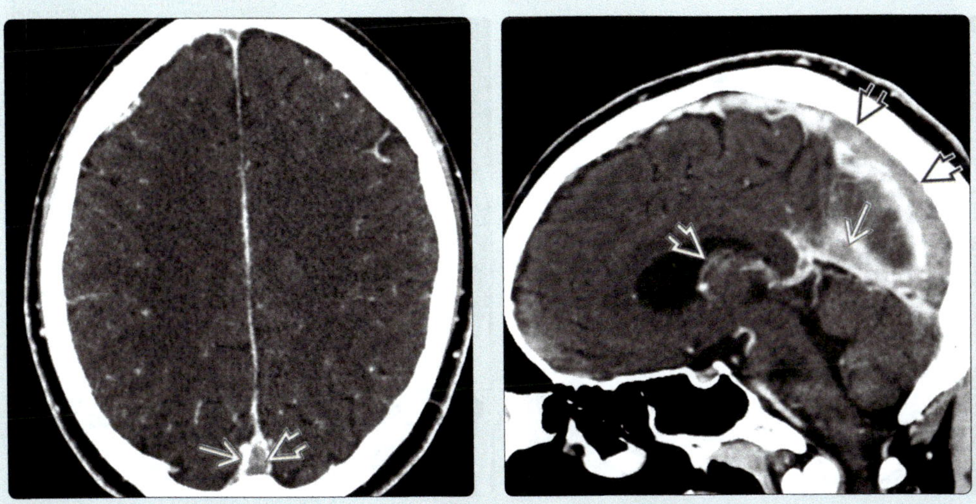

(Left) *Axial source image from a CTV in the same patient shows that the dura around the superior axial sinus enhances, but its clot-filled lumen does not (empty-delta sign).* **(Right)** *Sagittal reformatted view of the CTV in the same patient shows extensive nonenhancing thrombus in the superior sagittal and straight sinuses. The internal cerebral veins are occluded and do not enhance. Findings indicate extensive dural sinus, deep vein thrombosis.*

Cavernous Sinus Thrombosis/Thrombophlebitis

KEY FACTS

IMAGING

- CT
  - Bone CT
    - Look for sinus infection, erosive changes
  - CECT
    - Nonenhancing filling defects (clot) inside enhancing dural walls of cavernous sinus (CS)
    - CS margins convex (not flat/concave)
  - CTA/CTV
    - Filling defects in 1 or both CSs
- MR
  - T1WI
    - Convex, enlarged CS (isointense to gray matter)
    - Orbits: ± "dirty fat," enlarged EOMs, proptosis
  - T2WI
    - Clot heterogeneously hypointense
    - Look for absent carotid "flow void"
  - T2*: Thrombus "blooms"
  - T1 C+: Dura enhances; clot doesn't
    - Clot heterogeneous; ± absent carotid "flow void"

TOP DIFFERENTIAL DIAGNOSES

- Neoplasm (meningioma, schwannoma, lymphoma)
- Carotid-cavernous fistula
- Inflammatory pseudotumor (IgG4-related disease, sarcoid)

CLINICAL ISSUES

- Headache early
- Orbital/sinus pain, edema, chemosis
- Ptosis, ophthalmoplegia, visual loss
- Cranial neuropathy (typically V1 &/or V2)
- Prognosis
  - Spreads via communicating veins to contralateral CS, eye
  - Untreated CS thrombophlebitis can be fatal

DIAGNOSTIC CHECKLIST

- If initial CT negative and clinical suspicion high, CTA/CTV or MR/MRV

(Left) *Clinical photograph in a patient with septic cavernous sinus thrombosis shows ptosis of right eyelid and chemosis.* **(Right)** *Axial CECT in a 16-year-old boy with severe sphenoid sinusitis shows bilateral "filling defects" (nonenhancing clots) within the enhancing dura of the cavernous sinus. The left superior ophthalmic vein is also thrombosed.*

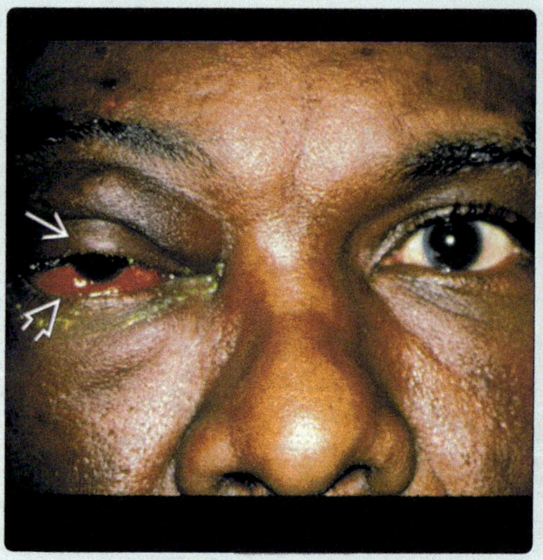

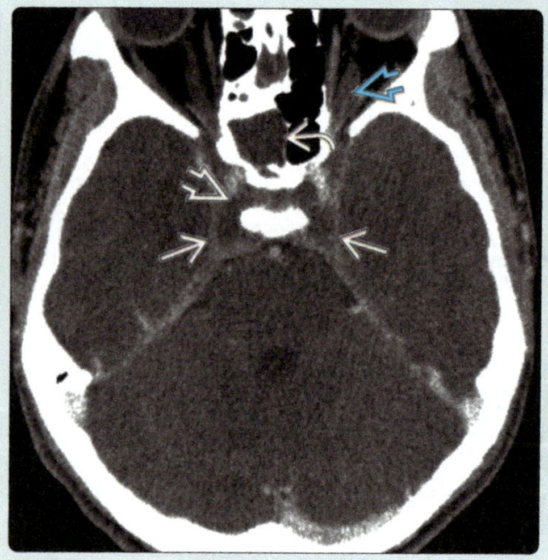

(Left) *Axial T1 C+ FS in the same case shows the nonenhancing thrombus within the intensely enhancing walls of the cavernous sinus.* **(Right)** *Coronal T2WI in the same case shows sphenoid sinusitis, heterogeneously hypointense thrombus bulging the cavernous sinus walls laterally.*

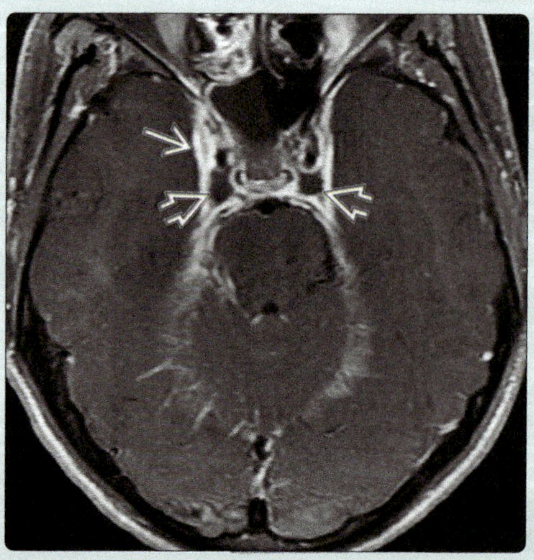

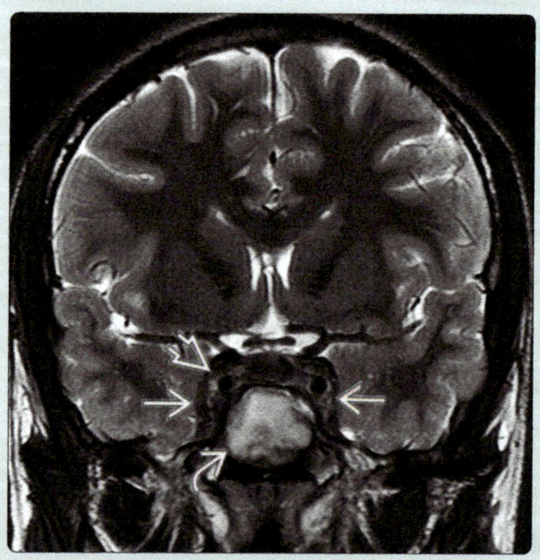

KEY FACTS

TERMINOLOGY

- Cortical/cerebral venous thrombosis (CVT)
- Dural sinus thrombosis (DST)
- CVT with DST > isolated CVT without DST

IMAGING

- NECT
  - Cord sign (hyperdense vein)
  - Involved veins usually enlarged (distended with clot), irregular
  - ± petechial parenchymal hemorrhage, edema
- CECT
  - If DST, empty-delta sign (25-30% of cases)
  - CTV: Thrombi may be seen as filling defects
- MR
  - Acute thrombus isointense on T1WI
  - Hypointense on T2WI (can mimic flow void)
  - T2* GRE best (clot usually blooms)
- 2D time of flight MRV
  - Thrombus seen as sinus discontinuity, loss of vascular flow signal
  - Subacute thrombus T1 hyperintense (mimics patent flow on maximum intensity projection)
- Imaging recommendations
  - NECT, CECT scans ± CTV
  - If CT negative → MR/MRV with T1WI C+, GRE
  - If MR is equivocal → DSA (gold standard)

TOP DIFFERENTIAL DIAGNOSES

- Normal (circulating blood slightly hyperdense)
- Anatomic variant (hypoplastic segment can mimic DST)

CLINICAL ISSUES

- Most common symptom is headache
- Seizure

DIAGNOSTIC CHECKLIST

- If "convexal" subarachnoid hemorrhage is seen, consider CVT

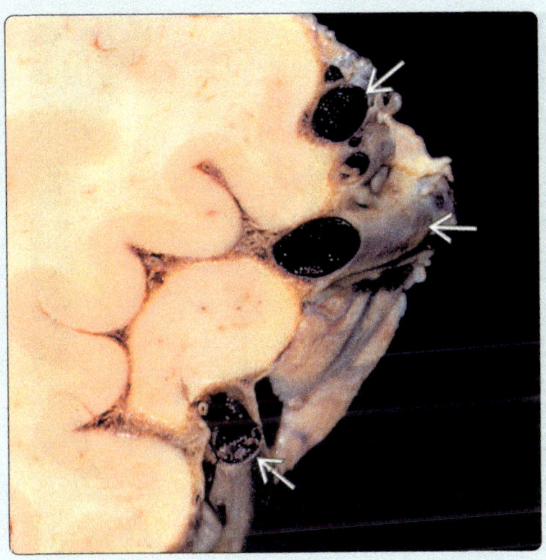

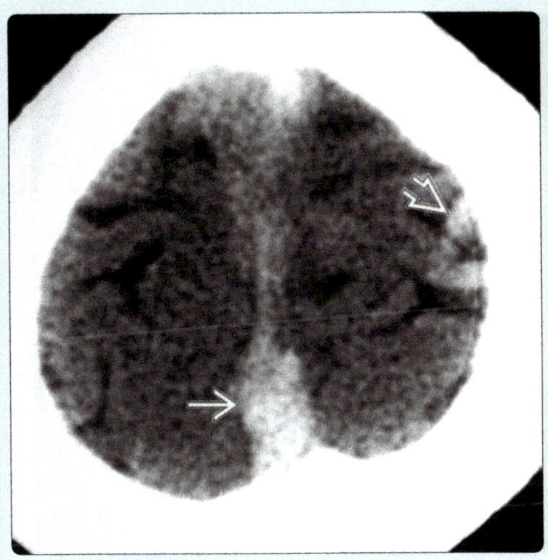

(Left) *Autopsy case shows thrombus in several cortical veins ➔, the pathologic basis for the cord sign. (Courtesy E.T. Hedley-Whyte, MD.)* **(Right)** *Axial NECT scan in a patient with thrombosis of the superior sagittal sinus shows dense clot ➔ filling and expanding of the superior sagittal sinus. Thrombus is seen in a vein ➔ over the cerebral convexity. Most (but not all) cortical vein thrombi occur as extension from clot in an adjacent dural venous sinus.*

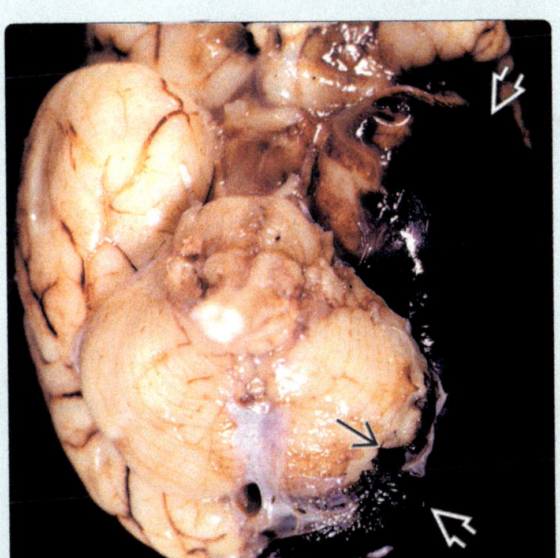

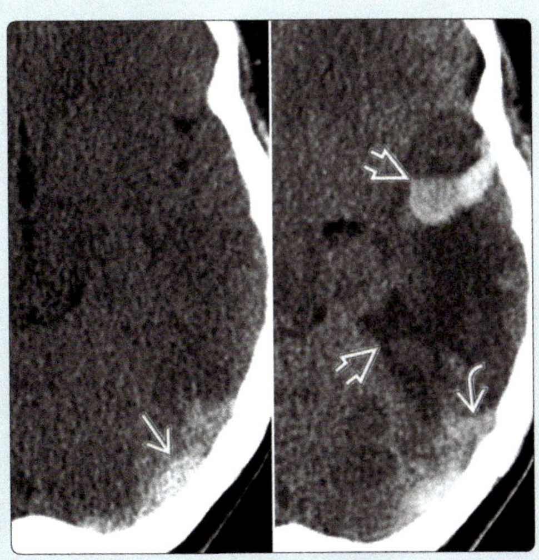

(Left) *Autopsy case of transverse sinus thrombosis ➔ that occluded the vein of Labbé shows extensive hemorrhagic venous infarction of the temporal, parietal, and occipital lobes ➔. (Courtesy R. Hewlett, MD.)* **(Right)** *This 23-year-old woman presented in the ER with "migraine headache." Initial NECT scan (L) was called normal. Note the hyperdense thrombus in left TS ➔. CT 1 day later (right) shows vein of Labbé thrombosis ➔ and a large left temporal lobe hemorrhagic venous infarct ➔.*

KEY FACTS

TERMINOLOGY

- Thrombotic occlusion of deep cerebral veins
  - Usually affects both internal cerebral veins (ICVs) ± vein of Galen (VOG), straight sinus (SS)
  - May occur with more widespread dural sinus thrombosis

IMAGING

- NECT
  - Hyperdense ICV ± VOG, SS
  - Hypodense thalami/basal ganglia (BG), loss of gray matter-white matter (WM) interfaces
    - Variable loss of deep gray-white interfaces; thalami seem to "disappear" into background WM hypodensity
  - ± petechial hemorrhages
- CECT
  - Loss of ICV enhancement, presence of enlarged collateral channels
  - "Shaggy," irregular veins (collateral channels) in deep WM, around tentorium
- MR
  - Acute clots hypointense on T2WI, "bloom" on T2*
  - Deep (medullary) WM veins prominent, tortuous on SWI
- Protocol advice
  - If CT/CECT/CTV scans negative → MR with MRV
  - If MRV equivocal → DSA

TOP DIFFERENTIAL DIAGNOSES

- Other bithalamic/basal ganglia lesions
  - Neoplasm (e.g., bithalamic astrocytoma)
  - Nonvenous ischemia (e.g., artery of Percheron infarct)
  - Toxic/metabolic disorders (e.g., CO poisoning)

CLINICAL ISSUES

- Venous thrombosis = 1-2% of strokes; ICV thrombosis = 10% of venous "strokes"
- Can present with headaches and coma

(Left) *Axial graphic depicts thrombosis of both internal cerebral veins (ICVs) and straight sinus (SS) ➡ with 2° hemorrhage in choroid plexus and thalami ➡. Edema in the thalami, basal ganglia, and deep cerebral white matter (WM) are common findings. Linear WM medullary veins ➡ may become engorged and enhance.* **(Right)** *NECT in a 32-year-old woman with severe headache shows hyperdense ICVs ➡. Both thalami are edematous, symmetrically isodense ➡ (normally hyperdense) compared to the surrounding WM.*

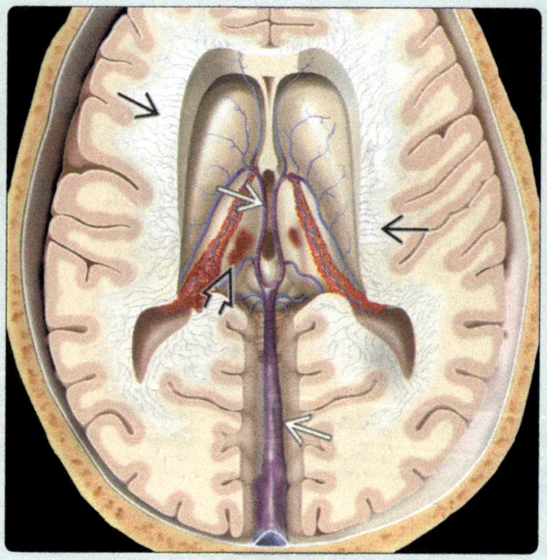

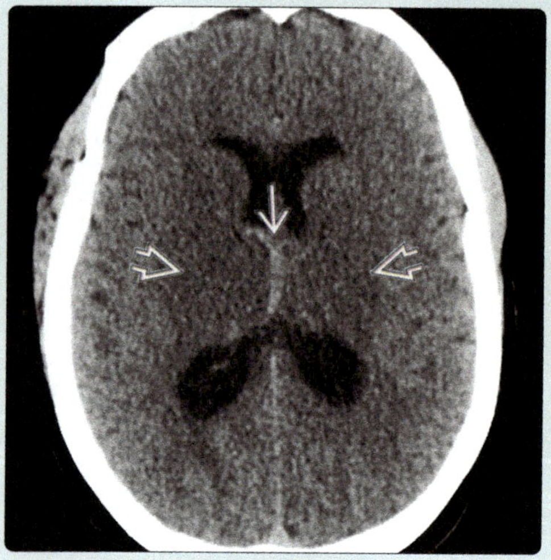

(Left) *Lateral DSA, venous phase, in the same patient shows normal opacification of the superior sagittal sinus ➡, transverse sinus ➡, and vein of Labbé ➡. The ICVs, vein of Galen, and SS are thrombosed and do not fill with contrast. Contrast with normal DSA with deep venous system filling is shown on right.* **(Right)** *Normal DSA, lateral view, venous phase, shows opacification of the ICV ➡, vein of Galen ➡, and SS ➡.*

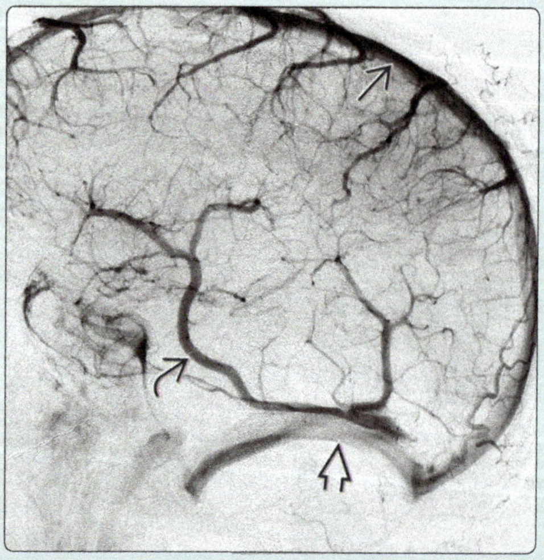

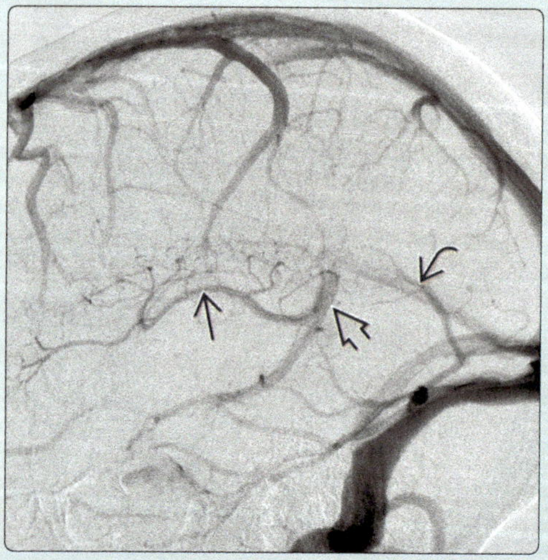

Subarachnoid Hemorrhage

Overview: The subarachnoid spaces (SASs) are cerebrospinal fluid (CSF)-filled spaces between the arachnoid (on the outside) and the pia (on the inside). Focal expansions of the SASs at the base of the brain and around the brainstem, tentorial incisura, and foramen magnum form the brain cisterns.

The SASs are anatomically unique, as they surround the entire brain, spinal cord, and spinal nerve roots and contain all the major brain arteries and cortical veins.

Acute extravasation of blood into the CSF spaces between the arachnoid membrane and pia can be caused by arterial leaks or torn veins. Blood can also extend into the SASs from parenchymal hemorrhage that ruptures through the cortex and pia, spilling into the adjacent SAS.

Trauma, "burst" aneurysm, vascular malformations, and amyloid angiopathy are potential causes of subarachnoid hemorrhage (SAH). The most common cause of SAH is trauma. Traumatic SAH (tSAH) occurs when hemorrhage from contused brain or lacerated cortical vessels extends into sulci adjacent to the injury.

Aneurysmal SAH (aSAH): Nontraumatic "spontaneous" SAH represents about 5% of all acute "strokes." The most common cause of nontraumatic SAH is a ruptured intracranial saccular ("berry") aneurysm (aSAH). Because most saccular aneurysms (SAs) are located either on the circle of Willis or at the middle cerebral artery bifurcation, the most common locations for aSAH are the suprasellar cistern and sylvian fissures.

aSAH can be focal or diffuse. Attempts to determine the precise anatomic location of a suspected intracranial aneurysm based on the distribution of SAH are necessarily imprecise. Anterior interhemispheric aSAH is typically associated with rupture of a superiorly directed anterior communicating artery aneurysm. aSAH seen primarily in the posterior fossa cisterns &/or 4th ventricle suggests a posterior inferior cerebellar artery aneurysm. Middle cerebral artery bi- or trifurcation aneurysm may cause focal hemorrhage in the adjacent sylvian fissure.

Perimesencephalic nonaneurysmal SAH (pnSAH): An uncommon but important cause of SAH, pnSAH, is a clinically benign variant that is probably venous in origin. pnSAH is confined to the cisterns around the midbrain and anterior to the pons.

Convexal SAH (cSAH): An uncommon subset of nontraumatic SAH occurs over the dorsolateral surface ("convexity") of the cerebral hemispheres. The basal and perimesencephalic cisterns are typically spared. cSAH typically affects just 1 sulcus or a grouping of adjacent sulci. Common etiologies in older adults are amyloid angiopathy or vasculitis, whereas vasculitis and reversible cerebral vasoconstriction syndrome are common causes in patients < 60 years old. Cortical vein occlusion with cSAH occurs at all ages.

Superficial siderosis (SS): Chronic, recurrent SAH results in hemosiderin deposition on the pia and cranial nerves. The brain, brainstem, cerebellum, and spinal cord can all be affected, although the posterior fossa is most commonly involved.

The classic clinical presentation of SS is in an adult with a history of trauma or surgery, who presents with ataxia and bilateral sensorineural hearing loss. A history of aSAH is uncommon. SS is best identified on T2* (GRE or SWI).

Aneurysms and Arterial Ectasias

Terminology and overview: The word "aneurysm" comes from the combination of 2 Greek words meaning "across" and "broad." Hence, brain arterial aneurysms are widenings or dilatations of intracranial arteries.

Intracranial aneurysms are generally classified by their phenotypic appearance. Saccular or "berry" aneurysms are the most common type. Fusiform aneurysms are focal dilatations that involve the entire circumference of a vessel and extend for relatively short distances. Ectasias refer to generalized arterial enlargement without focal dilatation and are not true aneurysms.

Saccular aneurysm (SA): As the name implies, SAs are focal sac- or berry-like arterial dilatations. The vast majority are acquired lesions, the result of an underlying genetically based susceptibility plus superimposed mechanical stresses on vessel walls. SAs lack the 2 strongest layers of blood vessel walls, the internal elastic lamina and the muscular layer. The aneurysm sac itself consists of only intima and adventitia.

Most SAs arise at major blood vessel bifurcations, where hemodynamic stresses are highest. The vast majority of intracranial aneurysms are located on the circle of Willis plus the middle cerebral artery bi- or trifurcation. 90% are "anterior circulation" aneurysms, i.e., on the internal carotid artery and its branches. The posterior communicating artery is considered part of the anterior circulation; the vertebrobasilar artery and branches constitute the "posterior circulation."

Pseudoaneurysm (PA): PAs are focal arterial dilatations not contained by layers of the normal arterial wall. They are often irregularly shaped and generally arise on vessels distal to the circle of Willis.

A PA develops when a completely disrupted blood vessel hemorrhages. A paravascular hematoma forms and then cavitates, establishing a communication with the parent vessel wall. The wall of a PA thus consists only of organized clot. PAs are much less common than either SAs or fusiform aneurysms. PAs are acquired lesions caused by trauma, infection, or inflammation ("mycotic" aneurysm), drug abuse, and neoplasm ("oncotic" aneurysm).

Blood blister-like aneurysm (BBAs): BBAs are eccentric hemispherical outpouchings that can develop at any location. Most commonly found on the greater curvature of the supraclinoid internal carotid artery, they are lined only by a thin layer of adventitia. They are difficult to detect, difficult to treat, and prone to rupture at smaller size and younger age than typical SAs.

Fusiform aneurysms: Fusiform aneurysms can be atherosclerotic (common) or nonatherosclerotic (rare). They involve long, nonbranching vessel segments and are seen as more focal circumferential outpouchings from an ectatic vessel. Fusiform aneurysms are more common in the vertebrobasilar (posterior) circulation.

Vertebrobasilar dolichoectasia: Fusiform enlargement or ectasia, also called arteriectasis, is commonly seen in patients with advanced atherosclerotic disease. Less commonly, fusiform ectasias occur with collagen-vascular disorders and non-atherosclerotic vascular disease arteriopathies.

(Left) *Diagram depicts the circle of Willis with relative prevalence of intracranial saccular aneurysms (SAs). Most are "anterior circulation" with 1/3 occurring on the ACoA and 1/3 at the internal carotid/PCoA junction; 15-20% are found at the middle cerebral artery (MCA) bi- or trifurcation. 10% occur on the "posterior circulation."* **(Right)** *Autopsied Circle of Willis shows a classic unruptured SA arising from the junction of the internal carotid artery and the PCoA. (Courtesy B. Horten, MD.)*

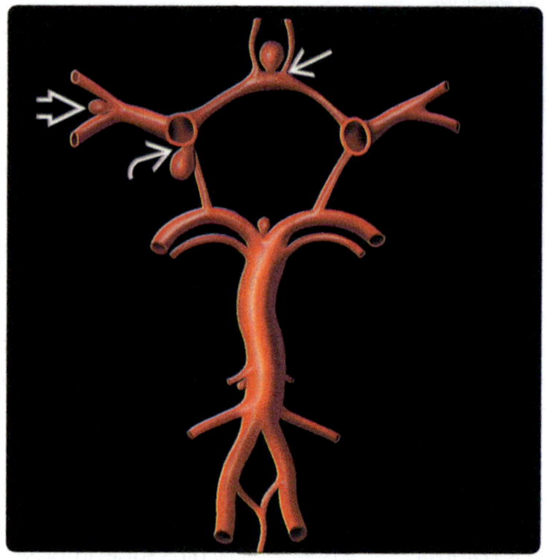

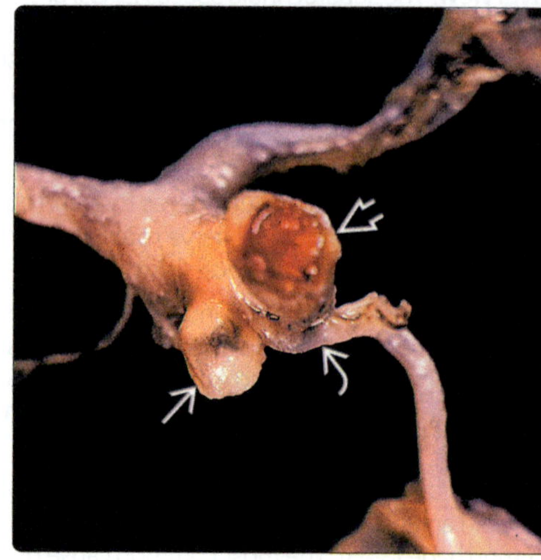

(Left) *Autopsied brain shows a small ruptured ACoA aneurysm with extensive focal clot in the interhemispheric fissure. Diffuse subarachnoid hemorrhage is also present. (Courtesy B. Horten, MD.)* **(Right)** *This patient died of cerebral ischemia several days after rupture of a MCA SA, which is surrounded by clot in the sylvian fissure. Note the extreme narrowing of the M1 MCA segment and both posterior cerebral arteries, indicative of severe vasospasm. (Courtesy R. Hewlett, MD.)*

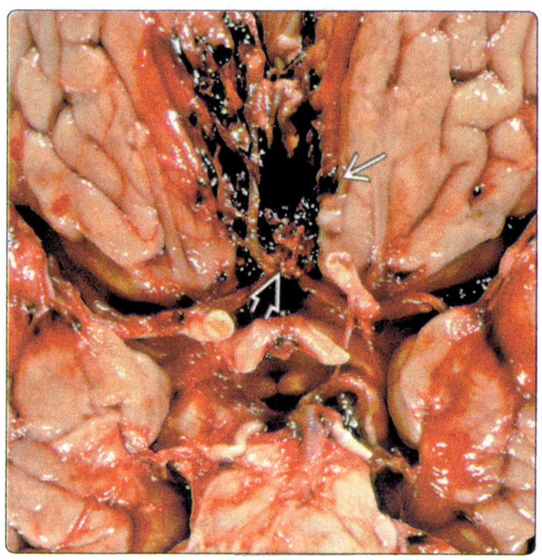

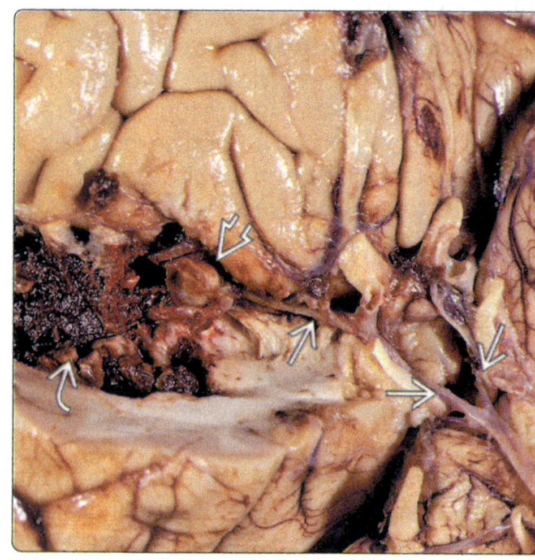

(Left) *Gross pathology shows atherosclerotic fusiform ectasias of the vertebrobasilar system, as well as both internal carotid arteries and M1 MCA segments. Focal enlargement of the basilar artery represents a fusiform aneurysm caused by atherosclerotic vascular disease. (Courtesy R. Hewlett, MD.)* **(Right)** *Nonatherosclerotic fusiform ectasias of the M1, A1/A2, and PCoAs are seen in a patient with HIV-associated vasculopathy. (Courtesy L. Rourke, MD.)*

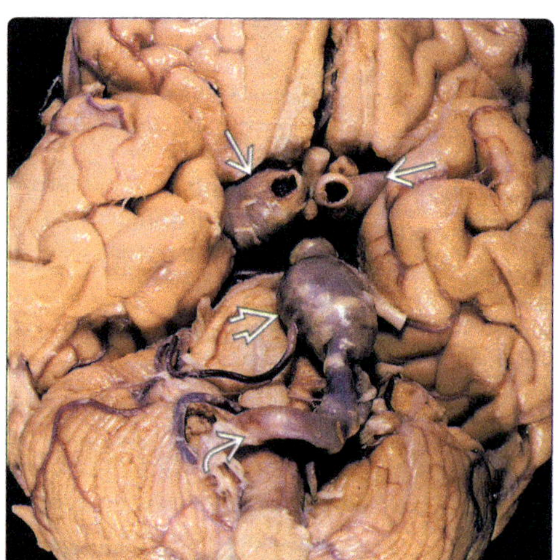

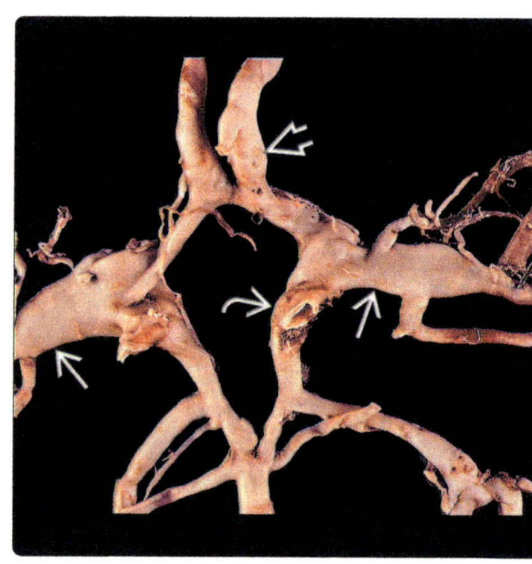

KEY FACTS

TERMINOLOGY

- Subarachnoid hemorrhage (SAH) caused by ruptured aneurysm (aSAH)
  - Saccular aneurysm (SA) > > dissecting aneurysm (DA)

IMAGING

- CT/CTA
  - Hyperdense sulci on NECT
  - Distribution varies with aneurysm location
  - Suprasellar cistern (IC-PCoA, ACoA aneurysms)
  - Sylvian fissure (middle cerebral artery bifurcation)
  - Prepontine, cerebellopontine angle cisterns (posterior inferior cerebellar artery, blood blister artery bifurcation SA or vertebral DA)
  - CTA 90-95% positive if aneurysm ≥ 2 mm
- MR/MRA
  - FLAIR hyperintense sulci, cisterns (nonspecific)
  - "Blooms" on T2* GRE
  - TOF MRA 85-95% sensitive for aneurysms ≥ 3 mm
- DSA
  - Used if CTA negative
  - If endovascular treatment is option

TOP DIFFERENTIAL DIAGNOSES

- Nonaneurysmal SAH
- Pseudo-SAH
- Reversible cerebral vasoconstriction syndrome

CLINICAL ISSUES

- Sudden onset severe headache
  - "Thunderclap/worst headache of life"
- 50% mortality
  - Vasospasm 1-3 weeks post aSAH
- 20% rebleed within 1st 2 weeks
- Treatment: Coil embolization ("coiling") generally > clipping

DIAGNOSTIC CHECKLIST

- Diffuse low-density brain makes normal arteries look hyperdense, can mimic aSAH

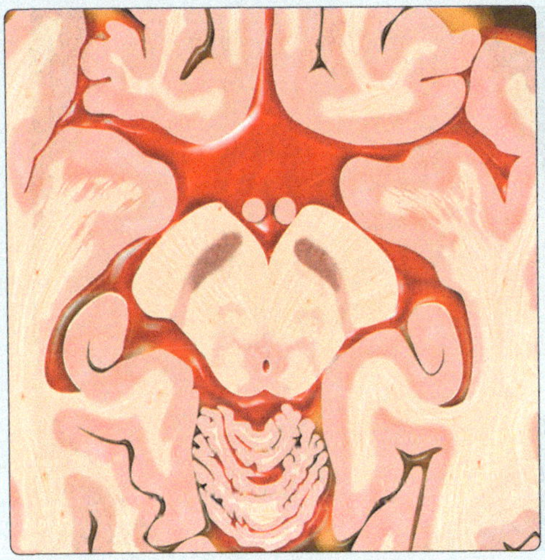
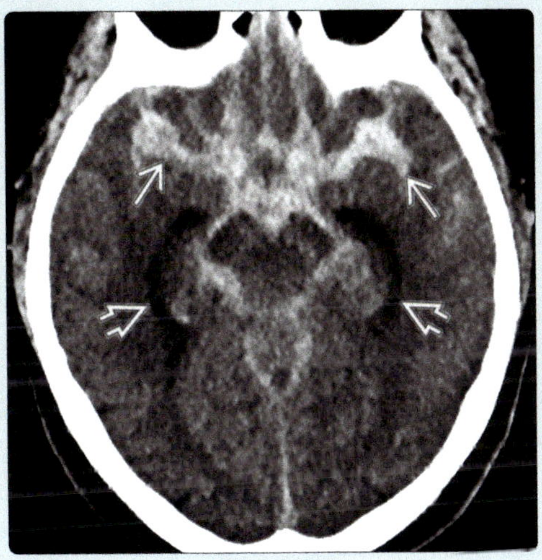

(Left) *Axial graphic through the midbrain depicts subarachnoid hemorrhage (SAH) in red throughout the basal cisterns. Given the diffuse distribution of SAH without focal hematoma, the most likely location of the ruptured aneurysm is the ACoA.* **(Right)** *Axial NECT scan in a 63-year-old man found down in a parking lot shows diffuse SAH ➡ throughout the basal cisterns. Note the enlargement of both temporal horns of the lateral ventricles ⇨ consistent with early extraventricular obstructive hydrocephalus.*

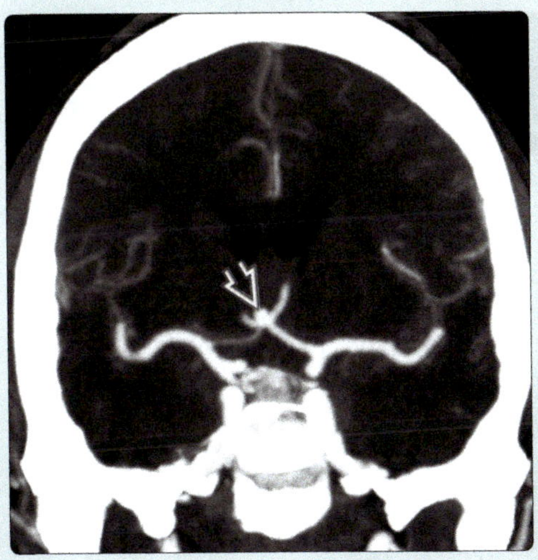
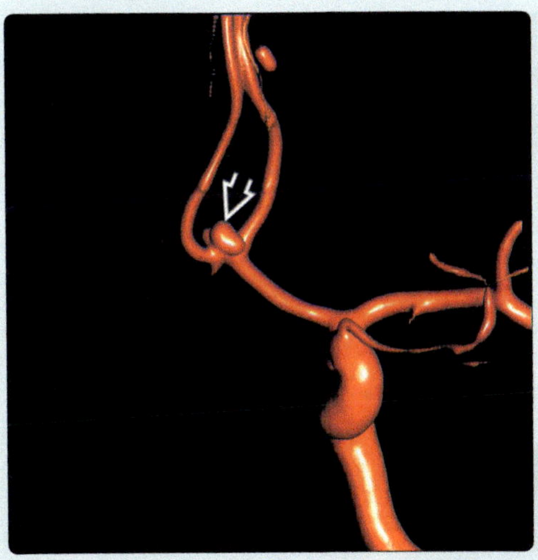

(Left) *Coronal maximal intensity projection image of the CTA obtained in the same patient shows a saccular aneurysm ⇨ projecting superiorly from the anterior communicating artery.* **(Right)** *Coronal shaded surface display of the DSA obtained in the same patient nicely demonstrates the "culprit" aneurysm ⇨. The lesion was successfully coiled after this diagnostic DSA was performed.*

Perimesencephalic Nonaneurysmal Subarachnoid Hemorrhage (pnSAH)

KEY FACTS

TERMINOLOGY

- Subarachnoid hemorrhage (SAH) centered immediately anterior to midbrain ± pons
- No source demonstrated at CTA/DSA/MRA

IMAGING

- NECT: Hyperdense prepontine, perimesencephalic cerebrospinal fluid (CSF)
  - Often involves interpeduncular, ambient, quadrigeminal cisterns
  - ± thin extension into posterior suprasellar, proximal sylvian/interhemispheric fissures
  - Does not extend into distal sylvian, interhemispheric fissures
- CTA used to exclude basilar tip aneurysm
- MR
  - T1: Iso- to hyperintense
  - T2 variable (iso- to hyper-) intensity compared with CSF
  - FLAIR: Hyperintense prepontine, perimesencephalic CSF

TOP DIFFERENTIAL DIAGNOSES

- Aneurysmal SAH
- Traumatic SAH
- Artifact (incomplete CSF suppression on FLAIR)

PATHOLOGY

- Most likely from ruptured perimesencephalic/prepontine vein
  - More common if basal vein of Rosenthal small, drains into veins other than Galen
- 5% of pnSAHs have other etiologies
  - Basilar bifurcation aneurysm, dissection most common
  - Other: Trauma, dural arteriovenous fistula, spinal cord vascular malformation, vascular neoplasm

CLINICAL ISSUES

- Benign course: Rebleed rare (< 1%); no vasospasm

(Left) *Axial graphic shows a classic pnSAH. Hemorrhage is confined to the interpeduncular fossa and ambient (perimesencephalic) cisterns ➔. The source is usually venous in pnSAHs, unlike in aneurysmal SAHs.* **(Right)** *Axial NECT of a 49-year-old woman in the ER with a "thunderclap" headache shows SAH around the midbrain in the perimesencephalic cisterns ➔. Note the absence of blood in the sylvian fissures and anterior suprasellar subarachnoid space.*

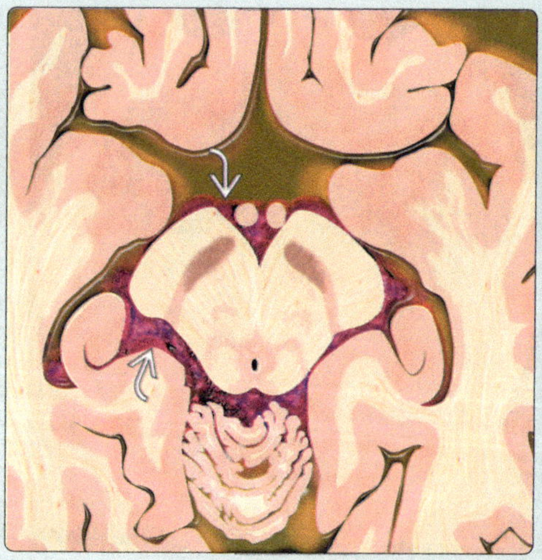

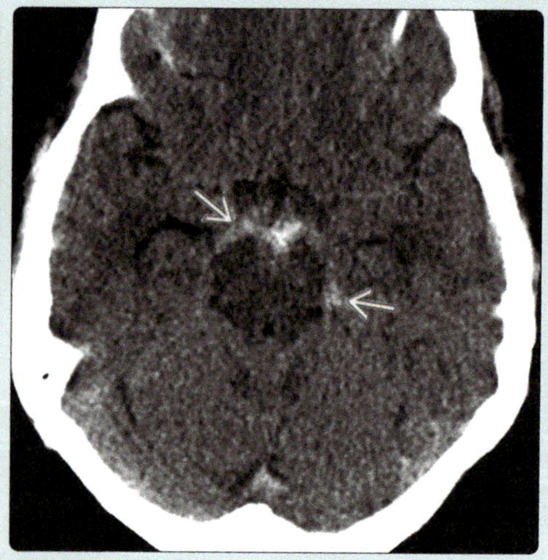

(Left) *Axial NECT in the same patient shows that the subarachnoid blood ➔ extends inferiorly in front of the pons.* **(Right)** *Coronal CTA in the same patient with reconstructed view through the basilar artery bifurcation shows no evidence for aneurysm. The high density in the vessels is easily discernible even with the presence of significant SAH. DSA (not shown) confirmed the absence of aneurysm. This case illustrates classic findings in pnSAH.*

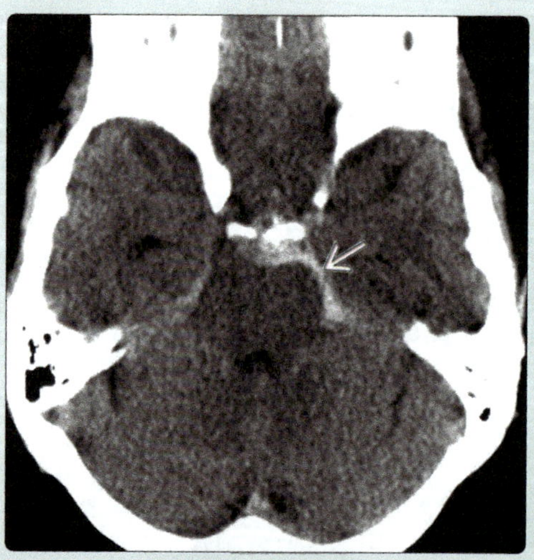

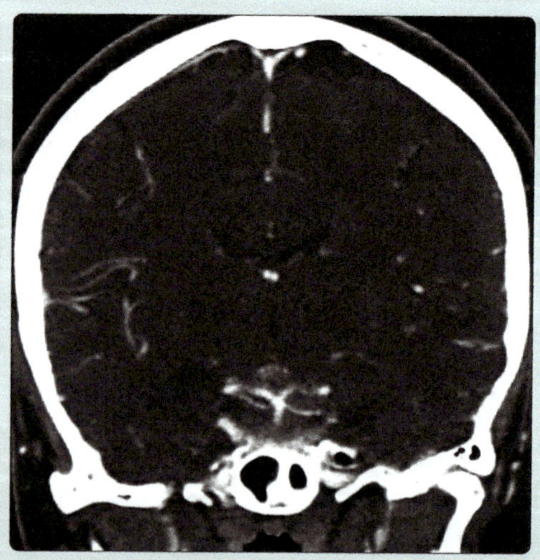

Convexal Subarachnoid Hemorrhage (cSAH)

KEY FACTS

TERMINOLOGY

- Unique type of subarachnoid hemorrhage (SAH)
  - Localized to sulci over top ("convexity") of brain

IMAGING

- NECT: Hyperdensity in 1 or several adjacent dorsolateral convexity sulci
  - Spares basal, perimesencephalic cisterns
- MR
  - Sulcal cerebrospinal fluid (CSF) replaced by isointense fluid in convexity sulcus ("dirty CSF")
  - Hyperintense sulcus on FLAIR
  - GRE, SWI show "blooming" in affected sulci

TOP DIFFERENTIAL DIAGNOSES

- Aneurysmal SAH
- Perimesencephalic nonaneurysmal SAH
- Traumatic SAH

PATHOLOGY

- Most common etiology varies with age
  - Elderly patients: Amyloid angiopathy, venous thrombosis, vasculitis
  - Middle aged: Reversible cerebral vasoconstriction syndrome (RCVS), vasculitis, vein thrombosis
  - Young adults, children: Drugs, vasculitis, vein/dural sinus thrombosis

CLINICAL ISSUES

- 7% of all spontaneous (nontraumatic) SAH
- Most common: Middle-aged women
- Presentation varies with age
  - < 60 years of age: Sudden "thunderclap" headache (e.g., RCVS)
  - > 60 years of age: Transient sensory, motor symptoms, less intense headache (cerebral amyloid angiopathy)

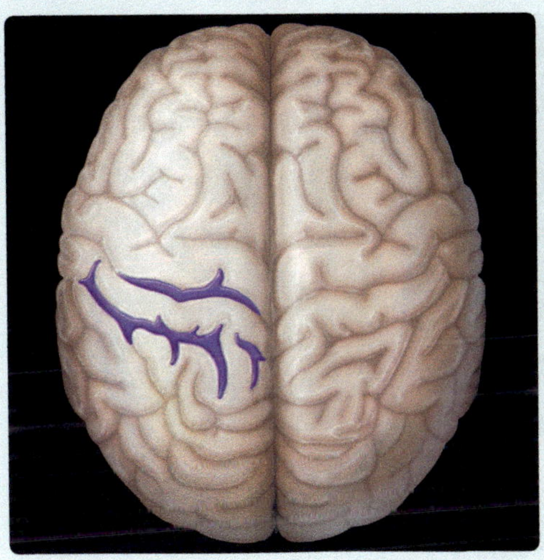

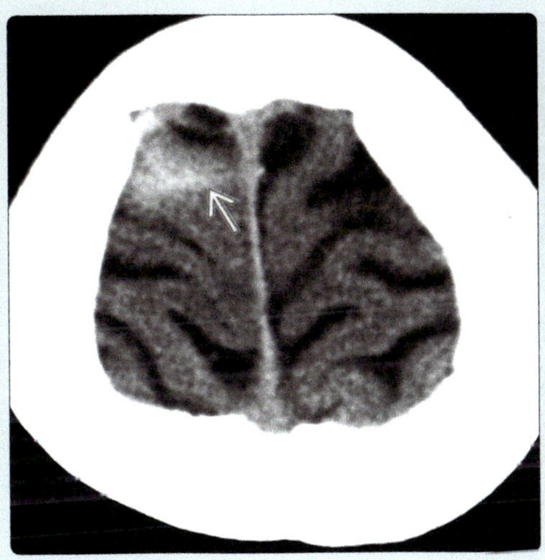

(Left) *Graphic of brain seen from above shows convexal subarachnoid hemorrhage in purple affecting adjacent sulci but sparing the basal cisterns.* **(Right)** *Axial NECT in a 28-year-old woman with severe headache following delivery shows focal subarachnoid hemorrhage ➡ over the right cerebral convexity.*

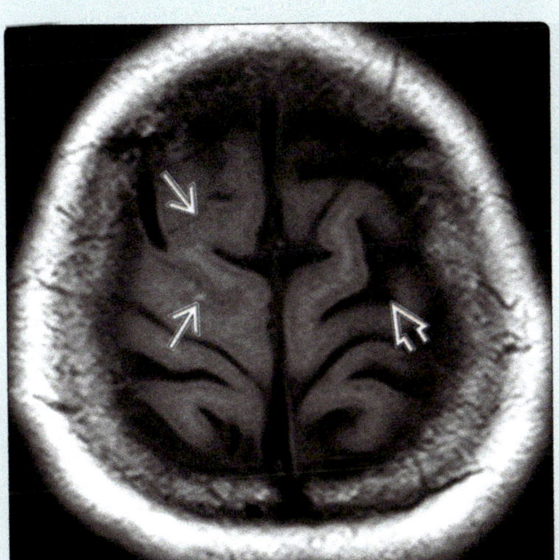

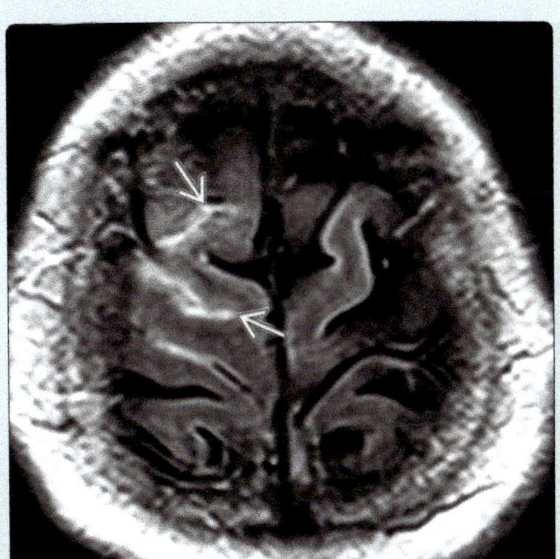

(Left) *Axial T1WI MR in the same patient shows "dirty" fluid filling, effacing the normal sulcal cerebrospinal fluid (CSF) in the right convexity sulci ➡ (compare to normal hypointense signal intensity in the contralateral sulci ➡).* **(Right)** *Axial FLAIR MR in the same patient shows hyperintense right convexity sulci ➡ (contrast with the normal suppressed hypointense CSF over the left convexity). Postpartum vasculopathy was diagnosed at DSA (not shown).*

KEY FACTS

TERMINOLOGY

- Intracranial saccular aneurysm (SA)
- Outpouching affecting only part of arterial circumference
  - Lacks internal elastic lamina ± tunica media

IMAGING

- Round/lobulated arterial outpouching
  - Usually arises from bifurcations of circle of Willis (COW), supraclinoid internal carotid and middle cerebral arteries
  - 90% occur in anterior circulation
  - 10% posterior circulation: Basilar tip, cerebellar arteries (posterior inferior cerebellar artery most common)
  - Rare (< 1%): Trigeminal artery, vertebrobasilar junction fenestration
- Ruptured SAs result in subarachnoid hemorrhage (SAH)
- May have mural Ca++
- Screening in suspected aneurysmal SAH
  - Multislice CTA sensitivity > 95% for SA > 2 mm
  - 3D TOF: > 90% sensitive for aneurysms ≥ 3 mm
  - DSA still considered "gold standard" but usually performed only if CTA negative or endovascular treatment contemplated

TOP DIFFERENTIAL DIAGNOSES

- Vessel loop
- Vessel infundibulum

CLINICAL ISSUES

- Vast majority of unruptured SAs are asymptomatic
  - 2-6% incidental finding at autopsy, imaging
- 80-90% of nontraumatic SAH caused by ruptured SA
- Treatment
  - Endovascular coiling vs. surgical clipping still controversial
  - 22.6% relative, 6.9% absolute risk ↓ for coiling vs. surgery for ruptured aneurysms
  - ↓ morbidity, mortality, and hospital costs; quicker recovery for unruptured aneurysms

(Left) *Most common sites for saccular aneurysms (SAs) are anterior communicating artery (ACoA) and IC-PC junction. Middle cerebral artery (MCA) bifurcation and basilar tip are other frequent sites.* **(Right)** *Graphic illustrates rupture of an ACoA aneurysm with active extravasation from a superiorly directed bleb (Murphy teat). An additional posterior communicating artery SA and tiny bleb at the left MCA bifurcation are seen. Patients with SAs have a 20% chance of having > 1 aneurysm.*

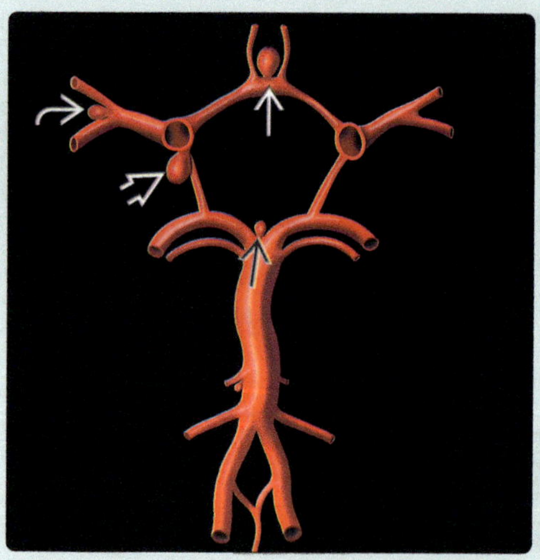

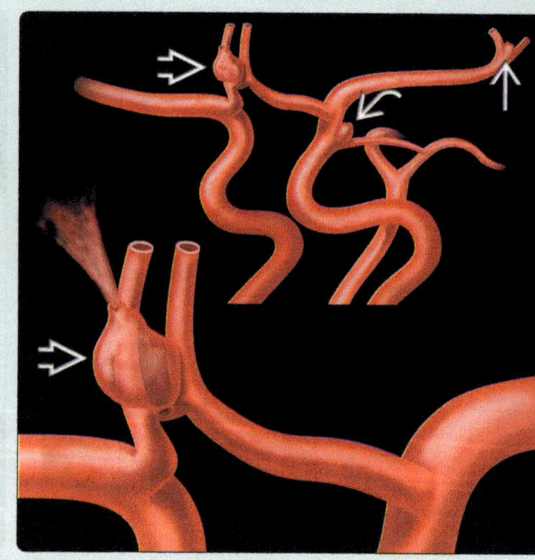

(Left) *A 63-year-old man was found down in a parking lot and brought to the ER. Axial NECT scan showed diffuse subarachnoid hemorrhage with a focal hematoma in the anteroinferior aspect of the interhemispheric fissure.* **(Right)** *Coronal MIP of the CTA in the same patient shows a 4-mm SA projecting upward from the ACoA.*

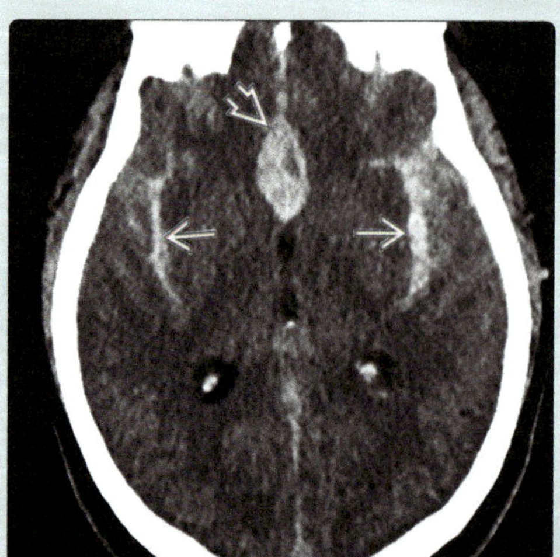

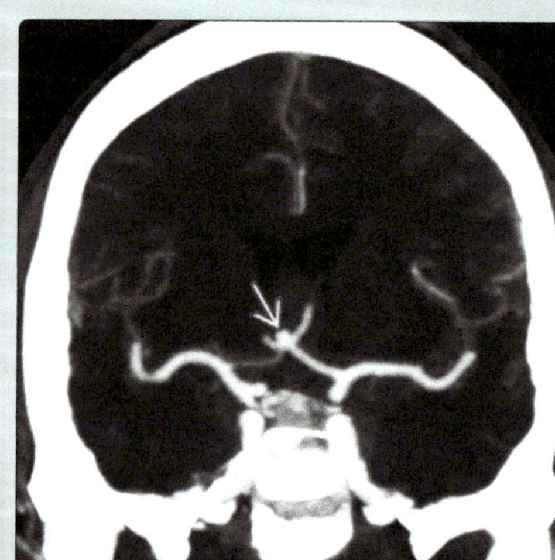

KEY FACTS

TERMINOLOGY

- Extensive ectatic, elongated vertebrobasilar artery (VBA)
- Usually associated with decreased blood flow velocity

IMAGING

- General findings
  - Irregular, elongated, tortuous VBA
  - Usually 6-12 mm, can be giant (> 2.5 cm)
  - Focal arterial dilatation = fusiform aneurysm
- CT
  - Hyperdense tortuous enlarged vessel, Ca++ common
  - Enlarged lumen enhances, intramural thrombus does not
- MR
  - Signal varies with flow, presence/age of thrombus
  - Dynamic CE MRA best
  - 3D TOF inadequate (slow flow saturation effects)

TOP DIFFERENTIAL DIAGNOSES

- Fusiform aneurysm, ASVD
- Giant serpentine aneurysm
- Nonatherosclerotic fusiform vasculopathy
- Dissecting aneurysm

CLINICAL ISSUES

- Peak age = 7th, 8th decades
- Often asymptomatic
  - Vertebrobasilar TIAs
  - Progressive cranial nerve compression less common
    - CN5, 7; hemifacial spasm
  - Rare: Hemorrhage, hydrocephalus

DIAGNOSTIC CHECKLIST

- Slow complex flow → heterogeneous signal, TOF artifact
- Dynamic contrast-enhanced CTA/MRA or DSA necessary to delineate true lumen

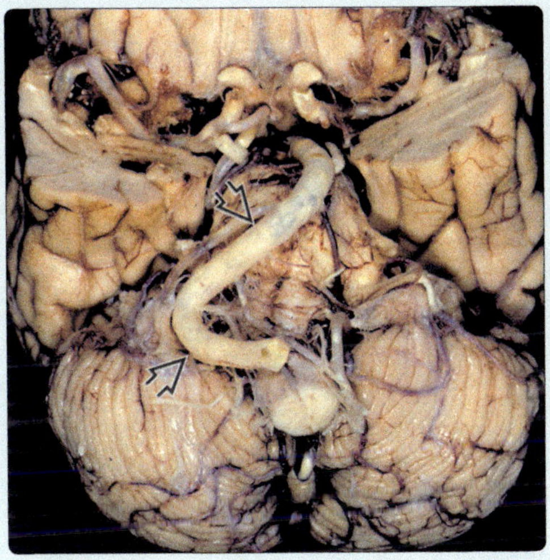

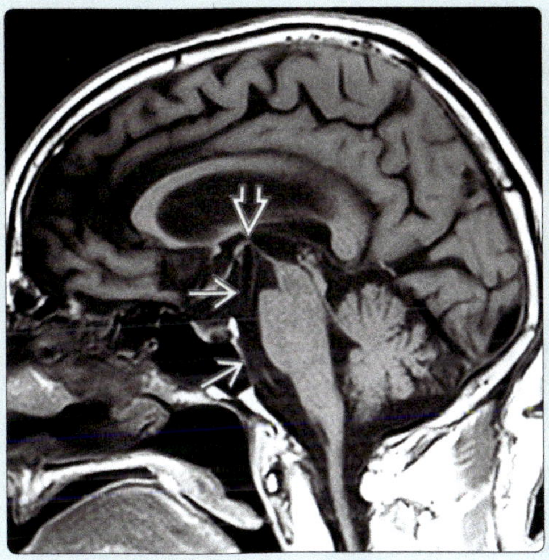

(Left) *Autopsied brain seen from below shows ectatic, very tortuous basilar artery ⇨ with extensive yellow plaques of atherosclerosis. No focal areas of dilatation are seen, so this is vertebrobasilar dolichoectasia, a relatively common finding in elderly patients. (Courtesy R. Hewlett, MD.)* **(Right)** *Sagittal T1WI MR in a 76-year-old man with headaches shows a very elongated, unusually ectatic basilar artery ➡. The basilar tip elevates and indents the 3rd ventricle ⇨.*

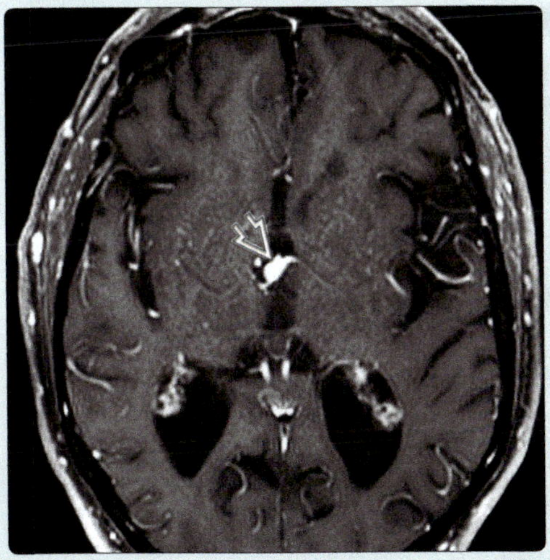

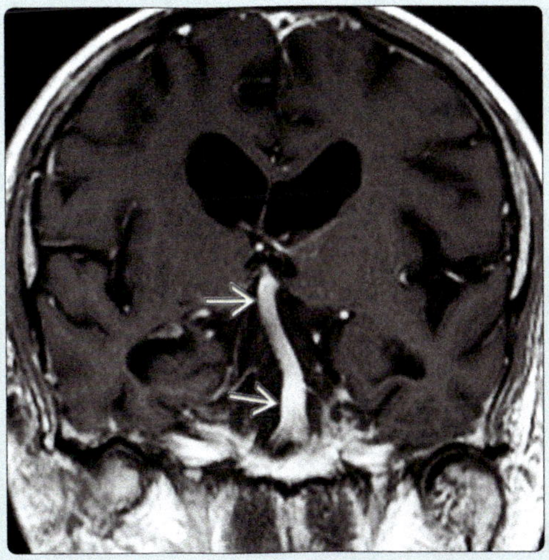

(Left) *Axial T1 C+ FS MR shows the strongly enhancing basilar bifurcation ⇨ as it indents the inferior 3rd ventricle.* **(Right)** *Coronal T1 C+ MR shows the extremely ectatic, elongated basilar artery ➡ characteristic of typical vertebrobasilar dolichoectasia.*

KEY FACTS

TERMINOLOGY

- Atherosclerotic vascular disease fusiform aneurysm (ASVD FA)
- ASVD → abnormal dilation, tortuosity of intracranial arteries
- Aneurysms with separate inflow, outflow ostia

IMAGING

- Exaggerated arterial ectasia(s) + focal fusiform/saccular enlargement
  - Long segment irregular fusiform or ovoid arterial dilatation
  - Usually large (> 2.5 cm), may be giant
  - Vertebrobasilar > carotid circulation
- CT: Hyperdense, Ca++ common
- MR: Signal varies flow, presence/age of hematoma
  - Lumen, intramural clot often heterogeneous
  - Residual lumen enhances; intramural clot does not
  - Prominent phase artifact common
- Noncontrast 3D TOF inadequate due to flow saturation, phase dispersion
- Dynamic contrast-enhanced MRA for aneurysm delineation, T2 for brainstem delineation

CLINICAL ISSUES

- Peak age: 7th to 8th decades
- Presentation: Ischemic stroke > compressive symptoms (cranial neuropathy)
- Unlike saccular aneurysms, rupture with subarachnoid hemorrhage and headache rare

DIAGNOSTIC CHECKLIST

- DSA or contrast-enhanced CTA/MRA necessary to delineate patent lumen
- Slow/complex flow in residual lumen → heterogeneous signal
- Consider dissecting aneurysm, non-ASVD etiology if younger patient

(Left) Autopsy shows a tortuous vertebrobasilar artery with an atherosclerotic vascular disease (AVD) fusiform aneurysm that extends from the vertebral artery junction to the distal basilar bifurcation. (Courtesy R. Hewlett, MD.) **(Right)** *Oblique DSA in same patient 2 yr later shows dolichoectasia of the proximal distal vertebral arteries. A fusiform ASVD aneurysm lies between the arterial ectasias; residual lumen is indicated, and aneurysm had enlarged but partially thrombosed, leading to mild TIAs.*

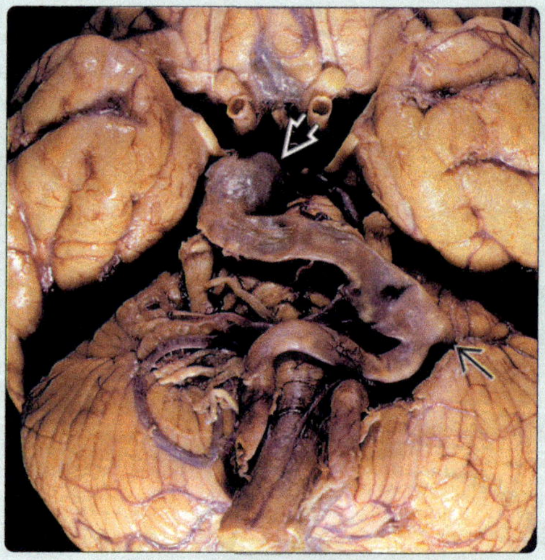

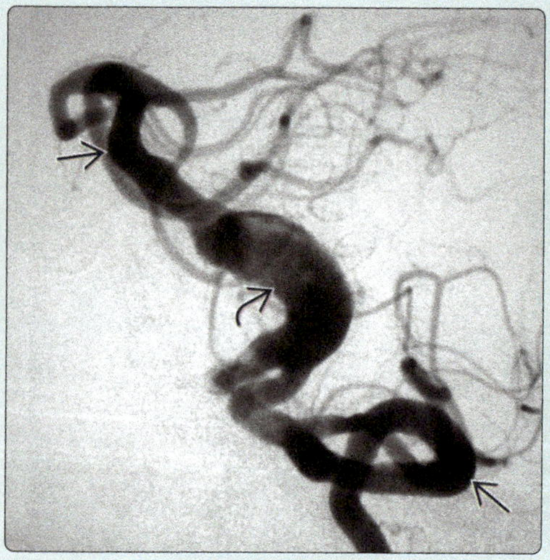

(Left) *NECT scan shows typical hyperdense atherosclerotic fusiform aneurysm with mural calcifications. Note extensive calcification of the internal carotid, right middle cerebral arteries.* **(Right)** *Series of MRs shows the bizarre appearance of classic atherosclerotic fusiform vertebrobasilar aneurysm. (Courtesy M. Hartel, MD.)*

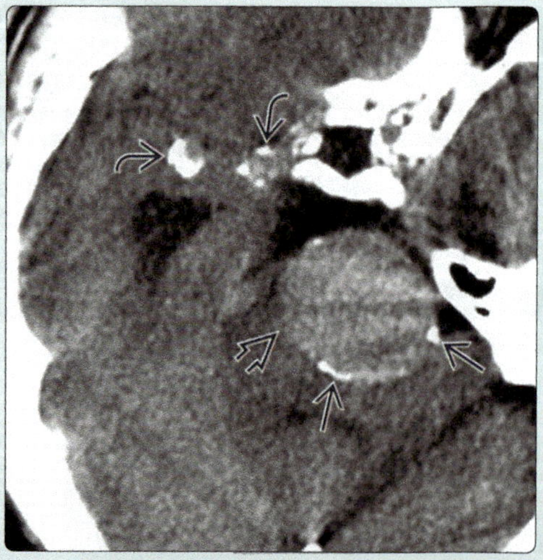

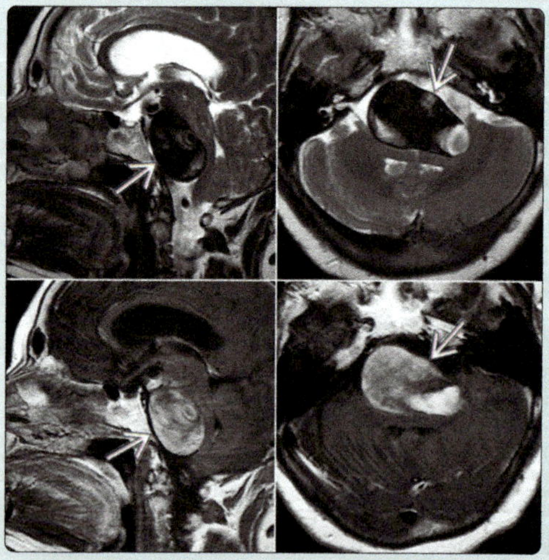

General Considerations

Cerebrovascular malformations (CVMs) of the brain are a heterogeneous group of disorders that represent morphogenetic errors affecting arteries, capillaries, veins, or various combinations of vessels.

The presentation, natural history, and management approaches to CVMs depend on their type, location, size, and hemodynamic characteristics. Some CVMs, such as venous or capillary malformations, are almost always clinically silent and therefore usually identified at imaging or autopsy. Others, such as arteriovenous malformations (AVMs) and cavernous malformations, may hemorrhage unexpectedly and without warning.

Terminology

Without a uniform consensus, there is much confusion regarding the nomenclature of brain CVMs. They have variously been called angiomas, hemangiomas, developmental anomalies, malformations, and hamartomas. For example, venous vascular malformations have been termed venous angiomas, venous anomalies, venous malformations, and developmental venous anomalies. Cavernous malformations have been called cavernous angiomas, cavernous hemangiomas, and "cavernomas" in the literature.

Using accurate terminology when discussing brain vascular malformations is important. Two major groups of vascular anomalies are recognized: Vascular malformations and hemangiomas. All CVMs ("angiomas") are malformative lesions. In contrast, "hemangiomas" are true proliferating, vasoformative neoplasms and, in the most recent WHO classification "Blue Book," are included with the mesenchymal, nonmeningothelial tumors.

Hemangiomas are benign vascular neoplasms, not malformations, and can be capillary or cavernous. Most intracranial hemangiomas are found in the skull, meninges, and dural venous sinuses, whereas most vascular malformations occur in the brain parenchyma. Therefore, the term hemangioma should be reserved for vasoproliferative neoplasms and not used to describe vascular malformations. In this text, CVMs are included in this section; hemangiomas are considered as neoplasms and included elsewhere.

Epidemiology

The overall prevalence of brain CVMs is difficult to estimate, as accurate epidemiologic data are scarce. Cushing and Bailey found that vascular anomalies constituted about 1% of all intracranial tumors. Using ICD-9 codes, hospital admission rates for CVMs have been calculated as ~ 1.5-1.8 cases per 100,000 person-years. CVMs are estimated to cause about 5% of all nontraumatic intracranial hemorrhages.

With modern imaging, and especially with contrast-enhanced MR, CVMs are found in up to 8-10% of imaged patients. Most (venous and capillary malformations) are asymptomatic and found incidentally.

Embryology

Development of the human fetal vascular system occurs via 2 related processes: Vasculogenesis and angiogenesis. Vasculogenesis begins with de novo differentiation of endothelial cells from mesoderm-derived precursors called hemangioblasts. Islands of hemangioblasts form an outer rim of endothelial cell precursors ("angioblasts") and an inner core of hematopoietic stem cells.

Angioblasts form capillary-like tubules that constitute the primitive vascular plexus. This embryonic vascular network is then remodeled by a process of sprouting, progressive anastomosis, and retrogressive differentiation. Endothelial cells differentiate into arterial and venous types, preceded, and guided by, migrating activated pericytes during definitive organization of the growing vessel wall.

Angiogenesis is regulated by a number of intercell signaling and growth factors. Some of these include Ang-1, Ang-2, Tie2, VEGF, PDGF, and TGF-β1, among others. Mutations in components of the angiogenetic system have been associated with the development of various CVMs.

Classification

In general, CVMs have been traditionally classified by histopathology and, more recently, by embryology and molecular genetics. With the advent of neurovascular interventional procedures, CVMs have also been classified by a practical, more functional approach.

Histopathologic Classification

Most neuropathology texts classify CVMs into 4 major types: (1) AVM, (2) venous angioma, (3) capillary telangiectasia, and (4) cavernous malformation. This histopathologic classification is used in this book.

Embryologic Classification

Some investigators have proposed an embryonic, "metameric" approach to classifying vascular malformations that accounts for the known relationship between some brain and cutaneous vascular malformations. They termed these "cerebral arterial metameric syndromes" or CAMS. For example, a CAMS1 syndrome links AVMs in the prosencephalon with those of the nose and orbit. Hence a CAMS1 patient may have a neurocutaneous AVM in the nose or retina and a brain parenchymal AVM.

Molecular Classification

The identification of underlying causal genes in familial forms of CVMs has allowed the definition of an ever-increasing number of these disorders at the molecular level. Specific mutations in some genes (e.g., *CCM1/KRIT1*, *CCM2/MGC4607*, *CCM3/PDCD10*) cause autosomal dominantly inherited cavernous malformation syndromes (CCM1, CCM2, and CCM3). Some patients with brain AVMs also have cutaneous capillary malformations attributable to *RASA1* gene mutations. Hereditary hemorrhagic telangiectasias (HHT) result from several mutations, among them the endoglin gene (*ENG*) in HHT1. Whether cavernous and venous malformations are "molecularly distinct" or only "phenotypically distinct" lesions that result from the same *CCM* gene mutations is controversial.

Functional Classification

Endovascular radiologists have proposed a functional, highly practical system that divides all CVMs into 2 basic categories: (1) CVMs that display arteriovenous shunting and (2) CVMs without AV shunting. The former category includes AVMs and arteriovenous fistulae; the latter is basically everything else (venous, capillary, cavernous malformations). The former are amenable to intervention; the latter are either left alone or treated surgically.

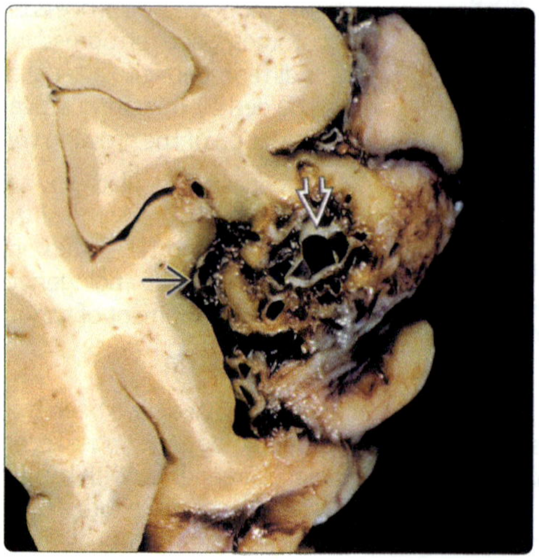

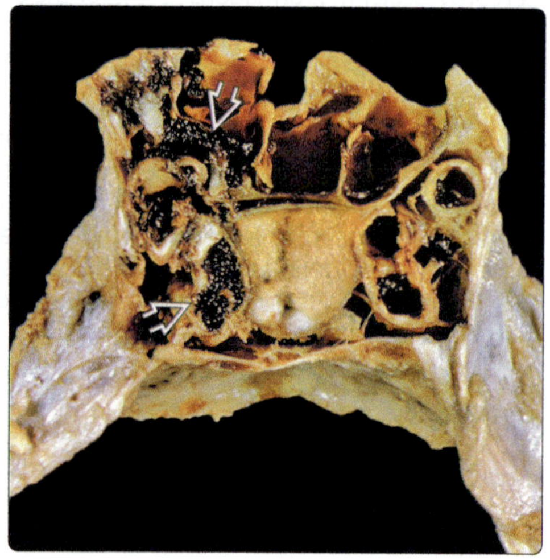

(Left) *Autopsied brain depicts an unruptured arteriovenous malformation (AVM). Multiple thin-walled vessels form the AVM nidus . A larger vessel may represent an intranidal aneurysm. (Courtesy R. Hewlett, MD.)* **(Right)** *Autopsy of a thrombosed carotid-cavernous fistula, another type of cerebrovascular malformation that displays arteriovenous shunting, shows multiple enlarged, arterialized venous channels . (Courtesy B. Horten, MD.)*

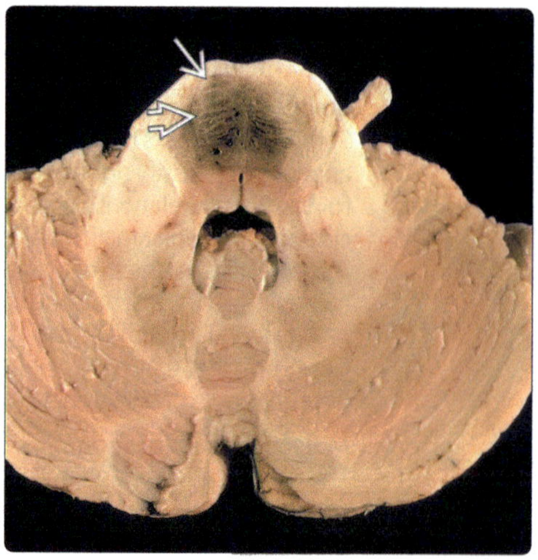

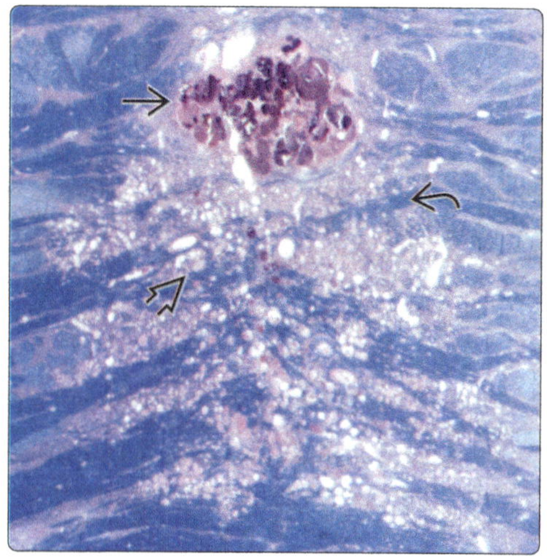

(Left) *Autopsied case cut in the axial plane shows a large pontine capillary telangiectasia . Note the transverse pontine fibers crossing through the telangiectasia without interruption or distortion. (Courtesy B. Horten, MD.)* **(Right)** *Low-power micropathology demonstrates a mixed pontine cavernous-capillary malformation. Normal white matter is interspersed with a cavernous malformation and multiple tiny thin-walled vessels . (Courtesy AFIP.)*

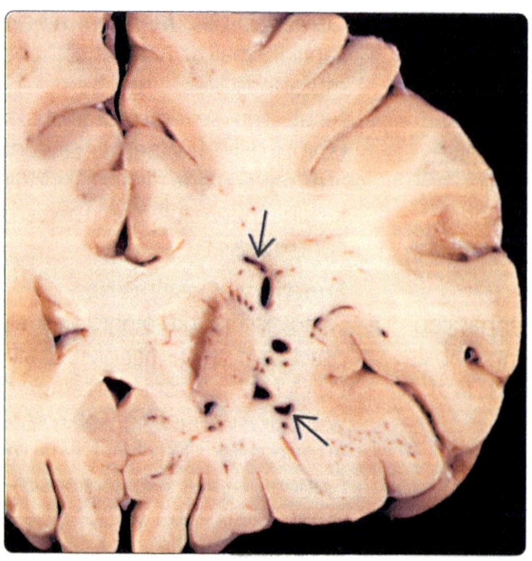

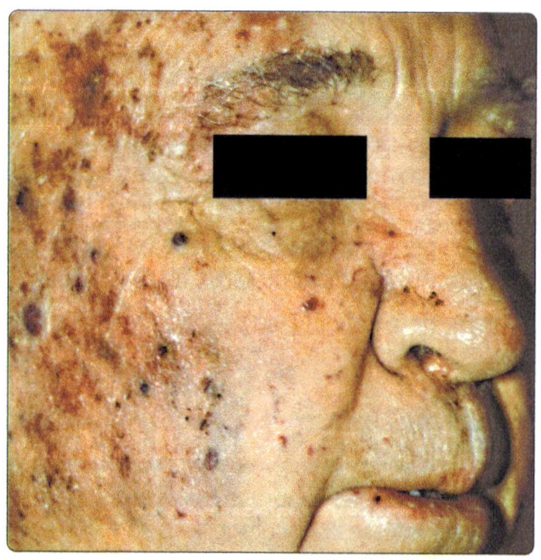

(Left) *Coronal autopsied brain shows an incidental developmental venous anomaly in the frontal lobe adjacent to the lateral ventricle. Note enlarged venous channels with normal white matter in between. (Courtesy M. Castillo, MD.)* **(Right)** *Clinical photograph of a patient with hereditary hemorrhagic telangiectasis and multiple episodes of severe epistaxis shows innumerable small capillary telangiectasias of the skin and scalp, nasal, and oral mucosa.*

KEY FACTS

TERMINOLOGY

- Pial vascular malformation of brain
  - Artery → vein shunting, no intervening capillary bed

IMAGING

- General features
  - Supratentorial (85%), posterior fossa (15%)
- CT/CTA
  - Iso-/hyperdense serpentine vessels ± Ca++
  - Arterial feeders, nidus, draining veins enhance
- MR
  - "Bag of worms"/tangle of serpiginous "honeycomb" flow voids
  - No intervening normal brain in arteriovenous malformation (AVM) nidus
  - Minimal/no mass effect
  - ± high signal (gliosis) on FLAIR
  - T2* GRE "blooming" if hemorrhage present
- DSA: Best delineates internal angioarchitecture, 3 components of AVM
  - Enlarged feeding arteries
  - Nidus of tightly packed vascular channels
  - Dilated draining veins
- Intranidal "aneurysm" > 50%
- Flow-related aneurysm on feeding artery (10-15%)

TOP DIFFERENTIAL DIAGNOSES

- Glioblastoma with arteriovenous shunting
- Dural arteriovenous fistula

CLINICAL ISSUES

- Annual hemorrhage risk varies widely
  - Overall annual hemorrhage risk 2-4% (cumulative)
  - However, ≤ 1% for unruptured, superficially-located nidi with superficial venous drainage
  - ≥ 30% for ruptured, deep-seated nidi with extensive deep venous drainage

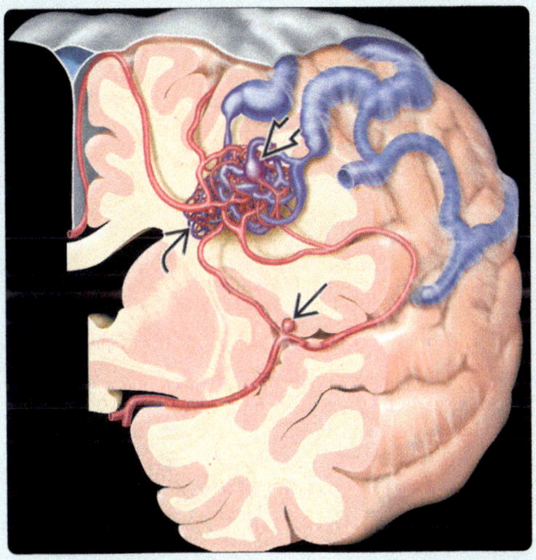

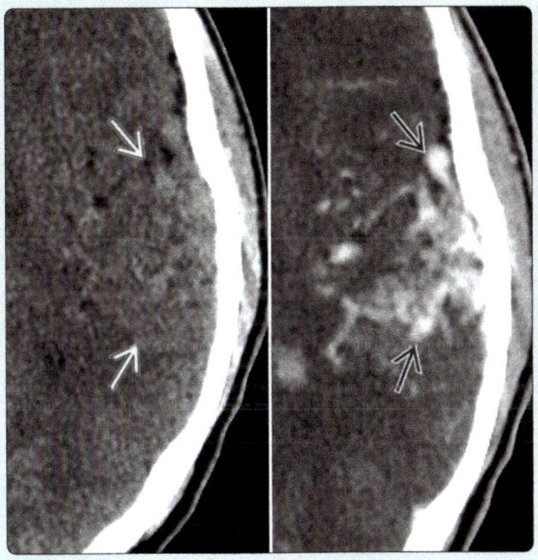

(Left) *Coronal graphic shows a classic cerebral arteriovenous malformation (AVM). Note the nidus ➡ with intranidal aneurysm ➡ and enlarged feeding arteries with a "pedicle" aneurysm ➡.* **(Right)** *Axial NECT (L) shows classic serpentine hyperdensities ➡ of an unruptured AVM. CECT (R) shows strong uniform enhancement ➡. Wedge-shaped configuration is typical.*

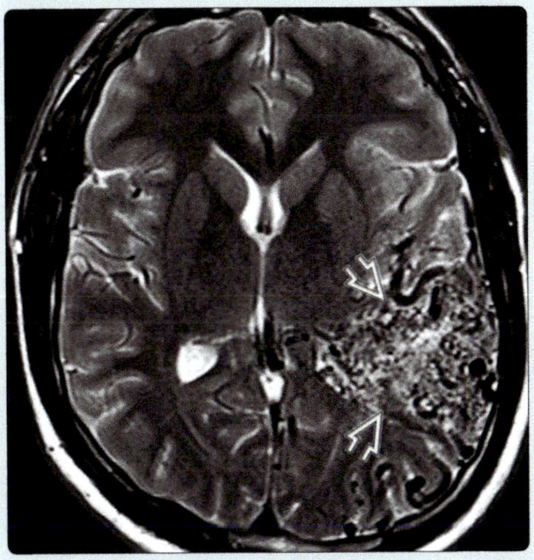

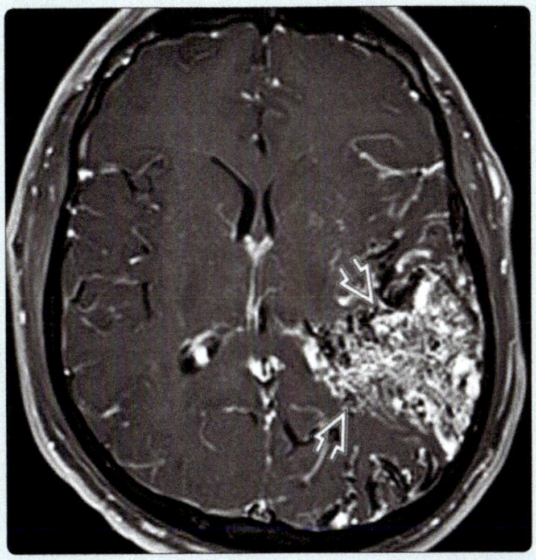

(Left) *Axial T2WI shows a classic AVM in the left parietal lobe. The AVM nidus is seen as a wedge-shaped mass of "flow voids" ➡ with its broad base at the cortical surface. There is no normal brain visible within the AVM.* **(Right)** *T1 C+ FS MR in the same case shows the tangle of vessels within the nidus enhances strongly ➡. Because AVMs are congenital lesions and replace (rather than displace) brain, there is almost no mass effect present.*

Dural Arteriovenous Fistula

KEY FACTS

IMAGING

- Location: Dural sinus wall
  - Posterior fossa >> supratentorial
  - Can involve any dural sinus (transverse/straight sinus most common)
- NECT
  - Usually normal; ICH if outlet vein thrombosed or flow-related aneurysm, venous pouch ruptures
- Bone CT
  - Dilated transosseous calvarial vascular channels, ± enlarged foramen spinosum
- MR
  - Isointense thrombosed sinus ± flow voids on T1/T2WI
  - Thrombosed dural sinus blooms on T2*
  - May show parenchymal hemorrhage in dAVF with cortical venous drainage
  - FLAIR: Isointense thrombosed sinus ± adjacent edema if venous congestion or ischemia present
- MR/CTA: Network of tiny (crack-like) vessels in wall of thrombosed dural venous sinus

TOP DIFFERENTIAL DIAGNOSES

- Hypoplastic transverse-sigmoid sinus; sigmoid sinus-jugular foramen pseudolesion; thrombosed dural sinus; dural sinus stenosis

PATHOLOGY

- Adult dAVFs are usually acquired, not congenital; can occur in response to trauma, venous sinus thrombosis; pathological activation of neoangiogenesis

CLINICAL ISSUES

- 10-15% of all cerebrovascular malformations with AV shunting
- Adult >> child
- Prognosis depends on location, venous drainage pattern
- Treatment options: Endovascular, surgery, stereotaxic XRT

(Left) *Clinical photograph in a patient with a "red eye" secondary to a dural arteriovenous fistula (dAVF) of the cavernous sinus. (Top) Note prominent scleral vessels ➔, focal hemorrhages ➔. (Bottom) After endovascular treatment of the cavernous dAVF, the eye appears normal.* **(Right)** *Graphic depicts dAVF with thrombosed transverse sinus ➔. Multiple transosseous branches ➔ from the external carotid artery supply innumerable tiny arteriovenous fistulae ➔ in the dural wall.*

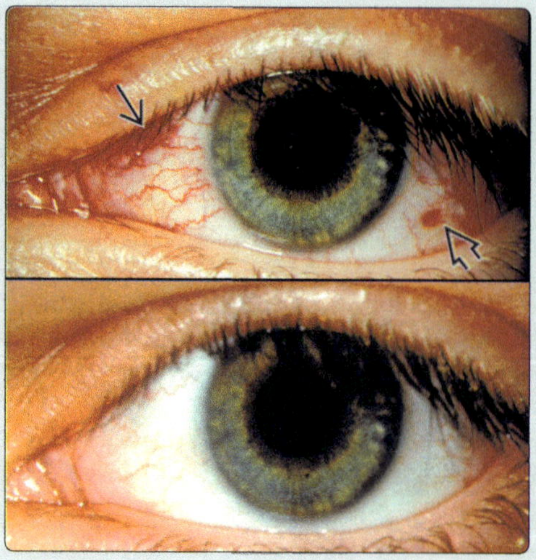

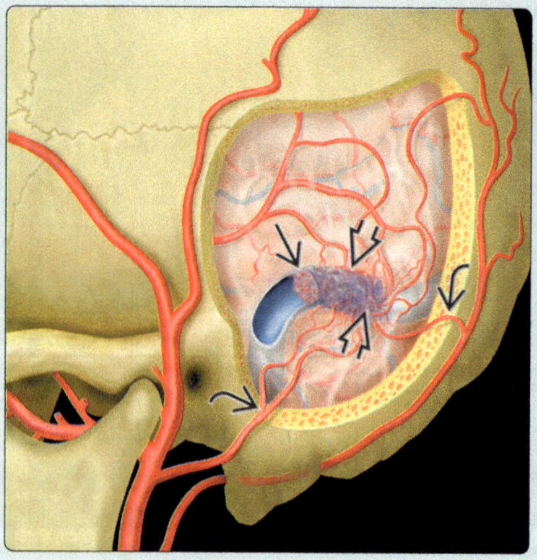

(Left) *Lateral view of an external carotid DSA depicts typical angiographic findings of dAVF. The ipsilateral transverse sinus is occluded ➔, and there are multiple prominent branches from the posterior auricular artery ➔ supplying a dAVF ➔ in the TS wall. The occipital artery ➔ is markedly enlarged.* **(Right)** *Selective injection of the OA in the same patient nicely demonstrates the mass-like dAVF ➔ in the occluded TS. Note innumerable enlarged transosseous branches ➔ that pass intracranially to supply the dAVF.*

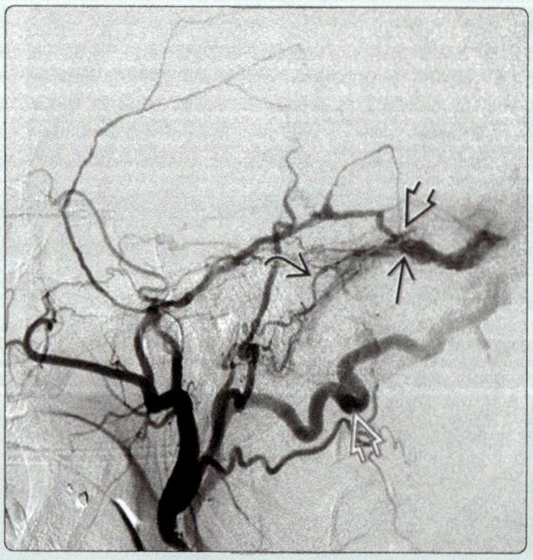

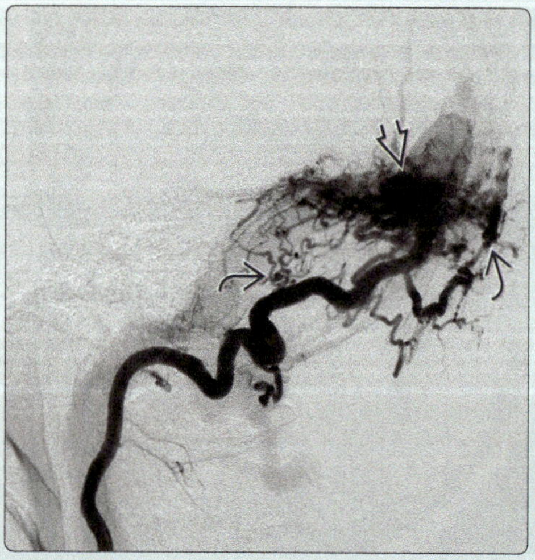

KEY FACTS

TERMINOLOGY

- Congenital cerebral vascular malformation with mature venous elements
- May represent anatomic variant of otherwise normal venous drainage

IMAGING

- General features
  - Umbrella-like collection of enlarged medullary (white matter) veins ("Medusa head")
  - At angle of ventricle
  - Numerous linear or dot-like enhancing foci
  - Converge on single enlarged "collector" vein
  - "Collector" vein drains into dural sinus/deep ependymal vein
  - Usually solitary, variable size (< 2-3 cm)
  - Hemorrhage may occur if mixed malformation or draining vein thromboses
- CT often normal; enlarged "collector" vein may appear hyperdense
- MR
  - Variable signal depending on size, flow; hypointense on SWI (BOLD effect in draining veins); strong enhancement

TOP DIFFERENTIAL DIAGNOSES

- Mixed vascular malformation (usually cavernoma)
- Vascular neoplasm
- Dural sinus thrombosis (chronic)

PATHOLOGY

- 15-20% coexisting cavernous &/or capillary malformations
- Blue rubber bleb nevus syndrome
- Sulcation-gyration disorders (may cause epilepsy)
- Cervicofacial venous or lymphatic malformation

CLINICAL ISSUES

- Can be asymptomatic or present with headaches &/or hemorrhage

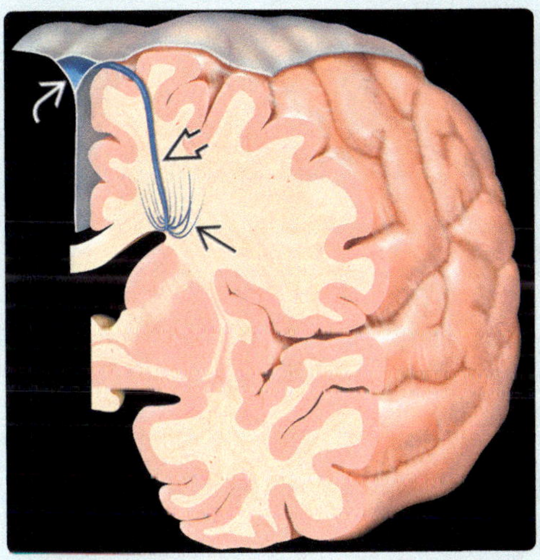

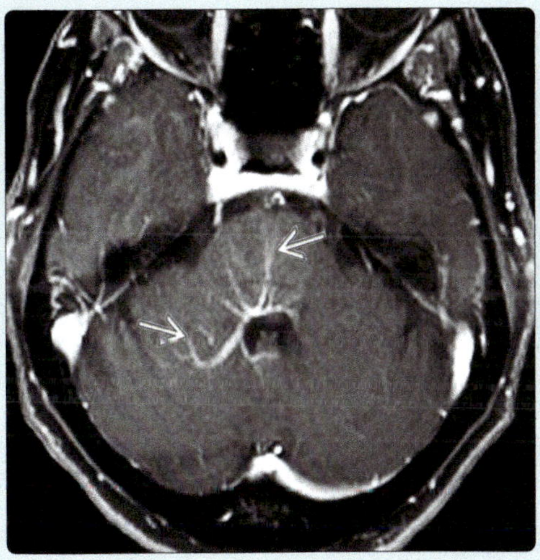

(Left) *Coronal oblique graphic depicts classic developmental venous anomaly (DVA) with umbrella-like "Medusa head" of enlarged medullary (deep WM) veins ➡ converging on a dilated transcortical "collector" vein ⇨, which drains into the superior sagittal sinus ↪.* **(Right)** *Axial T1 C+ FS in a 55-year-old man imaged for headache shows a large "Medusa head" ➡ of a DVA involving the pons and cerebellum.*

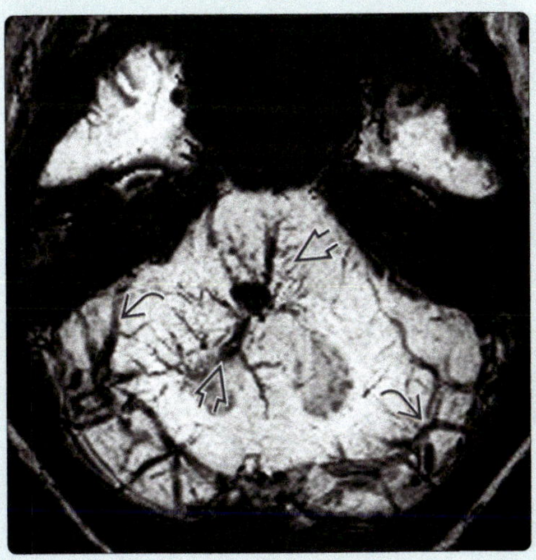

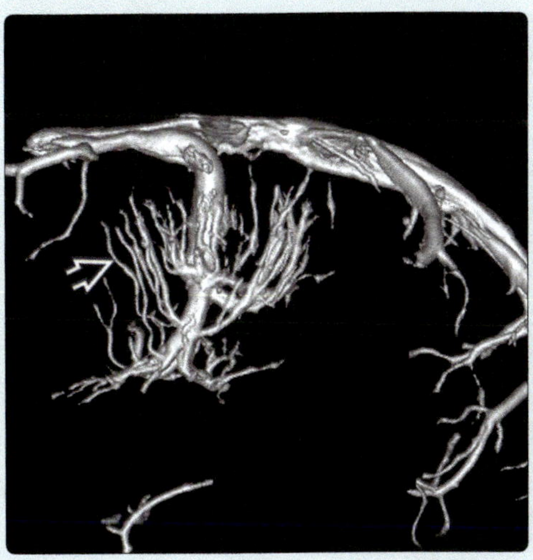

(Left) *T2* SWI in the same case shows multiple linear hypointensities ⇨ caused by slow flow, deoxyhemoglobin in the DVA. The hypointensities in the cerebellar fissures ↪ are normal peritentorial draining veins.* **(Right)** *3D shaded surface rendering of a venous-phase DSA in another case elegantly depicts the classic "Medusa head" of a DVA ⇨. (Courtesy P. Lasjaunias, MD.)*

KEY FACTS

TERMINOLOGY

- Cavernous malformation (CM)
- Benign vascular hamartoma
  - Contains masses of closely apposed immature blood vessels ("caverns"), no neural tissue
  - Intralesional hemorrhages of different ages

IMAGING

- General: Locules of variable size with blood at different stages of evolution
  - Variable appearance depending on hemorrhage/stage
  - CMs vary from microscopic to giant (> 6 cm)
- Classic MR: Popcorn-ball appearance with complete hypointense hemosiderin rim on T2WI MR
- DSA: Usually normal (angiographically occult vascular malformation) unless mixed with DVA
- Zabramski classification of CMs
  - Type 1 = subacute hemorrhage (may obscure underlying CM)
  - Type 2 = mixed signal intensity on T1, T2WI (classic "popcorn ball" lesion)
  - Type 3 = chronic hemorrhage (hypo- to isointense on T1, T2WI)
  - Type 4 = punctate microhemorrhages (blooming "black spots" on T2* GRE, SWI)

TOP DIFFERENTIAL DIAGNOSES

- Arteriovenous malformation
- Hemorrhagic neoplasm
- Calcified neoplasm
- Hypertensive microbleeds
- Amyloid angiopathy

CLINICAL ISSUES

- Variable behavior (enlarge, regress, form de novo)
- All ages (peak = 40-60 years)
- Can be cerebrum (most common) or posterior fossa (most serious); symptoms are neurological deficits

(Left) *Axial graphic depicts various stages of cavernous malformations with subacute hemorrhage and classic "popcorn ball" lesion with multiple blood-filled locules, surrounding hemosiderin rim. Multifocal "blooming black dots" are also depicted.* **(Right)** *Axial NECT scan shows a mixed-density right thalamic mass with edema. Note fluid-fluid level within the mass.*

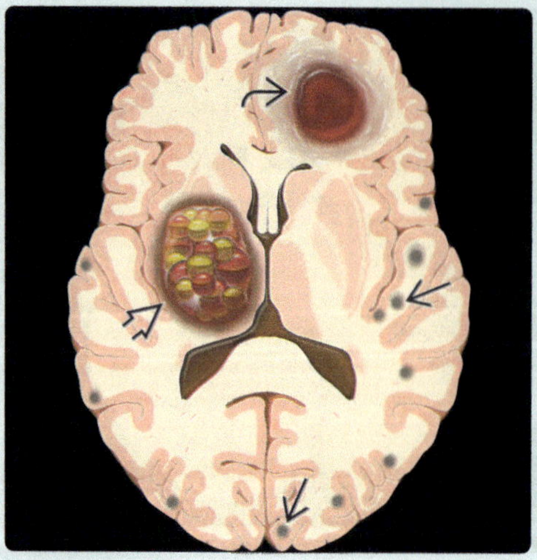

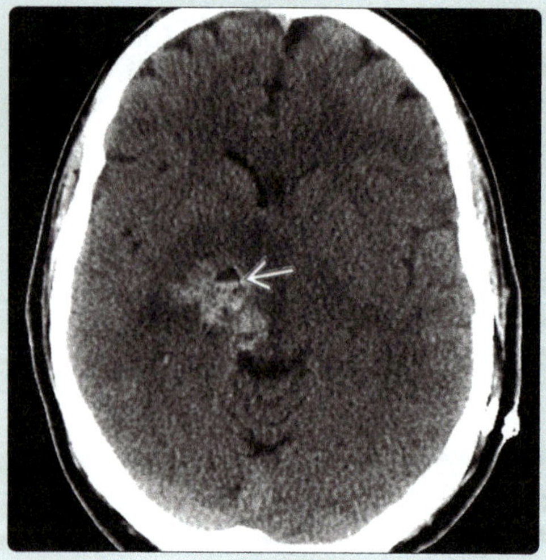

(Left) *Axial T2WI in the same case shows the classic popcorn-ball appearance of a cavernous malformation with multiple fluid-filled locules. A second, separate lesion is also present.* **(Right)** *T2* GRE scan in the same case shows striking "blooming" in and around the 2 lesions. A 3rd lesion in the right occipital lobe is present but was difficult to see on the standard FSE T2-weighted sequence.*

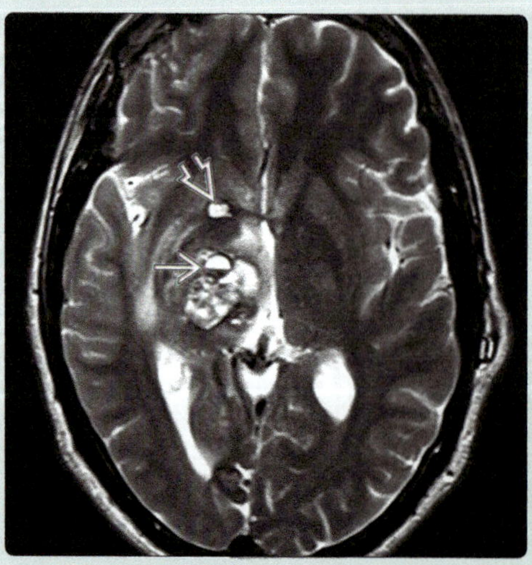

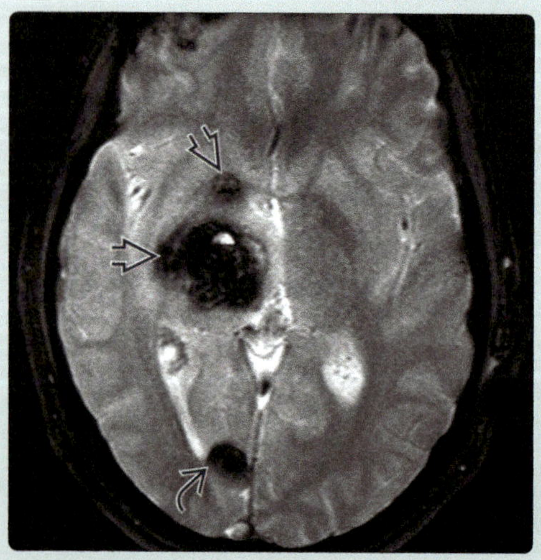

KEY FACTS

TERMINOLOGY

- Brain capillary telangiectasia (BCT)
- Cluster of enlarged, dilated capillaries interspersed with normal brain parenchyma

IMAGING

- General features
  - Common sites: Pons, cerebellum, spinal cord
  - Usually < 1 cm
- CT
  - Usually normal
- MR
  - T1WI usually normal
  - T2WI
    - 50% normal on T2WI
    - 50% show faint stippled foci of hyperintensity
  - Large BCTs may show ill-defined FLAIR hyperintensity
  - Moderately hypointense on GRE; profoundly hypointense on SWI
  - T1 C+ shows faint stippled or speckled brush-like enhancement
  - Large BCTs typically contain prominent linear draining vein(s)

TOP DIFFERENTIAL DIAGNOSES

- Developmental venous anomaly
- Metastasis
- Cavernous malformation
- Capillary hemangioma

CLINICAL ISSUES

- BCTs represent 15-20% of all intracranial vascular malformations
- Usually found incidentally at autopsy or imaging
- Rare: Headache, vertigo, tinnitus
- Clinically benign, quiescent
  - Unless histologically mixed (usually with capillary malformation)

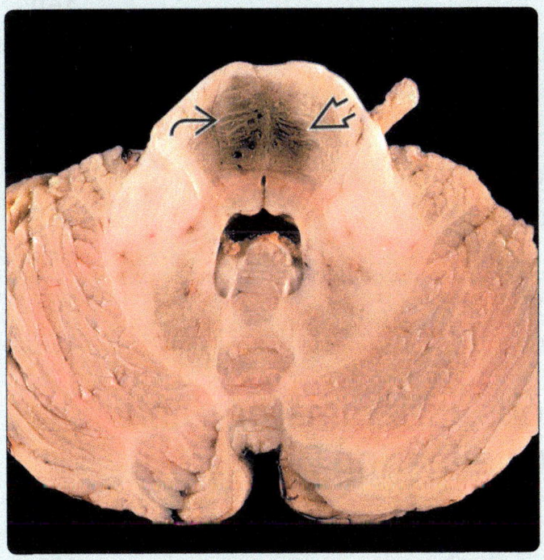

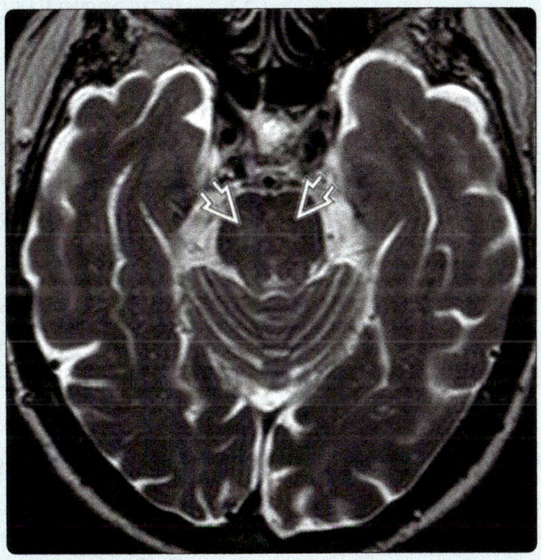

(Left) *Axial gross pathology shows a large capillary telangiectasia of the pons. The dusky color is caused by deoxygenated blood, not frank hemorrhage. Note undisturbed transverse pontine tracts crossing the telangiectasia.* **(Right)** *Axial T2WI in a neurologically normal patient with headaches shows very faint "stippled" hyperintensities in the central pons.*

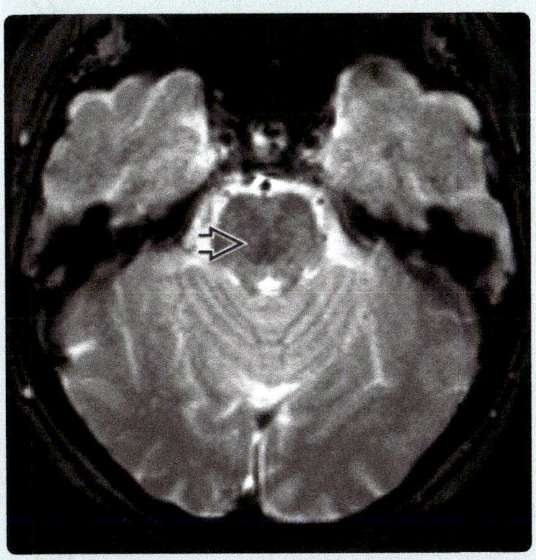

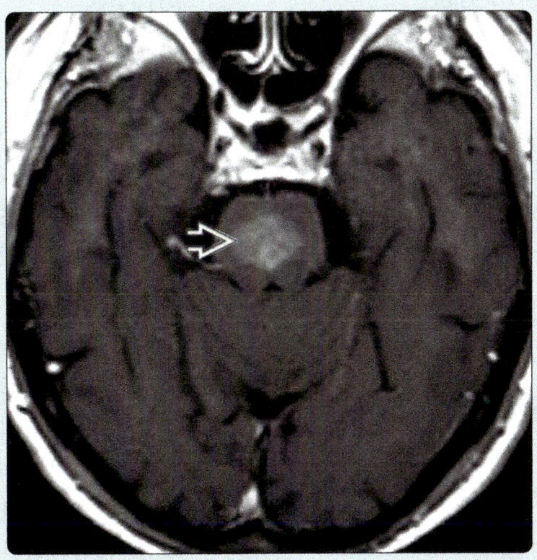

(Left) *Axial T2* GRE in the same patient shows faint hypointensity in the central pons.* **(Right)** *Axial T1 C+ MR in the same patient shows faint brush-like enhancement in the central pons, characteristic of a large capillary telangiectasia. (Courtesy P. Rodriguez, MD.)*

PART I: BRAIN
SECTION 2

Pathology-Based Diagnoses: Neoplasms, Cysts, and Disorders

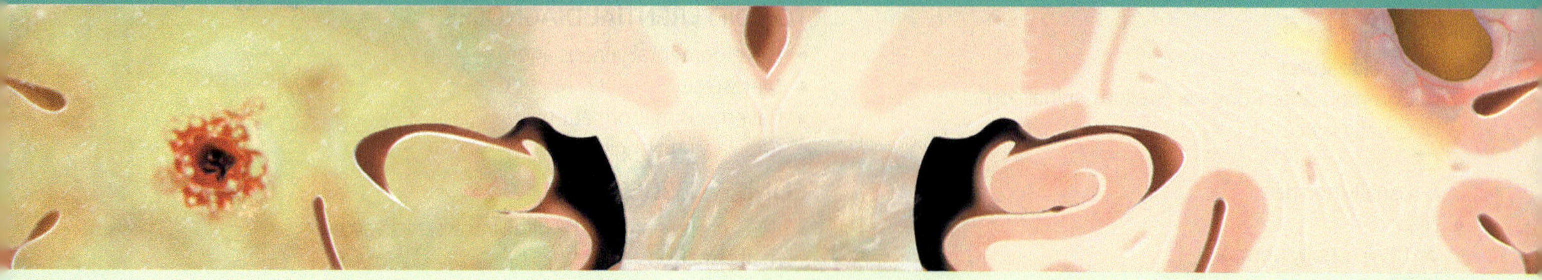

Neoplasms

Primary Nonneoplastic Cysts

Infectious, Inflammatory, and Demyelinating Disease

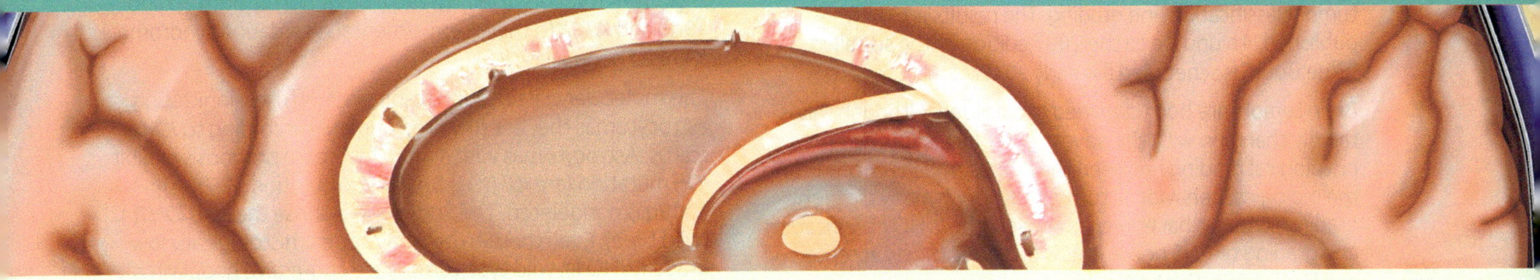

Introduction

The most widely accepted classification of brain neoplasms is sponsored by the World Health Organization (WHO). A working group of world-renowned neuropathologists periodically convenes for a consensus conference on brain tumor classification and grading. The results are then published. An update to the 2007 edition of the so-called "Blue Book" is scheduled for early 2017.

Brain tumors are both classified and graded. Although this is rapidly changing with the advent of molecular profiling, histological grading has been the primary means of predicting the biological behavior of tumors. Although many different grading schemas have been proposed, the WHO classification and grading of CNS neoplasms is the most widely accepted and is utilized in this text.

Classification/Grading of CNS Neoplasms

General Considerations

CNS neoplasms are divided into primary and metastatic tumors. Primary neoplasms are divided into 6 major categories. The largest by far is tumors of neuroepithelial tissue, followed by tumors of the meninges. Tumors of cranial and spinal nerves, lymphomas and hematopoietic neoplasms, and germ cell tumors are less common but important groupings. The final category of primary neoplasms, tumors of the sellar region, is identified by geographic region rather than histologic type.

Tumors of Neuroepithelial Tissue

This category is huge, and therefore it is divided into several discrete tumor subtypes. Once thought to arise from dedifferentiation of mature neurons or glial cells (e.g., astrocytes, oligodendrocytes, ependymal cells, etc.), it is now recognized that most brain tumors arise from neural stem cells.

Astrocytomas: There are many histologic types and subtypes of astrocytomas, ranging in biological behavior from benign, relatively circumscribed tumors, such as pilocytic astrocytoma (PA) and subependymal giant cell astrocytoma (SGCA), to the highly malignant, diffusely infiltrating glioblastoma (GBM).

Two of the localized astrocytomas (PA and SGCA) are designated as WHO grade I neoplasms. Neither displays a tendency to malignant progression, although a variant of PA called pilomyxoid astrocytoma may behave more aggressively and is classified as a WHO grade II tumor.

Diffusely infiltrating astrocytomas have no distinct border between tumor and normal brain, even though the tumor may look relatively discrete on imaging. The lowest grade is simply called "diffuse astrocytoma" and is designated as WHO grade II. Anaplastic astrocytoma is WHO grade III, and GBM is a grade IV neoplasm.

Patient age has a significant effect on astrocytoma type and location. For example, diffusely infiltrating astrocytomas are most common in the cerebral hemispheres of adults and the pons in children. PAs are tumors of children and young adults. They are common in the cerebellum and around the 3rd ventricle but only rarely occur in the hemispheres.

Oligodendroglial tumors: These vary from a diffusely infiltrating, but relatively well-differentiated, WHO grade II neoplasm (oligodendroglioma) to anaplastic oligodendroglioma (WHO grade III).

Low-grade gliomas (LGGs): LGGs have been distilled into 3 molecular subtypes, which yields a robust nonoverlapping, clinically relevant classification that is superior to traditional histologic methods in predicting biological behavior. LGG class is based on the fluorescence in situ hybridization status of 3 important markers: *IDH1*, 1p19q (codeletion of both 1p and 19q), and *ATRX* (α-thalassemia/mental retardation syndrome X-linked gene).

This molecular classification results in 2 diffusely infiltrating astrocytomas that are stratified primarily according to *IDH1* status. Astrocytomas with a more favorable prognosis exhibit *IDH* mutation {are *IDH1*(+)] &/or *ATRX* mutation [*ATRX*(+)]. 1p19q is nondeleted. The 2nd group is those that are *IDH1*(-) (wild-type). Even though they may appear histologically low grade (WHO II), wild-type tumors are aggressive neoplasms that behave more like GBMs. Oligodendrogliomas exhibit 1p19q codeletion and are typically *IDH1*(+). *ATRX* is nonmutated.

O-6-methylguanine-DNA methyltransferase (MGMT) promoter profiling is important for glioma treatment stratification. MGMT(+) tumors are typically more chemosensitive than wild-type neoplasms.

Gliomas in children vs. adults: Pediatric gliomas are often genetically different from their adult counterparts, even though they appear identical under the microscope. Intrinsic pediatric pontine gliomas, aggressive neoplasms that are almost always fatal, exhibit histone (*H3*) and *ACVR1* mutations. In contrast to adult oligodendrogliomas, pediatric oligodendrogliomas rarely exhibit 1p19q codeletion.

Ependymal tumors: Classic histologic criteria divide ependymal neoplasms into grade I subependymomas or myxopapillary ependymomas, grade II ependymomas (further subdivided into cellular, papillary, clear cell, and tanycytic types), and grade III (anaplastic) ependymomas.

DNA methylation profiling has recently identified 9 molecular subgroups of ependymoma. This molecular classification outperforms the current histopathological grading in the risk stratification of patients for treatment.

Choroid plexus tumors (CPTs): CPTs are papillary intraventricular neoplasms. Almost 80% are found in children. Classically, CPTs have been divided into choroid plexus papillomas (CPP) (WHO grade I), atypical choroid plexus papillomas (aCPP) (WHO grade III), and choroid plexus carcinomas (CPCa), designated as WHO grade III. Recent genomic analysis has shown aCPP is an immature variant of CPP with similar cytogenetic profiling and differs only by exhibiting increased proliferative activity. CPCa is a genetically distinct tumor group.

CPPs are 5-10x more common than CPCs. All CPTs can spread diffusely through the cerebrospinal fluid (CSF), so the entire neuraxis should be imaged prior to surgical intervention.

Other neuroepithelial tumors: These rare neoplasms include astroblastoma, chordoid glioma of the 3rd ventricle, and angiocentric glioma.

Neuronal and mixed neuronal-glial tumors: Neuroepithelial tumors with ganglion-like cells, differentiated neurocytes, or poorly differentiated neuroblastic cells are included in this heterogeneous group. Ganglion cell neoplasms (gangliocytoma, ganglioglioma), desmoplastic infantile ganglioglioma or astrocytoma (DIG/DIA), neurocytoma (central as well as the newly described extraventricular variant), dysembryoplastic neuroepithelial tumor, papillary glioneuronal tumor, rosette-forming glioneuronal tumor (of the 4th ventricle), and cerebellar liponeuroblastoma are included.

Pineal region tumors: Pineal region neoplasms account for < 1% of all intracranial neoplasms and can be germ cell tumors or pineal parenchymal tumors. Pineal parenchymal tumors are less common than germ cell tumors. Because germ cell neoplasms occur in other intracranial sites as well as the pineal gland, they are considered separately.

Pineocytoma is a very slowly growing, well-delineated tumor that is usually found in adults. Pineocytomas are WHO grade I. Pineoblastoma is a highly malignant primitive embryonal tumor mostly found in children. Highly aggressive and associated with early CSF dissemination, pineoblastomas are WHO grade IV neoplasms.

Pineal parenchymal tumor of intermediate differentiation (PPTID) is intermediate in malignancy, probably WHO grade II or III. Many so-called aggressive pineocytomas would probably be reclassified as PPTIDs. A newly described neoplasm, papillary tumor of the pineal region, is a rare neuroepithelia tumor of adults. No WHO grade has been assigned.

Embryonal tumors: This group includes medulloblastoma (MB), CNS primitive neuroectodermal tumors, and atypical teratoid-rhabdoid tumors (AT/RT). *SMARCB1* (INI1/hSNF5) mutation is diagnostic of AT/RT even in the absence of overtly rhabdoid cells.

MB, which has 1 classic and 3 histologic variants, is now divided into 4 groups based on molecular profiling (the 1st step in risk stratifying MB patients for therapy). Although all 4 groups are designated as WHO IV tumors, they behave quite differently, and 1 specific subgroup (Wnt) is associated with an especially favorable prognosis.

Meningeal Tumors

Overview: Meningeal tumors are the 2nd largest category of primary CNS neoplasms. They are divided into meningiomas and mesenchymal, nonmeningothelial tumors (i.e., tumors that are not meningiomas). Hemangiopericytomas (HPCs), hemangioblastomas (HGBLs), and melanocytic lesions are also considered part of the meningeal tumor grouping.

Meningiomas: Meningiomas arise from meningothelial (arachnoid cap) cells. Most are attached to the dura but can occur in other locations (e.g., choroid plexus of the lateral ventricles). Although meningiomas have many histologic subtypes (e.g., meningothelial, fibrous, psammomatous, etc.), the current WHO schema classifies them rather simply. Most meningiomas are benign and correspond to WHO grade I. Atypical meningioma, as well as the chordoid and clear cell variants, are WHO grade II tumors. Anaplastic (malignant) meningiomas correspond to WHO grade III.

Mesenchymal, nonmeningothelial tumors: Both benign and malignant mesenchymal tumors can originate in the CNS. Most correspond to tumors of soft tissue or bone. Generally, both a benign and malignant (sarcomatous) type occur. Lipomas and liposarcomas, chondromas and chondrosarcomas, osteomas and osteosarcomas are examples.

HPC is a highly cellular, vascular mesenchymal tumor that is almost always attached to the dura. HPCs are WHO II or III neoplasms. HGBL is a WHO grade I neoplasm, consisting of stromal cells and innumerable small blood vessels. It occurs both sporadically and as a part of von Hippel-Lindau syndrome. Primary melanocytic neoplasms of the CNS are rare. They arise from leptomeningeal melanocytes and can be diffuse or circumscribed, benign or malignant.

Tumors of Cranial (and Spinal) Nerves

Schwannoma: Schwannomas are benign, encapsulated nerve sheath tumors that consist of well-differentiated Schwann cells. They can be solitary or multiple. Multiple schwannomas are associated with neurofibromatosis type 2 (NF2) and schwannomatosis, a syndrome characterized by multiple schwannomas but lacking other features of NF2. Intracranial schwannomas are almost always associated with cranial nerves (CN8 is by far the most common) but occasionally occur as a parenchymal lesion. Schwannomas do not undergo malignant degeneration and are designated as WHO grade I neoplasms.

Neurofibroma (NF): NFs are diffusely infiltrating, extraneural tumors that consist of Schwann cells and fibroblasts. Solitary scalp NFs occur. Multiple NFs or plexiform NFs occur as part of NF1. NFs correspond histologically to WHO grade I. Plexiform NFs may degenerate into malignant peripheral nerve sheath tumors (MPNSTs). MPNSTs are graded from WHO II to IV, an approach similar to sarcoma grading.

Lymphomas and Hematopoietic Tumors

Primary CNS Lymphoma (PCNSL): As a result of HAART therapy in HIV/AIDS patients, as well as in other immunocompromised individuals, PCNSLs are dramatically increasing in prevalence. PCNSL can occur as both focal parenchymal and intravascular tumor. PCNSL can be single or multiple and is most commonly seen in the cerebral hemispheres. More than 95% of PCNSLs are diffuse large B-cell lymphomas.

Germ Cell Tumors

Intracranial germ cell tumors are morphologic homologues of germinal neoplasms that arise in the gonads and extragonadal sites. 80-90% occur in adolescents. Most occur in the midline (pineal region, around the 3rd ventricle).

Sellar Region Tumors

Craniopharyngioma: Craniopharyngioma is a benign (WHO grade I), often partially cystic neoplasm that is the most common nonneuroepithelial intracranial neoplasm in children. It shows a distinct bimodal age distribution, with the cystic adamantinomatous type seen mostly in children and a 2nd, smaller peak in middle-aged adults. The less common papillary type is usually solid and found almost exclusively in adults.

Miscellaneous sellar region tumors: Granular cell tumor of the neurohypophysis is a rare tumor of adults that usually arises from the infundibulum. Pituicytomas are glial neoplasms of adults that also usually arise within the infundibulum. Spindle cell oncocytoma of the adenohypophysis is a nonendocrine neoplasm of the adenohypophysis. These rare tumors are all WHO grade I.

Neuroepithelial Tumors

Neoplasm	Grade	Neoplasm	Grade	Neoplasm	Grade
Astrocytic		**Choroid plexus**		**Neuronal, mixed neuronal-glial**	
Pilocytic astrocytoma	I	Choroid plexus papilloma	I	Gangliocytoma	I
Pilomyxoid astrocytoma	II	Atypical choroid plexus papilloma	II	Ganglioglioma	I
Subependymal giant cell astrocytoma	I	Choroid plexus carcinoma	III	DIG/DIA	I
Pleomorphic xanthoastrocytoma	II			DNET	I
Anaplastic astrocytoma	III	**Pineal region**		Central neurocytoma	II
Glioblastoma	IV	Pineocytoma	I	Extraventricular neurocytoma	II
Gliosarcoma	IV	PPTID	II-III	Cerebellar liponeurocytoma	II
Gliomatosis cerebri	III, II-IV	Pineoblastoma	IV	Paraganglioma (spinal cord)	I
		Papillary tumor of pineal region	II-III	Papillary glioneuronal tumor	I
Oligodendroglial				Rosette-forming glioneuronal tumor	I
Oligodendroglioma	II	**Ependymal**			
Anaplastic oligodendroglioma	III	Subependymoma	I	**Other neuroepithelial**	
Oligoastrocytoma	Variable	Myxopapillary ependymoma	I	Astroblastoma	
		Ependymoma	II	Chordoid glioma of 3rd ventricle	II
Embryonal		Anaplastic ependymoma	III	Angiocentric glioma (angiocentric neuroepithelial tumor)	I
Medulloblastoma	IV				
Primitive neuroectodermal tumor	IV				
Atypical teratoid-rhabdoid tumor	IV				

Meningeal Tumors

Neoplasm	Grade	Neoplasm	Grade	Neoplasm	Grade
Meningothelial		**Nonmeningothelial mesenchymal**		**Primary melanocytic**	
Meningioma	I	Lipoma	I	Diffuse melanocytoma	
Atypical meningioma	II	Liposarcoma		Melanocytoma	
Anaplastic/malignant meningioma	III	Chondroma	I	Malignant melanoma	
		Chondrosarcoma		Meningeal melanomatosis	
Other related		Osteoma			
Hemangioblastoma	I	Osteosarcoma			
		Osteochondroma			
		Hemangioma	I		
		Hemangiopericytoma	II-III		

Other Tumors

Neoplasm	Grade	Neoplasm	Grade	Neoplasm	Grade
Cranial and spinal nerve tumors		**Germ cell tumors**		**Sellar region tumors**	
Schwannoma	I	Germinoma		Craniopharyngioma	I
Neurofibroma	I	Embryonal carcinoma		Adamantinomatous	
MPNST	II-IV	Yolk sac tumor		Papillary	
		Mixed germ cell tumor		Granular cell tumor of neurohypophysis	I
Lymphoma/hematopoietic		Teratoma		Pituicytoma	I
Malignant lymphoma				Spindle cell oncocytoma	I

Tables modified, adapted to conform to 2007 WHO Classification of Tumours of the CNS. MPNST= malignant peripheral nerve sheath tumor.

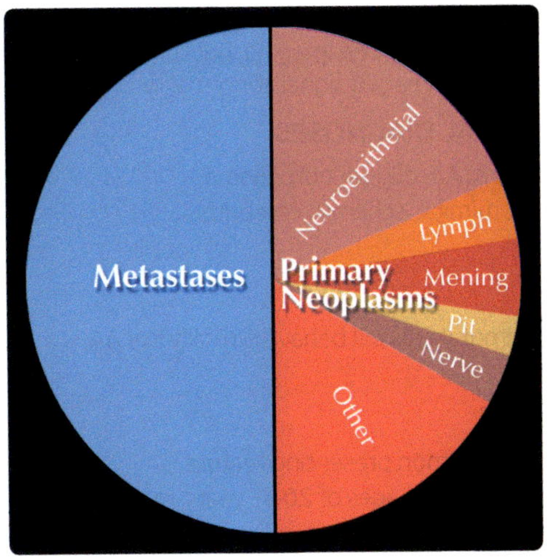

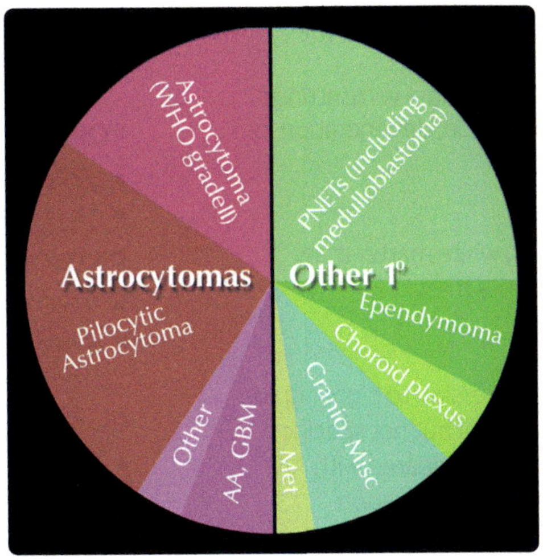

(Left) *Graphic depicts the relative prevalence of brain tumors in adults. Nearly 1/2 are metastases from systemic cancers; the other 1/2 are primary neoplasms.* **(Right)** *Graphic depicts brain tumors in children. Metastases, anaplastic astrocytoma (AA), and glioblastoma (GBM) are rare. Pilocytic astrocytoma and primitive neuroectodermal tumors (PNETs) in children are more common than in adults.*

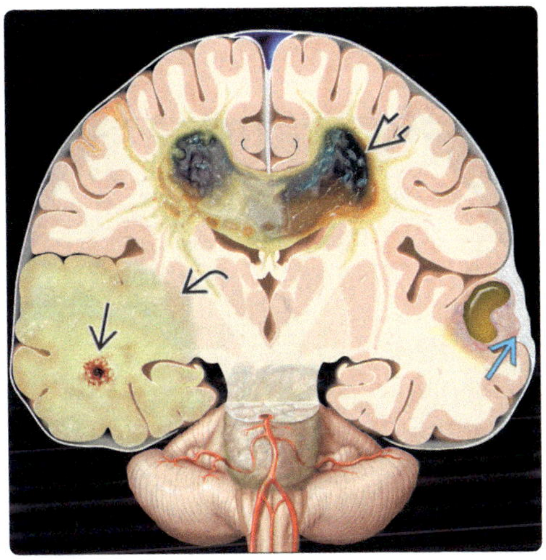

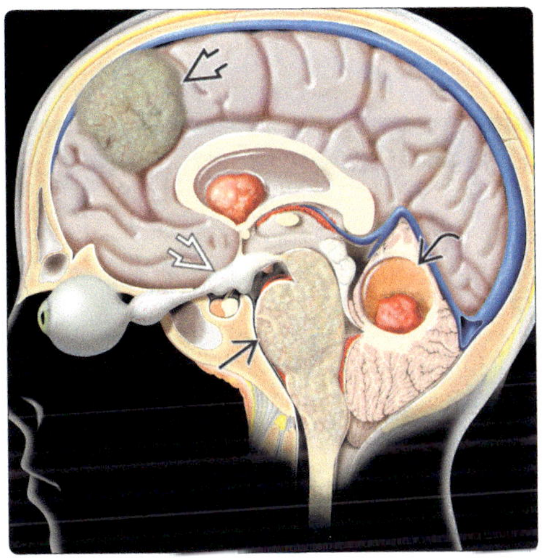

(Left) *Graphic depicts adult astrocytomas. Low-grade astrocytoma (WHO II) often becomes anaplastic. GBM is the most common (shown here in the corpus callosum). Pleomorphic xanthoastrocytoma is a cystic tumor with nodule abutting/thickening the meninges.* **(Right)** *Graphic shows childhood astrocytomas. Brainstem "gliomas", pilocytic astrocytoma (PA) are common. Except for PAs around the optic nerves/chiasm, supratentorial astrocytomas are less frequent.*

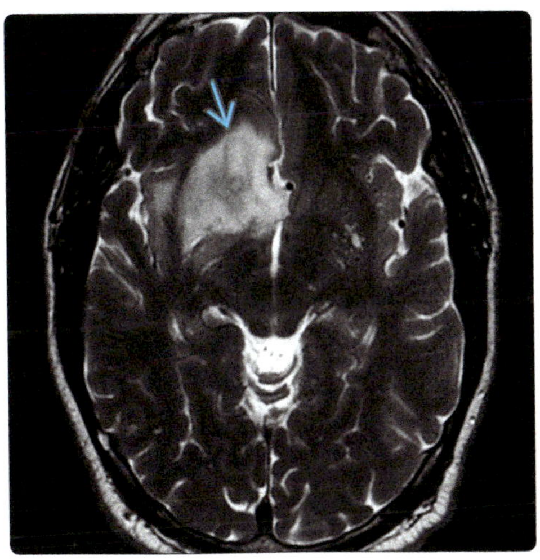

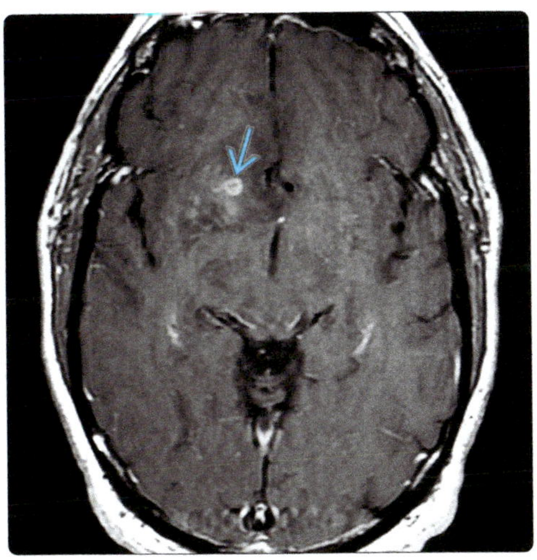

(Left) *Axial T2WI in a 58-year-old man with 2 seizures demonstrates a heterogeneously hyperintense mass infiltrating the right basal ganglia, frontal lobe, external capsule, and posterior limb of the internal capsule.* **(Right)** *T1WI C+ MR in the same patient shows a few enhancing foci in the center of the mass. Its location (frontal lobe) and large nonenhancing areas suggest this tumor is likely a secondary GBM. Biopsy disclosed IDH1(+), EGFR(-), MGMT(+), p53 70% (+), PTEN 25% (+), and MIB1 90%.*

Low-Grade Diffuse Astrocytoma

KEY FACTS

TERMINOLOGY

- Well-differentiated but infiltrating neoplasm, slow growth pattern
- Primary brain tumor of astrocytic origin with intrinsic tendency for malignant progression, degeneration into anaplastic astrocytoma (AA)

IMAGING

- Focal or diffuse nonenhancing white matter mass
- T2 homogeneously hyperintense mass
- May expand adjacent cortex
- Usually no enhancement
  - Enhancement suggests progression to higher grade
- MRS: High choline, low NAA typical but not specific
- Perfusion: Relatively lower rCBV compared with AA
- Cerebral hemispheres most common location
  - Supratentorial 2/3: Frontal and temporal lobes
- Infratentorial 1/3: Brainstem (50% of brainstem "gliomas" are low-grade astrocytoma)
- Low-grade astrocytoma may be indistinguishable from other tumors
- May appear circumscribed on imaging, but tumor cells are often found beyond imaged signal abnormality

TOP DIFFERENTIAL DIAGNOSES

- Other neoplasms: AA, oligodendroglioma
- Nonneoplastic mimics: Ischemia, cerebritis

PATHOLOGY

- WHO grade II
- If IDH-1(-) (nonmutated), will behave clinically like AA, glioblastoma

CLINICAL ISSUES

- Seizure is most common presenting feature
- Majority occur between ages of 20-45 years, mean: 34 years
- Median survival: 6-10 years
- Increased survival: Young age, gross total resection
- More favorable prognosis: *IDH1*(+), *ATRX*(+), *MGMT*(+)

(Left) *Coronal graphic shows an infiltrative mass centered in the white matter expanding the left temporal lobe. Axial insert shows mild mass effect upon the midbrain. Low-grade astrocytomas typically affect young adults.* **(Right)** *Axial T2 MR in a 34-year-old man with seizures shows a hyperintense infiltrative mass → centered in the right temporal lobe white matter with extension to the overlying cortex. No enhancement was present on contrast-enhanced images. WHO grade II astrocytoma was diagnosed at resection.*

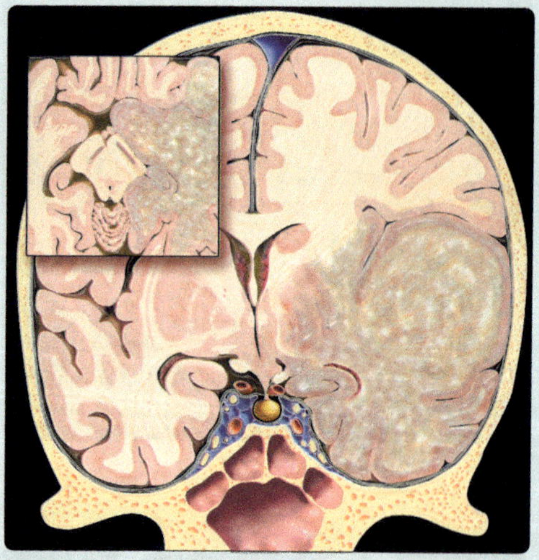

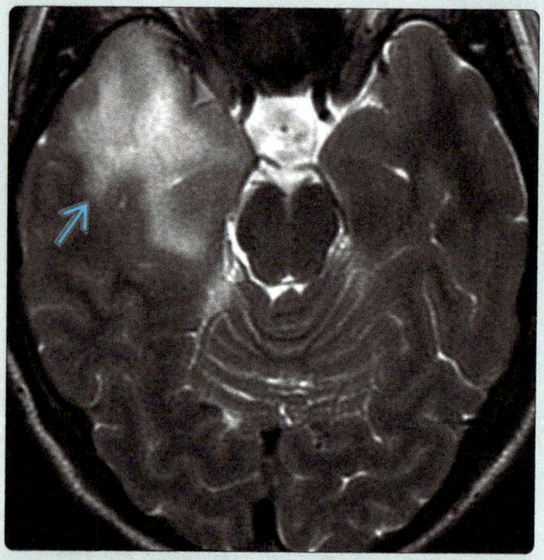

(Left) *Axial FLAIR MR shows a relatively homogeneous hyperintense mass with mild local mass effect, typical of a WHO grade II diffuse astrocytoma. These infiltrative tumors may be focal or diffuse. Fibrillary astrocytoma is the most frequent histologic variant.* **(Right)** *Axial MR perfusion in the same patient shows a low relative cerebral blood volume ➡ in the frontotemporal mass, suggesting a low-grade tumor. Perfusion MR has been shown to be helpful in preoperative tumor grading, predicting survival, and guiding biopsy.*

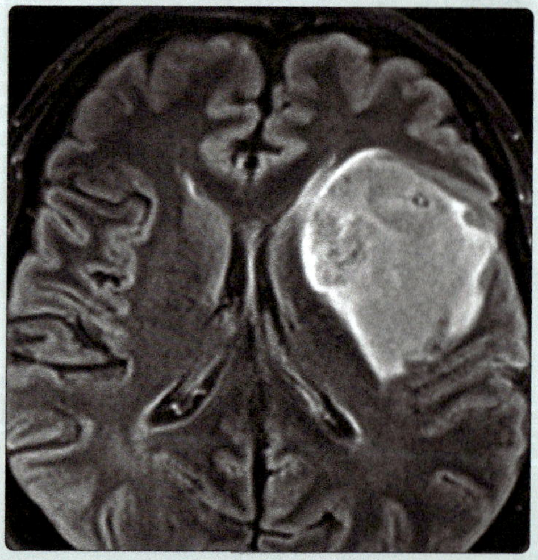

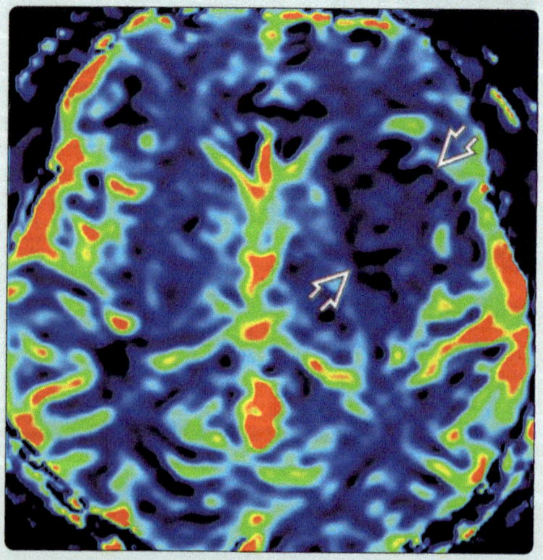

KEY FACTS

TERMINOLOGY

- Diffusely infiltrating malignant astrocytoma with anaplasia, marked proliferative potential

IMAGING

- Infiltrating mass that predominately involves white matter with variable enhancement
- T2 heterogeneously hyperintense
- Neoplastic cells almost always found beyond areas of abnormal signal intensity
- May involve and expand overlying cortex
- Usually no enhancement; focal, nodular, homogeneous, patchy enhancement less common
  - Ring enhancement is suspicious for glioblastoma (GBM)
- MRS: Increased Cho/Cr ratio, decreased *N*-acetylaspartate
- MRP: Elevated maximum regional cerebral blood volume
- Anaplastic astrocytomas have histologic and imaging characteristics along spectrum between low-grade astrocytoma and GBM

TOP DIFFERENTIAL DIAGNOSES

- Low-grade diffuse astrocytoma
- GBM
- Oligodendroglioma
- Cerebritis
- Ischemia

PATHOLOGY

- WHO grade III
- Usually evolves from low-grade (diffuse) astrocytoma (WHO grade II) (75%)

CLINICAL ISSUES

- Occurs at all ages, most common 40-50 years; 1/3 of astrocytomas
- Prognosis: Median survival: 2-3 years
  - *IDH1*(+) and *MGMT*(+) associated with increased survival
  - *IDH1, ATRX* wild-type (not mutated) = poor prognosis

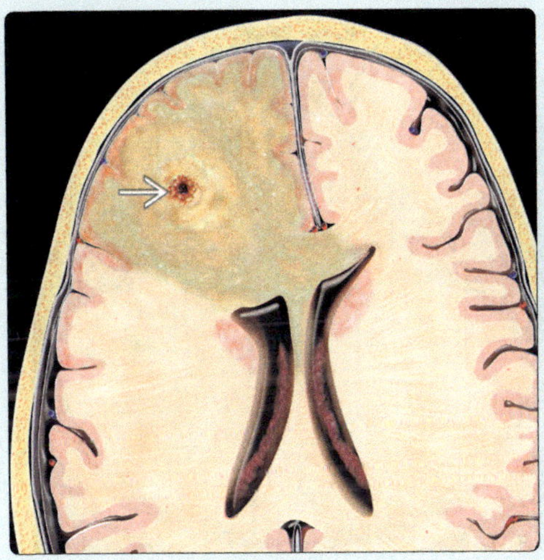

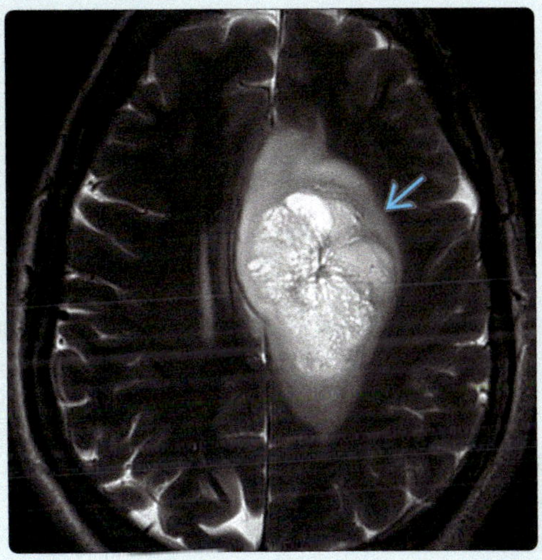

(Left) *Axial graphic shows an infiltrative white matter mass with extension along the corpus callosum, focal hemorrhage ➡, and local mass effect. White matter extension is typical of anaplastic astrocytoma (AA). They are most commonly located in the cerebral hemispheres.* **(Right)** *Axial T2 MR shows a heterogeneously hyperintense mass with local mass effect ➡ in the frontal lobe. AA, WHO grade III, was diagnosed at resection. These high-grade gliomas have a tendency to degenerate into glioblastomas (GBM).*

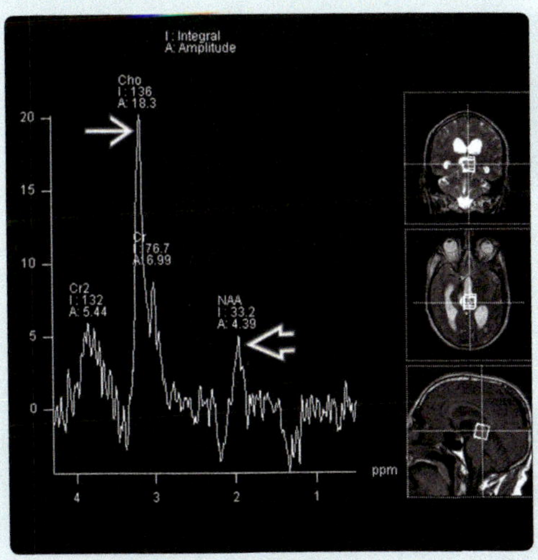

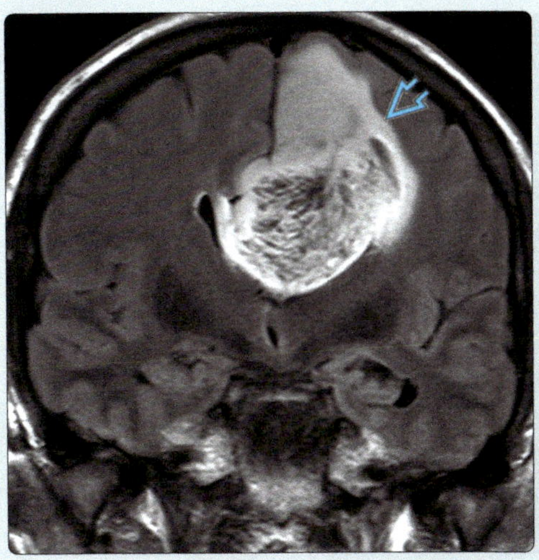

(Left) *MRS image in a patient with a tectal anaplastic astrocytoma shows a typical malignant tumor spectrum with a high choline peak ➡ and a low N-acetylaspartate peak ➡.* **(Right)** *Coronal FLAIR MR in a 47-year-old man shows a heterogeneously hyperintense mass ➡ centered in the frontal lobe white matter. Anaplastic astrocytomas represent 1/3 of all astrocytomas. Anaplastic astrocytomas are intermediate between low-grade (diffuse) astrocytoma (WHO grade II) and GBM (WHO grade IV).*

KEY FACTS

TERMINOLOGY

- Pilocytic astrocytoma (PA): Well-circumscribed, slow-growing tumor, often with cyst and mural nodule

IMAGING

- Cystic cerebellar mass with enhancing mural nodule
  - Arises from cerebellar hemisphere and compresses 4th ventricle
- Enlarged optic nerve/chiasm/tract with variable enhancement
- Cerebellum (60%) > optic nerve/chiasm (25-30%) > adjacent to 3rd ventricle > brainstem
- Well circumscribed with little to no edema
- Aggressive appearance (enhancement and MRS) of tumor is misleading

TOP DIFFERENTIAL DIAGNOSES

- Medulloblastoma (primitive neuroectodermal tumor)
- Ependymoma
- Ganglioglioma
- Hemangioblastoma
- Demyelination

PATHOLOGY

- WHO grade I
- 15% of neurofibromatosis type 1 (NF1) patients develop PAs, most commonly in optic pathway
- Up to 1/3 of patients with optic PAs have NF1
- Most common primary brain tumor in children

CLINICAL ISSUES

- Clinical presentation varies with location
  - Headache, nausea, vomiting most common
  - Visual loss (optic pathway lesions)
  - Ataxia, cerebellar signs (cerebellar lesions)
- Peak incidence: 5-15 years of age
- Slowly growing tumor with very good prognosis
- Median survival rates at 20 years > 70%

(Left) *Axial graphic shows the characteristic cyst with mural nodule appearance of a posterior fossa pilocytic astrocytoma (PA). These WHO grade I tumors most commonly arise in the cerebellar hemispheres and compress the 4th ventricle.* **(Right)** *Axial FLAIR MR shows a classic cyst with mural nodule appearance → of a cerebellar PA in a child. Note the typical lack of surrounding edema in the adjacent cerebellum. Mass effect on the 4th ventricle ➡ with associated hydrocephalus is common.*

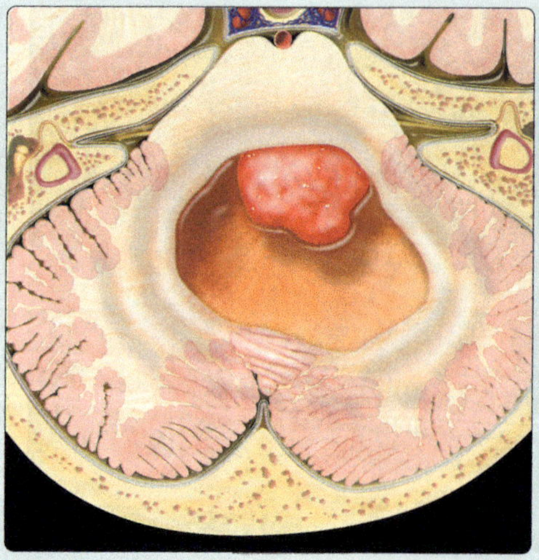

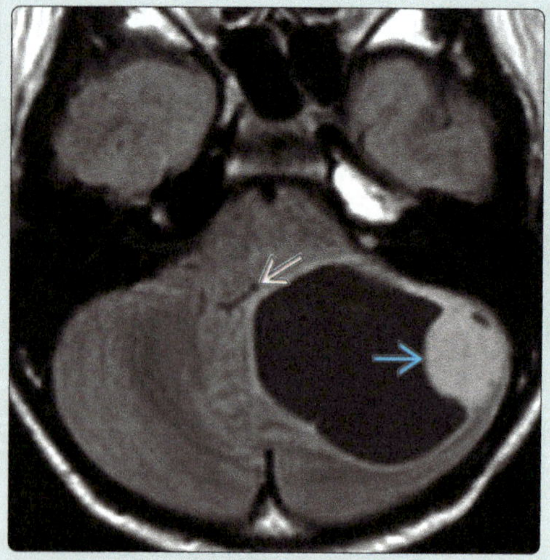

(Left) *Axial NECT shows a cystic and solid isodense posterior fossa mass → causing obstructive hydrocephalus. The lack of increased density helps to differentiate this PA from a medulloblastoma.* **(Right)** *Coronal T2WI MR shows a hyperintense hypothalamic/chiasmatic mass → with no surrounding edema. PAs in this location have variable enhancement. Optic pathway PAs are highly associated with neurofibromatosis 1 (NF1): ≤ 1/3 of patients with an optic pathway PA have NF1.*

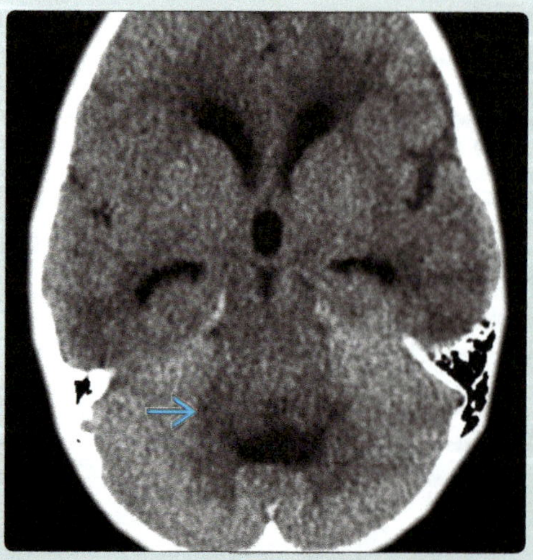

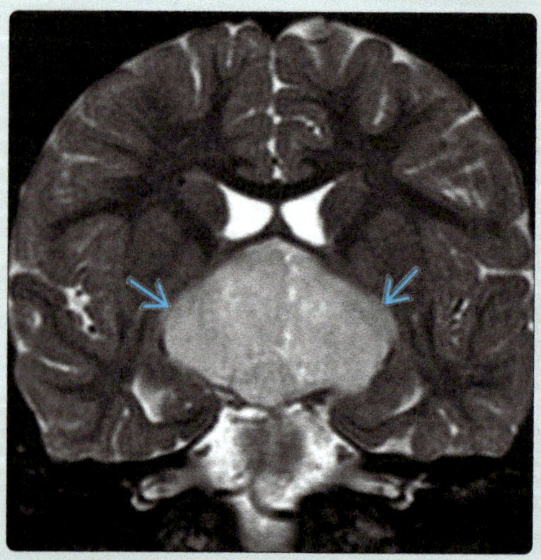

KEY FACTS

TERMINOLOGY

- Rapidly enlarging malignant astrocytic tumor characterized by necrosis and neovascularity
- Most common of all primary intracranial neoplasms

IMAGING

- Best imaging clue: Thick, irregularly enhancing rind of neoplastic tissue surrounding necrotic core
- Heterogeneous, hyperintense mass with adjacent tumor infiltration/vasogenic edema
- Necrosis, cysts, hemorrhage, fluid/debris levels, flow voids (neovascularity) may be seen
- Supratentorial white matter most common location
  - Cerebral hemispheres > brainstem > cerebellum
- Viable tumor extends far beyond signal changes

TOP DIFFERENTIAL DIAGNOSES

- Neoplasms: Anaplastic astrocytoma, lymphoma, metastasis
- Tumefactive demyelination, subacute ischemia

PATHOLOGY

- Histology: Necrosis, microvascular proliferation, WHO IV
- Genetically heterogeneous
  - 4 major subtypes = classic, mesenchymal, proneural, neural
  - Can be primary or secondary
    - Primary (de novo) glioblastoma (GBM)
      - 95% of GBMs; most are classical; *EGFR* amplified, *IDH1*(-) (wild-type)
    - Secondary (arises from lower grade astrocytoma)
      - Younger patient; often proneural; *IDH1, TP53* often mutated

CLINICAL ISSUES

- Seizures, focal neurologic deficits common
- Peak: 45-75 years, but may occur at any age
- 12-15% intracranial neoplasms, 2/3 of astrocytomas
- Relentless progression, survival often < 1 year
  - Varies with genetic, other factors (e.g., MGMT status)

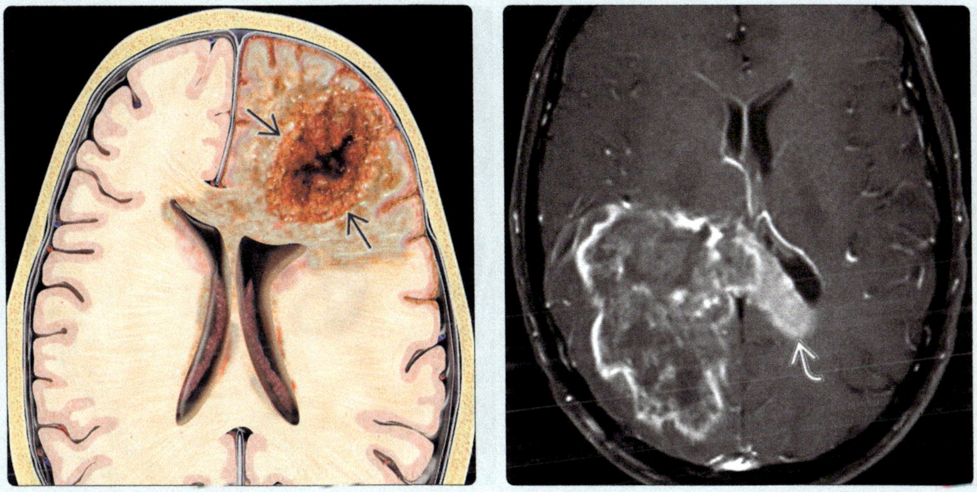

(Left) *Axial graphic shows a centrally necrotic infiltrating mass with extension across the corpus callosum; a peripheral rind of tumor* → *is seen surrounding the necrotic core, typical of glioblastoma (GBM).* **(Right)** *Axial T1WI C+ FS MR in a 60-year-old man with acute onset of seizures shows a heterogeneously enhancing occipital lobe mass with central necrosis and extension across the splenium of the corpus callosum* ↩*, characteristic of GBM. The frontal and temporal lobes are the most common locations for GBM.*

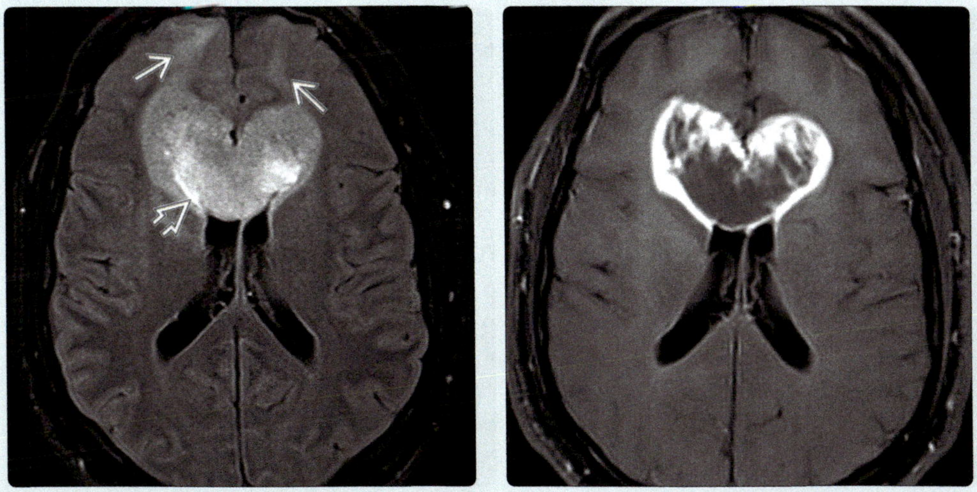

(Left) *Axial FLAIR MR shows a heterogeneously hyperintense mass* ⇨ *crossing the corpus callosum genu with signal abnormality extending into the frontal lobe subcortical white matter* →*. Viable tumor cells may extend beyond the area of MR signal abnormality.* **(Right)** *Axial T1 C+ FS MR in the same patient shows a thick enhancing rind of tumor that surrounds the necrotic tumor core, characteristic of GBM. Other lesions including lymphoma and demyelination may also involve the corpus callosum.*

Gliomatosis Cerebri

KEY FACTS

TERMINOLOGY

- Diffusely infiltrating, frequently bilateral glial tumor involving at least 3 lobes
- Infiltrative extent of tumor is out of proportion to histologic and clinical features

IMAGING

- T2 hyperintense infiltrating mass with enlargement of involved structures
  - Typical cerebral hemispheres (75%)
  - Brain architecture enlarged, distorted, but preserved
- Typically no or minimal enhancement
- Enhancement may indicate malignant progression or focus of malignant glioma
- MRS: Increased choline, decreased NAA

TOP DIFFERENTIAL DIAGNOSES

- Arteriolosclerosis
- Vasculitis
- Anaplastic astrocytoma
- Viral encephalitis
- Demyelination

PATHOLOGY

- Usually WHO grade III; range grade II-IV
- Shares many features of diffusely infiltrating astrocytoma
- Rarely, oligodendroglioma is predominant cell type
- Diagnosis typically made on basis of histology and imaging

CLINICAL ISSUES

- Presenting symptoms: Mental status changes, dementia, headaches, seizures, lethargy
- Treatment: Biopsy for diagnosis, ± radiation and chemotherapy
- Peak incidence between 40-50 years, occurs at all ages
- Relentless progression
- Survival ranges from weeks to years
  - Median survival ~ 14 months

(Left) *Axial graphic shows infiltrating tumor involving frontal lobes, insulae, basal ganglia with preservation of the underlying cerebral architecture. Note the focal malignant degeneration →.* **(Right)** *Axial T2 MR shows abnormal hyperintensity in the left cerebral peduncle → and left temporal and left frontal lobes with blurring of the corticomedullary junctions →. There is subtle expansion of the involved structures with relative preservation of the underlying architecture, typical of gliomatosis cerebri (GC).*

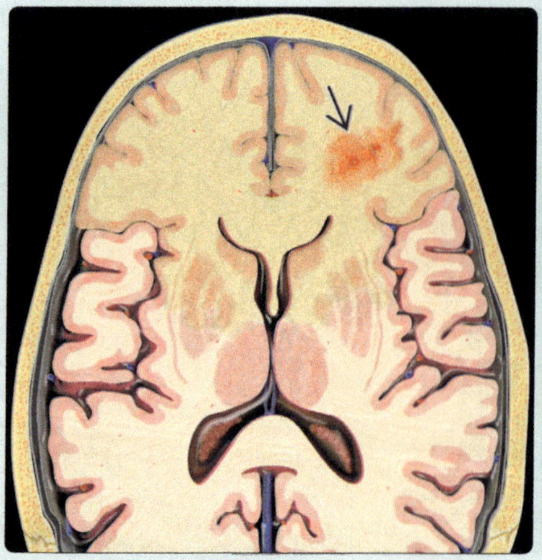

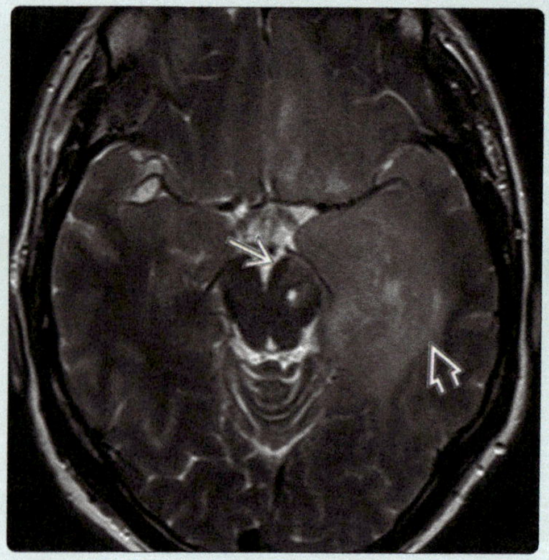

(Left) *Axial FLAIR MR in a 73-year-old man shows diffuse hyperintensity throughout the supratentorial white matter →, thickening the corpus callosum → but preserving the underlying anatomy. GC may mimic a nonneoplastic white matter disease including arteriolosclerosis.* **(Right)** *Axial T1 C+ MR in the same patient shows no enhancement, typical of GC. Enhancement often correlates with focal anaplasia or disease progression. Mild sulcal effacement is present →. These infiltrative tumors may be WHO grade II through IV.*

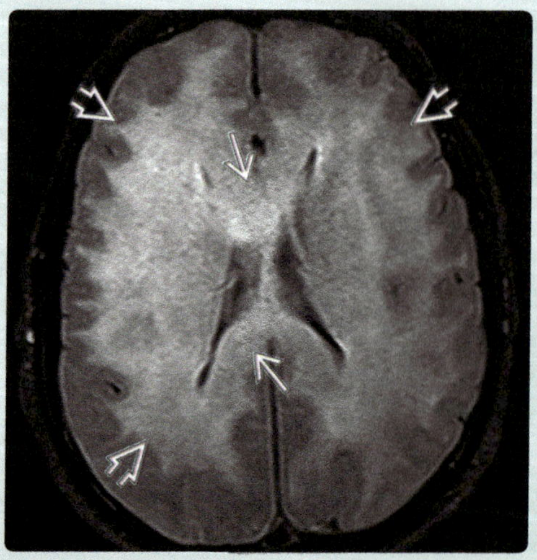

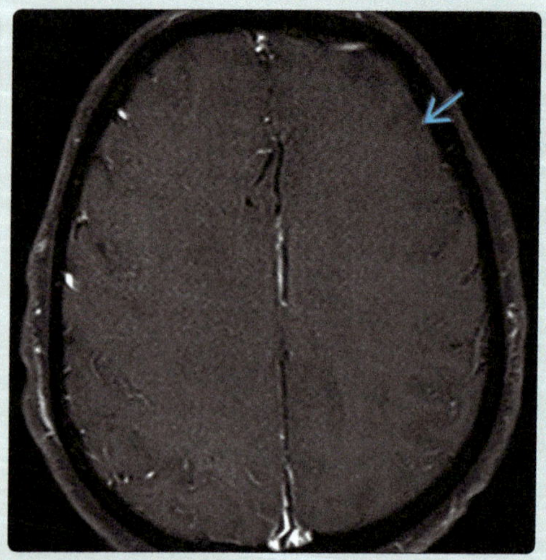

Oligodendroglioma

KEY FACTS

TERMINOLOGY

- Well-differentiated, slowly growing but diffusely infiltrating cortical/subcortical tumor

IMAGING

- Most common site is frontal lobe (50-65%)
- Best diagnostic clue: Partially calcified subcortical/cortical frontal mass in middle-aged adult
  - Typically T2 heterogeneous, hyperintense mass
- ~ 50% enhance
  - Heterogeneous enhancement is typical
- New enhancement in previously nonenhancing oligodendroglioma suggests malignant progression

TOP DIFFERENTIAL DIAGNOSES

- Anaplastic oligodendroglioma
- Low-grade diffuse astrocytoma
- Ganglioglioma
- Dysembryoplastic neuroepithelial tumor
- Pleomorphic xanthoastrocytoma
- Cerebritis
- Cerebral ischemia

PATHOLOGY

- Loss of heterozygosity for 1p and 19q (50-70%)
- WHO grade II
- Anaplastic oligodendroglioma = WHO grade III
- Oligodendrogliomas carry better prognosis than astrocytomas of same grade

CLINICAL ISSUES

- 5-10% of primary intracranial neoplasms
- Seizures, headaches, and focal neurologic deficits are most common presentations
- Peak incidence: 4th and 5th decades
- Median survival time = 10 years
- 1p, 19q deletions and *IDH1*(+) associated with more favorable prognosis

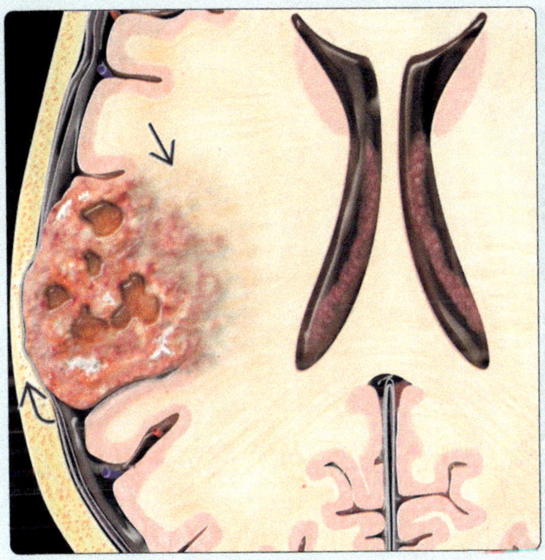

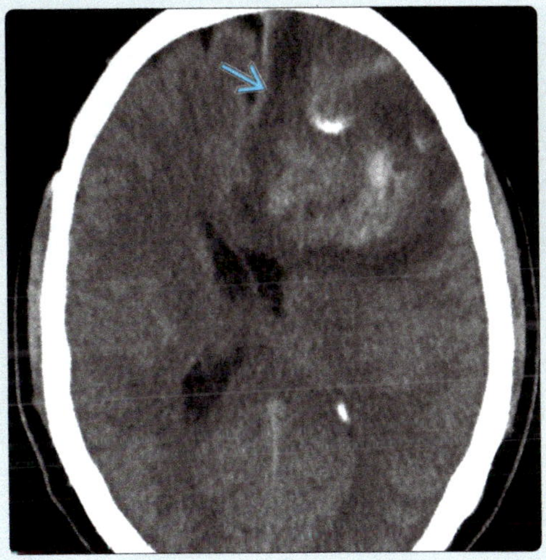

(Left) *Axial graphic shows a heterogeneous cystic and solid mass involving the cortex and subcortical white matter, typical of oligodendroglioma. Note the deep infiltrative margin* → *and calvarial remodeling* ↷. **(Right)** *Axial NECT in a 20-year-old man shows a large, calcified, left frontal lobe mass* →*, typical of oligodendroglioma. The vast majority (70-90%) of oligodendrogliomas show calcification. The calcification helps distinguish this tumor from other gliomas, particularly astrocytomas.*

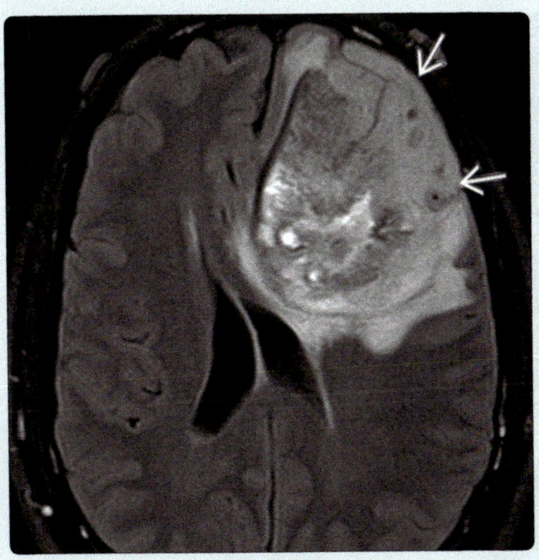

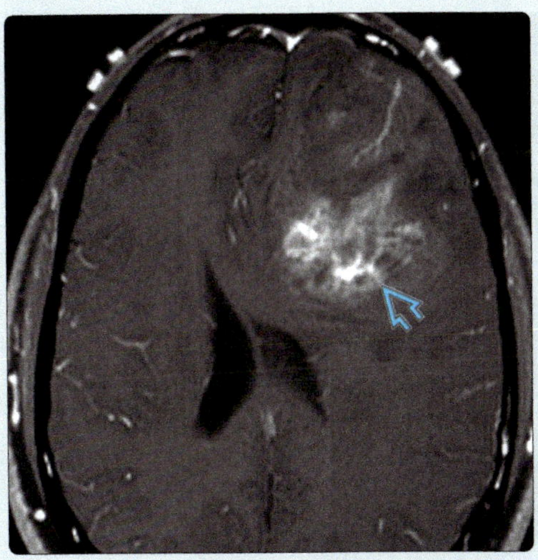

(Left) *Axial FLAIR MR in the same patient shows a heterogeneous, hyperintense infiltrative mass expanding the frontal gyri* →*. The frontal lobe location and involvement of both cortex and subcortical white matter are typical of oligodendroglioma.* **(Right)** *Axial T1WI C+ MR in the same patient shows heterogeneous enhancement* ⇨ *in this grade II oligodendroglioma. Differentiating a grade II from a grade III oligodendroglioma is difficult on conventional imaging. MRS and MR perfusion may help predict the tumor grade preoperatively.*

Anaplastic Oligodendroglioma

KEY FACTS

TERMINOLOGY

- Oligodendroglioma with focal or diffuse histologic features of malignancy

IMAGING

- Best diagnostic clue: Calcified frontal lobe mass involving cortex and subcortical white matter
  - Frontal lobe is most common location, followed by temporal lobe
- Majority have nodular or clumped calcification
- May see hemorrhage or necrosis
- Variable enhancement
  - Anaplastic oligodendroglioma more likely to enhance than low-grade oligo
- Neoplastic cells almost always found beyond areas of abnormal signal intensity
- MRS and MR perfusion may help distinguish grade II from grade III oligos

TOP DIFFERENTIAL DIAGNOSES

- Oligodendroglioma
- Anaplastic astrocytoma
- Glioblastoma multiforme
- Cerebritis
- Ischemia

PATHOLOGY

- WHO grade III
- Oligos: Better prognosis than astrocytomas of same grade

CLINICAL ISSUES

- Headache, seizures are most common presentations
- Occurs at all ages; mean is 49 years
- 20-50% of oligodendrogliomas are anaplastic
- Median survival: 4 years
- 5-year survival: 40-45%; 10-year survival: 15%
- 1p and 19q deletions associated with prolonged survival

(Left) *Axial graphic shows a heterogeneous frontal cortical and subcortical mass with areas of necrosis and hemorrhage. Note the mass effect and infiltrative margins, typical of anaplastic grade III oligodendroglioma. These malignant gliomas have a poor prognosis.* **(Right)** *Axial CT image in a 43-year-old man with seizures shows a calcified, cystic, and solid frontal lobe mass →. There is associated intraventricular obstructive hydrocephalus with ventricular enlargement and transependymal CSF flow (interstitial edema) ⇨.*

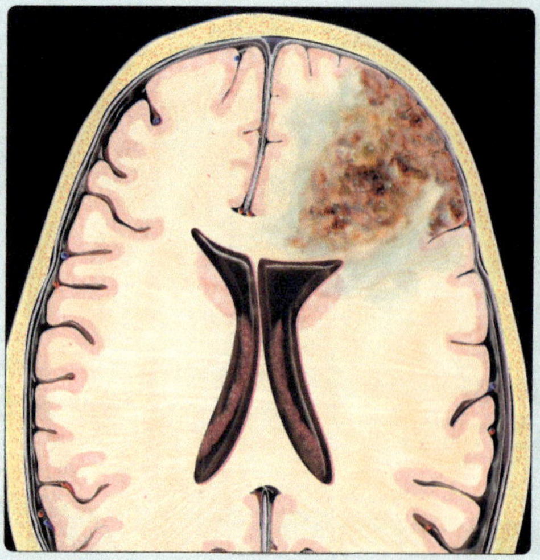

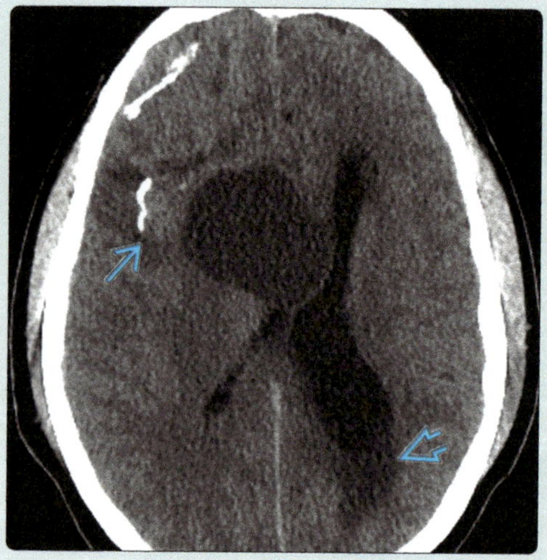

(Left) *Axial T2 MR in the same patient shows the heterogeneously hyperintense mass → with significant mass effect and associated hydrocephalus. The T2 heterogeneity is related to cystic change ⇨ and calcification. The calcification is better seen on CT or T2* MR.* **(Right)** *Axial T1 C+ MR in the same patient shows heterogeneous enhancement ⇨ of the mass. WHO grade III anaplastic oligodendroglioma was diagnosed at resection. Enhancement is more common in grade III than in grade II oligodendrogliomas.*

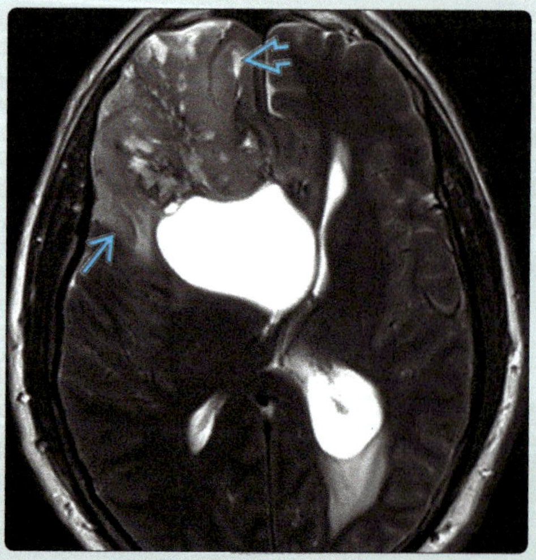

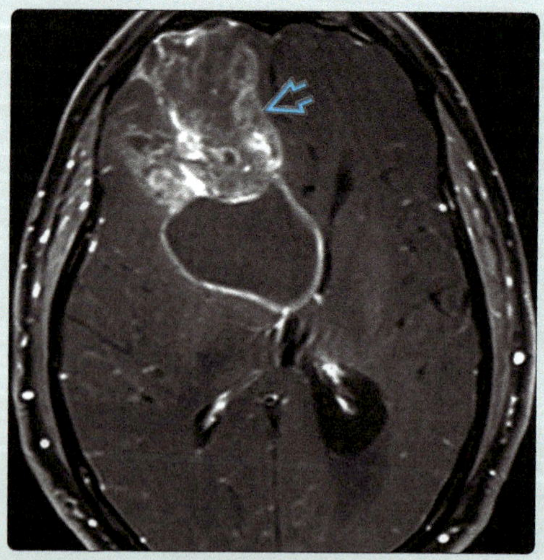

KEY FACTS

TERMINOLOGY

- Posterior fossa ependymoma (PF-EPN)

IMAGING

- Ependymoma can occur anywhere in neuraxis
- Most common site: Posterior fossa (2/3 of cases)
  - Lobulated mass in body/inferior 4th ventricle
    - Soft or "plastic" tumor
      - Accommodates to shape of ventricle
      - Squeezes through foramen of Magendie into cisterna magna
      - ± extension through foramina of Luschka into cerebellopontine angle cisterns
- NECT
  - Ca++ common (50%)
  - ± cysts, hemorrhage
  - Obstructive hydrocephalus common
- MR
  - Variable enhancement; usually does not restrict on DWI

PATHOLOGY

- 3 posterior fossa ependymoma molecular subtypes
  - Posterior fossa ependymoma subtype A (PF-EPN-A)
    - Most common (50%)
    - Predominately infants
    - Poor prognosis
  - PF-EPN-B
    - 10% of PF-EPNs
    - Older children, adults
    - Better prognosis
  - Subependymoma (PF-SE)

CLINICAL ISSUES

- Signs of increased intracranial pressure
- 3-17% cerebrospinal fluid dissemination

DIAGNOSTIC CHECKLIST

- Much less common than primitive neuroectodermal tumor-medulloblastoma or pilocytic astrocytoma

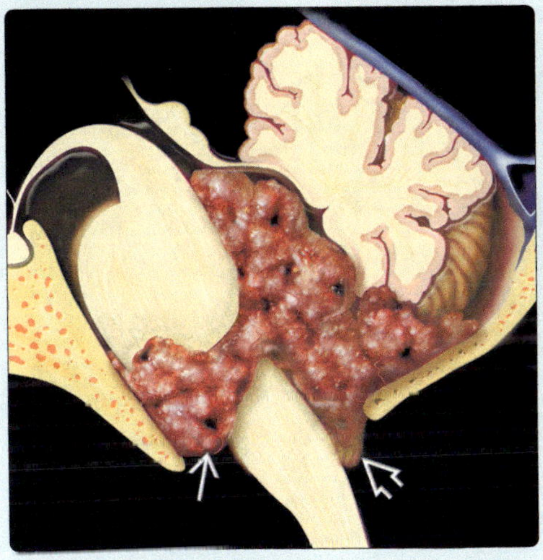

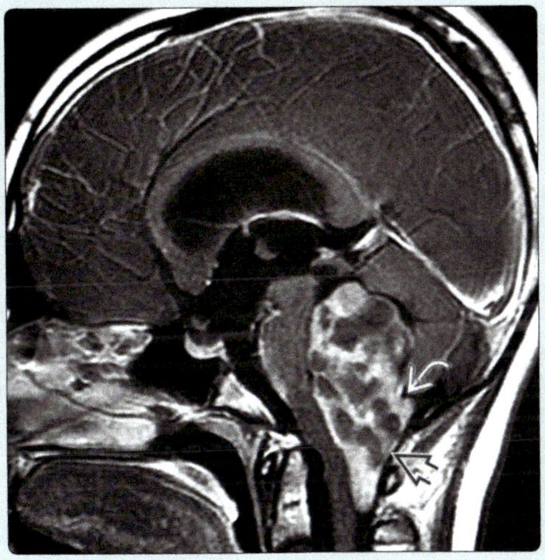

(Left) *Posterior fossa ependymoma (PF-EPN) extends through the 4th ventricle outlet foramina into the cisterna magna and CPA cistern; "plastic" pattern of growth is typical of ependymoma in this location, increases the difficulty of surgical resection.* **(Right)** *Sagittal T1 C+ MR shows classic PF-EPN as a lobulated mixed cystic/solid enhancing mass displacing the brainstem anteriorly, expanding the 4th ventricle. Tumor extrudes posteroinferiorly through the foramen of Magendie into the cisterna magna.*

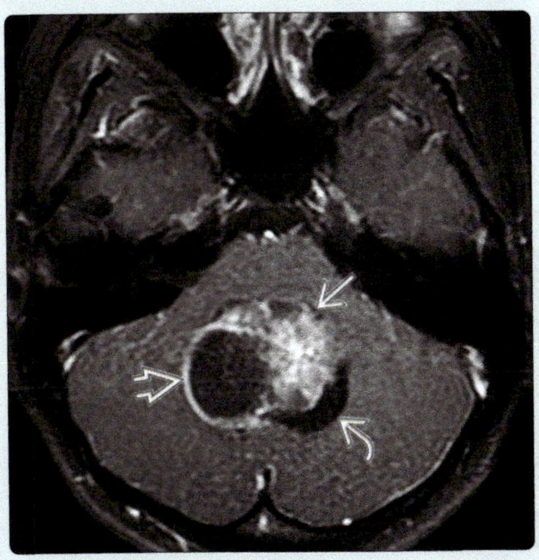

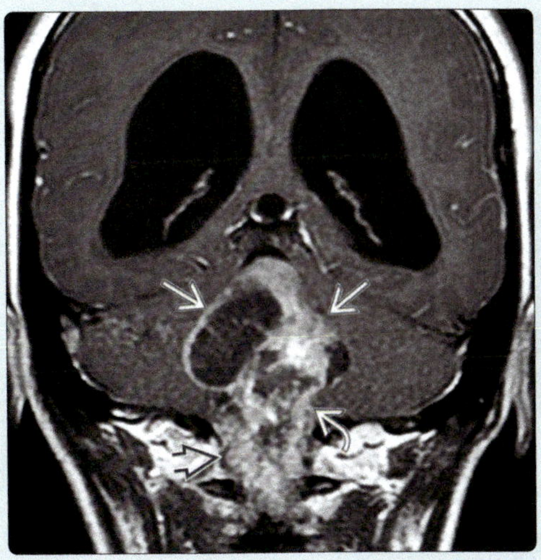

(Left) *Axial T1 C+ FS MR scan in the same case shows the enhancing mixed cystic and solid tumor expanding, filling the 4th ventricle.* **(Right)** *Coronal T1 C+ MR scan in the same case again shows the mixed cystic/solid enhancing mass conforming to the shape of the expanded 4th ventricle. The tumor extrudes inferiorly through the enlarged foramen of Magendie and extends into the upper cervical spinal canal. WHO II cellular ependymoma was found at surgery.*

KEY FACTS

TERMINOLOGY

- Rare, benign, well-differentiated, intraventricular ependymal tumor, typically attached to ventricular wall

IMAGING

- Intraventricular, inferior 4th ventricle typical (60%)
- Other locations: Lateral > 3rd ventricle > spinal cord
- T2/FLAIR hyperintense intraventricular mass
  - Heterogeneity related to cystic changes; blood products or Ca++ may be seen in larger lesions
- Variable enhancement, typically none to mild
- T2WI and FLAIR are often most sensitive sequences

TOP DIFFERENTIAL DIAGNOSES

- Ependymoma
- Central neurocytoma
- Subependymal giant cell astrocytoma
- Choroid plexus papilloma
- Hemangioblastoma
- Metastases

PATHOLOGY

- WHO grade I

CLINICAL ISSUES

- 40% become symptomatic, often supratentorial
  - Related to increased intracranial pressure, hydrocephalus
- Present in middle-aged/elderly adults (typically 5th-6th decades)
- Treatment: Conservative management with serial imaging if asymptomatic patient
- Surgical resection is curative in most cases
- Excellent prognosis for supratentorial lesions
  - Recurrence is extremely rare

DIAGNOSTIC CHECKLIST

- If 4th or lateral ventricular hyperintense mass in elderly man, think subependymoma

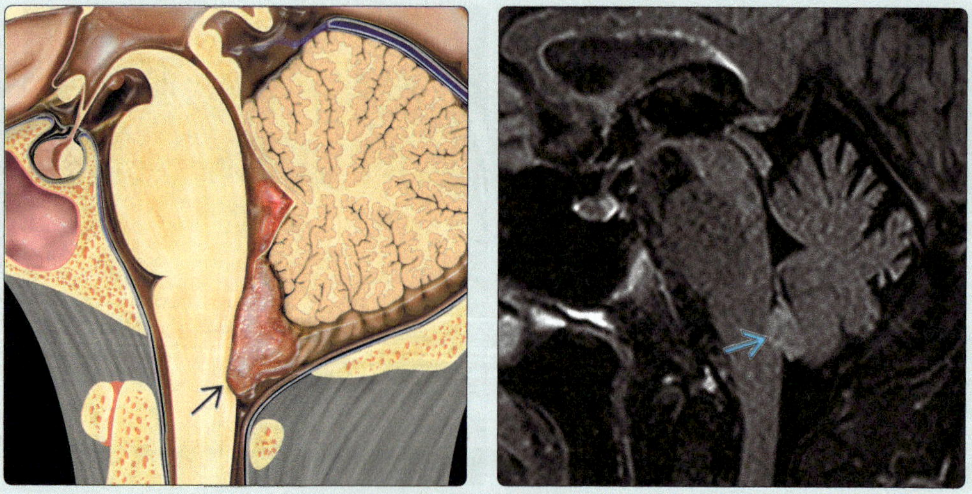

(Left) *Sagittal graphic shows a solid, well-circumscribed mass arising from the floor of the 4th ventricle with mild mass effect ➔. Note the lack of hydrocephalus, typical of subependymoma.* **(Right)** *Sagittal FLAIR MR shows a solid, hyperintense mass along the inferior 4th ventricle ➔ in a 64-year-old man with headaches. Subependymoma was found at resection. These 4th ventricular tumors are often asymptomatic. T2 and FLAIR are typically the most sensitive sequences to identify this WHO grade I tumor.*

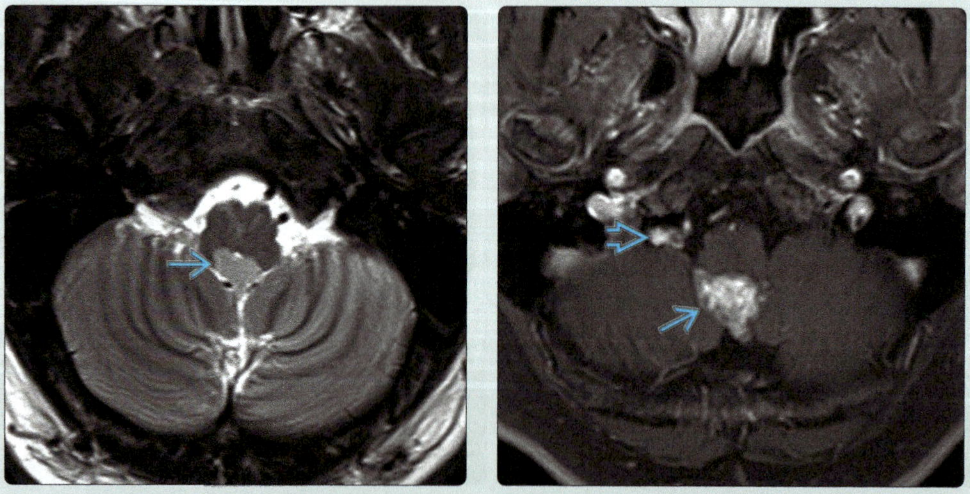

(Left) *Axial T2WI MR shows a hyperintense mass ➔ along the inferior 4th ventricle at the level of the medulla (classic imaging of a subependymoma).* **(Right)** *Axial T1 C+ MR shows an enhancing mass in the 4th ventricular outflow tract ➔. The moderate enhancement is uncommon. Subependymomas classically have no or minimal enhancement. They can protrude through the foramen of Magendie. In this case, tumor is also present anterior to the cerebellar hemisphere ➔ through the foramen of Luschka.*

Typical Choroid Plexus Papilloma

KEY FACTS

TERMINOLOGY

- Choroid plexus tumor (CPT)
  - 3 types of CPTs
    - Choroid plexus papilloma (CPP) (WHO grade I)
    - Atypical CPP (aCPP) (grade II)
    - Choroid plexus carcinoma (CPCa) (grade III)

IMAGING

- Classic: Child with enhancing lobulated (cauliflower-like) mass in atrium of lateral ventricle
- CPPs occur in proportion to amount of choroid plexus
  - 50% in lateral ventricle (usually atrium)
  - 40% in 4th ventricle &/or foramina of Luschka
  - 5% in 3rd ventricle (roof)
- Hydrocephalus (overproduction, obstructive)

TOP DIFFERENTIAL DIAGNOSES

- aCPP
- CPCa
- Physiologic choroid plexus enlargement
- Choroid plexus xanthogranuloma
- Meningioma
- Intraventricular metastasis
- Medulloblastoma
- Ependymoma

CLINICAL ISSUES

- Most common brain tumor in children < 1 year old
  - 13.1% of all brain tumors in 1st year of life
  - 7.9% of fetal brain tumors diagnosed by ultrasound
- Benign, slowly growing
  - ± cerebrospinal fluid spread (does not distinguish CPP from CPCa)
  - Malignant progression rare

DIAGNOSTIC CHECKLIST

- Consider CPP if intraventricular mass in child < 2 years old
- Imaging cannot reliably distinguish CPP from aCPP, CPCa

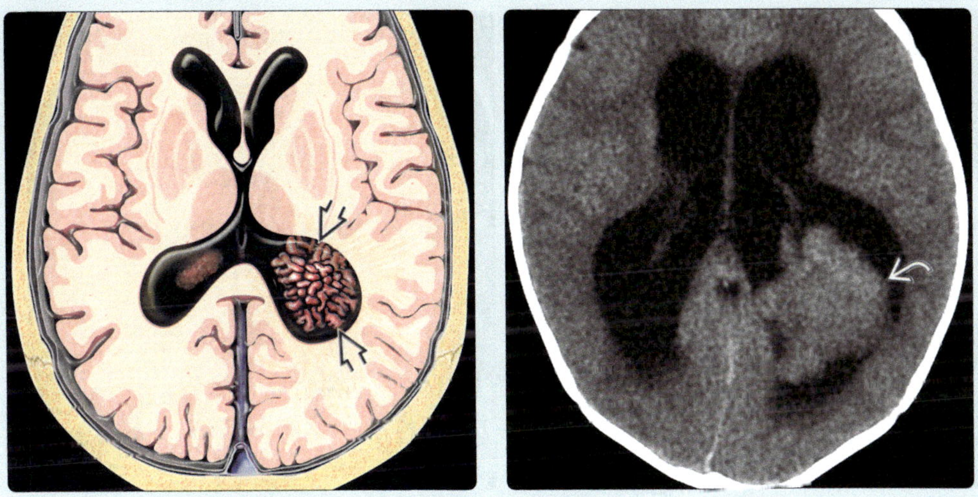

(Left) *Axial graphic shows a choroid plexus papilloma (CPP) arising from the glomus of the left lateral ventricular trigone. Note the characteristic frond-like surface projections. CPPs are most common in the lateral ventricles of a child.* **(Right)** *Axial NECT in a child with macrocephaly shows hydrocephalus with a lobulated mass in the atrium of the left lateral ventricle.*

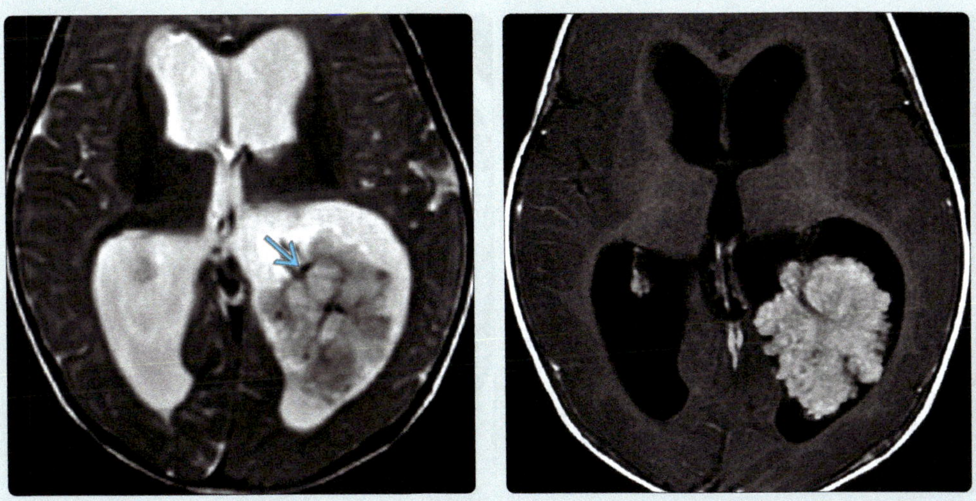

(Left) *Axial T2WI MR in the same patient shows a heterogeneously hyperintense lateral ventricle mass with scattered hypointense flow voids, indicating high vascularity. The lobulated nature of the mass is striking.* **(Right)** *Axial T1WI C+ MR in the same case shows marked enhancement of the lobular mass with frond-like projections, characteristic of CPP. CPP cannot be reliably differentiated from atypical CPP by conventional imaging alone.*

Ganglioglioma

KEY FACTS

TERMINOLOGY

- Well-differentiated, slowly growing neuroepithelial tumor composed of neoplastic ganglion cells and neoplastic glial cells
- Most common neoplastic cause of temporal lobe epilepsy (TLE)

IMAGING

- Best diagnostic clue: Partially cystic, enhancing, cortically based mass in child/young adult with TLE
- Can occur anywhere, but most commonly superficial hemispheres, temporal lobe (> 75%)
- Circumscribed cyst with mural nodule most common
- May be solid and appear well circumscribed
- Calcification is common (up to 50%)
- Superficial lesions may expand cortex, remodel bone
- ~ 50% enhance
- Protocol advice: Contrast-enhanced MR to include coronal T2 images for better evaluation of temporal lobes

TOP DIFFERENTIAL DIAGNOSES

- Pleomorphic xanthoastrocytoma
- Dysembryoplastic neuroepithelial tumor
- Astrocytoma
- Oligodendroglioma
- Neurocysticercosis

PATHOLOGY

- WHO grade I or II (80% grade I)
- Uncommon: Anaplastic ganglioglioma (WHO III)
- Rare: Malignant with glioblastoma multiforme-like glial component (WHO IV)

CLINICAL ISSUES

- Occurs at all ages (peak: 10-20 years)
- Most common mixed neuronal-glial tumor
- Cortical dysplasia is commonly associated with ganglioglioma
- Excellent prognosis if surgical resection complete

(Left) *Coronal graphic shows a discrete cystic and solid temporal lobe mass expanding the overlying cortex. Calvarial remodeling is seen, typical of a superficially located ganglioglioma. Gangliogliomas are the most common tumors to cause temporal lobe epilepsy.* **(Right)** *Coronal T1WI C+ MR in a young adult with temporal lobe epilepsy shows a circumscribed, cystic, and solid temporal lobe mass with intense enhancement of the mural nodule ➡. This is the classic enhancement pattern of a ganglioglioma.*

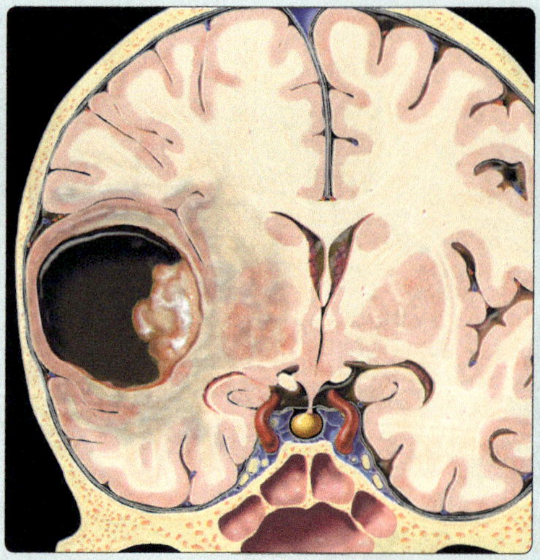

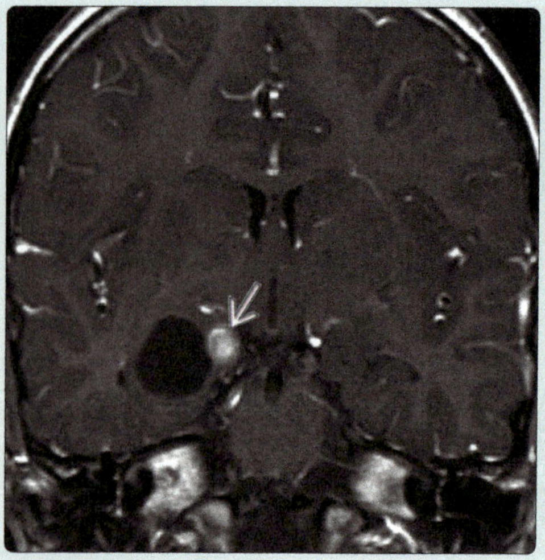

(Left) *Axial CT shows a partially calcified frontal lobe mass ➡ in a 25-year-old patient with headaches and seizures. The lack of surrounding edema is typical for ganglioglioma. Imaging mimics an oligodendroglioma. Calcification is seen in 30-50% of gangliogliomas.* **(Right)** *Coronal T1WI C+ MR shows subtle enhancement ➡ within a right temporal lobe ganglioglioma in a female patient with seizures. The differential diagnosis for this lesion includes DNET, astrocytoma, PXA, and oligodendroglioma.*

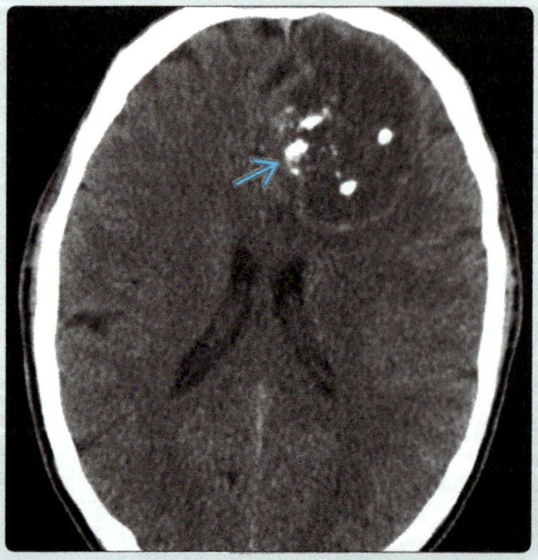

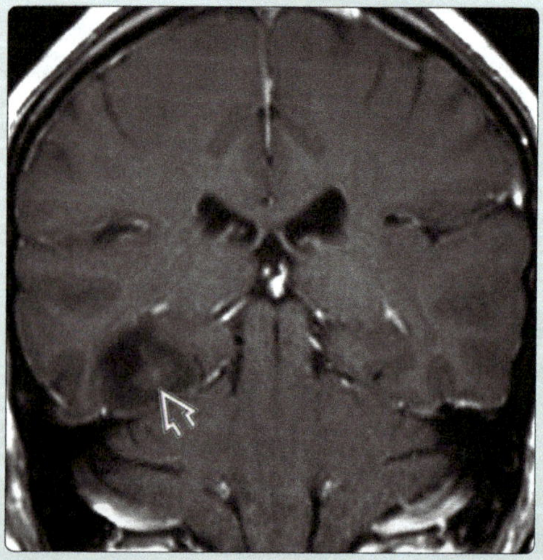

Dysembryoplastic Neuroepithelial Tumor (DNET)

KEY FACTS

TERMINOLOGY

- Dysembryoplastic neuroepithelial tumor (DNET)
  - Benign mixed glial-neuronal neoplasm
  - Frequently associated with cortical dysplasia

IMAGING

- May occur in any region of supratentorial cortex
  - Temporal lobe most common, followed by frontal lobe
  - Mass frequently "points" toward ventricle
- Sharply demarcated, wedge-shaped
  - Cystic ("bubbly") intracortical mass
  - Minimal/no mass effect
  - No surrounding edema
- Slow growth over years
- Usually does not enhance
- Faint focal punctate or ring enhancement in 20-30%
  - Higher rate of recurrence if enhancement

TOP DIFFERENTIAL DIAGNOSES

- Focal cortical dysplasia type II (Taylor type)
- Neuroepithelial cyst
- Ganglioglioma
- Pleomorphic xanthoastrocytoma
- Angiocentric glioma

PATHOLOGY

- WHO grade I
- Hallmark = specific glioneuronal element

CLINICAL ISSUES

- Longstanding drug-resistant partial complex seizures in child/young adult
- Surgical resection usually curative
- Histology usually remains benign even if tumor recurs, enhances

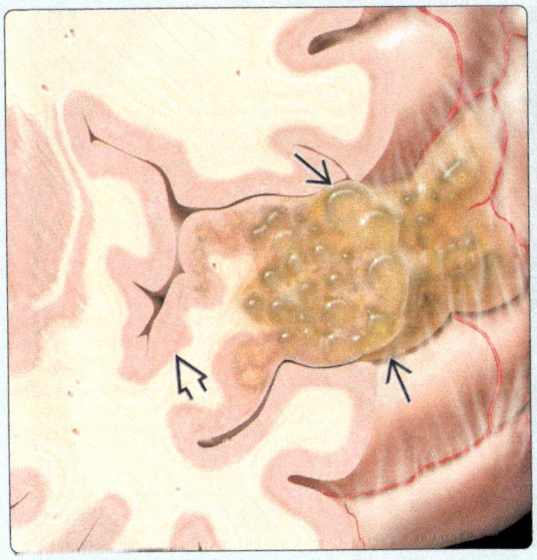
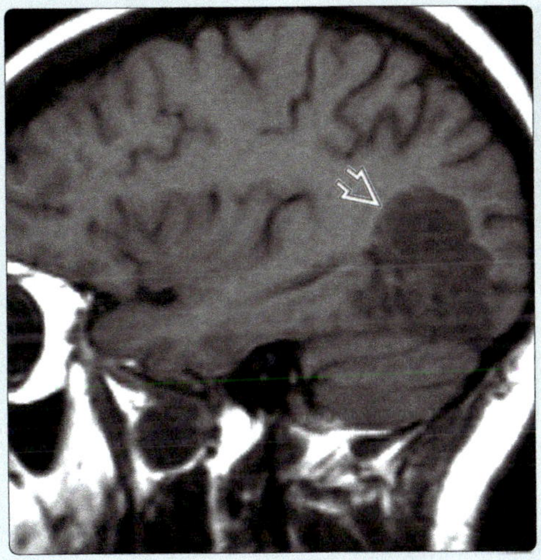

(Left) *Coronal oblique graphic shows typical appearance of a cystic cortical dysembryoplastic neuroepithelial tumor (DNET), which present in children or young adults with seizures. The gyrus is expanded by the multicystic tumor ➔; cortical dysplasia ➔ is common in adjacent brain.* **(Right)** *Sagittal T1 MR in a young adult with seizures shows characteristic "bubbly" appearance of DNET (WHO grade I neoplasm). Note low T1 signal within the wedge-shaped cortical mass ➔; there's excellent prognosis with surgical resection.*

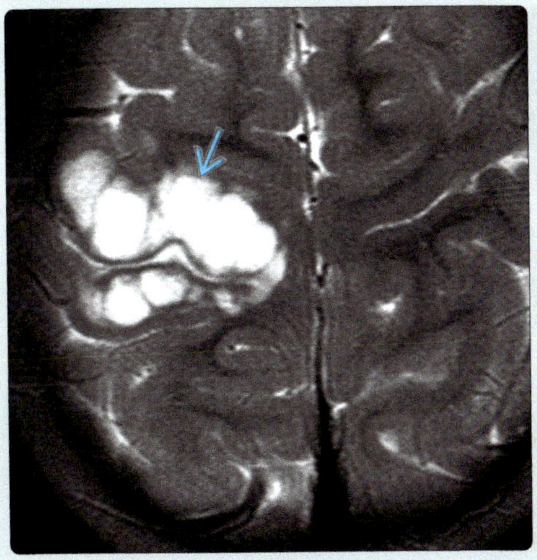
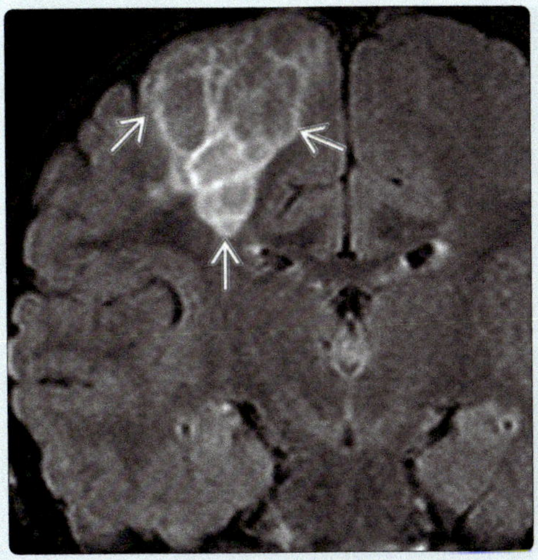

(Left) *Axial T2WI MR shows a multilobular, wedge-shaped cystic cortically based mass ➔ in the right posterior frontal lobe. Note the lack of edema and mass effect, given the size of the tumor, which is typical of a DNET.* **(Right)** *Axial FLAIR MR in the same patient shows the characteristic appearance of a DNET. Note the cortically based, sharply demarcated, wedge-shaped mass with a hyperintense rim ➔. The tumor points toward the ventricle, and there is no surrounding edema. (Courtesy L. Loevner, MD.)*

Central Neurocytoma

KEY FACTS

TERMINOLOGY

- Central neurocytoma (CN) = intraventricular neuroepithelial tumor with neuronal differentiation

IMAGING

- Best diagnostic clue: "Bubbly" mass in frontal horn or body of lateral ventricle
  - May involve 3rd ventricle
- CT: Usually mixed solid and cystic mass with calcification
  - Hydrocephalus common
  - Rarely complicated by hemorrhage
- MR: Heterogeneous, T2 hyperintense, "bubbly" appearance
  - May be predominantly solid mass
  - Moderate to strong heterogeneous enhancement
- MRS: ↑ Cho, ↓ *N*-acetylaspartate; glycine peak at 3.55 ppm
- If "bubbly," "feathery," or solid intraventricular mass near foramen of Monro in young adult, consider CN

TOP DIFFERENTIAL DIAGNOSES

- Subependymoma
- Subependymal giant cell astrocytoma
- Intraventricular metastasis
- Ependymoma
- Choroid plexus papilloma

CLINICAL ISSUES

- Young adults, commonly 20-40 years of age
- Usually benign, local recurrence is uncommon
  - Surgical resection is typically curative
  - If incomplete resection, radiation therapy, chemotherapy, &/or radiosurgery may be helpful
- 5-year survival rate: 90%
- MIB-1 (Ki-67 labeling) index > 2-3% = poorer prognosis
- Headache, increased intracranial pressure, mental status changes, seizure are most common presenting features
  - Hydrocephalus secondary to foramen of Monro obstruction

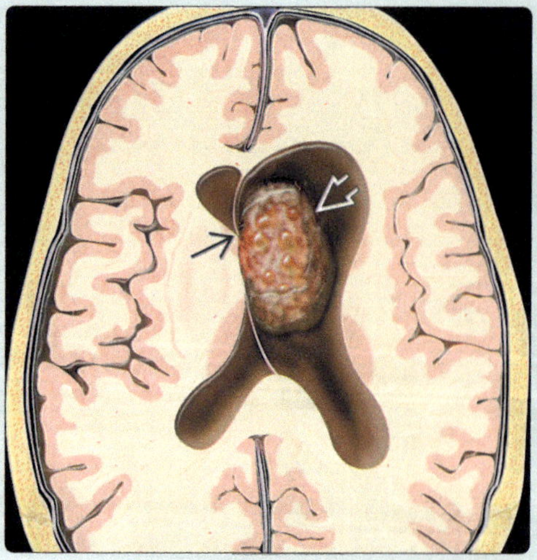

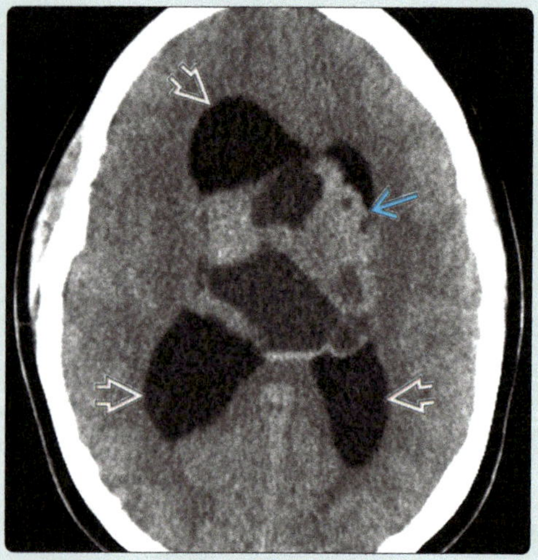

(Left) *Axial graphic shows a circumscribed, lobular, "bubbly" mass ➡ attached to the septum pellucidum ➡. Ventricular dilatation is related to foramen of Monro obstruction. This is the classic appearance of a central neurocytoma. Complete surgical resection is often curative for these WHO grade II tumors.* **(Right)** *Axial NECT shows a heterogeneous mixed cystic/solid mass ➡ in the lateral ventricles attached to the septum pellucidum. There is associated obstructive hydrocephalus ➡, typical for central neurocytoma.*

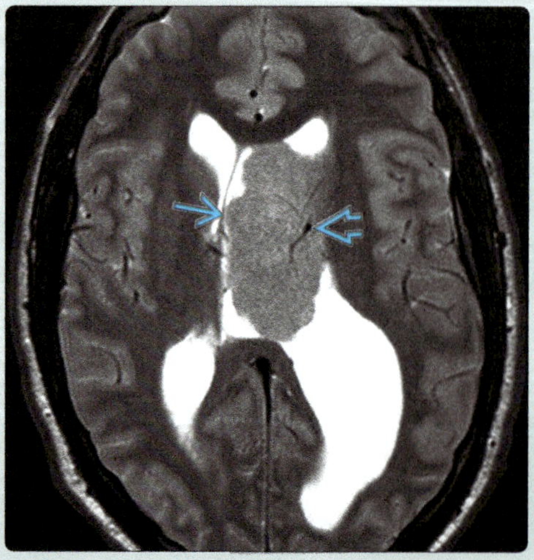

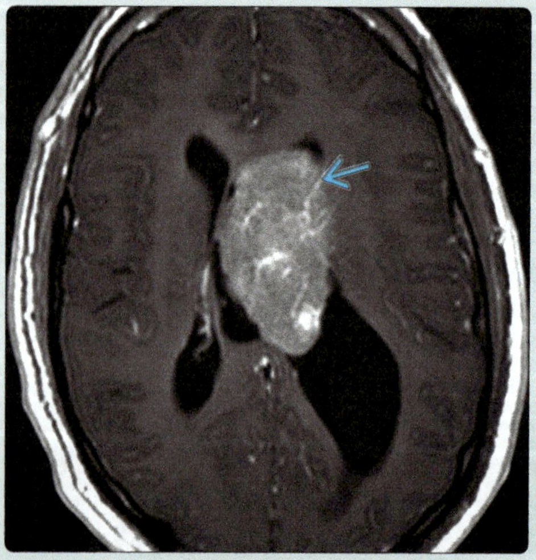

(Left) *Axial T2WI MR in a 20 year old with headaches shows a predominantly solid ventricular mass in the body of the lateral ventricle ➡ attached to the septum pellucidum with prominent flow voids ➡.* **(Right)** *Axial T1WI C+ MR in the same patient shows diffuse enhancement ➡. Central neurocytoma was diagnosed at resection. Imaging differential considerations include subependymal giant cell astrocytoma, subependymoma, and meningioma. (Courtesy S. van der Westhuizen, MD.)*

KEY FACTS

TERMINOLOGY

- Pineocytoma (PC), pineal parenchymal tumor (PPT)
- PCs are composed of small, uniform, mature cells
  - Cells resemble pineocytes

IMAGING

- General features: Circumscribed, enhancing pineal mass
  - May mimic benign pineal cyst or PPT of intermediate differentiation (PPTID)
  - Typically < 3 cm
  - May compress adjacent structures
  - Rarely extends into 3rd ventricle, rarely invasive
  - Can compress aqueduct → hydrocephalus
- CT
  - Circumscribed iso-/hypodense pineal region mass
  - Peripheral ("exploded") Ca++ common
  - CECT: Enhances (solid, ring, nodular)
- MR (most sensitive)
  - Cystic change may be present
  - Enhancement may be solid or peripheral

TOP DIFFERENTIAL DIAGNOSES

- Nonneoplastic pineal cyst
- PPTID
- Pineoblastoma
- Germinoma, other germ cell tumors

CLINICAL ISSUES

- Headache, dorsal midbrain (Parinaud) syndrome most common features
- Increased intracranial pressure, ataxia, hydrocephalus, mental status changes may occur
- Most common in adults, mean 40 years
- Stable or slow-growing tumor
- Germ cell markers (α-fetoprotein, hCG) absent
- Surgical excision or stereotactic biopsy is primary treatment
  - Complete surgical resection generally curative

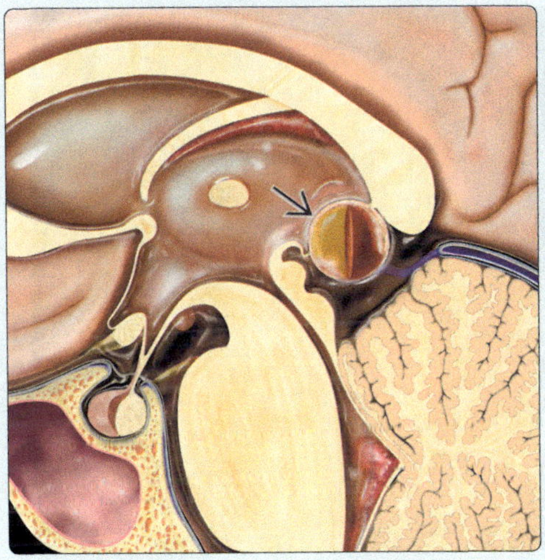

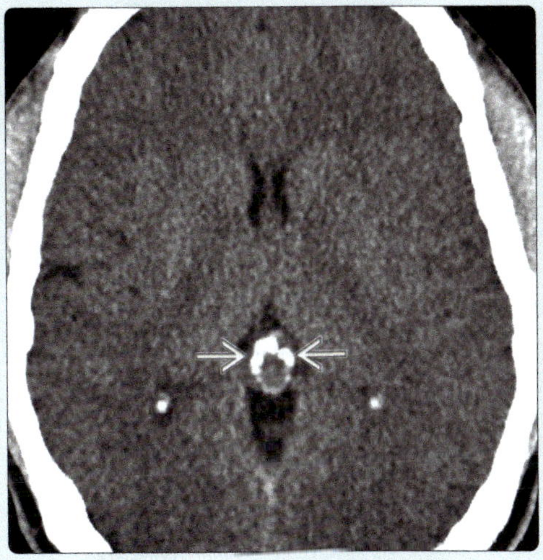

(Left) *Sagittal graphic shows a cystic pineal gland mass ➡ with a fluid-fluid level and nodular tumor along the periphery of the mass, typical of pineocytoma. No significant mass effect is present. Pituicytomas may be found incidentally or present with hydrocephalus.* **(Right)** *Axial NECT shows a classic example of a pineocytoma. Note the "exploded" peripheral calcification ➡ in this small mass that arises from the pineal region. The tumor is just over 1 cm in size. There is no hydrocephalus.*

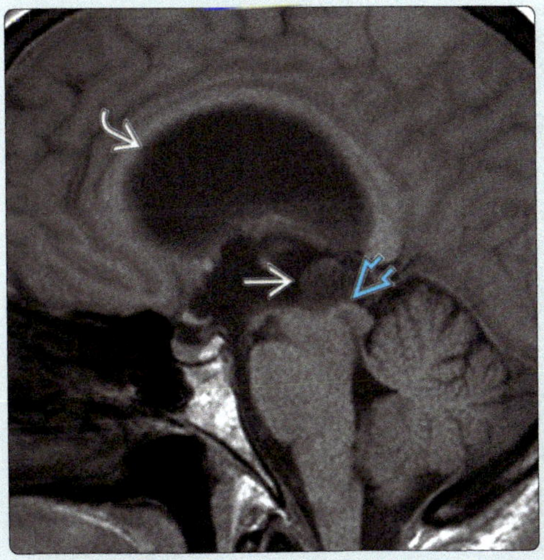

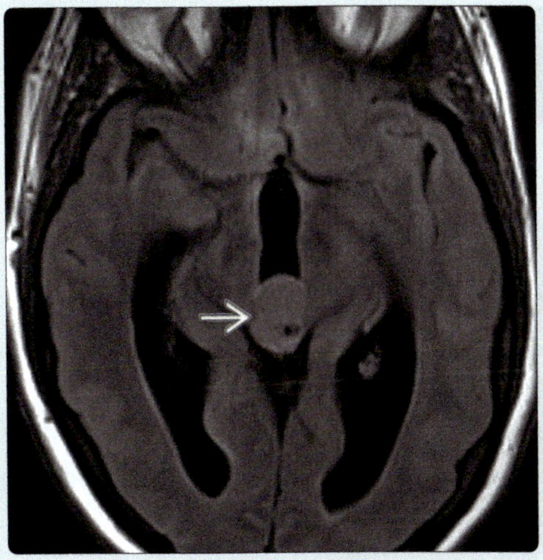

(Left) *Sagittal T1 MR of a 50-year-old woman with headache shows a cystic pineal region mass ➡ with associated ventriculomegaly ➡ and local mass effect on the tectum ➡. Mass effect on the superior tectum often results in dorsal midbrain (Parinaud) syndrome.* **(Right)** *Axial FLAIR MR in the same patient shows the hyperintense, lobular pineal region mass ➡ with associated ventriculomegaly. Pineocytoma was diagnosed at resection. These WHO grade I tumors are often stable for years.*

Pineal Parenchymal Tumor of Intermediate Differentiation (PPTID)

KEY FACTS

TERMINOLOGY

- Primary parenchymal neoplasm of pineal gland
  - Intermediate in malignancy between pineoblastoma and pineocytoma

IMAGING

- General features
  - Aggressive-looking pineal mass in adult
  - Extension into adjacent structures (ventricles, thalami) is common
  - Lobulated, moderately vascular
  - Size varies from small (< 1 cm) to large (~ 6 cm)
- CT
  - Hyperdense mass centered in pineal region
  - Engulfs pineal gland Ca++
  - Hydrocephalus
- MR
  - T1: Mixed iso-/hypointense mass
  - T2: Isointense with gray matter, + small hyperintense foci
  - FLAIR: Hyperintense
  - Strong, heterogeneous enhancement
  - MRS: Elevated Cho, decreased NAA
- If aggressive-looking pineal region tumor in middle-aged, older adult, consider PPTID

TOP DIFFERENTIAL DIAGNOSES

- Germinoma
- Pineocytoma
- Pineoblastoma
- Papillary tumor of pineal region

PATHOLOGY

- Neuroepithelial neoplasm
  - Arises from pineocytes or their precursors
- WHO grade II or III

CLINICAL ISSUES

- Dorsal midbrain (Parinaud) syndrome, headache
  - Upgaze paralysis, convergence-retraction nystagmus

(Left) *Sagittal T1WI MR in a 21-year-old man with headache shows a pineal region mass with obstructive hydrocephalus, enlargement of the 3rd ventricle, and cerebellar tonsillar descent. Imaging differential considerations include PPTID, pineoblastoma, and germinoma.* **(Right)** *Axial T2WI MR shows a very large PPTID with extension into the ventricular system. Note the heterogeneous T2 appearance of the mass with multiple cystic regions, typical of PPTID. (Courtesy L. Loevner, MD.)*

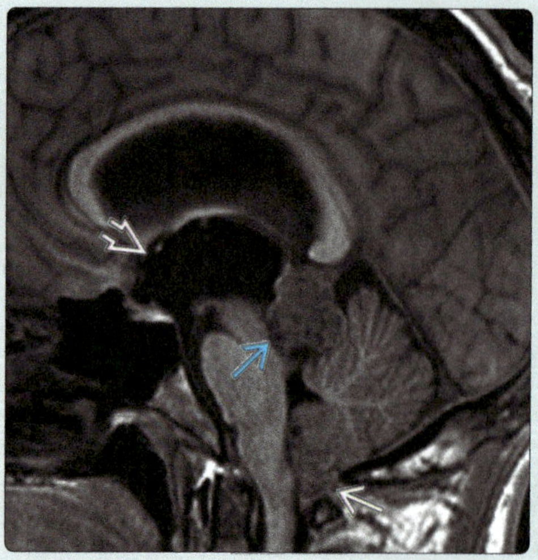

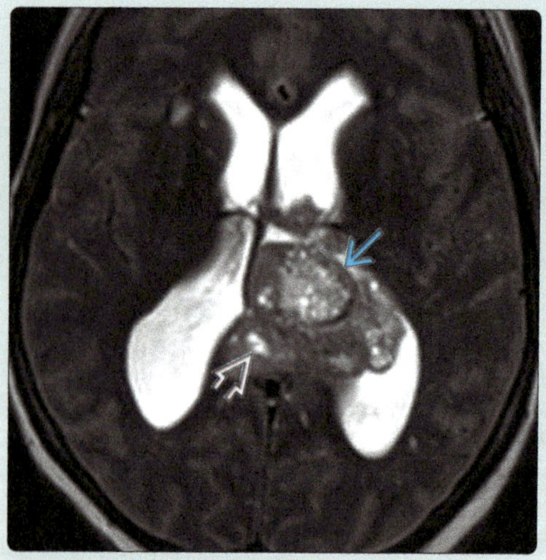

(Left) *Coronal T1WI C+ MR shows a large, peripherally enhancing pineal mass in a 24-year-old man. PPTID was diagnosed at resection.* **(Right)** *MRs in a 48-year-old woman shows elevated choline, decreased NAA, and a lactate doublet. Imaging is too aggressive for a pineocytoma. Germinomas are rare in middle-aged women. Imaging is most suggestive of a PPTID, although a papillary tumor of the pineal region would be a possible diagnosis. PPTID was confirmed at histologic examination.*

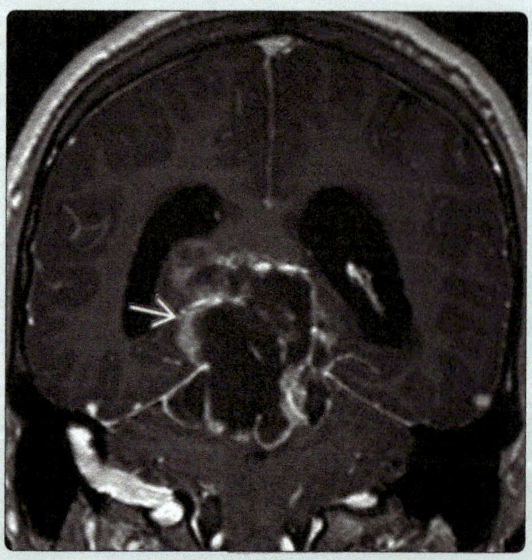

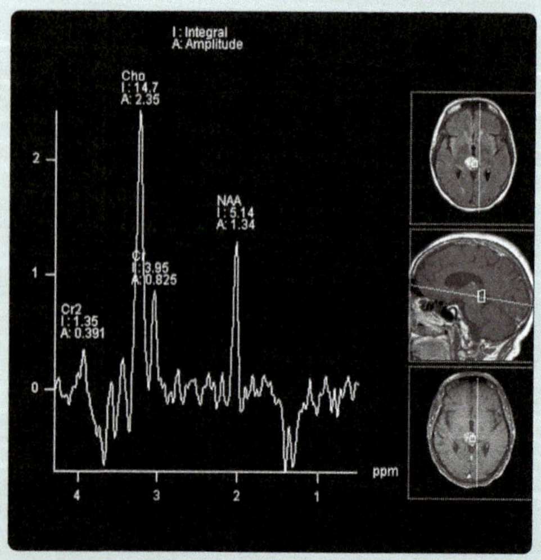

KEY FACTS

TERMINOLOGY

- Intracranial germ cell tumor (iGCT)
- iGCTs are intracranial homologue of gonadal germinomas (ovarian dysgerminoma, testicular seminoma)

IMAGING

- Most common: In/near midline (80-90%)
  - Pineal region ~ 50-65%
  - Suprasellar ~ 25-35%
- Less common: Basal ganglia/thalami ~ 5-10%
- 20% multiple
  - Most common = pineal with suprasellar
- Pineal germinoma
  - Hyperdense pineal region mass engulfs pineal Ca++
  - Strong, often heterogeneous enhancement
  - T2/FLAIR hyperintensity in surrounding brain = inflammation/granulomatous change
- Suprasellar germinoma
  - Absent posterior pituitary "bright spot"
  - "Fat" stalk/pituitary gland
  - Strong, relatively uniform enhancement
  - May have cysts, hemorrhage (rare)
- Basal ganglia germinoma
  - Rare; hemorrhage common

TOP DIFFERENTIAL DIAGNOSES

- Pineal germinoma
  - Pineocytoma, other pineal GCTs
- Suprasellar germinoma ("fat" infundibulum)
  - Adult = neurosarcoid, metastases
  - Child = Langerhans cell histiocytosis (LCH)

CLINICAL ISSUES

- 90% of patients < 20 years old
  - Pineal region germinoma: M:F ~ 10:1
  - Causes dorsal midbrain syndrome

DIAGNOSTIC CHECKLIST

- Child with diabetes insipidus? Think germinoma or LCH!

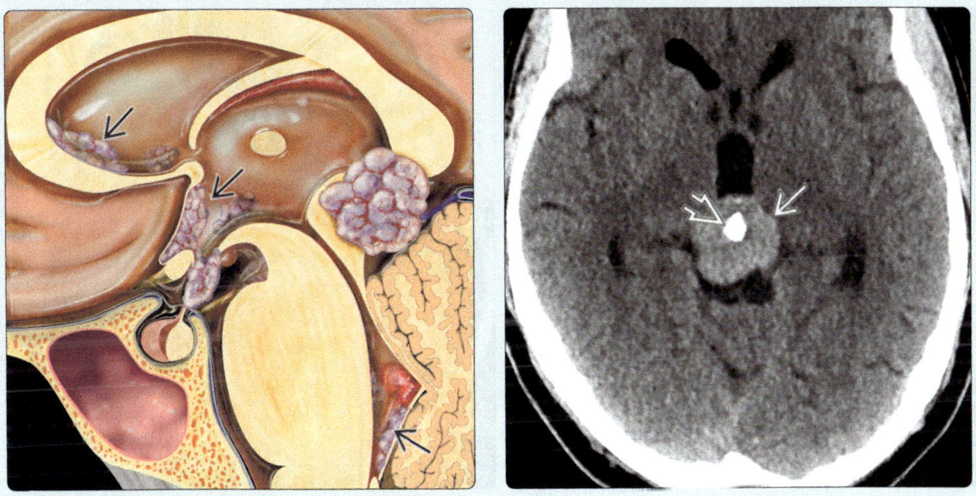

(Left) *Sagittal graphic shows synchronous germinomas in the suprasellar and pineal regions. Note the cerebrospinal fluid spread of tumor in the lateral, 3rd, and 4th ventricles →.* **(Right)** *Axial NECT scan shows typical findings of pineal germinoma with a well-demarcated slightly hyperdense mass → engulfing the calcified pineal gland →.*

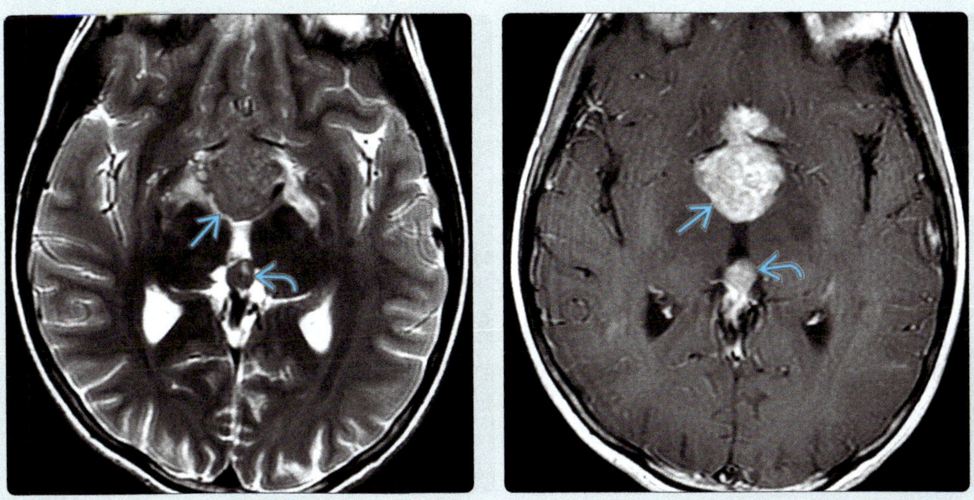

(Left) *Axial T2WI in a 14-year-old boy with visual symptoms shows a suprasellar mass → that is slightly hypointense relative to gray matter. A 2nd, smaller mass ↩ is present in the pineal gland.* **(Right)** *T1 C+ MR in the same patient shows that the lobulated suprasellar mass → enhances strongly. The pineal mass ↩ also enhances uniformly. The combination of suprasellar and pineal mass (sometimes called "double midline" germinoma) occurs in ~ 20% of cases.*

KEY FACTS

TERMINOLOGY

- Medulloblastoma (MB)
  - Malignant, invasive, highly cellular embryonal tumor
- 4 distinct MB molecular subgroups
  - Wingless (WNT)
  - Sonic hedgehog (SHH)
  - Group 3
  - Group 4

IMAGING

- MB subgroups arise in different locations
  - Midline (4th ventricle)
    - Predominately (but not exclusively) groups 3 and 4
  - Cerebellar peduncle/CPA cistern: WNT
  - Cerebellar hemispheres (lateral): SHH
- NECT: 90% hyperdense (Ca++, hemorrhage uncommon)
- MR: > 90% enhance (group 4 minimal/no enhancement)
  - Restricted diffusion, low ADC
  - T1 C+ essential to detect CSF dissemination

TOP DIFFERENTIAL DIAGNOSES

- Atypical teratoid/rhabdoid tumor
- Ependymoma
- Cerebellar pilocytic astrocytoma

PATHOLOGY

- WHO grade IV (overstates risk of WNT MB)
- Microscopy
  - "Small round blue cell" tumor
  - Neuroblastic (Homer Wright) rosettes (40%)
- Most common histologic type = classic MB
- Less common subtypes: Desmoplastic, MB with extensive nodularity, large cell/anaplastic

CLINICAL ISSUES

- Most common malignant pediatric brain tumor
- Prognosis varies with subgroup, mutations
  - WNT best, group 3 worst

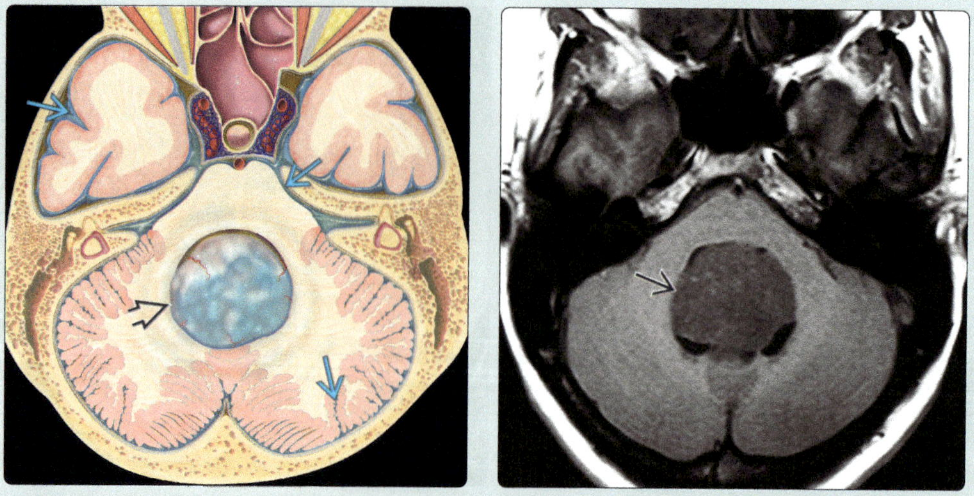

(Left) *Axial graphic shows a spherical tumor centered in the 4th ventricle ⇨, typical of classic medulloblastoma (MB). Cerebrospinal fluid (CSF) dissemination ("sugar icing") is common at initial diagnosis and is shown in blue ➔.* **(Right)** *Axial T1WI shows imaging findings of classic MB, with a rounded, slightly hypointense mass ⇨ in the 4th ventricle.*

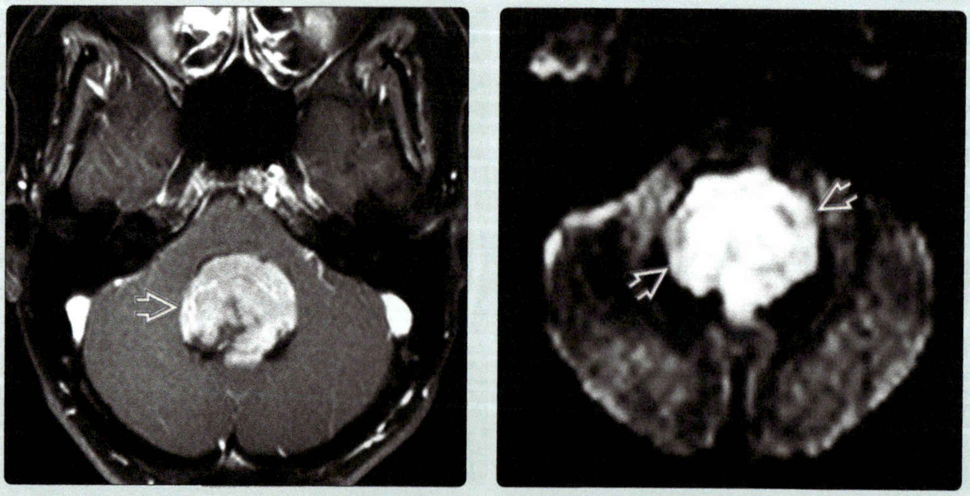

(Left) *Axial T1 C+ FS in the same case shows the mass mass ➡ enhances strongly, somewhat heterogeneously. No CSF spread is identified.* **(Right)** *DWI in the same case shows strongly restricted diffusivity ➡. Surgery disclosed MB, desmoplastic subtype. The midline 4th ventricle is the 2nd most common location for desmoplastic MBs and the most common site for classic MBs. Histopathology disclosed desmoplastic MB, Sonic hedgehog subtype.*

KEY FACTS

TERMINOLOGY

- Hemangioblastoma (HGBL): Highly vascular tumor of adults most commonly found in posterior fossa (PF), spinal cord
  - 25-40% of HGBLs in von Hippel-Lindau disease (VHL)

IMAGING

- Best diagnostic clue: Adult with cerebellar mass with cyst and enhancing mural nodule
- General features
  - 50-60% cyst + "mural" nodule; 40% solid enhancing mass
  - 90-95% in posterior fossa
  - 5-10% supratentorial (around optic pathways, hemispheres; usually in VHL)

TOP DIFFERENTIAL DIAGNOSES

- Metastasis (most common posterior fossa parenchymal mass in adults)
- Pilocytic astrocytoma (most common neoplasm with cyst + nodule in child)
- Cavernous malformation
- Hereditary hemorrhagic telangiectasia

PATHOLOGY

- WHO grade I
- Red or yellowish, well-circumscribed, unencapsulated, highly vascular mass that abuts leptomeninges
- Histology shows stromal cells, innumerable small vessels

CLINICAL ISSUES

- Headache is most common presenting symptom
- Primary therapy = surgical resection
- Begin MR screening of patients from VHL families after 10 years of age

DIAGNOSTIC CHECKLIST

- Most common posterior fossa intraaxial mass in middle-aged/older adult is metastasis, not HGBL

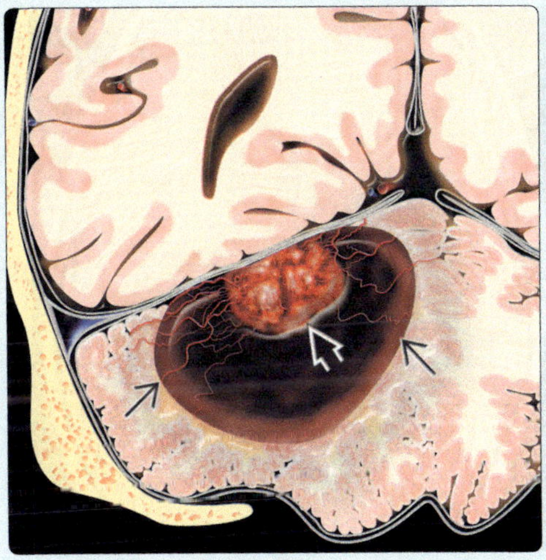

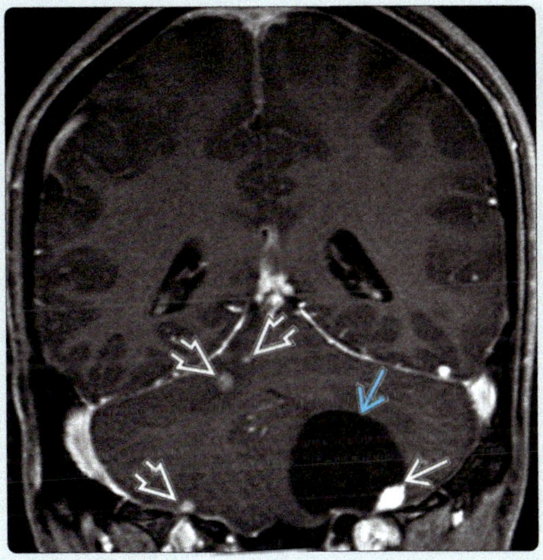

***(Left)** Coronal graphic shows a classic cerebellar hemangioblastoma as largely cystic mass with a vascular tumor nodule that abuts the pial surface. These low-grade tumors are the most common primary posterior fossa tumor in adults. **(Right)** Coronal T1 C+ MR shows a large cyst and mural nodule in a VHL patient with multiple hemangioblastomas. Note the lack of enhancement of the cyst wall, which consists of compressed but normal cerebellum. The other hemangioblastomas have a solid enhancing appearance.*

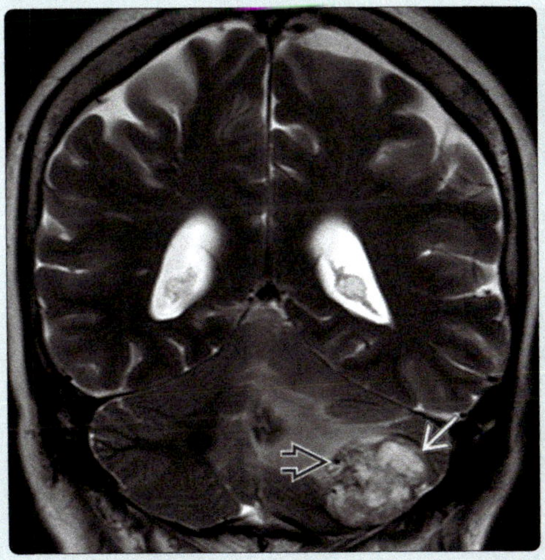

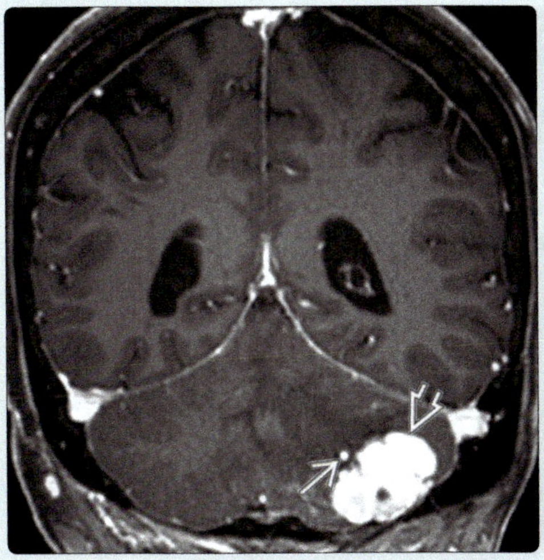

***(Left)** Coronal T2 MR in a 60-year-old woman with headaches shows a heterogeneous cerebellar mass with prominent flow voids and surrounding edema. **(Right)** Coronal T1 C+ MR in the same patient shows marked enhancement of the mass and a prominent adjacent vessel. Hemangioblastoma was found at surgical resection. The main imaging differential diagnosis in this adult was metastatic disease. These WHO grade I tumors have an excellent prognosis in sporadic cases.*

KEY FACTS

TERMINOLOGY

- Malignant primary CNS neoplasm primarily composed of B lymphocytes (PCNSL)

IMAGING

- Best diagnostic clue: Enhancing lesion(s) within basal ganglia &/or periventricular white matter
- 60-80% supratentorial
  - Often involve, cross corpus callosum
  - Frequently contact, extend along ependymal surfaces
- Classically hyperdense on CT (helpful for diagnosis)
- Diffusely enhancing periventricular mass in immunocompetent patients
- May see hemorrhage or necrosis in immunocompromised patients
- DWI: Low ADC values
- PWI: Low relative cerebral blood volume ratios
- Periventricular location and subependymal involvement is characteristic of PCNSL
- Corpus callosum involvement may be seen with PCNSL, glioblastoma (GBM), and rarely metastases or demyelination

TOP DIFFERENTIAL DIAGNOSES

- Acquired toxoplasmosis
- GBM
- Abscess
- Progressive multifocal leukoencephalopathy

PATHOLOGY

- 98% diffuse large B-cell, non-Hodgkin lymphoma

CLINICAL ISSUES

- Imaging and prognosis vary with immune status
- 6.6% of primary brain tumors, incidence rising
- Poor prognosis
- Stereotactic biopsy, followed by chemotherapy, ± XRT

(Left) *Axial graphic shows multiple periventricular lesions with involvement of the basal ganglia, thalamus, and corpus callosum, typical of primary CNS lymphoma (PCNSL). Note the extensive subependymal spread of the disease ➔. PCNSL typically extends along ependymal surfaces.* **(Right)** *Axial T1 C+ MR in a 63 year old shows the classic appearance of PCNSL. Note the multiple homogeneously enhancing masses in the basal ganglia along the ependymal lining of the ventricular system ➔.*

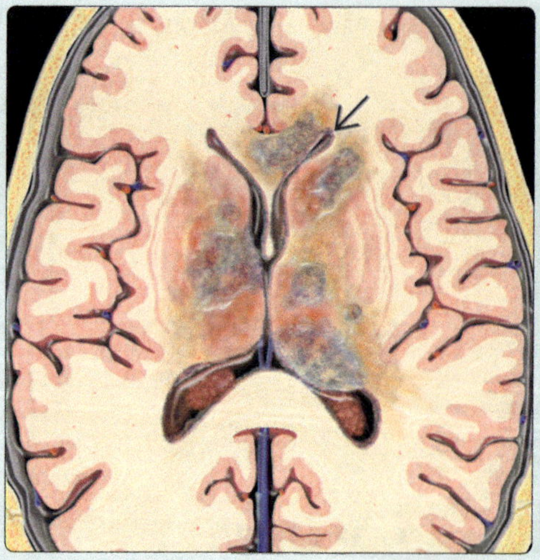

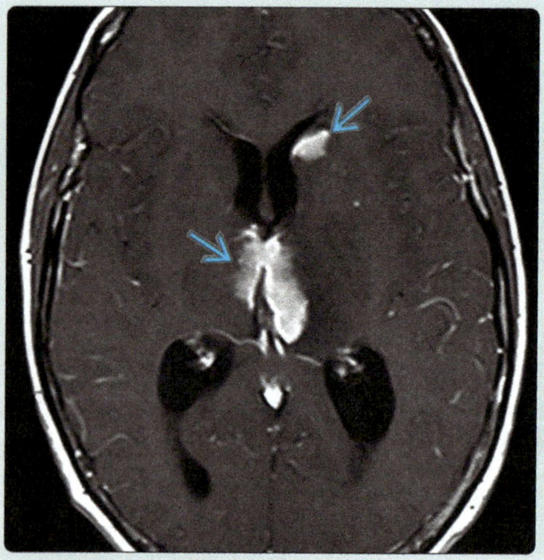

(Left) *Axial T1 C+ MR shows a homogeneously enhancing mass crossing the corpus callosum splenium ➔ typical of PCNSL in this 76-year-old man with a headache. The main differential consideration would be a glioblastoma, which typically has a more heterogeneous appearance.* **(Right)** *Axial T1WI C+ MR in an AIDS patient shows a ring-enhancing mass with a target sign ➔, suggestive of toxoplasmosis. Hemorrhage, necrosis, and ring-enhancing lesions are typical of PCNSL in AIDS patients.*

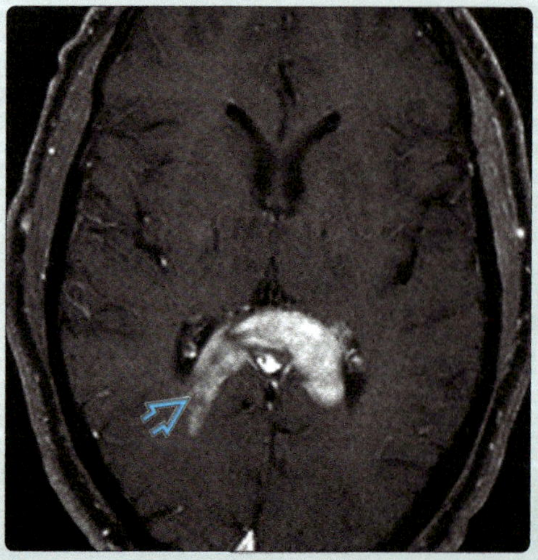

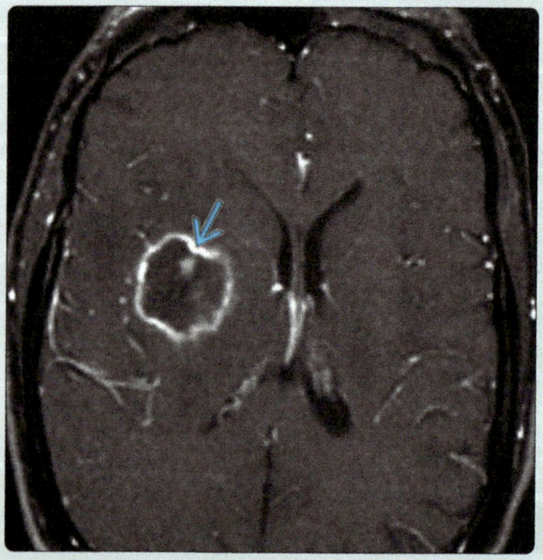

KEY FACTS

TERMINOLOGY

- Rare malignancy characterized by intravascular proliferation of lymphoid cells with predilection for CNS and skin

IMAGING

- T2/FLAIR multifocal hyperintensities in deep white matter, cortex, and basal ganglia
  - May mimic infarct
- Diffusion restriction common
- GRE/SWI: Multifocal hemorrhage often seen
- Linear and punctate enhancement typical
  - May see meningeal &/or dural enhancement
- Often mimics vasculitis

TOP DIFFERENTIAL DIAGNOSES

- Vasculitis
- Multi-infarct dementia
- Primary CNS lymphoma
- Neurosarcoid

PATHOLOGY

- Malignant lymphoid cells occlude and distend small arteries, veins, and capillaries

CLINICAL ISSUES

- Dementia is most common presenting feature
- May present with multiple stroke-like episodes
- Presents in 5th-7th decades; mean: 60-65 years
- Diagnosis may be made by skin or brain biopsy
- Rapidly progressive disease with high mortality rate
  - Mean survival: 7-13 months
- Rare, but underdiagnosed
  - CNS involved in up to 75% of cases

DIAGNOSTIC CHECKLIST

- Imaging of intravascular lymphoma (IVL) is nonspecific, but IVL should be considered in patients with dementia, multifocal lesions, and enhancement

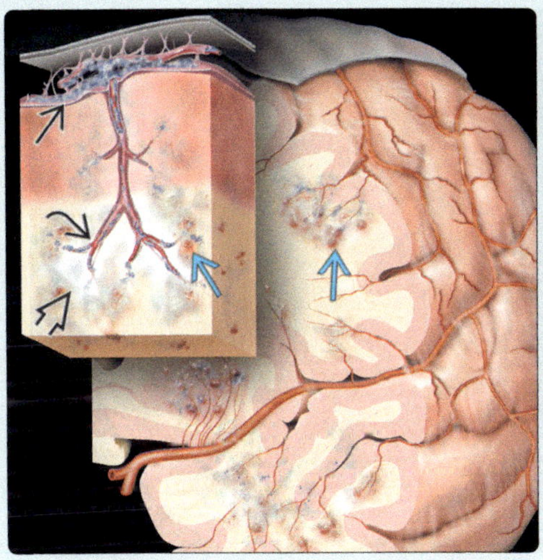

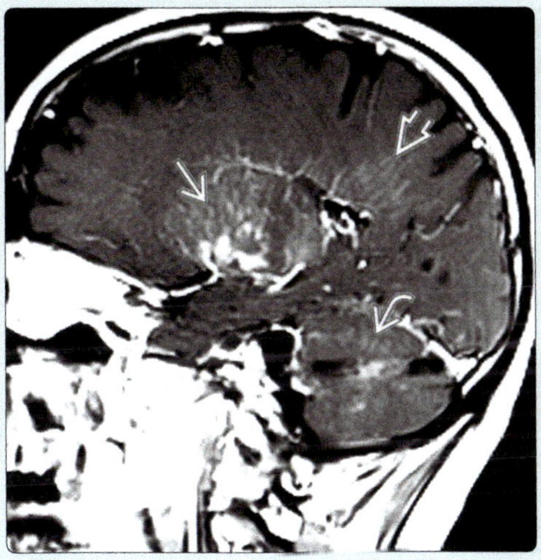

(Left) *Malignant lymphoid cells occlude and distend small arteries →, veins, and capillaries, resulting in ischemic lesions → and microbleeds →. Meningeal involvement → is typical of intravascular lymphoma (IVL).* **(Right)** *Sagittal T1 C+ MR in a 61-year-old man with known systemic diffuse large B-cell lymphoma and a 1-month history of lethargy and altered mental status shows diffuse linear enhancing foci throughout the basal ganglia →, hemispheric white matter →, and cerebellum →.*

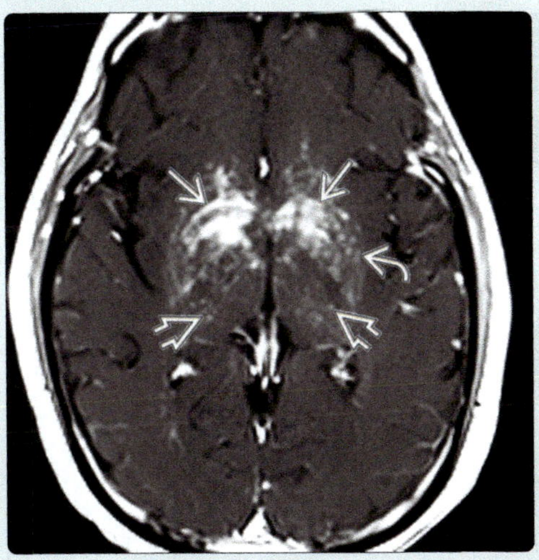

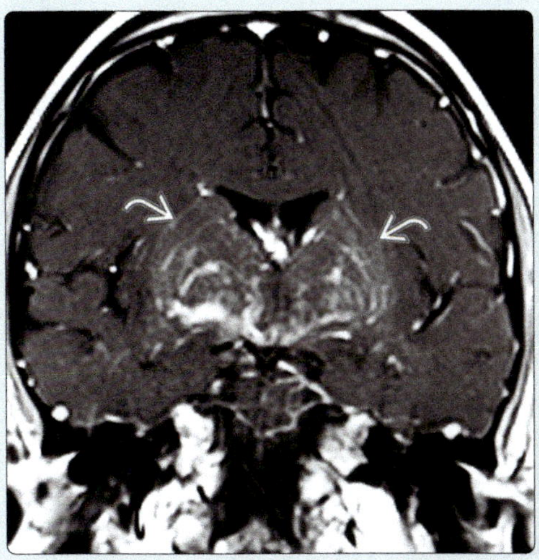

(Left) *Axial T1 C+ MR in the same case shows intense, nearly symmetric enhancement in the inferior basal ganglia →. Note numerous punctate enhancing foci in the putamina → and thalami →.* **(Right)** *Coronal T1 C+ MR in the same case shows curvilinear enhancement → following the course of the penetrating lenticulostriate arteries. Intravascular (angiocentric) lymphoma was found at autopsy.*

Leukemia

KEY FACTS

TERMINOLOGY

- Extramedullary leukemic tumors
- Synonyms: Granulocytic sarcoma, chloroma

IMAGING

- Best diagnostic clue: Homogeneous enhancing tumor(s) in patients with known or suspected myeloproliferative disorder
- Meningeal (dural-based or pial) > intraparenchymal lesions
- NECT: Hyperdense
- CECT: Moderate uniform enhancement
- MR
  - T2/FLAIR iso- to hypointense
  - Restricted diffusion on DWI

TOP DIFFERENTIAL DIAGNOSES

- Metastatic neuroblastoma
- Meningioma
- Extraaxial hematoma
- Extramedullary hematopoiesis
- Langerhans cell histiocytosis

PATHOLOGY

- CNS leukemia presents in 3 forms
  - Meningeal disease (usually with acute lymphoblastic leukemia)
  - Intravascular aggregates (leukostasis): Can rupture, hemorrhage with markedly ↑ leukocyte counts
  - Tumor masses (chloroma)
- Multiple other intracranial manifestations, complications of leukemia/treatment
  - Posterior reversible encephalopathy syndrome (PRES)
  - Posttransplant lymphoproliferative disease after bone marrow transplantation
  - Invasive fungal infection
  - Venous thrombosis associated with chemotherapy
  - Late development of cavernous angiomas after radiation therapy

(Left) *Coronal graphic shows multiple foci of leukemic infiltrates in the skull base/paranasal sinuses ➡, hypothalamus/infundibulum ➡, basal ganglia ⇨, and dura ➡. Green color observed at pathology results in the name "chloroma." The accepted term is "granulocytic sarcoma."* **(Right)** *Axial NECT scan in a child with acute myelogenous leukemia (AML) and a palpable scalp mass shows a hyperdense intra- ➡ and extracranial mass ➡ that centers on the calvaria.*

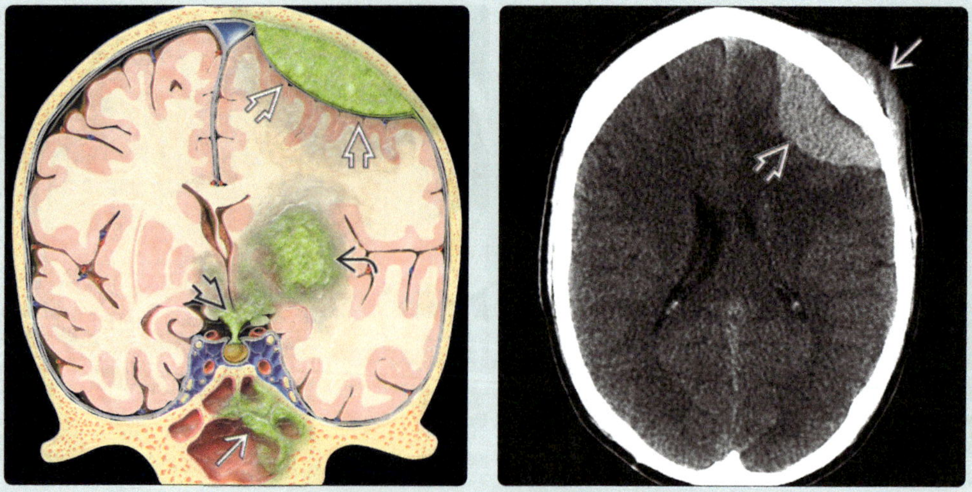

(Left) *Axial T2WI in a child with AML demonstrates a hypointense parietal mass ➡ surrounded by a collar of edema ➡. AML with parenchymal metastasis (cerebral granulocytic sarcoma) is rare.* **(Right)** *NECT scan in a 5-year-old girl with AML shows chloroma infiltrating both trigeminal nerves, enlarging the cisternal ⇨ and Meckel cave segments ⇨. (Courtesy N. Aggarwal, MD.)*

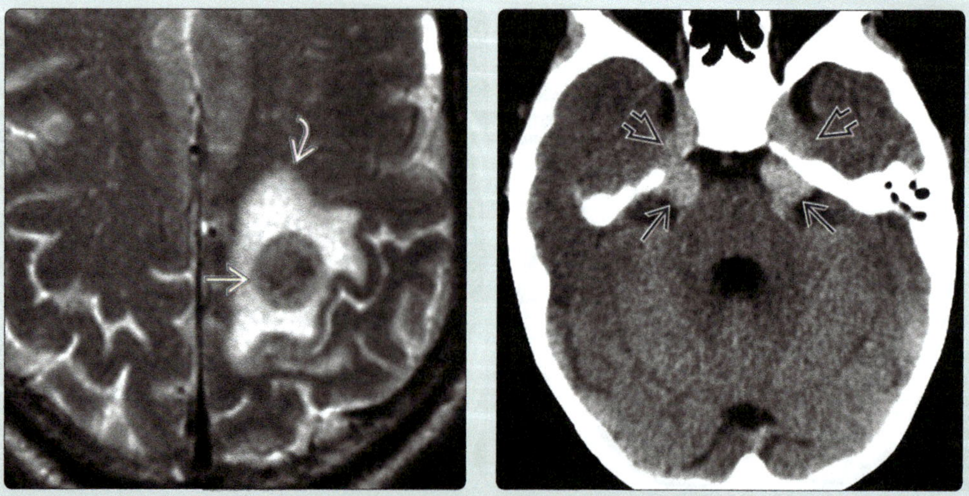

KEY FACTS

TERMINOLOGY

- Secondary brain tumors (metastases) arise from
  - Tumors outside CNS spreading to CNS (usually via hematogenous dissemination)
  - Primary CNS neoplasms spreading from 1 site to another (usually geographic extension, e.g., along WM tracts)

IMAGING

- General features
  - Round enhancing lesion(s) at gray-white interface (arterial border zones)
  - Most metastases are circumscribed/discrete > > infiltrating, spherical > > linear
  - 50% are solitary; 20% have 2 metastases
  - 30% of patients have 3 or more
- MR signal intensity varies with
  - Cellularity, nuclear:cytoplasmic ratio
  - Presence/absence of hemorrhage
- Usually no restriction on DWI
  - Exception: Densely cellular metastases may restrict

TOP DIFFERENTIAL DIAGNOSES

- Abscess (solitary or multiple)
- Glioblastoma multiforme
- Cerebral infarction (multiple embolic)
- Demyelinating disease (e.g., tumefactive MS)

PATHOLOGY

- Metastases represent at least 50% of all brain tumors
- In 10% of cases, brain is only site

CLINICAL ISSUES

- Progressive increase in size and numbers is typical
- Median survival with whole-brain XRT = 3-6 months
- Stereotactic radiosurgery alone > whole-brain XRT
- Survival advantage, if 1-4 metastases, avoids deleterious effects of whole-brain XRT on quality of life, cognition
- Resection of solitary metastasis may improve survival

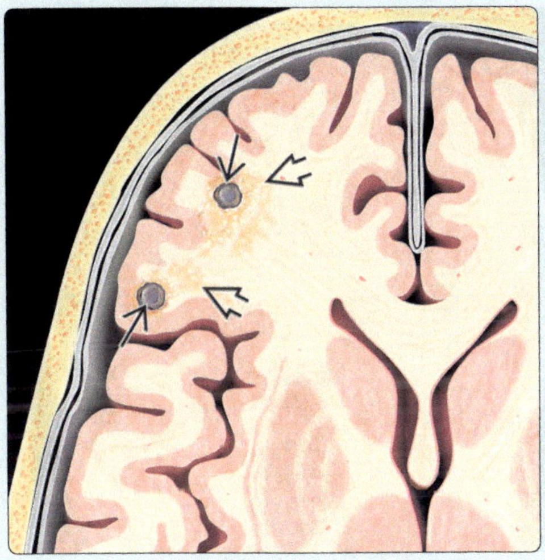

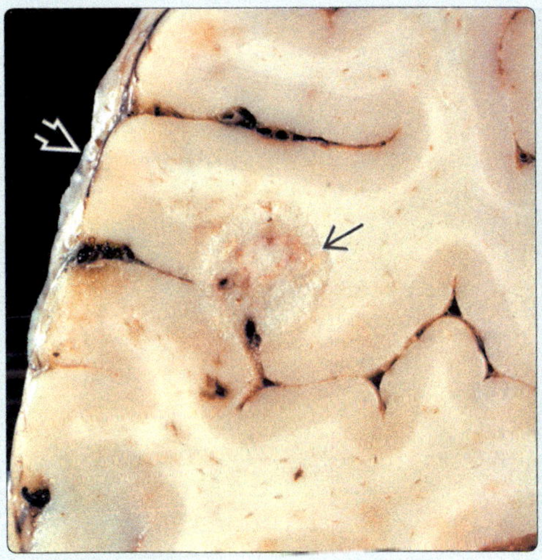

(Left) *Axial graphic shows parenchymal metastases → with surrounding edema ⇨. The gray-white matter junction is the most common location. Most metastases are round, not diffusely infiltrating.* **(Right)** *Close-up view of an axial section through an autopsied brain shows a classic metastasis → in the classic location, the gray-white matter junction. Note the round shape, central necrosis, and relative lack of edema. Diffuse leptomeningeal metastatic spread ⇨ is also present.*

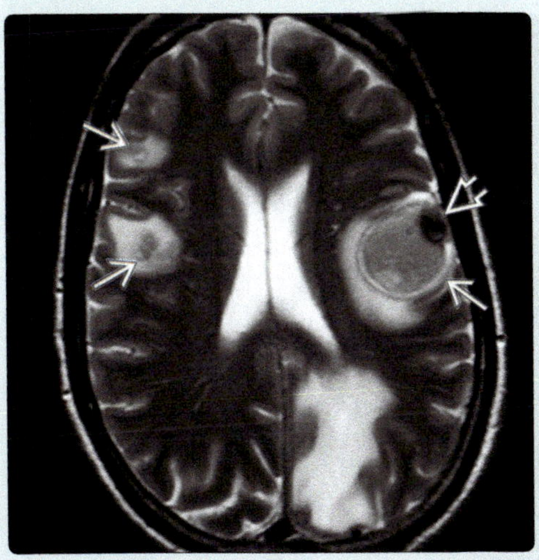

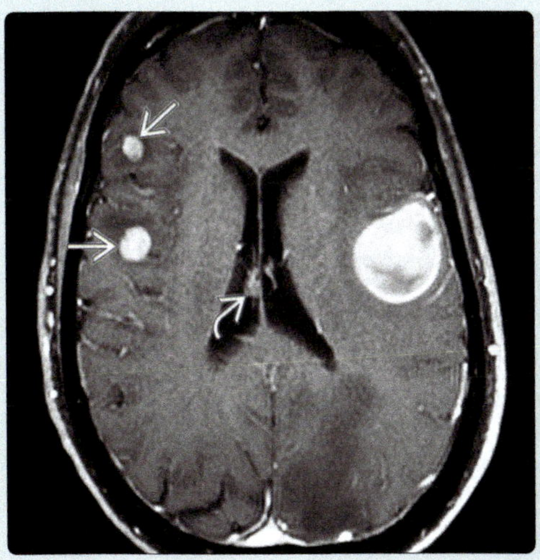

(Left) *Axial T2WI MR in a 52-year-old man with a seizure, history of melanoma, shows multiple lesions → at the gray-white matter interfaces. Moderate edema surrounds the lesions. One of the lesions has a hypointense nodule ⇨, suggesting that at least 1 is a hemorrhagic metastasis.* **(Right)** *T1 C+ FS MR (same case) shows that the lesions enhance →. Note small metastasis ↪ in the right ventricle choroid plexus that was not appreciated on T2WI. The extensive occipital edema is also from a metastasis (not seen on this image).*

Miscellaneous Intracranial Metastases

KEY FACTS

TERMINOLOGY

- Brain metastases in locations other than skull/meninges or parenchyma

IMAGING

- General features
  - > 95% of brain metastases parenchymal
  - Only 1-2% in ventricles, pituitary gland, etc.
  - Sites generally very vascular
  - Extraventricular metastases more diffuse, infiltrative than parenchymal metastases (usually round)
- Location
  - Choroid plexus ± ventricular ependyma
  - Pituitary gland infundibulum
  - Eye (choroid)
  - Cranial nerves
  - Pineal gland
  - Preexisting neoplasm ("collision tumor")
- Best imaging tool: MR with T1WI C+ FS
  - Metastases almost always enhance

TOP DIFFERENTIAL DIAGNOSES

- Varies with location
- Choroid plexus, ventricle = meningioma
- Pituitary gland, infundibular stalk
  - Pituitary macroadenoma
  - Lymphocytic hypophysitis
  - Lymphoma
- Cranial nerves = neurofibromatosis type 2, lymphoma
- Eye (globe)
  - Ocular melanoma
  - Retinal or choroidal detachment
  - Choroidal hemangioma

DIAGNOSTIC CHECKLIST

- Look for "secret sites" outside parenchyma when imaging brain for possible metastatic disease

(Left) *Submentovertex graphic shows the typical sites for miscellaneous nonparenchymal CNS metastases. These include the choroid plexus and ventricles, pituitary gland, infundibular stalk, and eye (choroid of the retina).* **(Right)** *Coronal T1WI C+ MR in an elderly woman with known breast carcinoma shows a thickened, enhancing infundibular stalk. This was the only intracranial metastasis identified in this patient.*

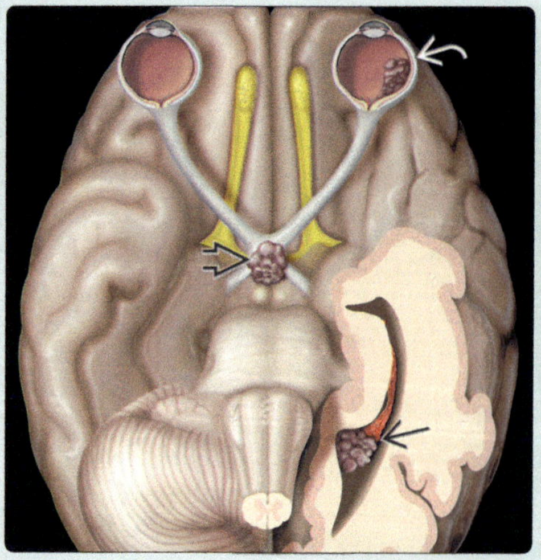

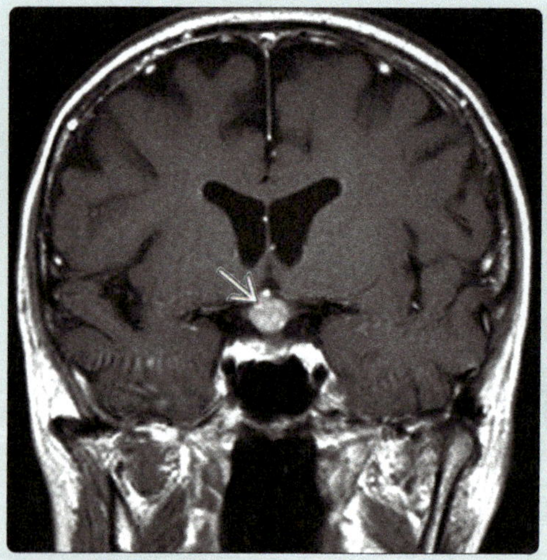

(Left) *Axial T1 C+ FS in a patient with diplopia and known esophageal cancer shows an enhancing nodule on the left 3rd cranial nerve, as well as on the left optic nerve/sheath. Cranial nerve metastases from extracranial tumors are less common than from hematopoietic neoplasms (e.g., lymphoma).* **(Right)** *Axial T1 C+ FS in a patient with systemic B-cell lymphoma shows multiple metastases to the choroid plexus. Subtle ependymal metastases are present along with diffuse dura-arachnoid thickening.*

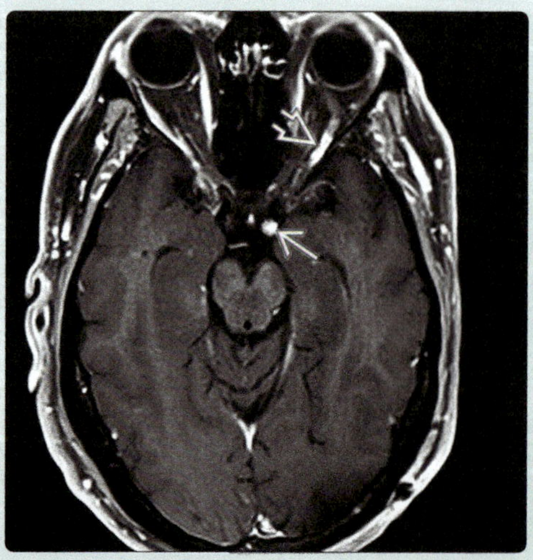

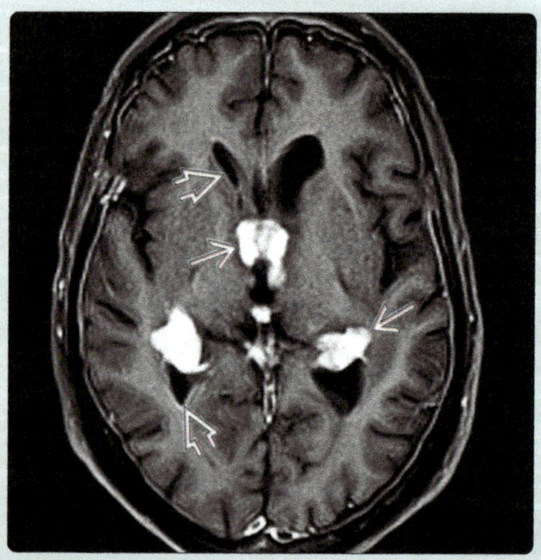

KEY FACTS

TERMINOLOGY

- Secondary CNS involvement in patients with systemic lymphoma (SCNSL)

IMAGING

- Secondary CNS lymphoma: Skull, dura, leptomeninges > > parenchymal mass
- Best diagnostic clue: Diffusely enhancing dural mass ± bone involvement
  - May see leptomeningeal enhancement or nonsupression of cerebrospinal fluid on FLAIR; CT hyperdensity
- Lower relative cerebral blood volume than other tumors

TOP DIFFERENTIAL DIAGNOSES

- Meningioma
- Meningeal metastases
- Primary CNS lymphoma
- "Tumefactive" demyelinating disease (MS, ADEM)

CLINICAL ISSUES

- Prognostic markers suggestive of CNS relapse
  - Elevated serum lactate dehydrogenase levels
  - Presence of B symptoms
  - Extranodal involvement at > 1 site
  - Advanced stage
- Aggressive histologic features increase risk for SCNSL
- Involvement of liver, bladder, testis, or adrenals also increases risk of CNS spread
- CNS involvement of lymphoma almost always fatal
- Prophylactic CNS chemotherapy recommended for patients considered at high risk of CNS recurrence

DIAGNOSTIC CHECKLIST

- Occult lymphoma found in 8% of patients presenting with CNS lymphoma
- SCNSL commonly mimics meningioma or other metastatic disease

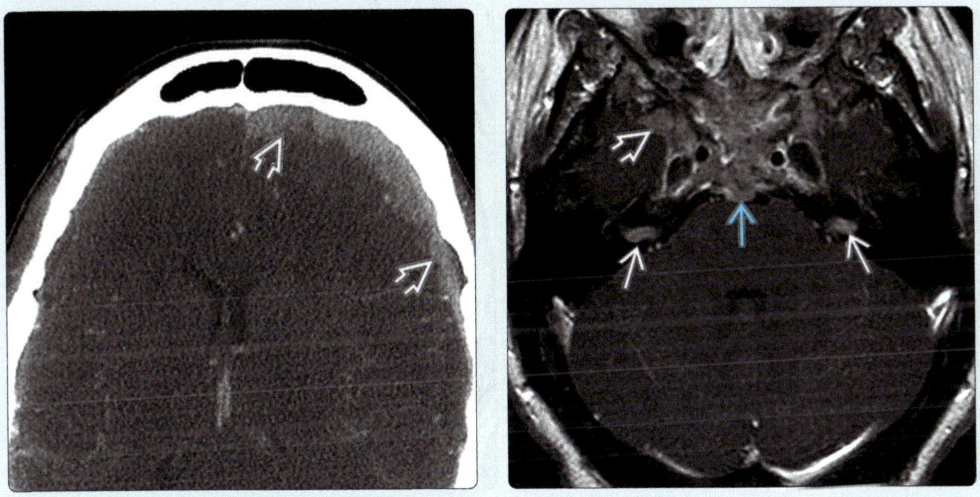

(Left) *Axial CECT shows extensive dural enhancement ⇨ related to metastatic intracranial lymphoma. Secondary lymphoma has a propensity for the meninges. About 1/3 of systemic lymphoma patients develop CNS disease.* **(Right)** *Axial T1 C+ MR shows an enhancing central skull base mass → with associated dural ⇨ and leptomeningeal enhancement ⇨ within the internal auditory canals. The clivus is often involved by metastatic disease, particularly breast cancer and lymphoma.*

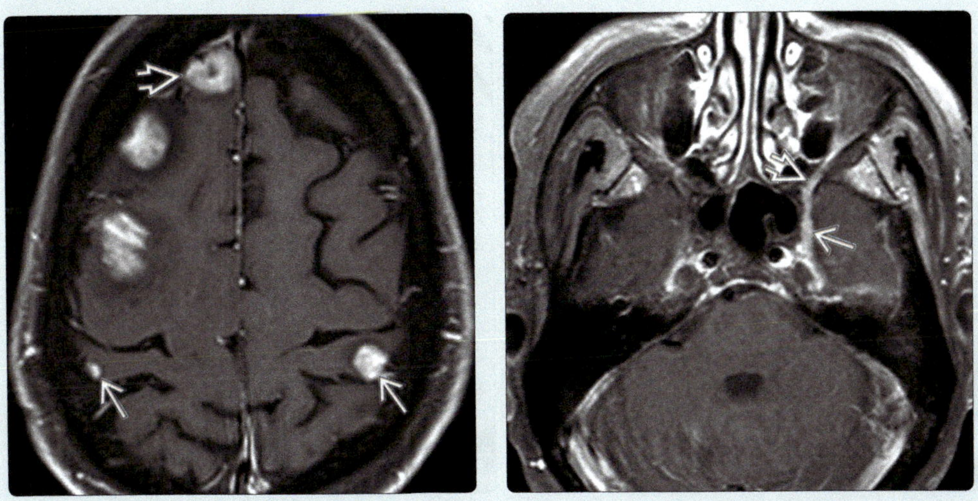

(Left) *Axial T1 C+ MR in a 54-year-old man with systemic lymphoma shows multiple enhancing masses. Some lesions involve the dura ⇨, whereas others are parenchymal ⇨. Metastatic intracranial lymphoma often involves the dura and may mimic a meningioma.* **(Right)** *Axial T1WI C+ FS MR shows enhancement along the maxillary division (V2) of CN5 ⇨, extending from the cavernous sinus into the pterygopalatine fossa ⇨, in this patient with systemic lymphoma and new facial paresthesias.*

KEY FACTS

TERMINOLOGY

- Remote neurological effects of cancer, associated with extra-CNS tumors
  - Most common tumor: Small cell lung carcinoma
- Limbic encephalitis (LE) is most common clinical paraneoplastic syndrome

IMAGING

- Limbic encephalitis: Hyperintensity in mesial temporal lobes, limbic system
  - Mimics herpes encephalitis but subacute/chronic
- Paraneoplastic cerebellar degeneration (PCD): Cerebellar atrophy
- Brainstem encephalitis: T2 hyperintensity in midbrain, pons, cerebellar peduncles, basal ganglia
- Most paraneoplastic syndromes do not have associated imaging findings

TOP DIFFERENTIAL DIAGNOSES

- Herpes encephalitis
- Low-grade (grade II) diffuse astrocytoma
- Status epilepticus
- Gliomatosis cerebri

CLINICAL ISSUES

- < 1% of patients with systemic cancers develop paraneoplastic syndrome
- Immune mediated by autoantibodies or cytotoxic T cell-related mechanisms
  - 60% have circulating serum autoantibodies
- LE: Memory loss, cognitive dysfunction, dementia, psychological features, seizures
- PCD: Ataxia, incoordination, dysarthria, nystagmus
- Brainstem encephalitis: Brainstem dysfunction including cranial nerve palsies, visual changes
- Treatment of primary tumor may improve symptoms

(Left) *Axial FLAIR MR shows abnormal hyperintensity in the bilateral medial temporal lobes ➔, characteristic of limbic encephalitis, the most common paraneoplastic syndrome. Bilateral involvement is typical of limbic encephalitis.* **(Right)** *Axial T1WI C+ MR in the same patient shows no significant enhancement in the medial temporal lobes. Enhancement is often present in limbic encephalitis. The patient's symptoms often improve after treatment of the primary tumor.*

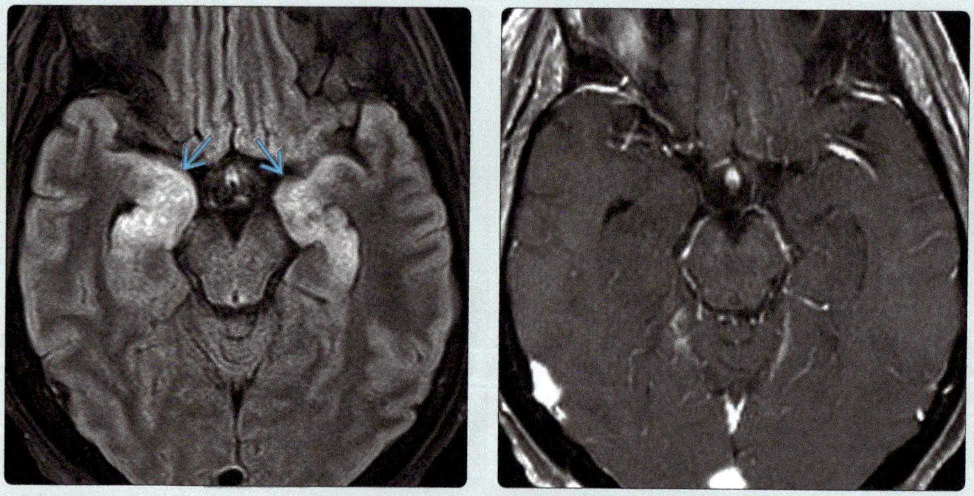

(Left) *Axial FLAIR MR in an older adult with small cell lung cancer and subacute dementia shows striking hyperintensity in the right insula ➲.* **(Right)** *Coronal T2WI in the same patient shows abnormal hyperintensity in both medial temporal lobes ➔ and right insular cortex ➲. Imaging of limbic encephalitis mimics that of herpes encephalitis; however, patients with limbic encephalitis have a subacute presentation. Hemorrhage suggests herpes rather than limbic encephalitis.*

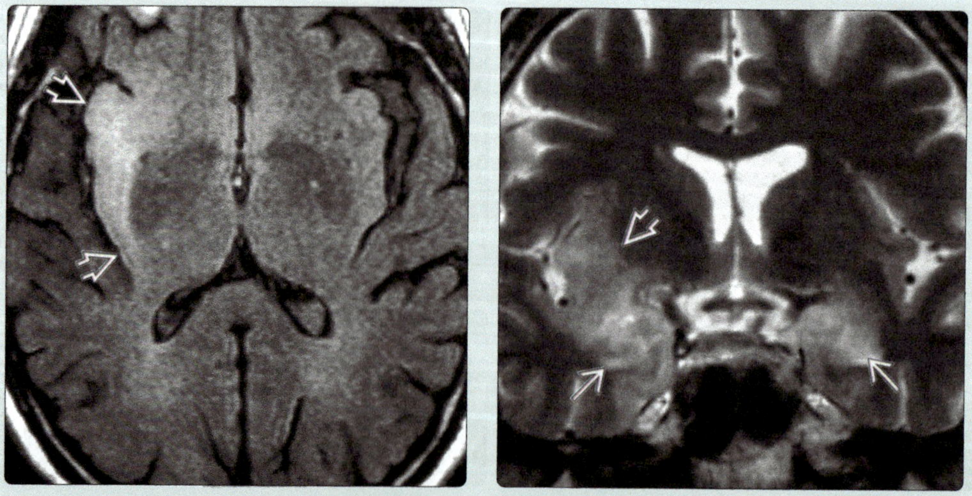

KEY FACTS

TERMINOLOGY

- Radiation-induced injury may be divided into acute, subacute/early delayed, late injury

IMAGING

- **Radiation injury**: Mild vasogenic edema to necrosis
- **Radiation necrosis**: Irregular enhancing lesion(s)
    - MRS: Markedly ↓ metabolites (NAA, Cho, Cr), ± lactate/lipid peaks
    - Perfusion MR: ↓ relative cerebral blood volume compared with tumor
- **Leukoencephalopathy**: T2 white matter (WM) hyperintensity, spares subcortical U fibers
- **Mineralizing microangiopathy**: Basal ganglia, subcortical WM Ca++, atrophy
- **Necrotizing leukoencephalopathy**: WM necrosis
- **PRES**: Posterior circulation subcortical WM edema
- MRS, MR perfusion, PET, or SPECT may help delineate recurrent tumor from radiation necrosis

TOP DIFFERENTIAL DIAGNOSES

- Neoplasm
- Abscess
- Multiple sclerosis
- Vascular dementia
- Progressive multifocal leukoencephalopathy

PATHOLOGY

- 2nd neoplasms: Meningiomas (70%), gliomas (20%), sarcomas (10%)
    - More aggressive tumors, highly refractory
    - Incidence: 3-12%
- Radiation-induced vascular malformations: Capillary telangiectasias ± cavernomas

CLINICAL ISSUES

- Overall incidence of radionecrosis: 3-9%
- Worse prognosis: Younger patient at treatment

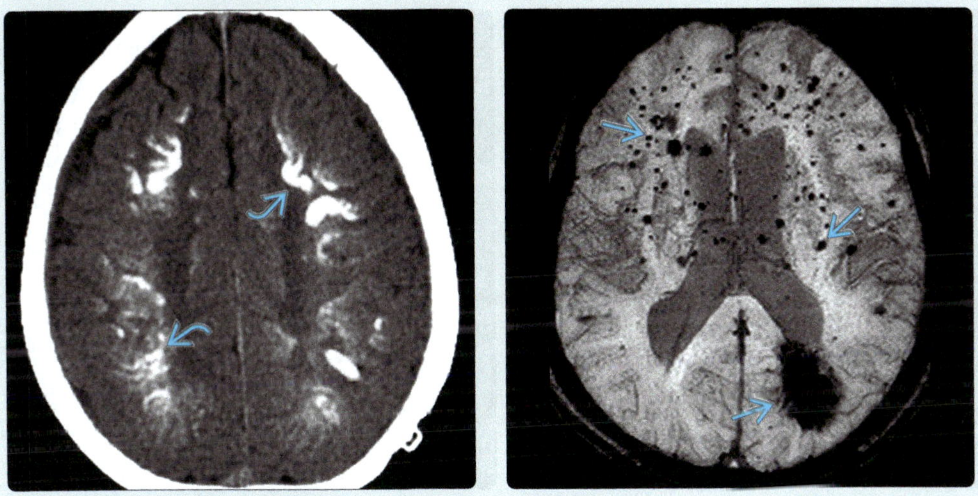

(Left) *Axial NECT shows extensive calcification in the subcortical white matter (WM) → in a 20-year-old patient. Mineralizing microangiopathy usually results after a combination of radiation therapy and chemotherapy 2 or more years after treatment.* **(Right)** *Axial SWI in an adult patient with neurofibromatosis and optic nerve glioma status post radiation therapy in childhood shows innumerable "blooming" hypointense foci → consistent with radiation-induced vascular malformations.*

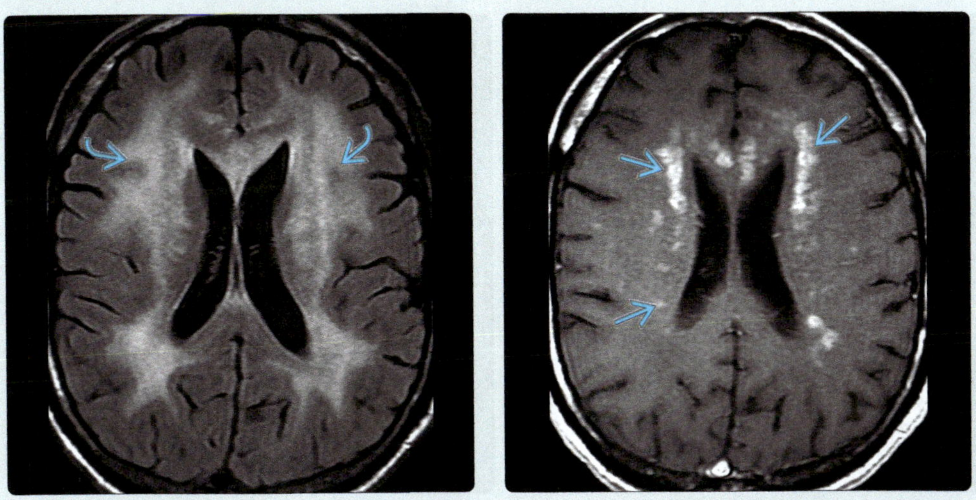

(Left) *Axial FLAIR MR in a 22 year old with acute leukemia treated with intrathecal methotrexate shows confluent periventricular and deep WM hyperintensities → with sparing of the subcortical WM.* **(Right)** *Axial T1 C+ MR in the same patient shows multiple nodular enhancing lesions in the WM →. Findings are consistent with chemotherapy-induced necrotizing leukoencephalopathy. Leukoencephalopathy is a potentially serious complication of chemotherapy.*

KEY FACTS

TERMINOLOGY

- Treatment-related increase in contrast enhancement mimics tumor progression
- Classically described after treatment with chemoradiation (temozolomide with radiation therapy)
- Typically occurs within 3-6 months after conclusion of radiation therapy (XRT)

IMAGING

- New enhancing lesion + ↑ FLAIR hyperintensity in treated malignant glioma at 3-4 months after XRT completion
- T2/FLAIR: Increased hyperintensity with mass effect
- DWI: Higher ADC values in PsP compared with tumor
- DSC MR
  - Lower mean rCBV values in PsP compared with tumor
- DCE MR
  - Mean K trans (volume transfer constant) is lower in PsP compared with true progression
- MRS: No significant elevation of choline in PsP
- Best imaging: Contrast-enhanced MR, DWI, ± MRS, MRP
- Follow-up studies may be necessary to make accurate diagnosis of PsP
- Knowing clinical history and timing of therapy is key to accurate brain tumor imaging

TOP DIFFERENTIAL DIAGNOSES

- Recurrent malignant glioma
- Radiation necrosis

CLINICAL ISSUES

- Current standard of care for malignant gliomas is surgical resection followed by concurrent XRT and chemotherapy with temozolomide (Temodar)
  - PsP occurs in ~ 35-50% of patients
- PsP is self-limited, enhancing lesions resolve without new treatment
- PsP has been associated with **improved survival**
- Important to recognize that not all new enhancement in patient with treated glioblastoma is progressive tumor

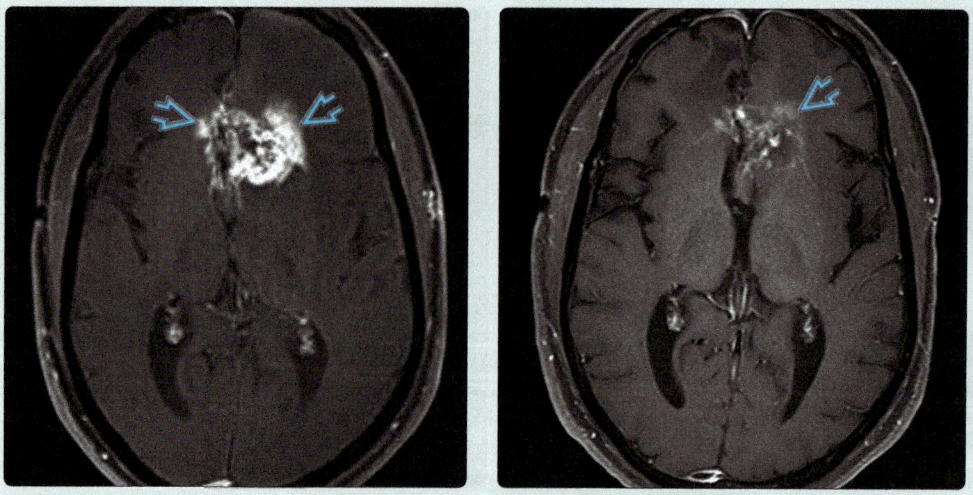

(Left) *Axial T1 C+ MR in a 48-year-old man treated with radiation therapy and Temodar for 3 months for his malignant glioma shows new enhancement ⇨ in the frontal lobes bilaterally. His initial postoperative MR study showed no enhancement. He was clinically doing well.* **(Right)** *Axial T1 C+ MR in the same patient 4 weeks later shows a marked decrease in the enhancement ⇨ without a change in therapy. Imaging findings are related to pseudoprogression, not true progression, likely related to an inflammatory response.*

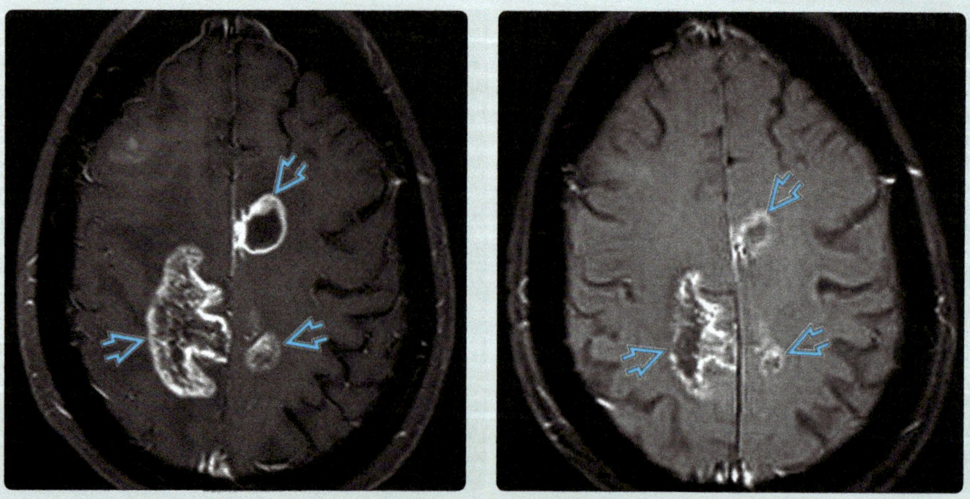

(Left) *Axial T1 C+ MR in a 62-year-old woman with a multifocal glioblastoma treated with Temodar and radiation therapy shows new enhancement ⇨ in the hemispheres on her 4-month scan, concerning for progressive tumor.* **(Right)** *Axial T1 C+ MR in the same patient 8 weeks later with no therapy change shows a marked decrease in the enhancing lesions ⇨. The new enhancement was related to pseudoprogression, which is associated with an increased survival.*

KEY FACTS

TERMINOLOGY

- Antiangiogenic agents may substantially reduce contrast enhancement in glioblastoma multiforme related to reduced vascular permeability rather than actual tumor response
  - **Bevacizumab** (Avastin): Anti-VEGF is main antiangiogenic agent currently used for treatment of recurrent malignant gliomas
  - **Cediranib**: VEGF receptor tyrosine kinase inhibitor has been tested in recent high-grade glioma treatment trials

IMAGING

- Decreased enhancement in patient with malignant glioma treated with anti-VEGF agent
  - May see persistent FLAIR and diffusion restriction, despite decreased enhancement
- DWI and ADC have been proposed as imaging markers for tumor response in presence of antiangiogenic agents to address pseudoresponse
- Beware, decreased enhancement in tumor follow-up study may be true treatment response or pseudoresponse in setting of newer therapies
- DSC: Early changes in relative cerebral blood volume after initiation of antiangiogenic therapy may distinguish pseudoresponse from true treatment response

TOP DIFFERENTIAL DIAGNOSES

- Treatment response
- Steroid effect

CLINICAL ISSUES

- Antiangiogenic agents normalize hyperpermeable tumor vasculature and restore blood-brain barrier
- Local response to tumor growth is controlled, but diffuse infiltration and distant metastases are common
- Antiangiogenic agents significantly improve 6-month progression-free survival but may not affect overall survival

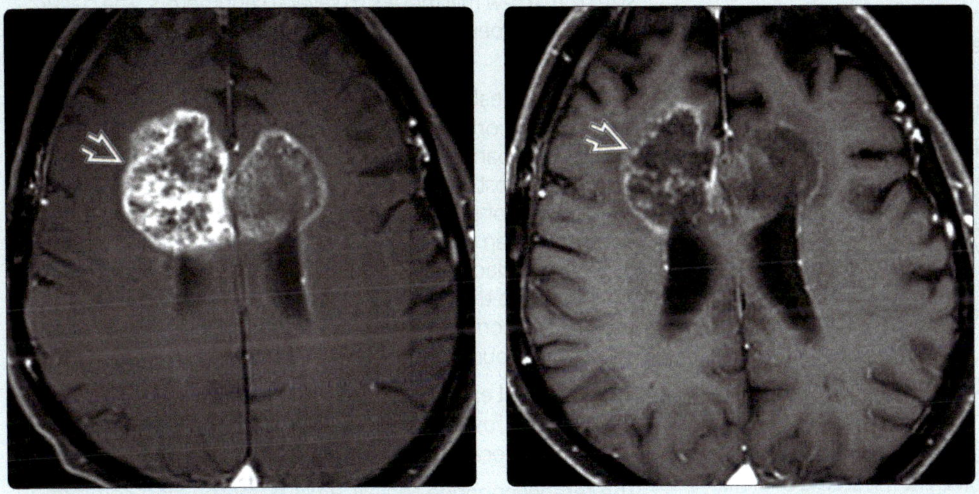

***(Left)** Axial T1 C+ MR in a GBM patient who progressed on standard therapy with radiation and Temodar shows there is a heterogeneously enhancing mass involving the genu of the corpus callosum ➔. Avastin therapy was started immediately after this MR examination. **(Right)** Axial T1 C+ MR in the same patient 4 weeks after the start of Avastin shows a marked decrease in the enhancing mass involving the genu of the corpus callosum ➔. The FLAIR and DWI showed stable hyperintensity and mass effect.*

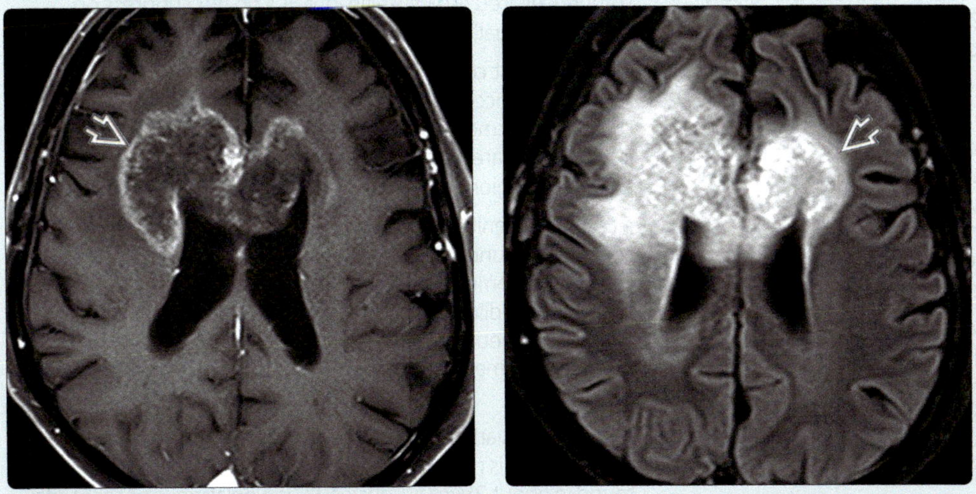

***(Left)** Axial T1 C+ MR in the same patient 8 weeks later shows an increase in the size of the corpus callosum enhancing mass ➔. **(Right)** Axial FLAIR MR in the same patient shows a marked increase in the size ➔ and associated mass effect of the corpus callosum mass related to progressive tumor. Decreased enhancement on the prior MR is a result of pseudoresponse from the antiangiogenic therapy, rather than true tumor response. Diffuse tumor infiltration is common after antiangiogenic therapy.*

General Approach to Brain Cysts

General Considerations

Overview: Cysts are common findings on MR and CT brain scans. There are many types of intracranial cysts, some significant, some incidental. In this section, we exclude cystic neoplasms (such as pilocytic astrocytoma and hemangioblastoma), solid neoplasms that commonly have intratumoral cysts (such as ependymoma), and tumors that often display central necrosis (e.g., glioblastoma).

We also exclude parasitic cysts (neurocysticercosis, hydatid disease) and cystic brain malformations (Dandy-Walker spectrum) from the discussion. Thus, the focus of this particular section is primary nonneoplastic cysts.

Because the etiology, pathology, and clinical importance of nonneoplastic cysts is so varied, classifying them presents a real challenge. Some neuropathologists typically classify cysts according to the histology of the cyst wall. Others group them according to putative origin or pathogenesis.

In a schema based on pathogenesis, cysts may occur as normal anatomic variants [e.g., enlarged perivascular (Virchow-Robin) spaces] (PVSs), congenital inclusion cysts [e.g., dermoid and epidermoid cysts (ECs)], or lesions derived from embryonic ecto-/endoderm [colloid cysts (CCs) and neurenteric cysts (NCs)]. Of course, there is a group of miscellaneous cysts [such as choroid plexus cysts (CPCs) and nonneoplastic tumor-associated cysts (TACs)] that does not fit nicely into any category.

Neurologists and their neuroradiology colleagues face a very real dilemma: A cystic-appearing lesion is identified on MR or CT. What is it? What else could it be? Histopathology of the cyst wall isn't a practical consideration. What **is** readily apparent is (1) the anatomic location of the cyst, (2) its imaging characteristics (density/signal intensity, presence or absence of calcification, enhancement, etc.), and (3) the patient's age. The recommended initial approach to analyzing brain cysts is anatomy based.

Anatomy-Based Approach to Brain Cysts

General Considerations

Key features: Four features help the diagnostic approach to cystic-appearing intracranial lesions. The 1st step is to determine whether the cyst is intra- or extraaxial. If it is extraaxial, is the cyst supra- or infratentorial? Is it midline or off midline? If a cyst is intraaxial, is it supra- or infratentorial? Is it parenchymal or intraventricular? Although many intracranial cysts certainly may occur in > 1 location, some sites are "preferred" by certain cysts.

Extraaxial Cysts

Supratentorial extraaxial cysts: Nonneoplastic, noninfectious extraaxial cysts can occur in the midline or off midline. Pineal and Rathke cleft cysts occur only in the midline. Although dermoid cysts seem to prefer a midline location like the suprasellar cistern, they also occur off midline. Look for rupture with fatty "droplets" in the subarachnoid cisterns.

Arachnoid cysts (AC) are usually off midline. In the supratentorial compartment, midline ACs are relatively rare. The most frequent midline locations are the suprasellar cistern, followed by the quadrigeminal cistern and velum interpositum. Large suprasellar ACs usually present in children and may cause obstructive hydrocephalus.

The most common off midline extraaxial supratentorial cyst is an AC. Although these can occur virtually anywhere, the middle cranial fossa is the location of at least 50% of all ACs. Occasionally, ACs occur over the cerebral convexities, most commonly over the parietal lobe. ACs follow cerebrospinal fluid (CSF) on all sequences and are differentiated from ECs using FLAIR and DWI. ACs suppress completely on FLAIR and do not show diffusion restriction.

Extraaxial tumors, such as meningioma, schwannoma, pituitary macroadenoma, and craniopharyngioma, may be associated with prominent extratumoral cysts. These nonneoplastic TACs occur in both the supra- and infratentorial compartments.

TACs are benign collections of fluid that vary from clear and CSF-like to proteinaceous. TACs are typically positioned between at the tumor-brain interface, between the mass and adjacent cortex. Whether TACs are true ACs, obstructed PVSs (Virchow-Robin), or fluid collections mostly lined by gliotic brain is debatable.

Scalp and skull cysts are less common than intracranial cysts. Sebaceous cysts [more accurately termed trichilemmal cysts (TCs)] are a common scalp mass in middle-aged and older patients. Most are identified incidentally on MR and CT scans. TCs can be solitary or multiple, are well delineated, and vary in size from a few millimeters to several centimeters. The classic finding is a subepidermal scalp tumor in a woman over the age of 60 years.

Leptomeningeal cysts, also known as "growing fractures," are a rare but important extraaxial cyst that is most commonly found in the parietal bone. An enlarging calvarial fracture adjacent to posttraumatic encephalomalacia is typical. The vast majority of patients are under 3 years of age. They present with an enlarging, palpable soft tissue mass. Fluid and encephalomalacic brain extrude through torn dura and arachnoid and then through the enlarging linear calvarial fracture. Leptomeningeal cysts are seen as linear lucent skull lesions with rounded, scalloped margins.

Infratentorial extraaxial cysts: Most nonneoplastic cysts in the posterior fossa occur off midline. The 2 major cyst types found in this location are ECs and ACs.

The cerebellopontine angle (CPA) is by far the most common posterior fossa sublocation of an EC. Occasionally, an EC occurs in the 4th ventricle. A 4th ventricular EC can mimic a trapped, dilated 4th ventricle, but ECs do not suppress on FLAIR and usually exhibit some degree of restricted diffusion.

The next most common posterior fossa cyst is AC. Although ACs can also occur in the midline cisterna magna, the CPS is the most common site. TACs sometimes occur in the CPA cistern. Most are associated with vestibular schwannoma, but a CPA meningioma may also cause formation of a TAC.

NEs are congenital endodermal cysts that are much more commonly found in the spinal canal. Intracranial NE cysts occur in the cerebromedullary cistern and are usually midline or slightly off midline, lying just anterior to the pontomedullary junction. Sometimes NE cysts occur off midline, in the lower CPA (cerebromedullary) cistern. Bony skull defects can occur but are rare.

An anatomic variant that can be confused with a posterior fossa NE cyst is retroclival ecchordosis physaliphora (EP), found in about 2% of autopsies. EP is a gelatinous notochordal remnant that can occur anywhere from the dorsum sellae to the sacrococcygeal region. Intracranial EPs typically occur in the prepontine cistern and are attached to a defect in the dorsal clivus by a thin, stalk-like pedicle. NE cysts and EPs are both hyperintense on T2WI. Chordomas are the malignant counterparts of ecchordosis.

Intraaxial Cysts

Supratentorial intraaxial cysts: Here, anatomic sublocation is key to the differential diagnosis. Parenchymal cysts represent a completely different group than intraventricular cysts. The most common parenchymal cysts in the brain are enlarged PVSs (Virchow-Robin). PVSs have a distinct predilection for the basal ganglia, where they tend to cluster around the anterior commissure. The midbrain is another common site. When they occur here, enlarged PVSs may cause obstructive hydrocephalus. Prominent PVSs also occur in the subcortical and deep white matter. They are pial-lined, interstitial fluid-containing structures that tend to occur in clusters of variably sized cysts. Most PVSs suppress completely; 75% are surrounded by normal-appearing brain, which helps distinguish them from porencephalic cysts.

Hippocampal sulcus remnant cysts (HSRCs) are common normal variants, seen as a "string" of small CSF-like cysts lying in the hippocampus just medial to the temporal horn of the lateral ventricle. They are caused by defective or incomplete fusion of the embryonic cornu ammonis and dentate gyrus and are of no clinical significance.

Porencephalic cysts are the 3rd most common supratentorial parenchymal cysts. They may communicate with the ventricles and are typically lined by gliotic white matter, not ependyma, and are caused by brain destruction (e.g., peri- or antenatal insult). The brain surrounding a porencephalic cyst is typically hyperintense on T2WI and FLAIR.

Periventricular cysts of newborns encompasses a wide, overlapping variety of periventricular cystic lesions that ranges from cystic periventricular leukomalacia to connatal and germinolytic cysts.

Neuroglial cysts, sometimes called neuroepithelial cysts, are benign glial lined cavities buried within the cerebral white matter. Although they can occur anywhere, the frontal lobe is the most common site. They tend to be solitary, whereas PVSs are usually collections of multiple cysts of different sizes. A choroid fissure cyst is a neuroglial cyst that occurs anywhere along the infolded choroid fissure. Most are found medial to the temporal horn of the lateral ventricle. HSRCs occur when there is incomplete fusion of the cornu ammonis and the dentate gyrus. HSRCs are often multiple, appearing like a string of small CSF-containing cysts along the lateral margin of the hippocampus.

Supratentorial intraventricular cysts are most often found in the atria of the lateral ventricles and foramen of Monro. CPCs are the most common of all intracranial neuroepithelial cysts, occurring in up to 50% of autopsies. Most CPCs are actually xanthogranulomas. Lipid accumulates in the choroid plexus from degenerating &/or desquamating choroid epithelium. CPCs are common incidental imaging findings in middle-aged and older adults. They are usually bilateral and are often multicystic. Most CPCs are small, measuring 2-8 mm in diameter. They typically do not suppress completely on FLAIR and may show moderately high signal intensity on DWI.

Ependymal cysts (ECs) are rare, benign, ependymal-lined cysts of the lateral ventricles. Most ECs, even large ones, are asymptomatic and incidental. EC patients presenting with headache, seizure, &/or obstructive hydrocephalus have been reported in the literature. They contain clear serous CSF-like fluid secreted from ependymal cells. ECs typically follow CSF on all sequences and suppress completely on FLAIR.

CCs occur almost exclusively in the foramen of Monro, attached to the anterosuperior portion of the 3rd ventricular roof. They are wedged into the foramen and are typically straddled by the fornices. CCs are endodermal in origin and contain viscous gelatinous material consisting of mostly mucin. CCs may also contain blood degradation products, foamy cells, and cholesterol crystals. Even relatively small CCs may suddenly obstruct the foramen of Monro, causing acute hydrocephalus. Occasionally brain herniation with rapid clinical deterioration ensues. The imaging appearance of a well-delineated, hyperdense mass at the foramen of Monro on NECT is virtually pathognomonic of a CC.

Infratentorial intraaxial cysts: Parenchymal infratentorial cysts are rare; most are PVSs. The only common site is in and around the dentate nuclei. Most are asymptomatic. Occasionally, large PVSs occur in the pons and can be a rare cause of cranial neuropathy.

Nonneoplastic, nonparasitic cysts in the 4th ventricle are uncommon. The most common cause is not a true cyst but an enlarged, "encysted" 4th ventricle. Infection or aneurysmal subarachnoid hemorrhage may cause outlet foraminal obstruction. When combined with superior obstruction near the aqueduct, the 4th ventricle can become completely encysted. Choroid plexus continues to produce CSF. With egress blocked, the 4th ventricle enlarges. ECs can arise in the 4th ventricle, a much less common posterior fossa location than the CPA. Some ECs are so similar to CSF that only FLAIR and DWI permit distinction of an EC from CSF in an enlarged but otherwise normal-appearing 4th ventricle.

Selected References

1. Aboud E et al: Giant intracranial epidermoids: is total removal feasible? J Neurosurg. 1-14, 2015
2. Ali M et al: Exploring predictors of surgery and comparing operative treatment approaches for pediatric intracranial arachnoid cysts: a case series of 83 patients. J Neurosurg Pediatr. 1-8, 2015
3. Culver SA et al: A Case for conservative management: characterizing the natural history of radiographically diagnosed Rathke cleft cysts. J Clin Endocrinol Metab. 100(10):3943-8, 2015
4. Din NU et al: Symptomatic surgically treated non-neoplastic cysts of the central nervous system: a clinicopathological study from Pakistan. J Coll Physicians Surg Pak. 25(8):588-91, 2015
5. Kalani MY et al: Pineal cyst resection in the absence of ventriculomegaly or Parinaud's syndrome: clinical outcomes and implications for patient selection. J Neurosurg. 1-5, 2015
6. Lauretti L et al: Treatment of giant congenital cysts of the midline in adults: report of two cases and review of the literature. Surg Neurol Int. 6(Suppl 13):S371-4, 2015
7. Bender B et al: MR imaging findings in colloid cysts of the sellar region: comparison with colloid cysts of the third ventricle and Rathke's cleft cysts. Acad Radiol. 20(11):1457-65, 2013
8. Osborn AG et al: Intracranial cysts: radiologic-pathologic correlation and imaging approach. Radiology. 239(3):650-64, 2006

Intracranial Cystic-Appearing Lesions

Extraaxial	Intraaxial
Supratentorial	Supratentorial
Midline	Parenchymal
Pineal cyst	Enlarged PVSs
Dermoid cyst	Neuroglial cyst
Rathke cleft cyst	Porencephalic cyst
Arachnoid cyst (suprasellar)	Connatal, germinolytic cysts
	Hippocampal sulcus remnants
Off midline	Intraventricular
Arachnoid cyst (middle cranial fossa, convexity)	Choroid plexus cysts
Epidermoid cyst	Ependymal cyst
TACs (macroadenoma, meningioma)	Colloid cyst
Sebaceous cyst (scalp)	
Leptomeningeal cyst ("growing fracture")	
Infratentorial	Infratentorial
Midline	Parenchymal
Neurenteric cyst	Enlarged PVSs (dentate nuclei)
Arachnoid cyst	
Off midline	Intraventricular
Epidermoid (CPA)	Epidermoid (4th ventricle, cisterna magna)
Arachnoid cyst (CPA)	Cystic ("trapped") 4th ventricle
TACs (schwannoma, meningioma)	

Nonneoplastic, noninfectious cystic brain lesions are classified by common anatomic locations. The 1st division is extra- vs. intraaxial, then supra- vs. infratentorial. Extraaxial cysts are further subdivided into midline and off midline lesions. Intraaxial cysts are subdivided into parenchymal and intraventricular. CPA = cerebellopontine angle; PVSs = perivascular (Virchow-Robin) spaces; TACs = tumor-associated cysts.

Intracranial Cysts by Type, Most Common Location(s)

Cyst Type	Common Location(s)
Arachnoid cyst	Middle cranial fossa, CPA, suprasellar cistern
Choroid fissure cyst	Choroid fissure, between temporal horn and suprasellar cistern
Choroid plexus cyst	Choroid plexus glomus
Colloid cyst	Interventricular foramen/anterosuperior 3rd ventricle
Connatal cyst(s)	Peri- or intraventricular, adjacent to frontal horn, body of lateral ventricle
Dermoid cyst	Suprasellar, frontonasal (anteroinferior interhemispheric fissure)
Enlarged PVSs	Basal ganglia, midbrain, cerebral white matter, dentate nuclei
Epidermoid cyst	CPA
Ependymal cyst	Lateral ventricle (atrium most common)
Germinolytic pseudocyst(s)	Periventricular, subependymal along caudothalamic groove
Hippocampal sulcus remnants	Hippocampus, just medial to lateral ventricle
Leptomeningeal cyst ("growing fracture")	Parietal bone
Neurenteric cyst	Prepontine at pontomedullary junction
Neuroglial cyst	Frontal/temporal subcortical white matter, choroid fissure
Pineal cyst	Pineal gland
Porencephalic cyst	Cerebral hemispheres, adjacent to lateral ventricles
Rathke cleft cyst	Suprasellar, intrasellar
Sebaceous (trichilemmal) cyst	Scalp (dermis or subcutaneous tissues)
Tumor-associated cyst	Between schwannoma, meningioma, macroadenoma, and brain

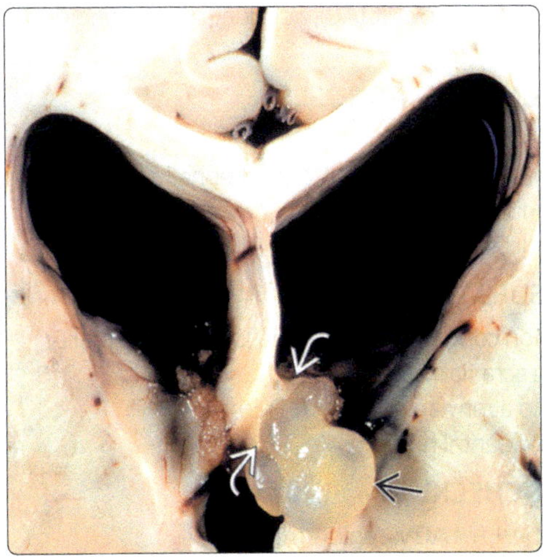

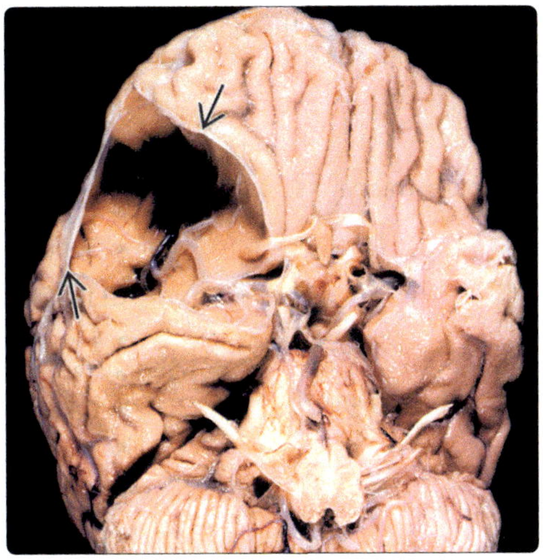

(Left) *Gross pathology shows an autopsied case of a colloid cyst, sectioned in the coronal plane through the foramen of Monro. Note the gelatinous-appearing lobulated cyst ➔ with the fornices ➔ straddling the cyst. This patient died of sudden obstructive hydrocephalus. (Courtesy J. Townsend, MD.)* **(Right)** *Gross pathology of an autopsied brain, seen from below, shows a large arachnoid cyst of the middle cranial fossa. The cyst contained cerebrospinal fluid within split layers of arachnoid ➔. (Courtesy J. Townsend, MD.)*

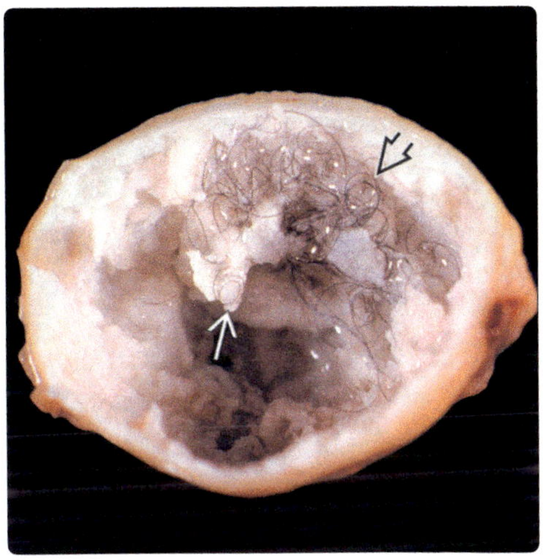

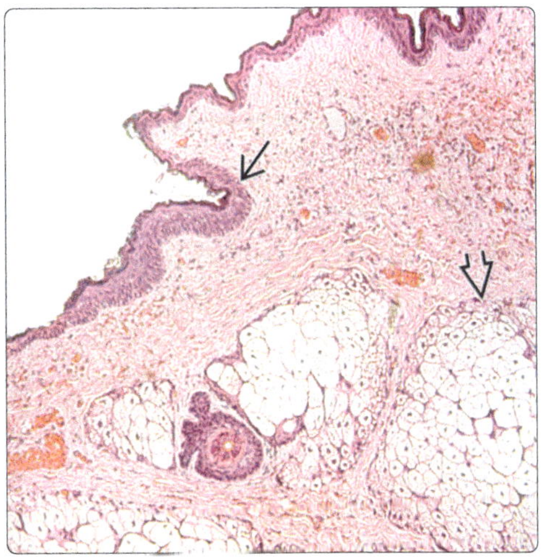

(Left) *Gross surgical specimen of a sectioned dermoid cyst shows the characteristic lining of stratified squamous epithelium plus intracystic keratin debris ➔. Matted, tangled hairs ➔ are present within the cyst, which contained thick, greasy sebaceous material when sectioned. (Courtesy R. Hewlett, MD.)* **(Right)** *Microscopy of a typical dermoid cyst shows squamous epithelium ➔ and sebaceous glands ➔ lining a cavity that contains desquamated keratinaceous debris.*

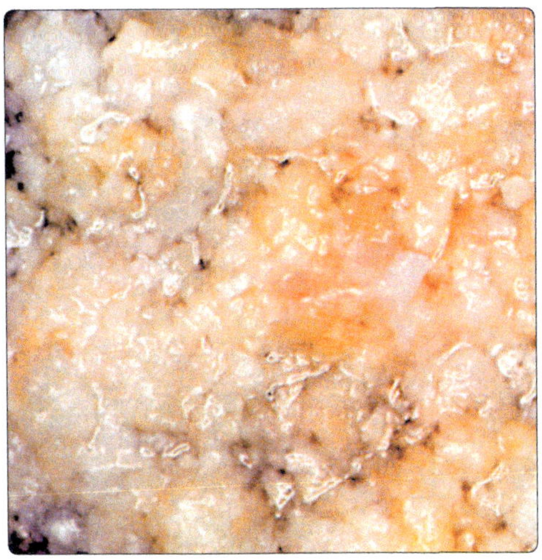

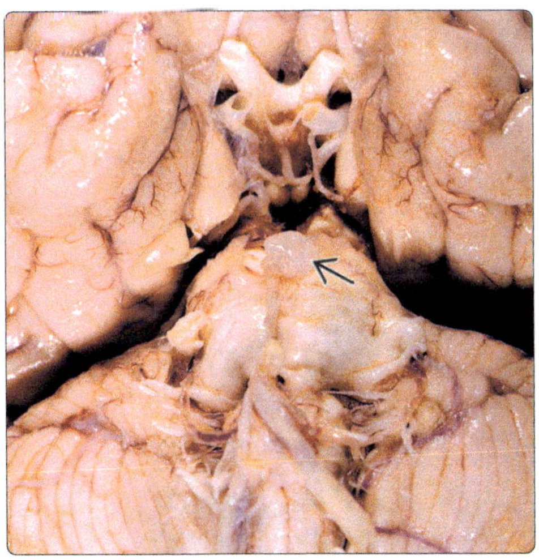

(Left) *Close-up view of an epidermoid cyst shows the cauliflower-like cyst surface that is composed of nodular masses of squamous epithelium and pearly white keratin.* **(Right)** *Autopsy specimen shows a small, gelatinous-appearing nodule ➔ just anterior to the pons. Ecchordosis physaliphora, a notochordal remnant, grossly appears similar to neurenteric cyst. (Courtesy R. Hewlett, MD.)*

Arachnoid Cyst

KEY FACTS

TERMINOLOGY

- Intraarachnoid cerebrospinal fluid (CSF)-filled sac that does not communicate with ventricular system

IMAGING

- General findings
  - Sharply demarcated round/ovoid extraaxial cyst
  - Isodense/isointense with CSF
- Location
  - Middle cranial fossa (50-60%)
  - Cerebellopontine angle (10%)
  - Suprasellar (10%)
  - Miscellaneous (10%) (convexity, quadrigeminal)
- MR
  - Isointense with CSF on all sequences
  - Suppresses completely with FLAIR
  - No restriction on DWI
  - CISS, FIESTA: Use to delineate cyst wall, adjacent structures
  - 2D cine phase contrast: Use to detect communication between arachnoid cyst (AC), adjacent subarachnoid space

TOP DIFFERENTIAL DIAGNOSES

- Epidermoid cyst
- Other nonneoplastic cysts (e.g., porencephalic)
- Chronic subdural hematoma
- Subdural hygroma

CLINICAL ISSUES

- Most common congenital intracranial cystic abnormality
- 1% of all intracranial masses
- Can be found at any age (75% in children)
- Usually an incidental finding

DIAGNOSTIC CHECKLIST

- FLAIR, DWI best for AC vs. epidermoid

(Left) *Graphic depicts the middle cranial fossa arachnoid cyst (AC). Note the arachnoid → splits and encloses CSF. The middle fossa is expanded, and the overlying bone is thinned. Note that the temporal lobe → is displaced posteriorly.* **(Right)** *Submentovertex view shows autopsied brain with incidental finding of middle cranial fossa AC. Note "splitting" of arachnoid → containing a large CSF collection (drained during removal). The temporal lobe is displaced posteriorly →, and the middle fossa is expanded. (Courtesy J. Townsend, MD.)*

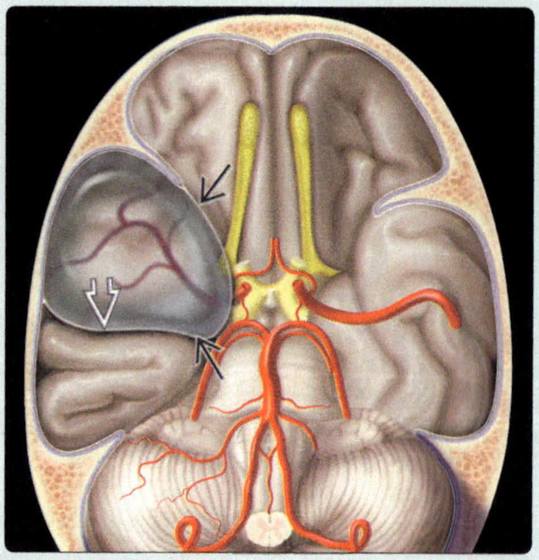

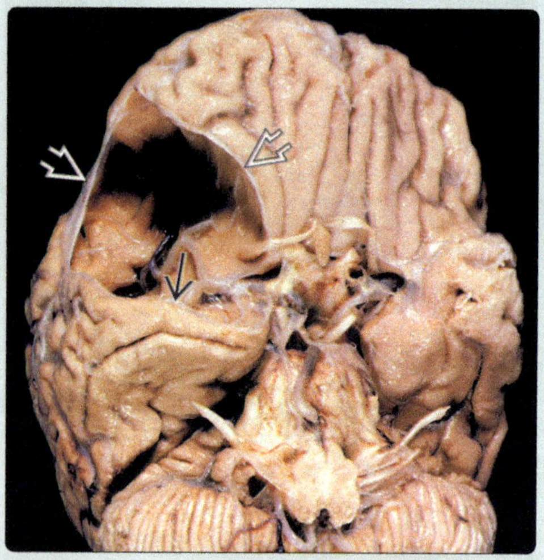

(Left) *Sagittal T1WI MR shows a classic middle fossa arachnoid cyst →. Note the expansion of the greater sphenoid wing → and posteriorly displaced temporal lobe →.* **(Right)** *Composite of axial T2, FLAIR, postcontrast T1WI, and coronal T1 C+ images shows the scalloped margins characteristic of ACs. ACs are CSF-like on T2WI →, suppress completely on FLAIR →, remodel the adjacent calvaria →, and do not enhance.*

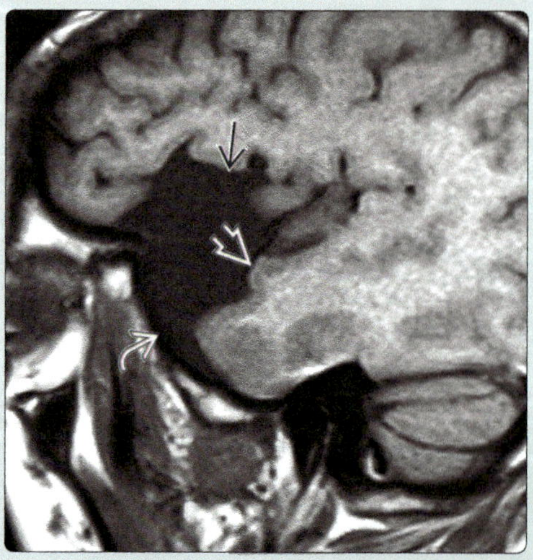

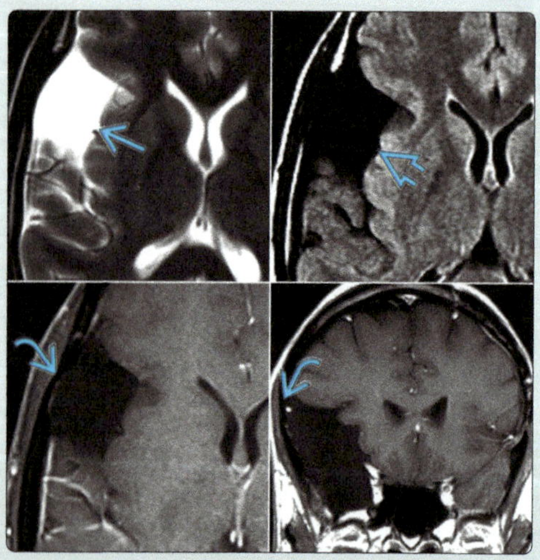

KEY FACTS

TERMINOLOGY

- Unilocular mucin-containing 3rd ventricular cyst

IMAGING

- > 99% are wedged into foramen of Monro
  - Pillars of fornix straddle, drape around cyst
  - Majority are hyperdense on NECT
  - Density correlates inversely with hydration state
- MR signal more variable
  - Generally reflects water content
  - Majority isointense to brain on T2WI (small cysts may be difficult to see)
  - 25% mixed hypo/hyper ("black hole" effect)
  - May show mild rim enhancement (rare)

TOP DIFFERENTIAL DIAGNOSES

- Neurocysticercosis
- Cerebrospinal fluid flow artifact (MR pseudocyst)
- Vertebrobasilar dolichoectasia/aneurysm
- Subependymoma
- Craniopharyngioma

PATHOLOGY

- From embryonic endoderm, not neuroectoderm
- Similar to other foregut-derived cysts (neurenteric, Rathke)

CLINICAL ISSUES

- 40-50% asymptomatic, discovered incidentally
- Headache (50-60%; can be periodic, intermittent)
  - Acute foramen of Monro obstruction may lead to rapid onset hydrocephalus, herniation, death
- Peak age = 3rd to 4th decade (rare in children)
- 90% stable or stop enlarging
- 10% enlarge

DIAGNOSTIC CHECKLIST

- Beware of flow artifact in 3rd ventricle mimicking colloid cyst

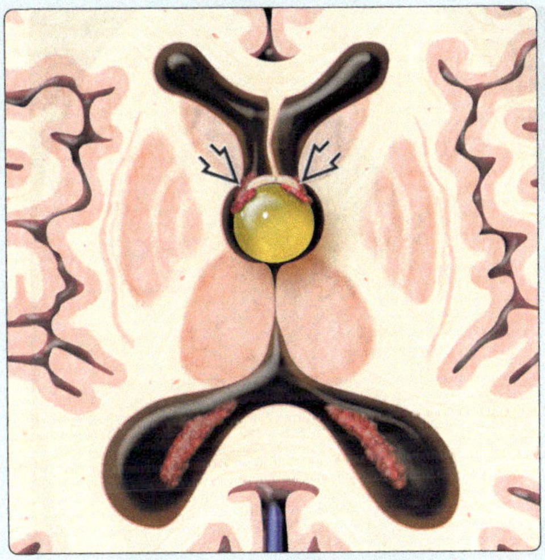
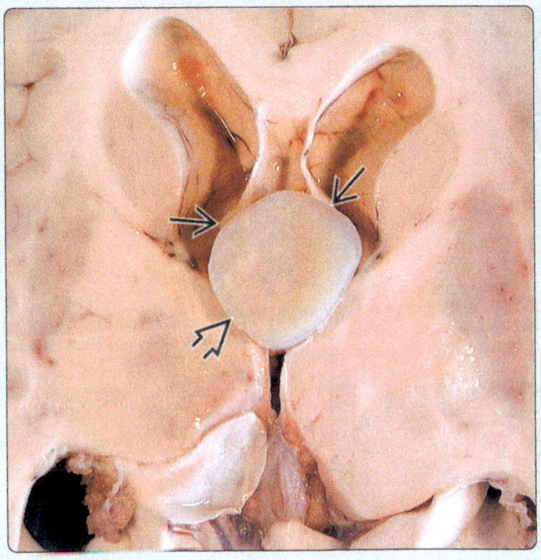

(Left) *Axial graphic shows a classic colloid cyst at the foramen of Monro causing mild/moderate obstructive hydrocephalus. Note that the fornices and choroid plexus are elevated and stretched over the cyst* ⇨. **(Right)** *Axial gross pathology in a patient who suddenly and inexplicably died shows a large colloid cyst* ⇨ *causing moderate obstructive hydrocephalus. A small cavum septi pellucidi is present. Fornices* → *are draped over the cyst. (Courtesy R. Hewlett, MD.)*

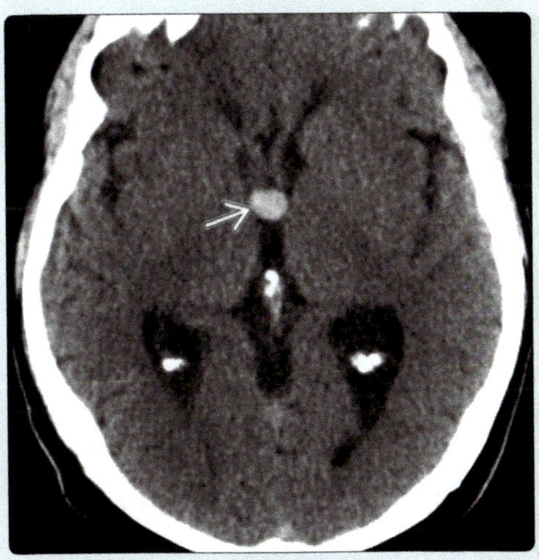
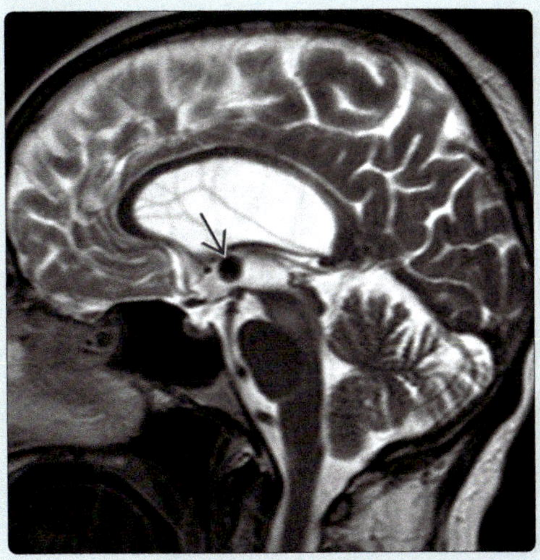

(Left) *Axial NECT in a 65-year-old man with "thunderclap" headache, obtained to look for a subarachnoid hemorrhage, shows a classic colloid cyst, seen here as a hyperdense mass* ➡ *wedged into the foramen of Monro and upper 3rd ventricle.* **(Right)** *Sagittal T2WI MR in the same patient shows the mass* → *to be very hypointense, indicating inspissated proteinaceous contents. Note the markedly enlarged lateral ventricle with a normal-sized 3rd ventricle. The colloid cyst was removed emergently.*

KEY FACTS

TERMINOLOGY

- Benign, ectopic, squamous epithelial cyst containing dermal elements, including hair follicles and sebaceous and sweat glands

IMAGING

- Midline unilocular cystic lesion with fat
  - Subarachnoid fatty droplets if ruptured
- Suprasellar or posterior fossa most common intracranial sites
- Extracranial sites = spine, orbit
  - May have fistulous connections to skin (dermal sinus tract)
- CT hypodensity (fat)
  - 20% capsular Ca++
- MR: T1 hyperintense
  - Fat-suppression sequence confirms lipid elements
  - Fat-fluid level in cyst and in ventricles (if ruptured)
- With rupture: Extensive leptomeningeal enhancement possible from chemical meningitis

TOP DIFFERENTIAL DIAGNOSES

- Epidermoid cyst
- Craniopharyngioma
- Teratoma
- Lipoma

CLINICAL ISSUES

- Rare: < 0.5% of primary intracranial tumors
- Intradural dermoid cysts 4-9x less common than epidermoid cysts
- Rupture can cause significant morbidity/mortality
- Dermoid + dermal sinus may cause meningitis, hydrocephalus
- Treatment: Complete surgical excision ± shunt for hydrocephalus

(Left) *Sagittal graphic of an inferior frontal dermoid ➔ shows a discrete, heterogeneous fat-containing mass with squamous epithelium and dermal appendages. There is a ventricular fat-fluid level ➔ and fat within the subarachnoid spaces ➔ related to the rupture.* **(Right)** *Axial NECT shows a hypodense midline fatty mass with focal calcification ➔ characteristic for ruptured dermoid cyst. Note fatty hypodense droplets in the sylvian fissures and subarachnoid spaces ➔.*

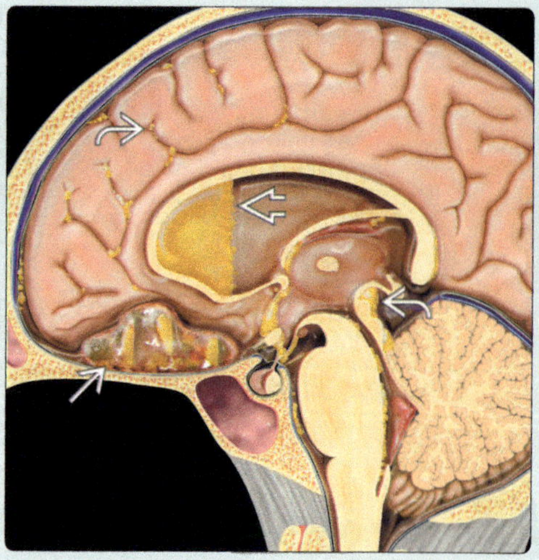

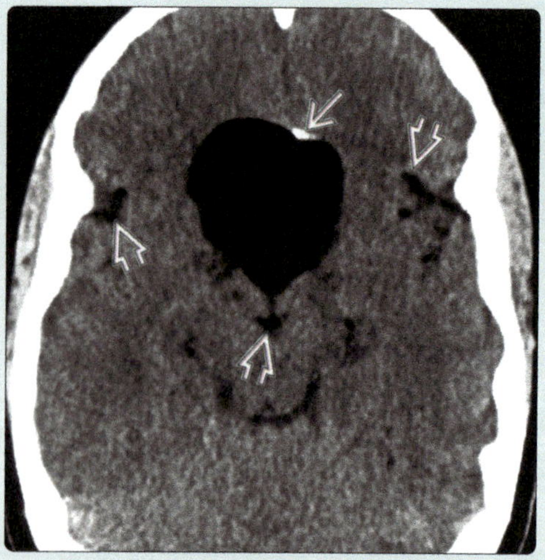

(Left) *T1WI shows classic dermoid cyst is hyperintense ➔. Note fatty droplets in adjacent sylvian fissure ➔ typical for ruptured dermoid.* **(Right)** *Axial FSE T2WI in the same patient shows that the mass ➔ is hyperintense but internally heterogeneous. Ruptured dermoid cyst was confirmed at surgery.*

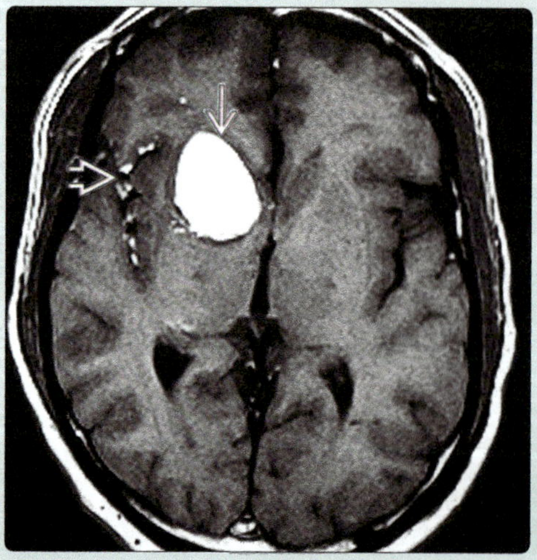

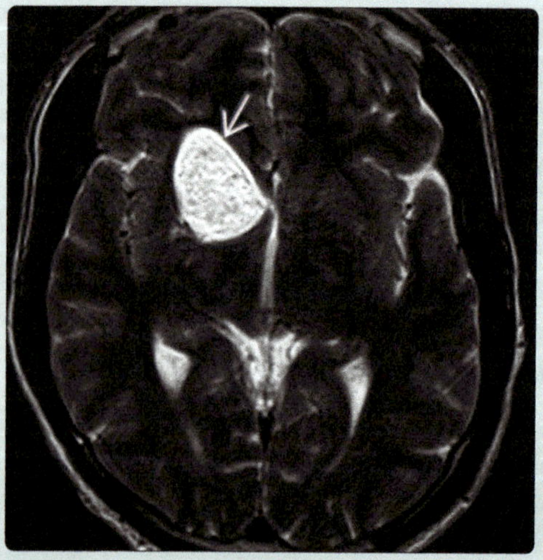

KEY FACTS

TERMINOLOGY

- Intracranial epidermoids: Congenital inclusion cysts

IMAGING

- Cerebrospinal fluid-like mass that insinuates cisterns and encases neurovascular structures
- Morphology: Lobulated, irregular, cauliflower-like mass with "fronds"
- FLAIR: Usually does not suppress completely
- DWI: Diffusion hyperintensity definitively distinguishes from arachnoid cyst

TOP DIFFERENTIAL DIAGNOSES

- Arachnoid cyst
- Inflammatory cyst (i.e., neurocysticercosis)
- Cystic neoplasm
- Dermoid cyst

PATHOLOGY

- Arise from ectodermal inclusions during neural tube closure, 3rd to 5th week embryogenesis

CLINICAL ISSUES

- Symptoms depend on location and effect on adjacent neurovascular structures
    - Most common symptom: Headache
    - Cranial nerve 5, 7, 8 neuropathy common
- 0.2-1.8% of all primary intracranial tumors
- Rare malignant degeneration into squamous cell carcinoma
- Treatment: Microsurgical resection
    - Recurrence common if incompletely removed

DIAGNOSTIC CHECKLIST

- Insinuates and surrounds rather than displaces cranial nerves, vessels
- FLAIR, DWI hyperintense

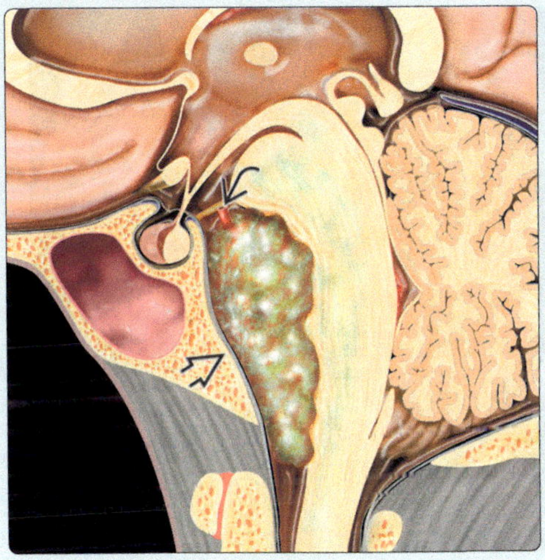

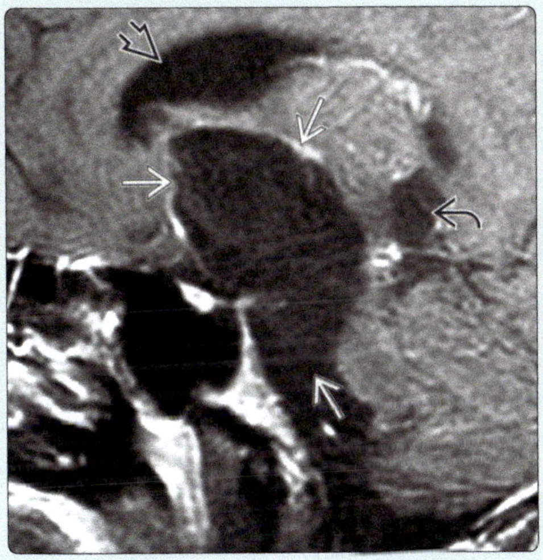

(Left) *Sagittal graphic illustrates a "pearly-appearing" epidermoid ⇨ within the prepontine cistern displacing the pons and medulla. The lobulated mass surrounds and encases the basilar artery ⤺.* **(Right)** *Sagittal T1WI C+ MR shows a nonenhancing epidermoid ➡ arising from the prepontine cistern with extensive mass effect upon the pons, midbrain, and hypothalamus. Its intensity is slightly greater than normal cerebrospinal fluid ⇨, and it has insinuated itself around the pons into the ambient cistern ⤺.*

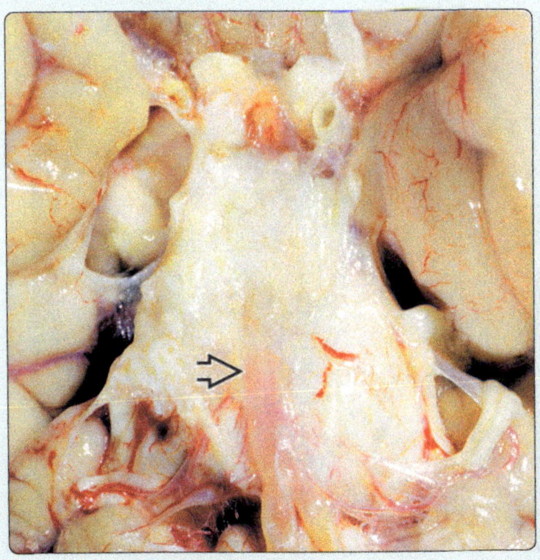

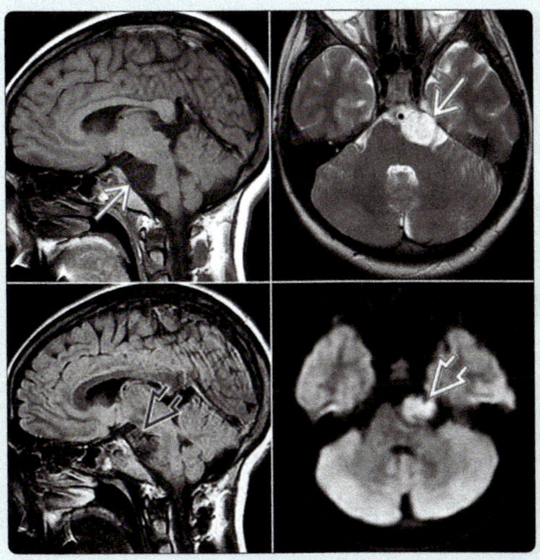

(Left) *Gross pathology shows an epidermoid cyst extending anterosuperiorly from the cerebellopontine angle cistern, insinuating within the prepontine cistern and encasing the basilar artery ⇨. Note its typical pearly appearance. (Courtesy E. Hedley-Whyte, MD.)* **(Right)** *Collage of images illustrates cerebellopontine angle epidermoid cyst that resembles cerebrospinal fluid on T1- and T2WI ➡ but typically does not suppress on FLAIR ⇨ and demonstrates moderate restricted diffusion ➡.*

Hippocampal Sulcus Remnant Cysts

KEY FACTS

TERMINOLOGY

- Synonyms: Hippocampal remnant cyst, hippocampal sulcal cavities
- Cyst or string of cysts along residual cavity of primitive hippocampal sulcus

IMAGING

- String of cysts along lateral margin of hippocampus
- Cysts follow cerebrospinal fluid signal on all MR sequences
  - T2: Hyperintense
  - FLAIR: Complete suppression
  - T1WI C+: No enhancement

TOP DIFFERENTIAL DIAGNOSES

- Mesial temporal sclerosis
- Choroid fissure cyst
- Arachnoid cyst
- Dysembryoplastic neuroepithelial tumor

PATHOLOGY

- Represent partially unfused hippocampal sulcus
- Embryology
  - Primitive hippocampal fissure is formed as cornu ammonis and dentate gyrus fold on each other to form cleft
  - Cornu ammonis and dentate gyrus then fuse, leaving shallow hippocampal sulcus
  - Defects in this fusion cause remnant cysts within primitive sulcus

CLINICAL ISSUES

- Incidental finding, not associated with pathology
- Often observed on high-resolution imaging for evaluation of seizure patients (10-15%)
- Have been noted to enlarge with temporal lobe atrophy in Alzheimer disease

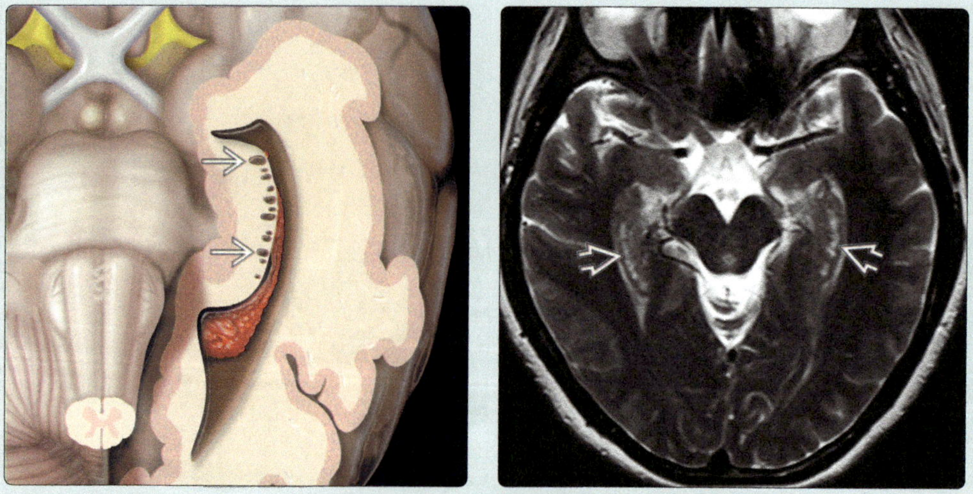

(Left) *Axial graphic of the normal temporal lobe shows a string of cysts within the lateral hippocampus, along the residual cavity of the primitive hippocampal sulcus ➡, representing hippocampal sulcus remnant cysts. These incidental findings have a characteristic appearance.* **(Right)** *Axial T2WI in an asymptomatic patient shows prominent hippocampal sulcus remnants ➡ in both medial temporal lobes.*

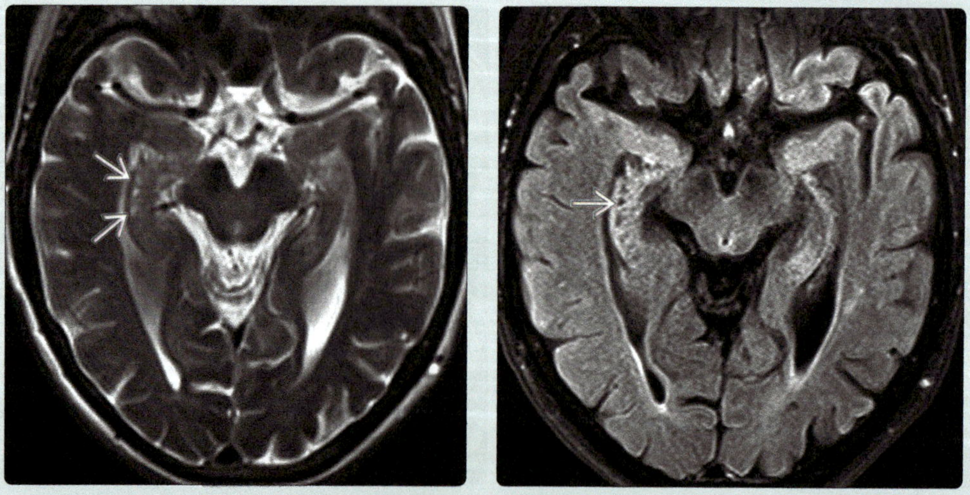

(Left) *Axial T2WI MR shows small hyperintense cysts in the hippocampus ➡. These unfused remnants of the embryonic hippocampal sulcus present as cerebrospinal fluid-like cysts, appearing as a "string of beads" coursing through the hippocampus.* **(Right)** *Axial FLAIR MR in the same patient shows complete suppression of the hippocampal sulcus remnant cysts ➡. The string of beads appearance is typical of these common normal variants. They have been found to enlarge in patients with temporal lobe atrophy.*

Enlarged Perivascular Spaces

KEY FACTS

TERMINOLOGY

- Perivascular spaces (PVSs)
  - Also known as Virchow-Robin spaces
- Pial-lined interstitial fluid-filled structures
  - Accompany penetrating arteries
  - Do not communicate with subarachnoid space

IMAGING

- Clusters of variably sized, well-delineated nonenhancing cysts
- PVSs occur in all locations, at all ages; easily seen in most patients on 3T imaging
- Most common site for normal PVSs = basal ganglia (clustered around anterior commissure)
  - Midbrain, thalami
  - Deep white matter (including corpus callosum, subinsular cortex, extreme capsule)
  - Almost never involve cortex (PVSs expand within subcortical white matter)
- PVSs usually 5 mm or less
  - Occasionally expand, attain large size
  - Most common location for expanded ("giant" or "tumefactive") PVSs = midbrain
  - May cause mass effect, obstructive hydrocephalus
- Isodense/isointense with cerebrospinal fluid

TOP DIFFERENTIAL DIAGNOSES

- Lacunar infarcts
- Cystic neoplasm (e.g., dysembryoplastic neuroepithelial tumor, cystic astrocytoma)
- Infectious/inflammatory cysts

CLINICAL ISSUES

- Should not be mistaken for serious disease
- Usually remain stable in size over years

DIAGNOSTIC CHECKLIST

- Prominent, but normal, PVSs are identified in nearly all patients, in virtually every location at 3T imaging

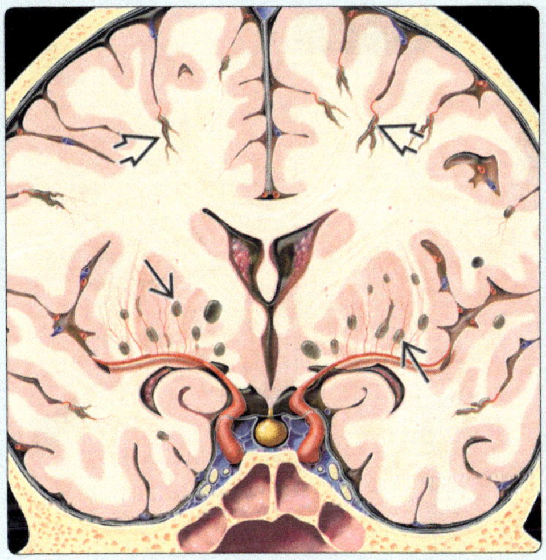

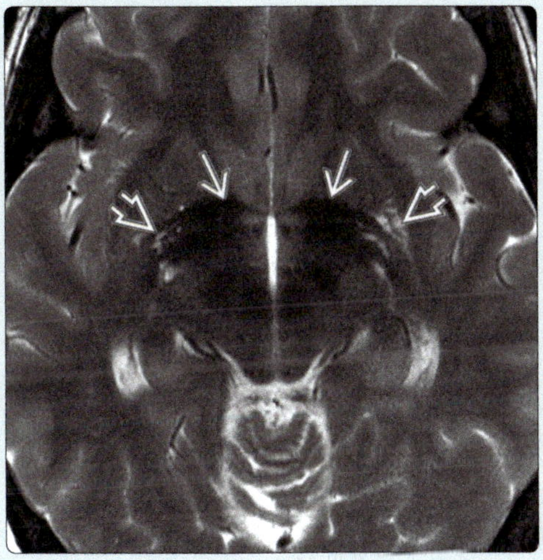

(Left) *Coronal graphic shows normal perivascular spaces as they accompany penetrating arteries into the basal ganglia ➔ and subcortical white matter ➔. Normal perivascular spaces cluster around the anterior commissure but occur in all areas.* **(Right)** *Axial T2WI 3T MR with thin sections shows multiple small perivascular spaces ➡ clustered around the anterior commissure ➡ in the inferior 1/3 of the basal ganglia. These are normal findings.*

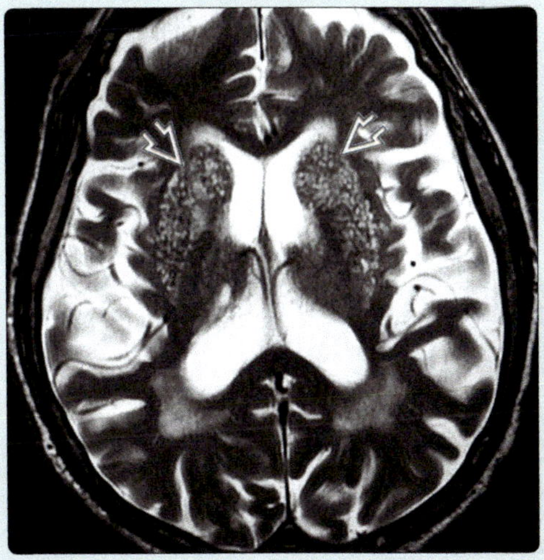

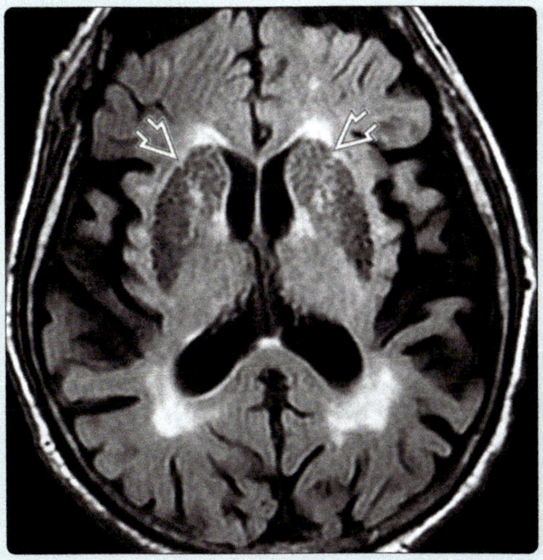

(Left) *Axial T2WI in an 88-year-old woman with mild cognitive decline shows innumerable tiny cerebrospinal fluid-like cysts in both basal ganglia ➡.* **(Right)** *Axial FLAIR in the same patient shows that almost all the basal ganglia cysts ➡ suppress, indicating they are filled with fluid similar to cerebrospinal fluid. The symmetry of the cysts and absence of FLAIR hyperintensity indicate these are enlarged perivascular spaces, sometimes called "état criblé" (cribriform state), and not lacunar infarcts.*

KEY FACTS

TERMINOLOGY

- Nonneoplastic intrapineal glial-lined cyst

IMAGING

- CT
  - Sharply demarcated, smooth cyst behind 3rd ventricle
  - 80% < 10 mm (can be large; reported up to 4.5 cm)
  - Fluid iso-/slightly hyperdense to cerebrospinal fluid (CSF)
  - 25% Ca++ in cyst wall
- MR
  - Slightly hyperintense to CSF (55-60%) on most sequences
  - Isointense (40%)
  - 1-2% hemorrhage (heterogeneous signal intensity)
  - Does not suppress on FLAIR

TOP DIFFERENTIAL DIAGNOSES

- Normal pineal gland
- Pineocytoma
- Epidermoid cyst
- Arachnoid cyst
- Pineal parenchymal tumor of intermediate differentiation

CLINICAL ISSUES

- Vast majority clinically silent, discovered incidentally
  - Occur at all ages
  - Found in 1-5% of normal MRs
  - May spontaneously resolve in children
- Headache (less common)
- "Pineal apoplexy" with intracystic hemorrhage (rare)
  - ± acute hydrocephalus, sudden death (very rare)

DIAGNOSTIC CHECKLIST

- Cannot distinguish benign PC from neoplasm (pineocytoma) on basis of imaging studies alone
  - Both may remain stable for many years
- Heterogeneous, nodular, or ring-like enhancing pineal mass may be benign cyst, not neoplasm

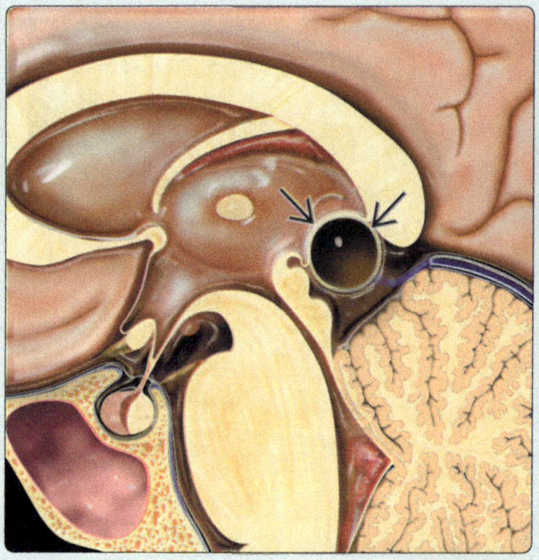

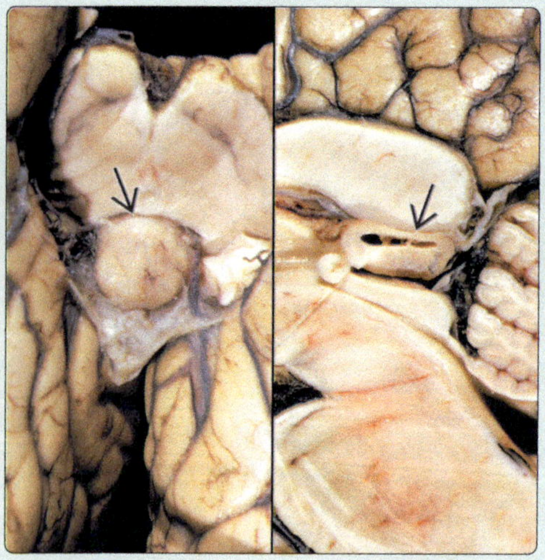

(Left) *Sagittal graphic shows a small cystic lesion within the pineal gland →. Small benign pineal cysts (PCs) are often found incidentally at autopsy or imaging.* **(Right)** *Submentovertex (L) and sagittal midline section (R) show a benign, nonneoplastic pineal gland cyst found incidentally at autopsy. The cyst → is very well delineated and has a moderately thick wall surrounding the cystic cavity. (Courtesy E. Tessa Hedley-Whyte, MD.)*

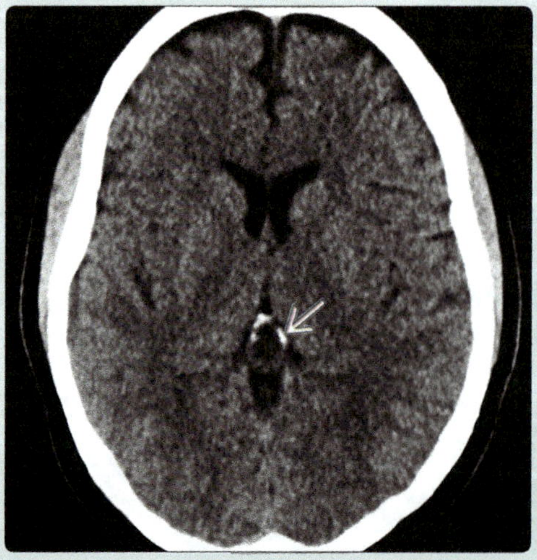

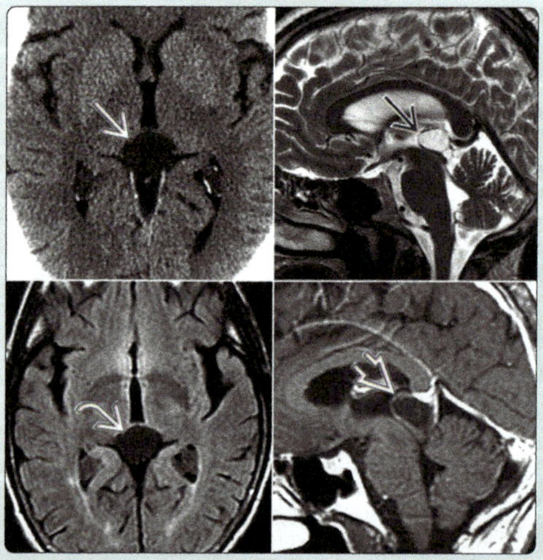

(Left) *Axial NECT scan in a patient with chronic nonspecific headaches and normal neurologic examination shows a 16-mm cystic pineal gland with rim calcifications →. The lesion is stable over several years and is a presumed nonneoplastic PC.* **(Right)** *Collage of images shows a 20-mm PC on NECT → that is slightly hyperdense to cerebrospinal fluid in the adjacent 3rd ventricle. The lesion is hyperintense on T2WI → and FLAIR →. A thin enhancing rim is present on T1C+ →. This is a surgically proven PC.*

Choroid Plexus Cyst

KEY FACTS

TERMINOLOGY

- Choroid plexus cysts (CPCs)
- Nonneoplastic, noninflammatory cysts
  - Contained within choroid plexus; lined by compressed connective tissue

IMAGING

- General
  - Typically in atria of lateral ventricle
  - Usually small (2-8 mm)
  - Rare: Large cysts (> 2 cm)
  - Usually multiple, often bilateral
- CT
  - Isodense or slightly hyperdense to CSF
  - Irregular, peripheral Ca++ common in adults
- MR
  - Isointense or slightly hyperintense compared with CSF on T1WI
  - 2/3 isointense, 1/3 hypointense on FLAIR
  - 60-80% "bright" on DWI
  - Enhancement (ring, nodular, solid) varies from none to strong

TOP DIFFERENTIAL DIAGNOSES

- Ependymal cyst
- Neurocysticercosis
- Epidermoid cyst
- Choroid plexus papilloma (CPP)
  - Purely cystic CPP very rare

CLINICAL ISSUES

- Found at both ends of age spectrum
  - Common in fetus, infants, older adults
  - Less common in children, young adults
- Clinically silent, discovered incidentally
- Associations: Aicardi syndrome, trisomy 18

DIAGNOSTIC CHECKLIST

- Most common choroid plexus mass in adults = CPC

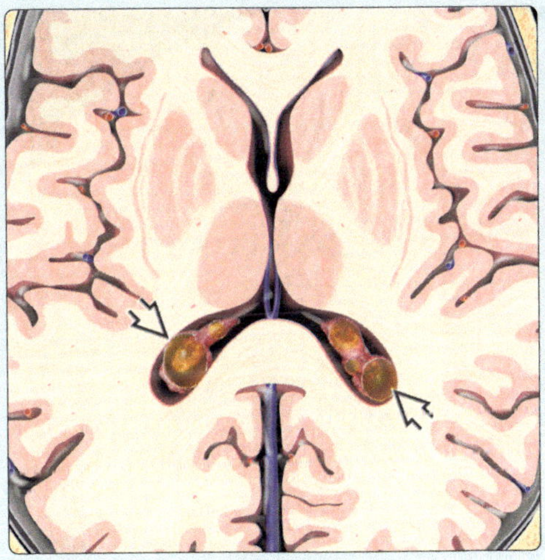

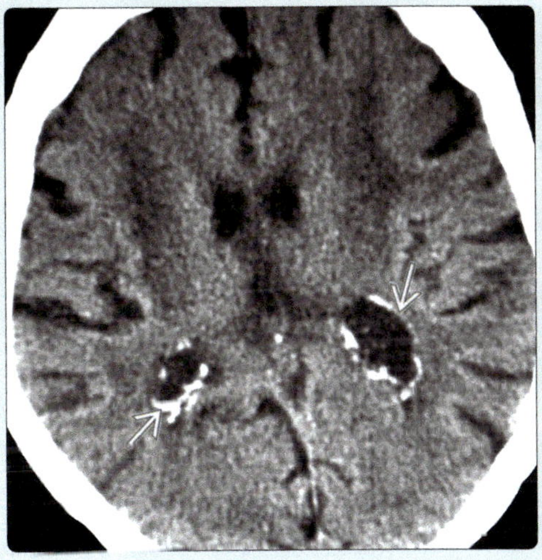

(Left) *Axial graphic shows multiple cystic masses in the choroid plexus glomi ➡, often seen incidentally on scans of middle-aged and older adults. Most are degenerative xanthogranulomas.* **(Right)** *Axial NECT obtained in an elderly adult with minor head trauma and a normal neurological examination shows dense peripheral calcifications ➡ around cystic masses in the atria of both lateral ventricles. This was an incidental finding with no clinical significance.*

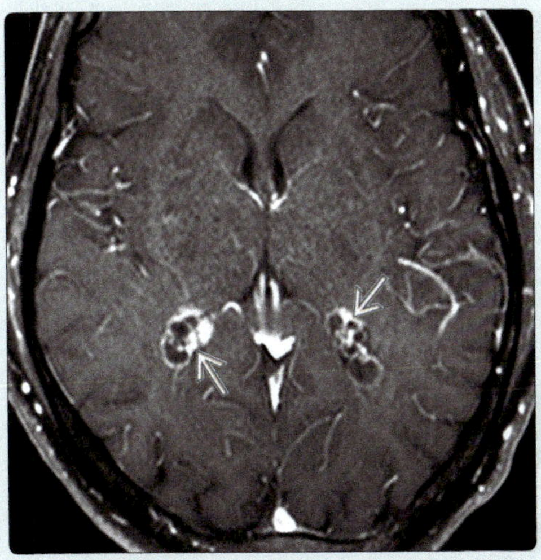

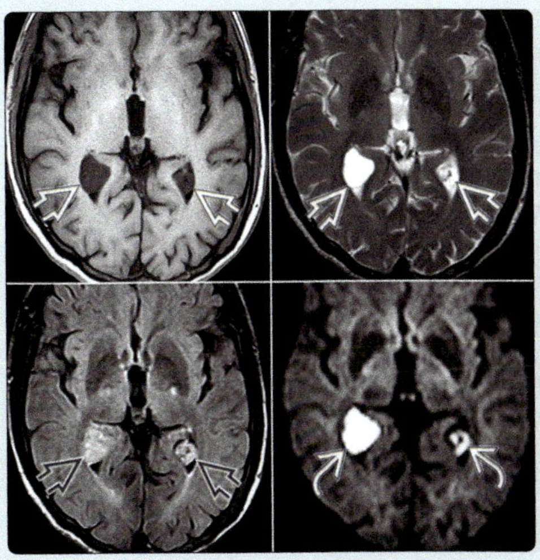

(Left) *Axial T1WI C+ FS MR in a 52-year-old man with headaches and no neurological abnormalities shows multiple mixed solid and ring-enhancing cysts in the atria of both lateral ventricles ➡.* **(Right)** *Series of axial MR scans show incidental finding of bilateral choroid plexus cysts in an older patient. Cysts are slightly hyperintense to cerebrospinal fluid on T1- and T2WIs ➡, typically do not suppress on FLAIR ➡, and frequently appear very bright on DWI ➡.*

Porencephalic Cyst

KEY FACTS

TERMINOLOGY

- Cerebrospinal fluid (CSF)-filled parenchymal cavity
  - Deep, unilateral/bilateral cavity/excavation
  - Usually communicates with ventricle &/or subarachnoid space
  - Lined by reactive gliosis/astrocytic proliferation
- Congenital (perinatal brain destruction) or acquired (trauma, infection, etc)

IMAGING

- Best diagnostic clue: CSF-filled cavities with enlarged adjacent ventricle
- MR: Smooth-walled cavity; CSF isointense; lined by gliotic white matter

TOP DIFFERENTIAL DIAGNOSES

- Consider arachnoid, ependymal, neoplastic, or inflammatory cyst
- Encephalomalacia
- Schizencephaly
- Dandy-Walker malformation
- Agenesis of corpus callosum with doral interhemispheric cyst
- Hydranencephaly

PATHOLOGY

- Congenital: In utero destructive process caused by cerebral vascular events or infectious injury
- Acquired: Injury later in life, following head trauma, surgery, vascular occlusion, or infection
- Genetics: Rare, autosomal dominant familial porencephaly → procollagen defect

CLINICAL ISSUES

- Spastic hemiplegia most common symptom
- Indications for therapy: Mass effect, localized/generalized refractory symptoms

(Left) *Coronal graphic illustrates an intraparenchymal CSF-filled cavity that communicates with the left lateral ventricle and subarachnoid space. Note the classic porencephalic cyst is lined with gliotic white matter.* **(Right)** *Lateral view of autopsied brain with a porencephalic cyst in the temporal lobe shows a CSF-filled cavity that extends from the brain surface to the ventricular ependyma of the temporal horn. The cyst is lined with gliotic white matter. (Courtesy J. Townsend, MD.)*

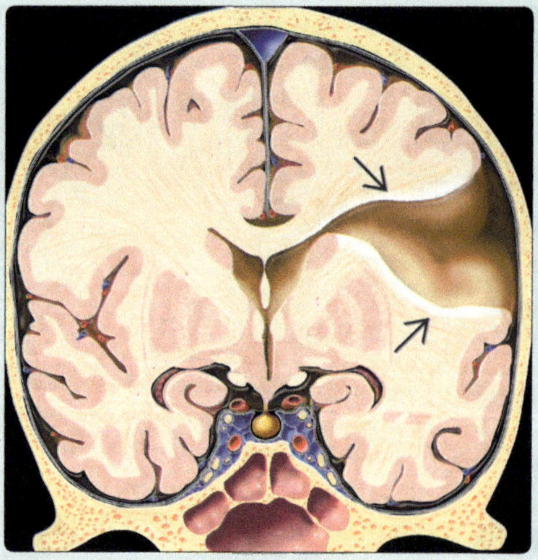

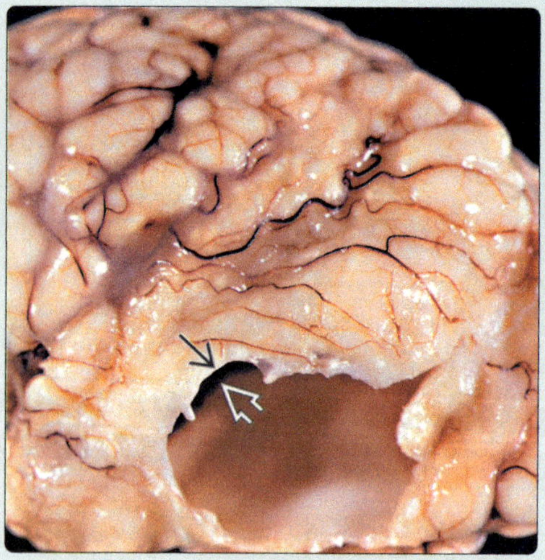

(Left) *Axial FLAIR of a porencephalic cyst shows a CSF intensity parenchymal defect, which was isointense to CSF on all sequences, including suppression on FLAIR. Note the small amount of associated white matter gliosis. Susceptibility artifact is secondary to a ventriculostomy shunt.* **(Right)** *Coronal T1 C+ MR in the same patient shows a CSF-density parenchymal defect, which communicates with the atrium of the left lateral ventricle with dilatation of the occipital horn. Classic porencephalic cyst is also seen.*

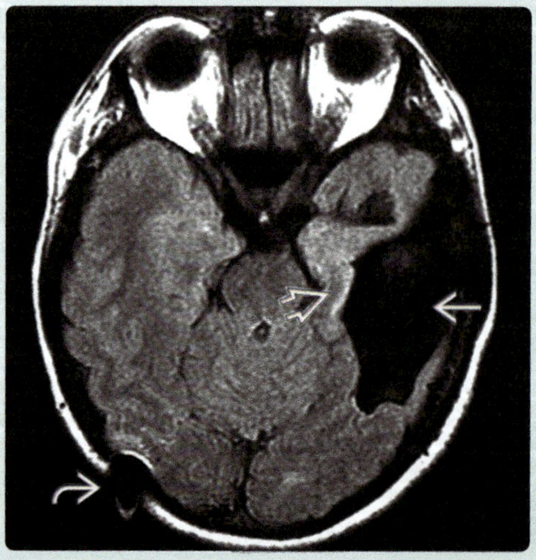

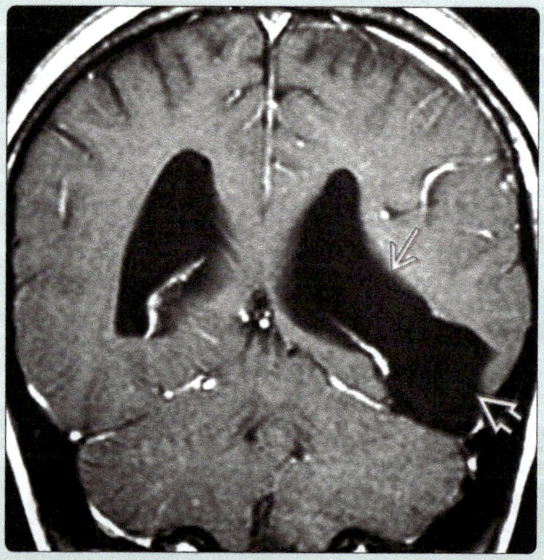

Overview of CNS Infections

General Considerations

Classification: Infectious diseases can be classified into congenital/neonatal and acquired infections. They can be further subdivided by etiology, i.e., bacterial, viral, fungal, parasitic, and rickettsial diseases.

Infectious diseases can have different manifestations depending on disease acuity. Some diseases like herpes encephalitis are typically acute and fulminant. Others are subacute or chronic [e.g., subacute sclerosing panencephalitis (SSPE) and Rasmussen encephalitis].

Congenital/Neonatal Infections

General Considerations

Terminology: Congenital brain infections are often grouped together and simply called TORCH infections (for **to**xoplasmosis, **r**ubella, **c**ytomegalovirus, and **h**erpes). If congenital syphilis is included, the grouping is called TORCH(S) or (S)TORCH.

Other congenital infections include HIV and lymphocytic choriomeningitis (LCM). Approximately 40% of HIV-positive mothers pass on their infection to the fetus, which has shown to be dramatically reduced with HAART treatment of mothers and delivery by cesarean section.

Etiology: Most congenital infections are transmitted to the fetus through the transplacental route, except for herpes, which is acquired during parturition. With 2 exceptions, toxoplasmosis and syphilis, most are viral. All are relatively rare with the possible exceptions of cytomegalovirus (CMV) and herpes encephalitis.

Pathology: Transplacental transmission of various pathogens results in a spectrum of findings depending on both the agent and timing of infection. When infections occur early in fetal development (e.g., the 1st trimester), they tend to result in miscarriage or birth defects. Malformations, such as migrational defects and schizencephaly, are seen in surviving neonates. When infections occur later, encephaloclastic manifestations predominate. Microcephaly with frank brain destruction and widespread encephalomalacia occur. Dystrophic parenchymal calcifications are characteristic of CMV, toxoplasmosis, HIV, and congenital rubella infections.

Acquired Infectious/Inflammatory Diseases

Bacterial Infections

Bacterial pathogens that commonly cause meningitis include *Streptococcus pneumoniae, Neisseria meningitidis, Haemophilus influenzae, Listeria monocytogenes*, Group B *Streptococcus*, and *Escherichia coli.*

Meningitis: Purulent exudates, predominately in the basal cisterns, are the common pathologic feature of meningitis, regardless of the specific infectious agent. Exudates may fill the cisterns and subarachnoid spaces. Pia-subarachnoid enhancement is the most common imaging finding. Complications, such as hydrocephalus, empyema, and vasculitis, with or without cerebral infarction, are common.

Abscess: Abscesses develop in 4 general stages, early and late cerebritis and early and late capsule. In early cerebritis, infection is focal but not yet localized. An unencapsulated mass of inflammatory cells, edema, necrotic foci, and petechial hemorrhage forms. In late cerebritis, the infection coalesces. Central necrosis with a poorly delineated rim of inflammatory cells, granulation tissue, and fibroblasts is seen. The early capsule stage follows late cerebritis. A well-defined collagenous capsule with a liquefied necrotic core forms 2-4 weeks after the initial infection. Eventually, the abscess cavity shrinks and collapses. This "late capsule" stage can last for months, with imaging findings still present long after symptoms resolve.

Ventriculitis: An abscess rim is thinnest on the paraventricular side. If the abscess ruptures into the ventricle, it causes ventriculitis ("pyocephalus") and choroid plexitis. Intraventricular abscess rupture is often fatal.

Viral Infections

Acute viral infections: Herpes simplex encephalitis is the most common nonepidemic viral encephalitis. Over 95% are caused by herpes simplex virus-1 (oral herpes virus). Currently the most common epidemic viral encephalitis is the West Nile virus.

Subacute and chronic viral infections: Many viruses have a slow incubation period and are characterized by symptoms that progress over months or even years. SSPE is an example. Progressive multifocal leukoencephalopathy, caused by JC virus (a ubiquitous polyomavirus), is another.

Miscellaneous Infections

Tuberculosis: With 8-10 million new cases each year and rising prevalence in developing countries, TB is a special public health concern. The emergence of multidrug-resistant TB and extremely drug-resistant TB makes early recognition and urgent treatment of TB even more important. The "deadly intersection" between HIV and TB, with each disease amplifying the lethality of the other, is of special concern.

Parasites: Neurocysticercosis (NCC) has become the most common CNS parasitic infection in the world and the most common worldwide cause of epilepsy. Although most parasites rarely infect the brain, CNS lesions eventually develop in most patients infected with NCC.

Fungal diseases: Fungi are ubiquitous organisms and endemic in many areas of the world. Most, such as *Aspergillus*, infect humans infrequently, usually through inhalation or puncture wounds. When fungal infections occur in immunocompetent patients, lung disease is more common than brain infection.

CNS and disseminated systemic fungal infections typically occur in immunocompromised patients. HIV/AIDS and immunosuppressive drugs are factors that increasingly predispose patients to opportunistic infections.

Rickettsial diseases: Rickettsial diseases, such as Rocky Mountain and Mediterranean spotted fever, usually have associated skin rashes. CNS infection is uncommon. When it occurs, Rickettsiae have a distinct predilection for the perivascular spaces and cause infarct-like lesions in the basal ganglia.

Spirochetes: Spirochetes are a phylum of gram-negative bacteria. Syphilis and Lyme disease, which are caused by *Treponema pallidum* and *Borrelia burgdorferi*, respectively, are the most common encountered diseases in this pathogen group. Lyme disease is the most common vector (tick)-borne disease in the USA. Lyme neuroborreliosis is neurologic involvement secondary to systemic infection by the spirochete *Borrelia burgdorferi.*

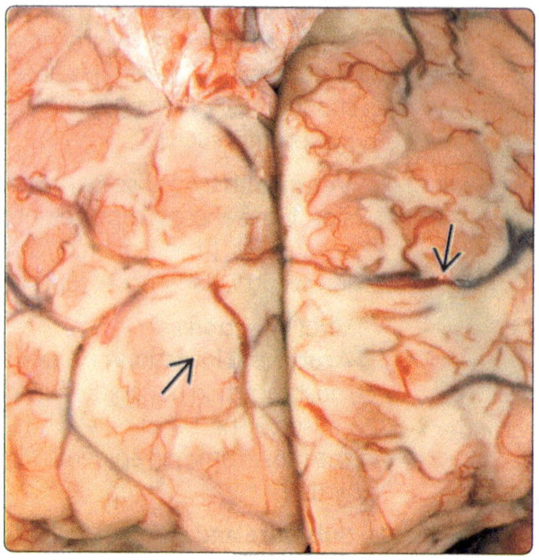

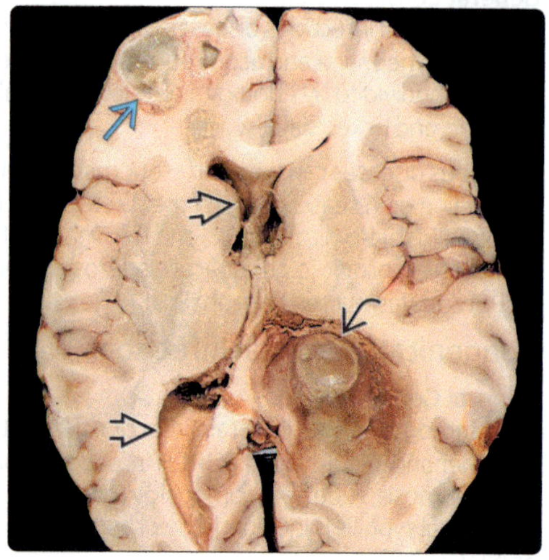

(Left) *Close-up view of the autopsied brain in a patient who died from acute bacterial meningitis. Note thick purulent exudate filling the sulci* ➔*. The underlying gyri are edematous and diffusely swollen. The pia is inflamed and congested, with prominent cortical vessels. (Courtesy R. Hewlett, MD.)* **(Right)** *Autopsy case shows multiple pyogenic abscesses* ➔*. A large abscess in the deep white matter* ➔ *has ruptured into the ventricles, causing ventriculitis* ⇨*. (Courtesy R. Hewlett, MD.)*

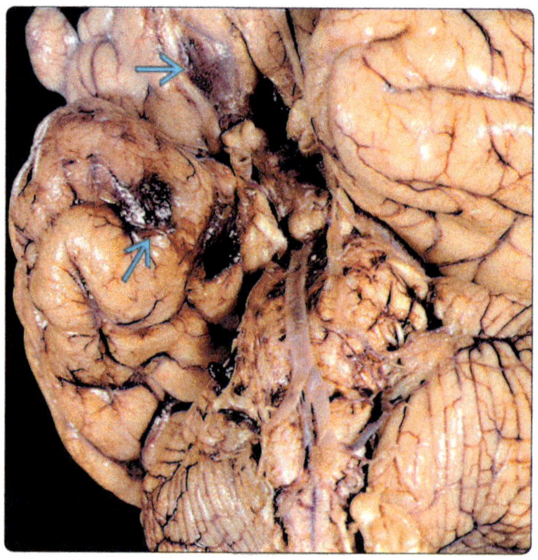

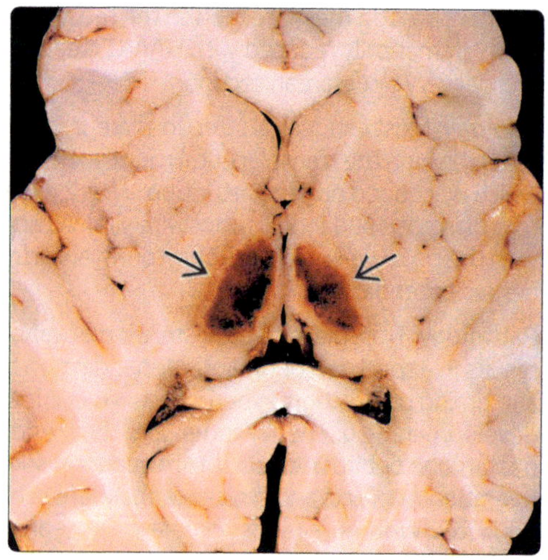

(Left) *Autopsied brain shows classic findings of acute herpes encephalitis. Note the predilection for the limbic system, seen here as hemorrhagic necrosis in the temporal lobe and subfrontal cortex* ➔*. (Courtesy R. Hewlett, MD.)* **(Right)** *Autopsy case of acute hemorrhagic, necrotizing encephalitis, probably viral. Many nonepidemic viral encephalitides have a predilection for the basal ganglia, thalami* ➔*, midbrain, and pons. (Courtesy R. Hewlett, MD.)*

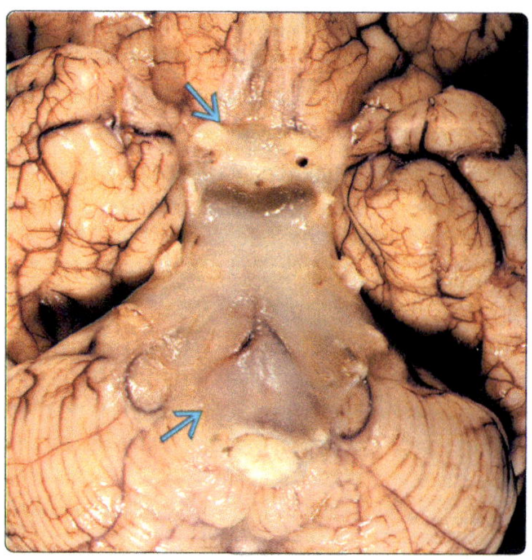

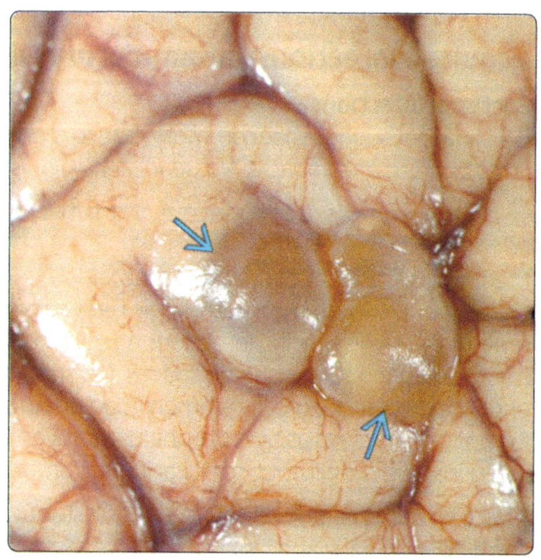

(Left) *Autopsy case demonstrates tuberculous meningitis (TBM). TBM* ➔ *typically causes thick, purulent-appearing exudates with a predilection for the basal cisterns. The imaging and pathologic appearance of meningitis is generally similar, regardless of the etiology. (Courtesy R. Hewlett, MD.)* **(Right)** *Autopsy case shows 2 neurocysticercosis (NCC) cysts* ➔ *lodged within the superficial sulci. The subarachnoid spaces are the most common location for NCC cysts in the brain. (Courtesy R. Hewlett, MD.)*

KEY FACTS

TERMINOLOGY

- Acute or chronic inflammatory infiltration of pia, arachnoid, and cerebrospinal fluid (CSF)
- Classified as acute pyogenic (bacterial), lymphocytic (viral), chronic (tuberculosis or granulomatous)

IMAGING

- Imaging best delineates complications: Empyema, ischemia, hydrocephalus, cerebritis/abscess, ventriculitis
- FLAIR MR: Hyperintense signal in sulci, cisterns
- T1WI C+: Exudate and brain surface (pia) enhance
- Delayed C+ FLAIR most sensitive sequence for leptomeningeal disease
- DWI: Invaluable for detecting complications
- Basilar meningitis typical of pyogenic infections, TB, cryptococcosis, neurosyphilis, sarcoid, lymphoma
- Meningitis is clinical/laboratory diagnosis, not imaging diagnosis
    - Can occur in presence of normal imaging

TOP DIFFERENTIAL DIAGNOSES

- Carcinomatous meningitis
- Neurosarcoidosis
- Increased FLAIR signal in CSF (subarachnoid hemorrhage, high inspired oxygen, artifact, venous congestion from stroke)

PATHOLOGY

- Hematogenous spread from remote infection (i.e., heart, teeth) is most common etiology

CLINICAL ISSUES

- Adults: Headache, fever, nuchal rigidity, ± altered mental status
- Children: Fever, irritability, nuchal rigidity
- Infants: Fever, lethargy, irritability
- Intravenous antibiotics are mainstay of therapy
- Empiric therapy based on age
- Specific therapy based on culture and sensitivity

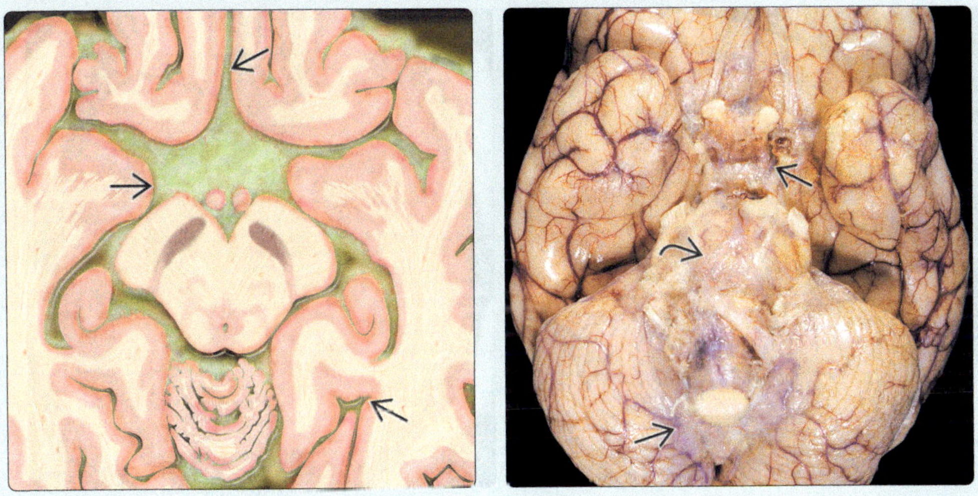

(Left) *Axial graphic shows diffuse inflammatory exudate that involves the leptomeninges and fills the basal cisterns and sulci ➔. This typically results in increased density on CT or T1 signal intensity on MR. It is important to remember that meningitis is a clinical/laboratory diagnosis, not an imaging diagnosis.* **(Right)** *Autopsy case shows changes of severe meningitis with dense purulent exudate covering the pons ↗ and filling the basal cisterns ➔. (Courtesy R. Hewlett, MD.)*

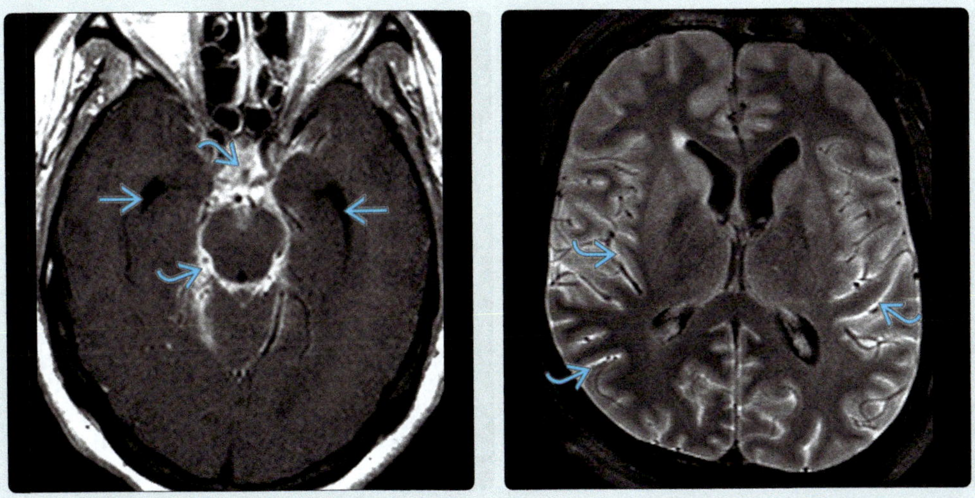

(Left) *Axial T1WI C+ MR in a patient with TB meningitis shows extensive cisternal enhancement ↗, as well as early hydrocephalus ➔.* **(Right)** *Axial FLAIR MR in a 24-year-old man with headache, fever, and vomiting demonstrates extensive high signal in the sulci ↗ due to a pyogenic meningitis. Axial FLAIR, T1 +C and DWI are important sequences in evaluation of a patient with suspected meningitis.*

KEY FACTS

TERMINOLOGY

- Focal pyogenic infection of brain parenchyma, typically bacterial; fungal or parasitic less common
- 4 pathologic stages: Early cerebritis, late cerebritis, early capsule, late capsule

IMAGING

- Ring-enhancing lesion with T2 hypointense rim and central diffusion restriction characteristic
- Imaging varies with stage of abscess development
  - Early cerebritis: Ill-defined T2 hyperintense mass
- Findings with contrast enhancement
  - Early cerebritis: Patchy enhancement
  - Late cerebritis: Intense, irregular rim enhancement
  - Early capsule: Well-defined, thin-walled, enhancing rim
  - Late capsule: Cavity collapses, capsule thickens
- MRS: Central necrotic area may show presence of amino acids (0.9 ppm), lactate (1.3 ppm), acetate (1.9 ppm), succinate (2.4 ppm)
- Multiplanar MR ± contrast, DWI, ± MRS, PWI
- Dual-rim sign on SWI (hypointense outside, hyperintense inside) helpful in from other ring-enhancing lesions

TOP DIFFERENTIAL DIAGNOSES

- Glioblastoma
- Parenchymal metastases
- Demyelinating disease
- Resolving intracerebral hematoma
- Subacute cerebral infarction

CLINICAL ISSUES

- Headache (up to 90%); may have seizures, altered mental status, focal deficits, nausea, vomiting
- Potentially fatal but treatable lesion

DIAGNOSTIC CHECKLIST

- DWI, MRS helpful to distinguish abscess from mimics

(Left) *Axial graphic shows the early capsule formation of an abscess with central liquified necrosis and inflammatory debris. Collagen and reticulin form the well-defined abscess wall* ➡ *are shown. Note the surrounding edema* ➡. **(Right)** *Axial T2WI in a 66-year-old woman with headaches, fever 4 weeks following a dental procedure, shows a mixed signal intensity mass in the left posterior temporal lobe* ➡. *The lesion has a "double rim" (hypointensity on the outside, hyperintensity on inside), commonly seen in pyogenic abscesses.*

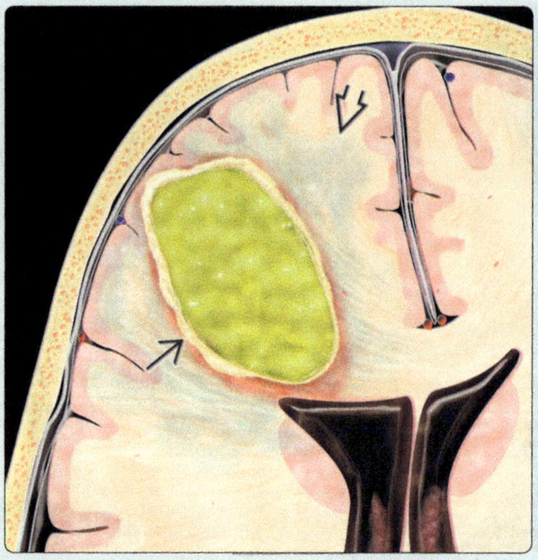

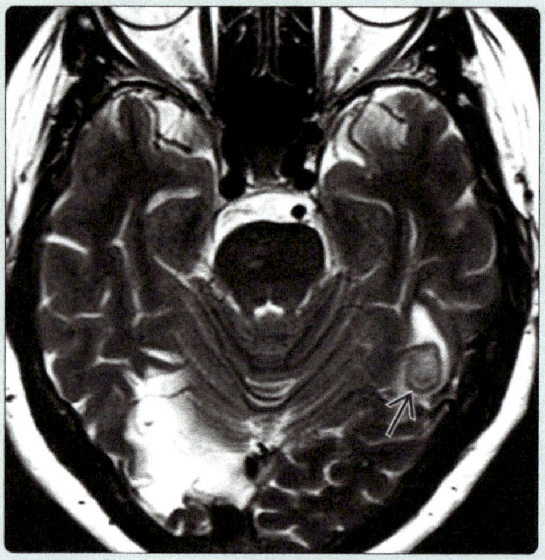

(Left) *T1 C+ FS in the same case shows irregular rim enhancement* ➡ *surrounding a nonenhancing center. Note: The lesion in the right occipital lobe* ➡ *is a remote infarct.* **(Right)** *DWI in the same case shows that the lesion strongly restricts. The imaging findings are very characteristic of a pyogenic abscess. Diffusion restriction in other rim-enhancing lesions such as metastasis, glioblastoma, and multiple sclerosis is uncommon.*

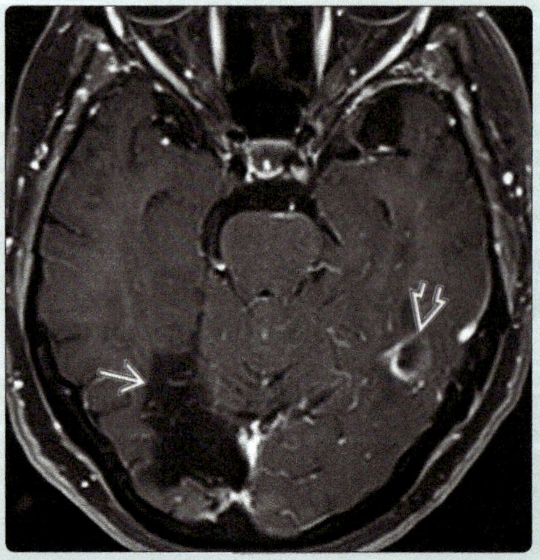

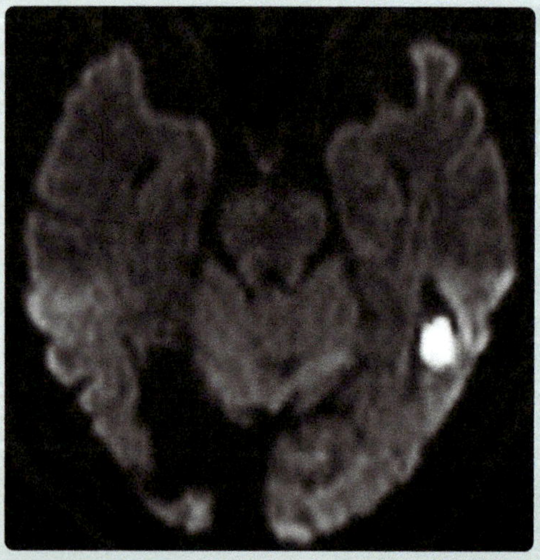

KEY FACTS

TERMINOLOGY

- Ventricular ependyma infection related to meningitis, ruptured brain abscess, or ventricular catheter

IMAGING

- Best imaging clue: Ventriculomegaly with debris level, abnormal ependyma, periventricular T2/FLAIR hyperintensity
- DWI
    - Restriction of layering debris with low ADC is characteristic
- T1WI C+
    - Marked ependymal enhancement with ventriculomegaly
- Ultrasound
    - Ventriculomegaly with echogenic ependyma and debris in infant
        - Can play important role in detection of postinfectious hydrocephalus

TOP DIFFERENTIAL DIAGNOSES

- Primary CNS lymphoma
- Ependymal tumor spread (e.g., glioblastoma multiforme, medulloblastoma, pineal and choroid plexus tumors, ependymoma)
- Intraventricular hemorrhage
- Prominent ependymal veins (e.g., arteriovenous malformation, developmental venous anomaly, cavernoma, Sturge-Weber)

CLINICAL ISSUES

- Bacterial ventriculitis may occur in healthy individuals after trauma or neurosurgical procedure
- Fungal or viral ventriculitis occurs most commonly in immunosuppressed patients
- Ventriculitis occurs in 30% of meningitis patients; up to 80-90% in neonates/infants
- High mortality rate: 40-80%
- Treatment: Surgical irrigation, drainage, &/or IV antibiotics

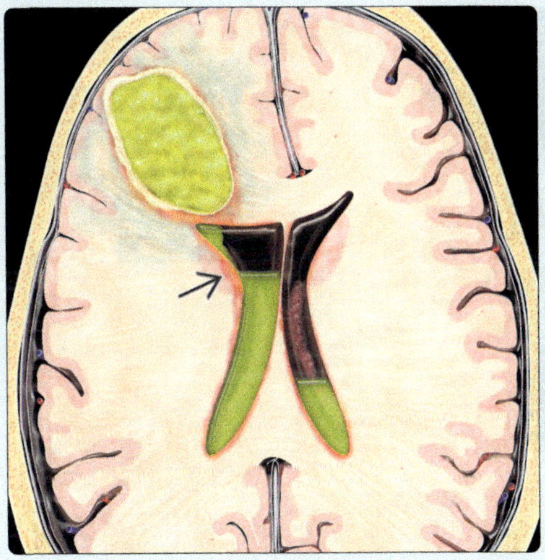

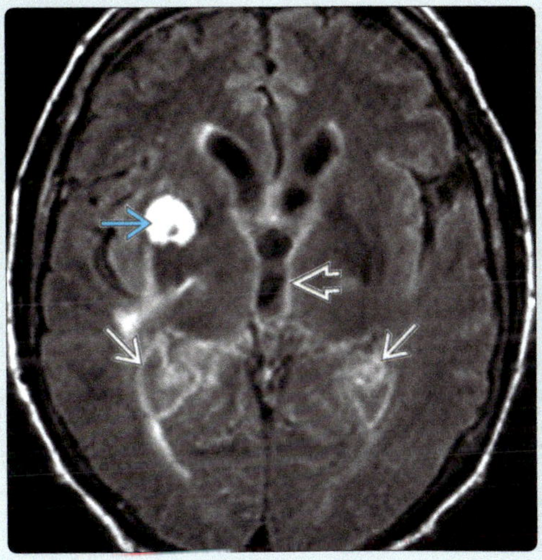

(Left) *Axial graphic shows a right frontal abscess that has ruptured into the ventricular system, resulting in ventriculitis. Note the characteristic debris level within the ventricles and the inflammation along the ventricular margins ➔.* **(Right)** *Axial FLAIR MR shows striking hyperintensity along the ventricular ependyma ➔ with hyperintense debris filling the atria of the lateral ventricles ➔. FLAIR and DWI are the most sensitive sequences to identify ventriculitis. Note the right basal ganglia abscess ➔.*

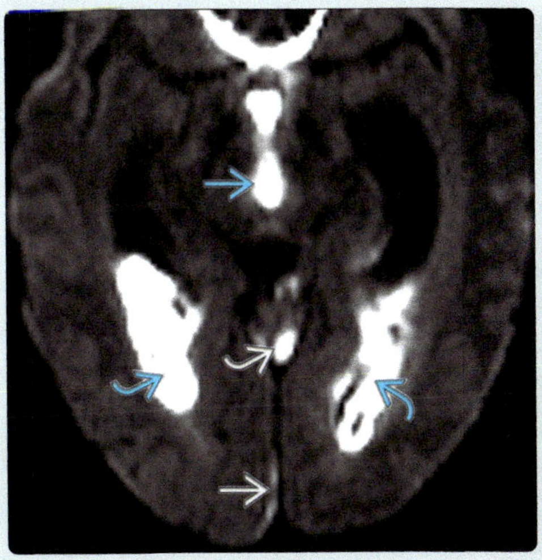

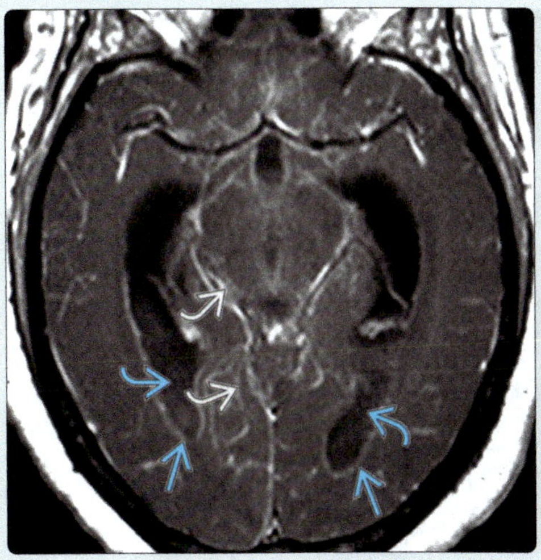

(Left) *Axial DWI MR in a patient with pneumococcal meningitis shows diffusion restriction in 3rd ventricle ➔ and lateral ventricular debris ➔ due to an associated ventriculitis. Exudates are in superior cerebellar cistern ➔ and a small subdural empyema ➔. DWI is invaluable in the diagnosis of ventriculitis.* **(Right)** *Axial T1WI C+ MR in the same patient shows dependent ventricular debris ➔, ependymal ➔ as well as leptomeningeal enhancement ➔.*

Empyema

KEY FACTS

TERMINOLOGY

- Collection of pus in subdural or epidural space, or both (15%); subdural much more common
- Subdural empyema (SDE), epidural empyema (EDE)

IMAGING

- Best diagnostic clue: Extraaxial collection with enhancing rim, DWI positive
- Supratentorial typical
  - EDE: Often adjacent to frontal sinus
  - SDE: Convexity in > 50%, parafalcine in 20%
- Infratentorial (up to 10%); related to mastoiditis
- T2 MR: Inwardly displaced dura seen as hypointense line between fluid and brain
- T1 C+ MR: Prominent enhancement at margin related to granulomatous tissue and inflammation
- MR with DWI best to demonstrate presence, nature, extent, and complications

TOP DIFFERENTIAL DIAGNOSES

- Chronic subdural hematoma
- Subdural effusion, subdural hygroma

PATHOLOGY

- Infants, young children: Complication of bacterial meningitis
- Older children, adults: Related to paranasal sinus disease (> 2/3)

CLINICAL ISSUES

- Sinus or ear infection in > 75% of cases
- EDE, SDE rare, yet highly lethal
- Complications common: Cerebritis, abscess, venous thrombosis, ischemia, hydrocephalus
- Mortality: 10-15%
- Surgical drainage is primary treatment
- Sinus drainage + antibiotics: Small sinus-related EDE

(Left) *Sagittal graphic depicts frontal sinus purulence with direct extension into the epidural space, resulting in an epidural empyema (EDE). Note the displaced dura and inflammation in the adjacent frontal lobe. EDE is often located adjacent to the frontal sinus.* **(Right)** *Sagittal T2WI MR shows an EDE with abnormal signal in the adjacent brain related to cerebritis. Note the inwardly displaced dura, seen as a hypointense line between the EDE and the brain, in this child with sinusitis.*

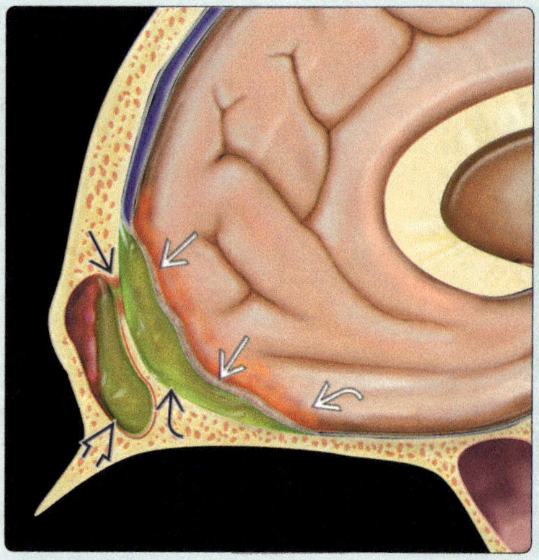

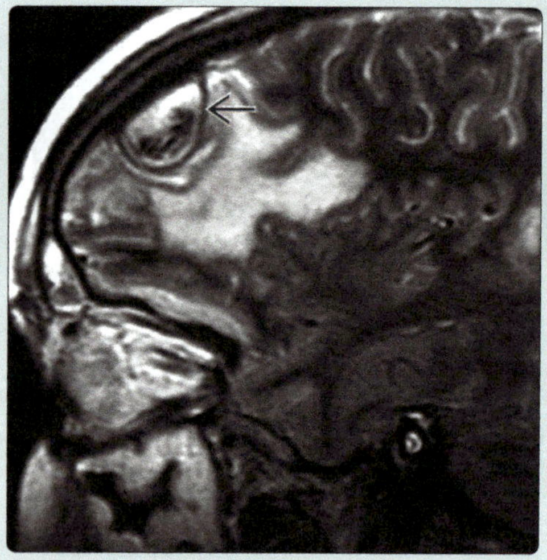

(Left) *Axial T1WI C+ FS MR in a patient presenting with headache and fever shows rim-enhancing parafalcine collections related to subdural empyemas.* **(Right)** *Axial DWI MR in the same patient shows bright diffusion restriction in the parafalcine and left frontal subdural empyemas. DWI is an important sequence to demonstrate the presence, extent, and complications of a subdural or epidural empyema.*

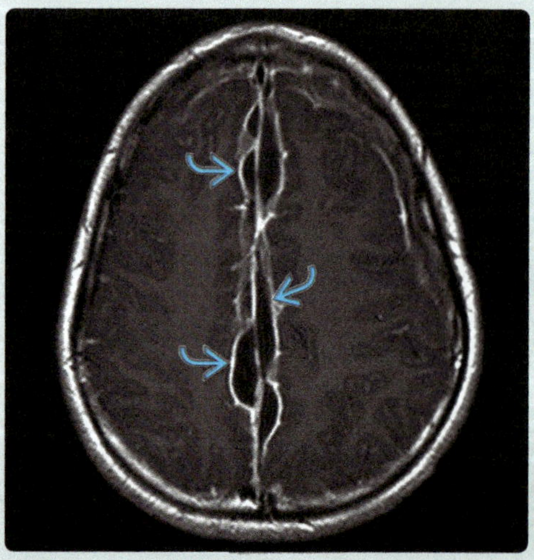

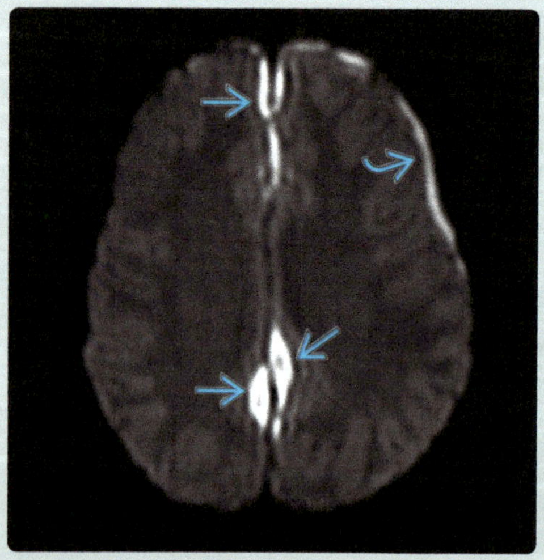

KEY FACTS

TERMINOLOGY

- Brain parenchyma infection caused by herpes simplex virus type 1 (HSV1)
- Typically reactivation in immunocompetent patients

IMAGING

- Best imaging clue: T2/FLAIR hyperintensity of limbic system (medial temporal and inferior frontal cortex) with DWI restriction
  - Typically bilateral disease, but asymmetric
  - Deep gray nuclei usually spared
- CT often normal early
- MR with DWI most sensitive for early diagnosis
- T2/FLAIR: Cortical, subcortical hyperintensity with relative white matter sparing
- GRE: If hemorrhagic, hypointensity "blooms" within edematous brain
- DWI: Restricted diffusion in limbic system
- T1WI C+: May see mild, patchy enhancement early
  - Gyriform enhancement usually seen 1 week after initial symptoms

TOP DIFFERENTIAL DIAGNOSES

- Acute cerebral ischemia-infarction
- Status epilepticus
- Limbic encephalitis
- Infiltrating neoplasm

CLINICAL ISSUES

- Common presentation: Fever, headache, seizures, ± viral prodrome
- Children often present with nonspecific symptoms
- PCR of cerebrospinal fluid most accurate diagnosis
- HSV1 causes 95% of all herpetic encephalitis
- Start IV acyclovir immediately if herpes simplex encephalitis suspected

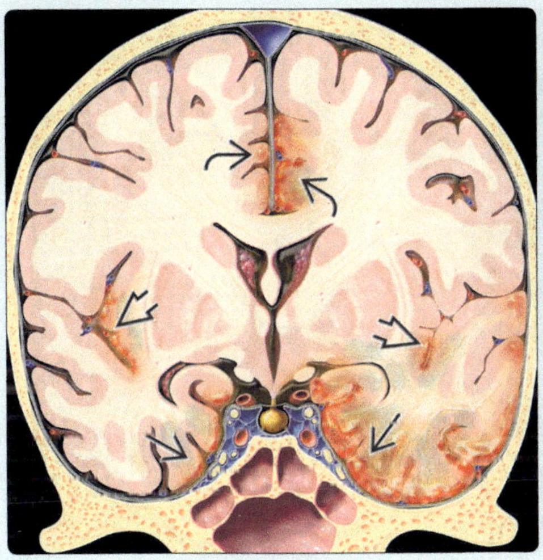

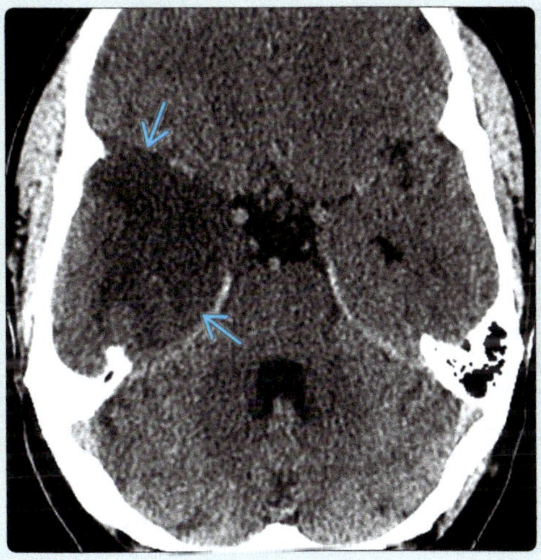

(Left) *Coronal graphic shows the classic features of herpes encephalitis with bilateral but asymmetric involvement of the limbic system. There is inflammation involving the temporal lobes →, cingulate gyri →, and insular cortices →.* **(Right)** *NECT in a 52-year-old man with herpes simplex encephalitis shows hypodensity → and mild mass effect in the right anteromedial temporal lobe. Hemorrhage and contrast enhancement appear 2-3 days later in the disease course.*

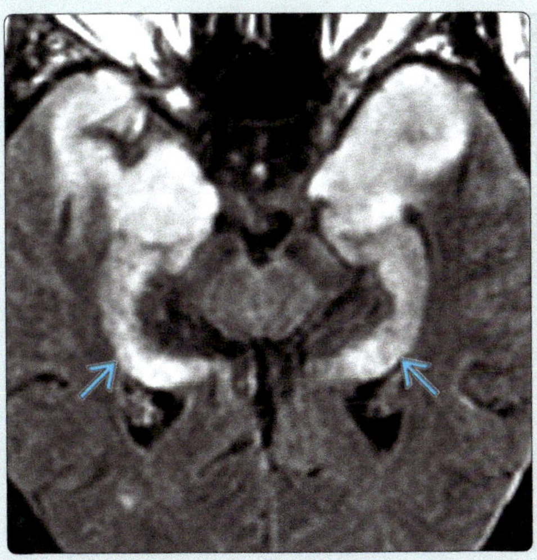

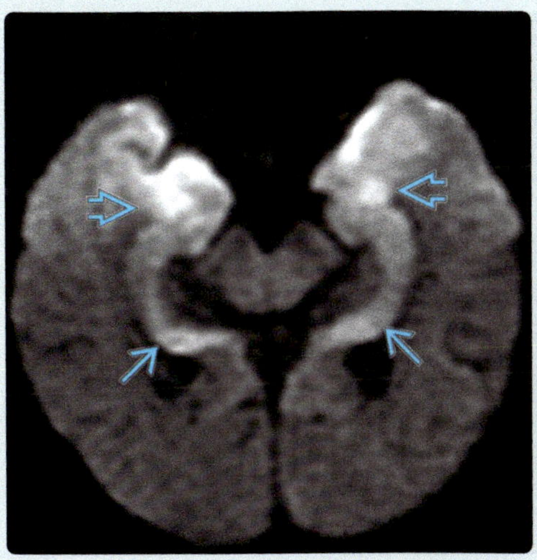

(Left) *Axial FLAIR MR shows classic bilateral but asymmetric abnormal hyperintense signal in the medial temporal lobes of this patient with herpes encephalitis. Note involvement of the hippocampi →.* **(Right)** *Axial DWI MR in the same patient shows diffusion restriction as a bright signal in the medial temporal lobes → and hippocampi →. DWI and FLAIR are the most sensitive sequences for detection of encephalitis. CT is often normal early in the course of herpes encephalitis.*

HHV-6 Encephalitis

KEY FACTS

TERMINOLOGY

- Encephalitis caused by human herpes virus 6 (HHV-6)

IMAGING

- Immunocompromised patient with abnormal signal medial temporal lobe(s)
  - Limbic system: Hippocampus, amygdala, parahippocampal gyrus
  - Insular region, inferior frontal lobe involvement less common than herpes simplex encephalitis
- Atypical pattern in infants/children (basal ganglia, thalami, cerebellum, brainstem)
- Best imaging: MR (coronal T2/FLAIR, DWI, T1 C+)

TOP DIFFERENTIAL DIAGNOSES

- Herpes simplex virus (HSV) encephalitis
  - Early HHV-6 exclusive involvement of mesial temporal lobes
  - Early extrahippocampal involvement common in HSV
- Paraneoplastic limbic encephalitis
- Status epilepticus

PATHOLOGY

- HHV-6: DNA virus belongs to herpes virus family
- 2 variants: HHV-6A and HHV-6B
- Reactivation in immunocompromised patients

CLINICAL ISSUES

- Mental status changes, short-term memory loss, fever, seizure, headache
- Febrile seizures in infants
- Post hemopoietic stem cell transplant, lung/liver transplant
- Antiviral drugs: Ganciclovir and foscarnet
- Mortality of HHV-6 encephalitis > 50%

DIAGNOSTIC CHECKLIST

- Consider HHV-6 encephalitis in immunocompromised patients with CNS symptoms + unilateral/bilateral medial temporal lobe signal changes

(Left) *Axial DWI MR in a 42-year-old patient post stem cell transplant who presented with altered sensorium demonstrates restricted diffusion in the hippocampi bilaterally ➯, more pronounced on the right.* **(Right)** *Axial FLAIR MR in the same patient shows corresponding high signal in the hippocampi bilaterally ➯, again more pronounced on the right. In this patient with immunosuppression, imaging findings are very typical for human herpes virus-6 (HHV-6) encephalitis*

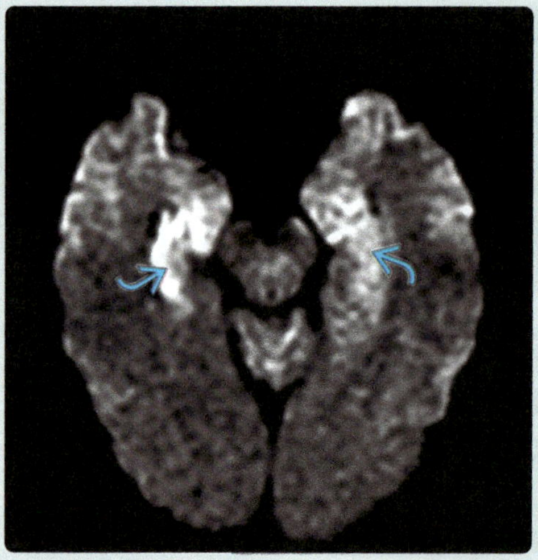

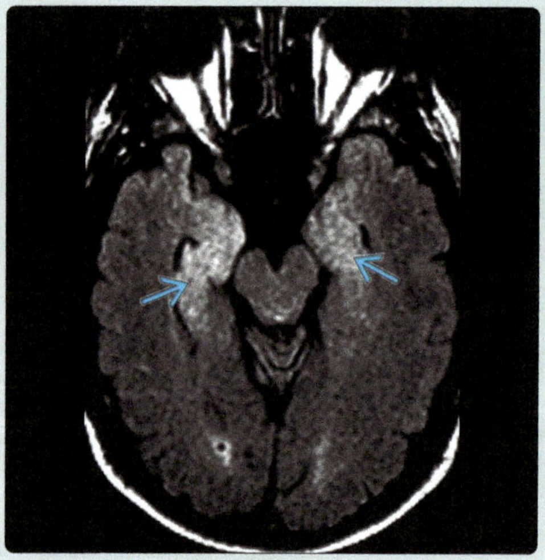

(Left) *Coronal T2WI MR in a 37-year-old man with immunosuppression, fever, and seizures shows hyperintense signal in the medial temporal lobes ➯, basal ganglia ➯, and subinsular white matter ➯.* **(Right)** *Axial T2WI MR in the same patient shows asymmetric hyperintense signal in the subinsular white matter ➯. Extrahippocampal involvement in HHV-6 encephalitis is less common than herpes simplex encephalitis.*

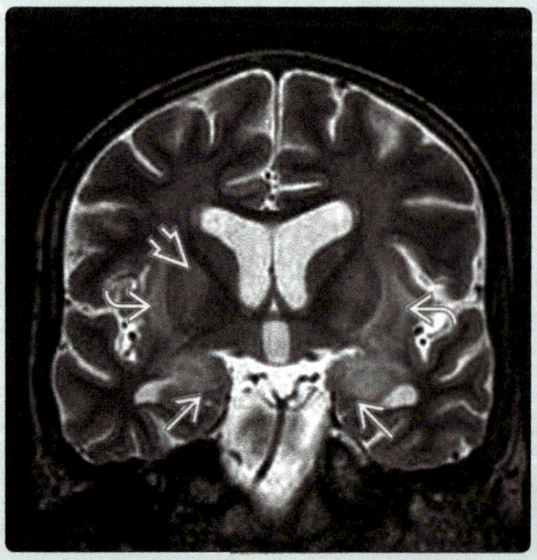

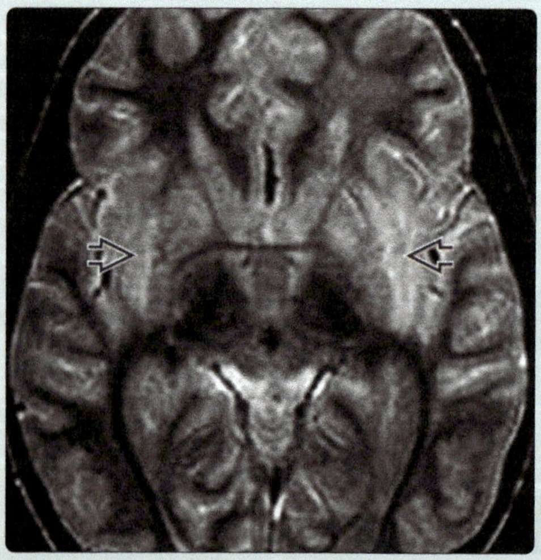

KEY FACTS

TERMINOLOGY

- West Nile virus (WNV), West Nile fever, West Nile neuroinvasive disease
- Mosquito-transmitted acute meningoencephalitis

IMAGING

- Head CT usually normal
- MR with DWI, T1 C+
  - Classic: Bilateral basal ganglia, thalamic hyperintensity
  - Patchy, poorly demarcated hyperintense foci in cerebral white matter on T2WI/FLAIR
  - Enhancement usually absent (has been reported)
  - DWI may show restricted diffusion
- Other sites of involvement
  - Brainstem
  - Corpus callosum splenium
  - Mesial temporal lobes
  - Cerebellum
  - Spinal cord, cauda equina

PATHOLOGY

- WNV: Flavivirus (like Japanese encephalitis)
- Arthropod-transmitted (mosquito)

CLINICAL ISSUES

- ~ 1/140 patients infected with WNV develop CNS symptoms
  - Incubation period: 3-14 days
- ~ 80% of infected individuals asymptomatic
  - Mild febrile syndrome (West Nile fever) in 20%
  - Meningoencephalitis in < 1%
  - Rare: Anterior myelitis
- CNS symptoms more common in diabetics, immunocompromised
- Treatment is supportive; hydration, antipyretics, airway and seizure management as indicated
- No human vaccine
  - Best way to prevent infection? Fight the bite
- Mortality rate is ~ 10%

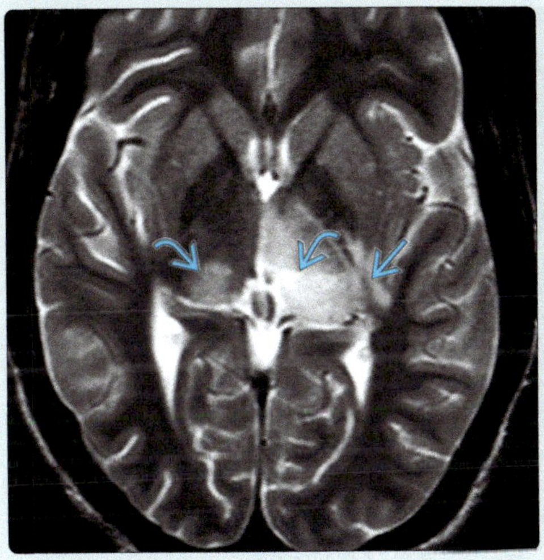

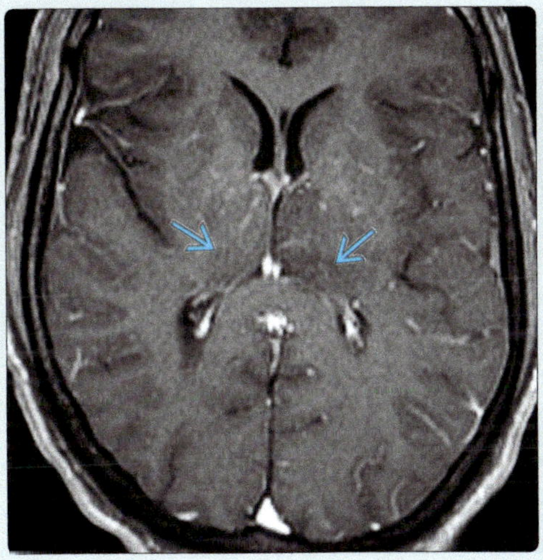

(Left) *Axial T2WI MR in a 24-year-old man with West Nile encephalitis demonstrates asymmetric T2 hyperintensity in the thalami. Posterior limb of left internal capsule is also involved.* **(Right)** *Axial T1 C+ MR in the same patient shows low signal in the thalami, more pronounced on the left with no abnormal enhancement. Anatomic areas commonly affected by West Nile encephalitis are basal ganglia, thalami, brainstem, mesial temporal structures, and cerebellum.*

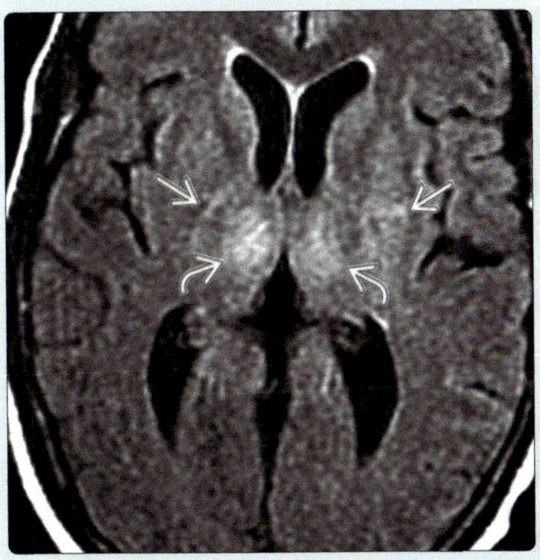

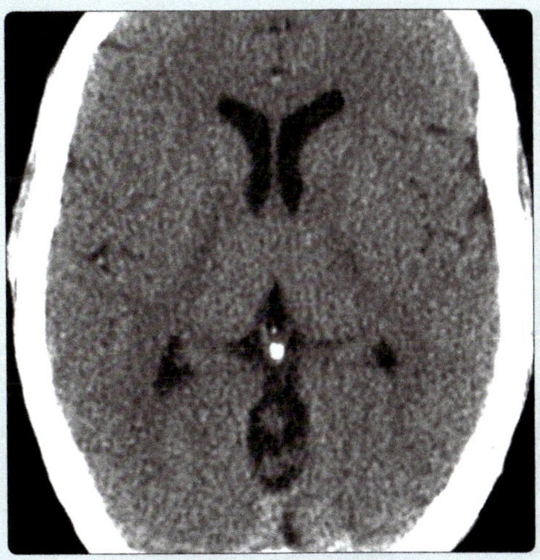

(Left) *Axial FLAIR MR in a patient with West Nile virus meningoencephalitis shows bilaterally symmetric high signal intensity in the thalami. There is subtle hyperintensity in the basal ganglia and right internal capsule.* **(Right)** *Axial NECT in the same patient performed 6 hours prior to the MR exam is normal. No edema is seen in the thalami or white matter. Indeed, early in the disease course, CT scans are frequently unremarkable.*

KEY FACTS

TERMINOLOGY

- Diffuse brain parenchymal inflammation caused by variety of pathogens, most commonly viruses
- Location dependent on etiology

IMAGING

- Abnormal T2 hyperintensity of gray matter ± white matter or deep gray nuclei
- Large, poorly delineated areas of involvement common, ± patchy hemorrhage
- Imaging is often nonspecific, mimics other etiologies

TOP DIFFERENTIAL DIAGNOSES

- Acute ischemia
- Autoimmune encephalitis
- Herpes encephalitis
- Status epilepticus
- Toxic/metabolic lesions

PATHOLOGY

- Most (but not all) are caused by viruses
- Spread of virus to CNS is hematogenous or neural

CLINICAL ISSUES

- Herpes: Most common cause of sporadic (nonepidemic) viral encephalitis
- Japanese encephalitis: Most common endemic encephalitis in Asia
- Many encephalitides have high morbidity, mortality
- Rapid diagnosis and early treatment with antiviral or antibacterial agents can decrease mortality, may improve outcome

DIAGNOSTIC CHECKLIST

- Clinical history often helpful for accurate diagnosis
- DWI may detect lesions earlier than conventional MR

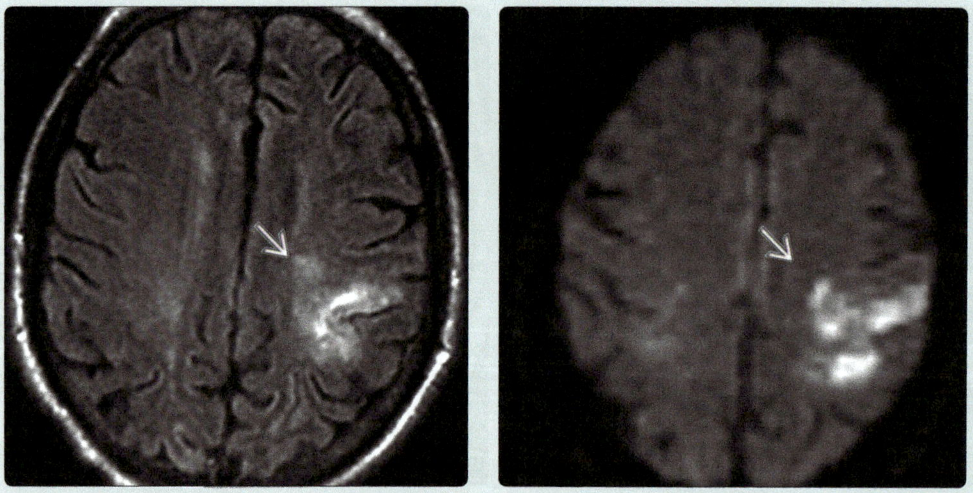

(Left) *Axial FLAIR MR shows hyperintense signal primarily in the left posterior frontal lobe → in an immunosuppressed patient with CMV meningoencephalitis. CMV typically involves the periventricular white matter.* **(Right)** *Axial DWI MR in the same patient shows restricted diffusion in the left posterior frontal lobe → with involvement of the gray and white matter. DWI is often positive in encephalitis and may be the most sensitive MR sequence.*

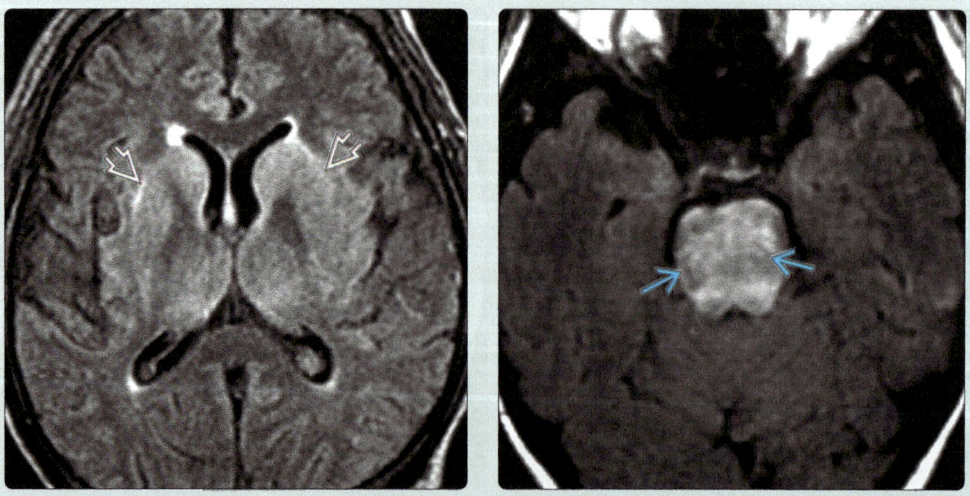

(Left) *Axial FLAIR MR shows symmetric abnormal hyperintensity in the basal ganglia → and thalami in this patient with West Nile virus encephalitis. Symmetric appearance of deep gray nuclei involvement mimics toxic and metabolic etiologies.* **(Right)** *Axial FLAIR MR in a patient with ataxia shows diffuse hyperintensity and enlargement of brainstem →. Rhombencephalitis is often caused by viruses; other pathogens include Listeria monocytogenes, Legionnaire, Mycoplasma, Lyme disease.*

Cerebellitis

KEY FACTS

TERMINOLOGY
- Acute cerebellitis

IMAGING
- Bilateral cerebellar hemispheric gray and white matter low attenuation (NECT), T2/FLAIR hyperintensity (MR); unilateral involvement less common
- Confluent regions of T2 prolongation, affecting gray and white matter
- ± pial or subtle parenchymal enhancement
- DWI/ADC → affected regions typically show increased diffusivity

TOP DIFFERENTIAL DIAGNOSES
- Acute disseminated encephalomyelitis (ADEM)
- Infiltrating cerebellar neoplasm
- Cerebellar infarct

PATHOLOGY
- Reported in association with varicella, Epstein-Barr, enterovirus, rotavirus, human herpesvirus-7, mumps, measles, influenza, and mycoplasma pneumoniae
- In most cases, definite etiology remains unknown
- Moderate to severe cerebellar swelling → vascular compression, upward transtentorial herniation, tonsillar herniation, brainstem compression, obstructive hydrocephalus

CLINICAL ISSUES
- Truncal ataxia, dysmetria, and headache
- Symptoms of ↑ intracranial pressure: Irritability, occipital headache, and vomiting may overshadow manifestations of cerebellar dysfunction
- Most symptoms and signs resolve completely over weeks to months
- Surgery rarely necessary to decompress herniating cerebellum, ventricular drain for hydrocephalus

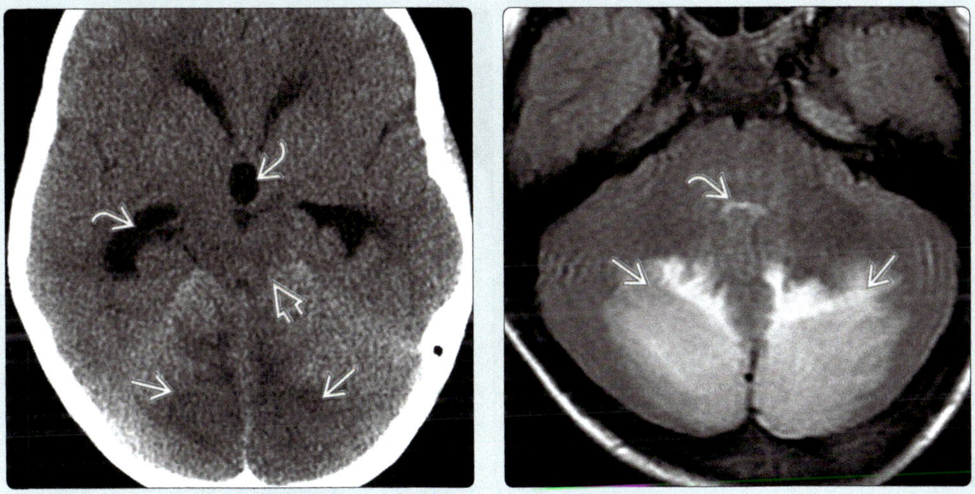

(Left) *Axial NECT in a 4-year-old girl with proven influenza A infection shows cerebellar hemispheric edema (low attenuation) ➡ involving both gray and white matter. The edema causes upward cerebellar herniation and effacement of the quadrigeminal plate cistern ➡. The resultant aqueductal compression causes hydrocephalus ➡.* **(Right)** *Axial T2WI MR demonstrates cerebellar edema (T2 hyperintensity) involving both gray and white matter ➡. Note the compressed 4th ventricle ➡.*

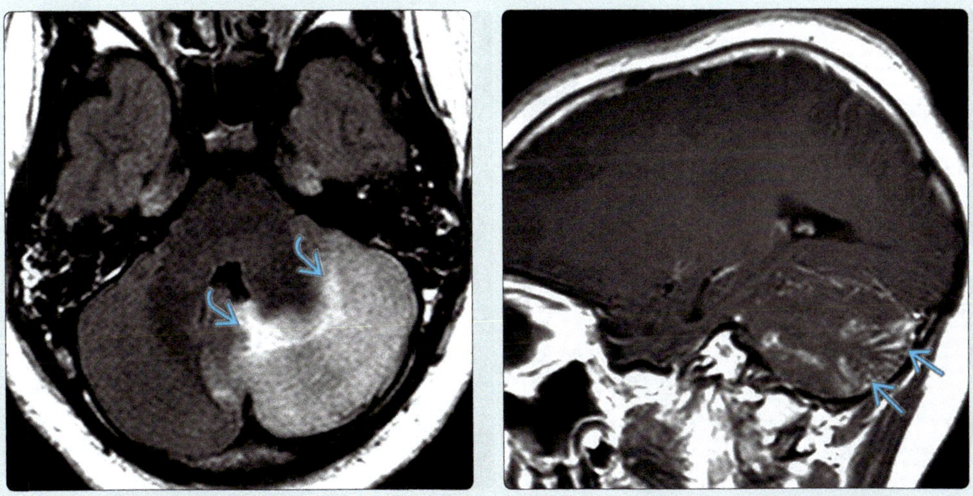

(Left) *Axial FLAIR MR in a 12-year-old patient with acute onset of cerebellar ataxia demonstrates high signal in the left cerebellar hemisphere ➡. Note mild mass effect on the 4th ventricle.* **(Right)** *Sagittal T1 C+ MR in the same patient shows patchy areas of pial enhancement ➡ along the left cerebellar hemisphere. In acute cerebellitis, unilateral involvement is far less common than bilateral.*

Tuberculosis

KEY FACTS

TERMINOLOGY

- Typically causes tuberculous meningitis &/or localized CNS infection, tuberculoma

IMAGING

- Basilar meningitis + extracerebral TB (pulmonary)
- Meningitis + parenchymal lesions highly suggestive
- Tuberculomas
  - Supratentorial parenchyma most common
  - Usually T2 hypointense
  - Enhances strongly (solid or ring enhancing)
- Tuberculous abscess: Multiloculated ring enhancement
- MR with FLAIR, DWI, T1 C+, ± MRA, MRS
- TB abscess has prominent lipid, lactate but no amino acid resonances

TOP DIFFERENTIAL DIAGNOSES

- Meningitis (pyogenic)
- Neurosarcoidosis
- Abscess
- Carcinomatous meningitis (pial, cerebrospinal fluid spread)
- Cryptococcosis (gelatinous pseudocysts in basal ganglia)

PATHOLOGY

- CNS TB almost always secondary (often pulmonary source)
- Meningitis = most frequent manifestation of CNS TB
  - More common in children

CLINICAL ISSUES

- Varies from mild meningitis with no neurologic deficit to coma
- Long-term morbidity in up to 80%: Mental retardation, paralysis, seizures, rigidity, or speech or visual deficits
- Mortality in 25-30% of patients; higher in AIDS patients
- Reemerging disease (immigration from endemic areas, AIDS, drug-resistant strains)

DIAGNOSTIC CHECKLIST

- TB often mimics other diseases, such as neoplasm

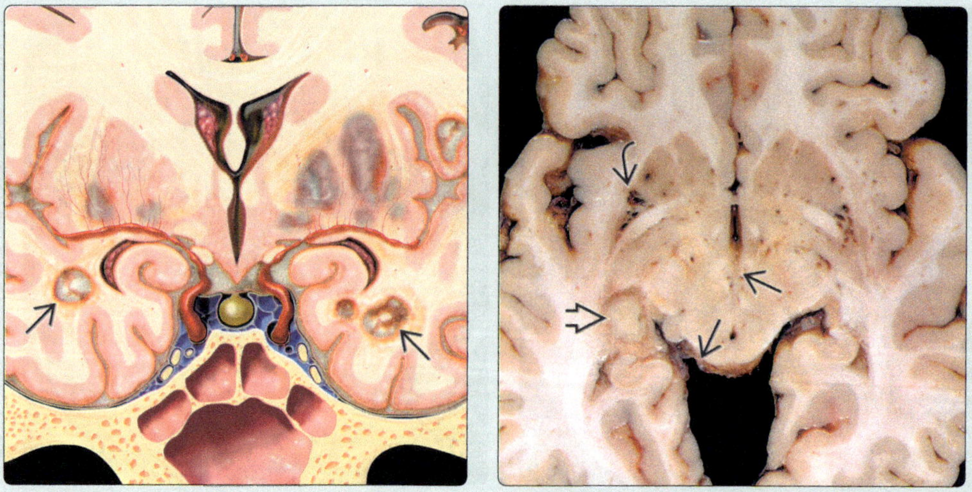

(Left) *Coronal graphic shows basilar TB meningitis and tuberculomas →, which often coexist. Note the vessel irregularity and early basal ganglia ischemia related to arteritis.* **(Right)** *Axial gross pathology section shows numerous features of CNS TB. Exudates with meningitis in the basilar cisterns →, tuberculoma →, and vasculitic changes → are all present in this autopsy specimen. (Courtesy R. Hewlett, MD.)*

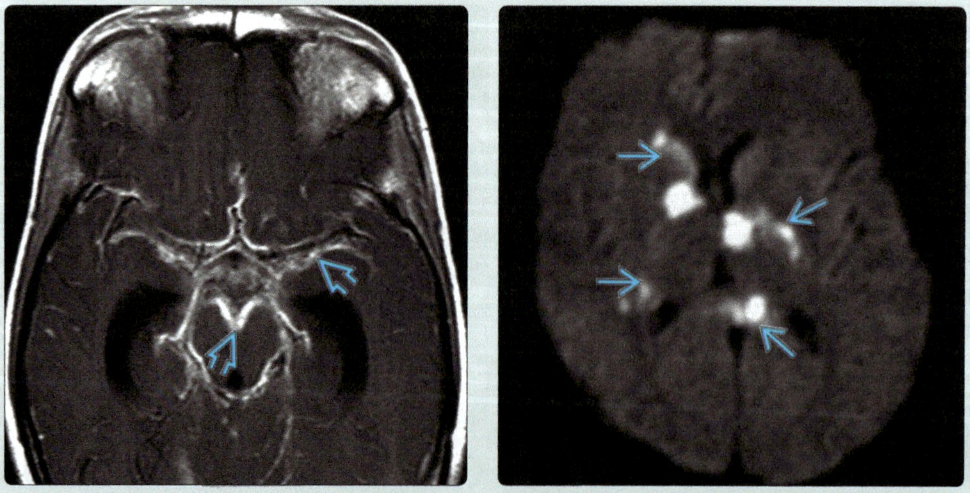

(Left) *Axial T1WI C+ MR in a child with documented TB meningitis shows thick, linear enhancement along the midbrain and temporal lobes →. Note the enlarged lateral ventricles and cerebral aqueduct.* **(Right)** *Axial DWI MR in a patient with TB meningitis shows multiple acute infarcts → in the basal ganglia, thalami, internal capsules, and splenium of the corpus callosum. Vasculitis is a common complication of TB meningitis involving small- and medium-sized vessels and causing cerebral infarction.*

KEY FACTS

TERMINOLOGY

- Intracranial parasitic infection caused by pork tapeworm *Taenia solium*
  - 4 pathologic stages: Vesicular, colloidal vesicular, granular nodular, and nodular calcified

IMAGING

- Best diagnostic clue: Cyst with "dot" inside
- Convexity subarachnoid spaces most common location
  - Inflammatory response around cyst may seal sulcus, making lesions appear intraaxial
- May involve cisterns > parenchyma > ventricles
- Intraventricular cysts are often isolated
- Basal cistern cysts may be racemose (grape-like)
- Imaging varies with development stage and host response
- Lesions may be at different stages in same patient
- FLAIR and T1 MR helpful to identify scolex and intraventricular lesions
- GRE/SWI helpful in young adults presenting with seizures

TOP DIFFERENTIAL DIAGNOSES

- Abscess
- Tuberculosis
- Neoplasm
- Arachnoid cyst
- Enlarged perivascular spaces

CLINICAL ISSUES

- Seizure, headaches, hydrocephalus common
  - Neurocysticercosis asymptomatic until larvae degenerate
- Cysticercosis is most common parasitic infection worldwide
  - CNS involved in 60-90% of cysticercosis cases
- Most common cause of epilepsy in endemic areas
- Increased travel, immigration have spread disease
- Diagnosis confirmed by ELISA of serum or CSF
- Oral albendazole (reduces parasitic burden, seizures)
- Steroids often required to decrease edema
- Consider excision or drainage of parenchymal lesions

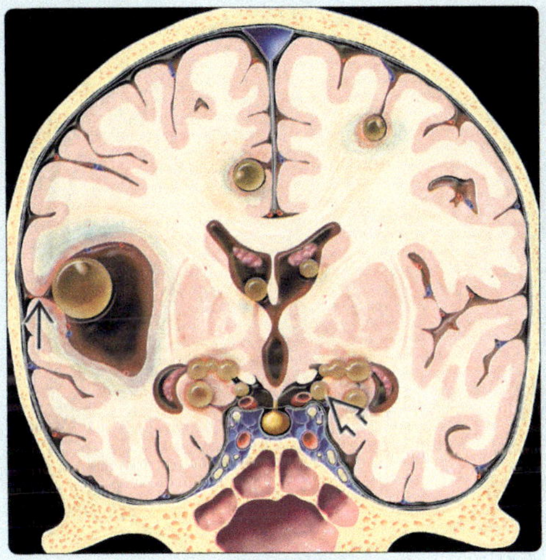

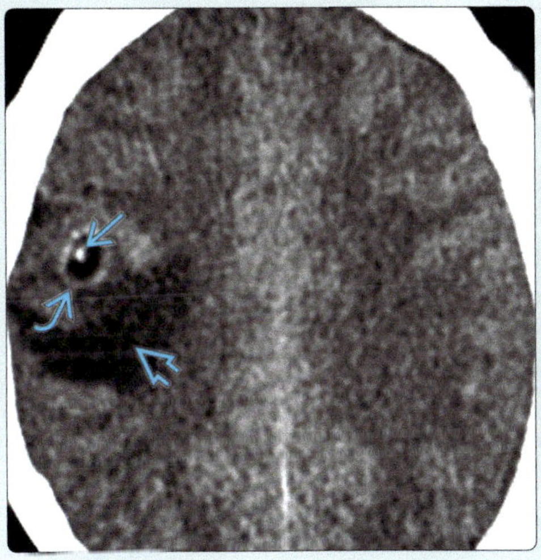

(Left) *Subarachnoid and ventricular cysts are shown; convexity cysts have a scolex and surrounding inflammation around the largest cyst that "seals" the sulcus and makes it appear parenchymal. Racemose cysts are multilocular, nonviable, seen in the basal cisterns, and typically lack a scolex.* **(Right)** *Axial CECT in a young male patient with first episode of seizure demonstrates a ring-enhancing lesion with an eccentric hyperdense "dot" typical for neurocysticercosis (NCC). Note surrounding edema.*

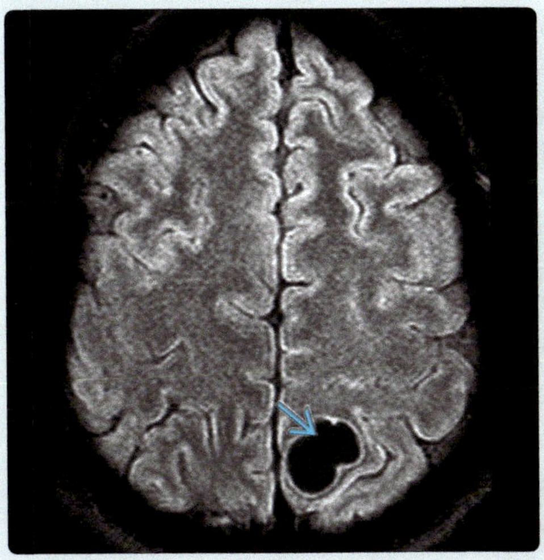

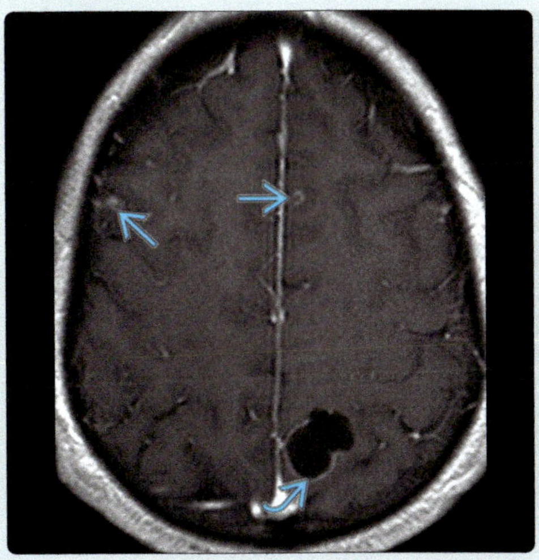

(Left) *Axial FLAIR MR shows a well-defined cyst in left parietal lobe, which follows cerebrospinal fluid signal. There is no edema surrounding this cyst.* **(Right)** *Axial T1+C MR in the same patient shows minimal rim enhancement of the cyst. Findings are typical for vesicular stage of NCC. Note nodular enhancing lesions in the frontal lobes due to granular nodular stage of NCC. It is important to remember that NCC lesions may be at different stages in same patient.*

KEY FACTS

TERMINOLOGY

- Lyme disease, Lyme neuroborreliosis (LNB)
- Multisystem inflammatory disease
  - Caused by spirochete *Borrelia burgdorferi* (USA)
  - Transmitted by *Ixodes* tick bite
  - Reservoirs = white tail deer/field mouse

IMAGING

- MS-like white matter (WM) lesions (may enhance)
  - 2-8 mm (large "tumefactive" lesions rare)
- ± multiple enhancing cranial nerves
- ± cauda equina, meningeal enhancement

TOP DIFFERENTIAL DIAGNOSES

- Demyelinating disease
- Vasculitis
- Sarcoidosis
- Bell's palsy (solitary CN 7 enhancement)
- Chronic fatigue syndrome

  - Bilateral WM atrophy with increased right anterior arcuate fractional anisotropy
  - May have abnormal resting-state functional connectivity

CLINICAL ISSUES

- Most common vector-borne disease in USA
  - Round, bull's-eye skin rash
  - ± flu-like symptoms
  - Meningopolyneuritis, radiculitis common
- Peak May-July; incubation varies (days to weeks)
- Progressive debilitating disorder if not treated early
- 10-15% of untreated patients develop neurologic manifestations

DIAGNOSTIC CHECKLIST

- Consider geography, recreational/travel history, season
- Consider LNB if MS-like lesions in patient with erythema migrans
  - ± enhancing cranial nerves, cauda equina

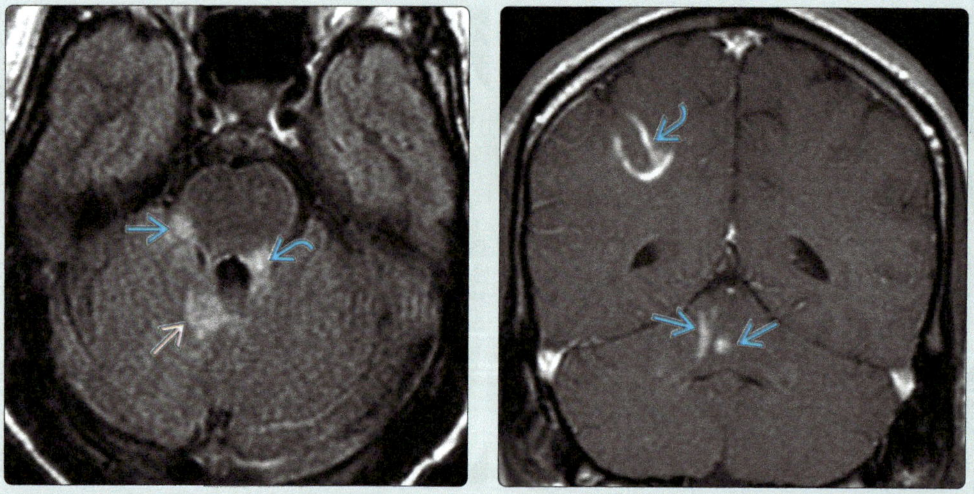

(Left) *Axial FLAIR MR in a patient with serologically documented Lyme disease shows multiple hyperintense foci in the left superior cerebellar peduncle, right lateral pons, and cerebellum.* **(Right)** *Coronal T1WI C+ MR in the same patient shows enhancement of a right cerebral white matter lesion, as well as posterior fossa lesions. Lyme disease generally manifests as foci of T2 hyperintensities, nerve root, or meningeal enhancement.*

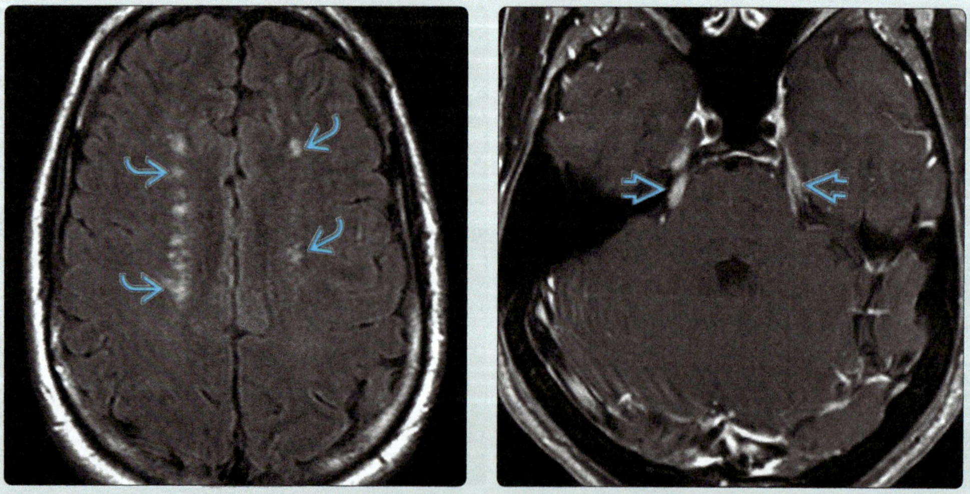

(Left) *Axial FLAIR in a patient with history of tick bite and erythema migrans demonstrates multiple white matter hyperintensities in the deep white matter. White matter lesions in Lyme may resemble multiple sclerosis plaques although involvement of callososeptal interface is less common.* **(Right)** *Axial T1 C+ MR in a 24-year-old man with recent history of camping shows enhancement of the cisternal segment of both trigeminal nerves. The 3rd, 5th, and 7th cranial nerve enhancement can be seen in Lyme neuroborreliosis.*

KEY FACTS

TERMINOLOGY

- HIV-1 encephalitis/HIV-1 encephalopathy
- HIV-associated neurocognitive disorders

IMAGING

- CT
  - Atrophy
  - Bilateral periventricular/diffuse WM hypointensities
  - Basal ganglia, cerebellum, brainstem hypodensity
- MR
  - Diffuse "hazy" hyperintense WM on T2/FLAIR
  - Nonenhancing (if enhancement present, consider opportunistic infections, immune reconstitution inflammatory syndrome)

PATHOLOGY

- HIV has ability to cause neurologic disease
  - Does not replicate within neural/glial cells
  - Microglial nodules with multinucleated giant cells
- WM pallor early, neocortical infection/atrophy late

CLINICAL ISSUES

- Moderate cognitive impairment common despite good virologic response to therapy
- Direct HIV infection of brain
  - Opportunistic infections absent
  - Cognitive, behavioral, motor abnormalities in 25-70%
  - Most frequent neurological manifestation of HIV infection

DIAGNOSTIC CHECKLIST

- Evidence of "cerebral atrophy" by CT/MR does not indicate AIDS dementia complex in HIV-positive patient
- Consider reversible causes 1st (dehydration, malnutrition, protein depletion, alcoholism)

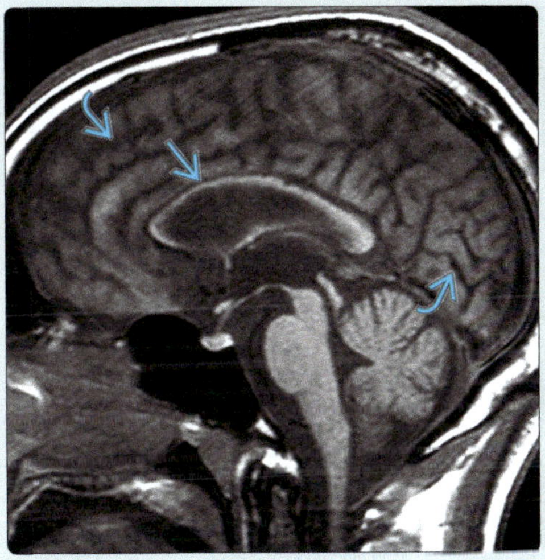

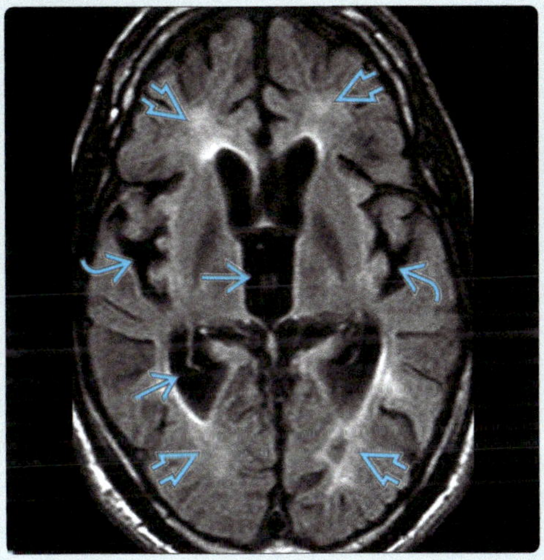

(Left) *Sagittal T1WI MR in a 35-year-old man with HIV shows generalized atrophy, enlarged sulci ➔, and severe atrophy of the corpus callosum ➔.* **(Right)** *Axial FLAIR MR in the same patient shows enlarged ventricles ➔ and sylvian fissures ➔ due to diffuse atrophy. There are hazy periventricular white matter hyperintensities ➔. These imaging findings are characteristic of HIV encephalitis.*

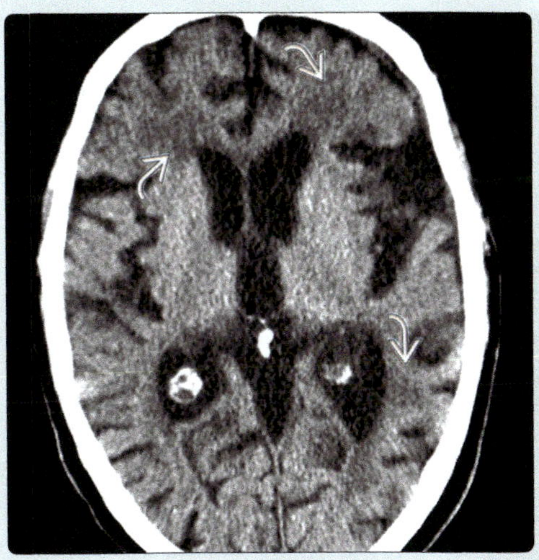

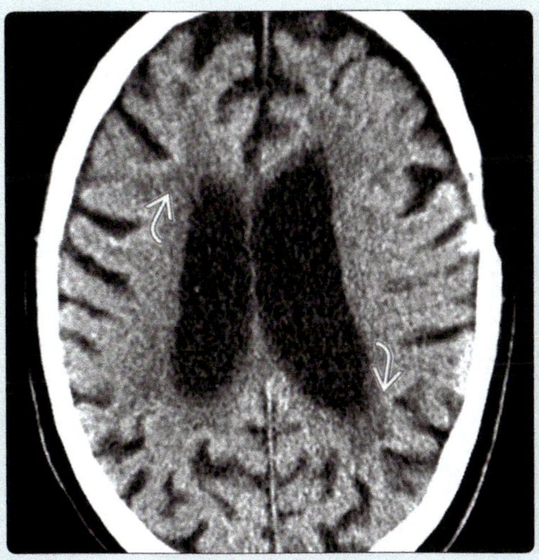

(Left) *Axial NECT in a 38-year-old man with longstanding HIV/AIDS, who was receiving HAART, was obtained for decreasing cognitive function. Note the gross atrophy and low density ➔ within the subcortical white matter.* **(Right)** *Axial NECT in the same patient shows characteristic low density in the periventricular white matter ➔ along with diffusely enlarged sulci and lateral ventricles.*

KEY FACTS

TERMINOLOGY

- Opportunistic infection
  - Caused by parasite *Toxoplasma gondii*
  - Most common opportunistic CNS infection in AIDS

IMAGING

- CT
  - Ill-defined, hypodense lesions and edema
  - Basal ganglia, thalamus, cerebellum
  - Rim, nodular, target enhancement
- MR
  - T2 hypointense
  - T1 C+ target sign highly suggestive
- Thallium-201 SPECT and 18F-FDG PET: Toxoplasmosis lesions are hypometabolic

TOP DIFFERENTIAL DIAGNOSES

- Lymphoma
  - Solitary mass in patient with HIV/AIDS? Lymphoma > toxoplasmosis
  - Lymphoma often restricts on DWI
  - Toxoplasmosis hypometabolic on PET, low relative cerebral blood volume on pMR
- Other opportunistic infections
  - Cryptococcosis, progressive multifocal leukoencephalopathy (usually does not enhance)

PATHOLOGY

- 20-70% of USA population seropositive for *T. gondii*
  - Usually reactivation of latent infection

CLINICAL ISSUES

- Fever, malaise, headache

DIAGNOSTIC CHECKLIST

- Multiple target lesions on T1WI C+ that are dark on T2WI
  - Consider toxoplasmosis encephalitis (TE)
- TE lesions usually resolve in 2-4 weeks

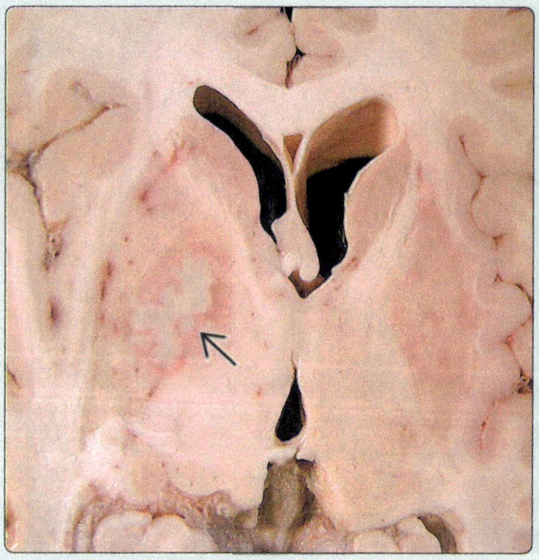

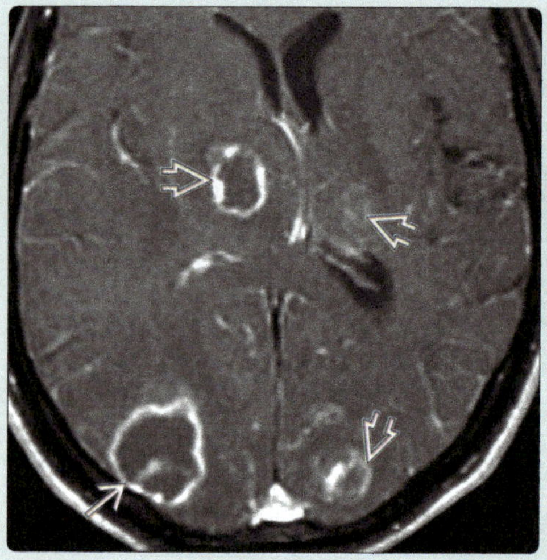

(Left) *Axial gross pathology specimen sectioned through the ventricles in a patient with HIV/AIDS shows a toxoplasmosis abscess in the right lentiform nucleus →. The lesion is necrotic and poorly demarcated. (Courtesy R. Hewlett, MD.)* **(Right)** *Axial T1WI C+ MR shows several ring-enhancing lesions in the thalami and left occipital lobe →. Note the large lesion showing a classic target appearance →. These lesions were hypointense on T2WI.*

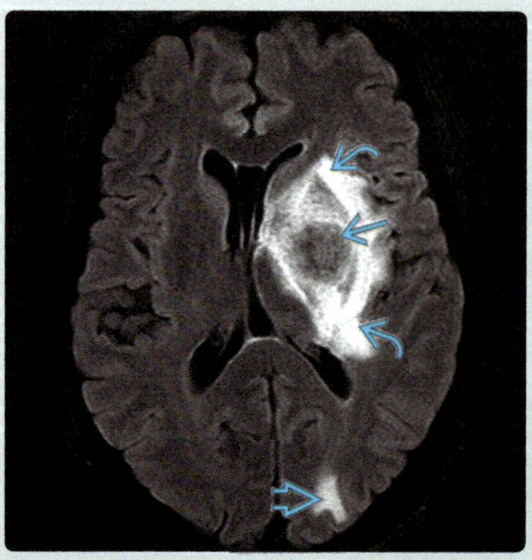

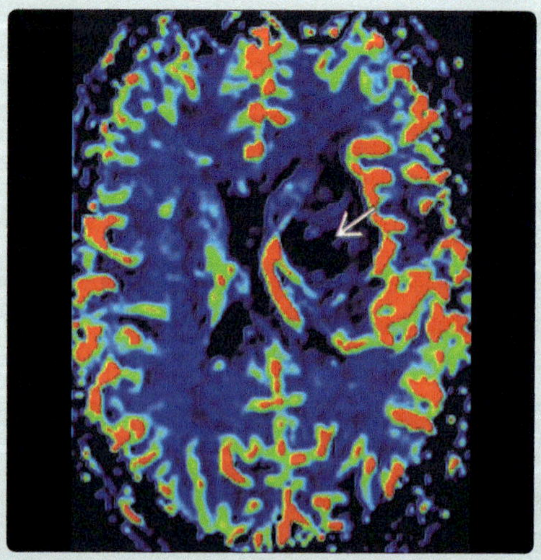

(Left) *Axial FLAIR MR in HIV patient demonstrates a large, hypointense lesion → in the left basal ganglia with extensive surrounding edema ↗. Another smaller lesion is seen in the left occipital region →. The left basal ganglia lesion showed rim and "target" enhancement on T1WI C+ MR. The most important differential consideration is toxoplasmosis vs. lymphoma.* **(Right)** *Axial CBV map from MR perfusion demonstrates low rCBV →, suggesting an infection (toxoplasmosis) rather than lymphoma.*

KEY FACTS

TERMINOLOGY

- Acquired CNS cytomegalovirus (CMV) infections: Meningitis, encephalitis, ventriculitis, transverse myelitis, radiculomyelitis, chorioretinitis
- Immunocompromised (AIDS, organ transplant) patients are at risk → reactivation of previously silent infection

IMAGING

- Best diagnostic clue: Ventriculitis with fluid-debris level and ependymal enhancement in immunocompromised patient
- Encephalitis: Ill-defined T2-hyperintense area, variable enhancement
- May mimic HIV encephalitis with patchy nonspecific T2-hyperintense lesions
- Contrast should be used for imaging of all immunocompromised patients

TOP DIFFERENTIAL DIAGNOSES

- HIV encephalitis
- Progressive multifocal leukoencephalopathy (PML)
- Toxoplasmosis
- Acute disseminated encephalitis

CLINICAL ISSUES

- Primary CMV infection is generally asymptomatic
- Infection may occur secondary to reactivation of latent viral infection or newly acquired via organ or bone marrow transplant from seropositive donor
  - CMV disseminates to CNS in late stages of HIV infection, low CD4(+) count (usually ≤ 50)
  - Clinically may mimic HIV encephalitis
- Disease manifestations vary in severity depending on degree of host immunosuppression
- HAART
  - Markedly ↓ incidence of CMV disease in AIDS
  - ↑ Immunocompetence against CMV

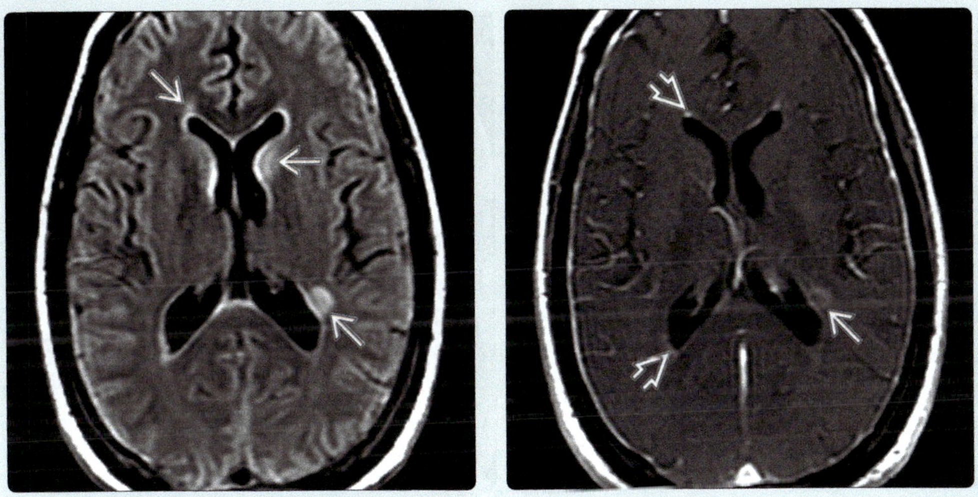

(Left) *Axial FLAIR MR shows mild ventriculomegaly and periventricular hyperintensities ➡ related to ventriculo-encephalitis.* **(Right)** *Axial T1WI C+ MR in the same patient shows ependymal ⇨ and periventricular ➡ enhancement. This patient was immunocompromised with ventriculitis and associated encephalitis. CMV encephalitis is commonly a ventriculo-encephalitis, involving the periventricular white matter. However, CMV may also cause hemorrhagic or necrotic lesions.*

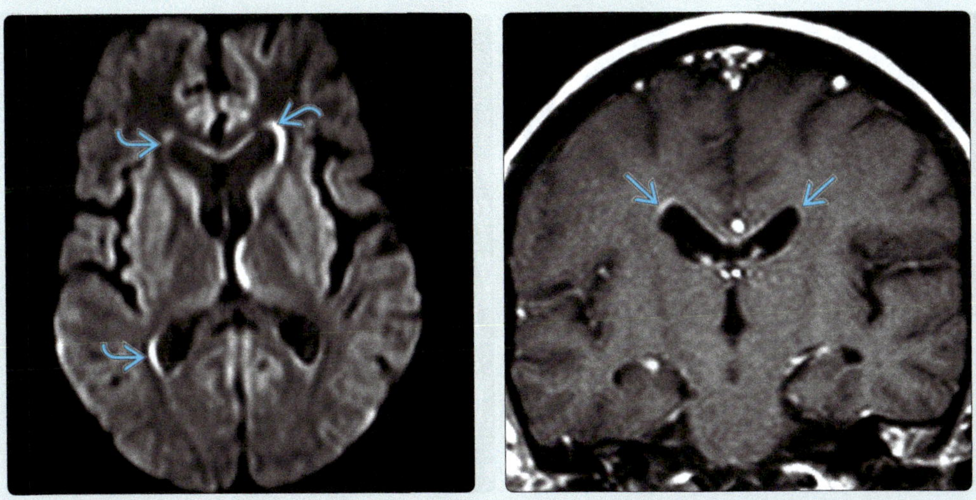

(Left) *Axial DWI MR in a 35-year-old HIV-positive patient with very low CD4(+) cell count demonstrates thin hyperintense rim along the ventricular margins ↪. There is mild enlargement of the ventricles and mild cortical atrophy.* **(Right)** *Coronal T1WI C+ MR in the same patient shows subtle ependymal enhancement along the frontal horns ⇨. Imaging findings are characteristic of CMV ventriculitis.*

KEY FACTS

IMAGING

- Varies with type, site of infection, immune status
  - MR ± contrast (add T2* for hemorrhage)
- Invasive fungal sinusitis
  - Most common in immunocompromised patient
  - Aspergillus, mucormycosis most common
  - Bone CT shows sinus/orbit/skull base involvement
  - Look for occluded carotid, thrombosed cavernous sinus
- Meningitis
  - Most common presentation of coccidioidomycosis
  - Meningeal enhancement, especially basal cisterns
- Vasculitis
  - Aspergillus, mucormycosis are angioinvasive
    - Especially in immunocompromised, diabetic patients
  - Multifocal parenchymal hemorrhagic lesions
  - May occlude vessels, cause multifocal lacunar or territorial infarcts
  - May cause mycotic pseudoaneurysm
- Fungal abscesses
  - Microabscesses, miliary granulomas common in candidiasis
  - Ring-enhancing foci with intracavitary projections, diffusion restriction

CLINICAL ISSUES

- General: Weight loss, fever, malaise, fatigue
- Other: Meningitis; acute neurologic deficit (cranial neuropathy, visual loss)

DIAGNOSTIC CHECKLIST

- Look for associated lung lesions (granulomas, airspace disease)
- Consider fungal infection in immunocompromised patient with acute neurologic deficit
- Consider fungal infection in immunocompromised patient with meningitis &/or multiple brain lesions

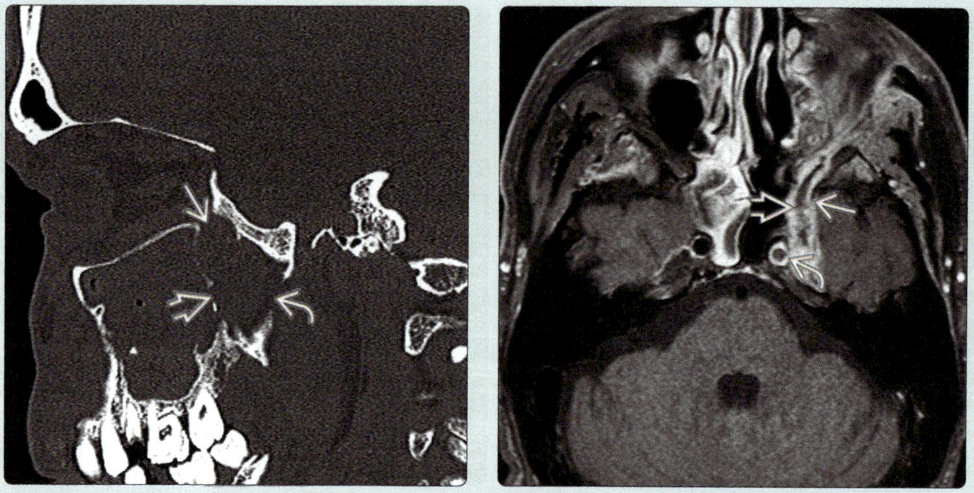

(Left) *Sagittal bone CT in a severe, poorly controlled diabetic patient shows an opacified left maxillary sinus with erosion of its posterior wall ➔ and destruction of the adjacent pterygoid plate ➔. The pterygopalatine fossa ➔ is expanded and deossified. Despite debridement, the patient developed a massive cerebral infarct.* **(Right)** *Follow-up T1 C+ FS MR shows left cavernous sinus thrombosis with enhancing dura ➔ surrounding the clot ➔. Note thrombosis with absent "flow void" of the left cavernous carotid artery ➔.*

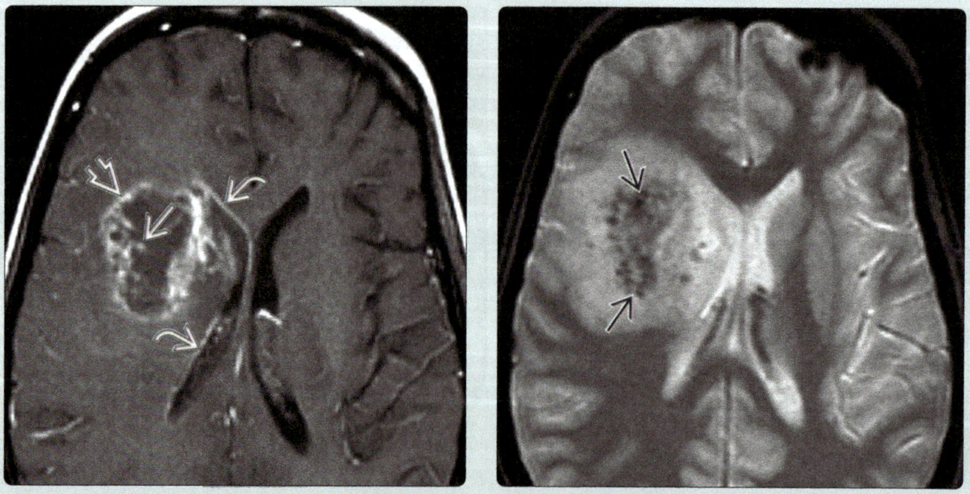

(Left) *Axial T1 C+ in an immunocompromised patient shows an irregular rim-enhancing mass ➔ with prominent intracavitary projections ➔. The adjacent ventricular ependyma is enhancing ➔, consistent with ventriculitis.* **(Right)** *T2* GRE scan in the same case shows multiple punctate "blooming" foci ➔ within the mass consistent with petechial hemorrhages. Aspergilloma was found at surgery.*

KEY FACTS

TERMINOLOGY

- *Cryptococcus neoformans* infection
- Opportunistic fungal infection that typically affects HIV and other immunosuppressed patients
- *Cryptococci* spread along perivascular spaces (PVS) to deep brain: Basal ganglia, thalamus, brainstem, cerebellum, dentate nucleus, periventricular WM

IMAGING

- Dilated PVS in deep gray nuclei of AIDS patient, often no enhancement
  - Degree of enhancement depends on cell-mediated immunity of host
- May see miliary or leptomeningeal enhancing nodules + gelatinous pseudocysts
- Cryptococcoma: Ring-like or solid enhancement
- Dilated PVS in AIDS patients → consider *Cryptococcus* infection
- 4 imaging patterns: Miliary enhancing parenchymal nodules, leptomeningeal-cisternal nodules, cryptococcoma, gelatinous pseudocysts

TOP DIFFERENTIAL DIAGNOSES

- Acquired toxoplasmosis
- Tuberculosis
- Primary CNS lymphoma

CLINICAL ISSUES

- Most common fungal infection in AIDS patients
  - 3rd most common infection seen in AIDS patients (HIV > toxoplasmosis > cryptococcosis)
- CNS infection related to hematogeneous dissemination from lungs
  - Headache most common symptom
- Diagnosis: India ink test highly specific
  - Antigen titers correspond to severity of illness
- Treatment: Amphotericin B, flucytosine/fluconazole

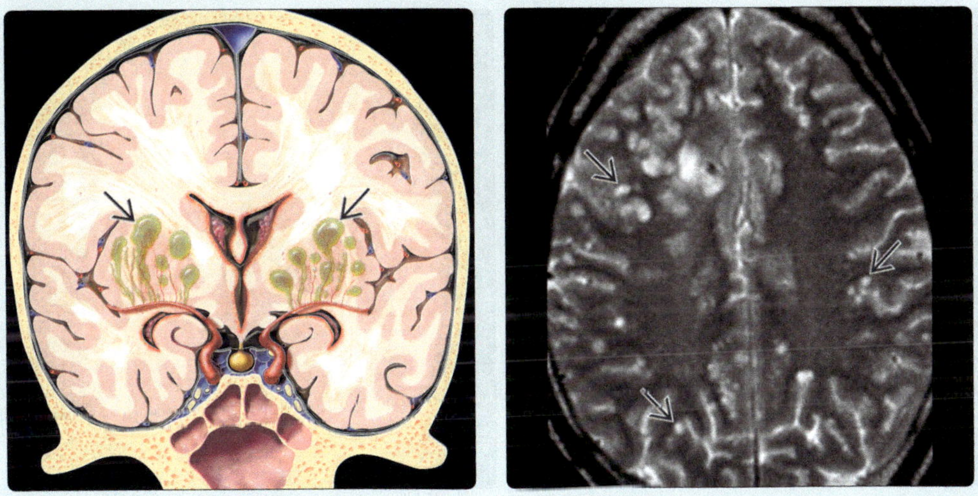

(Left) *Coronal graphic shows multiple dilated perivascular (Virchow-Robin) spaces ⇨, filled with fungi and mucoid material, resulting in gelatinous pseudocysts, which are characteristic of cryptococcal infection in AIDS.* **(Right)** *Axial T2WI MR shows multiple dilated perivascular spaces ⇨ in this immunocompromised patient with cryptococcal meningitis. Gelatinous pseudocysts are most commonly located in the basal ganglia and thalami but may be seen in the brainstem, cerebellum, and cerebral hemispheres.*

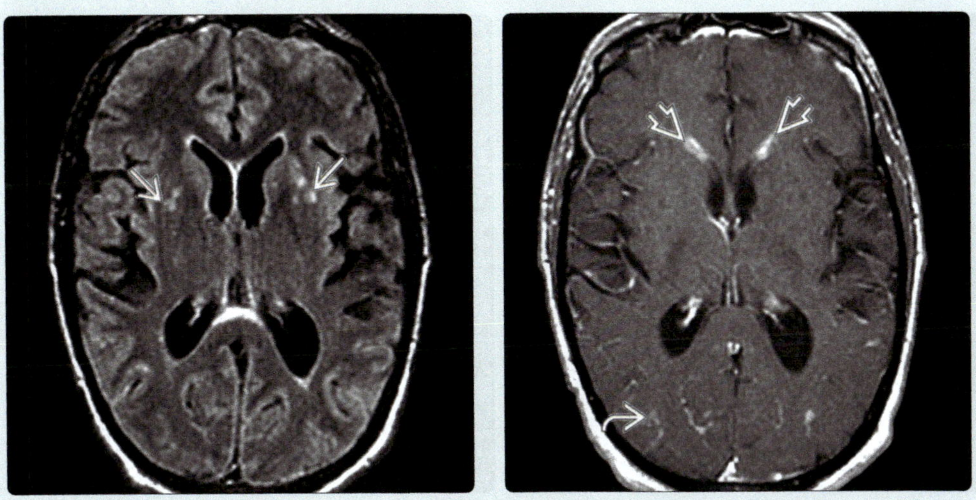

(Left) *Axial FLAIR MR shows bilateral dilated perivascular spaces ➡ with hyperintense rims in this AIDS patient with Cryptococcus meningitis. Hydrocephalus is a common complication of this infection.* **(Right)** *Axial T1WI C+ MR in the same patient shows subependymal enhancement ➡ along the frontal horns of the lateral ventricles as well as nodular leptomeningeal enhancement ➡. Enhancement in Cryptococcus infection is dependent on the cell-mediated immunity of the host.*

Progressive Multifocal Leukoencephalopathy (PML)

KEY FACTS

TERMINOLOGY

- Progressive multifocal leukoencephalopathy (PML)
- Subacute opportunistic infection caused by DNA virus JC polyomavirus (JCV)
- JCV infects oligodendrocytes, causes demyelination in immunocompromised patients
- Associated with immunosuppression, often AIDS
  - Organ transplant, cancer, chemotherapy, myeloproliferative disease, and steroid treatment
  - Reported in treatment for multiple sclerosis and in rheumatic diseases

IMAGING

- Multifocal T2-hyperintense demyelinating plaques involve subcortical white matter (WM), extend to deep WM; gray matter often spared until late stage
- Characteristic involvement of **subcortical U fibers**
- Generally no contrast enhancement or mass effect
- Late: Confluent WM disease, cystic changes
- Propensity for frontal and parietooccipital region, thalamus
  - May involve brainstem and cerebellum
- May be solitary, multifocal, or widespread confluent

TOP DIFFERENTIAL DIAGNOSES

- HIV encephalitis
- Acute disseminated encephalomyelitis
- Acquired CMV
- Immune reconstitution inflammatory syndrome

CLINICAL ISSUES

- Without treatment (plasma exchange): Poor prognosis, death in 2.5-4.0 months
  - HAART reported to improve survival
- Associated with natalizumab treatment

DIAGNOSTIC CHECKLIST

- Test for JCV before treatment with high-risk medications
- New multifocal WM lesions in AIDS or patient on high-risk medication? Consider PML!

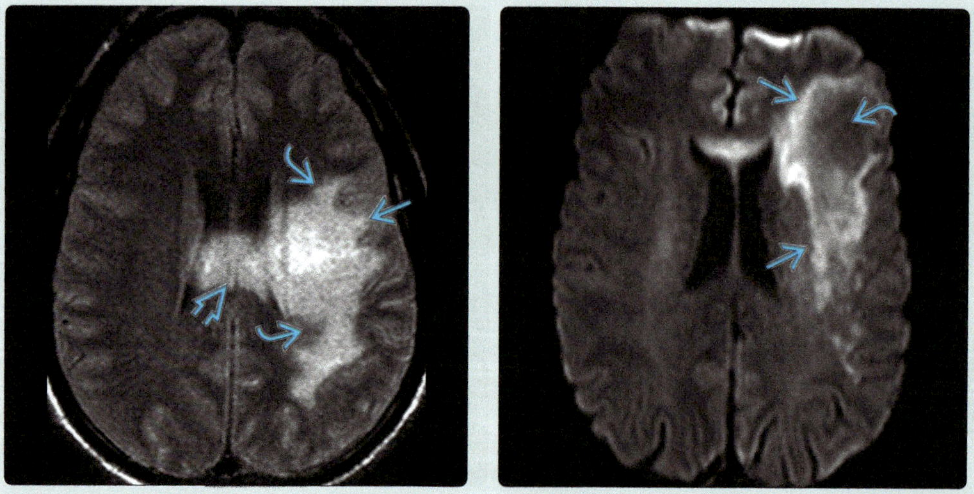

(Left) *Axial FLAIR MR in an AIDS patient who was somnolent at presentation shows scalloped hyperintensity in the left frontoparietal white matter. There is involvement of the subcortical U fibers, characteristic of PML. Note involvement of the corpus callosum but lack of mass effect.* **(Right)** *Axial DWI in an HIV patient with very low CD4(+) counts and PML demonstrates central core of low signal surrounded by rim of higher signal. Appearance of PML on DWI varies with disease stage.*

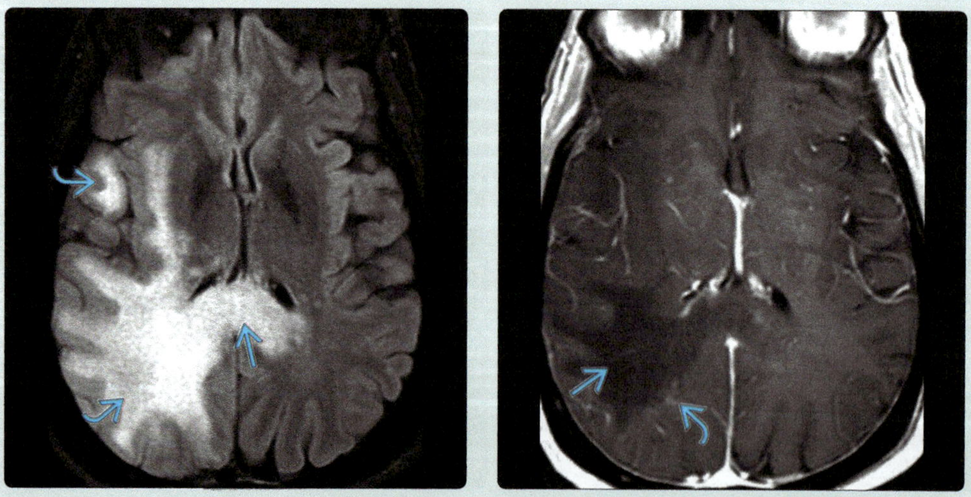

(Left) *Axial FLAIR MR in a patient with multiple sclerosis on natalizumab and developed PML demonstrates infiltrating hyperintensity involving the right temporal, parietal, and occipital white matter as well as the splenium.* **(Right)** *Axial T1C+ MR in the same patient shows white matter hypointensity with very faint enhancement at the margins. Monoclonal antibody therapy (like natalizumab) used in a wide spectrum of immunologic diseases may depress the immune system and predispose the patient to PML.*

KEY FACTS

TERMINOLOGY

- **I**mmune **R**econstitution **I**nflammatory **S**yndrome (IRIS)
  - Atypical/worsening opportunistic infection
  - HIV/AIDS patients following commencement of HAART
  - Patients with MS, immunomodulatory therapy

IMAGING

- Progressive multifocal leukoencephalopathy (PML)-IRIS
  - White matter (WM) hypodensities with ↑ mass
  - Patchy atypical enhancement
- TB-IRIS
  - ↑ leptomeningeal enhancement
  - ↑ size of ring-/nodular-enhancing tuberculomas
- Crypto-IRIS
  - ↑ nodular meningeal/subependymal enhancement
  - ↑ in size of "gelatinous" pseudocysts

TOP DIFFERENTIAL DIAGNOSES

- Diffuse/patchy WM abnormalities in AIDS
  - HIV encephalitis, PML, CMV infection
- Focal/multifocal brain lesions in AIDS
  - Lymphoma, toxo, tuberculoma, cryptococcosis

PATHOLOGY

- Reconstitution of immunity → abnormal immune response to infectious/noninfectious antigens
- IRIS is **not** caused by relapse/recurrence of preexisting disease

CLINICAL ISSUES

- 1/4 to 1/3 HIV-infected patients develop IRIS
- PML, TB common IRIS-associated pathogens

DIAGNOSTIC CHECKLIST

- IRIS if worsening/enhancing lesions in
  - HIV patient who recently started HAART
  - MS patient on immunomodulatory therapy

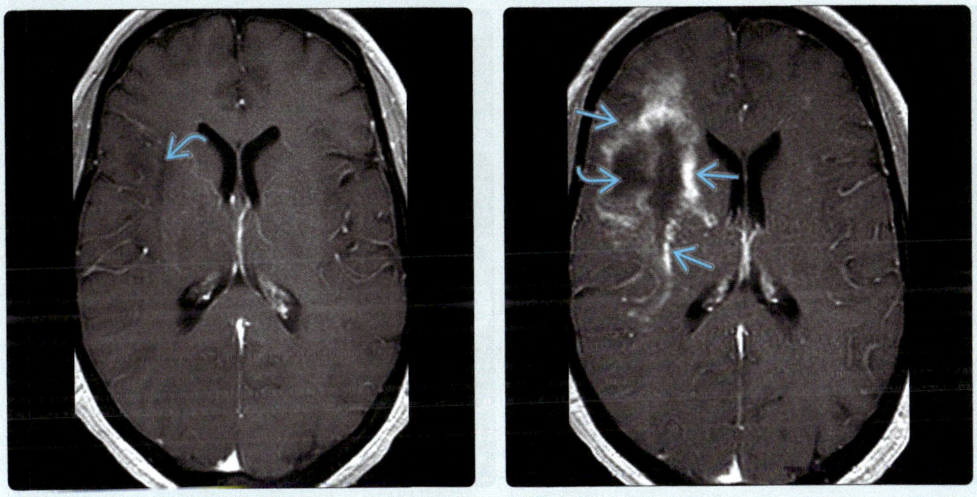

(Left) *Axial T1WI C+ MR in a patient with HIV and PML shows subtle hypodensity in right insular region without any abnormal enhancement. FLAIR images (not shown) demonstrated multifocal confluent white matter hyperintensities.* **(Right)** *Axial T1 C+ MR in the same patient after initiation of HAART therapy and significant clinical deterioration shows patchy nodular and linear foci of enhancement and worsening of the underlying hypodensity, findings typical for PML-IRIS.*

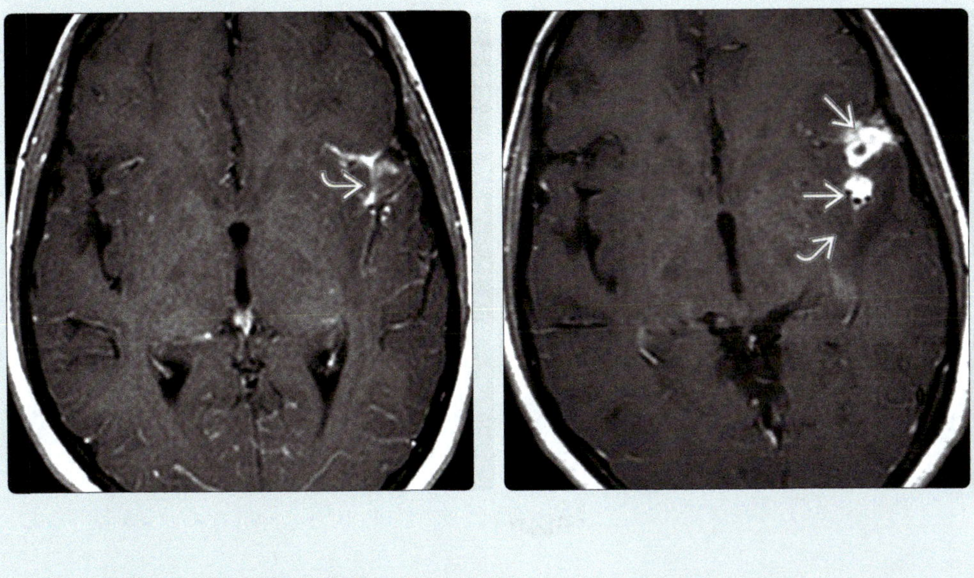

(Left) *Axial T1WI C+ MR demonstrates meningeal enhancement in the left sylvian fissure in an HIV-positive patient with tuberculous meningitis.* **(Right)** *Axial T1WI C+ MR in the same case shows worsening of imaging appearance after placement on HAART. There is an increase in enhancement, which appears more nodular, and there is development of surrounding edema. This worsening of disease could be due to drug resistance; however, the time course after starting HAART makes IRIS most likely.*

KEY FACTS

TERMINOLOGY

- HIV/AIDS-related opportunistic infections and neoplasms

IMAGING

- Findings
  - Primary CNS lymphoma: Enhancing lesions, often hemorrhagic/necrotic within basal ganglia, periventricular white matter
  - Kaposi sarcoma: Intense enhancing soft tissue mass in scalp
  - Bacterial abscesses: Ring-enhancing lesion with ↑ signal on DWI
  - Aspergillosis: Multiple ring-enhancing lesions
  - Neurosyphilis: Cortical/subcortical infarcts, granulomas, leptomeningeal enhancement
  - Benign lymphoepithelial lesions of HIV: Multiple cystic masses enlarging both parotid glands
- MR is most sensitive
- PET or thallium-201 SPECT helpful to differentiate from toxoplasmosis
- Immune reconstitution inflammatory syndrome: "Wild"-looking enhancing lesion(s)

TOP DIFFERENTIAL DIAGNOSES

- Toxoplasmosis
- Metastases
- Tuberculosis

DIAGNOSTIC CHECKLIST

- Consider using DWI, MRS, PET/SPECT to differentiate opportunistic infections from malignant lesions
- Bacterial abscess, aspergillosis, neurosyphilis may need surgical biopsy for diagnosis

(Left) *Axial graphic shows typical lymphoid and lymphoepithelial lesions of HIV/AIDS. Note hyperplastic tonsils ➡ and multiple cysts in both parotid glands ⇨.* **(Right)** *Axial CECT scan in a 33-year-old man with HIV/AIDS shows a large right parotid cyst with enhancing rim ↪ and enlarged Waldeyer ring ⇨ (the annular arrangement of lymphoid tissue in the pharynx, also known as the pharyngeal lymphoid ring).*

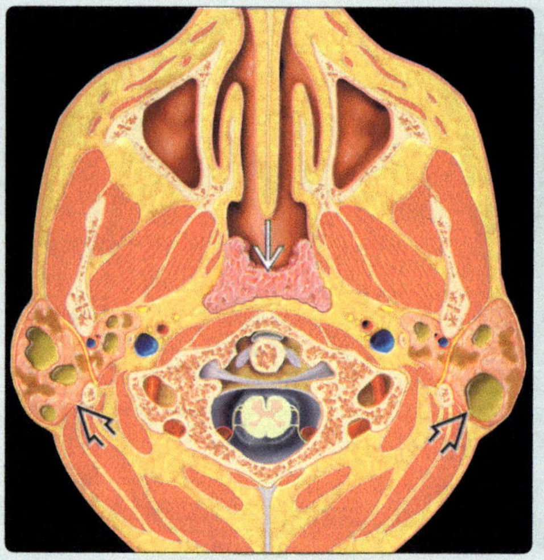

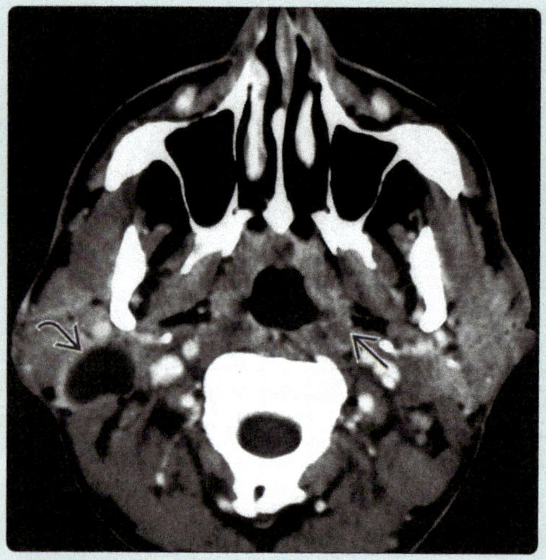

(Left) *T1 C+ scan in an HIV(+) man obtained prior to beginning HAART shows some nonenhancing periventricular hypointensities ⇨.* **(Right)** *The patient deteriorated 3 weeks following institution of HAART. T1 C+ scan now shows extensive patchy enhancing lesions ➡. Cerebrospinal fluid was positive for JC virus in this case of progressive multifocal leukoencephalopathy-immune reconstitution inflammatory syndrome (PML-IRIS). (Courtesy T. Hutchins, MD.)*

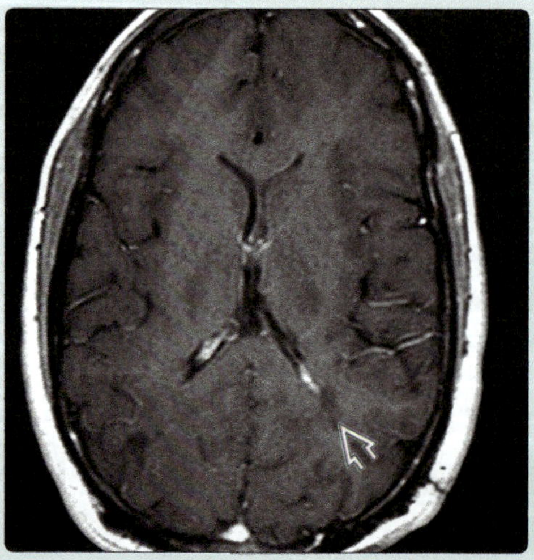

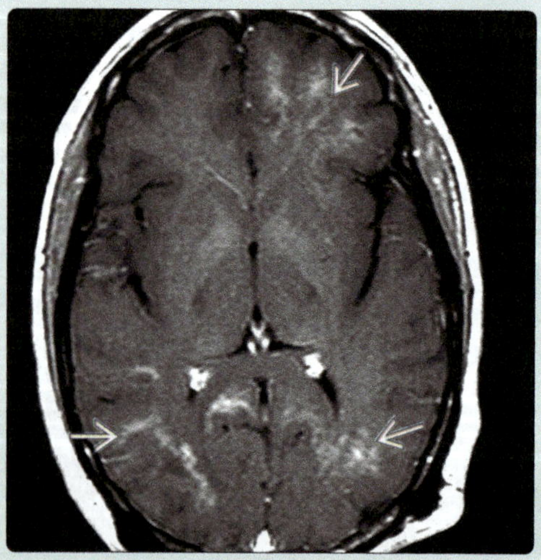

KEY FACTS

IMAGING

- Multiple perpendicular callososeptal T2 hyperintensities characteristic of multiple sclerosis (MS)
  - Perivenular extension: "Dawson fingers"
- Bilateral, asymmetric linear/ovoid FLAIR hyperintensities
  - > 85% periventricular/perivenular
  - 50-90% callososeptal interface
  - May also commonly involve subcortical U fibers, brachium pontis, brainstem, spinal cord common
- Transient enhancement during active demyelination
  - > 90% disappear within 6 months
- Rare: Large tumefactive enhancing rings
- T1: Hypointense lesions suggest worse prognosis
  - Correlate with disability, atrophy, progressive disease
- Advanced imaging techniques show disease in normal-appearing white matter

TOP DIFFERENTIAL DIAGNOSES

- Acute disseminated encephalomyelitis (ADEM)
- Neuromyelitis optica
- Autoimmune-mediated vasculitis
- CADASIL
- Lyme disease
- Susac syndrome

CLINICAL ISSUES

- Estimated 2.5 million people in world have MS
- Most common disabling CNS disease of young adults; 1:1,000 in Western world
- Age: 20-40 years
  - Peak onset = 30; 3-5% < 15, 9% > 50
- Adults: M:F = 1:2; adolescents: M:F = 1:3-5

DIAGNOSTIC CHECKLIST

- Requires dissemination in time and space in CNS for diagnosis
- McDonald criteria: Consensus statement for diagnostic criteria, last revised in 2010

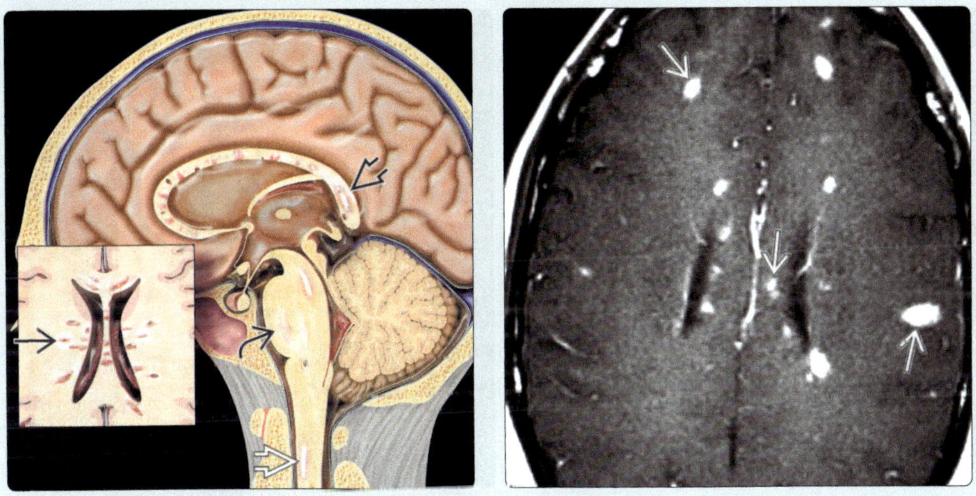

(Left) *Sagittal graphic illustrates multiple sclerosis (MS) plaques involving the corpus callosum, pons, and spinal cord. Note the characteristic perpendicular orientation of the lesions at the callososeptal interface along penetrating venules.* **(Right)** *Axial T1WI C+ MR shows numerous enhancing MS plaques that were present throughout the infratentorial and supratentorial brain. Lesions may show homogeneous enhancement but may also exhibit ring or an incomplete ring pattern of enhancement.*

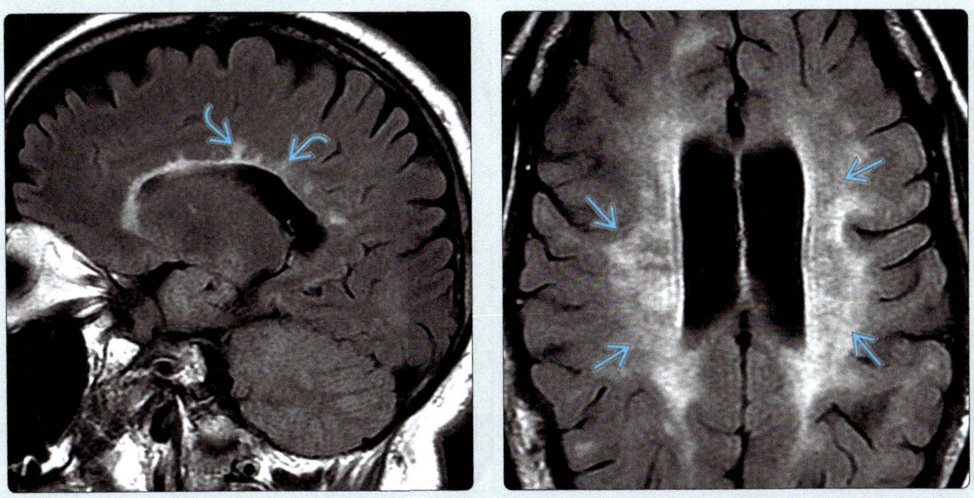

(Left) *Sagittal FLAIR shows callososeptal hyperintensities radiating from the lateral ventricles with a typical perpendicular orientation, characteristic of multiple sclerosis.* **(Right)** *Axial FLAIR in a 35-year-old woman with MS shows extensive confluent periventricular hyperintense lesions typical of advanced, longstanding MS with loss of discrete, linear, periventricular lesions. Note prominence of the ventricles and cortical sulci due to diffuse atrophy.*

KEY FACTS

TERMINOLOGY

- Neuromyelitis optica (NMO)
- NMO spectrum disorders
- Idiopathic inflammatory demyelinating disorder of CNS characterized by severe attacks of optic neuritis and myelitis

IMAGING

- Hyperintense, mildly enlarged optic nerves
- Expansile, hyperintense cord signal, ≥ 3 segments
- Long segment optic nerve enhancement
- Acute cord lesions show patchy enhancement
- Patchy enhancement with blurred margins ("cloud-like" enhancement) in cerebral lesions
- "Pencil-thin" ependymal enhancement

TOP DIFFERENTIAL DIAGNOSES

- Multiple sclerosis
  - Radially oriented, well-demarcated perivenular lesions
  - Patchy cord lesions > > long multisegmental
- Optic neuritis
- Transverse myelitis
- Syringomyelia
- Spinal cord neoplasm

PATHOLOGY

- Serum marker: **NMO-IgG**, targets water channel aquaporin-4 (AQP4)
- Seen in 70% of NMO patients, **99% specificity**

CLINICAL ISSUES

- Hallmark = severe optic neuropathy, myelopathy
  - May progress to blindness
- 20% present with brainstem symptoms at disease onset
- Relapsing course in 90% of patients
- Anti-AQP4 antibody positivity as prognostic marker
- Acute exacerbation: IV corticosteroids, immunosuppressives

(Left) *Axial T1WI C+ FS MR shows a markedly enhancing prechiasmatic right optic nerve and chiasm* ➡, *consistent with acute optic neuritis.* **(Right)** *Sagittal T2 PD FSE MR in the same patient shows a long segment of cord enlargement with hyperintensity. Ill-defined enhancement was also present in the cervical cord in this patient with myelopathy and vision loss. Patients with neuromyelitis optica (NMO) have a worse prognosis with more severe disability than multiple sclerosis, despite lack of brain involvement.*

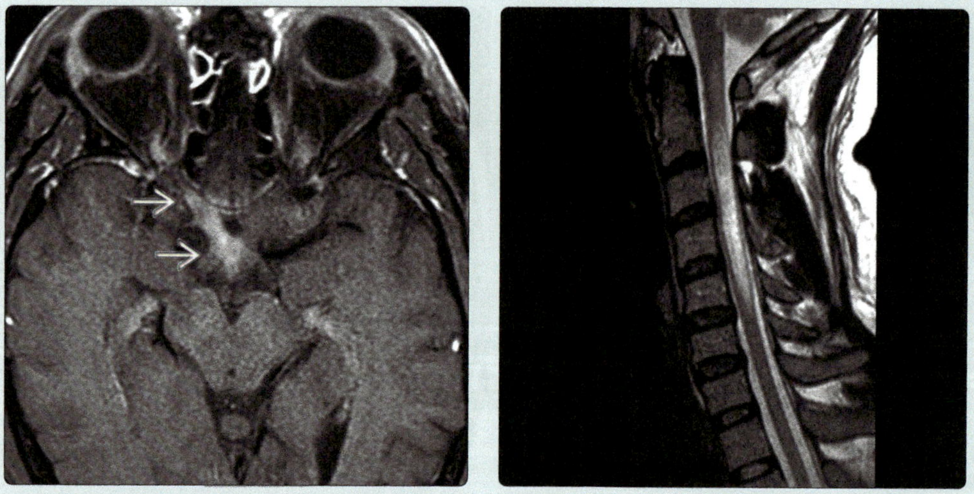

(Left) *Axial FLAIR MR in a patient with NMO spectrum disorder (NMOSD) shows characteristic periependymal lesions surrounding the 3rd ventricle, involving the thalamus* ↪ *and hypothalamus* ➡. **(Right)** *Axial T1+C MR in the same patient shows subtle rim enhancement in the lesion in the right thalamus* ➡. *Brain lesions in NMO/NMOSD are typically localized in the periependymal regions where aquaporin-4 is highly expressed.*

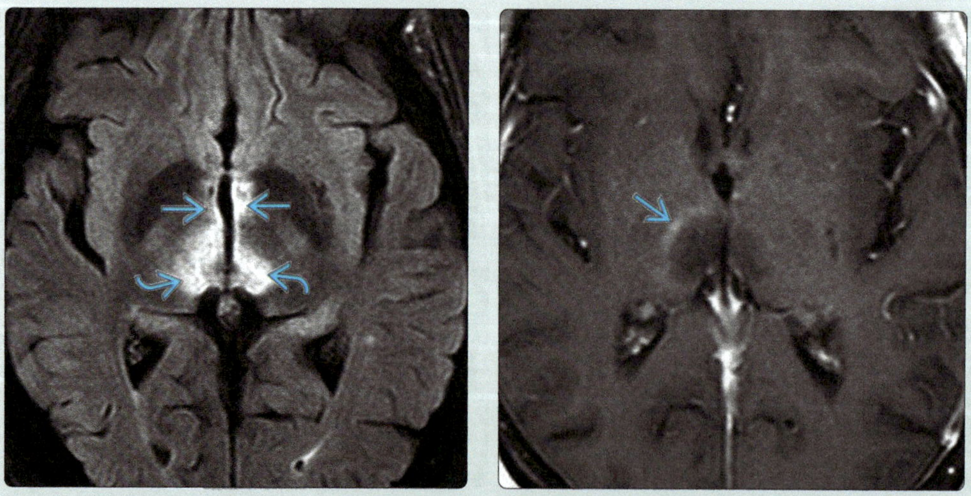

KEY FACTS

TERMINOLOGY

- Autoimmune-mediated white matter (WM) demyelination of brain &/or spinal cord, usually with remyelination

IMAGING

- Best diagnostic clue: Multifocal WM and deep gray lesions days to weeks following infection/vaccination
- May involve both brain and spinal cord; WM > gray matter, but usually both affected
- Deep/juxtacortical WM > periventricular WM
- Both supratentorial and infratentorial lesions
- Multifocal punctate to large flocculent FLAIR hyperintensities
- Do not usually involve callososeptal interface
- Most lesions show increased signal on DWI (T2 shine through)
- Punctate, ring, incomplete ring, peripheral enhancement
- Absence of enhancement does not exclude diagnosis
- MRS: ↓ NAA within lesions; may see ↑ Cho, ↑ lactate

TOP DIFFERENTIAL DIAGNOSES

- Multiple sclerosis (MS)
  - Incomplete rim enhancement most common in ADEM
- Neuromyelitis optica
- Autoimmune-mediated vasculitis
- Acute hypertensive encephalopathy, PRES
- Fabry disease
- Behçet disease

PATHOLOGY

- > 30 different infectious agents & immunizations reported

CLINICAL ISSUES

- Mean age is 5-8 years but can occur at any age
- Male predominance (M:F = 1.0:0.6-0.8), unlike MS
- Usually monophasic, self-limited
- Complete recovery within 1 month: 50-60%
- Mortality: 10-30%

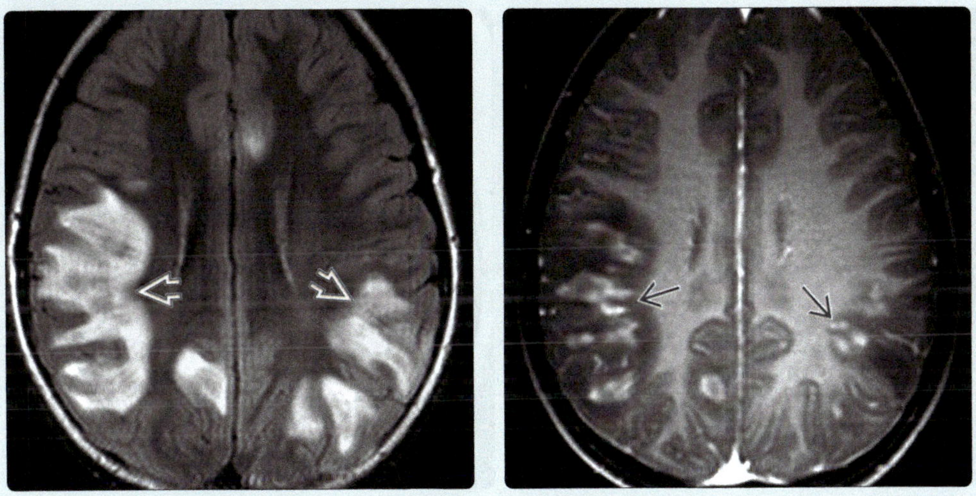

(Left) *Axial FLAIR MR shows peripheral, confluent areas of hyperintensity ➡ predominantly involving the subcortical white matter in this child with ADEM. The bilateral but asymmetric pattern is typical of ADEM.* **(Right)** *Axial T1WI C+ MR in the same patient shows marked, irregular enhancement of nearly all of the lesions ➡. Because ADEM is usually a monophasic illness, enhancement of the majority of lesions is typical, as the lesions all have a similar time course. Enhancement of MS lesions is more variable.*

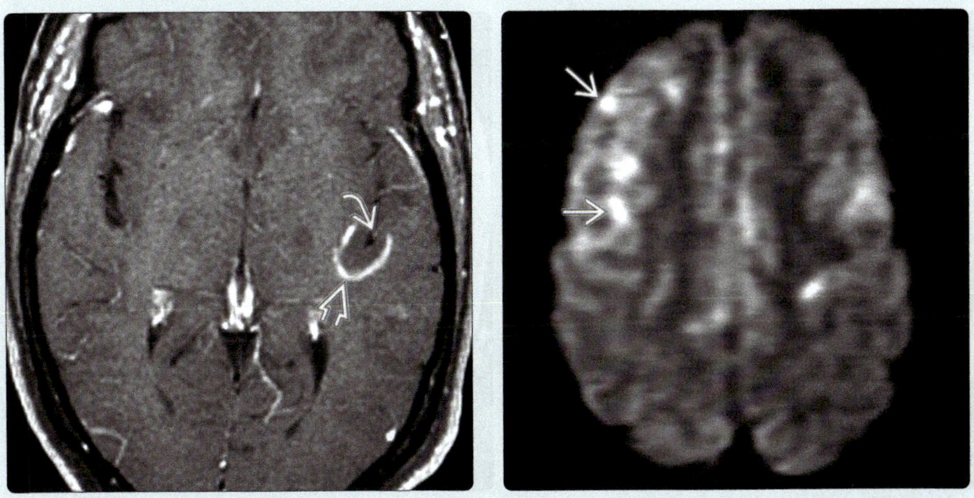

(Left) *Axial T1WI C+ MR shows an incomplete ring or "horseshoe" of peripheral enhancement ➡ with open ends pointing toward the cortex ➡, classic for a demyelinating process (ADEM > MS).* **(Right)** *Axial DWI MR in a patient with ADEM shows multiple foci of increased signal ➡. The foci were hypointense on ADC images (not shown), indicating diffusion restriction. White matter, gray matter involvement is present. Diffusion restriction is an uncommon finding, associated with a worse prognosis.*

KEY FACTS

TERMINOLOGY

- **C**hronic **l**ymphocytic **i**nflammation with **p**ontine **p**erivascular **e**nhancement **r**esponsive to **s**teroids (CLIPPERS)
  - Predominantly involving brainstem, adjacent rhombencephalic structures
  - Shows clinical, imaging response to glucocorticosteroids

IMAGING

- Location: Predominately pons
  - May extend into cerebellar peduncles, hemispheres
  - Caudally into medulla, spinal cord
  - Rostrally into midbrain
- MR
  - Classic: Enhancing punctate/curvilinear lesions; pons often appears "peppered"; may exhibit subtle radiating pattern
  - ± faint, patchy or "speckled" punctate hyperintensities on T2/FLAIR
  - Beware: May begin as isolated, enhancing mass in pons/cerebellar peduncle before exhibiting typical pattern of multifocal punctate pontine lesions

TOP DIFFERENTIAL DIAGNOSES

- Angiocentric (intravascular) lymphoma
- Neurosarcoidosis
- Demyelinating disease (multiple sclerosis, neuromyelitis optica spectrum)
- Vasculitis (primary, secondary, Behçet)
- Lymphomatoid granulomatosis
- CNS histiocytosis (Langerhans cell histiocytosis, Erdheim-Chester, hemophagocytic)

CLINICAL ISSUES

- Brainstem symptoms, gait ataxia, diplopia
  - Often relapsing-remitting course (without treatment)
  - Mean age at onset 40-50 years (range 13-86 years)
- Keep in mind: CLIPPERS is diagnosis of exclusion

(Left) *Sagittal FLAIR MR in a 56-year-old woman with weight loss and 3-week history of diplopia and disequilibrium shows confluent and punctate hyperintensities in the pons ➡ and medulla ➡.* **(Right)** *Axial T1 C+ scan in the same patient shows multiple punctate and curvilinear enhancing foci "peppering" the pons ➡. Additional lesions are present in both cerebellar peduncles, vermis, and the left cerebellar hemisphere.*

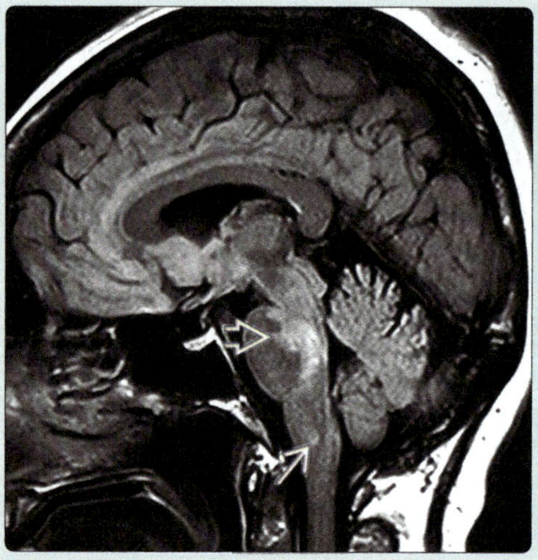

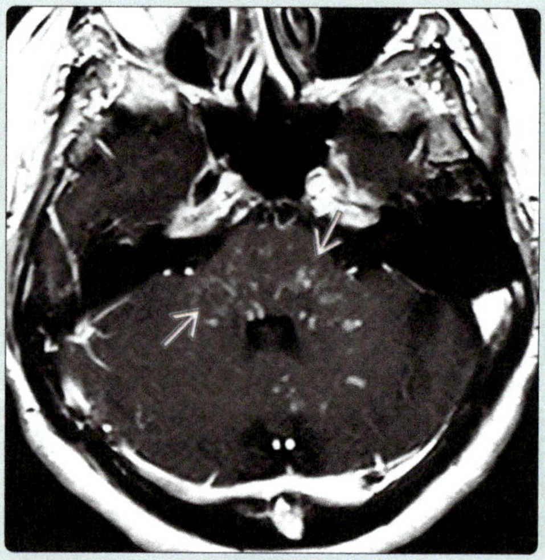

(Left) *More cephalad T1 C+ scan in the same patient shows the punctate ➡ and curvilinear ➡ lesions involving the upper pons.* **(Right)** *Coronal T1 C+ FS scan in the same patient shows the lesions "peppering" the pons. Note cephalad extension into the cerebral peduncles ➡ and inferior extension into the medulla ➡ and upper cervical cord ➡. DSA (not shown) was negative. The lesions resolved with corticosteroids, so this is a presumed case of CLIPPERS.*

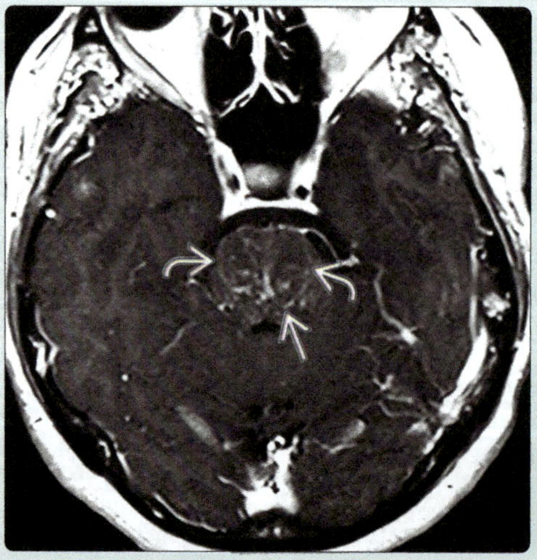

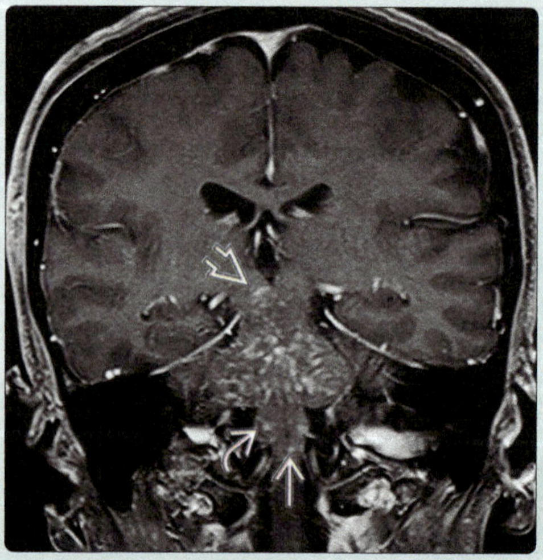

Overview

Inherited metabolic disorders (IMD) are very difficult to diagnose. Affected patients can present at any age; symptoms vary depending on age of onset and severity of the biochemical defect. Completely different parts of the brain may be involved in less severely affected patients compared with more severely affected patients. The same enzyme may perform different functions, in different parts of the brain, as the person matures from infancy to childhood to adulthood. Clearly, patients will have different symptoms if different parts of the brain are involved.

Adding to the confusion, IMDs have been **classified** in many different ways: Biochemical characteristics, the biochemical pathway that is affected, the cellular organelle in which the affected protein or affected biochemical pathway is located, characteristics of clinical presentation, and the gene that is affected. None of these classifications have been very successful, and it is likely that classification by the biochemical pathways affected will, ultimately, be the most useful.

The imaging features of inherited metabolic disorders can be equally confusing, particularly if not approached methodically. The imaging appearances of many disorders overlap and often vary with the stage and the variant of the disease. Imaging is most helpful early in the course of the disease, when it can help to narrow the differential diagnosis and reduce the amount of testing needed. From a neuroimaging perspective, it is most useful to classify disorders based on the **pattern of brain involvement on MR early in the course of the disease**. This pattern can be supplemented by the use of metabolic data (obtained from proton MR spectroscopy), diffusion data (obtained from diffusion-weighted imaging), and, occasionally, magnetization transfer.

First Analysis: White vs. Gray Matter

The first important determination is whether the disease involves primarily gray matter, primarily white matter, or both gray and white matter.

If the gray matter is primarily involved, scrutinize both the cortex and deep nuclei to determine whether involvement is primarily cortical, primarily deep nuclear, or both. Sometimes disorders that primarily affect cortical gray matter will show cortical swelling with effaced sulci early in the course of the disease; more commonly, diagnosis is made later, and cortical thinning is found, with prominent cortical sulci. In later stages, cortical thinning is the rule in all such disorders. The cerebral white matter will often have an abnormal appearance in patients with primary cortical disorders, as Wallerian degeneration of axons causes diminished white matter volume and sometimes mild hyperintensity on FLAIR and T2-weighted images. This appearance can be differentiated from that of primary white matter disorders if the study is performed early in the course of the disease; primarily affected white matter will typically be edematous and, therefore, brighter and more voluminous (causing compressed, smaller sulci) than the white matter that has undergone secondary degeneration. In the acute phase, disorders primarily affecting deep gray matter will typically show edema (FLAIR hyperintensity and prolonged T1 and T2 relaxation times) in the involved structures. In the chronic phase, volume loss with gliosis (resulting in T2 hyperintensity) is more typical.

Disorders primarily affecting white matter cause marked signal abnormality before any volume loss is apparent. Some white matter disorders cause spongiform changes, result in intramyelinic edema, or have an inflammatory component in the early stages. These conditions cause edema with accompanying mass effect on adjacent structures. Diffusion-weighted images can add specificity, as spongiform changes typically cause increased diffusivity, whereas intramyelinic edema and inflammation cause reduced diffusivity. Alternatively, many white matter disorders, such as X-linked adrenoleukodystrophy and fibrinoid leukodystrophy (Alexander disease), start locally and expand to involve adjacent areas. Neither of these appearances are seen in the white matter of gray matter disorders. White matter diseases can result in necrosis and cavitation of the affected regions and subsequent ex vacuo dilation of the ventricles, whereas the abnormal white matter in gray matter disorders appears less severely damaged.

Gray Matter Disorders

Gray matter disorders need to be further analyzed to determine whether the disorder primarily involves the cerebral cortex or the deep gray matter nuclei. If the pattern of the imaging study indicates that the metabolic disorder is **primarily one of cortical involvement** (cortical thinning with enlarged cortical sulci), consideration should be given to disorders such as the neuronal ceroid lipofuscinoses, the mucolipidoses, glycogen storage diseases, or GM1 gangliosidosis.

When **only deep gray matter is involved**, it is important to identify the specific structures that are affected and their signal intensities. Involvement of the striatum (caudate and putamen) is typically seen in mitochondrial disorders [primarily Leigh syndrome, mitochondrial encephalopathy with lactic acidosis and stroke-like symptoms (MELAS), and the glutaric acidurias], propionic acidemia, Wilson disease, juvenile Huntington disease, molybdenum cofactor deficiency, asphyxia, and childhood or adult hypoglycemia.

Associated white matter or cortical injury may be present in many disorders. If globi pallidi show isolated T2 prolongation, then succinate semialdehyde dehydrogenase deficiency, methylmalonic academia (cavitation of globi pallidi), guanidinoacetate methyltransferase deficiency (a creatine synthesis disorder), isovaleric acidemia, pyruvate dehydrogenase deficiency [due to mutation of the dihydrolipoamide acetyltransferase (E2) component], carbon monoxide poisoning, or the chronic phase of kernicterus should be considered. If T2 or FLAIR hyperintensity of the globi pallidi is associated with subcortical white matter demyelination, then sparing of the periventricular white matter and involvement of the cerebellar dentate nuclei, L-2-hydroxyglutaricaciduria, and Kearns-Sayre syndrome should be considered. When the MR shows atrophy of the dorsal brainstem, cerebellar nuclei, and subthalamic nuclei, one should consider Leigh syndrome secondary to *SURF1* mutation. If T1 hyperintensity of the globi pallidi is associated with normal T2 signal, and the patient is not receiving hyperalimentation, consider chronic hepatic disease. If both T1 and T2 hyperintensity are seen in a neonate or young infant, consider acute hyperbilirubinemia of infancy, systemic lupus erythematosus, and hemolytic-uremic syndrome; in the presence of edema involving the external and extreme capsules and the claustrum, hemolytic-uremic syndrome is the most likely. If the globi pallidi, the insula, and perirolandic cortex are all hyperintense on T2-weighted or FLAIR images, the diagnosis of hyperammonemia (frequently due to a urea cycle disorder) should be suggested. If the involvement of the globus pallidus is manifested on MR as T2 hypointensity with central T2 hyperintensity, the diagnosis of pantothenate kinase-associated neuropathy (formerly called Hallervorden-Spatz disease) can be made with some confidence.

White Matter Disorders

White matter disorders can be divided into disorders in which white matter never myelinates completely (**hypomyelination**) and disorders in which myelin forms and breaks down (demyelination) with or without cavitation of white matter. The pattern of a lack of myelination, or hypomyelination, is seen in very few disorders, called the hypomyelinating leukoencephalopathies. These should be differentiated from delayed myelination, which has a very different differential diagnosis. If a follow-up MR in 6 months shows no change or minimal change in myelination, a hypomyelinating disorder can be diagnosed. The appearance of the brain in these disorders is often that of a normal, much more immature brain. For example, the MR of a 5-year-old child with hypomyelination might be mistaken for that of a 5-month-old infant; diffusivity is normal, whereas magnetization transfer is reduced. Such disorders include Pelizaeus-Merzbacher and like diseases, leukodystrophies with trichothiodystrophy and photosensitivity, Tay syndrome, 18q syndrome (deletion of a large portion of the long arm of chromosome 18), sialic acidemia (Salla disease), hypomyelination with atrophy of basal ganglia and cerebellum, and hypomyelination with congenital cataracts. Cerebral or cerebellar atrophy may develop over time in many of these patients.

When myelin develops but is subsequently damaged, the condition is called **demyelination** to differentiate it from breakdown of abnormal myelin, sometimes called **dysmyelination**. By the use of diffusion tensor imaging, it may eventually be possible to differentiate these 2 entities, but the differentiation cannot currently be made. Myelin destruction can, however, be differentiated from white matter cavitation (cystic degeneration). Cystic degeneration has much lower signal on FLAIR sequences, significantly less magnetization transfer, and greater diffusivity than areas of myelin destruction without cavitation. In disorders where inflammation is associated with demyelination (typically peroxisomal disorders), the inflammatory infiltrate causes reduced diffusivity and blood-brain barrier breakdown (resulting in regions of contrast enhancement). When myelin breakdown occurs, the white matter becomes more hypointense on T1-weighted images and more hyperintense on T2-weighted images. In these situations, analyze the brain to determine whether the region primarily affected is the periventricular white matter, the deep white matter, or the subcortical white matter.

Disorders Affecting Gray and White Matter

Disorders involving both gray and white matter are first separated by the type of gray matter involvement: Those involving only the cerebral cortex and those involving deep gray matter (with or without cortical involvement).

Disorders involving only cortical gray matter can be subdivided depending on the involvement of long bones and the spinal column. If the long bones are normal, the cortex should be analyzed for malformations of cortical development (MCD). If an MCD is present in addition to a lack of myelination, the differential diagnosis includes the generalized peroxisomal disorders, congenital cytomegalovirus disease, and the so-called cobblestone cortical malformations. If no MCD is found, differential considerations include Alpers disease and Menkes disease, both of which cause considerable cerebral cortical destruction. If the bones are abnormal, the differential diagnoses include primarily storage diseases, such as the mucopolysaccharidoses and lipid storage disorders.

If deep gray matter is involved, determine precisely which nuclei are affected. If thalami are involved, differential considerations include Krabbe disease and the GM1 and GM2 gangliosidoses; the thalami in these disorders display high attenuation on CT and are hyperintense on T1-weighted images and hypointense on T2-weighted images. Krabbe disease is distinguished by the early presence of abnormal T2 hyperintensity along the corticospinal tracts and in the cerebellar dentate nuclei.

Another disorder with thalamic involvement is profound neonatal hypoxic-ischemic injury, which typically involves the ventrolateral thalami, posterior putamina, and perirolandic cortex; a characteristic history of perinatal distress and neonatal encephalopathy simplifies the diagnosis. Another consideration when thalamic involvement is identified is autosomal-dominant acute necrotizing encephalitis, particularly if T2 hyperintensity is also seen in the dorsal brainstem. Thalami may also be affected in mitochondrial disorders, Wilson disease, and Canavan disease; typically other deep gray matter nuclei will be affected as well (e.g., putamina in mitochondrial disorders and Wilson disease, globi pallidi in Canavan disease). Globus pallidus involvement in association with diffuse white matter disease including the subcortical, deep, and periventricular regions suggests a diagnosis of Canavan disease, particularly if associated with macrocephaly. Association of globus pallidus involvement with affected subcortical white matter but sparing of periventricular white matter suggests a later phase of Kearns-Sayre syndrome or L-2-hydroxyglutaric aciduria; the latter will often show involvement of the cerebellar dentate nuclei.

Globus pallidus injury with sparing of subcortical white matter in early stages suggests methylmalonic academia (look for cavitation), maple syrup urine disease, carbon monoxide toxicity, or cyanide toxicity. MR of maple syrup urine disease during the acute neonatal phase of the disease shows involvement of the centrum semiovale, internal capsules, cerebral peduncles, dorsal pons, and cerebellar white matter, reduced diffusivity in the affected regions, and a peak at 0.9 ppm on proton MR spectroscopy. Carbon monoxide and cyanide toxicity typically involve the cerebral cortex, globi pallidi, and cerebellum. White matter disease associated with striatal involvement suggests Leigh syndrome, MELAS, propionic acidemia, glutaric aciduria type 1, molybdenum cofactor deficiency, isolated sulfite oxidase deficiency, hypomyelination with atrophy of the basal ganglia and cerebellum, toxic exposure, later infantile or childhood profound hypoxic-ischemic injury, or childhood hypoglycemia. Proper analysis of the MR scans using this pattern system can facilitate the work-up of patients with inborn errors of metabolism.

Imaging Patterns

Metabolic Disorders With
T2 or FLAIR Hyperintensity of Corpus Striatum
Leigh syndrome (includes pyruvate dehydrogenase deficiency, respiratory complex I and complex II disorders)
Wilson disease
Glutaric aciduria type 1
Molybdenum cofactor deficiency
Propionic acidemia
T2 or FLAIR Hyperintensity of Globi Pallidi
Methylmalonic acidemia
Succinic semialdehyde dehydrogenase deficiency
Urea cycle disorders
Guanidinoacetate methyltransferase deficiency
Pyruvate dehydrogenase (E2) deficiency
Systemic lupus erythematosus
Hemolytic-uremic syndrome
Bilirubin toxicity
Isovaleric acidemia
Carbon monoxide or cyanide toxicity
Early Involvement of Subcortical White Matter
Alexander disease
Kearns-Sayre syndrome
Galactosemia
Mitochondrial disorders
Early Involvement of Periventricular and Deep White Matter With Sparing of Subcortical White Matter
X-linked adrenoleukodystrophy
Krabbe disease (globoid cell leukodystrophy)
Metachromatic leukodystrophy
GM2 gangliosidoses
Childhood ataxia with CNS hypomyelination (vanishing white matter disease)
Merosin-deficient congenital muscular dystrophy with cortical malformation
Damage from radiation or chemotherapy
Globus Pallidus and White Matter Involvement
Canavan disease
Methylmalonic acidemia
Kearns-Sayre syndrome
L-2-hydroxyglutaric aciduria
Maple syrup urine disease
Carbon monoxide or cyanide poisoning
Striatal (Caudate and Putaminal) and White Matter Involvement
Leigh syndrome
Mitochondrial encephalopathy with lactic acidosis and stroke-like symptoms (MELAS)
Other mitochondrial leukoencephalopathies
Propionic acidemia
Glutaric acidemia type 1
Isolated sulfite oxidase deficiency
Late infantile/childhood profound hypoxic-ischemic injury
Childhood hypoglycemia

(Left) *Axial T2WI MR in a patient with Kearns-Sayre syndrome shows bilateral globus pallidus hyperintensity* . **(Right)** *More cephalad T2WI MR in the same case shows involvement of subcortical white matter* *with sparing of periventricular regions.*

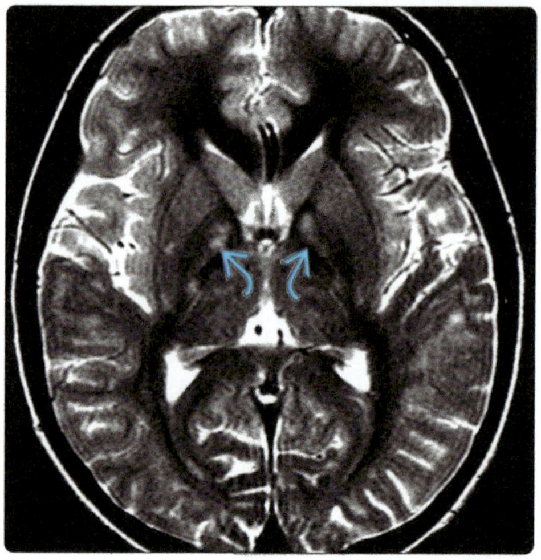

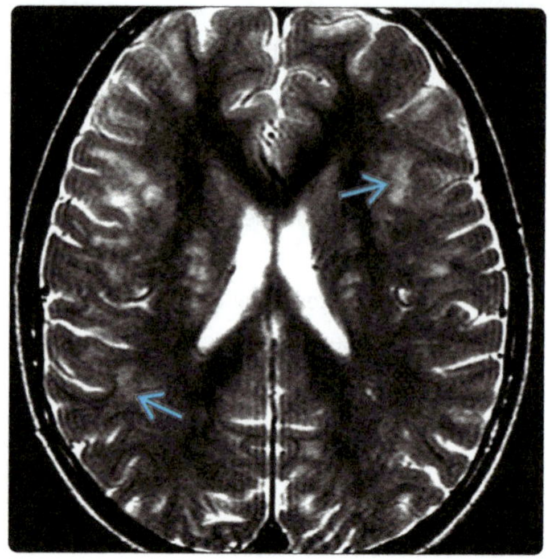

(Left) *Axial FLAIR MR in a 22-month-old child with macrocephaly and decreasing acquisition of developmental milestones shows large, bilateral temporal lobe cysts* *typical of megalencephaly with leukoencephalopathy and cysts (MLC). The hypomyelinated white matter is swollen and diffusely hyperintense.* **(Right)** *Axial FLAIR MR in a 2-year-old child with MLC shows swollen, hyperintense hypomyelinated white matter* *and numerous subcortical cysts* .

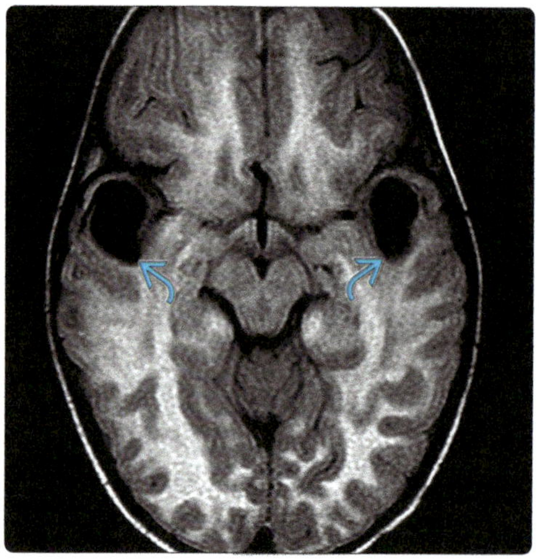

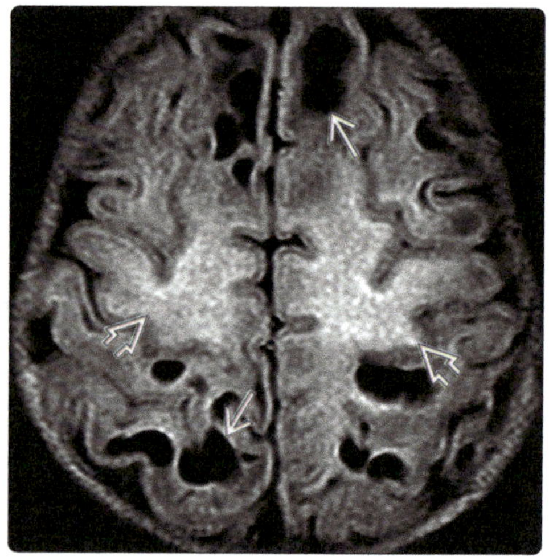

(Left) *Axial T2WI MR in a child with methylmalonic acidemia shows abnormal hyperintensity* *of the bilateral globi pallidi. The white matter is unaffected in this patient.* **(Right)** *Axial FLAIR MR shows multiple areas of hypointense cavitation* *in the cerebral white matter in this patient with vanishing white matter disease. The less affected subcortical white matter* *is hyperintense.*

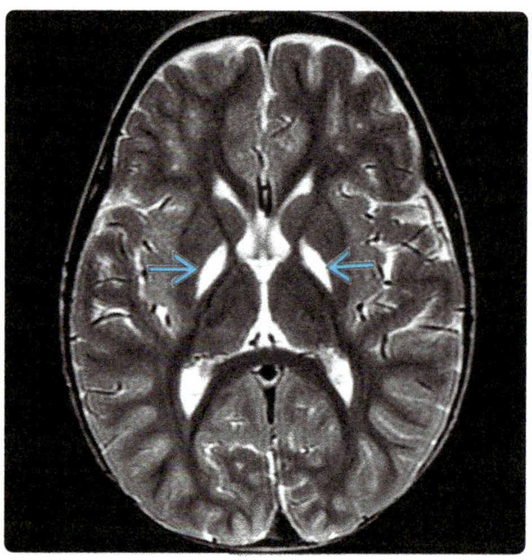

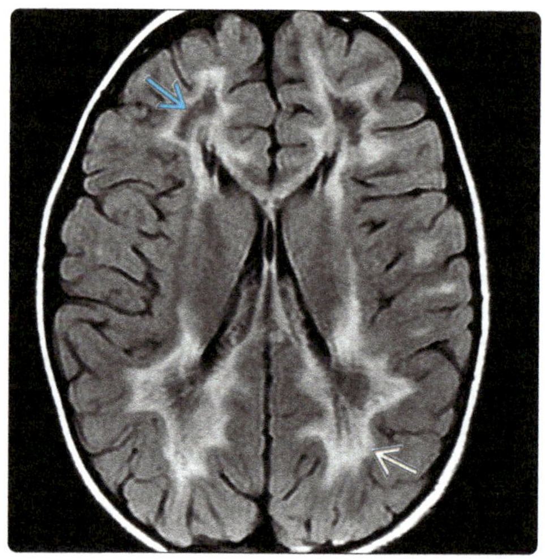

KEY FACTS

TERMINOLOGY

- a.k.a. subacute necrotizing encephalomyelopathy
- Genetically heterogeneous mitochondrial disorder characterized by progressive neurodegeneration

IMAGING

- Best imaging: MR with DWI/MRS
  - Bilateral, symmetric ↑ T2/FLAIR corpora striata (putamen > caudate) > globi pallidi, periaqueductal gray matter, substantia nigra/subthalamic nuclei, dorsal pons, cerebellar nuclei
  - Reduced diffusion in regions of acute disease
  - Lactate peak often present on MRS; may be large
  - Uncommon appearance: Predominant white matter disease (simulates leukodystrophy)

TOP DIFFERENTIAL DIAGNOSES

- Profound perinatal asphyxia
- Mitochondrial encephalopathy, lactic acidosis, stroke-like episodes (MELAS)
- Glutaric aciduria type 1
- Wilson disease

PATHOLOGY

- Bioenergetic failure (ATP loss) and production of reactive oxygen species likely key factors in mitochondria-mediated cell apoptosis
- 50-75% of patients with Leigh syndrome have detectable biochemical or molecular abnormality

CLINICAL ISSUES

- Presentation
  - Psychomotor delay/regression, dystonia/hypotonia, ataxia
  - Other: Ophthalmoplegia, seizures, lactic acidosis
- Prenatal diagnosis: Chorionic villus sampling (mutations and biochemical defects)
- Majority present by age 2 years

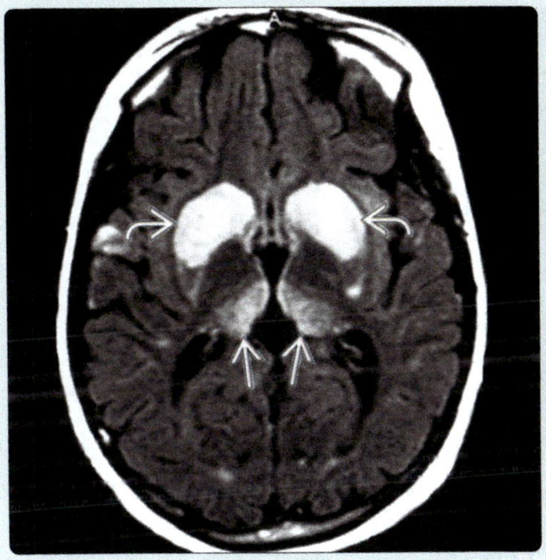

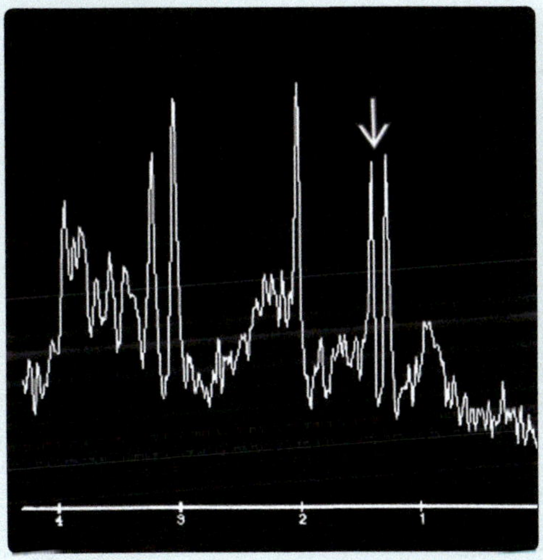

(Left) *Axial FLAIR MR shows swelling and abnormal hyperintensity in the caudate heads and putamina. Foci of hyperintensity are also present in the medial thalami, a typical location of involvement in Leigh syndrome.* **(Right)** *Single voxel proton MR spectroscopy (TE = 26 ms) of the same patient shows a large lactate doublet at 1.3 ppm. The identification of a lactate peak supports the diagnosis of mitochondrial disease but is variably present.*

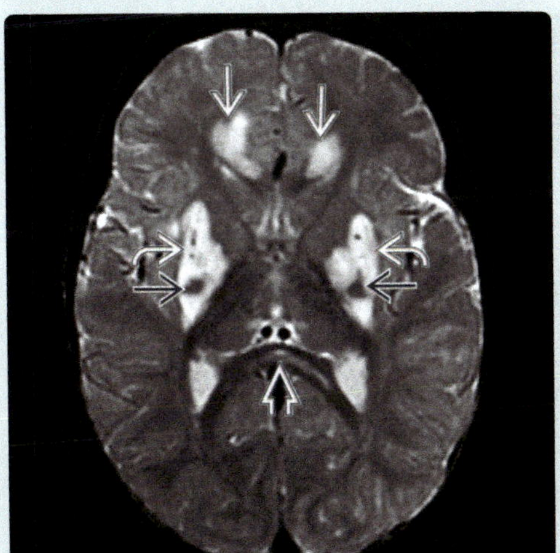

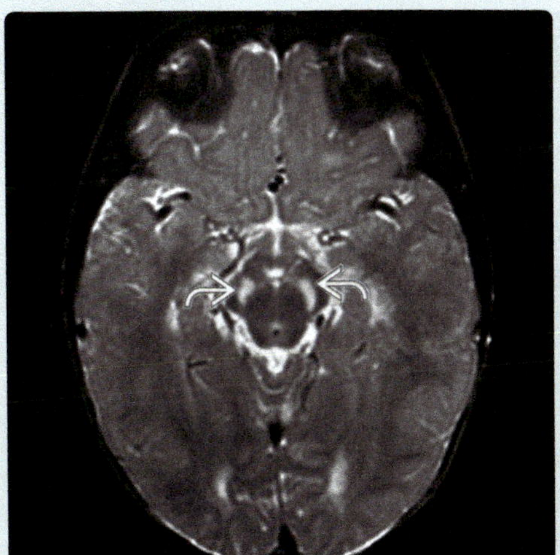

(Left) *Axial T2WI MR shows T2 hyperintensity and some swelling of the lentiform nuclei bilaterally. In addition, the genu and splenium of the corpus callosum are affected. Note that foci of unaffected tissue are present in the putamina; heterogeneous involvement is common.* **(Right)** *Axial T2WI MR in the same patient shows T2 hyperintensity of the cerebral peduncles. This is another common site of involvement in Leigh syndrome.*

KEY FACTS

TERMINOLOGY

- **M**itochondrial myopathy, **e**ncephalopathy, **l**actic **a**cidosis, and **s**troke-like episodes (MELAS)
- Inherited disorder of intracellular energy production caused by point mutation in mtDNA

IMAGING

- Stroke-like cortical lesions crossing vascular territories
  - Posterior location most common
- "Shifting spread" (appearance, disappearance, reappearance elsewhere) is classic
- Lactate "doublet" at 1.3 ppm in 60-65%
  - Elevated lactate in cerebrospinal fluid, "normal" brain on MRS
- Basal ganglia lesions and calcifications

PATHOLOGY

- mtDNA contribution to zygote exclusively maternal inheritance
- Caution: Relationship of phenotype to genotype complex, variable
- Mutations may present as MELAS but also as other mitochondrial phenotypes

CLINICAL ISSUES

- Classic MELAS triad: Lactic acidosis, seizures, stroke-like episodes
  - Onset of stroke-like episodes usually occurs in childhood/early adulthood
  - Also: Sensorineural hearing loss, diabetes, short stature

DIAGNOSTIC CHECKLIST

- Think
  - MELAS in patient with acute stroke-like cortical lesion that crosses usual vascular territories
- Consider
  - MELAS in adult presenting with unusual and recurrent stroke-like episodes

(Left) *Axial graphic shows pathology of MELAS. Acute gyriform cortical swelling that crosses vascular territories is depicted →. Note old lacunes →, generalized/focal atrophy with large sulci →.* **(Right)** *Axial FLAIR MR in an 8-year-old girl with short stature and new-onset stroke-like symptoms reveals a focus of abnormally increased signal intensity in the right thalamus → and extensive hyperintensity and abnormal thickening of the cerebral cortex → in the right occipital lobe. The underlying WM is largely spared.*

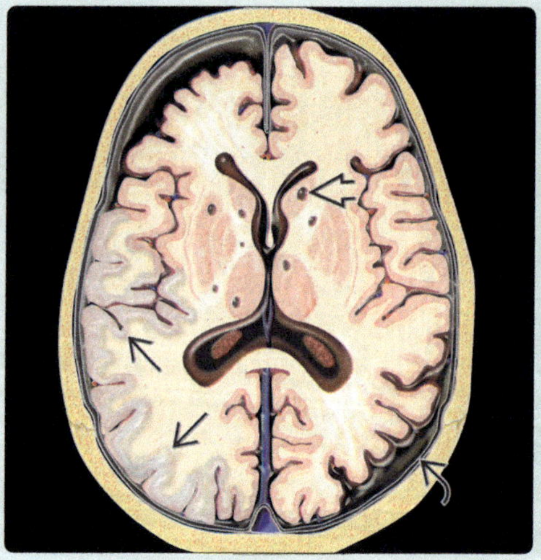

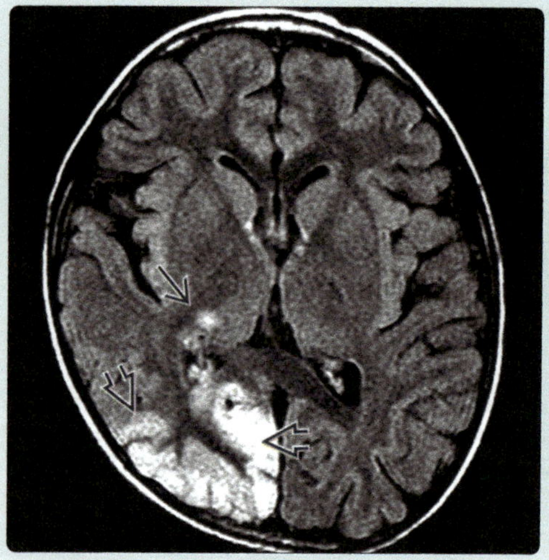

(Left) *Axial T2WI MR in the same patient shows similar abnormal signal hyperintensity lesions in the same thalamic focus of signal increase → and in the edematous right occipital cortex →. Note the prominent subarachnoid spaces, which may result from malnutrition, medications, or the disease process itself.* **(Right)** *Axial DWI MR demonstrates reduced diffusion in the affected regions of the brain →, confirming the acuity of the lesion.*

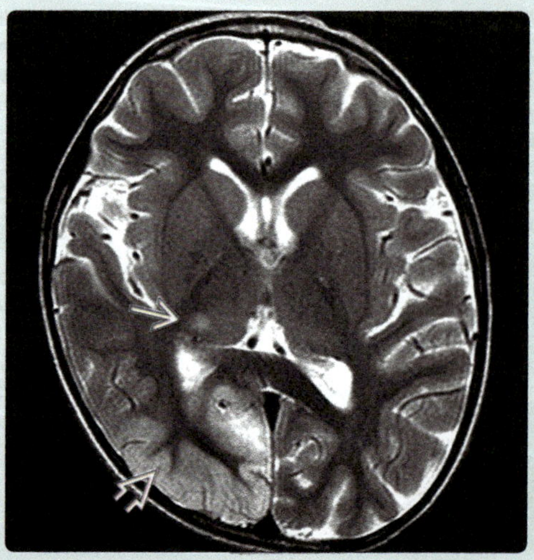

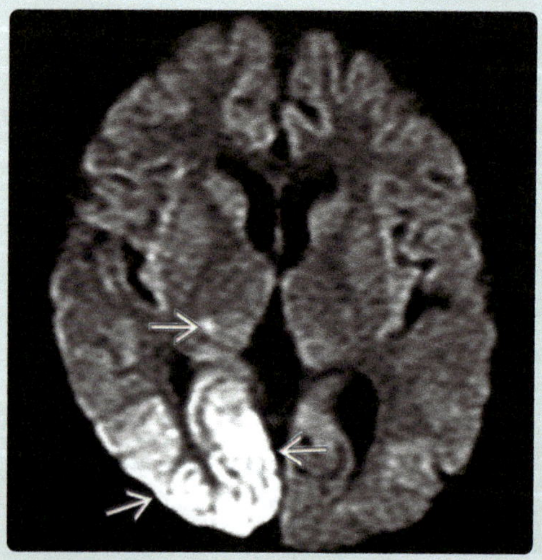

KEY FACTS

TERMINOLOGY

- Clinical phenotypes associated with single large-scale mtDNA deletions (SLSMDs)
  - Kearns-Sayre syndrome (KSS)
  - Chronic progressive external ophthalmoplegia
  - Pearson syndrome
    - Multisystem disorder characterized by bone marrow failure, pancreatic insufficiency
    - Children who survive develop KSS later in life
- SLSMDs often exhibit overlapping disease spectrum
  - Most common non-CNS disease; anemia, renal impairment, endocrine disturbance

IMAGING

- Can be normal (especially early in disease)
- Diffuse symmetric Ca++ in basal ganglia on NECT
- ↑ T2 signal in hemispheric subcortical WM, U fibers, corpus callosum, globi pallidi, substantia nigra, posterior brainstem
  - Early sparing of periventricular WM
  - Occasional radial stripes in hyperintense WM
- Posterior fossa lesions
  - Dorsal brainstem, bilateral brachium pontis; cerebellar WM

PATHOLOGY

- Polygenetic: Caused by various mtDNA rearrangements
- Status spongiosus, spongy myelinopathy
- Cerebellar atrophy
- Ragged-red fibers on muscle biopsy

CLINICAL ISSUES

- Common symptoms: Progressive external ophthalmoplegia, ataxia, retinitis pigmentosa, sensorineural hearing loss
- Additional symptoms: Short stature, proximal muscle weakness, diabetes
  - Cardiac abnormalities 1 of most feared complications
- Age of onset usually before 20 years

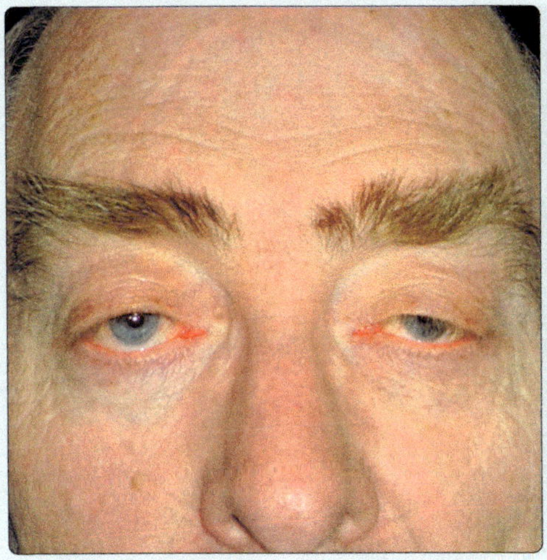
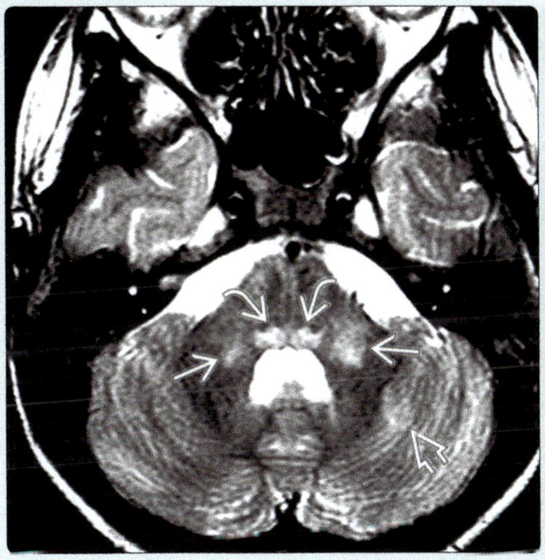

(Left) *Clinical photograph of a patient with chronic progressive external ophthalmoplegia (CPEO). He had weakness of eye closure and limitation of gaze in all directions.* **(Right)** *Axial T2WI MR in a teenager with symptomatic Kearns-Sayre syndrome demonstrates abnormal increased signal intensity bilaterally in the brachium pontis ➡, dorsal pons ➡, and cerebellum ➡. Widening of the interfoliate sulci results from mild cerebellar atrophy.*

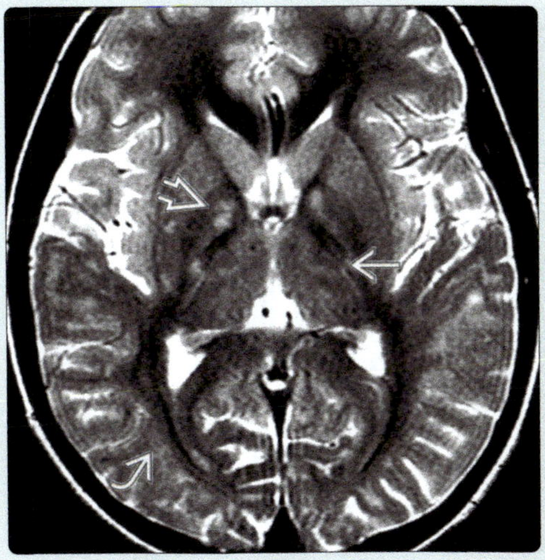
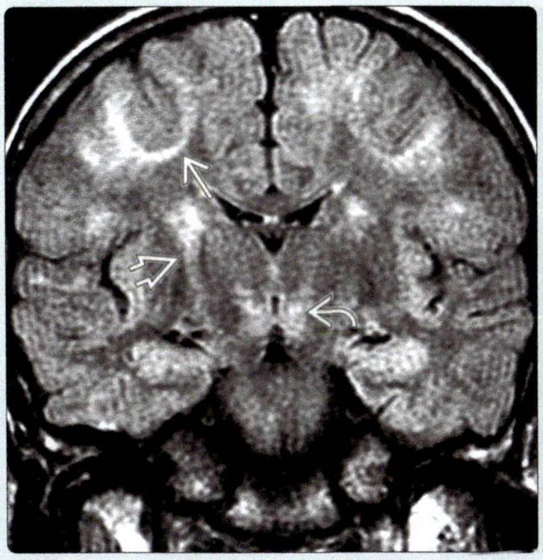

(Left) *Axial T2WI MR in the same teenager demonstrates foci of abnormal signal bilaterally within the globi pallidi ➡ and the corticospinal tracts ➡. Note the subtle loss of myelin arborization into the subcortical U fibers ➡.* **(Right)** *Coronal FLAIR MR in the same patient shows abnormal hyperintense signal in corticospinal tracts ➡, subcortical U fibers ➡, and thalami ➡.*

Mucopolysaccharidoses

KEY FACTS

TERMINOLOGY

- Mucopolysaccharidoses (MPS): 1-9
- Group of lysosomal storage disorders
  - Characterized by inability to break down glycosaminoglycans (GAGs)
  - Undegraded GAGs toxic, accumulate in multiple organs
  - Each type of MPS causes accumulation of particular GAG in lysosomes, extracellular matrix
  - 11 known enzyme deficiencies, resulting in 7 distinct forms of MPS
    - Prototype MPS = MPS 1H (Hurler)

IMAGING

- Perivascular spaces (PVS) dilated by accumulated GAG
- Favored sites of dilated PVSs in MPS: Corpus callosum, peritrigonal white matter (WM)
  - Can occur in other lobes
- Single to too many to count
- Dysostosis multiplex, broad ribs, trident hands
- Progressive odontoid dysplasia → risk atlantoaxial subluxation; some correction follows bone marrow transplant (BMT)

CLINICAL ISSUES

- Prognosis, deterioration rate depends on specific enzyme deficiency
- Treatment: BMT or IV recombinant human enzyme (e.g., MPS 1H: α-L-iduronidase)
- Significant correlation exists between WM alterations and mental retardation

DIAGNOSTIC CHECKLIST

- Always visualize foramen magnum on any CNS study for craniovertebral junction compression
- Airway: Major sedation and anesthesia risk
- Not all MPS have typical facial features, dilated Virchow-Robin spaces may still signal less common MPS
- Look at upper cervical spine on sagittal images; aids in making diagnosis

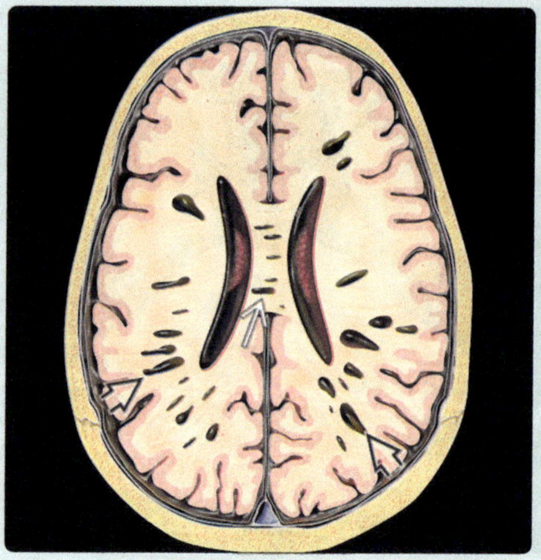

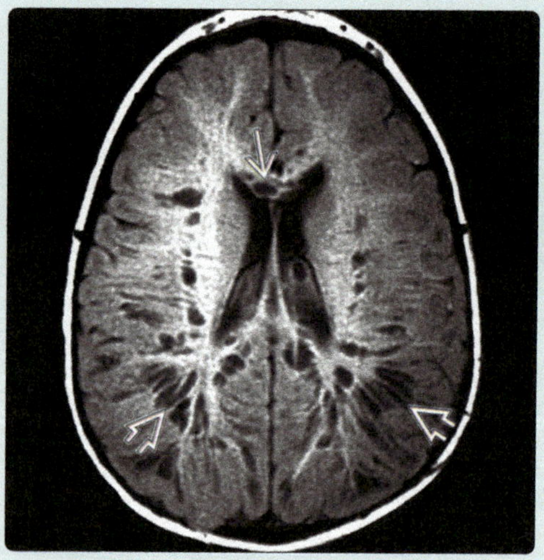

(Left) *Axial graphic of a prototype mucopolysaccharidosis (MPS) shows multiple dilated perivascular spaces radially oriented in the white matter (WM) of the brain. Note the posterior predominance and involvement of the corpus callosum* ➡ *and parietal WM* ➡. **(Right)** *Axial T1WI MR in a toddler with MPS 1H demonstrates prominent perivascular spaces involving the WM, including the corpus callosum* ➡. *Note the posterior predominance of involvement* ➡, *which is typical in MPS.*

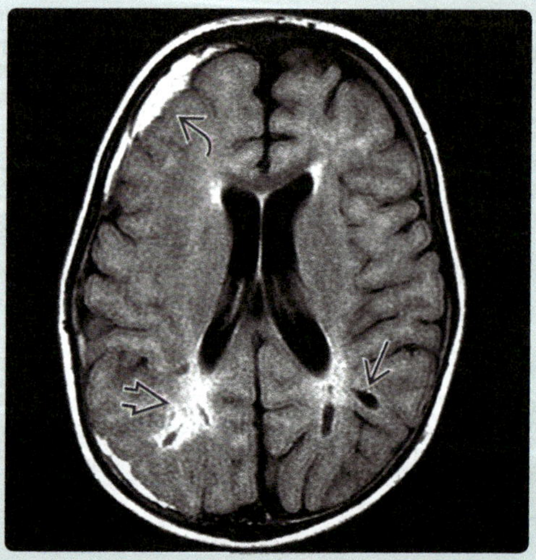

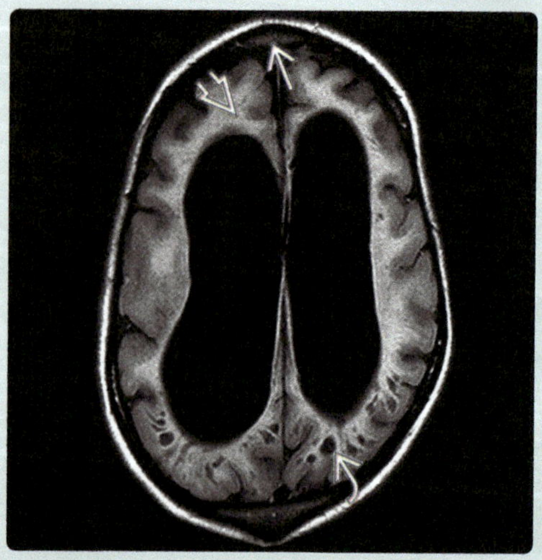

(Left) *Axial FLAIR MR in a boy with MPS 2 reveals a few dilated perivascular spaces* ➡ *surrounded by gliotic WM* ➡. *Note the unilateral subdural hematoma* ➡. *Extraaxial bleeds, while uncommon, have been reported in MPS with vasculopathy, trauma, or large subdural effusions.* **(Right)** *Axial FLAIR MR in a different boy with MPS 2 demonstrates dilated perivascular spaces* ➡, *hyperintense WM* ➡, *and hydrocephalus. Note the typical anterior beaking* ➡.

KEY FACTS

TERMINOLOGY

- Lysosomal storage disorder
  - Caused by ↓ arylsulfatase A
  - Results in CNS, PNS demyelination
- 3 clinical forms
  - Late infantile (most common), juvenile, adult

IMAGING

- Best diagnostic clue: Confluent butterfly-shaped ↑ T2 signal in deep cerebral hemispheric white matter (WM)
  - Early: Spares subcortical U fibers
    - Corpus callosum splenium, parietooccipital WM initially
    - Rapid centrifugal spread to frontal, temporal WM
  - Late: Involves subcortical U fibers
- Sparing of perivenular myelin = tigroid or leopard pattern
- No WM enhancement
  - Reports cranial nerve, cauda equina enhancement

TOP DIFFERENTIAL DIAGNOSES

- Pelizaeus-Merzbacher disease
- TORCH
- Pseudo-TORCH
- Periventricular leukomalacia
- Sneddon syndrome (arylsulfatase A pseudodeficiency)
- Krabbe disease
- Megalencephaly with leukoencephalopathy and cysts

CLINICAL ISSUES

- Clinical profile: Toddler with visuomotor impairment and abdominal pain

DIAGNOSTIC CHECKLIST

- Adult patients presenting with cryptic spasticity of legs should be screened for X-linked adrenoleukodystrophy/adrenomyeloneuropathy, lysosomal disorders (e.g., MLD)

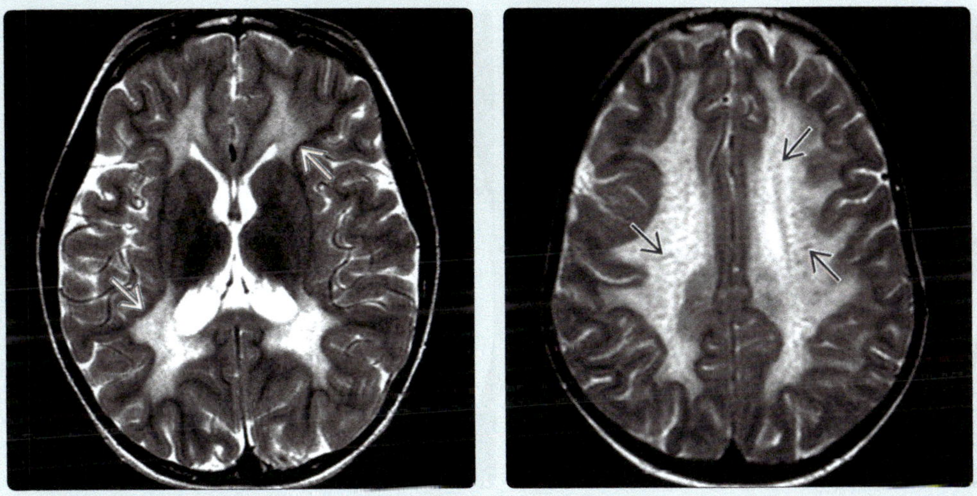

(Left) *Axial T2WI MR shows typical butterfly-shaped pattern of white matter (WM) involvement in metachromatic leukodystrophy (MLD). Note the sparing of internal/external capsules and subcortical U fibers ➡, typical of early disease.* **(Right)** *Axial T2WI MR shows confluent, symmetric WM hyperintensity with sparing of subcortical U fibers. Perivenular myelin sparing causes the hypointense lines and dots within the WM ➡, the characteristic tigroid or leopard pattern of MLD.*

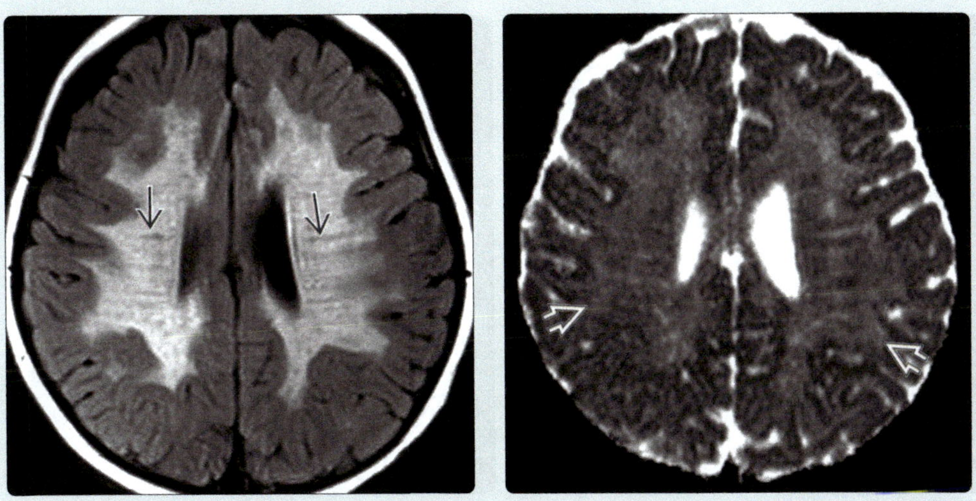

(Left) *Axial FLAIR MR demonstrates the characteristic confluent, symmetric, central WM involvement of MLD. The tigroid or leopard pattern of lines ➡ and dots within the cerebral hemispheric WM is evident.* **(Right)** *Axial ADC map in the same patient shows high signal intensity within the affected WM ➡ consistent with increased diffusivity and probable interstitial edema. Reduced diffusivity (cytotoxic edema) is sometimes seen in areas of active demyelination.*

KEY FACTS

TERMINOLOGY

- Fabry disease (FD)

IMAGING

- NECT
    - Ca++ in lateral pulvinar, globus pallidus, putamen, substantia nigra, dentate nuclei
- MR may show earlier changes
    - ↑ T1 signal in deep gray nuclei
    - T1 lateral pulvinar hyperintensity considered pathognomonic of FD
    - T2/FLAIR hyperintensities in periventricular white matter, deep gray matter

TOP DIFFERENTIAL DIAGNOSES

- Endocrinologic disorders
    - Hyperparathyroidism, hypoparathyroidism, pseudohypoparathyroidism, hypothyroidism
- HIV-associated mineralizing calcific microangiopathy
- Fahr disease

PATHOLOGY

- X-linked disorder of glycosphingolipid metabolism
- Deficient activity of α-galactosidase A
- Endothelial accumulation of glycosphingolipids
    - Compromises vessel lumen size
    - Leads to vascular events
        - Most common: Myocardial ischemia, strokes

CLINICAL ISSUES

- Angiokeratomas of skin
- Neurologic complications in 4th/5th decades
    - Lancinating pains early on
- Enzyme replacement therapy may help

DIAGNOSTIC CHECKLIST

- Consider FD in young male patients with white matter disease, basal ganglia/pulvinar calcification
- T1 hyperintensity in pulvinar is highly suggestive of FD

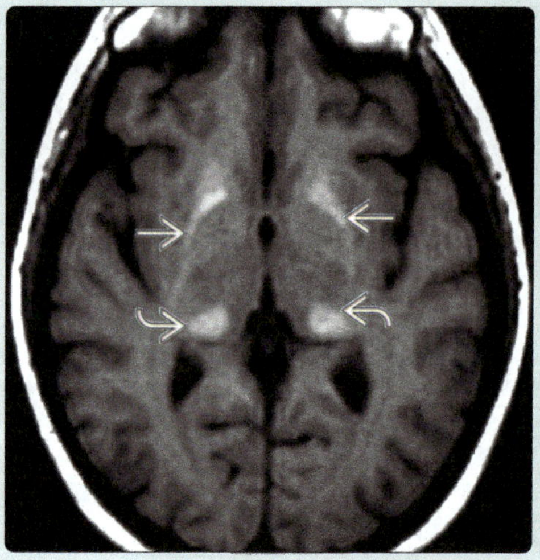

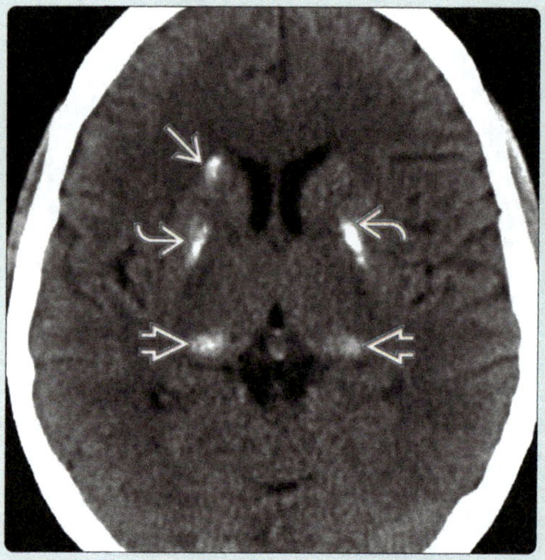

(Left) *Axial T1WI MR in a patient with Fabry disease shows bilateral hyperintense lesions in the lateral putamina and lateral aspects of both pulvinars. T1 hyperintensity in the lateral pulvinar is considered a virtually pathognomonic sign of Fabry disease.* **(Right)** *Axial NECT in the same patient shows calcifications in the right caudate and both putamina and lateral pulvinars, corresponding to the T1 hyperintensities seen on the previous MR scan.*

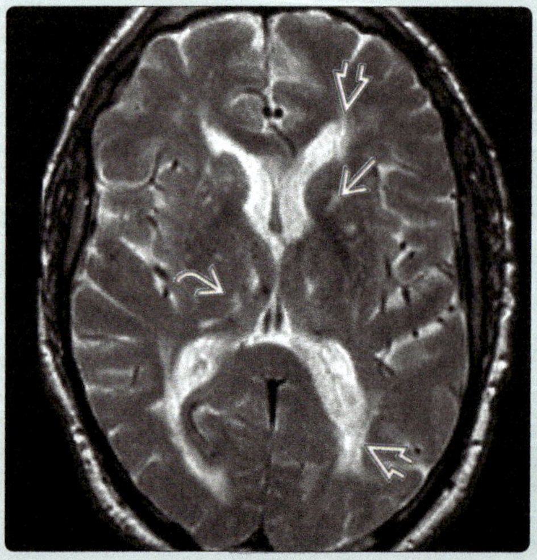

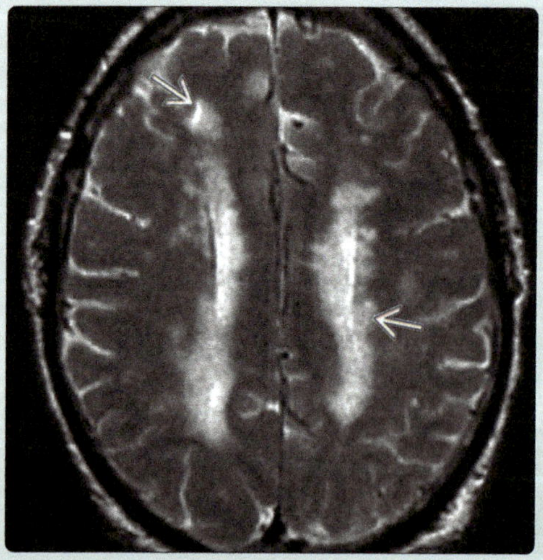

(Left) *Axial T2WI MR in a 50-year-old man with Fabry disease shows multifocal lacunar infarcts in the basal ganglia and thalami, as well as confluent hyperintensities in the deep periventricular white matter.* **(Right)** *Axial T2WI MR in the same patient shows multifocal, discrete, and confluent white matter hyperintensities in the deep cerebral white matter. Deep white matter and basal ganglia infarcts are due to large and small vessel involvement in Fabry disease.*

KEY FACTS

TERMINOLOGY

- Abbreviations
  - X-linked adrenoleukodystrophy (X-ALD)
  - Classic childhood ALD (CCALD)
- Inherited peroxisomal disorder
  - *ABCD1* mutation → impaired β-oxidation of very-long-chain fatty acids (VLCFAs)
  - Accumulation of VLCFAs in white matter causes severe inflammatory demyelination
- Several clinical forms of ALD and related disorders
  - Classic X-ALD
    - Severe form almost exclusively in boys 5-12 years old
  - At least 6 variants other than classic childhood X-ALD
    - Presymptomatic X-ALD, adolescent ALD, adult ALD, adrenomyeloneuropathy (AMN), Addison only, symptomatic female carriers
  - AMN
    - "Mild" adult (spinocerebellar) form, cerebral involvement in up to 50%
    - X-ALD and AMN account for 80% of cases

IMAGING

- 3 zones of myelin loss in CCALD
  - Innermost: Necrotic astrogliotic core
  - Intermediate: Enhancing active demyelination, inflammation
  - Peripheral: Advancing demyelination without inflammation

CLINICAL ISSUES

- X-ALD and variants = 1:16,800 North American births
- Common clinical features
  - Behavioral changes, learning disability
  - Blindness, quadriparesis
  - Seizures (progressive, generally late in course)

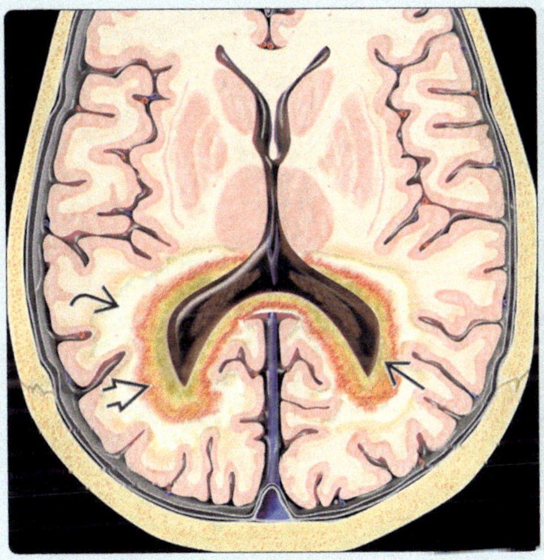

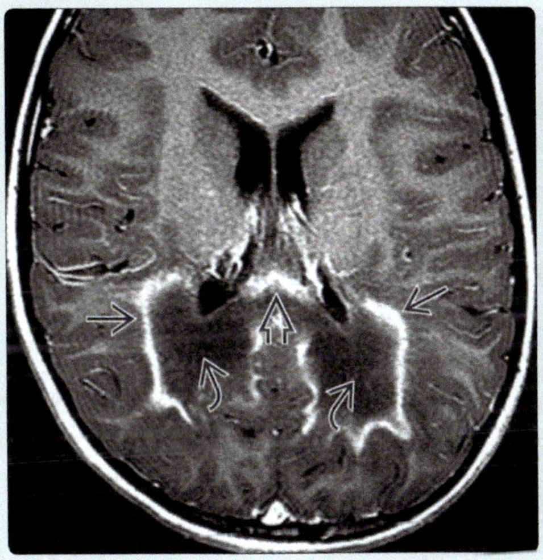

(Left) *Multiple layers of demyelination are shown. The layers correspond to 3 zones histopathologically. The outer layer consists of active destruction and the middle layer of active inflammation. Note that the central area is burnt out.* **(Right)** *Axial T1WI C+ MR reveals marked rim enhancement surrounding the most severely damaged parietal white matter (WM) and the splenium of the corpus callosum in a preteen boy with typical classic childhood adrenoleukodystrophy (CCALD) (Loes pattern 1).*

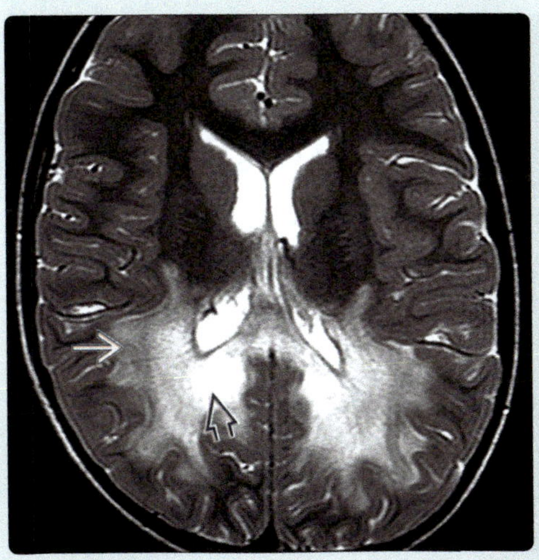

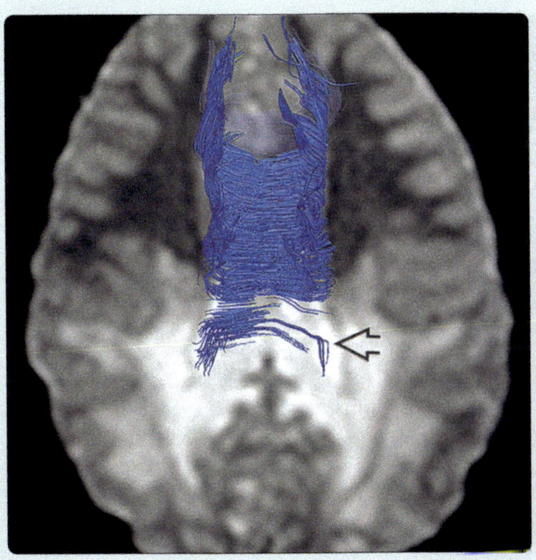

(Left) *Axial T2WI MR distinguishes the active inflammation of the outer zone from the innermost "burnt-out" zone of WM destruction in this preteen boy who presented with well-developed brain involvement.* **(Right)** *Axial tractograph of the corpus callosum from a DTI sequence demonstrates significant loss of WM tracts crossing the splenium of the corpus callosum and forceps major in another preteen symptomatic boy with CCALD.*

Canavan Disease

KEY FACTS

TERMINOLOGY

- Progressive autosomal-recessive spongiform leukodystrophy
    - a.k.a. spongy degeneration of infancy
- Aspartoacyclase deficiency (autosomal recessive)

IMAGING

- White matter
    - Involves subcortical U fibers
    - Spares internal capsule and corpus callosum
- Gray matter
    - Thalami, globi pallidi (GP), ± dentate nuclei
    - Spares caudate, putamen
- ↑ T2 + DWI signal, normal to ↓ apparent diffusion coefficient in involved areas
- MRS shows ↑ NAA/Cr, ↓ Ch/Cr

TOP DIFFERENTIAL DIAGNOSES

- Maple syrup urine disease
- Pelizaeus-Merzbacher disease
- Merosin-deficient congenital muscular dystrophy
- Alexander disease

PATHOLOGY

- Deficiency of aspartoacylase → NAA ↑ in brain and urine
- Spongiform degeneration of white matter; GP and thalami with swollen astrocytes

CLINICAL ISSUES

- Early severe hypotonia and macrocephaly
- Evident by 4 months
- ↑ risk for Ashkenazi Jewish patients (1 in 40 carriers)
- Relentless, progressive neurodegenerative disorder
    - Chronic vegetative state with autonomic crises
    - Death by end of 1st decade
- No proven treatment (gene therapy under evaluation)
    - Acetate supplementation

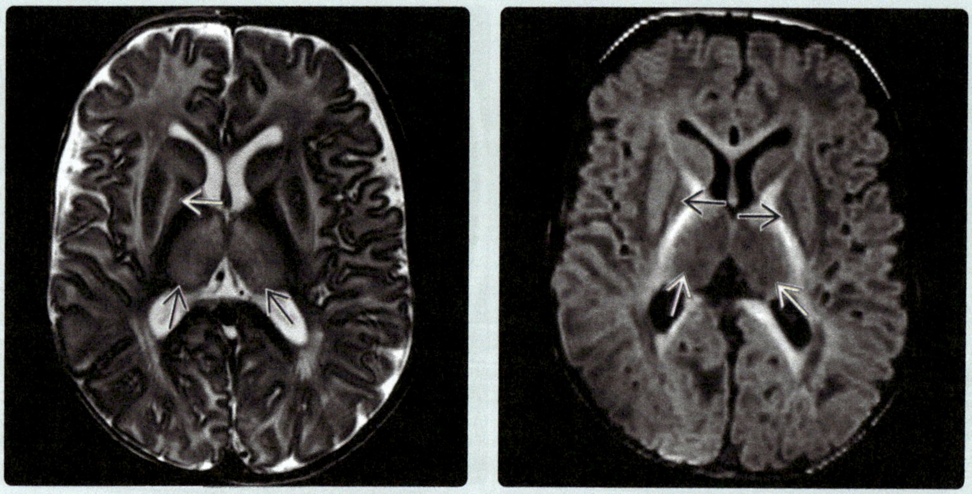

(Left) *Axial T2WI MR in a 6-month-old infant boy shows diffusely increased signal in the cerebral white matter, thalami ⇨, and right globus pallidus ➡ with relative sparing of the internal capsule, corpus callosum, caudate, and putamen.* **(Right)** *Axial T1WI MR in the same 6-month-old infant shows diffusely decreased signal in the white matter, thalami ➡, and globi pallidi ⇨. Normal signal intensity is present within the internal capsule, corpus callosum, caudates, and putamina.*

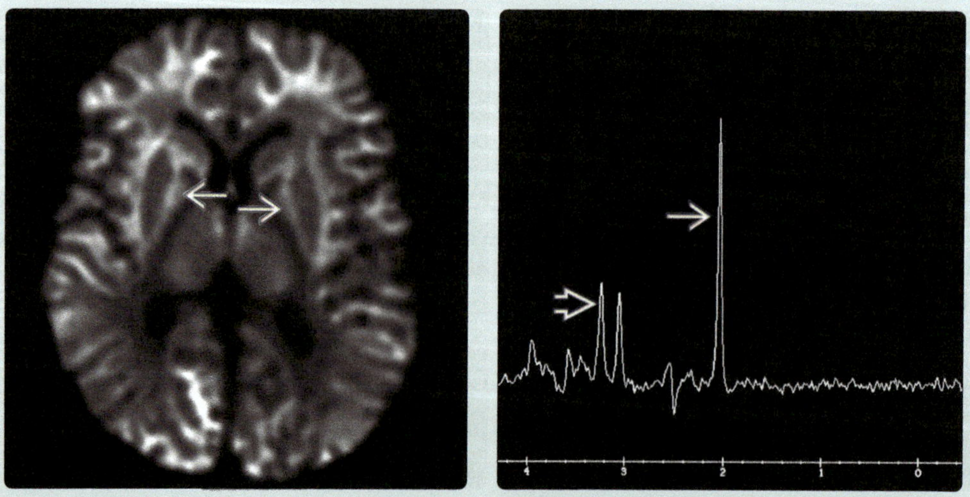

(Left) *Axial DWI MR in the same 6-month-old infant shows diffusely increased signal (reduced diffusivity) in the cerebral white matter and globi pallidi ➡. Normal diffusivity is seen in the myelinated internal capsule and corpus callosum. Caudates and putamina appear unaffected.* **(Right)** *Axial long echo (TE = 144 ms) proton MRS acquired in the centrum semiovale at 1.5T shows a marked relative increase in NAA ➡ and decrease in choline ➡ relative to Cr for age.*

KEY FACTS

TERMINOLOGY

- Rare inherited leukoencephalopathy characterized by Rosenthal fibers (eosinophilic intracytoplasmic inclusions)
- 3 clinical forms
  - Infantile (most common)
  - Juvenile
  - Adult

IMAGING

- Infantile: Symmetric ↑ T2 bifrontal white matter (WM) including subcortical U fibers
- Juvenile/adult: ↑ T2 brainstem (especially medulla), cerebellum, cervical cord
- Other findings: ↓ T2, ↑ T1 enhancing nodular periventricular rim
  - 1 of few metabolic disorders that enhance

TOP DIFFERENTIAL DIAGNOSES

- Canavan disease
- Megaloencephalic leukoencephalopathy with subcortical cysts
- Other: Glutaric aciduria type 1, mucopolysaccharidoses

PATHOLOGY

- Dominant mutations *GFAP* (17q21) (> 95% of cases)

CLINICAL ISSUES

- Clinical profile: Infant with macrocephaly, seizures
- Natural history: Variable rate of progression ultimately leading to death in all forms

DIAGNOSTIC CHECKLIST

- Enhancing, symmetric bifrontal WM disease in macrocephalic infant highly characteristic of Alexander disease (AD)
- Consider adult AD if ↑ T2 signal and atrophy in medulla (inferior olives and gracile nuclei) and cervical cord

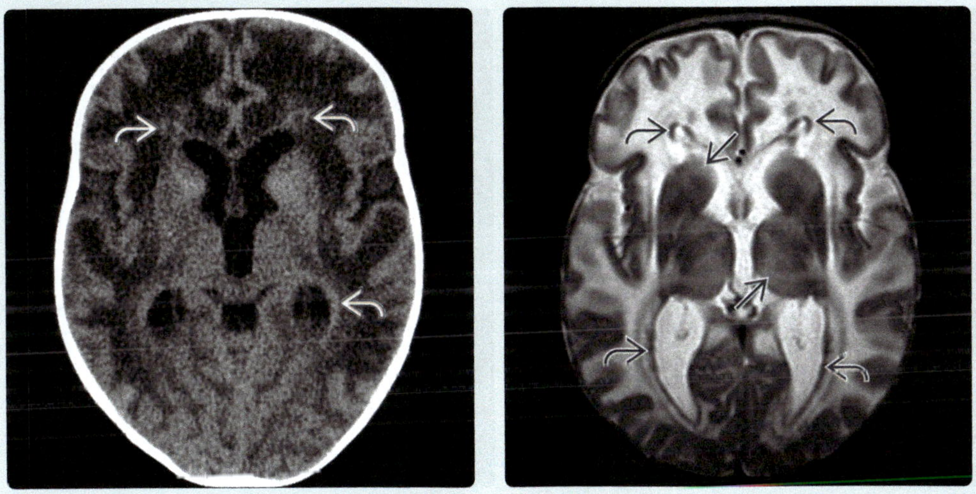

(Left) *Axial NECT shows the typical appearance of infantile Alexander disease. The striatum and periventricular rim are hyperdense. Note the symmetric, frontal predominant, white matter (WM) hypodensity.* **(Right)** *Axial T2WI MR shows a nodular, hypointense, periventricular rim with symmetric, mild hyperintensity in the striata and thalami. The cerebral WM is diffusely hyperintense, greatest in the frontal lobes, where it extends from the ventricular margin to the subcortical U fibers.*

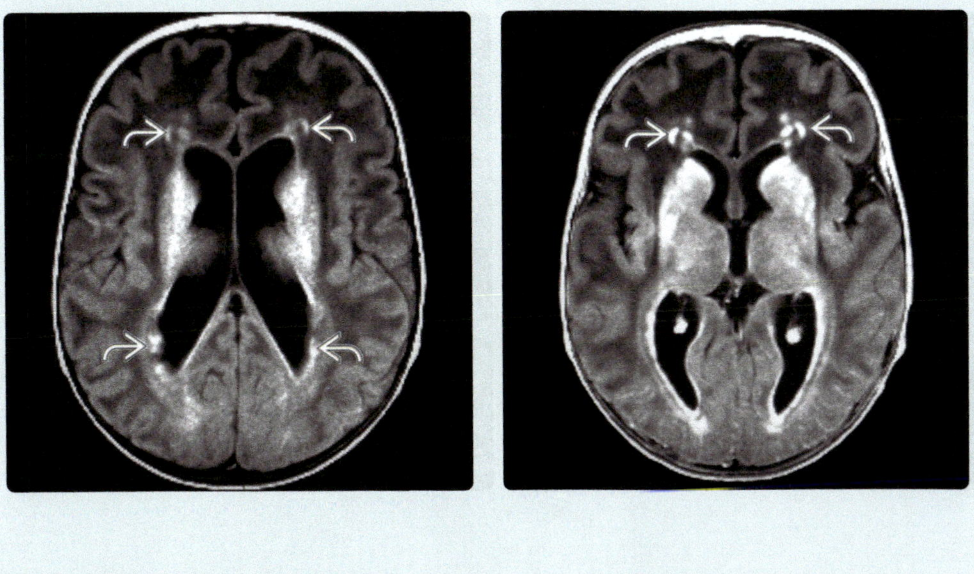

(Left) *Axial T1WI MR shows diffusely hypointense, swollen-appearing WM with a frontal to occipital gradient. Only the occipital WM appears myelinated. The nodular periventricular rim is hyperintense. The lateral ventricles are abnormally enlarged.* **(Right)** *Axial T1WI C+ MR shows enhancement of the periventricular rim, the caudate heads, and the putamina bilaterally. The nodular, rabbit ear appearance of the frontal periventricular rim is typical of Alexander disease.*

Neurodegeneration With Brain Iron Accumulation (NBIA)

KEY FACTS

TERMINOLOGY

- Group of neurodegenerative disorders characterized by dystonia, parkinsonism, and spasticity
  - Caused by mutations in L-ferritin gene *FTL*
  - All characterized by abnormal Fe accumulation in basal ganglia
    - Lewy bodies, axonal swellings, hyperphosphorylated tau in some subtypes
  - Includes (among others)
    - Pantothenate kinase-associated neurodegeneration (PKAN)
    - Infantile neuroaxonal dystrophy (INAD)
    - Aceruloplasminemia

IMAGING

- Globus pallidus (GP) T2 hypointensity with central hyperintensity of GP: Eye of the tiger sign
  - Specific to classic PKAN (*PANK2* mutations)
  - May also be seen in neuroferritinopathy
- GP ± substantia nigra, dentate nucleus, cortex, striatum, & thalamus T2 dark without eye of the tiger sign = other NBIA
- Caution: GP normally hypointense on T2 at 3T or above

PATHOLOGY

- Iron directly causes or facilitates cellular injury or is consequence of axonal disruption

CLINICAL ISSUES

- PKAN
  - Classic < 6 years, atypical during teenage years
- INAD
  - Classic < 2 years, atypical at 4-6 years
- Aceruloplasminemia and neuroferritinopathy
  - Mean age 40 years

DIAGNOSTIC CHECKLIST

- Look for: T2 hypointensity of GP in patient with movement disorder

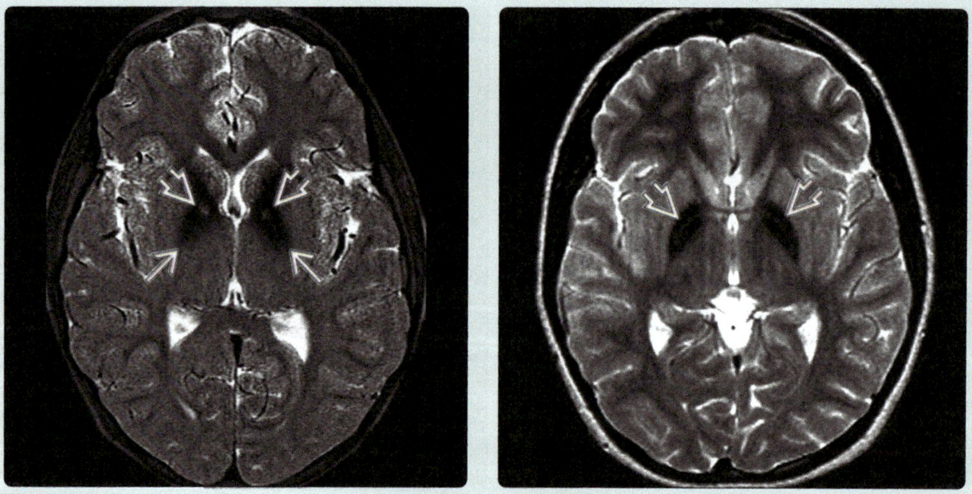

(Left) *Axial T2WI FS MR shows classic imaging of PKAN (Hallervorden-Spatz syndrome), which is within the spectrum of NBIA. Note the globus pallidi hypointensity ➡ related to iron deposition with central hyperintensity ➡, consistent with the eye of the tiger sign, highly specific for the PANK2 mutation.* **(Right)** *Axial T2WI MR shows symmetric hypointensity within the globus pallidi ➡. The eye of the tiger sign is absent; therefore, this is not PKAN. These findings are characteristic of NBIA.*

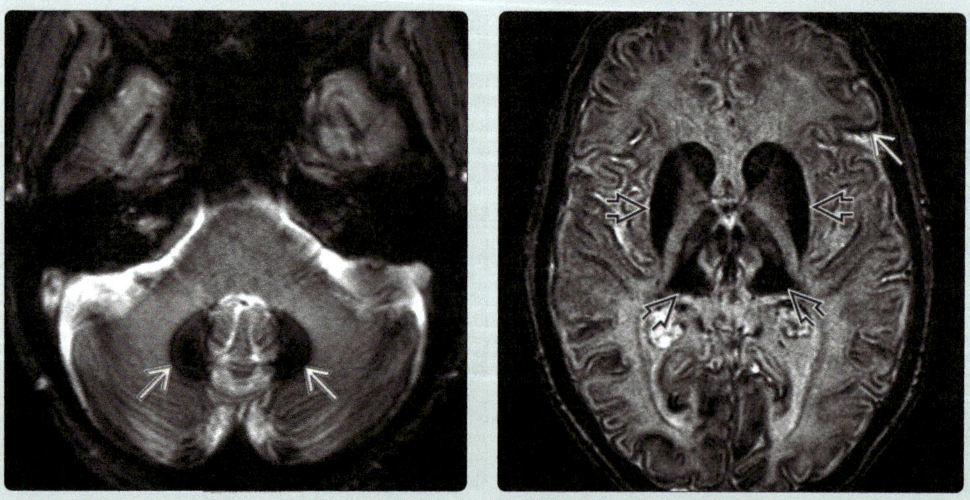

(Left) *Axial T2* GRE MR shows marked hypointensity related to iron deposition in the dentate nuclei ➡ of the cerebellum in this patient with aceruloplasminemia. Aceruloplasminemia and neuroferritinopathy occur in adults and have a similar imaging appearance.* **(Right)** *Axial T2* SWI MR in the same patient shows diffuse linear hypointensity in the cortex ➡ with marked "blooming" in the basal ganglia and thalami ➡ related to iron deposition. Substantia nigra involvement is also typical.*

Pantothenate Kinase-Associated Neurodegeneration (PKAN)

KEY FACTS

TERMINOLOGY

- Pantothenate kinase-associated neurodegeneration (PKAN)
  - Most common form of neurodegeneration with brain iron accumulation (NBIA)
  - Mutated pantothenate kinase 2 gene (*PANK2*)
  - Formerly known as Hallovorden-Spatz disease

IMAGING

- Best diagnostic clue
  - Highly suggestive of PKAN is eye-of-the-tiger sign
    - Diffuse pallidal T2 hypointensity with medial foci ↑ T2 signal

TOP DIFFERENTIAL DIAGNOSES

- Disorders with ↑ T2 signal globus pallidus
  - Metabolic
    - Methylmalonic acidemia, Kearns-Sayre, L-2-hydroxyglutaric aciduria, Canavan, neuroferritinopathy
  - Ischemic/toxic
    - Anoxic encephalopathy, carbon monoxide/cyanide poisoning, kernicterus

CLINICAL ISSUES

- Classic PKAN
  - Dystonia, dysarthria, rigidity, choreoathetosis in young child
- Atypical PKAN
  - Psychiatric, speech, pyramidal/extrapyramidal disturbances in older child/teenager
- Epidemiology
  - Rare; incidence unknown
- Prognosis
  - Classic PKAN: Fatal; mean disease duration after symptom onset is 11 years
  - Atypical PKAN: Eventual severe impairment/death
- No curative treatment

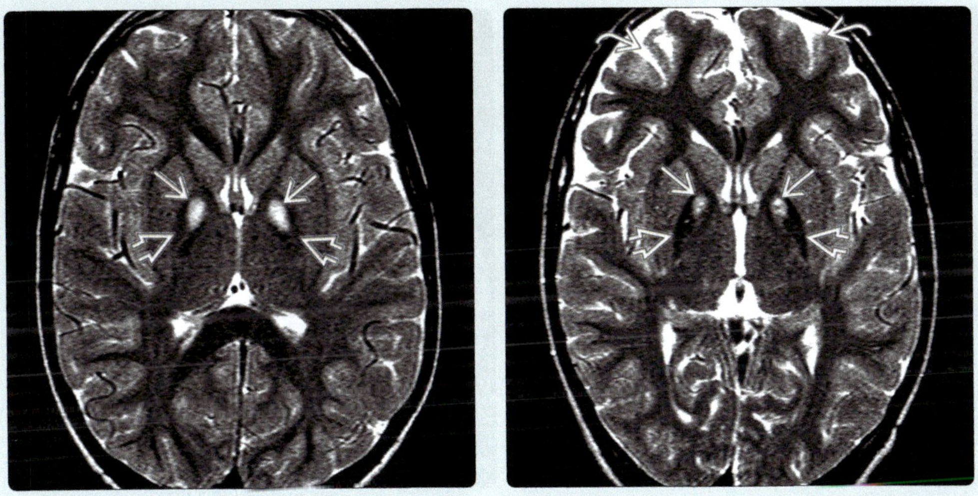

(Left) *Axial T2WI MR in a 5 year old with a diagnosis of cerebral palsy demonstrates an "eye of the tiger" typical of PKAN: Symmetric areas of high T2 signal ➡ within the medial globus pallidus with surrounding pallidal hypointensity ➡.* **(Right)** *Four years later, dystonia prompted repeat imaging in the same patient. Axial T2WI MR shows that the "eyes" ➡ have decreased in size and intensity; the surrounding pallidal hypointensity ➡ is more prominent. Volume loss is now seen, particularly frontal ➡.*

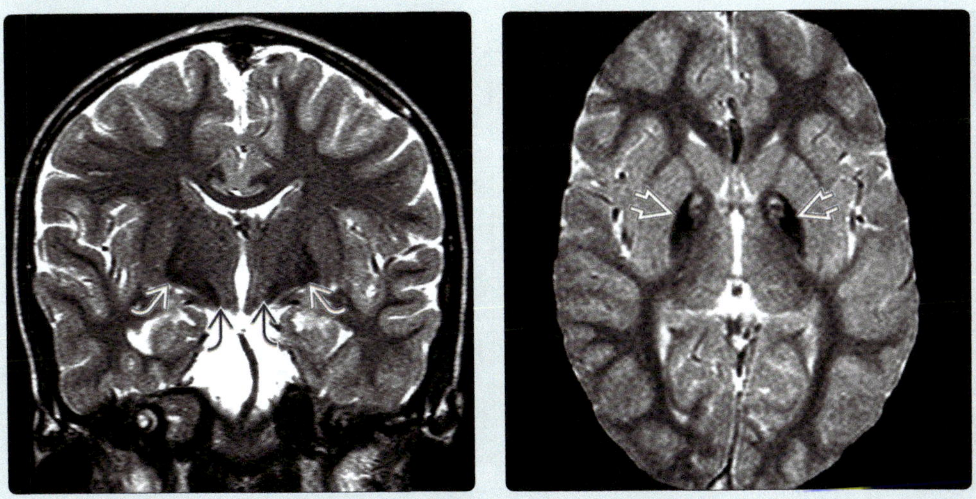

(Left) *Coronal T2WI MR of the same patient at 9 years of age shows abnormal hypointense signal in the globus pallidus ➡ and substantia nigra ➡.* **(Right)** *Axial T2* GRE MR in the same patient at 9 years of age shows "blooming" of hypointense signal in the globus pallidus secondary to the paramagnetic effect of iron ➡. The findings in this patient are typical of the evolution of classic PKAN: Diminishing caliber of the "eye," increasing surrounding pallidal hypointensity, and progressive volume loss.*

Huntington Disease

KEY FACTS

TERMINOLOGY

- Autosomal dominant neurodegenerative disease
  - Loss of GABAergic neurons of basal ganglia (BG)

IMAGING

- Diffuse cerebral atrophy
- Caudate nucleus (CN) atrophy → frontal horns enlarged
- ↑ "Bicaudate" ratio (BCR) or Evans ratio
  - Intercaudate distance divided by distance between inner tables of skull
  - BCR = 0.18 in Huntington disease (HD) vs. 0.09 controls
  - Most specific & sensitive anatomic measure for HD
- Hyperintense signal in CN, putamina in juvenile HD
- PET: ↓ FDG uptake in BG before any detectable atrophy
  - ± frontal lobe hypometabolism

TOP DIFFERENTIAL DIAGNOSES

- Leigh disease
- Wilson disease
- Pantothenate kinase-associated neurodegeneration (formerly called Hallervorden-Spatz)
- Carbon monoxide poisoning

PATHOLOGY

- Autosomal dominant with complete penetrance; CAG trinucleotide repeat disease affecting HD gene on chromosome 4p16.3

CLINICAL ISSUES

- Presents with chorea, psychiatric issues (depression, irritability), and loss of executive functions

DIAGNOSTIC CHECKLIST

- Rule out reversible dementias, movement disorders
- Caudate atrophy is main radiologic feature of HD
- ↑ bicaudate diameter: Sensitive for CN atrophy
- ↓ size of GP, putamen correlates with disease progression
- Consider HD in child with ↑ signal in CN/putamina on PD/T2WI

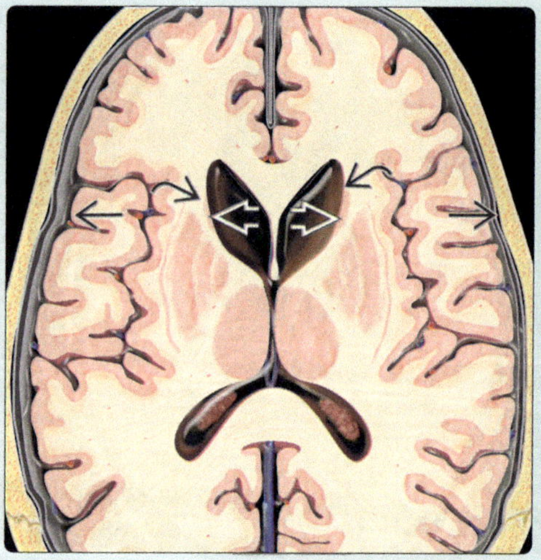

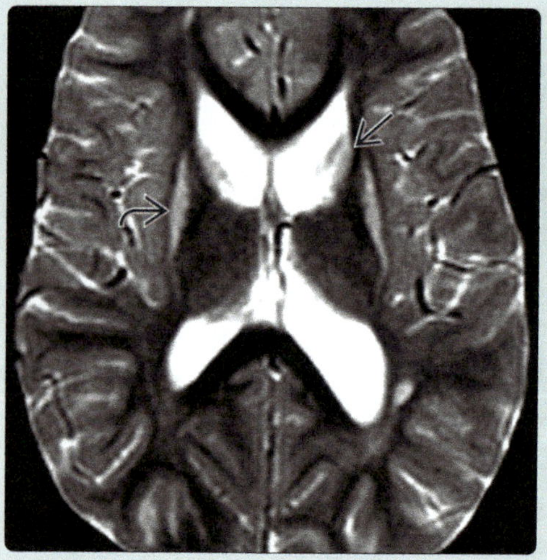

(Left) *Axial graphic shows the convex margins of the frontal horns with atrophy of the heads of the caudate nuclei. Bicaudate ratio = ratio between intercaudate distance vs. distance between inner tables of skull at same level.* **(Right)** *Axial T2WI MR in a patient with juvenile Huntington disease shows generalized volume loss and striking atrophy and hyperintensity of both caudate nuclei. The frontal horns of the lateral ventricles are enlarged, and there is atrophy and hyperintensity in the putamina.*

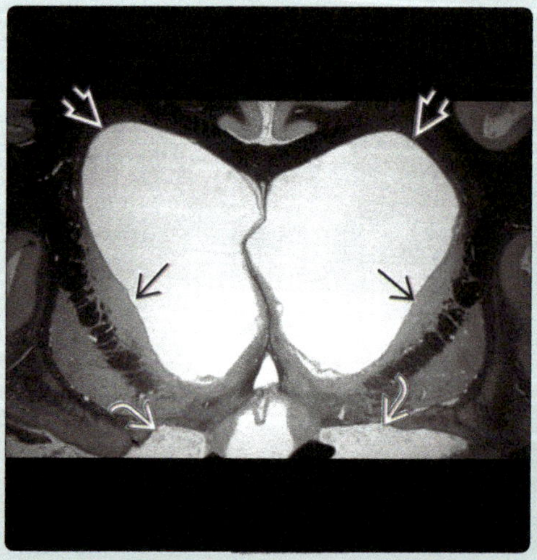

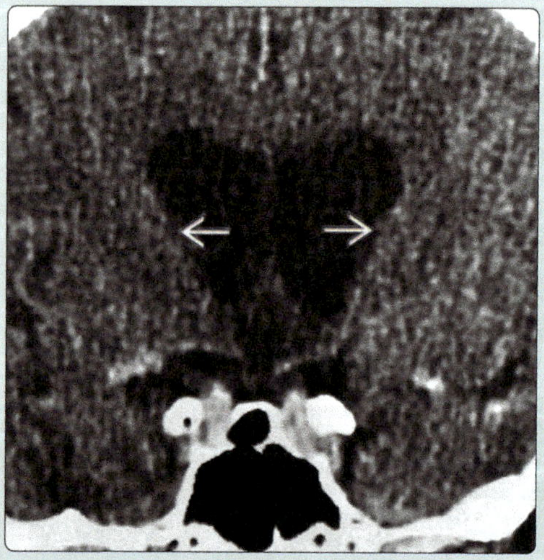

(Left) *Autopsy specimen sectioned in the coronal plane shows enlarged lateral ventricles and basal cisterns. Both caudate nuclei appear thinned and atrophic.* **(Right)** *Coronal CECT, cut in same plane to correspond to the autopsy specimen in the previous image, shows straightening of the lateral borders of the lateral ventricles due to caudate atrophy and increased intercaudate distance, which are characteristic findings of Huntington disease.*

KEY FACTS

TERMINOLOGY

- Wilson disease is also known as hepatolenticular degeneration
- Autosomal recessive disorder of copper metabolism
  - Abnormal accumulation of copper in various tissues
  - Particularly in liver, basal ganglia (BG), midbrain

IMAGING

- Usually normal MR in presymptomatic patients
- T1WI: Normal or BG hyperintensity (similar to chronic hepatic encephalopathy)
- T2/FLAIR: Symmetric hyperintensity in putamina (with hyperintense peripheral putaminal rim), caudate nuclei, ventrolateral thalami
  - Characteristic face of giant panda sign on axial sections at midbrain level
- Copper-chelating therapy may ↓ MR abnormalities

TOP DIFFERENTIAL DIAGNOSES

- Leigh disease
- PKAN
- Organic aciduria
- Menkes disease ("kinky hair")
- Hypoxic-ischemic encephalopathy

CLINICAL ISSUES

- Early onset (8-16 years): Liver disease
  - Kayser-Fleischer ring in cornea on slit-lamp
- Later onset 2nd, 3rd decades: Neurologic
  - Asymmetric tremor, ataxia, dyskinesia, dysarthria, dystonia (mainly face), behavioral disturbances
  - Chelation therapy prevents progression

DIAGNOSTIC CHECKLIST

- MR improvement correlated with clinical recovery

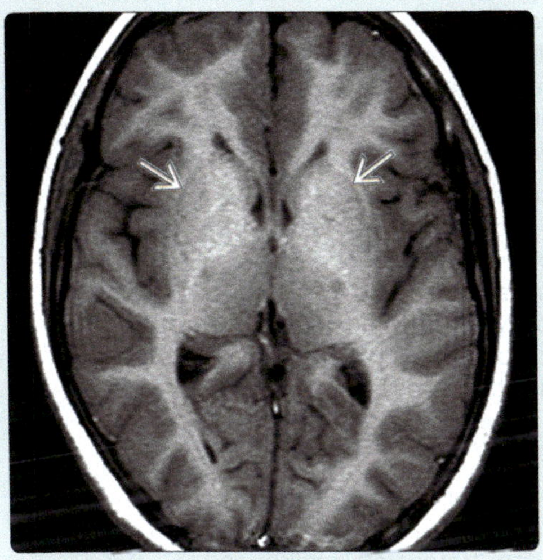

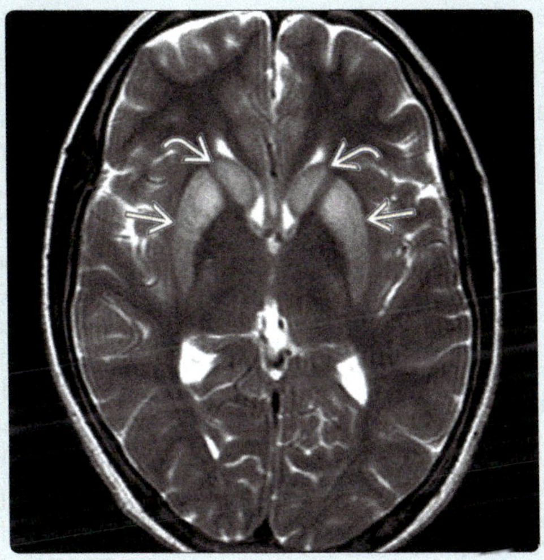

(Left) *Axial T1WI in a patient with Wilson disease shows basal ganglia hyperintensity* →. **(Right)** *Axial T2WI in the same case shows hyperintensity in the caudate nuclei* → *and putamen* →. *The globi pallidi are spared.*

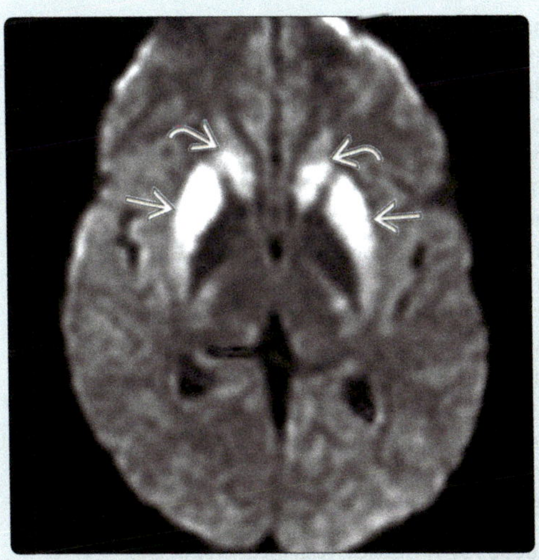

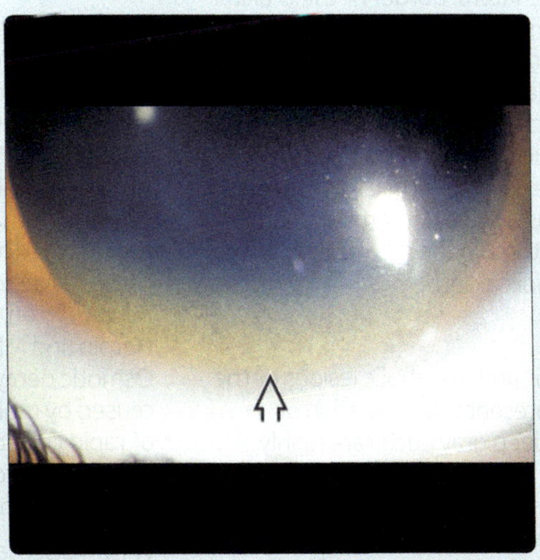

(Left) *Axial DWI in the same case shows restricted diffusion in the caudate nuclei* → *and putamina* →. *The lesions did not enhance on T1 C+ imaging. (Courtesy M. Ayadi, MD.)* **(Right)** *Slit-lamp examination shows a Kayser-Fleischer ring of the cornea* ⇨*, an important marker in Wilson disease that is almost always present in patients with neurological involvement.*

Approach to Toxic and Metabolic Disorders

Acquired toxic and metabolic disorders of the brain result from a wide variety of agents, including toxic exposures, substance abuse, radiation, and chemotherapy, as well as metabolic alterations, including hypertension, hepatic failure, hypoglycemia, and osmotic demyelination. The vast majority of toxic and metabolic disorders of the brain involve the deep gray nuclei (basal ganglia and thalamus) or the cerebral white matter. Typically, there is symmetric abnormality of the involved structures, which can provide a clue to the correct diagnosis. MR shows damage at both early and delayed phases of toxic and metabolic disorders. DWI and FLAIR are extremely valuable in differentiating among the various pathologies in this group and can help arrive at a correct diagnosis. Of course, clinical history of possible exposure or substance abuse is often the key to the patient's diagnosis.

Imaging Anatomy

Basal Ganglia

The basal ganglia (BG) are symmetric paired deep gray matter nuclei in cerebral hemispheres and form the core of the extrapyramidal system and regulate motor activity. The BG consists of caudate nucleus, putamen, and globus pallidus (GP). Caudate nucleus and putamen form the corpus striatum. The putamen and BG together are called the lentiform nuclei.

- **Caudate nucleus** is a C-shaped nucleus with a large head, tapered body, and down-curving tail. The head forms the floor and lateral wall of the anterior horn of the lateral ventricle. The caudate body parallels the lateral ventricles. The anterior limb of the internal capsule separates the caudate head from the putamen and GP.
- **Putamen** is the outermost part of the BG located lateral to GP and is separated by the lateral or external medullary lamina.
- **GP** consists of 2 segments, lateral (external) and medial (internal), separated by a thin layer of myelinated axons, the internal medullary lamina.

Thalamus

The thalamus is comprised of paired ovoid nuclear complexes that act as relay stations for most of the sensory pathways. The thalami extend from the foramen of Monro to the quadrigeminal plate of the midbrain. The medial aspect of the thalami form the 3rd ventricle lateral walls. The posterior limb of the internal capsule forms the lateral border of the thalami. The thalamus is subdivided into several nuclear groups, the anterior, medial, lateral, medial geniculate nuclei (part of the auditory system), lateral geniculate nuclei (part of the visual system), and pulvinar. These nuclear groups are further subdivided into 10 additional nuclei. The pulvinar is easily identified, as it is the most posterior of the thalamic nuclei and overhangs the superior colliculus. The subthalamic nucleus is small, lens-shaped, lies superolateral to the red nucleus, and is rarely involved in toxic or metabolic disorders.

Pathologic Issues

The mechanisms for various toxic and metabolic lesions of the brain are complex and often represent a combination of various pathways. Because the deep gray nuclei are highly metabolically active and require significant oxygenation, they are commonly affected by toxins, metabolic abnormalities, and hypoxic-ischemic injury. Often, as in carbon monoxide (CO) and cyanide poisoning, there is a component of hypoxic injury that helps explain the predilection for involvement of the GP, which is extremely sensitive to hypoxia. Selective vulnerability of the deep gray nuclei is also related to dysfunction of selected excitatory neuronal circuits, inhibition of mitochondrial function, and selective loss of dopaminergic neurons.

Differential Diagnosis

Most of the pathologies that affect the brain have a characteristic location, which helps the radiologist arrive at a correct diagnosis. The following differential diagnosis considerations will provide clues to the common toxic and metabolic processes that affect the deep gray nuclei and white matter.

Basal Ganglia Calcification

Basal ganglia calcification is the end result of many toxic, metabolic, inflammatory, and infectious insults. Fahr disease is a rare neurodegenerative disorder that results in extensive bilateral BG calcifications. The GP is most commonly involved, followed by the putamen, caudate, and thalamus. Additionally, there may be involvement of the cerebellum, particularly the dentate nuclei and cerebral white matter.

Other endocrinologic disorders, including hypothyroidism and hypoparathyroidism, may cause calcification, particularly involving the GP, putamen, dentate nuclei, thalami, and subcortical white matter. Radiation and chemotherapy may result in mineralizing microangiopathy that commonly causes BG and subcortical white matter calcifications and atrophy. Physiologic calcification as part of the normal aging brain typically occurs in the GP more than the putamen.

T1 Hyperintense Basal Ganglia

Basal ganglia T1 hyperintensity is usually symmetric, related to calcification or other mineralization. T1 hyperintensity is often seen in the GP and substantia nigra in patients with a history of liver disease or hyperalimentation related to abnormal manganese metabolism. Kernicterus, related to toxic unconjugated bilirubin in a newborn, results in increased T1 signal in the GP, as well as the substantia nigra, hippocampus, and dentate nucleus.

Many endocrine disorders that result in BG calcification will also cause T1 hyperintensity. These include hypothyroidism, hyperparathyroidism, hypoparathyroidism, and pseudohypoparathyroidism. Fahr disease also results in T1 hyperintensity, particularly in the GP.

T2 Hyperintense Basal Ganglia

T2 hyperintensity within the BG is typically symmetric in toxic and metabolic disorders. Often DWI helps to differentiate the various lesions of the BG. CO poisoning classically causes symmetric GP hyperintensity but occasionally also involves the putamen, thalamus, and white matter. DWI may be positive acutely. Methanol toxicity typically results in putaminal necrosis and may be hemorrhagic. Drug abuse is another cause for abnormalities of the basal ganglia, often in young adults. Often, drug abuse results in strokes or vasculitis. Heroin and MDMA (ecstasy) often result in GP ischemia. Osmotic demyelination syndrome is acute demyelination caused by rapid shifts in serum osmolality, often in the setting of rapid correction of hyponatremia. Extrapontine myelinolysis commonly affects the caudate and putamen, as well as the white matter.

Wilson disease causes symmetric hyperintensity in the putamen, GP, caudate, and thalami. It also results in a face of the giant panda sign at the midbrain level with T2 hyperintense white matter tracts. Acute hypertensive encephalopathy (posterior reversible encephalopathy syndrome, PRES) is caused by hypertension and may be related to chemotherapy. PRES typically affects the cortex and subcortical white matter of the posterior circulation. However, involvement of the BG may occur. The main considerations besides toxic and metabolic insults that may cause T2 hyperintense BG are hypoxic-ischemic encephalopathy, deep venous occlusion, and infectious etiologies.

Globus Pallidus Lesions

Lesions that often only involve the GP include CO poisoning, cyanide poisoning, heroin and MDMA (ecstasy) abuse, kernicterus, neurodegeneration with brain iron accumulation (NBIA)-pantothenate kinase-associated neurodegeneration (PKAN), hyperalimentation, hepatic encephalopathy, and methylmalonic acidemia. NBIA is a group of progressive neurodegenerative disorders with extrapyramidal motor impairment and brain iron accumulation, resulting in GP T2 hypointensity. PKAN, also known as Hallervorden-Spatz syndrome or NBIA-1, has a classic eye-of-the-tiger appearance with bilateral, symmetric GP T2 hyperintensity surrounded by hypointensity.

Other disorders that commonly affect the GP more prominently than the other BG nuclei include Fahr disease, hypothyroidism, and Wilson disease. As with other lesions of the BG, hypoxic-ischemic encephalopathy should also be considered.

Bilateral Thalamic Lesions

Thalamic lesions are most commonly caused by arterial or venous ischemia or hypoxic-ischemic encephalopathy. However, they are also involved in many toxic and metabolic processes. Alcoholic encephalopathy, particularly Wernicke encephalopathy, typically results in T2 hyperintense medial thalami, mammillary bodies, hypothalamus, and periaqueductal gray matter. Wernicke encephalopathy results from a vitamin B1 deficiency and is frequently associated with alcohol abuse. T1 hyperintensity in the pulvinar is a common and sensitive finding for Fabry disease and is considered by many as the T1 pulvinar sign. Fabry disease is a rare multisystem X-linked disorder that includes renal and cardiac dysfunction and strokes. Although Fahr disease most commonly causes extensive bilateral calcification of the BG, the thalami are frequently affected.

Other diseases that affect the thalami include PRES, vasculitis, osmotic demyelination, and acute disseminated encephalomyelitis. Additionally, many of the encephalitides affect the thalami, including Ebstein-Barr virus, Japanese encephalitis, and West Nile virus. Creutzfeldt-Jakob disease often affects the basal ganglia and thalami symmetrically.

Diffuse White Matter Abnormality

Toxic and metabolic disorders often cause a confluent T2 hyperintense leukoencephalopathy. Radiation and chemotherapy classically causes a leukoencephalopathy with T2 hyperintensity throughout the cerebral white matter. Sparing of the subcortical U fibers is typical. A diffuse necrotizing leukoencephalopathy may also result, commonly from a combination of radiation and chemotherapy, which causes white matter necrosis in addition to leukoencephalopathy. Heroin vapor inhalation, a.k.a. chasing the dragon syndrome, causes a toxic leukoencephalopathy that results in T2 hyperintense cerebellar white matter and the posterior limb of the internal capsule showing involvement of the posterior cerebral white matter, with relative sparing of the subcortical white matter.

Hypothyroidism related to Hashimoto thyroiditis may result in a diffuse confluent white matter encephalopathy that typically affects the anterior cerebral white matter. There is involvement of the subcortical U-fibers but relative sparing of the posterior hemispheres. Acute liver failure may also result in diffuse edema with T2 hyperintensity in the periventricular and subcortical white matter. Cortex involvement is typical. PRES typically involves the cortex and subcortical white matter in a posterior circulation. Alcoholic encephalopathy may rarely result in diffuse white matter T2 hyperintensity related to acute demyelination.

Selected References

1. Chokshi FH et al: Imaging of acquired metabolic and toxic disorders of the basal ganglia. Semin Ultrasound CT MR. 35(2):75-84, 2014
2. Bathla G et al: MRI and CT appearances in metabolic encephalopathies due to systemic diseases in adults. Clin Radiol. 68(6):545-54, 2013

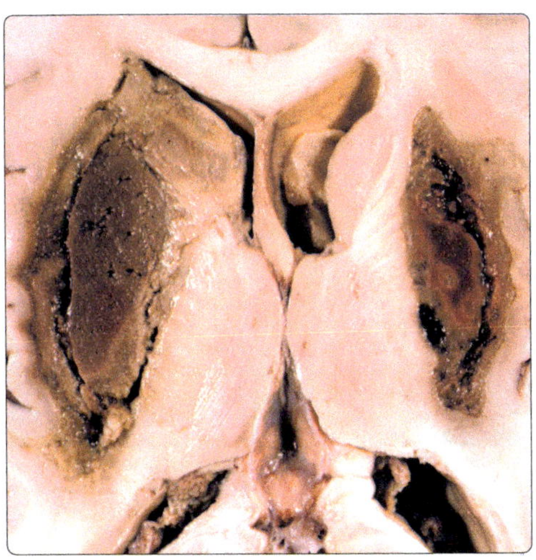

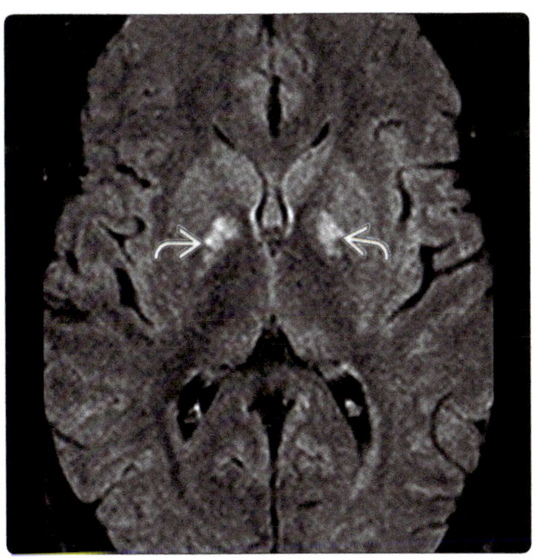

(Left) *Axial gross pathology section shows bilateral hemorrhagic necrosis in the putamen, characteristic of methanol injury to the brain. The right-sided injury extends to involve the globus pallidus and caudate head. (Courtesy R. Hewlett, MD.)* **(Right)** *Axial FLAIR MR shows acute carbon monoxide (CO) poisoning with symmetric hyperintensity in the globi pallidi* ➢*. Carbon monoxide has a propensity to affect the globus pallidus. In CO poisoning, delayed leukoencephalopathy and T1 shortening in the globus pallidus may be encountered.*

(Left) *Axial NECT shows extensive subcortical white matter, cerebellar, and basal ganglia calcifications ➡ in this patient with a history of radiation and chemotherapy for a posterior fossa medulloblastoma ➡. Mineralizing microangiopathy typically occurs 2 or more years after treatment.* **(Right)** *Coronal T1 C+ MR shows symmetric high signal in the globus pallidus ➡ in a patient with chronic cirrhosis. T1 hyperintense areas in globus pallidus and substantia nigra have been attributed to manganese deposition.*

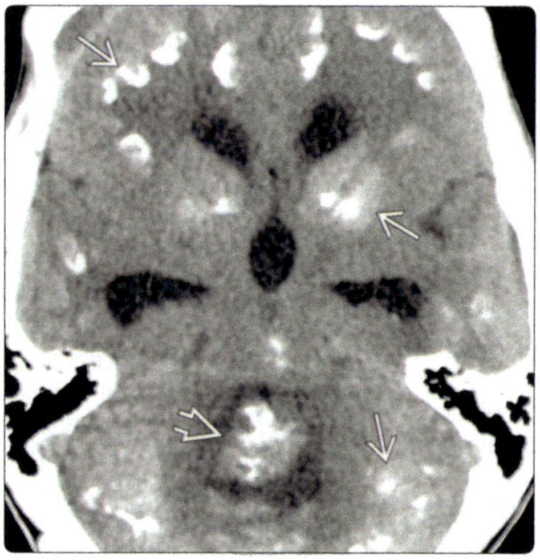

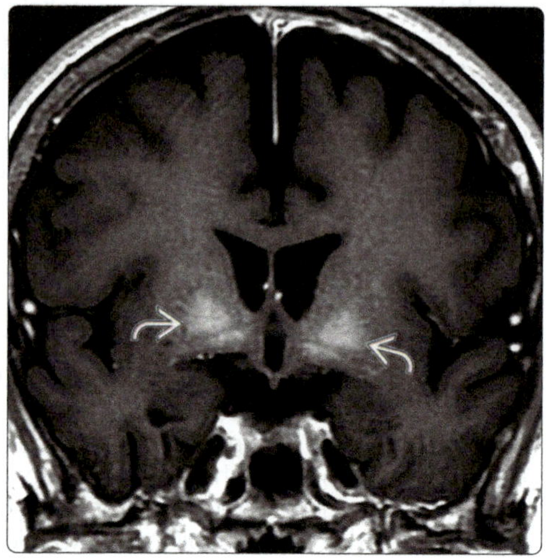

(Left) *Axial NECT shows symmetric calcifications in the caudate ➡, putamen ➡, and pulvinar nucleus of thalamus ➡ in a patient with Fahr disease. Numerous endocrine disorders can show similar calcifications.* **(Right)** *Axial FLAIR MR shows symmetric hyperintensity in both posteromedial thalami ➡ and in the region of the mammillary bodies related to Wernicke encephalopathy. DWI is often acutely positive. Wernicke encephalopathy is related to a thiamine deficiency and is often related to alcohol abuse.*

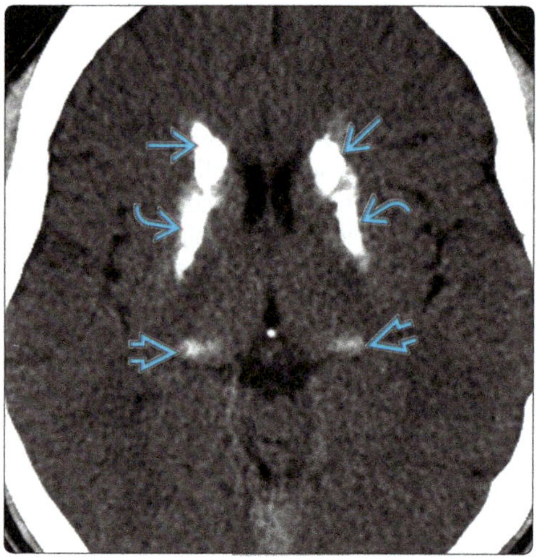

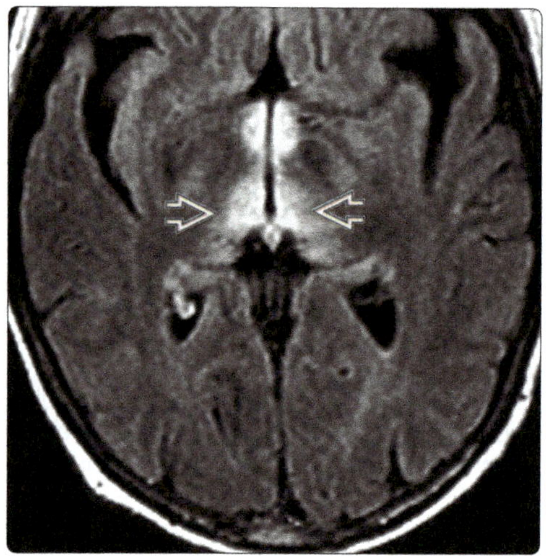

(Left) *Axial FLAIR MR shows symmetric hyperintensity in the caudate ➡ and putamen ➡ in this patient with both extrapontine and central pontine myelinolysis. Osmotic demyelination is often DWI positive and is typically related to a rapid correction of hyponatremia. Cerebral white matter demyelination may also occur.* **(Right)** *Axial gross pathology section shows bilateral necrosis of the putamen and globus pallidus ➡ with areas of cavitation related to neurotoxicity. (Courtesy R. Hewlett, MD.)*

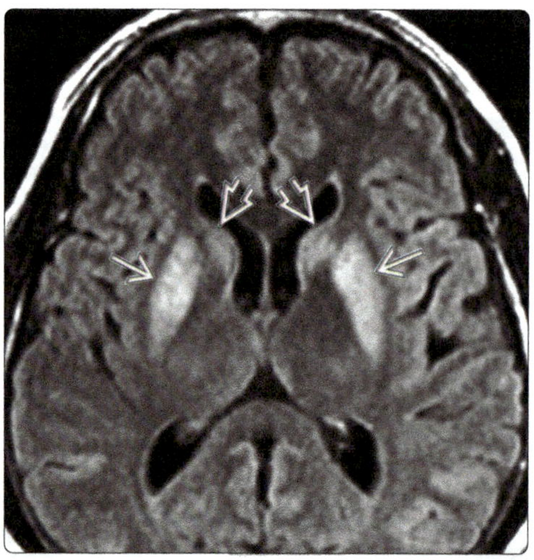

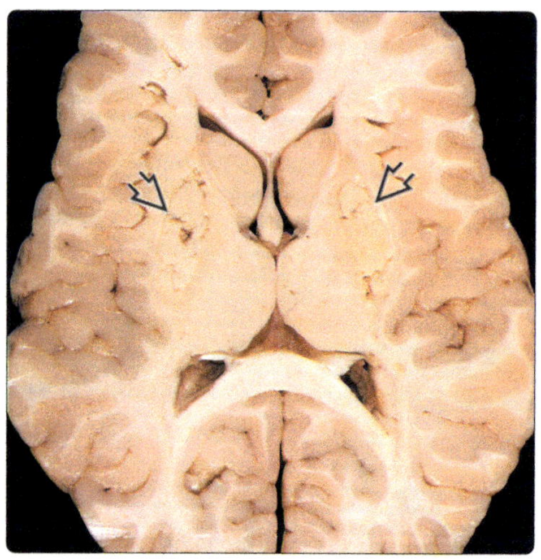

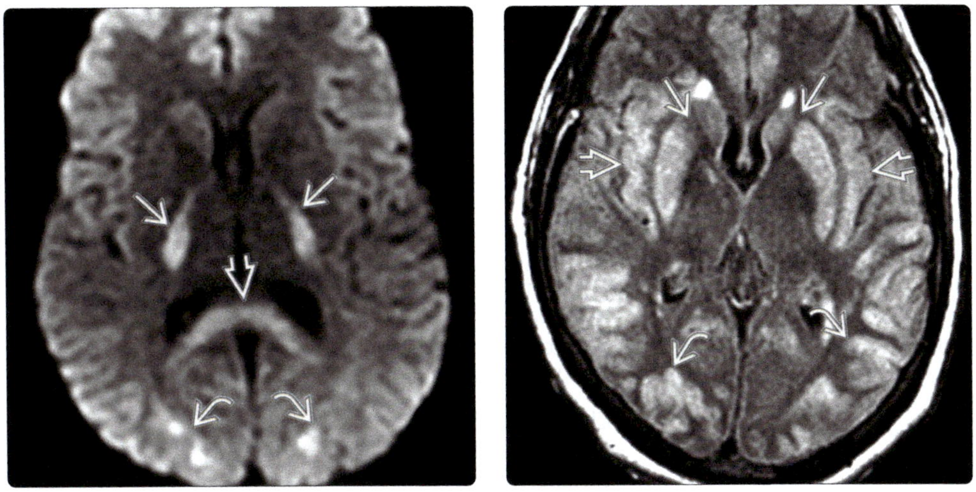

(Left) *Axial DWI MR shows hyperintensity in the internal capsule posterior limbs, corpus callosum splenium, and occipital white matter related to heroin-induced leukoencephalopathy, a.k.a. chasing the dragon syndrome.* **(Right)** *Axial FLAIR MR shows extensive, symmetric hyperintensity in the basal ganglia, cortex, and subcortical white matter related to profound hypoglycemia. Predilection for the parietal and occipital lobes is typical.*

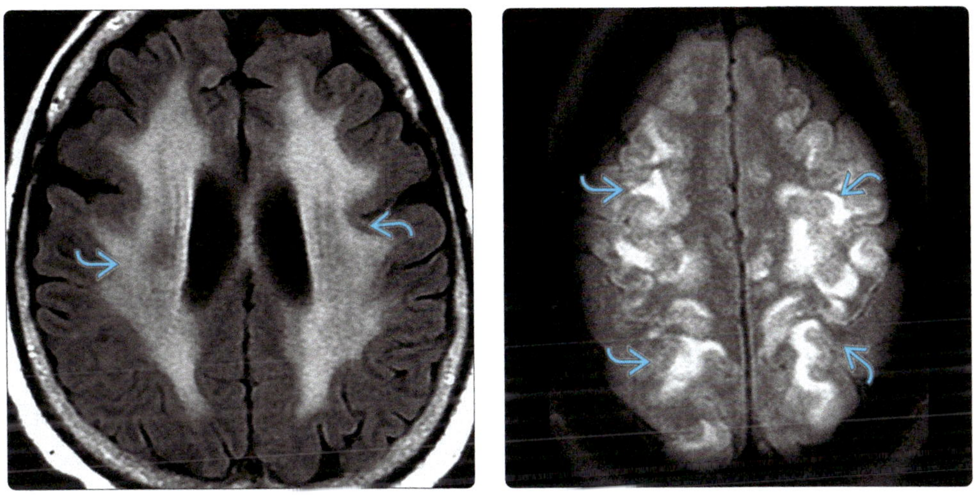

(Left) *Axial FLAIR MR in a patient with history of whole-brain radiation shows extensive hyperintensity throughout the white matter and sparing of the subcortical U fibers, typical of treatment-related leukoencephalopathy. Radiation and chemotherapy cause a variety of toxic injuries to the brain, with leukoencephalopathy being the most common.* **(Right)** *Axial FLAIR MR shows bilateral cortical and subcortical hyperintensities related to acute hypertensive encephalopathy or PRES.*

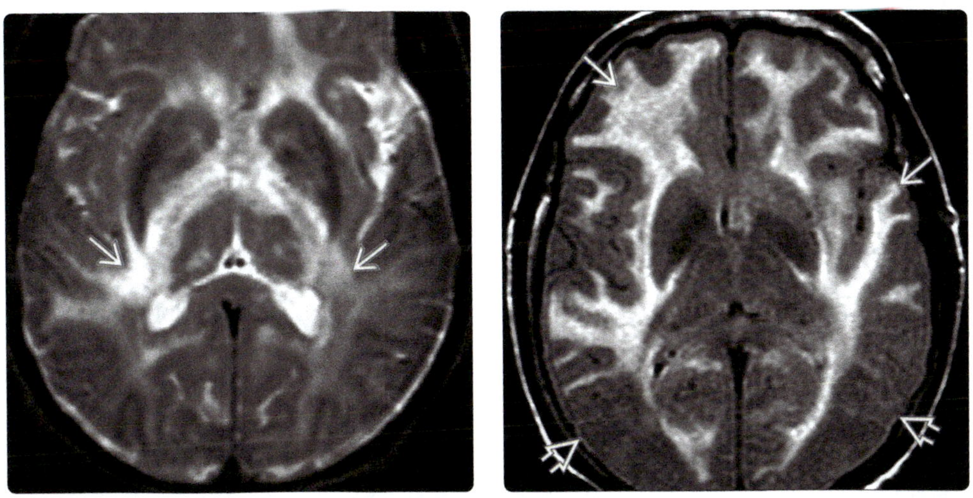

(Left) *Axial T2WI MR shows diffuse white matter hyperintensity related to severe alcohol poisoning from binge drinking and acute demyelination.* **(Right)** *Axial FLAIR MR in a 58-year-old woman with autoimmune thyroiditis shows diffuse, symmetric white matter hyperintensity with involvement of the subcortical U fibers. There is relative sparing of the occipital lobes, typical of Hashimoto encephalopathy, a rare complication of Hashimoto thyroiditis.*

KEY FACTS

TERMINOLOGY

- Adult hypoglycemic encephalopathy
- Imbalance between glucose supply, utilization → brain injury
- Hypoglycemia: Sudden decrease in serum glucose level < 50 mg/dL

IMAGING

- Stroke/coma in adult diabetic on insulin replacement therapy (IRT)
- Parietal/temporal/occipital lobes, basal ganglia, ± hippocampi
- Hyperintensity in parietooccipital cortex and basal ganglia
- Thalami, subcortical/deep white matter and cerebellum generally spared
- Restricted diffusion, ↓ ADC (may be transient)
- MRS shows ↓ NAA, ↑ lactate

TOP DIFFERENTIAL DIAGNOSES

- Acute cerebral ischemia/infarction
- Hypoxia, hypoperfusion
- Acute hypertensive encephalopathy (PRES)

PATHOLOGY

- Caused by IRT either without adequate glucose intake or excessive glucose utilization
- Ingestion of oral hypoglycemic medication, either accidental or intentional
- Accumulation/release of excitatory neurotransmitters increases glucose utilization
- Patchy or diffuse laminar necrosis
  - Varying severity, white matter generally spared

CLINICAL ISSUES

- Often elderly diabetic, altered dietary glucose intake
- Coma, depressed level of consciousness
- May be preceded by seizures

(Left) *Axial FLAIR MR in a diabetic patient with altered sensorium and a blood glucose of 36 mg/dL shows symmetric hyperintensity involving the hippocampus →, temporal and occipital cortex bilaterally ↪.* **(Right)** *Axial DWI in the same patient shows corresponding areas of restricted diffusion in the hippocampus →, temporal and occipital cortex ↪. Prognosis in adult hypoglycemic encephalopathy varies with severity and duration of hypoglycemia, as well as extent of brain injury.*

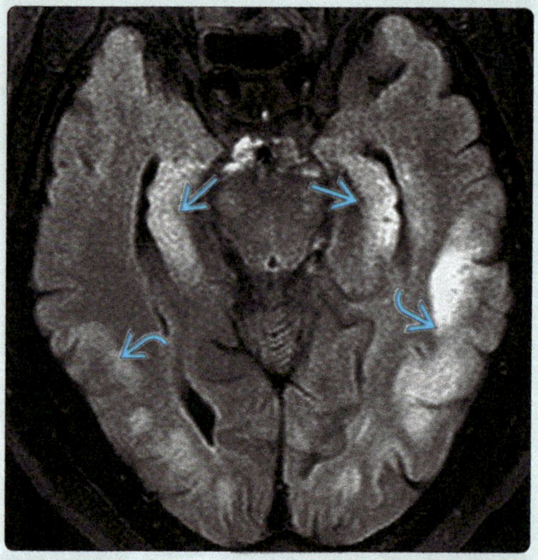

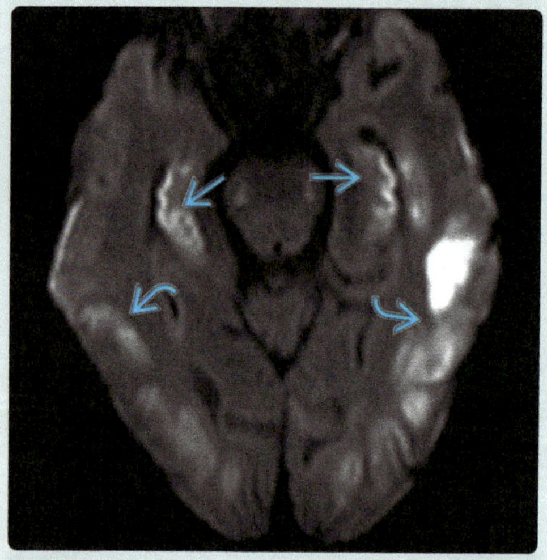

(Left) *Axial DWI in patient with overdose of glipizide and blood glucose level of 20 mg/dL shows severe changes of hypoglycemic encephalopathy. There is extensive symmetric diffusion restriction in the basal ganglia → and cerebral cortex ↪.* **(Right)** *Intermediate TE MRS in a hypoglycemic patient shows a relatively low NAA peak → and a prominent lactate peak ↪. Using an intermediate TE inverts only lactate, allowing it to be distinguished from lipid. Lactate is a marker of anaerobic metabolism with no peak seen in normal spectra.*

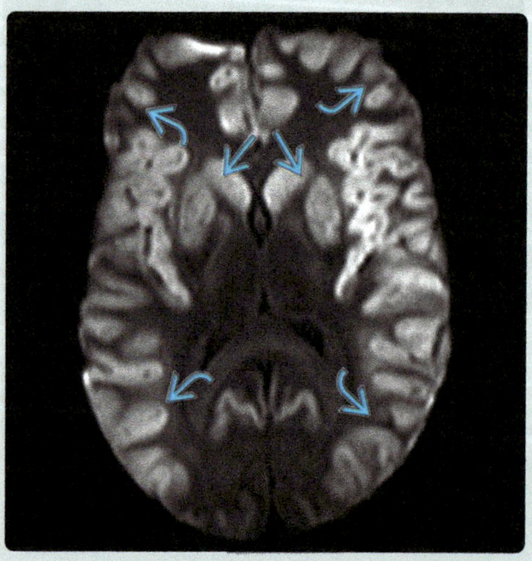

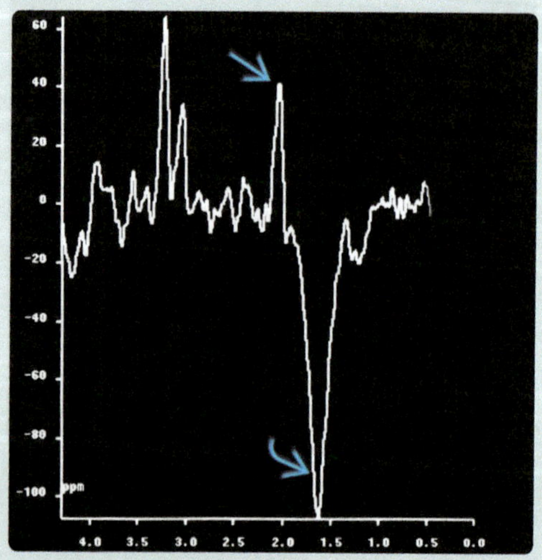

KEY FACTS

TERMINOLOGY

- Hashimoto encephalopathy (HE)
- HE synonym: Steroid-responsive encephalopathy associated with autoimmune thyroiditis

IMAGING

- Pituitary hyperplasia (PH): Symmetrical pituitary enlargement that is reversible with thyroid hormone replacement therapy
- Basal ganglia variably hyperintense (Ca++)
- HE: Bilateral patchy or confluent subcortical and periventricular white matter T2 hyperintensity with relative sparing of occipital lobes, bilateral and symmetric or unilateral mesial temporal lobe edema

TOP DIFFERENTIAL DIAGNOSES

- Pituitary macroadenoma
- Physiologic PH
- Confluent white matter lesions

PATHOLOGY

- Diffuse hyperplasia of anterior pituitary responds to treatment
- **HE**
  - High titers of antithyroglobulin or anti-thyroperoxidase (antimicrosomal) antibodies
  - Various studies reported no evidence of pathogenic role of antibodies in HE

CLINICAL ISSUES

- Hypothyroidism: Poor memory, psychomotor slowing, depression, reversible dementia
- In congenital hypothyroidism, thyroid hormone replacement ASAP (< 13 days)
- HE: 2 types of initial clinical presentation, acute stroke-like (vasculitic type) episode and gradual cognitive impairment
  - Confusion, focal/generalized seizure, focal neurological deficit, cognitive decline, dementia

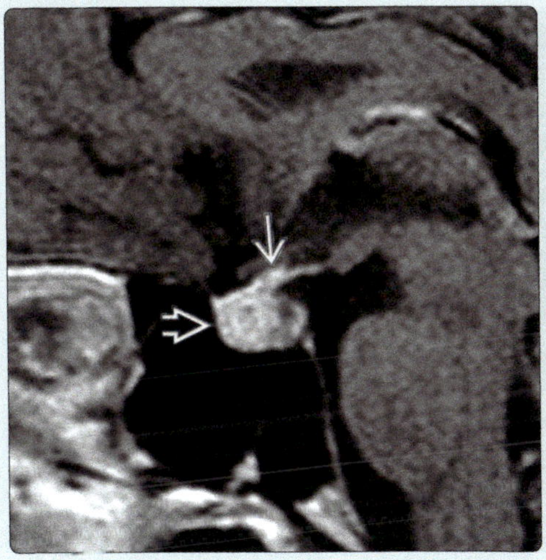

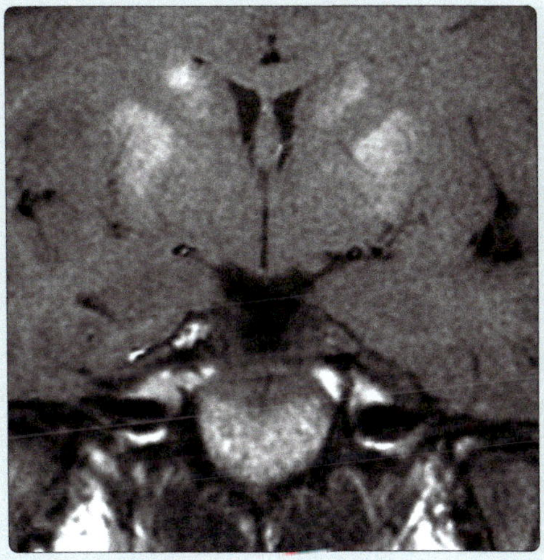

(Left) *Sagittal T1WI C+ MR shows an enlarged homogeneously enhancing pituitary gland* → *with infundibular thickening* → *related to hypothyroid-induced pituitary hyperplasia. The hyperplasia resolves with thyroid-replacement therapy.* **(Right)** *Axial T1WI MR shows a focal T1 hyperintensity related to hypothyroidism, involving the caudate heads and globus pallidus bilaterally. These changes are related to mineralization of the basal ganglia, which are hyperdense on CT.*

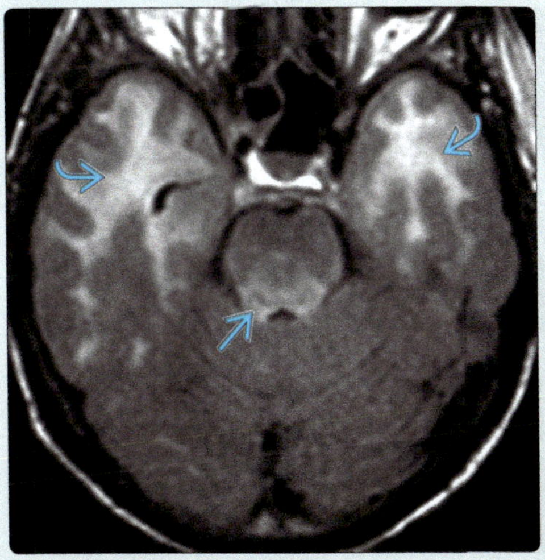

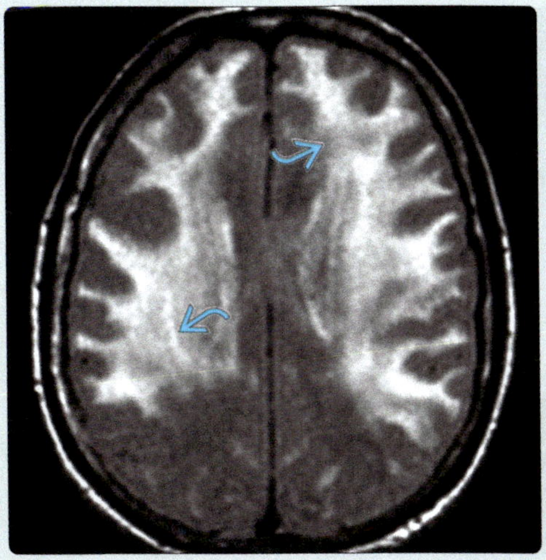

(Left) *Axial FLAIR MR shows extensive hyperintensity throughout the anterior temporal white matter* → *and dorsal pons* → *related to leukoencephalopathy in a patient with Hashimoto encephalopathy.* **(Right)** *Axial FLAIR MR in the same patient shows extensive involvement of the white matter* → *with relative sparing of the posterior cerebral hemispheres. Involvement of the subcortical U fibers is typical of Hashimoto encephalopathy.*

KEY FACTS

TERMINOLOGY

- CNS manifestations related to parathyroid hormone (PTH) metabolic abnormalities
  - Hyperparathyroid (HPTH); hypoparathyroid (HP)

IMAGING

- Bilateral symmetric calcifications in globi pallidi, putamen, caudate nuclei
- Diffuse patchy "salt & pepper" lesions in skull in primary HPTH
- Plaque-like dural calcification, "pipestem" calcifications of carotid arteries in secondary HPTH
- Brown tumors: Focal expansile lytic lesions with nonsclerotic margins in primary HPTH and secondary HPTH
- T2WI: Hypointensity involving basal ganglia, cerebral cortex, or dentate nucleus due to Ca++ deposition

TOP DIFFERENTIAL DIAGNOSES

- Fahr disease
- Physiologic calcification
- Congenital HIV
- Hypoxic-ischemic encephalopathy

PATHOLOGY

- Primary HPTH: Parathyroid adenoma (75-85%), parathyroid hyperplasia (10-20%), carcinoma (1-5%), ↑ PTH, ↑ Ca++
- Secondary HPTH: Chronic renal failure, kidney fails to convert vitamin D to active form and excrete phosphate
- HP: Parathyroids are absent or atrophied; genetic autoimmune syndrome or DiGeorge syndrome (total absence of PT glands at birth)
- PHP: Insensitivity of end-organ to PTH, rather than decreased production of PTH

CLINICAL ISSUES

- HPTH: ↑ Ca++ affects transsynaptic nerve conduction, fatigue, pain, nausea, osteoporosis
- HP: Carpal-pedal spasm, tetany, seizure, and hyperreflexia

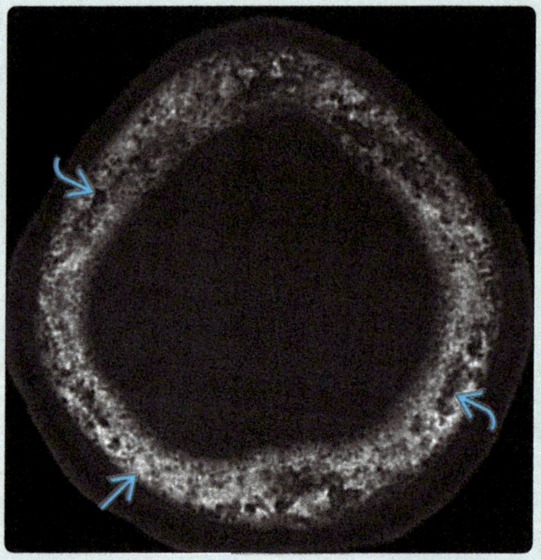
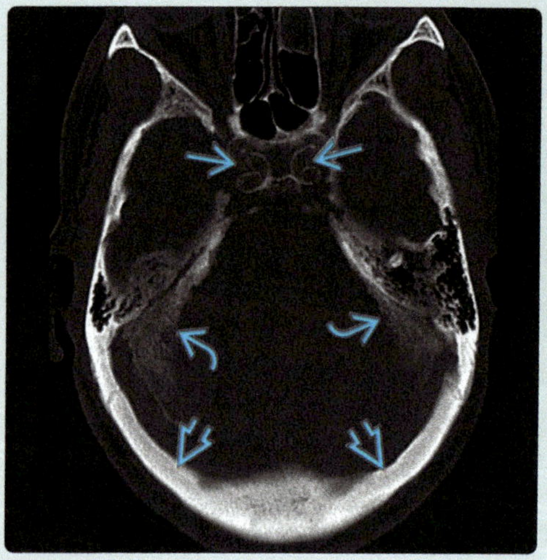

(Left) *Axial NECT in primary hyperparathyroidism shows extensive patchy lytic and sclerotic areas involving the calvaria. This gives a classic salt and pepper appearance of the calvaria.* **(Right)** *Axial NECT in a patient with a long history of dialysis for chronic renal failure demonstrates classic changes in skull due to secondary hyperparathyroidism. There is extensive calcification of the tentorium, sclerosis of calvaria, and pipe-like calcification of the internal carotid arteries.*

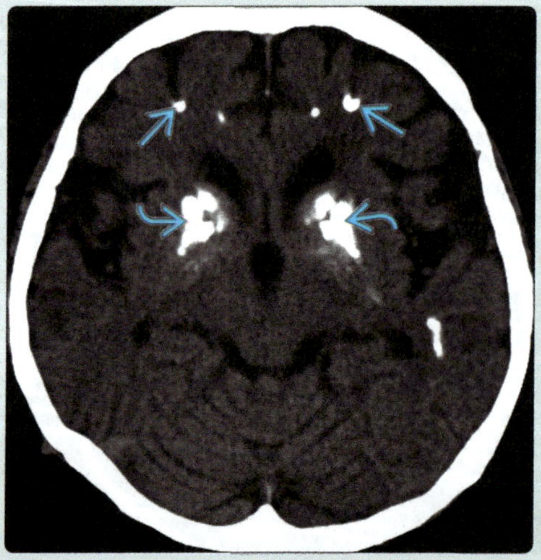
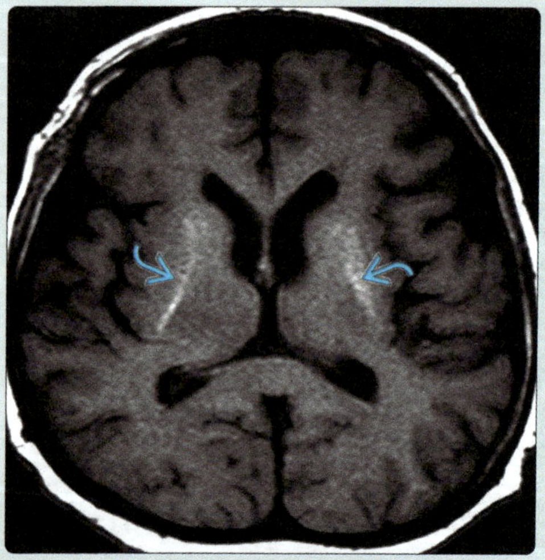

(Left) *Axial NECT in a patient with hypoparathyroidism shows symmetric bilateral basal ganglia calcifications. Focal calcifications are also seen in the subcortical white matter.* **(Right)** *Axial T1 MR in the same patient shows T1 shortening in the basal ganglia due to calcifications. Calcium deposition in the basal ganglia is seen in both hyper- and hypoparathyroidism. Additional sites for calcium deposition include thalamus, subcortical white matter, dentate nuclei, and dura.*

KEY FACTS

TERMINOLOGY

- Fahr disease (FD)
  - a.k.a. cerebrovascular ferrocalcinosis, bilateral striopallidodentate calcification
- Rare degenerative neurological disorder
  - Extensive bilateral basal ganglia (BG) calcifications (Ca++)
  - ± progressive dystonia, parkinsonism, neuropsychiatric manifestations

IMAGING

- Bilateral symmetric Ca++ in BG, thalami, dentate nuclei, and cerebral white matter on CT

TOP DIFFERENTIAL DIAGNOSES

- Normal (physiologic)
  - Symmetrical BG Ca++ in middle-aged, elderly patients
- Pathologic BG Ca++ (e.g., endocrinological)

PATHOLOGY

- FD is often familial yet heterogeneous
- Characteristic feature: Diffuse neurofibrillary tangles with calcification (a.k.a. Fahr-type calcification)

CLINICAL ISSUES

- Most common signs/symptoms
  - Neuropsychiatric disturbance
  - Cognitive impairment (subcortical dementia)
  - Extrapyramidal movement disorders
- Ca++/P metabolism, parathyroid hormone levels normal
- Bimodal pattern of clinical onset
  - Early adulthood (schizophrenic-like psychosis)
  - 6th decade (extrapyramidal syndrome, subcortical dementia)

DIAGNOSTIC CHECKLIST

- BG Ca++ if < 50 years old merits investigation

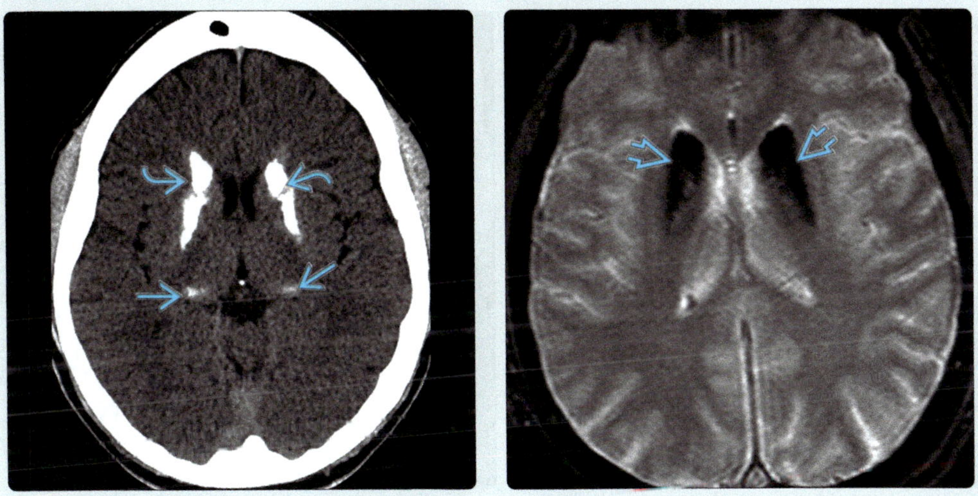

(Left) *Axial NECT in patient with Fahr disease demonstrates classic extensive calcifications in the basal ganglia and thalami.* **(Right)** *Axial T2* GRE MR in the same patient shows low signal in the basal ganglia. This appearance on T2* GRE is due to a combination of calcification and iron deposition.*

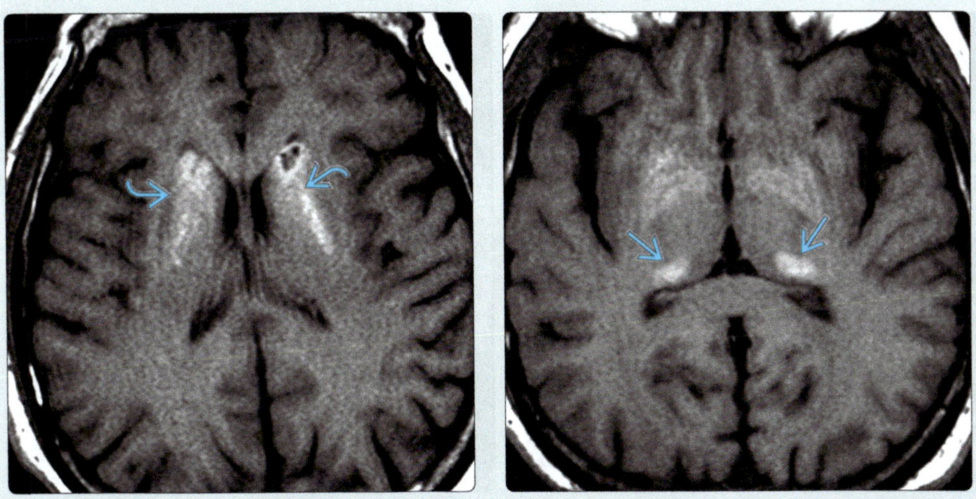

(Left) *Axial T1 MR in the same patient shows T1 shortening in the basal ganglia. T1 shortening is typical and is secondary to the presence of Fahr-type calcification.* **(Right)** *Axial T1 MR in the same patient shows similar T1 shortening in the thalami. This corresponds to the calcification seen on CT. Fahr disease is a degenerative neurological disorder that manifests as bilateral symmetric calcifications in the basal ganglia, thalami, dentate nuclei, and cerebral white matter.*

Alcoholic Encephalopathy

KEY FACTS

TERMINOLOGY

- Acute/subacute/chronic toxic effects of EtOH on CNS
  - Wernicke encephalopathy (WE)
  - Marchifava-Bignami disease (MBD)

IMAGING

- EtOH: Disproportionate superior vermian atrophy, enlargement of lateral ventricles, sulci with chronic EtOH
- WE: Mammillary body, medial thalamus, hypothalamus, periaqueductal gray abnormal signal/enhancement/diffusion restriction
- MBD: Abnormal signal and later necrosis in corpus callosum

TOP DIFFERENTIAL DIAGNOSES

- Nonalcoholic atrophy
- Demyelination (toxic, acquired/inherited metabolic)
- Corpus callosal hyperintensity
  - Status epilepticus
  - Drug toxicity
  - Encephalitis
  - Hypoglycemia

PATHOLOGY

- EtOH: Causes both direct/indirect neurotoxicity
- WE: Thiamine (vitamin B1) deficiency
- WE can be alcoholic or nonalcoholic
- MBD: Chronic EtOH abuse, anecdotal association with red wine

CLINICAL ISSUES

- WE: Triad of ataxia, oculomotor abnormalities, confusion
- Classic clinical triad present in only minority of patients
- EtOH: Cessation, establishment of adequate nutrition
- WE: Immediate administration of IV thiamine → quick response

DIAGNOSTIC CHECKLIST

- 50% of WE cases occur in nonalcoholics, including children!
  - Nutritional deficiency, after gastric bypass, etc.

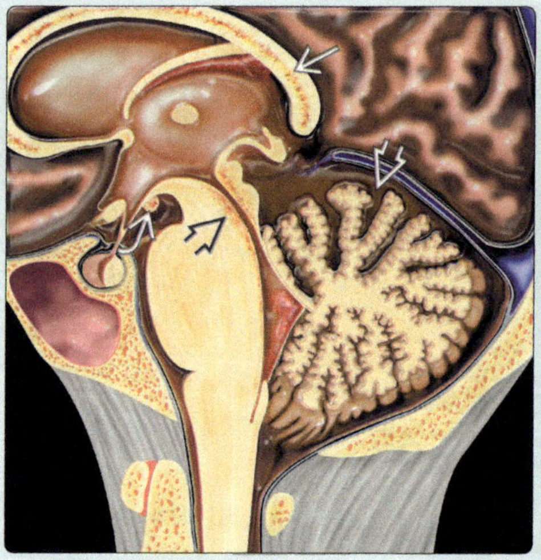

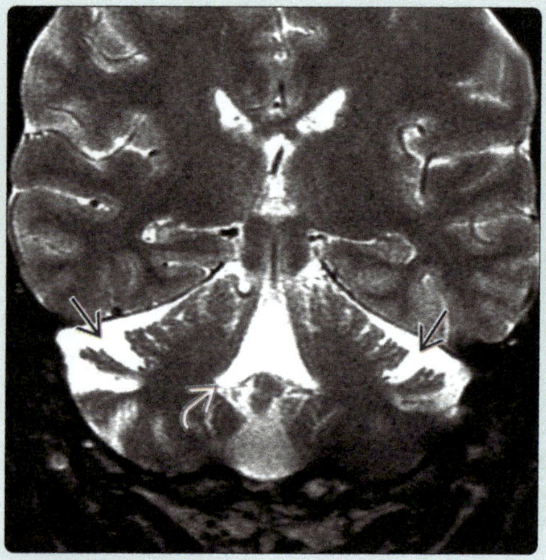

(Left) *Sagittal graphic shows generalized and superior vermian atrophy, as well as necrosis in the mid-corpus callosum related to alcoholic toxicity. Mammillary body, periaqueductal gray necrosis is seen with Wernicke encephalopathy.* **(Right)** *Coronal T2WI MR demonstrates pronounced cerebellar atrophy with enlarged 4th ventricle, markedly enlarged cerebellar fissures.*

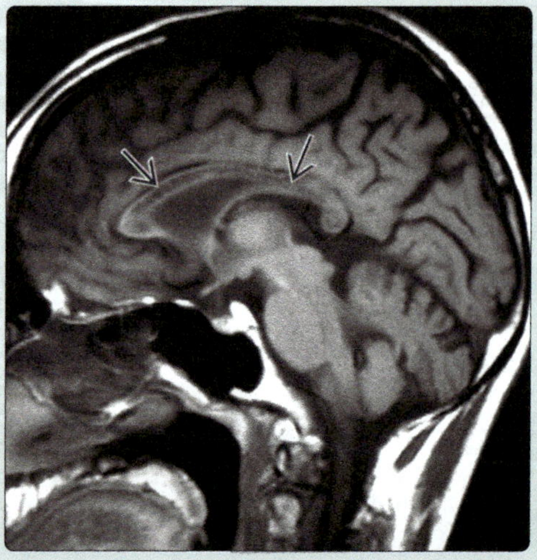

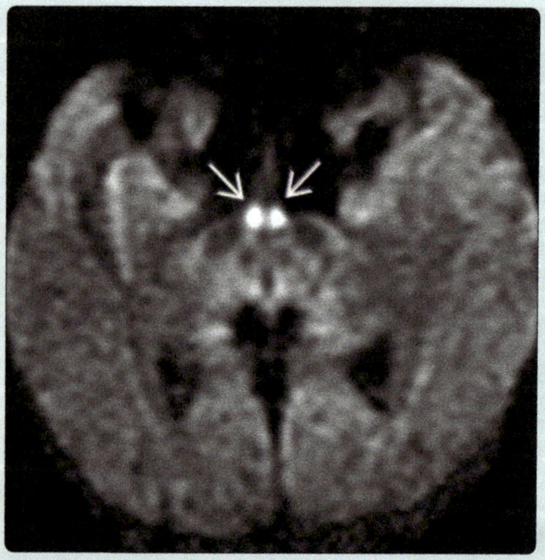

(Left) *Sagittal T1WI MR shows a classic finding for Marchiafava-Bignami disease with a thinned corpus callosum and hypointensity in the middle layers. Note that the genu, body, and splenium are all involved. (Courtesy A. Datir, MD.)* **(Right)** *Axial DWI MR shows restricted diffusion in the mammillary bodies in this patient with acute Wernicke encephalopathy.*

KEY FACTS

TERMINOLOGY

- Functional, potentially reversible clinical syndrome
  - Acute hepatic encephalopathy (AHE)
  - Chronic hepatic encephalopathy (CHE)
- Characterized by psychiatric, cognitive, and motor components

IMAGING

- AHE (hyperammonemia)
  - High T2 signal in most of cerebral cortex (preferential insular cortex and cingulate gyri) with diffusion restriction
  - Perirolandic/occipital regions relatively spared
- CHE
  - Bilateral T1WI hyperintensity in basal ganglia (BG), particularly globus pallidus
  - ↑ T1WI in pituitary gland/hypothalamus less common
- FLAIR: Diffuse high signal intensity along hemispheric white matter in or around corticospinal tract

TOP DIFFERENTIAL DIAGNOSES

- Cholestatic diseases
- Liver copper overload
- Hyperalimentation
- Other causes of T1 hyperintense BG
  - Hypoxic-ischemic encephalopathy
  - Fahr disease (idiopathic calcification of BG)
  - Carbon monoxide poisoning
  - Neurofibromatosis type 1

PATHOLOGY

- Brain accumulation of neurotoxic &/or neuroactive substances
- Ammonia, manganese, aromatic amino acids

DIAGNOSTIC CHECKLIST

- After therapy, clinical features and MRS abnormalities improve 1st, followed 3-6 months later by normalization of BG signal

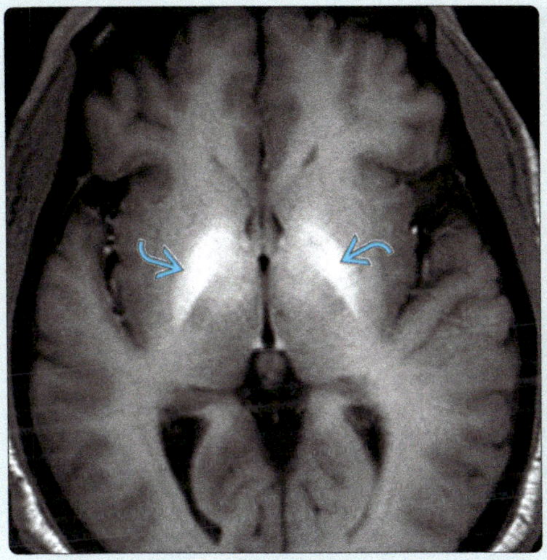
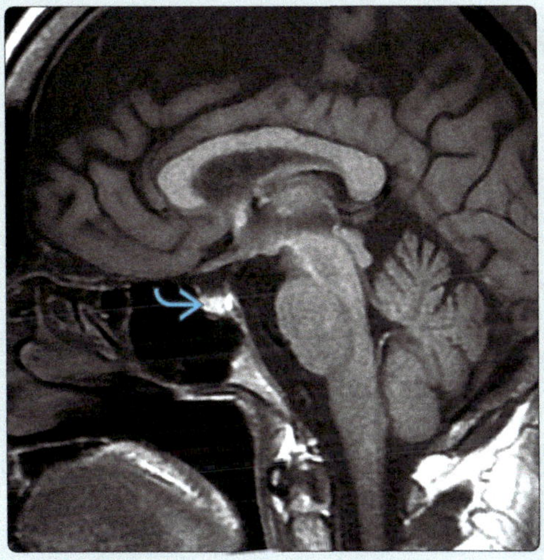

(Left) *Axial T1 MR in a patient with chronic liver disease demonstrates high T1 signal in the globus pallidus* ➔. **(Right)** *Sagittal T1 MR in the same patient shows a hyperintense anterior pituitary gland* ➔. *In patients with chronic liver disease, T1 hyperintensity is most commonly seen in the globus pallidus. The anterior pituitary and hypothalamus may also show similar T1 hyperintensity but is less common. T1 hyperintensity is thought to be due to manganese deposition.*

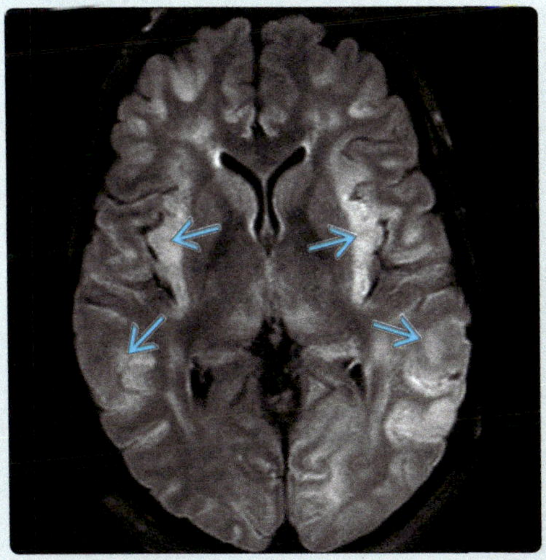
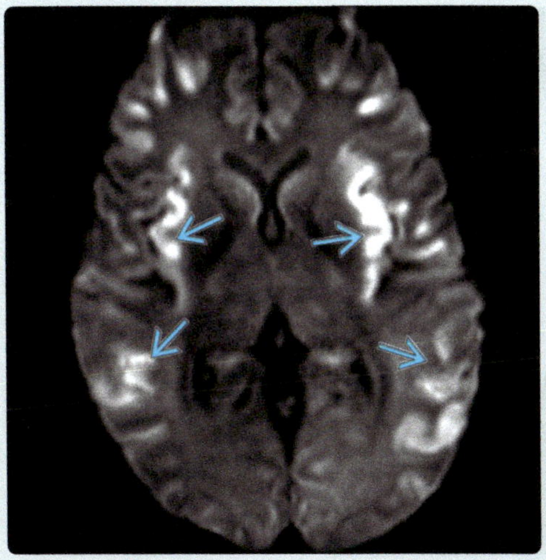

(Left) *Axial FLAIR MR in a patient with acute liver failure shows extensive cortical swelling and hyperintensity* ➔. *There is relative sparing of the occipital cortex.* **(Right)** *Axial DWI MR in the same patient shows corresponding high signal* ➔ *due to diffusion restriction. Note: Acute hepatic encephalopathy is caused by hyperammonemia. It is a life-threatening but potentially treatable disorder with high morbidity and mortality.*

Acute Hypertensive Encephalopathy, Posterior Reversible Encephalopathy Syndrome (PRES)

KEY FACTS

TERMINOLOGY

- Cerebrovascular autoregulatory disorder
- Many etiologies with HTN as common component
  - Preeclampsia, eclampsia
  - Drug toxicity (e.g., chemotherapy)
  - Uremic encephalopathies

IMAGING

- General
  - Patchy parietooccipital cortical/subcortical edema in patient with severe acute/subacute HTN
- CT
  - Bilateral nonconfluent hypodense foci
  - ± symmetric lesions in basal ganglia
- MR
  - Parietooccipital T2/FLAIR hyperintensities in 95%
  - ± basal ganglia, pontine, cerebellar involvement
  - 3 patterns of hemorrhage: Focal parenchymal hemorrhage, microhemorrhages, convexity SAH
  - Generally no restriction on DWI
  - Variable patchy enhancement
  - However, atypical imaging patterns common

TOP DIFFERENTIAL DIAGNOSES

- Acute cerebral ischemia-infarction
- Status epilepticus
- Hypoglycemia
- Thrombotic microangiopathies (DIC, TTP, malignant HTN)

PATHOLOGY

- Acute HTN damages vascular endothelium; failed autoregulation causes blood-brain barrier disruption
- Result = vasogenic (not cytotoxic) edema

CLINICAL ISSUES

- Headache, seizure, ↓ mental status, visual symptoms
- Caution: Some patients may be normotensive or have only minimally elevated BP

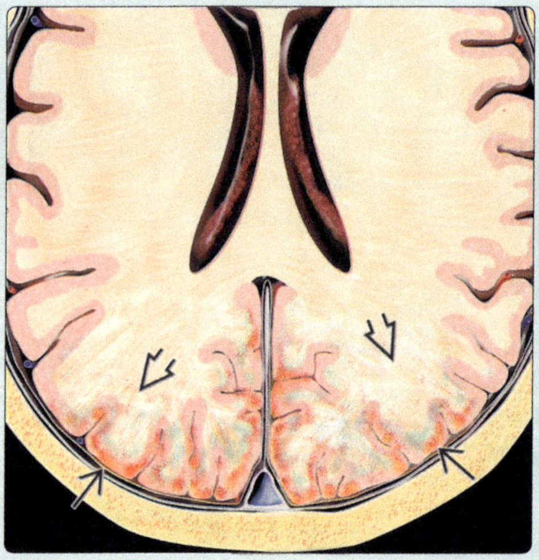

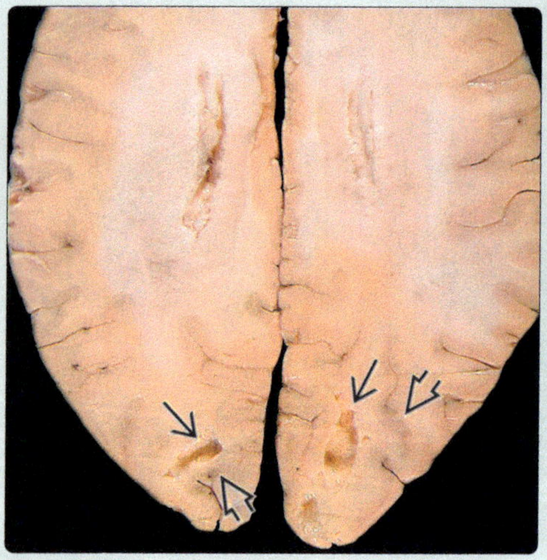

(Left) *Axial graphic shows the classic posterior circulation cortical/subcortical vasogenic edema ➡ characteristic of posterior reversible encephalopathy syndrome (PRES). Petechial hemorrhage ➡ occurs in some cases.* **(Right)** *Gross pathology of a patient with complicated PRES demonstrates diffuse cerebral edema with swollen gyri. Multifocal petechial microhemorrhages are present in the occipital cortex ➡ with several areas of focal encephalomalacia secondary to infarction ➡. (Courtesy R. Hewlett, MD.)*

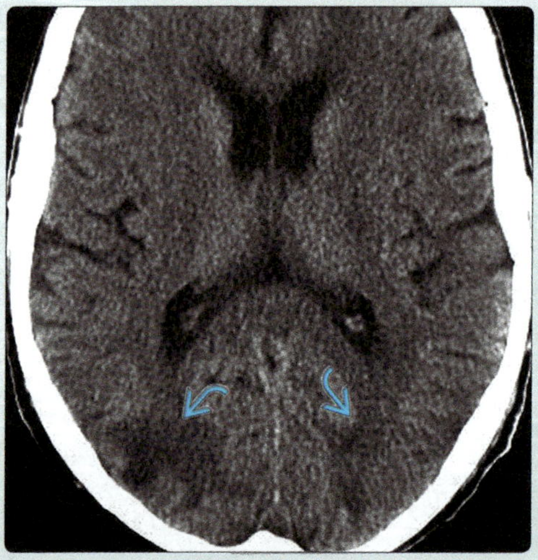

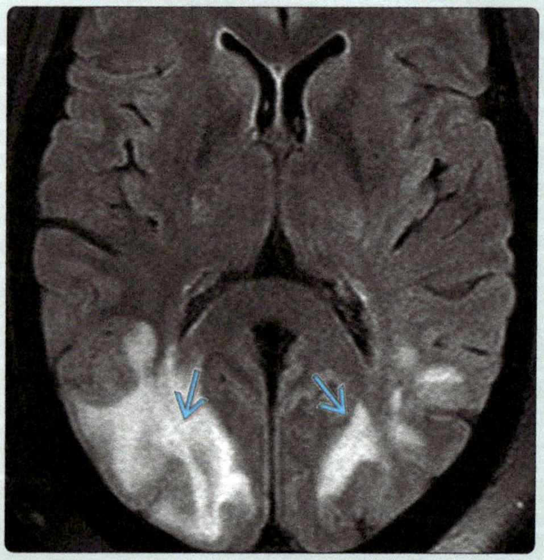

(Left) *Axial NECT in a 54-year-old patient with liver transplant on Tacrolimus FK 506 who presented with seizures demonstrates asymmetric subcortical edema in the occipital lobes bilaterally ➡. Findings are typical of PRES.* **(Right)** *Axial FLAIR MR in a 20-year-old eclamptic woman who presented with severe hypertension, seizures, and altered sensorium shows classic findings of PRES with occipital cortical/subcortical edema ➡. Her BP at presentation was 210/140.*

KEY FACTS

TERMINOLOGY

- Subcortical arteriosclerotic encephalopathy

IMAGING

- General features
  - Lacunae (lenticular nuclei, pons, thalamus, internal capsule, caudate)
  - Cerebral hemorrhage (basal ganglia/external capsule, thalamus)
  - Confluent white matter (WM) disease (centrum semiovale, corona radiata)
- CT
  - Diffuse WM hypodensity on CT
  - Lacunar infarcts [basal ganglia (BG), thalamus/brainstem]
- MR
  - Hyperintense lesions within corona radiata, centrum semiovale, BG
  - Multiple microhemorrhages (GRE, SWI)
    - Predilection for BG/thalami, brainstem, cerebellum
  - Acute WM lesions may restrict

TOP DIFFERENTIAL DIAGNOSES

- Amyloid angiopathy
- CADASIL
- Dementing disorders
  - Alzheimer dementia
  - Multiinfarct dementia
- Antiphospholipid antibody syndrome
- Neuropsychiatric systemic lupus erythematosus
- Vasculitis

PATHOLOGY

- Chronic HTN is associated with hyaline deposition within small arteries (so-called lipohyalinosis)

CLINICAL ISSUES

- Stepwise/gradual mental deterioration
- Acute strokes, lacunar syndrome

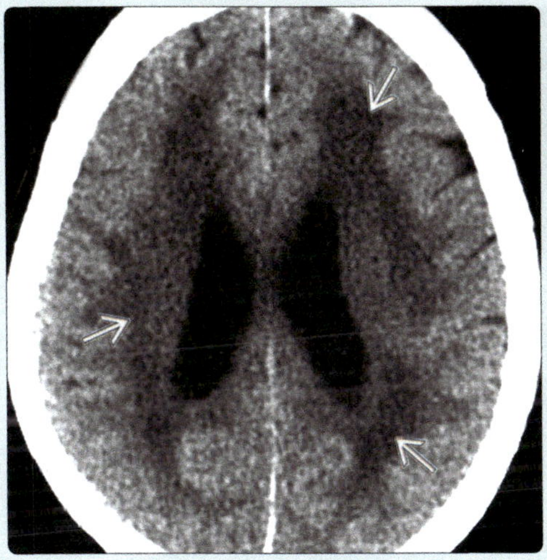

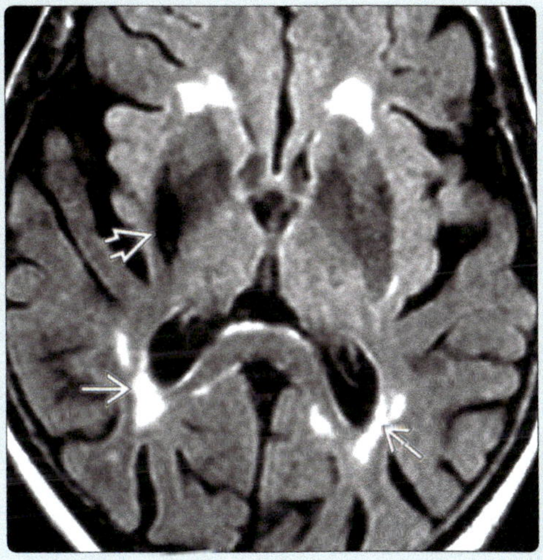

(Left) *Axial NECT shows the typical appearance of chronic hypertensive encephalopathy, seen here as diffuse confluent periventricular white matter hypodensity →.* **(Right)** *Axial FLAIR in a 72-year-old woman with longstanding systemic HTN demonstrates multifocal discrete and confluent hyperintensities scattered throughout the deep periventricular white matter, especially near the atria and occipital horns →. Note the old, hypertensive, basal ganglionic hemorrhage →.*

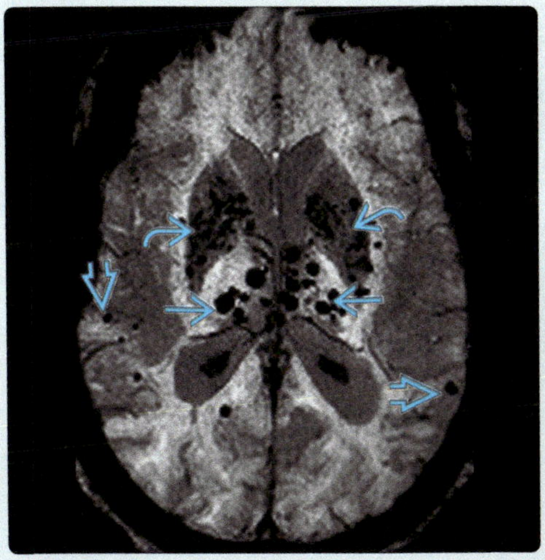

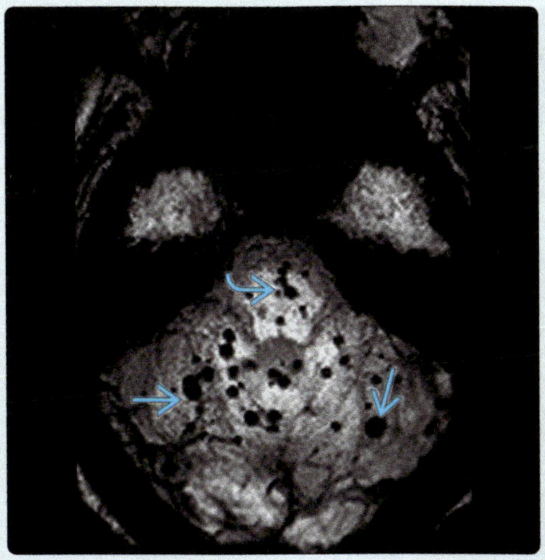

(Left) *Axial SWI in a patient with long-standing poorly controlled HTN shows numerous microhemorrhages in the basal ganglia → and thalami →. A few microhemorrhages are also seen in the subcortical white matter →.* **(Right)** *Axial SWI in the same patient shows more microhemorrhages in the brainstem → and both cerebellar hemispheres →. The distribution of these microhemorrhages is typical for chronic hypertensive encephalopathy.*

Idiopathic Intracranial Hypertension

KEY FACTS

TERMINOLOGY

- Idiopathic intracranial hypertension (IIH)
- Pseudotumor cerebri
- "Benign intracranial hypertension"
- ↑ intracranial pressure (ICP) without identifiable cause

IMAGING

- Empty or partially empty sella
- Posterior globe flattening
- Intraocular protrusion of optic nerve head
- Optic nerve sheath enlargement: Widened ring of cerebrospinal fluid around optic nerve
- Optic nerve tortuosity
- Slit-like ventricles, rare: Poor neuroimaging sign of IIH
- MRV: Often shows transverse sinus stenosis and "flow gaps"
  - Whether this is cause or consequence of raised ICP is controversial
- Best imaging tool: MR brain + T2 coronal fat-sat orbit + MRV

TOP DIFFERENTIAL DIAGNOSES

- Secondary pseudotumor syndromes
  - Cerebral venous thrombosis, dural sinus stenosis
- Idiopathic or postinflammatory (i.e., multiple sclerosis) optic nerve atrophy
- Idiopathic empty sella (normal variant)

CLINICAL ISSUES

- Obese woman age 20-44 years most common
  - Headache in 90-95%
  - Papilledema (bilateral optic nerve head swelling) virtually universal
- Progressive visual loss ± CN6 paresis, diplopia
- Chief hazard: Vision loss from chronic papilledema
- Treatment: Medical or surgical (LP and VP shunt, optic nerve sheath fenestration)

(Left) *Funduscopy in a patient with IIH, severe papilledema shows swelling/blurred margins of the optic disc, striking venous engorgement, and focal hemorrhages adjacent to the disc.* **(Right)** *Axial T2WI MR shows dilated CSF spaces around the optic nerves and protrusion of the optic nerve papilla into the posterior globes. Opening CSF pressure in this 32-year-old woman was 45 cm of H_2O. Prominent CSF space in the suprasellar cistern represents an empty sella. Note the tortuosity of the left optic nerve.*

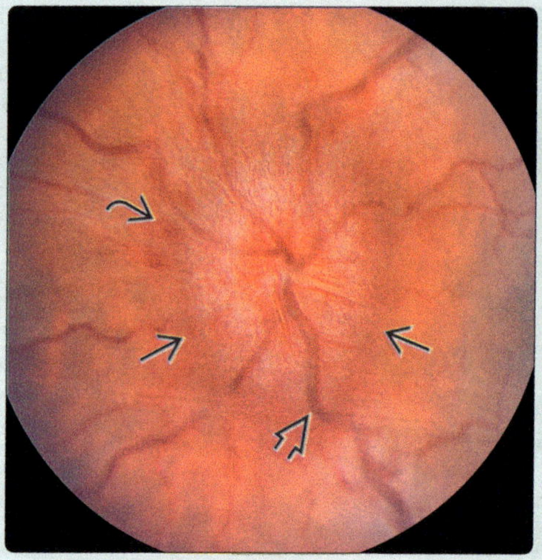

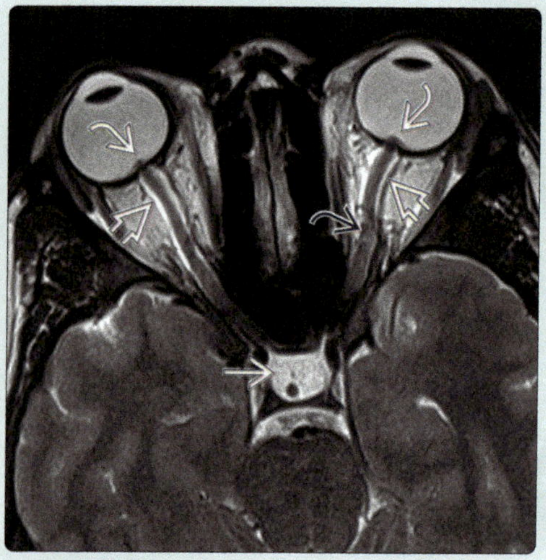

(Left) *Axial T1WI C+ MR in the same patient demonstrates enhancement, as well as protrusion of prelaminar optic nerves bilaterally. Mild diffuse optic nerve sheath enhancement is also present.* **(Right)** *Coronal T1WI C+ FS MR in the same patient shows diffuse enhancement of the optic nerve sheaths associated with prominent subarachnoid spaces along the optic nerves. Treatment for IIH includes weight loss and medications (i.e., diuretics), as well as lumbar punctures, shunt, and optic nerve fenestration.*

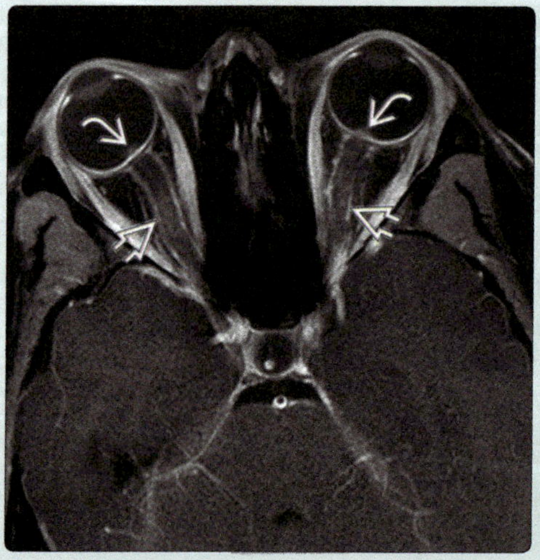

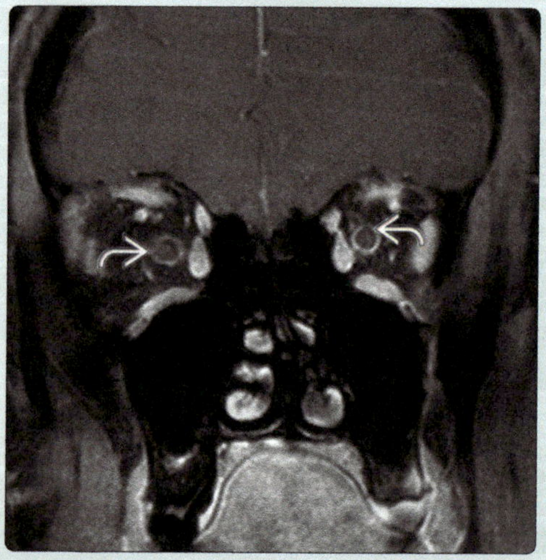

KEY FACTS

TERMINOLOGY

- Anoxic-ischemic encephalopathy, usually with bilateral lesions, caused by inhalation of carbon monoxide (CO) gas

IMAGING

- Best diagnostic clue: Globi pallidi (GP) T2/FLAIR hyperintensity
- T1 MR: Both hypointensity in GP (likely necrosis) and hyperintensity in GP (likely hemorrhage) reported
- T2 MR: Ischemia/infarct of GP
  - Cerebral hemispheric white matter (WM): Bilateral confluent hyperintense WM (periventricular, centrum semiovale)
  - Cortical hyperintensity (commonly temporal lobe)
  - Medial temporal lobe hyperintensity (uncommon despite frequent pathologic findings)
- DWI MR: Acute restriction is common
- MRS: Progressively ↓ NAA/Cr with time; ↑ Cho/Cr
  - Progressively ↑ Lac/Cr with time

TOP DIFFERENTIAL DIAGNOSES

- Wilson disease
- Japanese encephalitis
- Creutzfeldt-Jakob disease

PATHOLOGY

- Impairs ability of erythrocytes to transport oxygen, causing hypoxia and reducing cellular oxygen metabolism
- CO-induced parkinsonism
- Demyelination, edema, and hemorrhagic necrosis

CLINICAL ISSUES

- Acute toxicity: Nausea, vomiting, headache
- Neuropsychological sequelae
- Hyperbaric oxygen therapy: Treatment of choice in acute carbon monoxide poisoning (within 6 hours for best effect)
- Delayed neurologic sequelae (10-30% of victims)

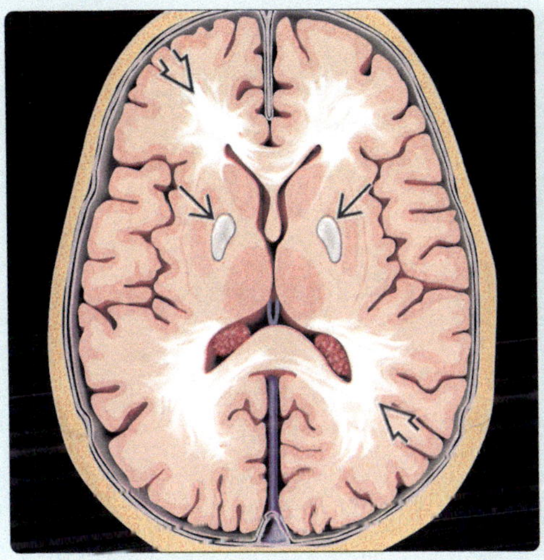

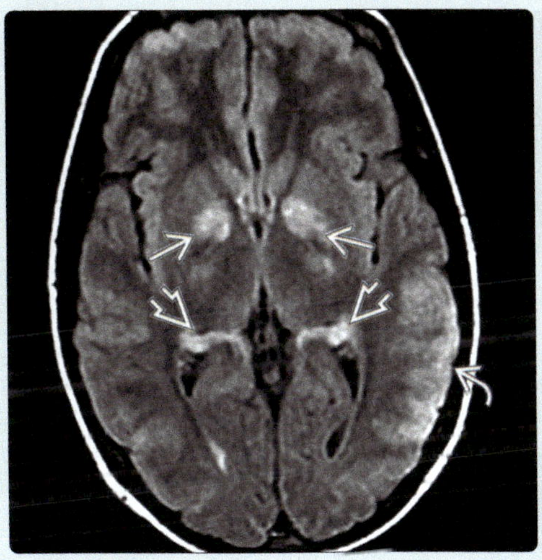

(Left) *Axial graphic shows the typical involvement of the brain by CO poisoning. The globi pallidi (GP) ➡ are most affected, followed by the cerebral white matter. Pathologically, there is necrosis of the GP with variable areas of necrosis and demyelination in the white matter ➡.* **(Right)** *Axial FLAIR MR in this patient with acute CO poisoning shows the classic appearance with symmetric GP hyperintensity ➡. Note the additional involvement of the posterior temporal cortex ➡ and hippocampi ➡, a less common finding.*

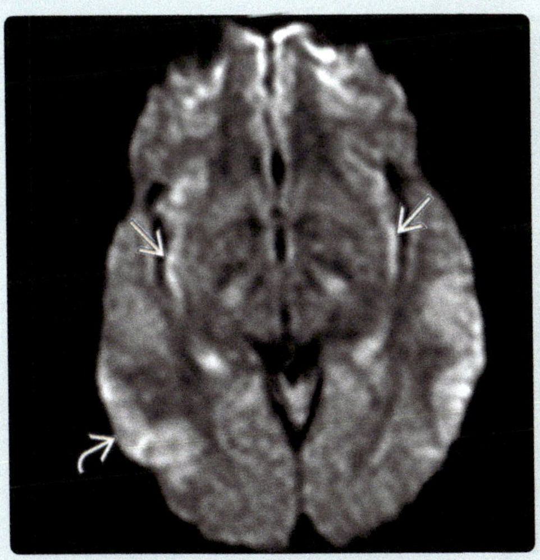

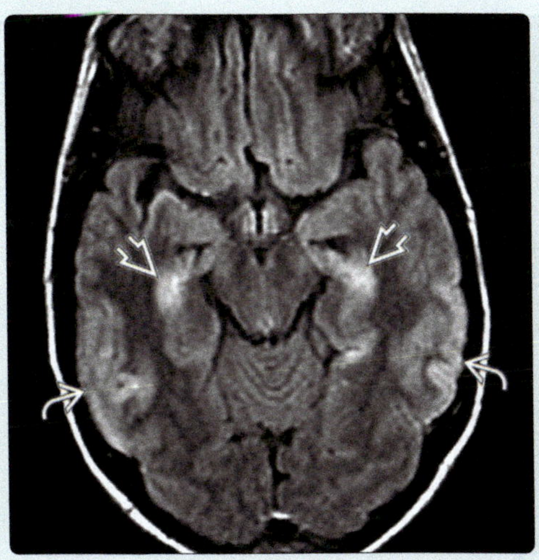

(Left) *Axial DWI MR in the same patient shows areas of restricted diffusion involving the posterior temporal cortex ➡, hippocampal tail, and insular cortex ➡ bilaterally. DWI often shows the affected areas more readily than corresponding T2 or FLAIR MR.* **(Right)** *Axial FLAIR MR in the same patient shows symmetric hyperintensity involving the bilateral hippocampi ➡ and posterior temporal cortex ➡.*

KEY FACTS

TERMINOLOGY

- Many drugs (prescription, illicit, or street) have adverse CNS effects
  - Illicit drug use often causes cerebrovascular disease
  - Amphetamines, cocaine > opioids, cannabis
- Polydrug abuse (including EtOH) is common
- Nitrous oxide (NO_2) abuse → vitamin B12 inactivation → subacute combined degeneration

IMAGING

- Best imaging clue: Young/middle-aged adult with ischemic or hemorrhagic stroke after recent drug administration
  - Hemorrhage: Intracranial, subarachnoid, intraventricular
  - Nonhemorrhagic ischemic stroke: Middle cerebral artery territory most common
- Heroin, MDMA: Globus pallidus ischemia
- Amphetamines: Hemorrhage, vasculitis, pseudoaneurysm, infarcts
- NECT for suspected hemorrhage indicated: If NECT reveals hemorrhage, consider CTA/MRA/DSA
- Consider drug abuse or dissection in young/middle-aged stroke patient

TOP DIFFERENTIAL DIAGNOSES

- Intracranial hemorrhage in young adults
  - Vascular malformations; dural sinus thrombosis with hemorrhagic infarct; severe posterior reversible encephalopathy syndrome with secondary hemorrhage
- Vasculitis

PATHOLOGY

- 40-50% of drug-related intracranial hemorrhage is related to underlying vascular malformation (cerebral aneurysm, arteriovenous malformation)

CLINICAL ISSUES

- 30% of strokes in patients < 45 years old are drug related
- Cocaine, MDMA, amphetamines: Stroke, headache, seizures

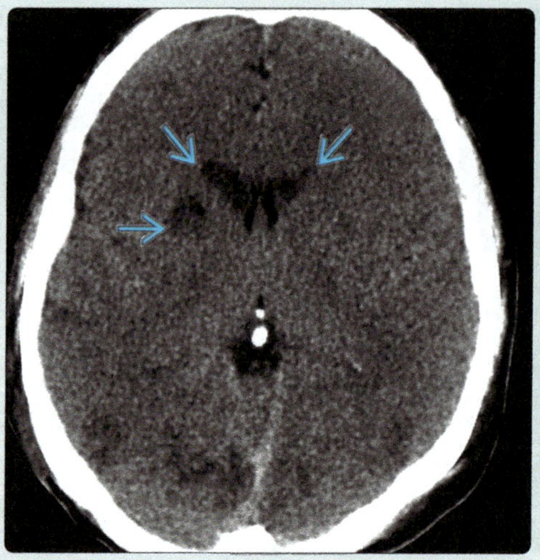

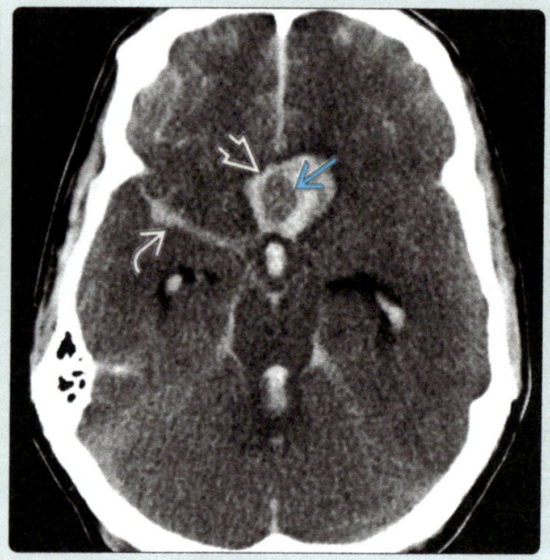

(Left) *Axial NECT in comatose patient after cocaine abuse shows focal hypodensities ➔ in basal ganglia related to ischemia. Diffuse loss of corticomedullary differentiation is due to severe anoxia.* **(Right)** *A 32-year-old woman methamphetamine abuser had sudden severe headache followed by coma. NECT shows diffuse subarachnoid ➔, intraventricular hemorrhage. Focal interhemispheric hematoma ➔ surrounds a ruptured anterior communicating artery aneurysm ➔.*

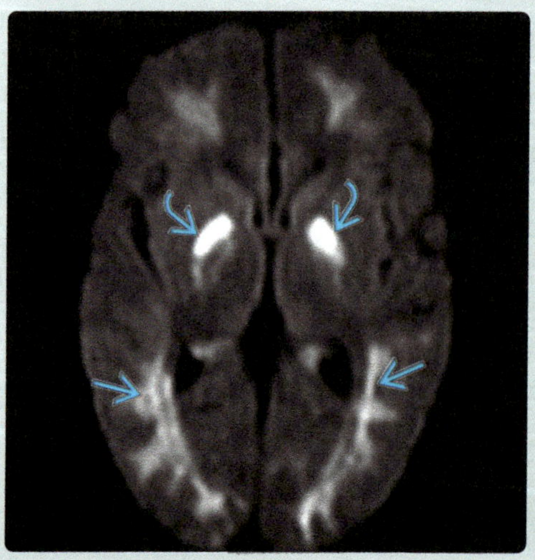

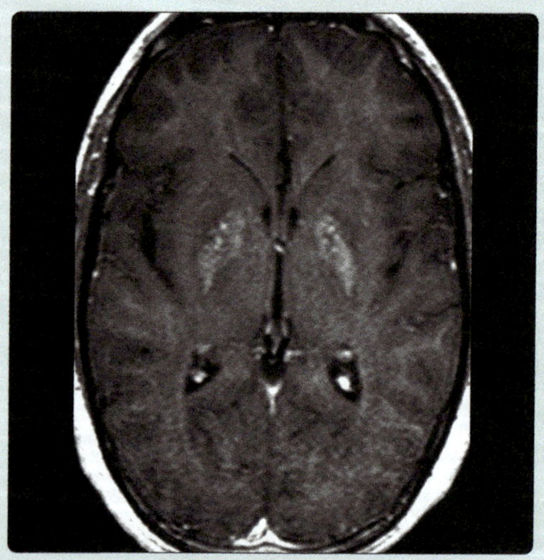

(Left) *Axial DWI MR in a young male patient following ingestion of ecstasy (MDMA) shows symmetric diffusion restriction in the globi pallidi ➔ and deep white matter ➔.* **(Right)** *Axial T1 C+ MR in the same patient shows enhancement within the globi pallidi due to necrosis. MDMA causes rapid release of 5-hydroxytryptamine, which is 1 of the most potent vasoconstrictors in the brain, and it ultimately leads to necrosis of the involved regions of the brain. The occipital cortex and globi pallidi are most vulnerable.*

KEY FACTS

TERMINOLOGY

- Osmotic demyelination syndrome (ODS)
  - Formerly called central pontine myelinolysis (CPM) &/or extrapontine myelinolysis (EPM)
- Acute demyelination from rapid shifts in serum osmolality
  - Classic setting: Rapid correction of hyponatremia
  - ODS may occur in normonatremic patients

IMAGING

- Central pons T2 hyperintensity with sparing of periphery
- 50% in pons (CPM); 50% in extrapontine sites (EPM)
  - Central fibers involved; peripheral fibers spared
  - Basal ganglia
  - Cerebral white matter
- CPM + EPM = almost pathognomonic for ODS
- Acute: Confluent hyperintensity in central pons with sparing of periphery and corticospinal tracts
- Round, triangular, or batwing-shaped
- DWI earliest and sensitive for ODS
- Subacute: Hyperintensity often normalizes
- Best imaging tool: MR > > CT

TOP DIFFERENTIAL DIAGNOSES

- Pontine ischemia/infarction
- Demyelinating disease
- Pontine neoplasm (astrocytoma, metastasis)
- Metabolic disease (Wilson, Leigh, diabetes, hypertensive encephalopathy)

PATHOLOGY

- Heterogeneous disorder with common etiology: Osmotic stress

CLINICAL ISSUES

- Alcoholic, hyponatremic patient with rapid correction of serum sodium
- ODS symptoms emerge 2-8 days (occasionally weeks) after correction of hyponatremia
- "Comorbid" conditions common, poorer prognosis

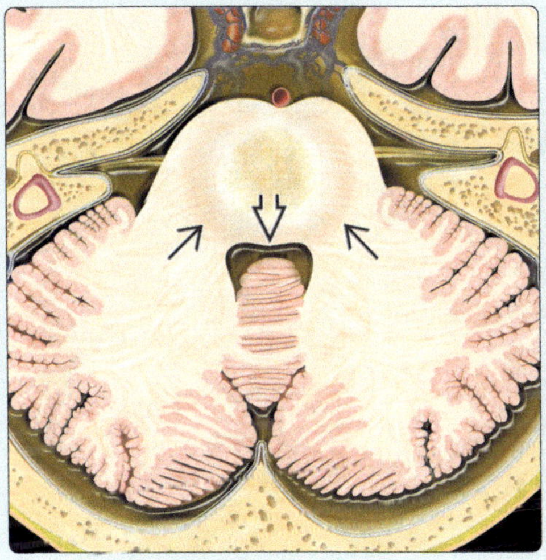

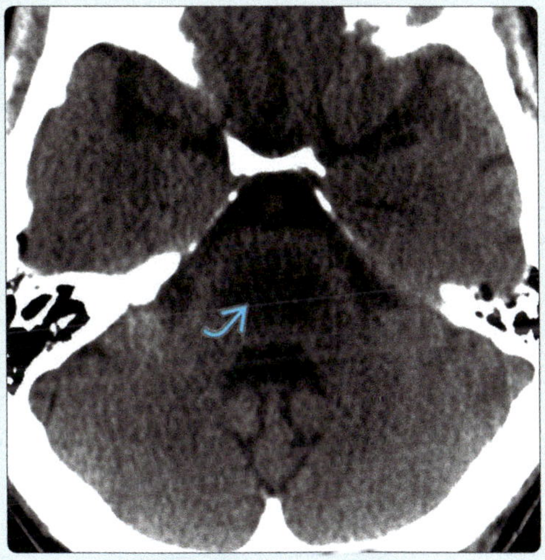

(Left) *Axial graphic shows acute osmotic demyelination affecting the central pons →. The pons is slightly swollen with mild mass effect on the 4th ventricle →.* **(Right)** *Axial NECT in a chronic alcoholic patient who presented with altered sensorium demonstrates central pontine hypodensity → due to osmotic demyelination syndrome. Osmotic demyelination syndrome is an acute demyelination caused by rapid shifts in serum osmolality.*

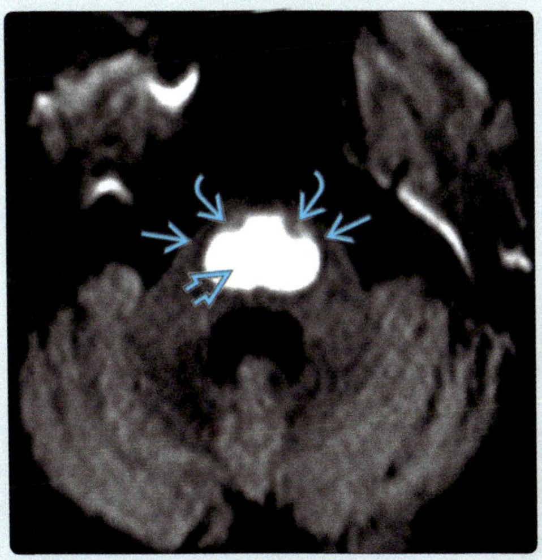

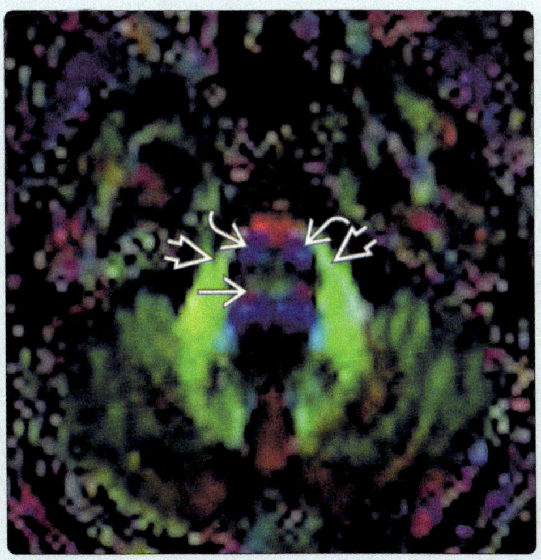

(Left) *Axial DWI in the same patient shows restricted diffusion in the pons → corresponding to the hypodensity on CT. There is sparing of the corticospinal tracts → and peripheral pontine pons →.* **(Right)** *Axial DTI in the same patient shows disruption of the central pontine white matter → with preservation of the corticospinal tracts → and peripheral pontine fibers →. Pontine osmotic demyelination is round, triangular, or batwing-shaped.*

Mesial Temporal Sclerosis

KEY FACTS

TERMINOLOGY

- Seizure-associated neuronal loss and gliosis in hippocampus and adjacent structures

IMAGING

- Primary features: Abnormal T2 hyperintensity, hippocampal volume loss/atrophy, obscuration of internal architecture
- Secondary signs: Ipsilateral fornix and mammillary body atrophy, enlarged ipsilateral temporal horn, and choroidal fissure
- ↑ hyperintensity on DWI (T2 shine through)
- ↓ NAA in hippocampus, temporal lobe

TOP DIFFERENTIAL DIAGNOSES

- Status epilepticus
- Low-grade astrocytoma
- Choroidal fissure cyst
- Hippocampal sulcus remnant

PATHOLOGY

- Prolonged febrile seizures may produce acute hippocampal injury → subsequent atrophy
- Coexistent 2nd developmental lesion in 15% of mesial temporal sclerosis (MTS) patients

CLINICAL ISSUES

- Partial complex seizures
- Often history of childhood febrile or medically intractable seizures
- Surgical temporal lobectomy reserved for medically intractable seizures, intolerable drug side effects

DIAGNOSTIC CHECKLIST

- Most common cause of partial complex epilepsy in adult age group
- Low-grade neoplasms and cortical dysplasia more common causes of partial complex epilepsy than MTS in pediatric age group

(Left) *Coronal graphic depicts the characteristic appearance of mesial temporal sclerosis. The right hippocampus is small (atrophic) with loss of normal internal architecture reflecting neuronal loss and gliosis. Note concordant atrophy of the ipsilateral fornix and widening of the ipsilateral temporal horn and choroidal fissure.* **(Right)** *Coronal STIR MR at 3.0 tesla in a normal nonepileptic patient imaged for headaches demonstrates normal bilateral hippocampal anatomy, size, and signal intensity.*

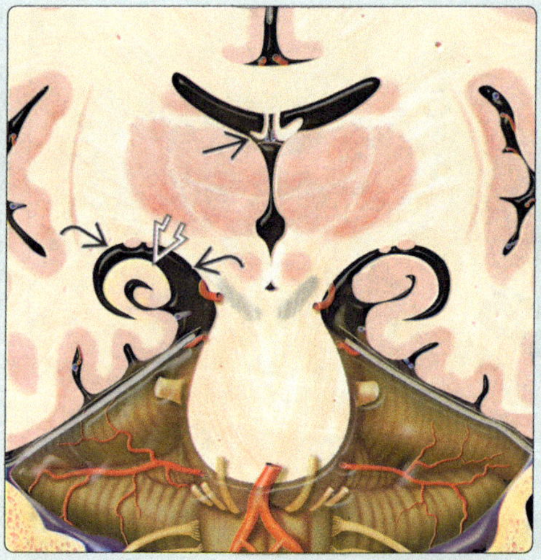

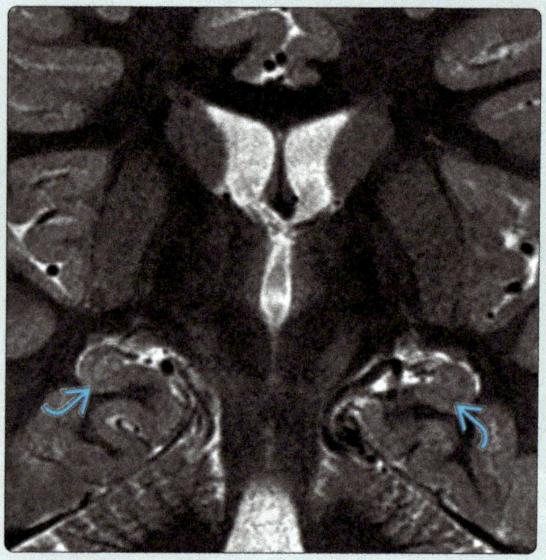

(Left) *Coronal T1-weighted true inversion recovery MR at 3.0 tesla shows asymmetric right hippocampal volume loss and obscuration of normal internal gray-white differentiation. The ipsilateral fornix is smaller than the normal left fornix.* **(Right)** *Coronal T2-weighted MR at 3.0 tesla in the same patient with right hippocampal sclerosis shows hippocampal volume loss and obscuration of normal internal architecture but normal T2 signal intensity. FLAIR better shows the increase in signal intensity.*

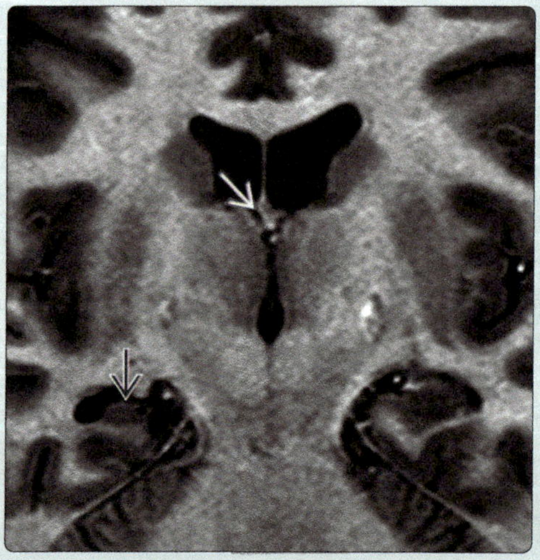

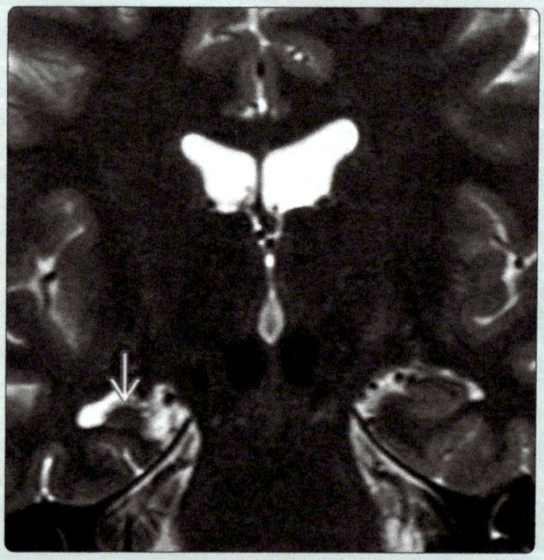

KEY FACTS

TERMINOLOGY

- Status epilepticus: > 30 minutes of continuous seizures (SZs) or ≥ 2 SZs without full recovery of consciousness between seizures
- Synonyms: Transient seizure-related MR changes, reversible postictal cerebral edema

IMAGING

- Best diagnostic clue: T2 hyperintensity in gray matter &/or subcortical white matter (WM) with mild mass effect
  - Supratentorial, related to epileptogenic focus
  - Typically cortex &/or subcortical WM
  - May involve hippocampus, corpus callosum, thalamus (particularly pulvinar nucleus)
- Swelling and increased volume of involved cortex
- DWI: Restricted diffusion acutely
- T1WI C+: Variable enhancement, none to marked
- PWI: Marked hyperemia, ↑ relative cerebral blood flow and volume

TOP DIFFERENTIAL DIAGNOSES

- Cerebritis
- Cerebral ischemia-infarction
- Herpes encephalitis
- Hypoglycemia (usually bilateral, multifocal)
- Astrocytoma

CLINICAL ISSUES

- Active SZs &/or status epilepticus
- Other signs/symptoms: Location dependent

DIAGNOSTIC CHECKLIST

- Acute SZs or status epilepticus may mimic other pathology, such as tumor progression or cerebritis
- Clinical information and follow-up imaging often differentiates from other etiologies
- Look for underlying mass that may have caused SZs/status epilepticus
- SZ-related changes usually resolve within days to weeks

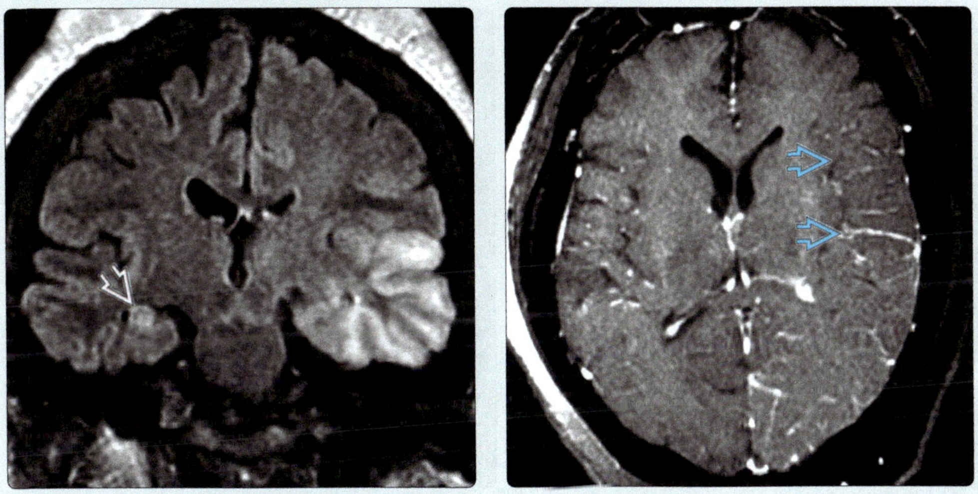

(Left) *Coronal FLAIR was performed shortly after a long episode of status epilepticus hyperintensity involving the left temporal lobe cortex and subcortical white matter. Note "mirror focus" in the right hippocampus ➡.* **(Right)** *Axial T1WI C+ FS MR in the same patient shows mild edema and vascular congestion in the left temporal lobe ➡. Imaging 1 month later showed near complete resolution of the signal abnormalities. Status epilepticus may result in MR changes that are likely related to transient cerebral edema.*

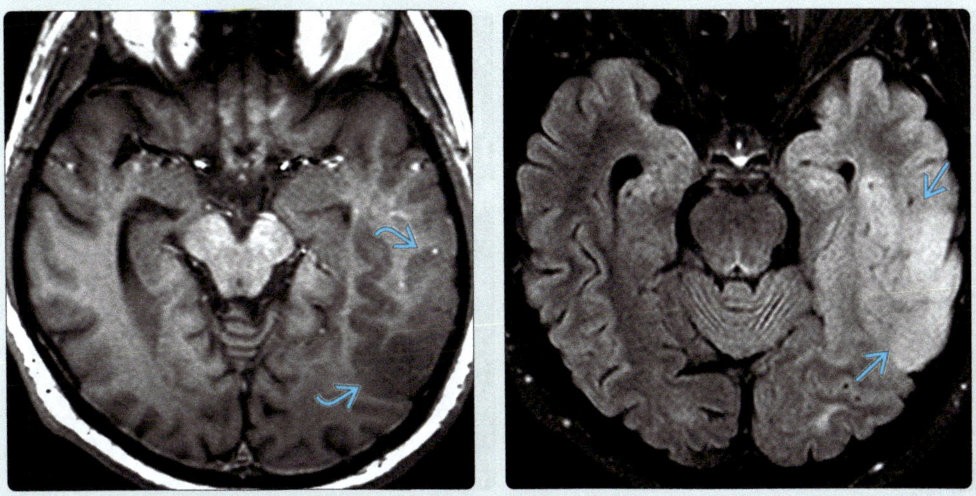

(Left) *Axial T1WI MR in a patient with status epilepticus shows mild thickening of the left temporal cortex ➡.* **(Right)** *Axial FLAIR MR in the same patient shows cortical and subcortical white matter edema ➡. MR signal abnormalities are related to transient vasogenic &/or cytotoxic edema. Follow-up imaging in such cases usually shows resolution of the acute imaging abnormalities in treated patients. Atrophy may be seen chronically.*

KEY FACTS

TERMINOLOGY

- Sudden memory loss without other signs of cognitive or neurologic impairment; usually resolves within 24 h

IMAGING

- NECT, CECT almost invariably normal
- MR
  - T2/FLAIR usually normal
  - DWI: Focal dot-like area of diffusion restriction in hippocampus
    - Single (55%)
    - Multiple (45%)
    - Unilateral (50-55%)
    - Bilateral (45-50%)
  - DWI abnormalities increase with time
    - From 35% at 0-6 h to 65-70% by 12-24 h
    - Complete resolution by day 10
- PWI, PET/CT may show hippocampal hypoperfusion/hypometabolism

TOP DIFFERENTIAL DIAGNOSES

- Cerebral ischemia-infarction
- Seizure/postictal state
- Hypoglycemia

PATHOLOGY

- Underlying pathophysiology still unknown
- Functional, reversible modification of hippocampus

CLINICAL ISSUES

- Most common in middle aged, elderly patients (rare < 40 years)
  - Younger patients with physical/emotional stress, trauma, migraine (rare)
- Abrupt onset of massive episodic memory impairment
  - Both anterograde and retrograde
  - Often accompanied by repetitive questioning
  - Other neurologic functions intact
- Self-limited (spontaneous resolution within 24 h)

(Left) *Axial T2WI in a 54-year-old man with sudden onset of amnesia is normal.* **(Right)** *Axial FLAIR MR shows no abnormalities. Both temporal horns ➡ are well visualized and are normal. The hippocampi, just medial to the cerebrospinal fluid-filled temporal horns, also appear completely normal.*

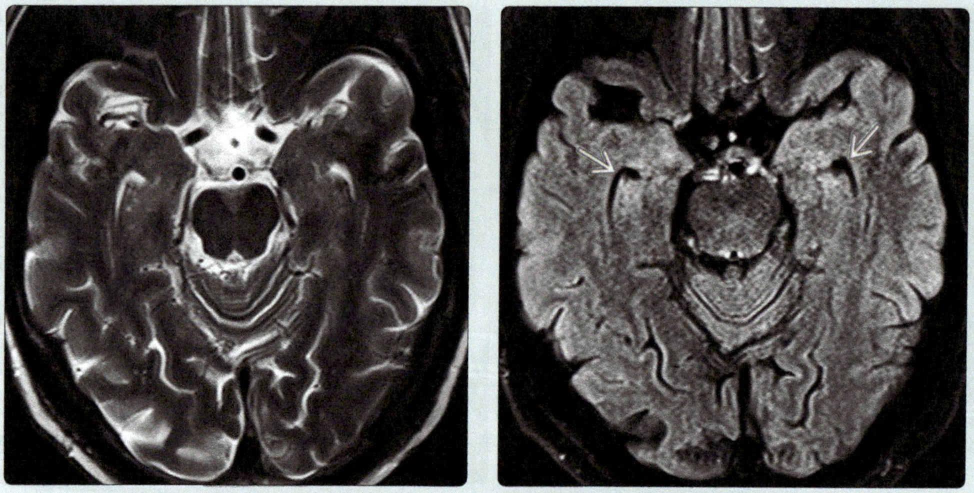

(Left) *Axial DWI in the same patient shows a dot-like focus of restricted diffusion in the right hippocampus ➡, just inside the temporal horn of the lateral ventricle ➡.* **(Right)** *The hyperintense focus seen on the DWI image is dark on ADC (hypointense to the adjacent parenchyma) ➡, confirming the reduced diffusivity. The patient's memory recovered within 24 hours. This is a classic case of transient global amnesia with the classic findings on DWI.*

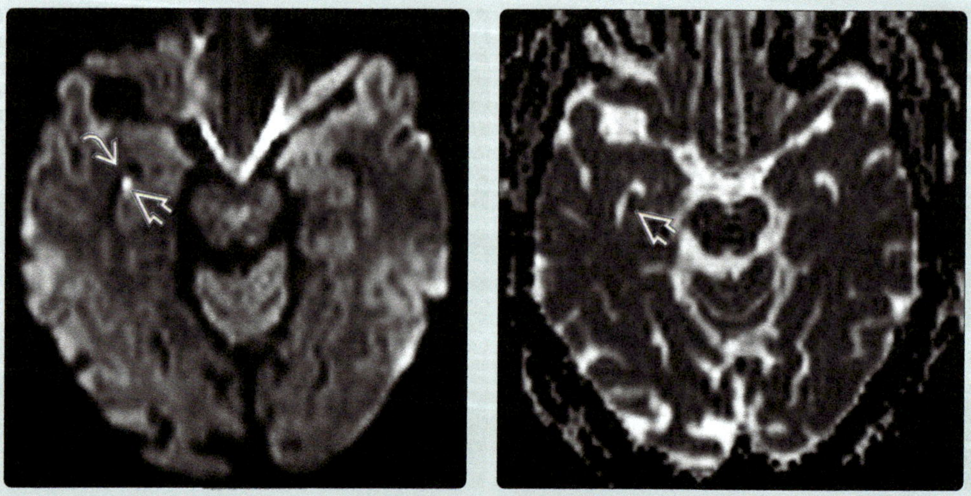

KEY FACTS

TERMINOLOGY

- ↓ overall brain volume with advancing age
  - Reflected in relative ↑ cerebrospinal fluid spaces

IMAGING

- Broad spectrum of "normal" on imaging in elderly patients
- "Successfully aging brain"
  - Smooth, thin, periventricular, high signal rim on FLAIR is normal
  - White matter hyperintensities (WMHs) absent/few
- Decreased total brain volume
  - Selective atrophy of white matter (not gray matter) predominates
- WMHs
  - ↑ In number/size after 50 years
  - Approximately universal after 65 years
- GRE/SWI
  - Increasing mineralization of basal ganglia with age
  - Microbleeds are not characteristic of successful aging brain
- Age-related shift from anterior to posterior cortical metabolism

TOP DIFFERENTIAL DIAGNOSES

- Mild cognitive impairment
- Alzheimer disease
- Sporadic subcortical arteriosclerotic encephalopathy
- Vascular dementia
- Frontotemporal lobar degeneration (Pick disease)

CLINICAL ISSUES

- WMHs correlate with age, silent stroke, hypertension, female sex

DIAGNOSTIC CHECKLIST

- Cannot predict cognitive function from CT/MR
  - Imaging only roughly correlates with cognitive function
  - Significant overlap with dementias

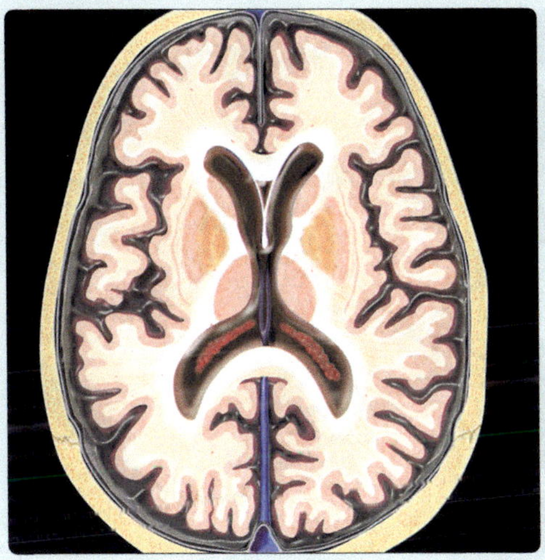

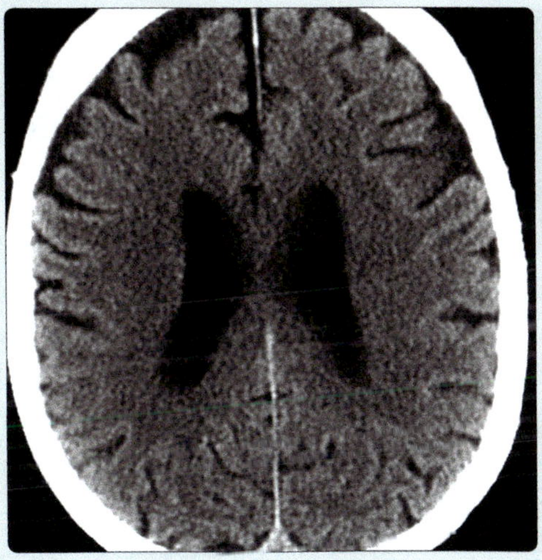

(Left) *Axial graphic depicts a normally aging brain in an 80-year-old patient. Note the widening of sulci and ventricles in the absence of any brain parenchymal abnormalities.* **(Right)** *Axial NECT demonstrates mild sulcal enlargement and mild ventriculomegaly in a 70-year-old patient. The white matter appears completely normal, without periventricular hypodensities or white matter lacunar infarcts.*

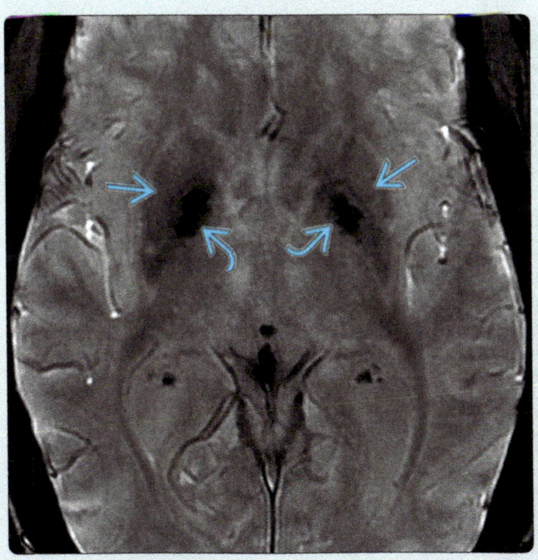

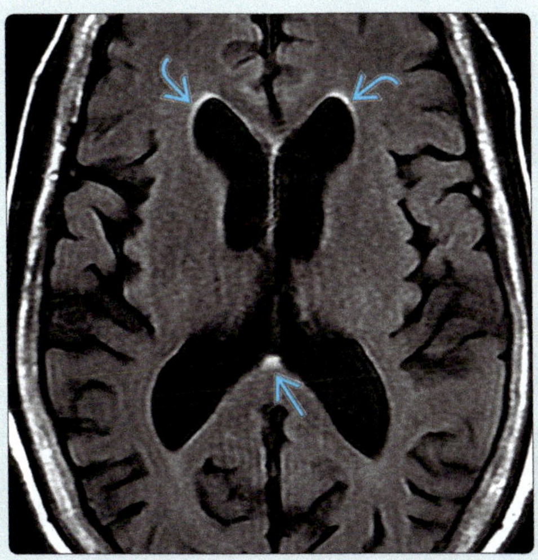

(Left) *Axial SWI in a 67-year-old woman shows striking hypointensity in the globi pallidi ➙ with less prominent hypointensity in the putamina ➙ due to iron deposition.* **(Right)** *Axial FLAIR MR in a 79-year-old man shows enlargement of ventricles and sulci due to age-related volume loss. Smooth, thin, periventricular hyperintense rim ➙ and subtle hyperintensity in the splenium ➙ of corpus callosum are common and normal.*

KEY FACTS

TERMINOLOGY

- Alzheimer disease (AD)
  - Slowly progressive neurodegenerative disease

IMAGING

- Current role of imaging in AD
  - Exclude other causes of dementia
  - Identify region-specific patterns of brain volume loss
  - Identify imaging markers of coexistent disease such as amyloid angiopathy
  - Identify early AD for possible innovative therapy
- Best imaging = volumetric MR, FDG-18 PET
- Thinned gyri, widened sulci, and enlarged ventricles
- Medial temporal lobe particularly hippocampus and entorhinal cortex disproportionately affected
- FDG-18 PET
  - Early stage AD: ↓ metabolism in parietotemporal association cortices, posterior cingulate, and precuneus regions
  - Moderate to severe AD: Additional frontal lobe involvement
- Amyloid PET imaging: High sensitivity in detecting amyloid plaques and vascular amyloid in vivo

TOP DIFFERENTIAL DIAGNOSES

- Frontotemporal lobar degeneration
- Dementia with Lewy bodies
- Normal pressure hydrocephalus
- Vascular dementia
- Normal aging

CLINICAL ISSUES

- Most common cause of dementia over age 65
- Age is biggest risk factor
  - 1-2% prevalence at age 65
  - Incidence doubles every 5 years after age of 60

DIAGNOSTIC CHECKLIST

- Look for reversible causes of dementia

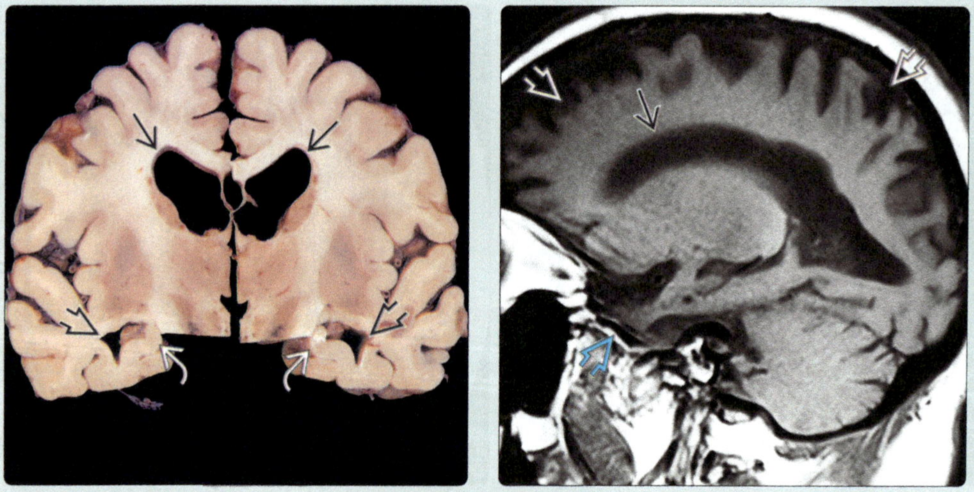

(Left) *Coronal autopsied brain from a patient with histologically proven early-onset Alzheimer disease shows enlarged lateral ventricles ➔ and temporal horns ➔ with shrunken hippocampi ➔.* **(Right)** *Sagittal T1WI in a 59-year-old man with progressive dementia of unclear etiology over 4-5 years with some language difficulties shows an enlarged lateral ventricle ➔, prominent sulci ➔, and a remarkably atrophic temporal lobe ➔.*

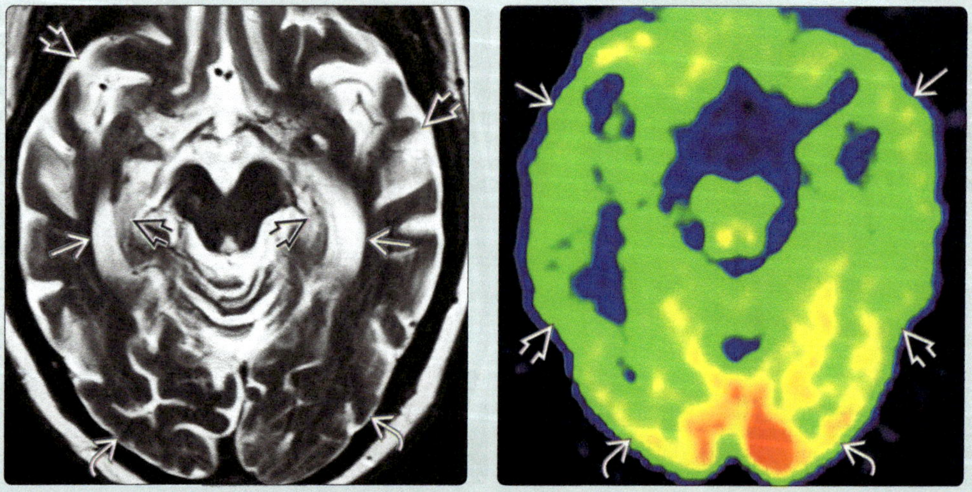

(Left) *Axial T2WI in the same case shows enlarged temporal sulci ➔ with relative occipital sparing ➔. Note shrunken hippocampi ➔ and unusually large temporal horns ➔.* **(Right)** *FDG-PET was requested to differentiate frontotemporal dementia from Alzheimer disease. Markedly reduced FDG metabolism is noted in both temporal ➔ and parietal ➔ lobes. Note occipital sparing ➔. The right hemisphere is significantly more involved than the left. Findings were most consistent with severe Alzheimer disease.*

Vascular Dementia

KEY FACTS

TERMINOLOGY

- Vascular dementia (VaD), multiinfarct dementia (MID)
- Stepwise progressive ↓ in cognitive function
- Heterogeneous group of disorders with varying etiologies, pathologic subtypes
  - VaD often mixed etiology
  - Can occur alone or in association with Alzheimer disease (AD)
  - MID secondary to repeated cerebral infarctions

IMAGING

- General features
  - Multifocal infarcts [cortical gray matter, subcortical white matter (WM)]
  - Basal ganglia, pons
  - Territorial as well as lacunar lesions
  - Coexisting microvascular WM disease common
  - Multiple remote microhemorrhage
- CT
  - Multifocal infarcts
  - Single or multiple, lacunar to territorial
  - WM hypointensities (discrete to confluent)
- FDG PET
  - Multifocal regions ↓ metabolism in cortex, WM

TOP DIFFERENTIAL DIAGNOSES

- AD
- Frontotemporal lobar degeneration
- CADASIL
- Dementia with Lewy bodies

CLINICAL ISSUES

- 2nd most common dementia (after AD)
- Mood and behavioral changes more typical than memory loss

DIAGNOSTIC CHECKLIST

- Report strategically placed infarcts
- Look for hemorrhage, DWI abnormalities

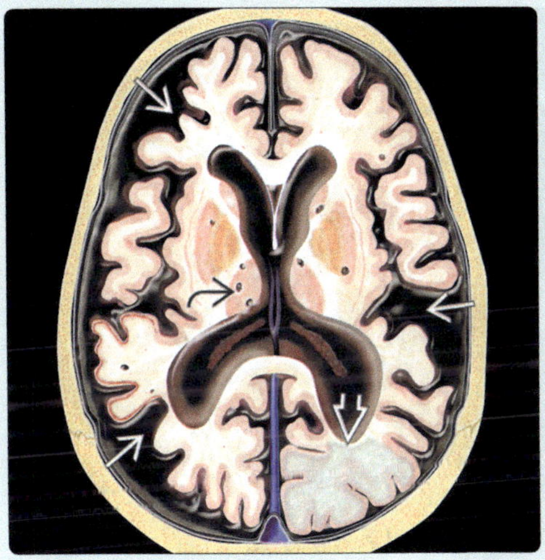
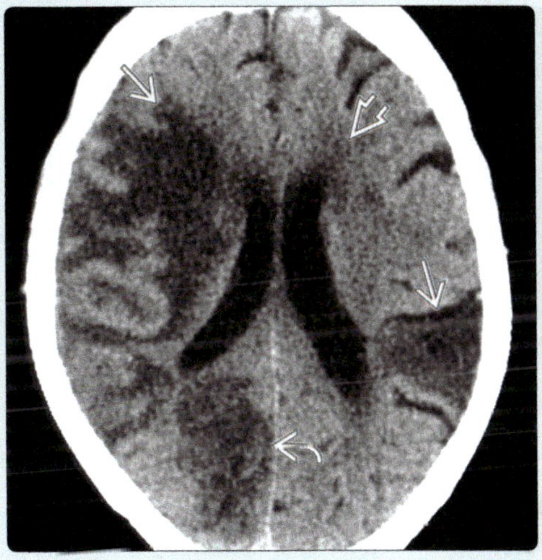

(Left) *Axial diagram of vascular dementia shows diffuse cerebral atrophy, focal volume loss due to multiple chronic infarcts, an acute left occipital lobe infarct, and small lacunar infarcts in the basal ganglia/thalami.* **(Right)** *Axial NECT demonstrates periventricular white matter hypodensity, as well as bilateral MCA and right PCA infarcts, in a patient with vascular dementia. The clinical history plus findings of infarcts in multiple separate vascular distributions are consistent with vascular dementia.*

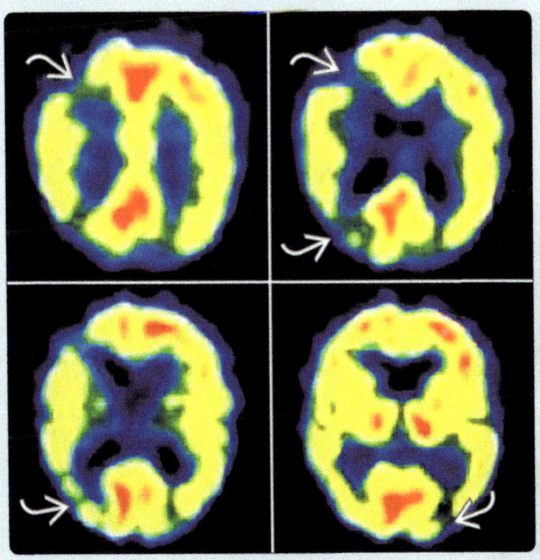
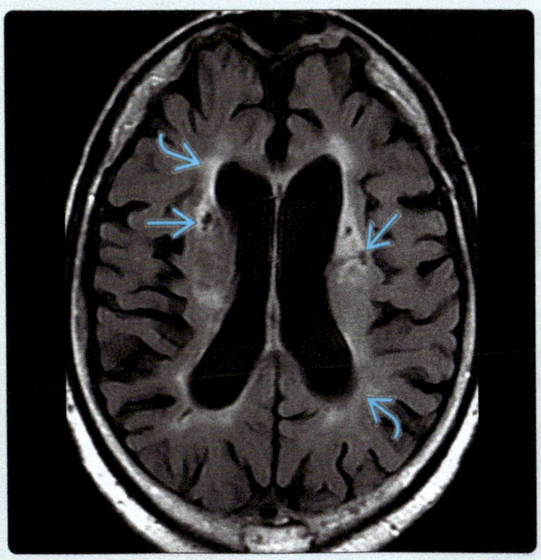

(Left) *Axial FDG PET in a patient with multiinfarct dementia demonstrates multiple wedge-shaped areas of hypometabolism due to chronic infarcts. (Courtesy A. Ali, MD.)* **(Right)** *Axial FLAIR MR in a 72-year-old man with chronic hypertension and diabetes presenting with mood and behavioral changes shows confluent white matter hyperintensities in the periventricular regions. Note the multiple chronic lacunar infarcts in the basal ganglia as well as enlargement of the ventricles and cortical sulci.*

KEY FACTS

TERMINOLOGY

- Clinical subtypes
  - Behavioral-variant frontotemporal dementia (bvFTD)
  - Primary progressive aphasia syndromes (PPA)
    - Semantic variant (sv-PPA)
      - Previously known as semantic dementia
    - Nonfluent/agrammatic variant (nfv-PPA)
      - Previously known as progressive nonfluent aphasia
    - Logopenic variant (lv-PPA)
  - Frontotemporal dementia with motor symptoms

IMAGING

- Early
  - PET shows frontotemporal ↓ glucose metabolism
- Late
  - Frontotemporal atrophy with knife-like gyri on MR
- Subtypes have characteristic cortical atrophy patterns

TOP DIFFERENTIAL DIAGNOSES

- Alzheimer dementia
- Vascular dementia
- Corticobasal ganglionic degeneration
- Dementia with Lewy bodies

CLINICAL ISSUES

- Clinical syndromes (some overlap)
  - **bvFTD**: Marked changes in personality & behavior, mixture of apathy & disinhibition
  - **sv-PPA**: Progressive loss of "semantic" knowledge about words, objects & concepts, fluent speech
  - **nfv-PPA**: Effortful speech production & orofacial apraxia
  - **lv-PPA**: Word finding pauses & poor sentence repetition
- Younger age group than Alzheimer disease
- Frontotemporal lobar degeneration most common cause of early-onset (< 65 years) dementia
- Median survival: 6-11 years from symptom onset & 3-4 years from diagnosis

(Left) *Graphic depicts the classic disproportionate frontal lobe atrophy of late-stage frontotemporal dementia (FTD). The sulci are widened, and gyri are knife-like ➔. Parietal occipital lobes are spared. Gyri around the central sulcus are normal.* **(Right)** *Parasagittal image (3D-MP-RAGE) was obtained as part of the initial evaluation in a patient with suspected FTD. Note the frontal lobe knife-like gyri ➔ with markedly widened sulci and preservation of the parietal and occipital lobes.*

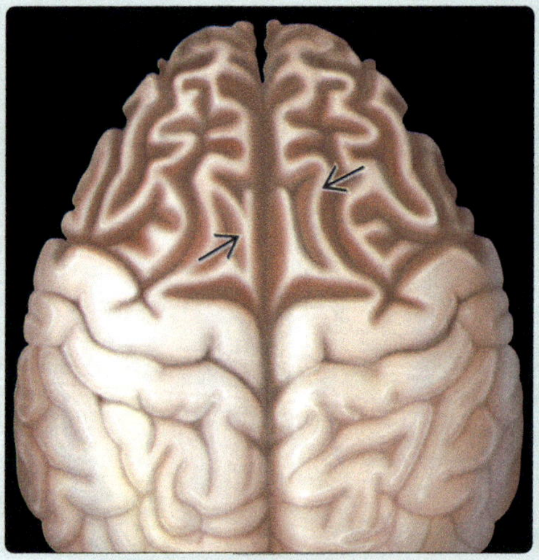

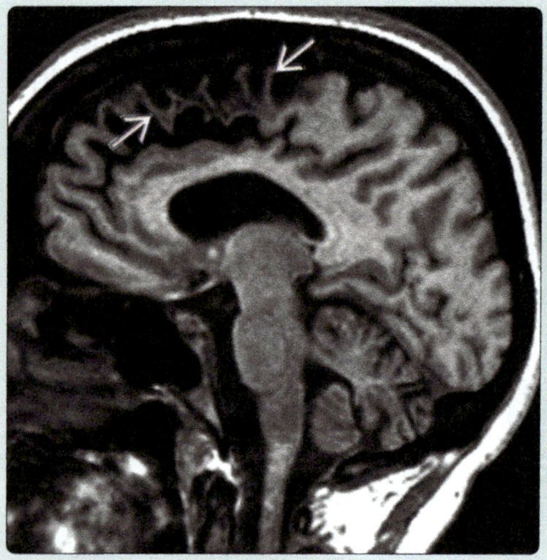

(Left) *Sagittal SSP FDG PET scan in a 72-year-old man with FTD shows a normal elderly control map (2nd row), the patient's glucose metabolism (3rd row), and Z-score statistical map (bottom row). The frontal lobes ➔ are strikingly hypometabolic. The temporal lobes ➔ are somewhat less severely affected.* **(Right)** *Axial T2WI MR in a patient with semantic dementia subtype of FTLD shows marked atrophy of anterolateral temporal lobes ➔. Note the relative preservation of the hippocampi ➔.*

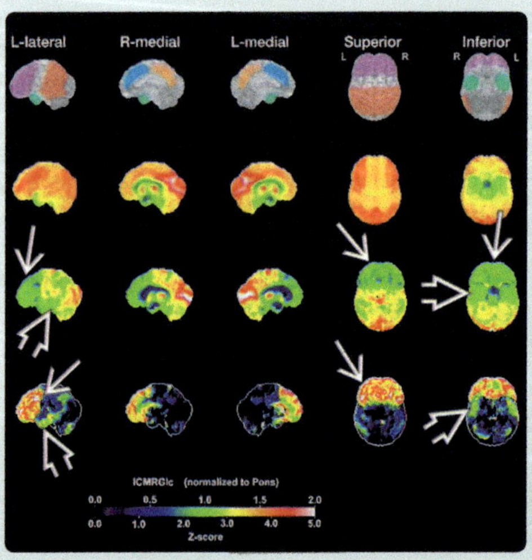

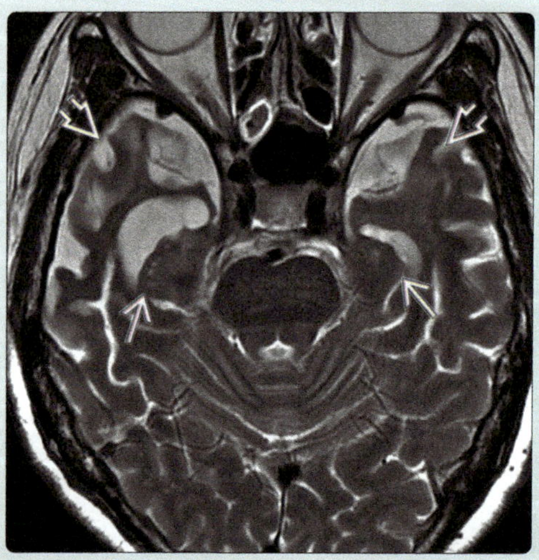

Dementia With Lewy Bodies

KEY FACTS

TERMINOLOGY

- Progressive neurodegenerative dementia caused by pathologic aggregation of α-synuclein protein in neurites (Lewy bodies)

IMAGING

- MR may differentiate Alzheimer disease (AD) from dementia with Lewy bodies (DLB)
- Voxel-based morphometry
  - Relatively preserved hippocampal/medial temporal lobe volume in DLB compared with AD
  - Reduced volume of hypothalamus, substantia innominata, and putamen in DLB compared with AD
- fMRI may show loss of inhibition in visual system
- PET, SPECT most useful for DLB diagnosis
- FDG PET
  - ↓ in glucose metabolism in occipital cortex, especially primary visual cortex
  - 18F-DOPA-PET: ↓ striatal dopamine uptake in DLB vs. AD
- SPECT: ↓ perfusion in anterior cingulate, orbitofrontal, cuneus in DLB with visual hallucinations
- 123FP-CIT-SPECT: ↓ uptake in striatum in DLB vs. AD

TOP DIFFERENTIAL DIAGNOSES

- Parkinson disease-associated dementia
  - Similar clinical, pathological, imaging features with DLB
- AD
- Frontotemporal lobar degeneration
- Vascular dementia

CLINICAL ISSUES

- Presents with loss of executive functions, Parkinsonian features, and vivid visual hallucinations

DIAGNOSTIC CHECKLIST

- Unlike AD, medial temporal lobe atrophy not prominent feature

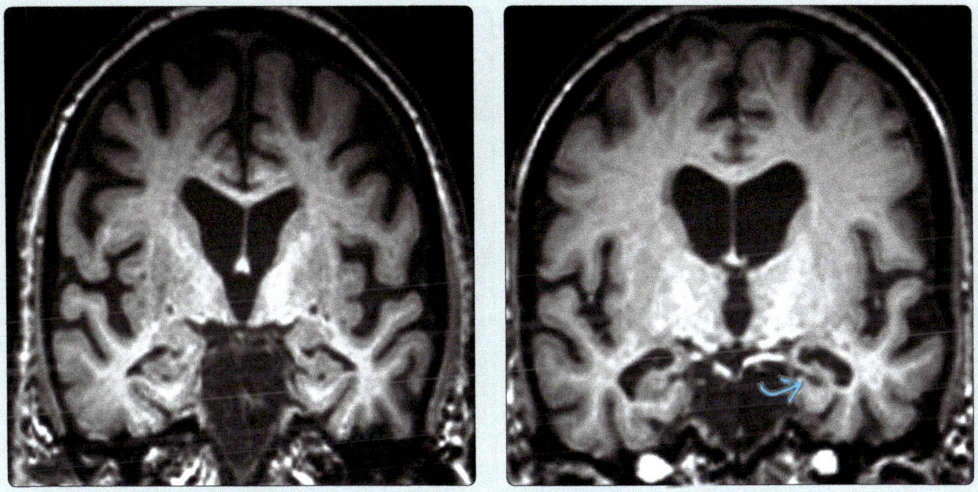

(Left) *Coronal T1WI MR in a patient with dementia with Lewy bodies (DLB) shows prominent frontal lobe volume loss with relative sparing of hippocampal volume. (Courtesy M.J. Firbank, MD, and J.T. O'Brien, MD.)* **(Right)** *Coronal T1WI MR in a patient with Alzheimer disease (AD) shows marked hippocampal volume loss and relative sparing of frontal lobes. (Courtesy M.J. Firbank, MD, and J.T. O'Brien, MD.)*

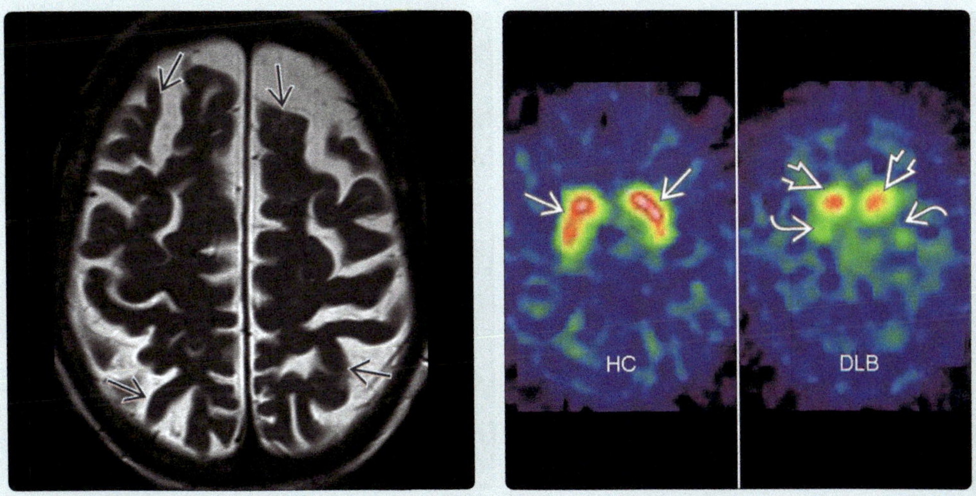

(Left) *Axial T2WI MR in a patient with DLB shows nonspecific diffuse cortical atrophy. Conventional MR findings are frequently nonspecific in DLB.* **(Right)** *123FP-CIT-SPECT, DAT imaging (dopamine transporter) shows normal symmetric uptake in the striatum of a healthy control (HC). In DLB, there is marked reduced update in the putamen, mild in the caudate nuclei. Using DAT imaging, it isn't possible to distinguish DLB from atypical parkinsonian syndromes like MSA, PSP, and CBD.*

KEY FACTS

TERMINOLOGY

- Creutzfeldt-Jakob disease (CJD): Rapidly progressing, fatal, potentially transmissible dementia caused by prion

IMAGING

- Best imaging clue: Progressive T2 hyperintensity of basal ganglia, thalamus, and cerebral cortex
- Predominantly gray matter: Caudate and putamen > globus pallidus
  - Thalamus: Common in variant CJD (vCJD)
  - Cerebral cortex: Frontal, parietal, and temporal
- Heidenhain variant: Occipital lobe
- 2 signs seen in 90% of vCJD but can also occur in sporadic CJD (sCJD)
  - Pulvinar sign: Symmetric T2 hyperintensity of pulvinar of thalamus
  - Hockey-stick sign: Symmetric pulvinar and dorsomedial thalamic nuclear hyperintensity
- Best imaging tool: MR with DWI

TOP DIFFERENTIAL DIAGNOSES

- Hypoxic-ischemic injury
- Osmotic demyelination syndrome
- Other causes of dementia
  - Alzheimer, frontotemporal, multiinfarct dementia, dementia in motor neuron disease
- Leigh syndrome
- Corticobasal degeneration

CLINICAL ISSUES

- Definite CJD diagnosed by brain biopsy or autopsy
- Progressive dementia associated with myoclonic jerks and akinetic mutism; variable constellation of pyramidal, extrapyramidal, and cerebellar signs
- Cerebrospinal fluid (CSF) protein biomarkers: 14-3-3 protein, total tau (t-tau), and neuron-specific enolase
- DWI MR has higher diagnostic accuracy, 97% than any or all of these 3 CSF biomarkers
- Death usually ensues within months of onset

(Left) *Axial DWI in a 67-year-old man with rapidly progressing dementia shows typical findings of sporadic Creutzfeldt-Jakob disease (sCJD). There is symmetric restricted diffusion involving the caudate nuclei and putamina.* **(Right)** *Axial FLAIR MR in the same patient shows corresponding high signal in the caudate nuclei and putamina. CJD is a rapidly progressing, fatal, neurodegenerative disorder caused by a prion. MR with DWI is the imaging procedure of choice.*

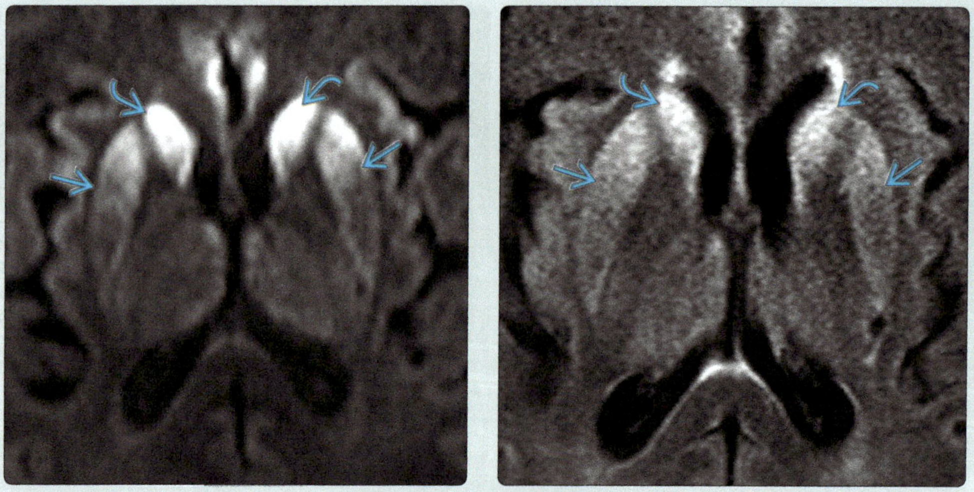

(Left) *Axial DWI in a patient with sCJD demonstrates restricted diffusion involving the caudate nuclei and putamina. There is also involvement of the posteromedial thalami, giving the classic hockey-stick sign.* **(Right)** *Axial DWI in a patient with variant CJD (vCJD) shows classic pulvinar sign with symmetric hyperintensity in the posterior thalami. The hockey-stick and pulvinar signs are seen in 90% of vCJD but can also occur in sCJD.*

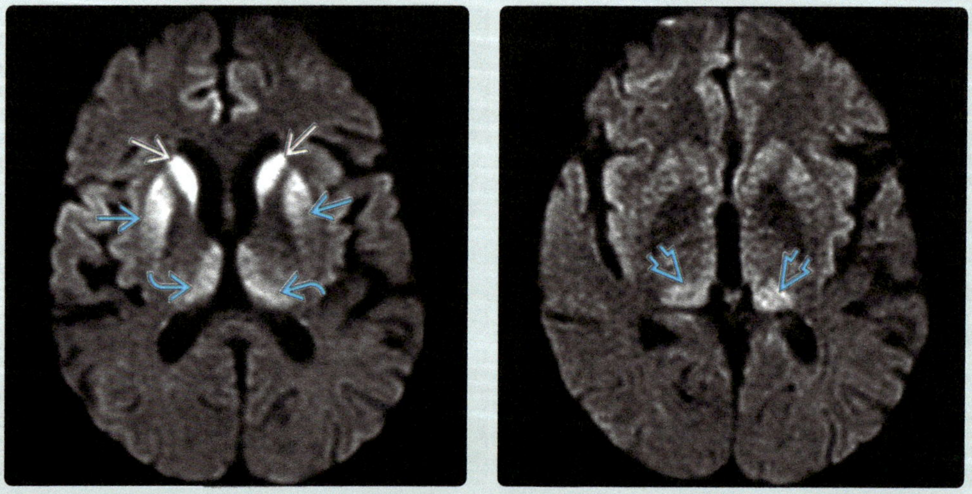

KEY FACTS

TERMINOLOGY

- Important clinicopathologic Creutzfeldt-Jakob disease (CJD) variants
  - Heidenhain variant CJD
    - Visual variant of CJD
    - Early isolated visual symptoms
  - Brownell-Oppenheimer variant (rare)
    - Pure cerebellar syndrome

IMAGING

- FLAIR
  - Subtle cortical hyperintensity in occipital lobes ("cortical ribbon")
  - Basal ganglia usually normal
- DWI
  - Most sensitive for early detection (look for restriction in "cortical ribbon")
  - Occipital cortex hyperintensity
- T1 C+: No enhancement
- FDG-PET occipital hypometabolism

TOP DIFFERENTIAL DIAGNOSES

- Heidenhain variant CJD
  - Posterior cerebral artery ischemia/infarction
    - Typically involves both cortex, white matter
  - Posterior cortical atrophy
    - Does not restrict on DWI
- Brownell-Oppenheim variant of CJD
  - Other cerebellar degeneration syndromes

CLINICAL ISSUES

- Heidenhain variant CJD
  - Visual field defects
  - Abnormal color or visuospatial perception
  - Visual hallucinations
  - Visual neglect, agnosia
  - Dementia, ataxia, or myoclonus later
  - Rare: Isolated eye-movement abnormalities

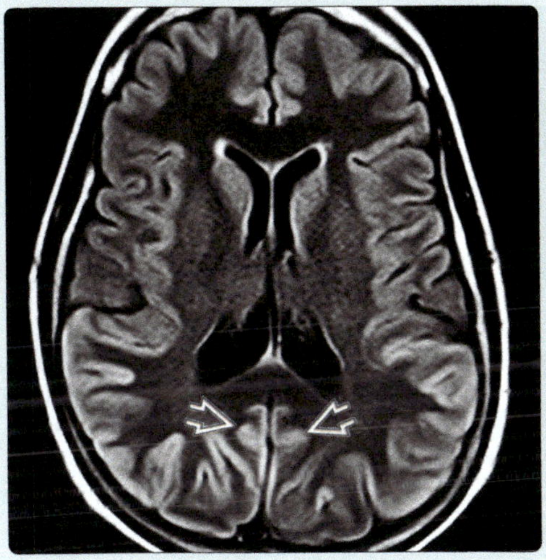

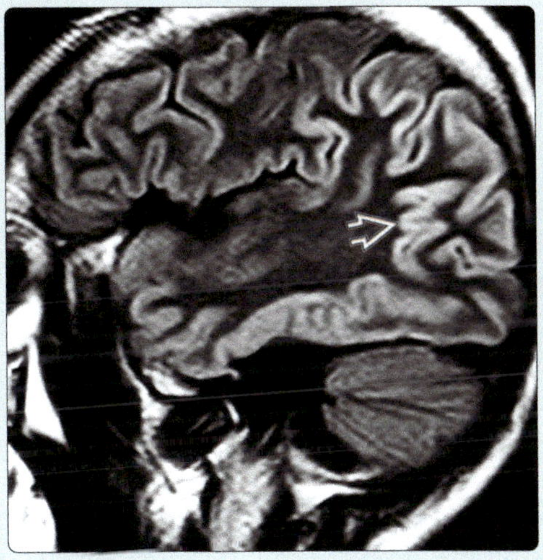

(Left) *Axial FLAIR MR in a 59-year-old woman with visual agnosia shows subtle hyperintensity in both parietooccipital lobes with definite involvement of the calcarine cortex ➡.* **(Right)** *Sagittal FLAIR in the same case shows hyperintensity ➡ of the left parietal, occipital, and inferior temporal cortex. This is an excellent example of an abnormal "cortical ribbon" in CJD.*

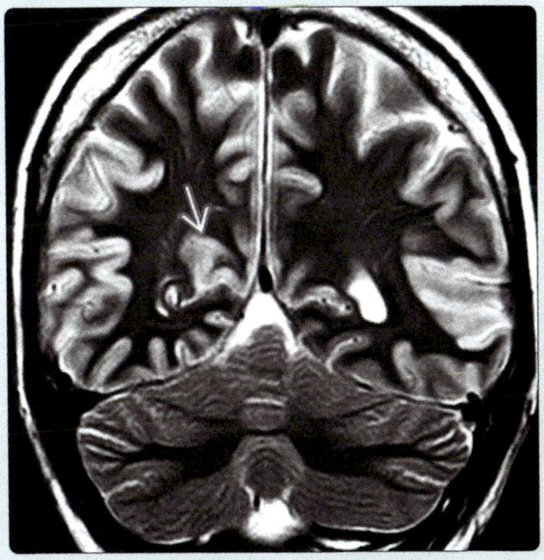

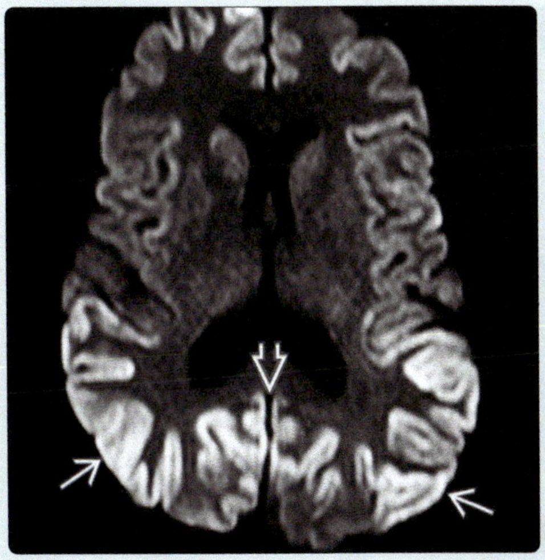

(Left) *Coronal T2WI in the same patient shows striking hyperintensity in the parietooccipital lobes, particularly in the right calcarine cortex ➡.* **(Right)** *DWI in the same case shows swelling, restricted diffusion in both parietooccipital lobes ➡, including both calcarine cortices ➡. Note the absence of abnormality in the frontal and temporal lobes, basal ganglia, and thalami. This is a classic case of Heidenhain variant Creutzfeldt-Jakob disease.*

KEY FACTS

TERMINOLOGY

- Parkinson disease (PD)
  - Progressive neurodegenerative disease
  - Primarily affects pars compacta of substantia nigra (SNpc)

IMAGING

- MR
  - SNpc narrowed/inapparent (T2WI)
  - SNpc progressively loses normal hyperintensity (from lateral to medial)
  - Border between SNpc, red nucleus blurred in PD
  - ↑ R2' relaxation at 3T in SNpc, caudal putamen (reflects ↑ iron content)
  - DWI may differentiate PD from progressive supranuclear palsy, parkinsonian variant of multiple system atrophy (MSA-P)
  - MRS: Nonspecific, ↓ NAA/Cr and NAA/choline ratios in basal ganglia
- PET/SPECT helpful for distinction from "Parkinson-plus" syndromes
- ↑ ADC in putamen and caudate nucleus

TOP DIFFERENTIAL DIAGNOSES

- MSA or MSA-P
- Progressive supranuclear palsy
- Corticobasal ganglionic degeneration
- Dementia with Lewy bodies

PATHOLOGY

- Lewy bodies (eosinophilic intracytoplasmic inclusions with peripheral halos and dense cores), gliosis

CLINICAL ISSUES

- Resting tremor
- "Cogwheel" rigidity
- Bradykinesia
- Shuffling gate
- "Masked" facies

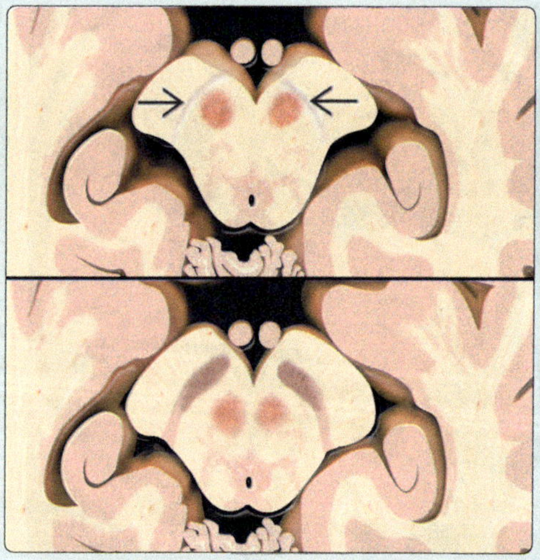

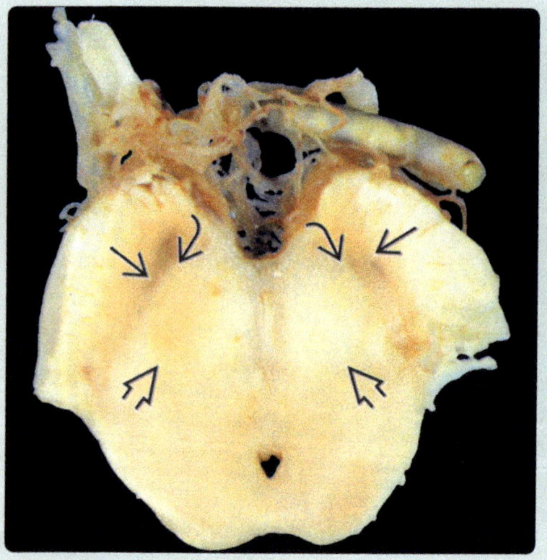

(Left) *Axial midbrain diagram shows narrowing and depigmentation of the substantia nigra ➔ in Parkinson disease (top) relative to normal anatomy (bottom).* **(Right)** *Axial slice through the midbrain of a patient with severe Parkinson disease shows gross pathologic changes. Note the striking narrowing and depigmentation of the pars reticulata ➔ of the substantia nigra. The pars compacta ➔, which is the region between the pars reticulata and the red nucleus ➔, is markedly narrowed.*

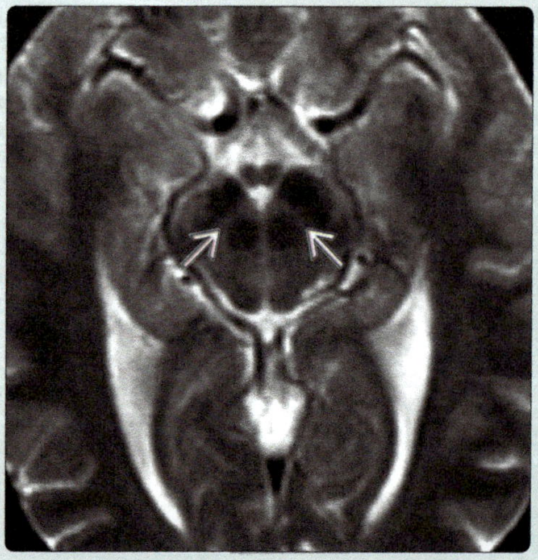

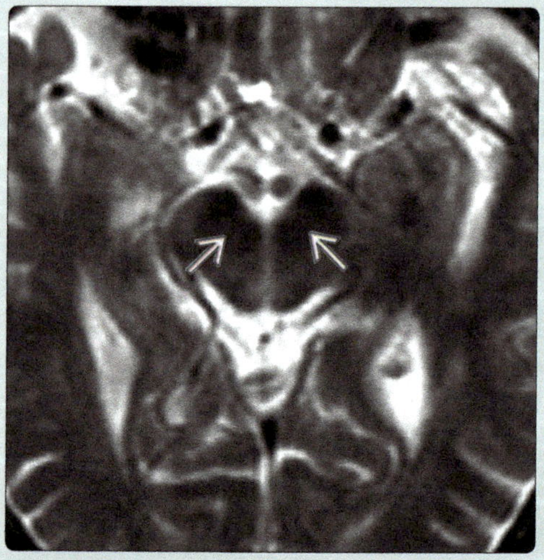

(Left) *Axial T2WI MR in a normal individual shows the appropriate width of the pars compacta ➔, a striking contrast to the abnormal findings seen in a patient with Parkinson disease.* **(Right)** *Axial T2WI MR in a patient with Parkinson disease shows classic midbrain findings. Note the "blurring" and thinning of pars compacta ➔ between 2 hypointense structures (i.e., the pars reticulata of substantia nigra and red nucleus). As a result, the red nuclei and substantia nigra are almost touching.*

KEY FACTS

TERMINOLOGY

- Adult-onset fatal neurodegenerative disease
- Multiple system atrophy (MSA) has 3 clinical subtypes
- Cerebellar (MSA-C)
  - Sporadic olivopontocerebellar (OPCA) atrophy
- Extrapyramidal (MSA-P)
  - Parkinson subtype
  - Striatonigral degeneration
- Autonomic (MSA-A)
  - Shy-Drager syndrome

IMAGING

- General findings
  - ↓ ("flat") pons/medulla
  - Cerebellar vermis/hemispheres atrophic
- MSA-C
  - Selective atrophy of lower pons, medulla, middle cerebellar peduncles (MCPs), cerebellar hemispheres
    - ↑ T2 signal in pons, MCPs, cerebellar WM
    - Cruciform pontine hyperintensity ("hot cross bun")
- MSA-P
  - ↓ T2 signal in dorsolateral putamen
  - ± ↑ T1 signal in lateral putamen rim
- FDG PET shows ↓ metabolism in putamen in MSA-P & ↓ FDG activity in cerebellar hemispheres and MCPs in MSA-C

TOP DIFFERENTIAL DIAGNOSES

- Parkinson, Parkinson-plus syndromes
- Friedreich ataxia (spinocerebellar ataxia)
- Progressive nonfamilial adult-onset cerebellar degeneration
- Hereditary spinal cerebellar ataxia or OPCA
- Hereditary cerebellar atrophy

DIAGNOSTIC CHECKLIST

- MR features may overlap
- All MR findings may be observed in every MSA subtype

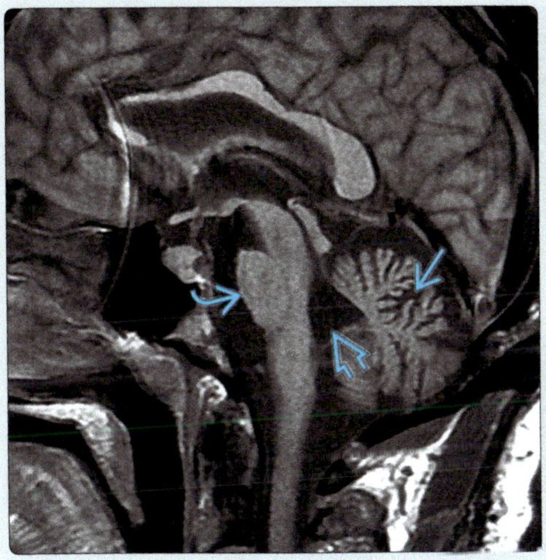
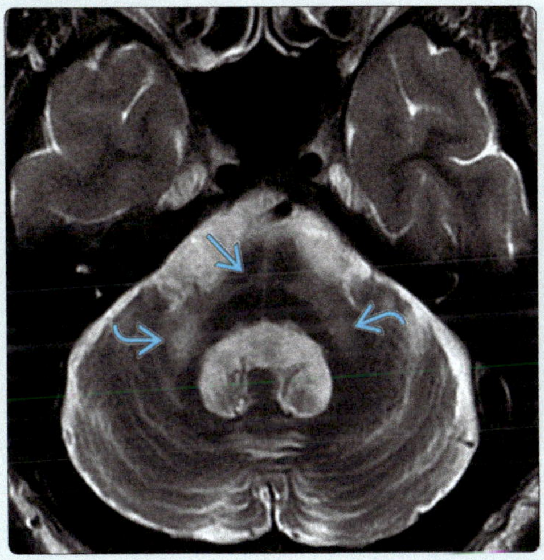

(Left) *Sagittal T1 MR in a patient with cerebellar multiple system atrophy (MSA-C) shows atrophy with flattening of the belly of pons. There is atrophy of the cerebellar vermis with prominence of the 4th ventricle.* **(Right)** *Axial T2 MR in the same patient shows characteristic pontine hot cross bun sign as well as symmetric hyperintensity in the middle cerebellar peduncles. The hot cross bun sign is caused by loss of myelinated transverse pontocerebellar fibers in the pontine raphe.*

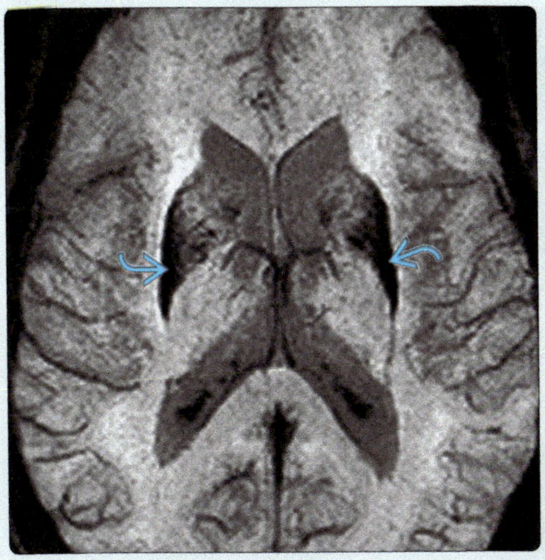
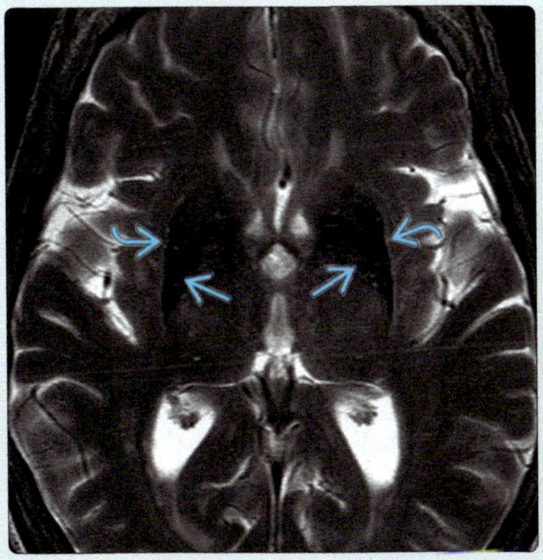

(Left) *Axial SWI in a patient with extrapyramidal (MSA-P) type shows abnormal putaminal hypointensity with greater involvement of the lateral putamen. This is caused by higher iron deposition in MSA.* **(Right)** *Axial T2 MR in the same patient shows putaminal hypointensity due to iron deposition. In addition, there is subtle T2 hyperintensity at the lateral margin of the putamen hyperintense putaminal rim sign.*

Posterior Cortical Atrophy

KEY FACTS

TERMINOLOGY

- Posterior cortical atrophy (PCA)
  - Rare neurodegenerative disorder of posterior cerebral cortex/connecting white matter (WM)
  - Considered subtype of Alzheimer disease (AD)
  - Results in impairment of ventral, dorsal visual perception pathways
  - Typically precedes memory, executive impairment

IMAGING

- Sagittal T1WI, axial FLAIR show posterior > frontal, temporal volume loss
  - Cortical thinning
  - Left typically > right
- ↓ fractional anisotropy in inferior/superior longitudinal fasciculi
- FDG-PET
  - Hypometabolism/hypoperfusion of posterior parietal, occipital regions

TOP DIFFERENTIAL DIAGNOSES

- Other Alzheimer clinical variants
  - Primary progressive aphasia
  - Biparietal syndrome
- Frontotemporal lobar dementia
- Diffuse Lewy body disease
- Creutzfeldt-Jakob disease (Heidenhain variant)

PATHOLOGY

- Atrophy of posterior portions of cerebral cortex
- ↓ integrity of corresponding WM tracts

CLINICAL ISSUES

- PCA patients usually younger than patients with typical AD
- May initially present for ophthalmologic evaluation
- Visuospatial symptoms common
  - Visual field defect
  - Visual hallucinations
- Visual symptoms often precede onset of dementia

(Left) *Parasagittal T1WI in a 64-year-old woman with visual agnosia and left cortical blindness shows disproportionate atrophy of the parietal* ⇨ *and occipital* ➡ *lobes.* **(Right)** *Axial FLAIR MR in the same case shows relatively normal frontal lobes but atrophic left parietal* ➡ *and occipital lobes* ➡*.*

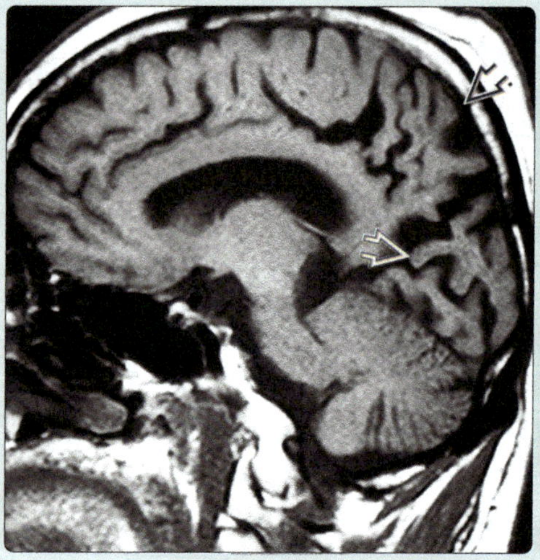

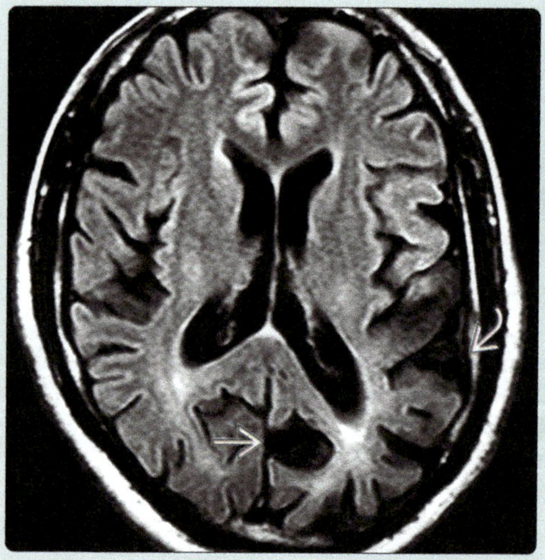

(Left) *Color-difference map comparing the same patient's cortical volume with age-matched control shows normal frontal lobes (blue) but markedly abnormal left parietal (green) and occipital lobes. The left occipital lobe (orange/red) is more affected than the right (yellow). These findings are typical of posterior cortical atrophy.* **(Right)** *Axial T2WI in a 62-year-old woman with dementia and visual neglect shows striking atrophy of both posterior parietal lobes* ⇨*.*

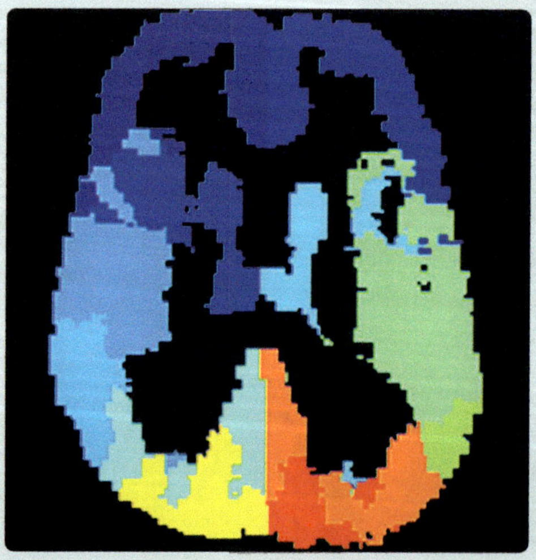

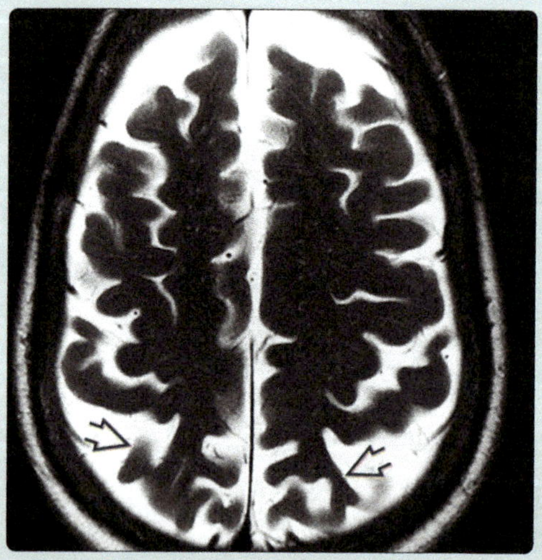

KEY FACTS

TERMINOLOGY

- Corticobasal degeneration
  - Progressive neurodegenerative disease
  - Presents with cognitive dysfunction, "asymmetrical" parkinsonism

IMAGING

- Severe focal asymmetric cortical atrophy
  - Perirolandic (posterior frontal, parietal cortex)
  - Relative sparing of temporal, occipital regions
- ↑ signal intensity in frontal &/or parietal subcortical white matter
- Marked T2 hypointensity
  - Putamen, globi pallidi
- FDG-18 PET decreased uptake in cortical and subcortical regions (frontal, temporal, sensorimotor, and parietal association cortices), caudate, lentiform nucleus, and thalamus
- SPECT: Asymmetric hypoperfusion in frontoparietal lobes, basal ganglia (putamen), thalamus, and cerebellar hemispheres

TOP DIFFERENTIAL DIAGNOSES

- Progressive supranuclear palsy
- Frontotemporal lobar dementia/degeneration
- Alzheimer disease
- Dementia with Lewy bodies
- Amyotrophic lateral sclerosis

PATHOLOGY

- Hyperphosphorylated tau/abnormal filamentous inclusions accumulate in neurons/glia

CLINICAL ISSUES

- Unilateral or asymmetrical parkinsonism
  - Dystonia, tremor
  - Ideomotor apraxia, "alien limb" phenomenon
- Cognitive decline

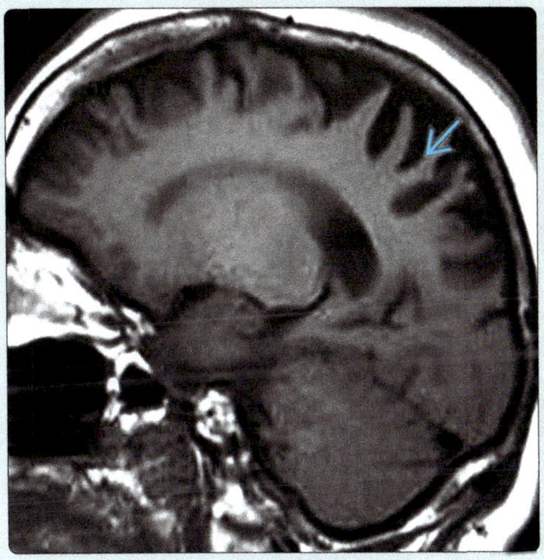

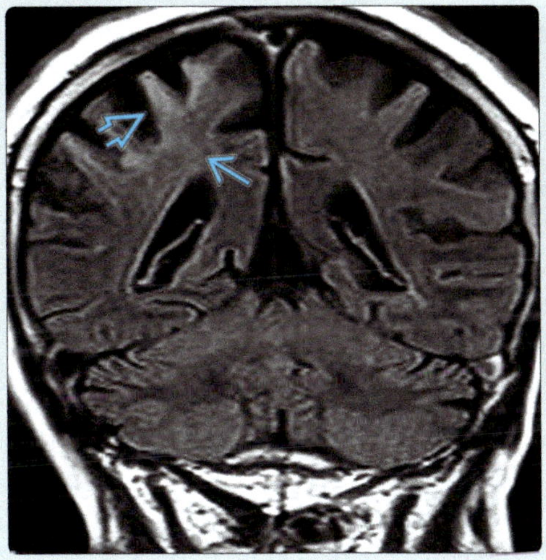

(Left) *Parasagittal T1WI MR through the right hemisphere in a 63-year-old man with corticobasal degeneration shows prominent volume loss in the posterior frontal and parietal cortex ➔. The anterior frontal lobe cortex is normal in appearance.* **(Right)** *Coronal FLAIR MR in the same patient shows asymmetric parietal atrophy, worse on the right ⇨, with subcortical white matter hyperintensity ➔. (Courtesy A. Erbetta, MD.)*

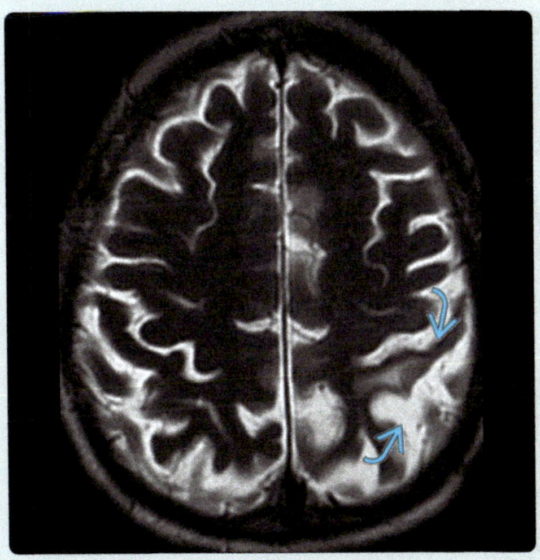

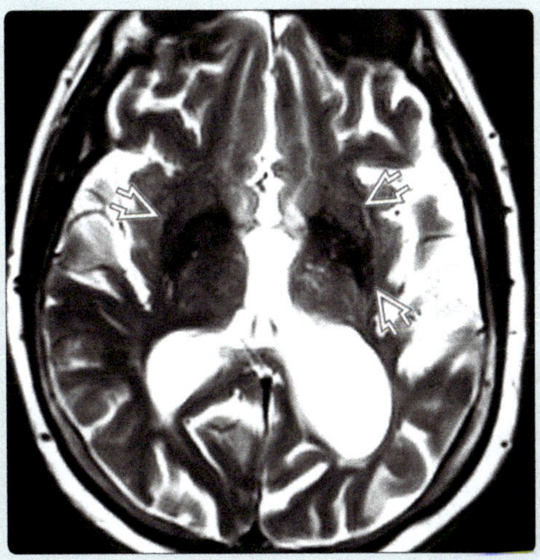

(Left) *Axial T2 MR in a 71-year-old man with corticobasal degeneration demonstrates asymmetric atrophy and thin cortex in the left perirolandic region ➔.* **(Right)** *Axial T2WI in a 72-year-old woman with corticobasal degeneration shows the hyperintense putaminal rim ⇨ suggestive of the disease.*

KEY FACTS

TERMINOLOGY

- Neurodegenerative disease characterized by supranuclear palsy, postural instability, mild dementia

IMAGING

- Midbrain atrophy (penguin or hummingbird sign)
  - Sagittal T1WI shows concave/flat upper border of midbrain (normally convex)
  - Axial T1WIs show abnormal concavity of lateral margins of midbrain tegmentum (morning glory or Mickey Mouse sign)
  - Thinning of superior colliculus
- Midsagittal 3D-MP-RAGE or FS-PGR images
  - Voxel-based morphometry used to calculate ratio of midbrain to pons area
  - Midbrain area < 70 mm² (50% of normal)
  - Midbrain to pons ratio < 0.15 strongly suggests PSP
  - MR Parkinsonism index: Allows discrimination of PSP from MSA-P, Parkinson disease, and control

TOP DIFFERENTIAL DIAGNOSES

- Multiple system atrophy, Parkinsonian type; corticobasal degeneration; dementia with Lewy bodies; Parkinson disease

PATHOLOGY

- Neurofibrillary tangles and neuropil threads in globus pallidus, subthalamic nucleus, substantia nigra; cerebral cortex relatively preserved except for perirolandic cortex; neuronal loss, gliosis

CLINICAL ISSUES

- PSP-RS (Richardson syndrome)
- Lurching gait, axial dystonia, vertical supranuclear palsy
- PSP-P (Parkinsonian type)
- Bradykinesia, rigidity, normal eye movements
- 2nd most common neurodegenerative cause of Parkinsonism overall

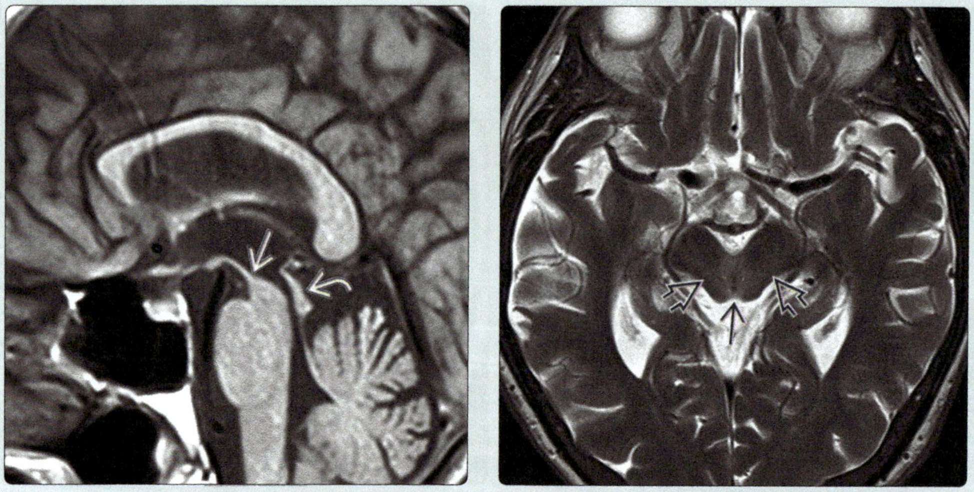

(Left) *Sagittal T1WI MR in a patient with bradykinesia and suspected Parkinson disease shows the classic penguin or hummingbird sign of progressive supranuclear palsy (PSP). Note thinning of the midbrain ➡ with atrophy of the tectum ↪, also consistent with PSP. In contrast to the strikingly abnormal midbrain findings, here the pons appears normal.* **(Right)** *Axial T2WI MR in the same patient shows volume loss of the midbrain with thinned tectum ➡ and concave lateral midbrain margins ⇨.*

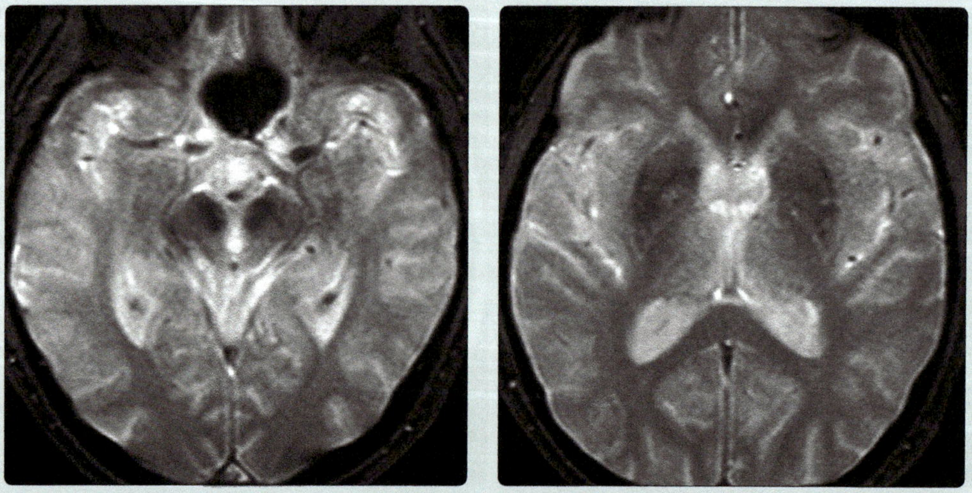

(Left) *Axial T2* GRE MR in the same patient shows no evidence for abnormal iron accumulation in the midbrain, which helps to distinguish PSP from Parkinson disease.* **(Right)** *Axial T2* GRE MR shows no evidence for abnormal iron accumulation in the striatum, another location in which iron is commonly found in Parkinson disease.*

Amyotrophic Lateral Sclerosis (ALS)

KEY FACTS

TERMINOLOGY

- Amyotrophic lateral sclerosis (ALS)
- Selective degeneration of somatic motor neurons of brainstem/spinal cord and large pyramidal neurons of motor cortex
  - Eventual loss of corticospinal tract (CST) fibers

IMAGING

- Small percentage demonstrate CST hyperintensity
- As CST is normally slightly hyperintense, especially at 3.0 T, this finding lacks sensitivity & specificity
- T2 hyperintense CST may be specific for ALS when seen on corresponding proton density (PD) images
- Consider FLAIR and PD in suspected ALS
- DWI hyperintensity (↓ diffusivity) in CST
- Hypointense gray matter in precentral gyrus (motor cortex)

TOP DIFFERENTIAL DIAGNOSES

- Primary lateral sclerosis
- Wallerian degeneration
- Hypertrophic olivary degeneration
- Metabolic diseases involving bilateral CSTs
- Demyelinating and inflammatory diseases
- Neoplasms: Brainstem glioma, malignant lymphoma
- CST can appear hyperintense on 3T MR normally

PATHOLOGY

- Majority of ALS cases are sporadic (sALS)
- 15-20% are familial (fALS)

CLINICAL ISSUES

- Upper motor neuron signs: Babinski sign, spasticity, hyperreflexia
- Lower motor neuron signs: Asymmetric muscle weakness, atrophy, fasciculations, hyporeflexia
- Bulbar signs: Slurred speech, dysphagia
- Onset usually between 4th-7th decades of life
- Complete disability and death within 10 years

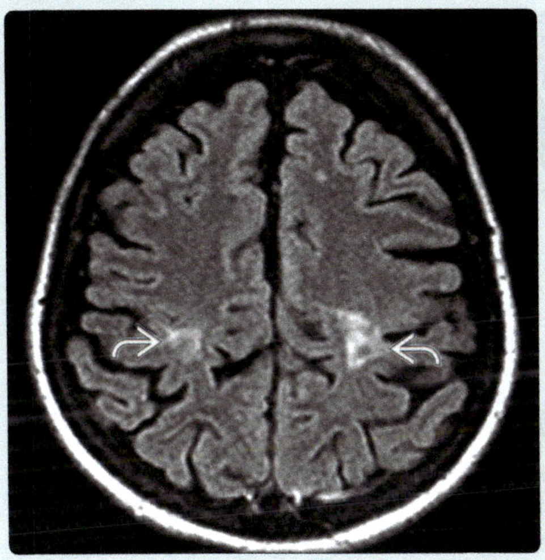

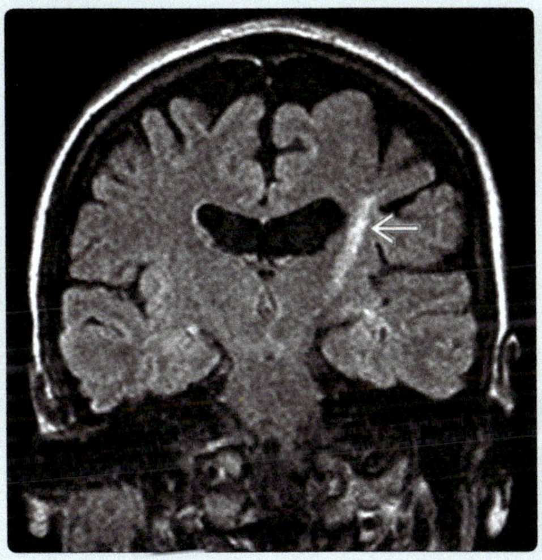

(Left) *Axial FLAIR MR shows increased signal in the precentral gyri in a amyotrophic lateral sclerosis (ALS) patient. There is also atrophy of bilateral motor cortices.* **(Right)** *Coronal FLAIR MR shows linear hyperintensity along the corticospinal tract (CST) from the precentral gyrus to the cerebri crus; right CST signal abnormality is out of this slice. Hyperintensity of the precentral gyrus subcortical WM on FLAIR is a potentially useful and specific sign of ALS not seen in healthy, asymptomatic patients.*

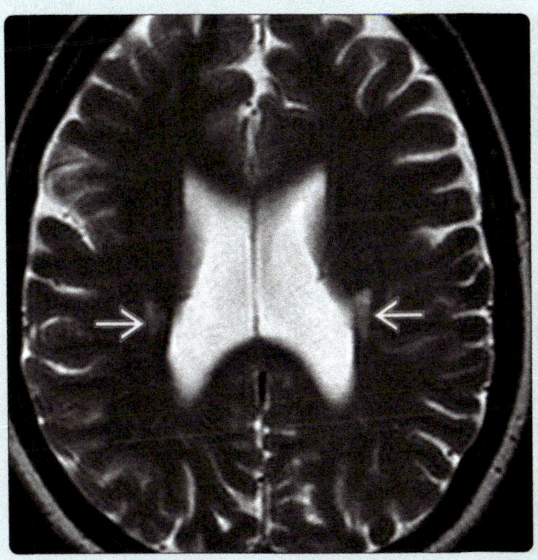

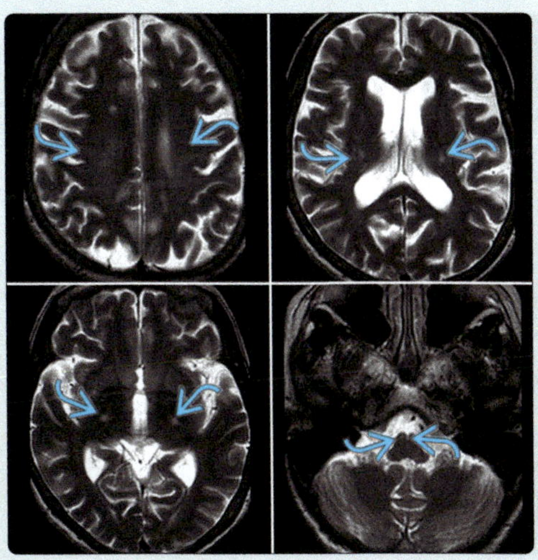

(Left) *Axial T2WI FS MR demonstrates ovoid hyperintensity along the CSTs bilaterally. The atrophy and hyperintensity are due to myelin loss and gliosis. There is frequently involvement of the prefrontal motor neurons, which play a role in planning or orchestrating the work of the upper and lower motor neurons.* **(Right)** *Axial T2 MR in a patient with ALS shows hyperintensity along the course of the CST bilaterally. It is important to note that CST is typically slightly hyperintense on T2, especially at 3.0 T.*

KEY FACTS

TERMINOLOGY

- Wallerian degeneration (WaD)
- Secondary anterograde degeneration of axons and their myelin sheaths caused by interruption of the axonal integrity or damage to neuron

IMAGING

- Primary lesion is cortical or subcortical with WaD in descending white matter tracts ipsilateral to neuronal injury
  - WaD can be seen in fibers crossing the corpus callosum, fibers of optic radiations, fornices, and cerebellar peduncles
- CT is not sensitive for WaD in acute-subacute stages
  - Detects atrophy of corticospinal tracts (CSTs) in chronic stage
- Time-dependent changes in CSTs on MR
  - Strong correlation between WaD detected on T2WI and DWI and long-term morbidity
  - DWI findings precede development of WaD assessed by conventional MR
- DTI may distinguish between primary lesion and associated WaD
  - Reduced fractional anisotropy (FA) with increased mean diffusivity (MD) in infarct
  - Reduced FA with preserved MD in CST

TOP DIFFERENTIAL DIAGNOSES

- Neurodegenerative diseases
- Brainstem glioma
- Demyelinating and inflammatory diseases
- Hypertrophic olivary degeneration
- Metabolic diseases
- Intoxication (heroin inhalation)
- Normal appearance of hyperintensity on high-field-strength MR

(Left) *Axial NECT shows encephalomalacia in the left frontal and temporal opercula ➔ related to a chronic stroke. Hypodensity and volume loss in the thalamus ➔ is likely due to wallerian degeneration of the corticothalamic fibers.* **(Right)** *Axial NECT in the same patient shows atrophy of the left cerebral peduncle ➔ due to chronic wallerian degeneration of the corticospinal tracts. NECT is not sensitive for acute-subacute stages but detects atrophy of the pyramidal tracts in the chronic stage of wallerian degeneration.*

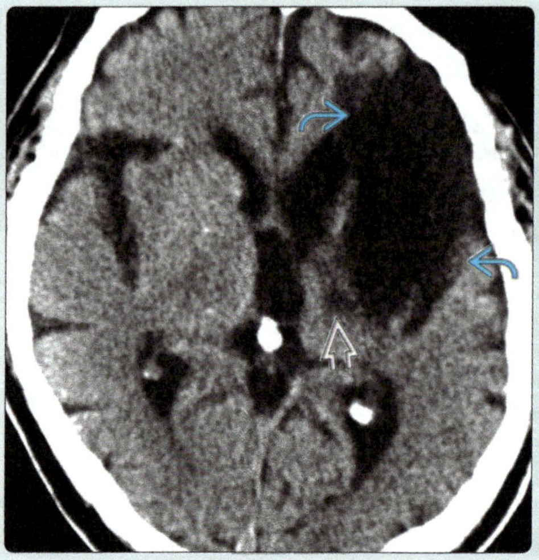

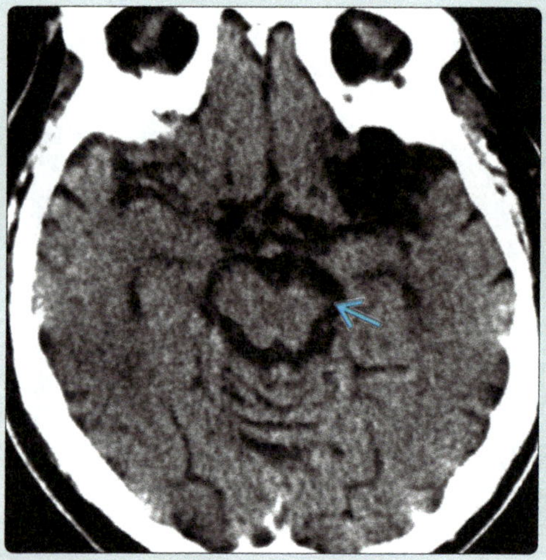

(Left) *Axial DWI demonstrates restricted diffusion ➔ in the right frontal and parietal lobes due to an acute infarct in the right middle cerebral artery distribution.* **(Right)** *Axial DWI in the same patient demonstrates restricted diffusion in the ventral medulla ➔ in the region of the corticospinal tract due to acute wallerian degeneration. DWI is more sensitive at detecting early wallerian degeneration compared with standard MR sequences.*

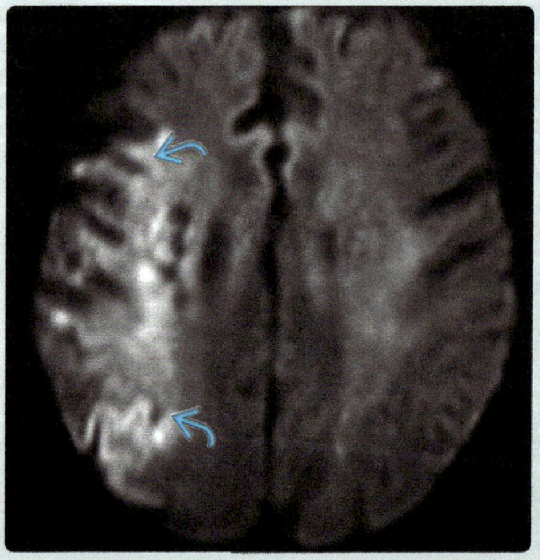

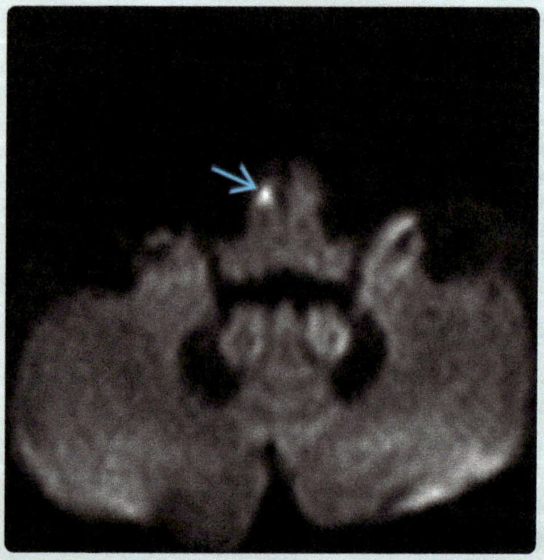

KEY FACTS

TERMINOLOGY

- Spinocerebellar ataxias (SCAs)
  - Spinocerebellar atrophy; spinocerebellar degeneration
  - Previously known as Marie ataxia, inherited olivopontocerebellar atrophy, spinocerebellar degeneration
- Inherited progressive neurodegenerative disorders
  - Clinically, genetically very heterogeneous (> 60 types)
    - SCA 3 most frequent subtypes
  - 2 groups: Autosomal dominant, autosomal recessive

IMAGING

- General features
  - Atrophy of cerebellum, brainstem with normal cerebral hemispheres
  - Cerebellar atrophy = hallmark of cerebellar ataxias but can be mild or even absent in some
- Autosomal recessive ataxias
  - Most common = Friedreich ataxia (often not imaged)
    - Cerebellum generally normal
    - Spinal cord/brainstem atrophic
- Autosomal-dominant ataxias
  - Findings vary with type
  - Brainstem (pontine) > > cerebellar atrophy (often only vermis)
    - Pons in SCA1, total brainstem SCA3, cerebellum in SCA6

CLINICAL ISSUES

- Autosomal-recessive ataxias (onset < 20 years)
  - Peripheral sensorimotor neuropathy
    - Extra-CNS involvement common
  - Slowly progressive course despite early onset
- Autosomal-dominant ataxias
  - Mean age at onset = 3rd, 4th decades
  - Gait disorders, abnormal eye movements, macular degeneration
  - Progressive, often fatal (brainstem failure)

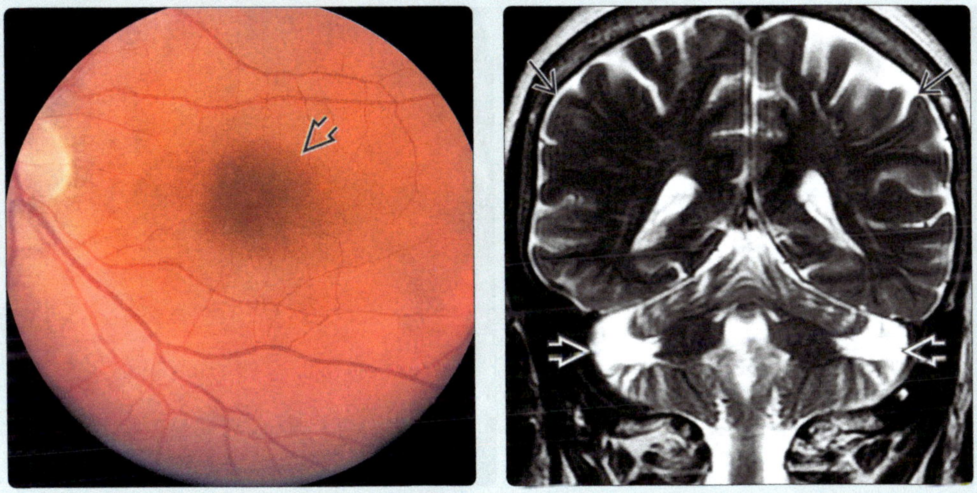

(Left) *Funduscopic examination in a patient with proven SCA7 shows striking pigmented maculopathy →. The patient presented with changes in visual acuity and color vision (tritanopia).* **(Right)** *Coronal T2WI in a 65-year-old woman with progressive cerebellar ataxia since her early 40s shows that the great horizontal fissures of the cerebellum are grossly widened →. The parietal and occipital lobes of the hemispheres appear normal →. Spinocerebellar ataxia is shown (specific genetic type is currently unknown).*

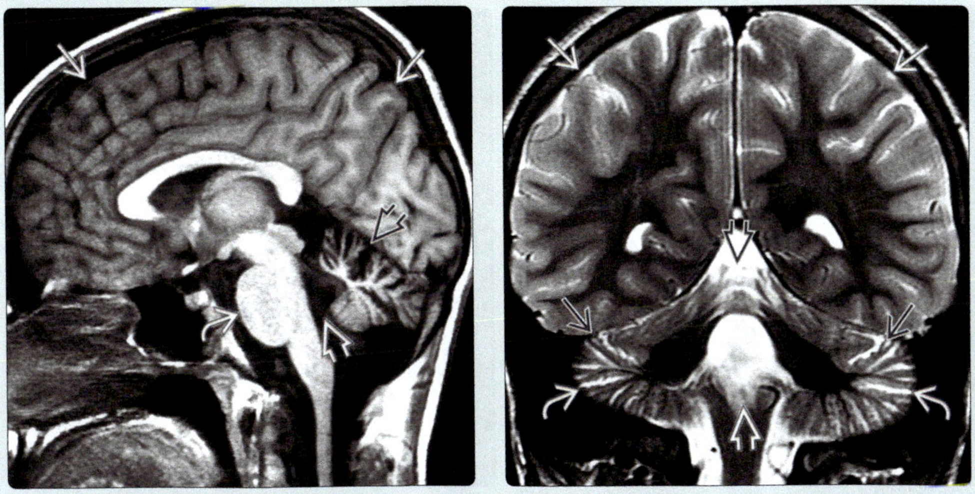

(Left) *Sagittal T1WI in a 13-year-old boy with autosomal-recessive spastic ataxia of Charlevoix-Saguenay shows normal cerebral hemispheres → and pons →. The vermis is grossly atrophic →, and the 4th ventricle → is markedly enlarged.* **(Right)** *Coronal T2WI in the same case shows the normal cerebral hemispheres →. The 4th ventricle → is markedly enlarged, the vermis atrophic →, and the cerebellar fissures → appear prominent because the folia are thinned →.*

KEY FACTS

TERMINOLOGY

- Diaschisis = sudden loss of function in brain connected to (but at distance from) damaged area
- Crossed cerebellar diaschisis (CCD) = decreased blood flow/metabolism in cerebellar hemisphere contralateral to supratentorial infarct

IMAGING

- Acute: CT/MR perfusion shows ↓ cerebral blood flow (CBF) in cerebellar hemisphere opposite acute hemispheric infarct
  - ↑ Time to peak, ↓ CBF in cerebellum contralateral to infarct
  - Add DTI as subtle cases may show ↓ fractional anisotropy when conventional MR normal
  - FDG-18 PET/CT shows diffusely reduced uptake in contralateral cerebellar hemisphere
- Chronic: CT or MR shows atrophic cerebellar hemisphere opposite old cerebral hemispheric infarct

TOP DIFFERENTIAL DIAGNOSES

- Superior cerebral artery infarct
  - CCD involves > just superior cerebral artery territory
- Encephalomalacia
  - Trauma, infection, surgery
- Cerebellitis
  - Cerebellum swollen, hyperintense (not shrunken, atrophic)

PATHOLOGY

- Corticopontocerebellar (CPC) tract
  - Input to cerebellum via CPC tracts 40x all other afferent sources combined
  - Injury at any point along CPC can result in ↓ CBF, metabolism in contralateral cerebellar hemisphere
  - Most common cause = middle cerebral artery infarct
  - Others = status epilepticus, neoplasm, trauma, surgery,migraine, Rasmussen encephalitis, etc.

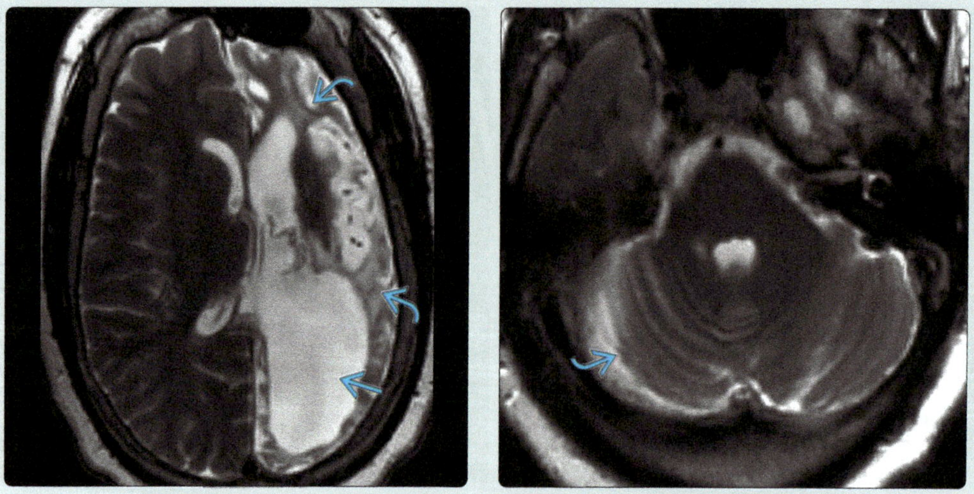

(Left) *Axial T2WI MR in a patient with a remote left middle cerebral artery infarct shows the typical changes of encephalomalacia and volume loss ➢. The ipsilateral ventricle is enlarged ➢.* **(Right)** *Axial T2 MR in the same patient shows volume loss with enlarged horizontal sulci in the contralateral cerebellar hemisphere ➢. These findings are consistent with chronic crossed cerebellar diaschisis (CCD).*

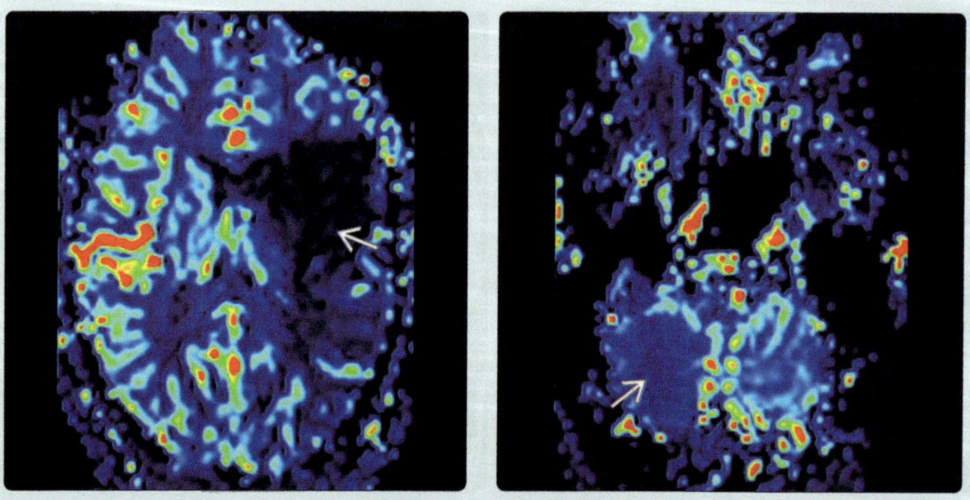

(Left) *MR perfusion study cerebral blood flow (CBF) map in a patient with acute right hemiparesis shows diminished blood flow ➡ (blue area) in the left middle cerebral artery distribution.* **(Right)** *CBF map in the same patient demonstrates reduced CBF in the right cerebellar hemisphere ➡ consistent with acute CCD. CCD is caused by an interruption of the corticopontocerebellar fibers. As a result of ↓ afferent input, there is a ↓ in cerebellar metabolism, coupled with a ↓ in cerebellar perfusion.*

KEY FACTS

TERMINOLOGY

- Inferior olivary nucleus (ION) degeneration
  - Unique type of transsynaptic neuronal degeneration
  - Olivary deafferentation thought to be source of ensuing hypertrophic olivary degeneration (HOD)
- Usually caused by primary lesions in dento-rubro-olivary pathway (anatomical triangle of Guillain-Mollaret)
- Triangle of Guillain-Mollaret defined by 3 anatomic structures
  - Dentate nucleus (DN) of cerebellum
  - Ipsilateral red nucleus (RN)
  - ION ipsilateral to RN

IMAGING

- ION initially hypertrophies rather than atrophies
- 3 distinct MR stages in HOD
  - Hyperintense signal without hypertrophy of ION: Within 1st 6 months of ictus
  - Increased signal + ION hypertrophy: Between 6 months and 3-4 years after ictus
  - Only ION hyperintensity: Begins when hypertrophy resolves (can persist indefinitely)
- MR also detects primary lesion located in ipsilateral central tegmental tract or contralateral DN

TOP DIFFERENTIAL DIAGNOSES

- Vertebrobasilar perforating artery infarct
- Demyelination (MS, microvascular disease)
- Amyotrophic lateral sclerosis
- HIV/AIDS
- Rhombencephalitis

CLINICAL ISSUES

- Oculopalatal myoclonus (palatal "tremor")
- Usually develops 10-11 months after primary lesion
- Clinical symptoms (tremors) rarely improve

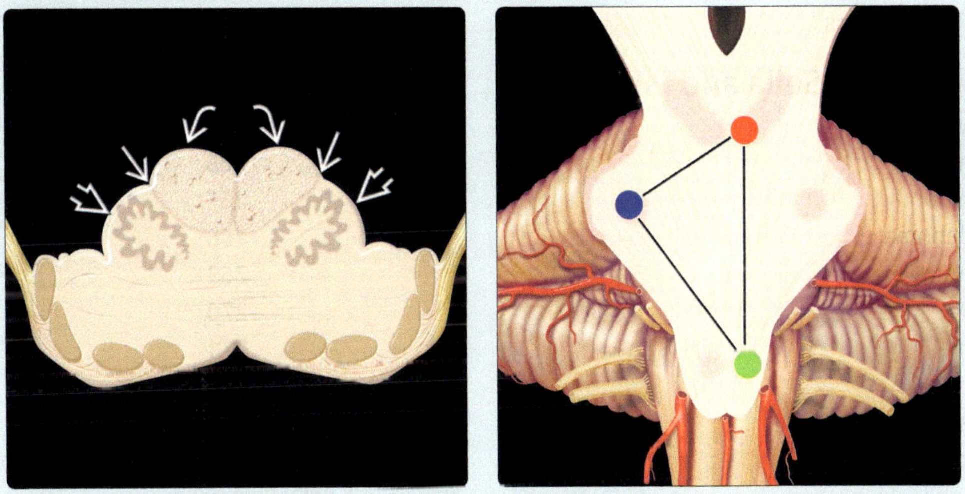

(Left) *Axial graphic of the upper medulla shows the medullary pyramids* → *on each side of the ventral median fissure. The olives* → *lie just posterior to the preolivary sulci* →. **(Right)** *Coronal graphic of the midbrain, pons, and medulla is sectioned to depict the Guillain-Mollaret triangle. The triangle of Guillain-Mollaret is composed of the ipsilateral inferior olivary nucleus (green), dentate nucleus (blue) of the contralateral cerebellum, and the ipsilateral red nucleus (red).*

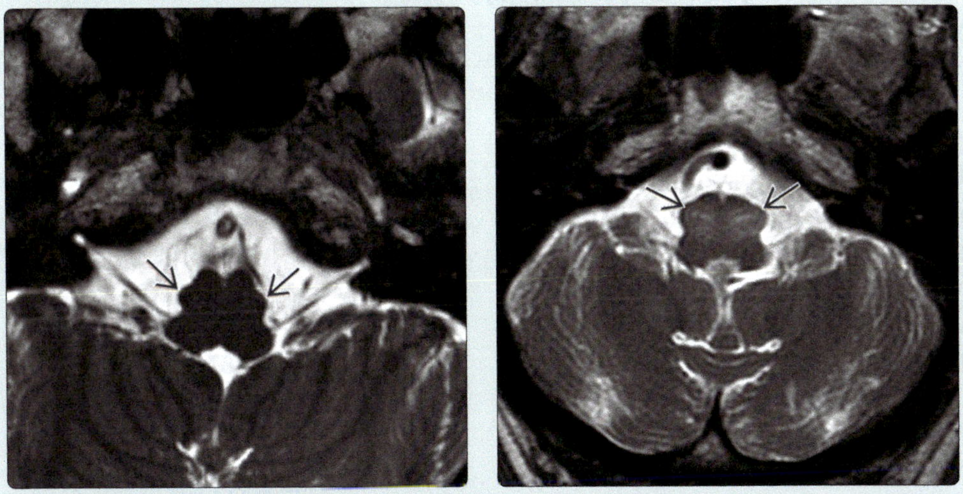

(Left) *Axial T2WI MR (CISS) shows the normal shape of the medullary olives* →. **(Right)** *Axial T2WI MR in a patient who developed palatal myoclonus ~ 6 months after resection of a midbrain cavernous malformation shows hyperintensity and enlargement of both olives* →. *This pattern is typical in the subacute stage of hypertrophic olivary degeneration, which typically appears between 6 months and 3-4 years after injury to the dento-rubro-olivary pathway.*

PART I: BRAIN
SECTION 3
Anatomy-Based Diagnoses

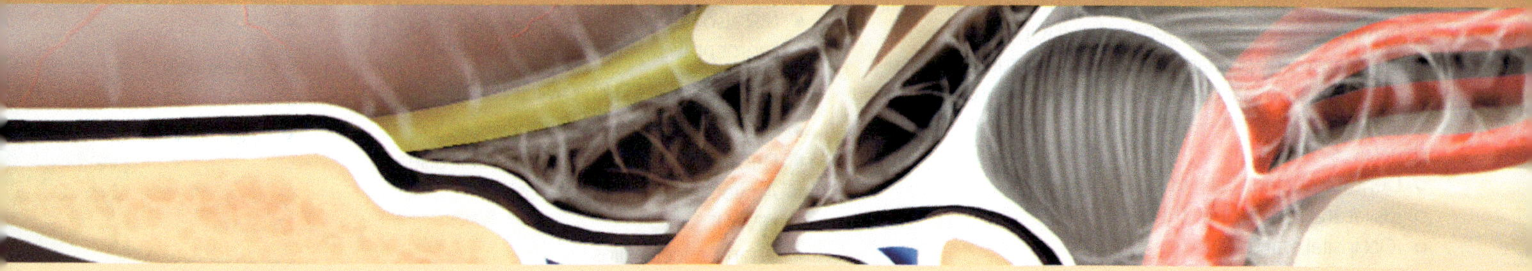

Ventricles and Cisterns

Sella and Pituitary

Cerebellopontine Angle and Internal Auditory Canal (CPA-IAC)

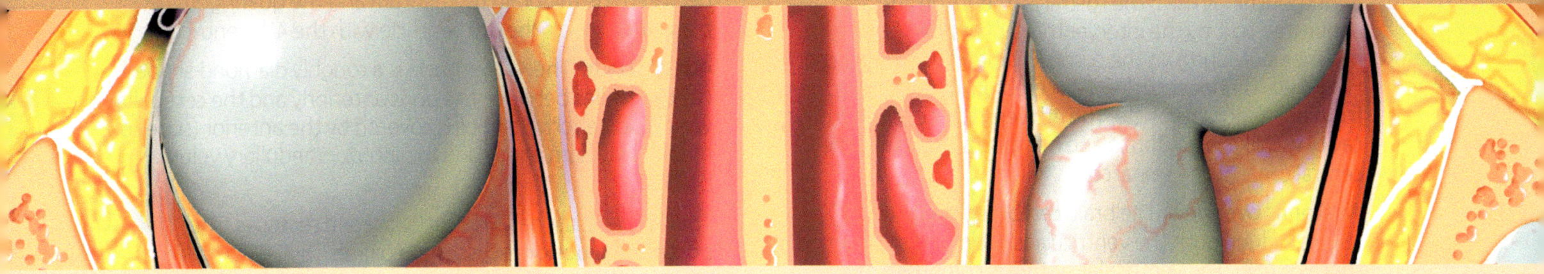

Skull, Scalp, and Meninges

Eye, Orbit, and Optic Nerve

Gross and Imaging Anatomy

Ventricles and Choroid Plexus

Basic embryology: Early in embryonic development, the forebrain cavity divides into 2 lateral ventricles, which develop as outpouchings from the rostral 3rd ventricle and are connected to it by the interventricular foramen (a.k.a. foramen of Monro). In the coronal plane, these form a central H-shaped "monoventricle." The cerebral aqueduct develops from the midbrain vesicle. The 4th ventricle develops from a cavity within the hindbrain and merges caudally with the central canal of the spinal cord.

Anatomic overview: The brain cerebrospinal fluid (CSF) spaces include both the ventricular system and subarachnoid spaces (SASs). The ventricular system is comprised of 4 interconnected CSF-filled, ependymal-lined cavities that lie deep within the brain. The paired **lateral ventricles** communicate with the 3rd ventricle via the Y-shaped **foramen of Monro**. The **3rd ventricle** communicates with the 4th ventricle via the **cerebral aqueduct** (of Sylvius). In turn, the **4th ventricle** communicates with the SAS via its outlet foramina (the midline **foramen of Magendie** and the 2 lateral **foramina of Luschka**).

Lateral ventricles: Each lateral ventricle has a body, atrium, and 3 projections ("horns"). The roof of the **frontal horn** is formed by the corpus callosum genu. It is bordered laterally and inferiorly by the head of the caudate nucleus. The septi pellucidi is a thin, bilayered membrane that extends from the corpus callosum genu anteriorly to the foramen of Monro posteriorly and forms the medial borders of both frontal horns.

The **body** of the lateral ventricle passes posteriorly under the corpus callosum. Its floor is formed by the dorsal thalamus, and its medial wall is bordered by the fornix. Laterally, it curves around the body and tail of the caudate nucleus.

The **atrium** contains the choroid plexus glomus and is formed by the confluence of the body with the temporal and occipital horns. The **temporal horn** extends anteroinferiorly from the atrium and is bordered on its floor and medial wall by the hippocampus. Its roof is formed by the tail of the caudate nucleus. The **occipital horn** is surrounded entirely by white matter fiber tracts, principally the geniculocalcarine tract and the forceps major of the corpus callosum.

Foramen of Monro is a Y-shaped structure with 2 long arms extending toward each lateral ventricle and a short inferior common stem that connects with the roof of the 3rd ventricle.

3rd ventricle: The 3rd ventricle is a single, slit-like, midline, vertically oriented cavity that lies between the thalami. Its roof is formed by the tela choroidea, a double layer of invaginated pia. The lamina terminalis and anterior commissure lie along the anterior border of the 3rd ventricle.

The floor of the 3rd ventricle is formed by several critical anatomic structures. From front to back these include the optic chiasm, hypothalamus with the tuber cinereum and infundibular stalk, mammillary bodies, and roof of the midbrain tegmentum.

The 3rd ventricle has 2 inferiorly located CSF-filled projections: The slightly rounded **optic recess** and the more pointed **infundibular recess**. Two small recesses, the **suprapineal and pineal recesses**, form the posterior border of the 3rd ventricle. A variably sized interthalamic adhesion (also called the **massa intermedia**) lies between the lateral walls of the 3rd ventricle. The massa intermedia is not a true commissure.

Cerebral aqueduct is an elongated tubular conduit that lies between the midbrain tegmentum and the quadrigeminal plate. It connects the 3rd ventricle with the 4th ventricle.

4th ventricle: The 4th ventricle is a roughly diamond-shaped cavity that lies between the pons anteriorly and the cerebellar vermis posteriorly. Its roof is covered by the anterior (superior) medullary velum above and the inferior medullary velum below.

The 4th ventricle has 5 distinctly shaped recesses. The **posterior superior recesses** are paired, thin, flat, CSF-filled pouches that cap the cerebellar tonsils. The **lateral recesses** curve anterolaterally from the 4th ventricle, extending under the brachium pontis (major cerebellar peduncle) into the lower cerebellopontine angle (CPA) cisterns. The lateral recesses transmit choroid plexus through the foramina of Luschka into the adjacent SAS. The **fastigium** is a triangular, blind-ending, dorsal midline outpouching that points toward the cerebellar vermis. The 4th ventricle gradually narrows as it courses inferiorly, forming the **obex**. Near the cervicomedullary junction, the obex becomes continuous with the central canal of the spinal cord.

Choroid plexus and the production of CSF: The choroid plexus is comprised of highly vascular papillary excrescences with a central connective tissue core coated by an ependyma-derived secretory epithelium. The embryonic choroid plexus forms where the infolded tela choroidea contacts the ependymal lining of the ventricles, thus developing along the entire choroidal fissure.

The largest mass of choroid plexus, the **glomus**, is located in the atrium of the lateral ventricles. The choroid plexus extends anteriorly along the floor of the lateral ventricle, lying between the fornix and thalamus. It then dives through the interventricular foramen (of Monro) and curves posteriorly along the roof of the 3rd ventricle. The choroid plexus, in the body of the lateral ventricle, curls around the thalamus into the temporal horn, where it fills the choroidal fissure and lies superomedial to the hippocampus.

CSF is predominantly, but not exclusively, secreted by the choroid plexuses. Brain interstitial fluid, ependyma, and capillaries may also play a poorly defined role in CSF secretion. The choroid plexus epithelium secretes CSF at the rate of about 0.2-0.7 mL/min or 600-700 mL/day. The mean CSF volume is 150 mL, with 25 mL in the ventricles and 125 mL in SASs. CSF flows through the ventricular system and passes through the exit foramina of the 4th ventricle into the SASs. The bulk of CSF resorption is through the arachnoid villi along the superior sagittal sinus. CSF also drains into lymphatic vessels around the cranial cavity and spinal canal.

Not all CSF is produced in the choroid plexus. Drainage of brain interstitial fluid is a significant extrachoroidal source.

CSF plays an essential role in the maintenance of brain interstitial fluid homeostasis and regulation of neuronal functioning.

Cisterns and SAS

Overview: The SASs lie between the pia and arachnoid. The sulci are CSF-filled spaces between the gyral folds. Focal expansions of the SASs form the brain CSF cisterns. These cisterns are found at the base of the brain around the brainstem, tentorial incisura, and foramen magnum. Numerous pial-covered septa cross the SAS from the brain to the arachnoid. All SAS cisterns communicate with each other and the ventricular system, providing natural pathways for disease spread (e.g., meningitis, neoplasms).

The brain cisterns are conveniently grouped into supra-, peri-, and infratentorial cisterns. All contain numerous important critical structures, such as vessels and cranial nerves.

Supratentorial/peritentorial cisterns: The **suprasellar cistern** lies between the diaphragma sellae and the hypothalamus. Critical contents include the infundibulum, optic chiasm, and circle of Willis.

The **interpeduncular cistern** is the posterior continuation of the suprasellar cistern. Lying between the cerebral peduncles, it contains the oculomotor nerves as well as the distal basilar artery and proximal segments of the posterior cerebral arteries. Important perforating arteries, the thalamoperforating and thalamogeniculate arteries arise from the top of the basilar artery and cross the interpeduncular cistern to enter the midbrain.

The **perimesencephalic (ambient) cisterns** are thin wings of CSF that extend posterosuperiorly from the suprasellar cistern to the quadrigeminal cistern. They wrap around the midbrain and contain the trochlear nerves, P2 PCA segments, superior cerebellar arteries, and basal vein of Rosenthal.

The **quadrigeminal cistern** lies under the corpus callosum splenium, behind the pineal gland and tectal plate. It connects with the ambient cisterns laterally and the superior cerebellar cistern inferiorly. The quadrigeminal cistern contains the pineal gland, trochlear nerves, P3 PCA segments, proximal choroidal arteries, and vein of Galen. An anterior extension, the **velum interpositum**, lies below the fornix and above the 3rd ventricle. The velum interpositum contains the internal cerebral veins and medial posterior choroidal arteries.

Infratentorial cisterns: The unpaired posterior fossa cisterns that lie in the midline are the prepontine, premedullary, and superior cerebellar cisterns, as well as the cisterna magna. The lateral cisterns are paired and include the cerebellopontine and cerebellomedullary cisterns.

The **prepontine cistern** lies between the upper clivus and the "belly" of the pons. It contains numerous important structures including the basilar artery, the anterior inferior cerebellar arteries (AICAs), and the trigeminal and abducens nerves (CN5 and CN6).

The **premedullary cistern** is the inferior continuation of the prepontine cistern. It lies between the lower clivus in front and the medulla behind. It extends inferiorly to the foramen magnum and contains the vertebral arteries and branches (e.g., posterior inferior cerebellar arteries, PICAs) and the hypoglossal nerve (CN12).

The **superior cerebellar cistern** lies between the straight sinus above and the vermis below. It contains the superior cerebellar arteries and veins. It connects superiorly through the tentorial incisura with the quadrigeminal cistern and inferiorly with the cisterna magna. The **cisterna magna** lies below the inferior vermis between the medulla and the occiput. It contains the cerebellar tonsils and the tonsillohemispheric branches of the PICA. The cisterna magna merges imperceptibly with the SAS of the upper cervical spinal canal.

The CPA **cisterns** lie between the pons/cerebellum and the petrous temporal bone. Their most important contents are the trigeminal, facial, and vestibulocochlear nerves (CN5, CN7, and CN8). Other structures found here include the petrosal veins and AICAs. The CPA cisterns are contiguous inferiorly with the cerebellomedullary cisterns, sometimes termed the "lower" CPA cisterns.

The **cerebellomedullary cisterns** extend laterally around the medulla and are continuous with the cisterna magna below and the CPAs above. They contain the vagus, glossopharyngeal, and spinal accessory nerves (CN9, CN10, and CN11). A tuft of choroid plexus exits each foramen of Luschka into the cerebellomedullary cistern. The flocculus of the cerebellum that projects into this cistern can appear very prominent. The flocculus and choroid plexus are normal contents of the cerebellomedullary cisterns and should not be mistaken for pathology.

Imaging Recommendations

MR: Thin-section 3D T2WI or FIESTA/CISS best details CSF within the ventricular system, SASs, and basal cisterns and exquisitely delineates their contents. Whole-brain FLAIR is especially useful for evaluating potential abnormalities in the SASs. Spin dephasing with pulsatile CSF flow is common and can mimic intraventricular pathology, especially in the basal cisterns and around the interventricular foramen. Incomplete CSF suppression with "bright" CSF can mimic pathologic SASs.

Differential Diagnosis Approach

Ventricles and Choroid Plexus

Overview: Approximately 10% of intracranial neoplasms involve the cerebral ventricles, either primarily or by extension. An anatomy-based approach is most effective, as there is a distinct predilection for certain lesions to occur in 1 ventricle or cistern and not others. Age is also a helpful consideration. Specific imaging findings, such as signal intensity, enhancement, and the presence or absence of calcification, are relatively less important than location and age.

Normal variants: Asymmetry of the lateral ventricles is a common normal variant, as is flow-related CSF pulsation artifact. A cavum septi pellucidi (CSP) is a common normal variant, seen as a CSF cleft between the 2 leaves of the septum pellucidum. An elongated, finger-like posterior continuation of the CSP between the fornices, a cavum vergae, may be associated with a CSP.

Lateral ventricle mass: Choroid plexus cysts (xanthogranulomas) are a common, generally age-related, degenerative finding with no clinical significance. They are nonneoplastic noninflammatory cysts, usually bilateral with rim calcification. They may be hyperintense on FLAIR, and 60-80% appear quite bright on DWI. A strongly enhancing choroid plexus mass in a child is most likely a choroid plexus papilloma. With the exception of the 4th ventricle, a choroid plexus mass in an adult is usually meningioma or metastasis, not a choroid plexus papilloma.

Some lateral ventricle lesions display a distinct predilection for specific sublocations within the lateral ventricles. An innocent-appearing frontal horn mass in a middle-aged or older adult is most often a subependymoma. A bubbly mass in the body of the lateral ventricle is usually a central neurocytoma. Neurocysticercosis cysts can occur in all ages and in virtually every CSF space.

Foramen of Monro mass: The most common "abnormality" here is a pseudolesion caused by CSF pulsation artifact. Colloid cyst is the only relatively common pathology here. It is rare in children and typically a lesion of adults. Flow artifact can mimic a colloid cyst, but mass effect is absent. In a child with an enhancing mass in the interventricular foramen, tuberous sclerosis with subependymal nodule &/or giant cell astrocytoma should be a consideration. Masses such as ependymoma, papilloma, and metastasis are rare.

3rd ventricle mass: Again, the most common "lesion" in this location is either CSF flow artifact or a normal structure (the massa intermedia). Colloid cyst is the only common lesion that occurs in the 3rd ventricle; 99% are wedged into the foramen of Monro. Extreme vertebrobasilar dolichoectasia can indent the 3rd ventricle, sometimes projecting upward as high as the interventricular foramen, and should not be mistaken for colloid cyst.

Primary neoplasms in children are uncommon here but include choroid plexus papilloma, germinoma, craniopharyngioma, and a sessile-type tuber cinereum hamartoma. Primary neoplasms of the 3rd ventricle in adults are also uncommon, although an intraventricular macroadenoma and chordoid glioma are examples. Neurocysticercosis occurs here but is uncommon.

Cerebral aqueduct: Other than aqueductal stenosis, intrinsic lesions of the cerebral aqueduct are rare. Most are related to masses in adjacent structures (e.g., tectal plate glioma).

4th ventricle mass: Pediatric masses are the most common intrinsic abnormalities of the 4th ventricle. Medulloblastoma, ependymoma, and astrocytoma predominate. Atypical teratoid/rhabdoid tumor is a less common neoplasm that may occur here. It usually occurs in children under the age of 3 and can mimic medulloblastoma.

Metastases to the choroid or ependyma are probably the most common 4th ventricle neoplasm of adults. Primary neoplasms are rare. Choroid plexus papilloma does occur here, as well as in the CPA cistern. Subependymoma is a lesion of middle-aged adults that is found in the inferior 4th ventricle, lying behind the pontomedullary junction. A newly described rare neoplasm, rosette-forming glioneuronal tumor, is a midline mass of the 4th ventricle. It has no particular distinguishing imaging features and, although it may appear aggressive, it is a benign (WHO grade I) lesion. Hemangioblastomas are intraaxial masses but may project into the 4th ventricle. Epidermoid cysts and neurocysticercosis cysts can be found in all ages.

SASs and Cisterns

Overview: The SASs are a common site of pathology that varies from benign congenital lesions (such as arachnoid cyst) to infection (meningitis) and neoplastic involvement ("carcinomatous meningitis"). Anatomic location is key to the differential diagnosis, as imaging findings, such as enhancement and hyperintensity on FLAIR, are often nonspecific. Patient age is also helpful although generally of secondary importance.

Normal variants: CSF flow-related artifacts are common, especially in the basal cisterns on FLAIR imaging. Mega cisterna magna may be considered a normal variant, as is a cavum velum interpositum (CVI). A CVI is a thin, triangular-shaped CSF space between the lateral ventricles that lies below the fornices and above the 3d ventricle. Occasionally a CVI may become quite large.

Suprasellar cistern mass: Common masses in adults are upward extensions of macroadenoma, meningioma, and aneurysm. The 2 most common suprasellar masses in children are astrocytoma of the optic chiasm/hypothalamus and craniopharyngioma.

CPA mass: In adults, vestibular schwannoma accounts for almost 90% of all CPA-internal auditory canal masses. Meningioma, epidermoid cyst, aneurysm, and arachnoid cyst **together** represent about 8% of lesions in this location. All other less common entities, such as lipoma, schwannomas of other cranial nerves, metastases, neurenteric cysts, etc., account for about 2%.

In the absence of neurofibromatosis type 2, vestibular schwannomas are very rare in children. CPA epidermoid and arachnoid cysts may occur in children. Extension of ependymoma laterally through the foramina of Luschka may involve the CPA.

Cystic-appearing CPA masses comprise their own special differential diagnosis. Although vestibular schwannoma with intramural cysts can occur, it is less common than epidermoid and arachnoid cysts. Neurocysticercosis may occasionally involve the CPA. Large endolymphatic sac anomaly shows a CSF-like mass within the posterior wall of the temporal bone. Hemangioblastoma and neurenteric cysts are other less common cystic masses that occur in the CPA.

Cisterna magna mass: Tonsillar herniation, whether congenital (Chiari 1) or secondary to posterior fossa mass effect or intracranial hypotension, is the most common "mass" in this location. Nonneoplastic cysts (arachnoid, epidermoid, dermoid, neurenteric) may also occur here.

Neoplasms in and around the cisterna magna, such as meningioma and metastasis, are typically anterior to the medulla. Subependymoma of the 4th ventricle originates in the obex and lies behind the medulla.

FLAIR hyperintensity: Hyperintense sulci and SASs are seen with MR artifacts, as well as a variety of lesions. Pathologic FLAIR hyperintensity is typically related to blood (e.g., subarachnoid hemorrhage), protein (meningitis), or cells (pia-SAS metastases). Less commonly, gadolinium-based contrast agents in patients with blood-brain barrier leakage or renal failure can cause FLAIR hyperintensity.

Rare causes of FLAIR hyperintensity include ruptured dermoid cyst, moyamoya (ivy sign), and acute cerebral ischemia. Contrast enhancement helps distinguish meningitis and metastases from subarachnoid hemorrhage and CSF artifacts.

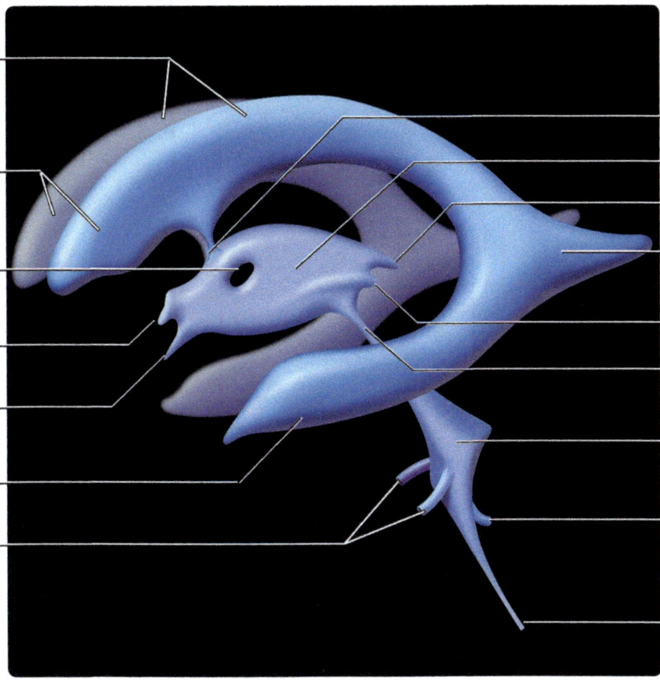

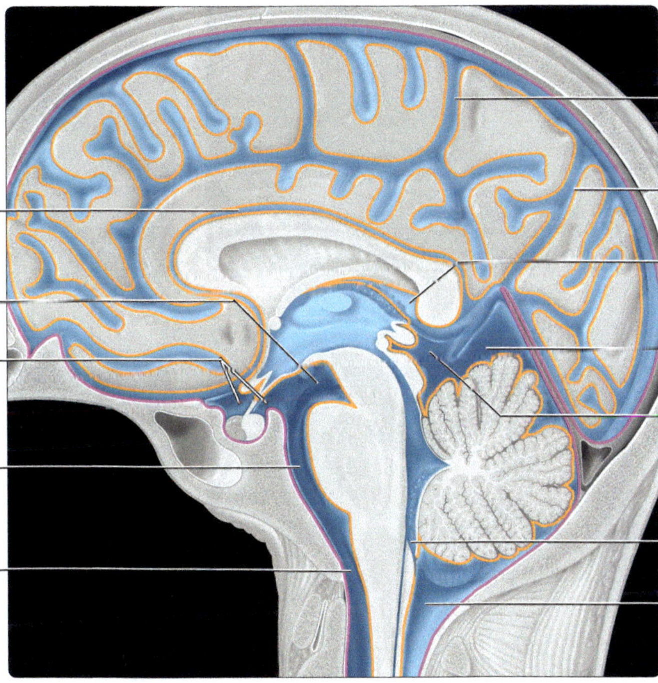

(Top) *Schematic 3D representation of the ventricular system, viewed in the sagittal plane, demonstrates the normal appearance and communicating pathways of the cerebral ventricles.* **(Bottom)** *Sagittal midline graphic through the interhemispheric fissure depicts subarachnoid spaces (SASs) with cerebrospinal fluid (CSF) (blue) between the arachnoid (purple) and pia (orange). The central sulcus separates the frontal lobe (anterior) from the parietal lobe (posterior). The pia mater is closely applied to the brain surface, whereas the arachnoid is adherent to the dura. The ventricles communicate with the cisterns and SAS via the foramina of Luschka and Magendie. The cisterns normally communicate freely with each other.*

(Left) *Axial T2 MR demonstrates normal anatomy at the level of the lateral ventricles. The frontal horns of the lateral ventricle are separated by a tiny septi pellucidi. Note the foramen of Monro connecting the lateral ventricles to the 3rd ventricle.* **(Right)** *Axial T2 MR at the level of the cerebral aqueduct demonstrates the infundibular recess of the 3rd ventricle, mammillary bodies, interpeduncular cistern, and the quadrigeminal cisterns.*

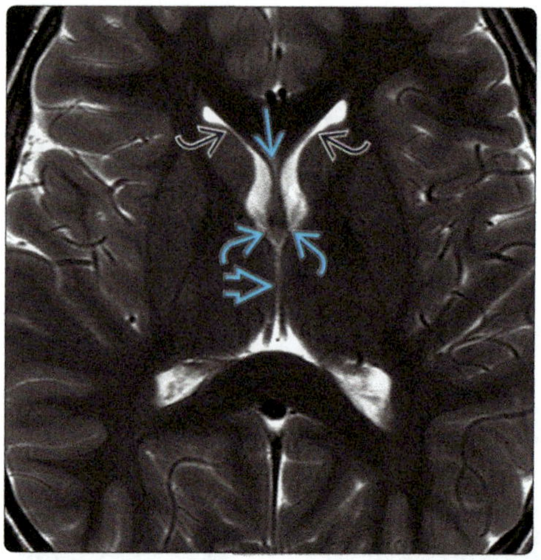

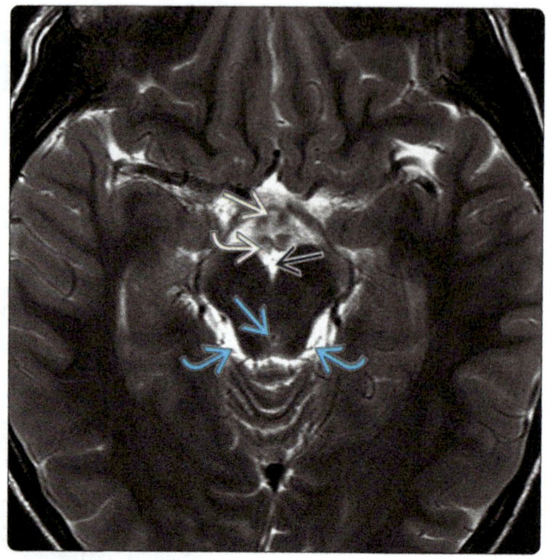

(Left) *Axial T2 MR at the level of the 4th ventricular outlet shows the foramen of Magendie and foramina of Luschka.* **(Right)** *Sagittal T2 SPACE MR shows the normal flow void due to CSF flow at the cerebral aqueduct and foramen of Magendie. Note the chiasmatic and infundibular recesses of the 3rd ventricle and fastigium of the 4th ventricle.*

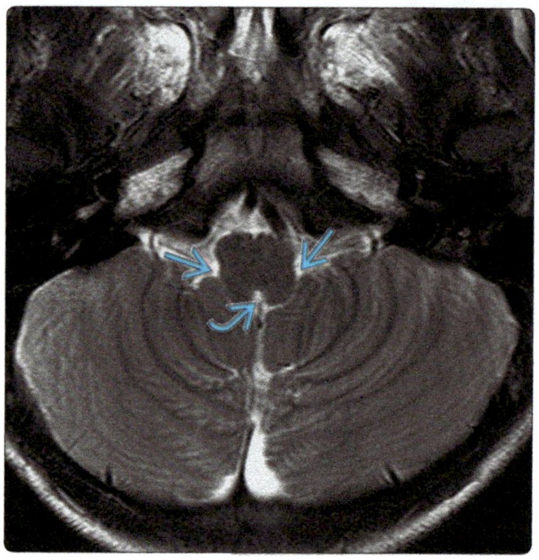

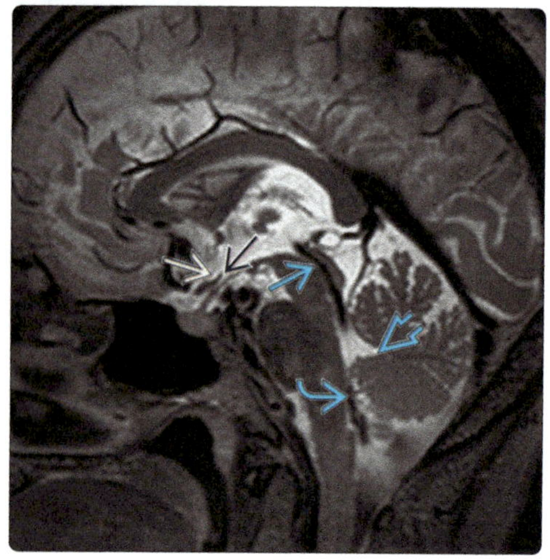

(Left) *Axial T2 MR shows normal asymmetry of the lateral ventricles with the right being larger than the left. The septi pellucidi are slightly bowed and displaced across the midline. When there is lateral ventricular asymmetry, it is important to scrutinize the region of foramen of Monro to exclude any obstructing pathology.* **(Right)** *Axial FLAIR in a patient with hydrocephalus demonstrates a prominent pseudomass of the 3rd ventricle caused by pulsatile CSF.*

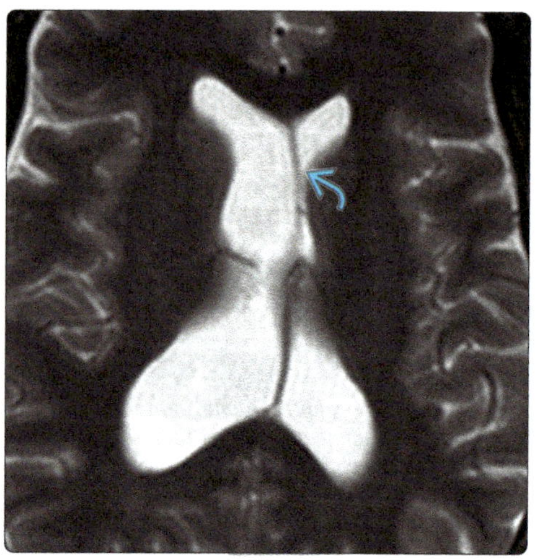

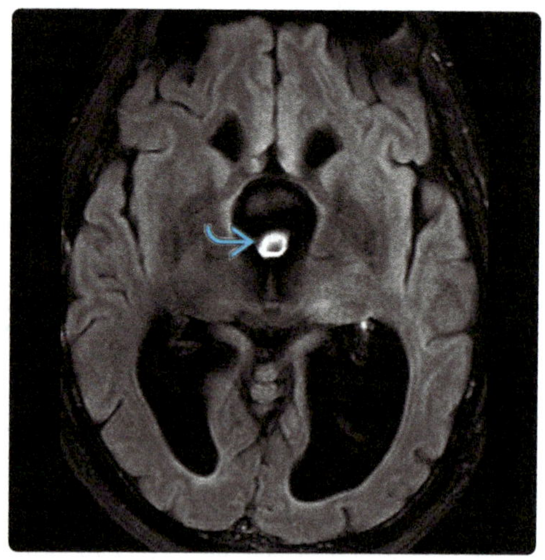

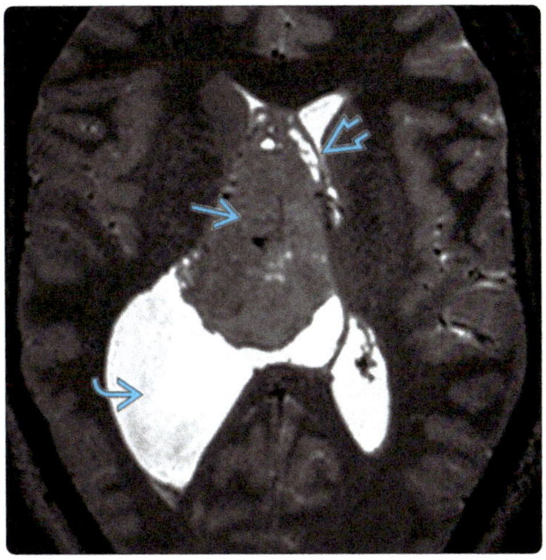

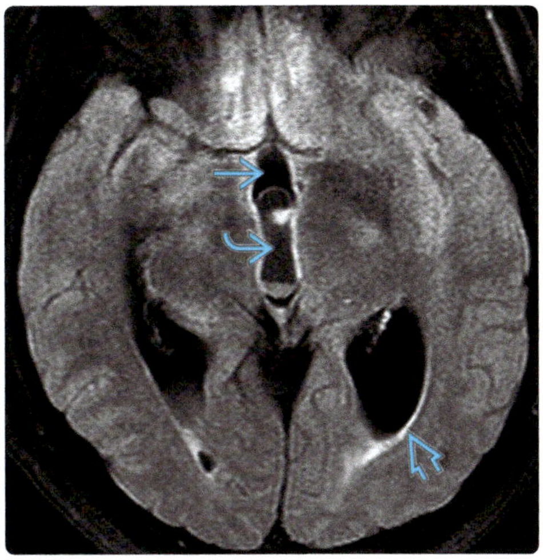

(Left) *Axial T2 MR shows a large ventricular mass ➡ in the frontal horn and anterior body of the right lateral ventricle. There is dilatation of the posterior body of the right lateral ventricle ➡ and displacement of the septi pellucidi ➡ to the left. On histopathology, this was a central neurocytoma.* **(Right)** *Axial FLAIR MR demonstrates an intraventricular neurocysticercosis ➡ in the posterior 3rd ventricle with dilatation of the anterior 1/3 ➡ and lateral ventricles. Note the mild periventricular interstitial edema ➡.*

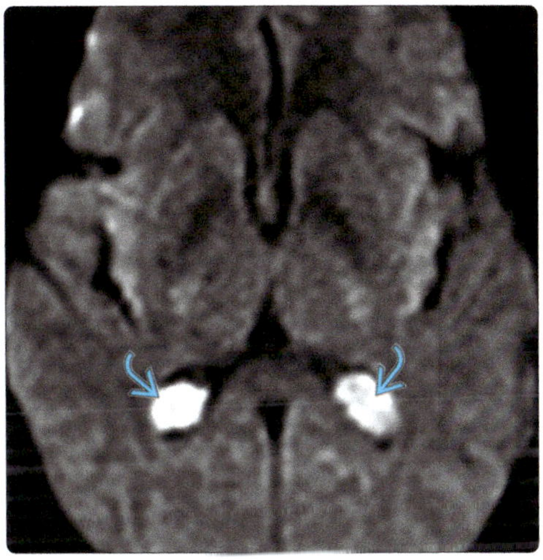

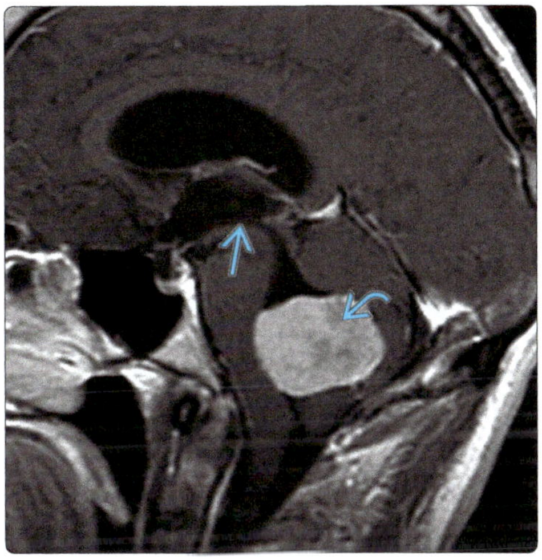

(Left) *Axial DWI shows characteristic large choroid plexus cysts ➡ in the atria of both lateral ventricles, within the choroid plexus glomi. Choroid plexus cysts, often called choroid plexus xanthogranuloma, are nonneoplastic noninflammatory cysts. Between 60-80% appear quite bright on DWI, as in this case.* **(Right)** *Sagittal T1 C+ shows a homogenously enhancing 4th ventricular mass ➡, which on pathology was a meningioma. Note dilatation of the ventricular system ➡ proximal to the mass.*

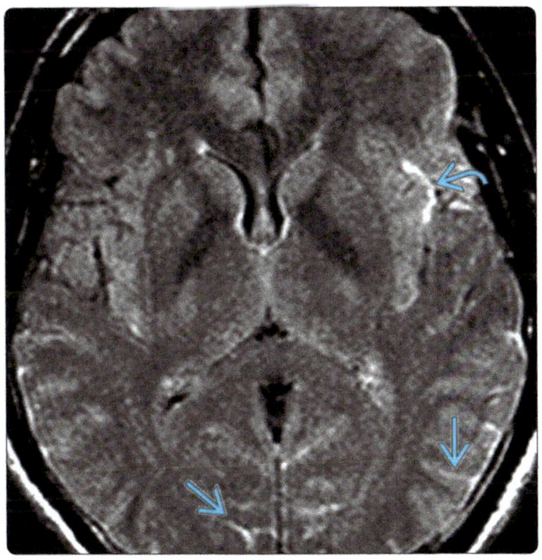

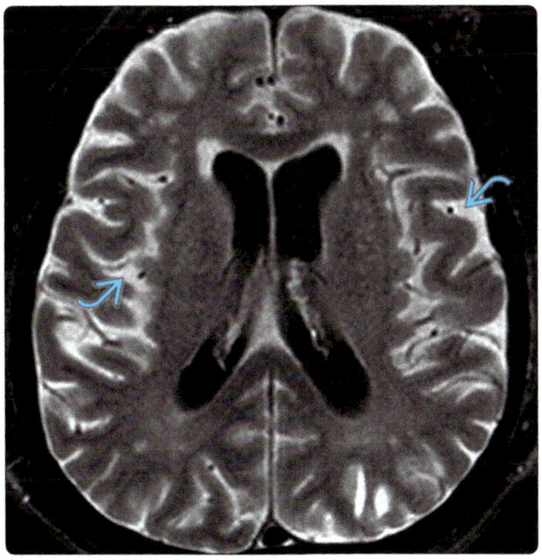

(Left) *Axial FLAIR MR in a patient with acute subarachnoid hemorrhage due to aneurysm rupture shows high signal in the left sylvian fissure ➡ and posterior cortical sulci ➡.* **(Right)** *Axial FLAIR MR in a patient with chronic renal disease who received IV gadolinium 48 hours prior shows marked FLAIR hyperintensity ➡ in the cortical sulci. Sulcal hyperintensity on FLAIR can be caused by pia-subarachnoid metastases, blood, protein (meningitis), high oxygen content, and retained contrast (renal failure as in this case).*

Cavum Septi Pellucidi (CSP)

KEY FACTS

TERMINOLOGY

- Cystic CSF cavity of septum pellucidum (SP)
  - Occurs ± cavum vergae (CV)

IMAGING

- Elongated finger-shaped CSF collection between lateral ventricles
  - Cavum septi pellucidi (CSP): Between frontal horns of lateral ventricles
  - CV: Posterior extension between fornices
  - CV is posterior extension of CSP
- Size varies from slit-like to several mm, occasionally > 1 cm
- SP invariably cystic in fetus
  - Width of fetal CSP increases between 19-27 weeks
  - Plateaus at 28 weeks
  - Gradually closes in rostral direction between 28 weeks and term
  - CSP present in 100% of premature, 85% of term infants
- CSP seen in up to 15-20% of adults

TOP DIFFERENTIAL DIAGNOSES

- Asymmetric lateral ventricles
- Cavum velum interpositum
- Ependymal cyst
- Absent SP

PATHOLOGY

- CSP forms if fetal SP fails to obliterate
- CSP is not "5th ventricle"
- CV is not "6th ventricle"

CLINICAL ISSUES

- Usually asymptomatic, incidental
- Headache (relationship to cyst unclear)
- CSP frequent among athletes with history of repeated traumatic brain injury, such as boxers

DIAGNOSTIC CHECKLIST

- CV almost never occurs without CSP

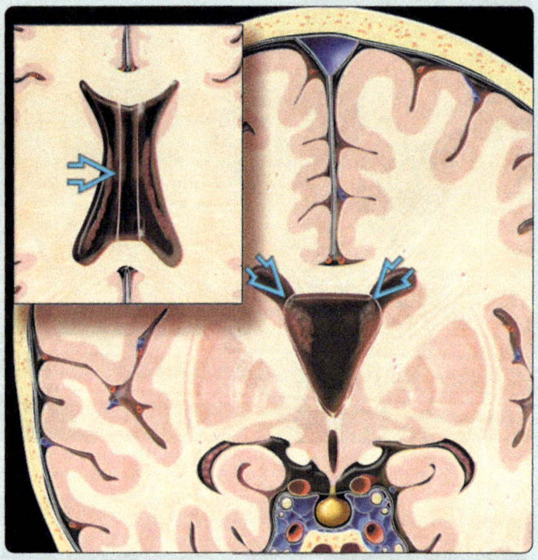

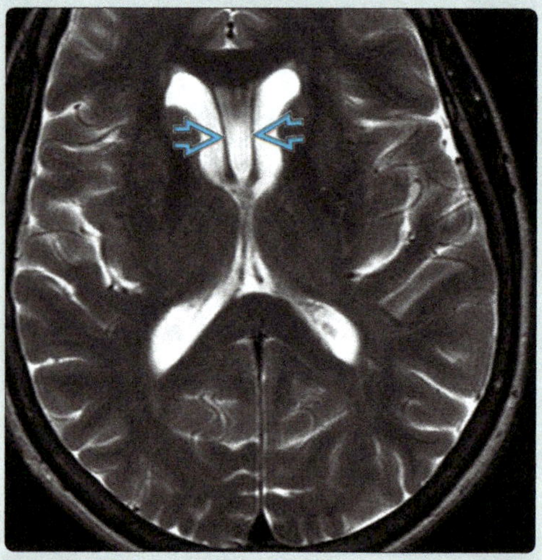

(Left) *Coronal graphic with axial insert shows classic cavum septi pellucidi (CSP) with cavum vergae (CV). Note the finger-like cerebrospinal fluid (CSF) collection between the lateral ventricles.* **(Right)** *Axial T2WI MR shows CSP as a CSF collection between the leaves of the septum pellucidum. Although seen incidentally, some studies have reported that CSP is frequent among athletes with a history of repeated traumatic brain injury, such as boxers and American professional football players.*

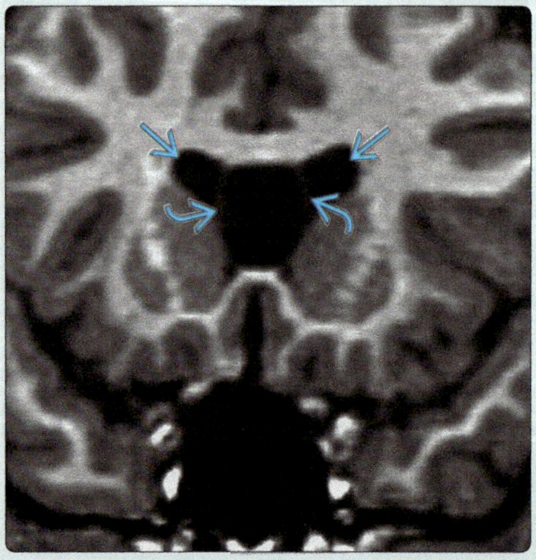

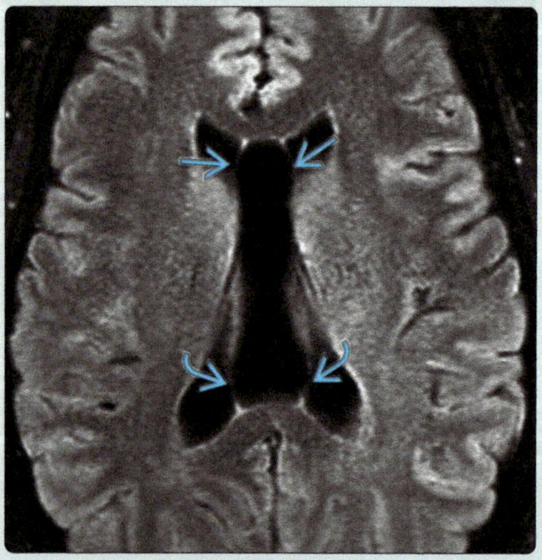

(Left) *Coronal T1WI MR shows a classic large CSP between the frontal horns bowing the leaves of the septum pellucidum laterally.* **(Right)** *Axial FLAIR MR shows a large CSP with CV as a large CSF collection between the leaves of the septum pellucidum, continuing directly posteriorly with the CSF collection, splaying the fornices laterally.*

Intraventricular Obstructive Hydrocephalus

KEY FACTS

TERMINOLOGY

- Intraventricular obstructive hydrocephalus (IVOH) = obstruction proximal to foramina of Luschka, Magendie
  - Acute (aIVOH)
  - Chronic "compensated" (cIVOH)

IMAGING

- aIVOH = "ballooned" ventricles plus indistinct ("blurred") margins
  - "Fingers" of CSF extend into periventricular white matter
  - Most striking around ventricular horns (periventricular "halos")
  - After decompression, corpus callosum may show hyperintensity
- cIVOH = "ballooned" ventricles without periventricular "halo"

TOP DIFFERENTIAL DIAGNOSES

- Ventricular enlargement secondary to parenchymal loss
- Normal pressure hydrocephalus
- Extraventricular obstructive hydrocephalus
- Choroid plexus papilloma
- Longstanding overt ventriculomegaly in adults

PATHOLOGY

- Intraventricular obstruction to CSF flow
  - CSF production continues, ventricular pressure ↑
- Ventricles expand, compress adjacent parenchyma
- Periventricular interstitial fluid increases
  - Leads to myelin vacuolization, destruction
- Pathology varies depending on obstruction etiology

CLINICAL ISSUES

- Headache, papilledema (aIVOH)
- Nausea, vomiting, diplopia (6th nerve palsy)

DIAGNOSTIC CHECKLIST

- Size of ventricles generally correlates poorly with intracranial pressure

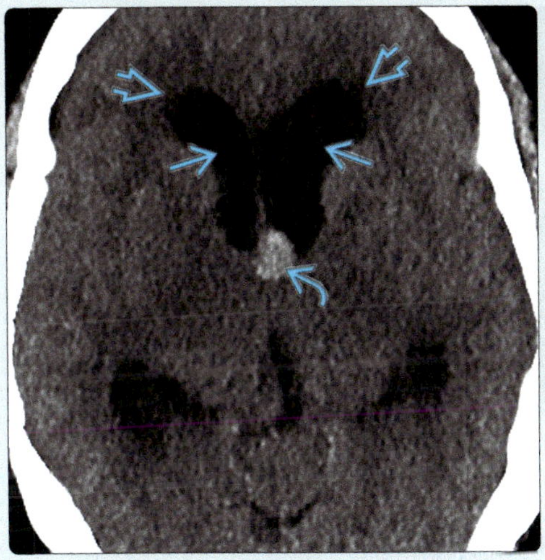
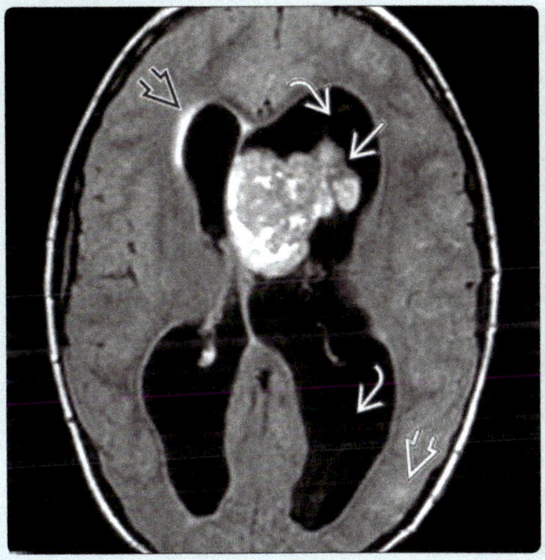

(Left) *Axial NECT in a patient with headache demonstrates a classic colloid cyst at the foramen of Monro causing intraventricular obstructive hydrocephalus with dilatation of both lateral ventricles. Note the periventricular hypodensities due to transependymal leakage of CSF.* **(Right)** *Axial FLAIR in a patient with tuberous sclerosis shows large subependymal giant cell astrocytoma causing obstructive hydrocephalus with mild periventricular edema. Note the subtle hyperintensity in the occipital lobe tuber.*

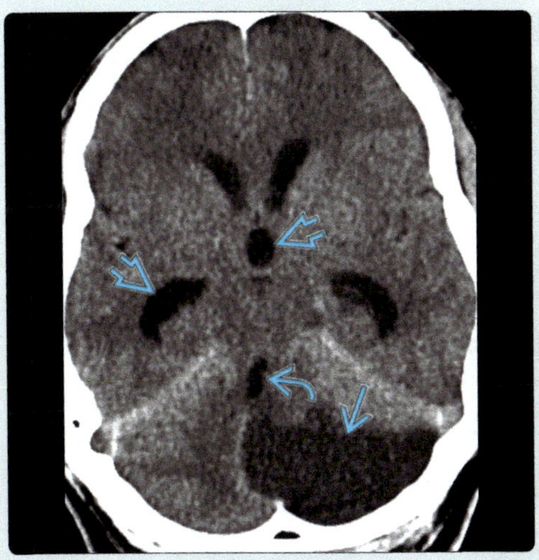
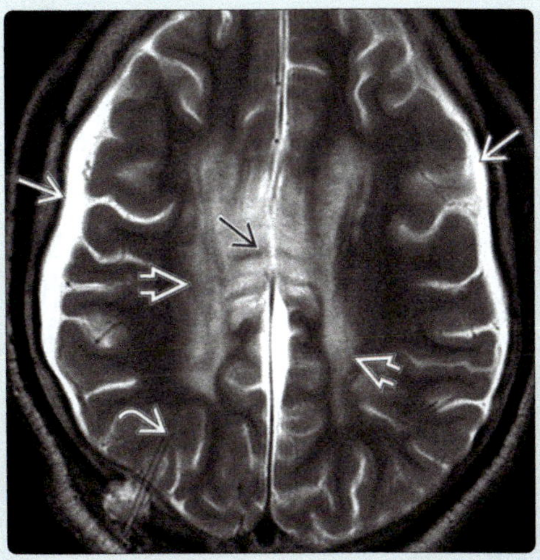

(Left) *Axial CECT demonstrates a subacute left posterior inferior cerebellar infarct causing mass effect on the 4th ventricle and resulting in obstructive hydrocephalus.* **(Right)** *Axial T2WI MR in a patient with corpus callosum impingement syndrome, after shunting for severe IVOH, shows a shunt tube, bilateral subdural fluid collections, and "striated" hyperintensity in the corpus callosum with somewhat less striking changes in the periventricular WM. (Courtesy S. Candy, MD.)*

KEY FACTS

TERMINOLOGY

- Extraventricular obstructive hydrocephalus (EVOH): Enlarged ventricles due to mismatch between cerebrospinal fluid (CSF) formation, absorption
- Synonym: "Communicating" hydrocephalus

IMAGING

- Impaired absorption of CSF distal to 4th ventricle outlet foramina
- Ventricular size varies with duration of obstruction
- All ventricles enlarged with no intraventricular obstructive cause
- Lateral, 3rd, and 4th ventricles dilated
- ± periventricular white matter interstitial edema
- ± abnormal density/intensity of cisternal CSF ± leptomeningeal enhancement

TOP DIFFERENTIAL DIAGNOSES

- Intraventricular obstructive hydrocephalus
- Ventricular enlargement secondary to parenchymal loss
- Normal pressure hydrocephalus

PATHOLOGY

- Hemorrhage → fibrosis/obstruction of subarachnoid space
  - Most common cause of EVOH
- Other etiologies include suppurative meningitis, neoplastic or inflammatory exudates
- Subarachnoid hemorrhage, exudates may fibrose/occlude subarachnoid space, reduce CSF pulsations

CLINICAL ISSUES

- Headache, papilledema
- Nausea, vomiting, diplopia (cranial nerve palsy)

DIAGNOSTIC CHECKLIST

- EVOH: Generalized ventricular enlargement with abnormal density/intensity in basal cisterns ± leptomeningeal enhancement

(Left) *Axial NECT shows acute subarachnoid hemorrhage in the basal cisterns ➔ and sylvian fissures ➔. There is early extraventricular obstructive hydrocephalus with mild periventricular hypodensity ➔ due to interstitial edema.* **(Right)** *Axial T1WI C+ MR shows extensive leptomeningeal enhancement of the basal cisterns in neurosarcoidosis ➔. Notice the early communicating hydrocephalus with the dilated 3rd ventricle ➔ and temporal horns ➔.*

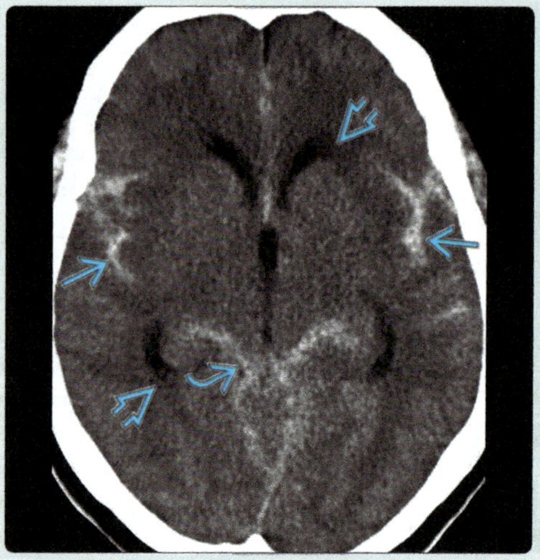

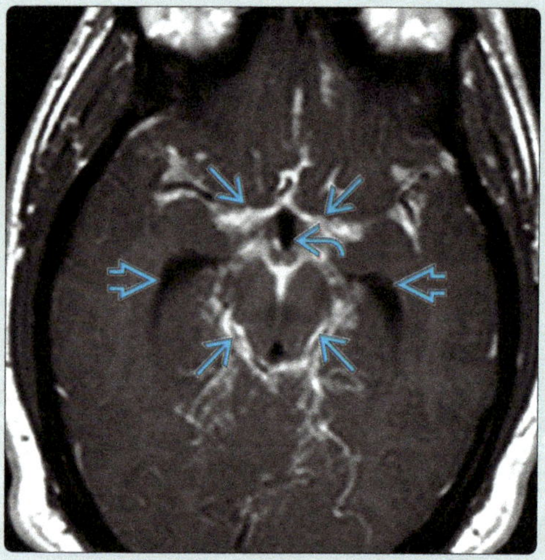

(Left) *Axial T2 MR in a 21-year-old patient with a remote history of meningitis shows chronic "compensated" extraventricular communicating hydrocephalus with marked dilatation of the lateral ➔ and 3rd ventricles ➔.* **(Right)** *Sagittal T1 MR in the same patient shows a patent widened cerebral aqueduct ➔ and foramen of Magendie ➔ with dilatation of 4th ventricle ➔. In long-standing "compensated" hydrocephalus, there is no periventricular interstitial edema around the ventricles, as in this case.*

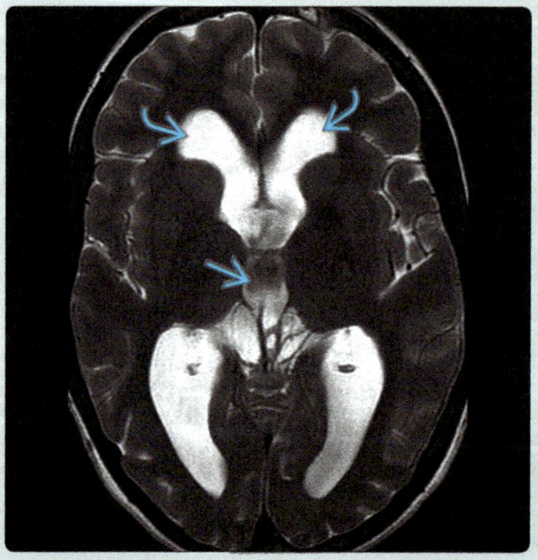

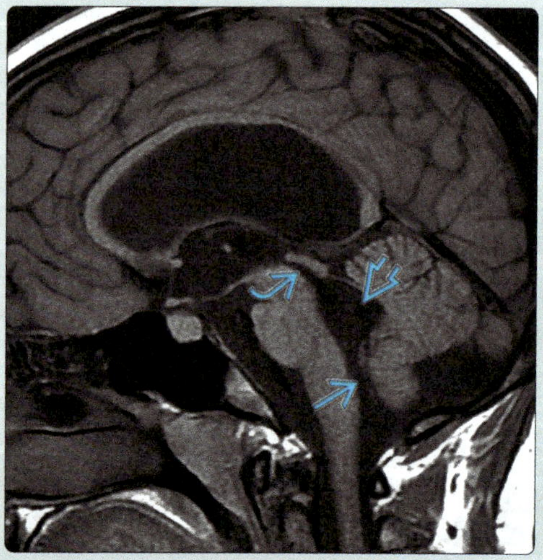

KEY FACTS

TERMINOLOGY

- Focal reduction of cerebral aqueduct diameter

IMAGING

- Ventriculomegaly of lateral and 3rd ventricles with normal-sized 4th ventricle
- ± periventricular interstitial edema (uncompensated hydrocephalus)
- Multiplanar MR with sagittal 3D-heavy T2WI sequences and sagittal cardiac-gated cine MR

TOP DIFFERENTIAL DIAGNOSES

- Obstructing extraventricular pathology
    - Neoplasm
    - Vein of Galen malformation
    - Quadrigeminal cistern arachnoid cyst
- Obstructing intraventricular (aqueductal) pathology
- Postinflammatory gliosis (aqueductal gliosis)
- Rhombencephalosynapsis

PATHOLOGY

- Congenital aqueductal stenosis is common cause of fetal hydrocephalus
- Aqueductal web and fork are pathological subsets

CLINICAL ISSUES

- Symptoms depend on patient age at time of diagnosis
- Onset often insidious, may occur at any time from birth to adulthood
- Headache, papilledema, 6th nerve palsy, bulging fontanelle
- Parinaud syndrome (sun-setting eyes, lid retraction, and tonic downgaze), convergence retraction nystagmus

DIAGNOSTIC CHECKLIST

- Consider postinflammatory gliosis (aqueductal gliosis), particularly if history of prematurity or meningitis
- Carefully scrutinize posterior 3rd ventricle, tectum, and tegmentum for obstructing neoplastic mass

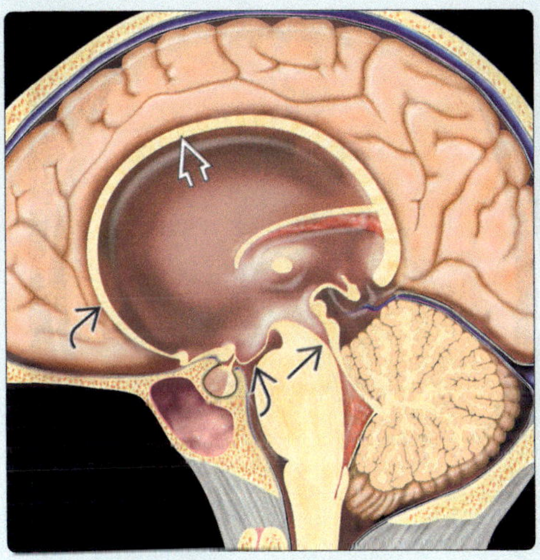

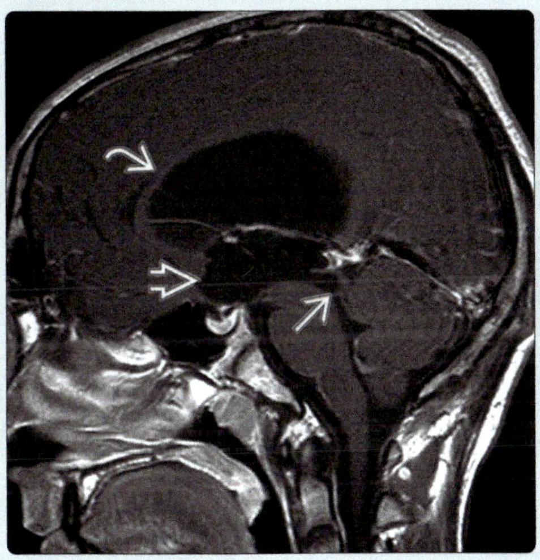

(Left) *Sagittal graphic shows obstructive hydrocephalus with markedly enlarged lateral and 3rd ventricles, stretched (thinned) corpus callosum, and a funnel-shaped cerebral aqueduct related to distal obstruction. Note the normal size of the 4th ventricle and herniation of the floor of the 3rd ventricle from the hydrocephalus.* **(Right)** *Sagittal T1WI C+ MR demonstrates aqueductal web causing dilation of the proximal cerebral aqueduct, 3rd and lateral ventricles. The 4th ventricle below the web is normal.*

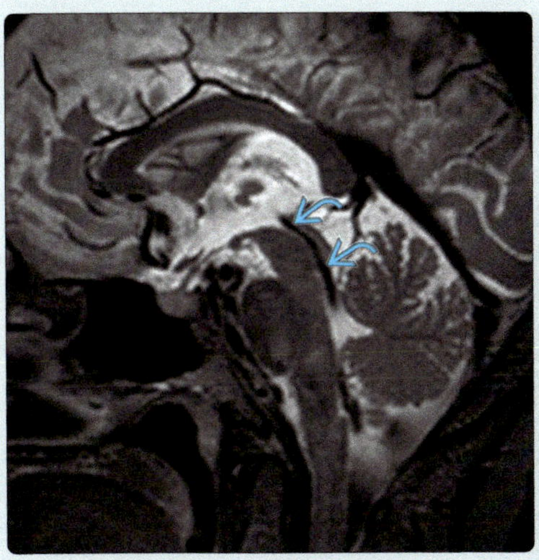

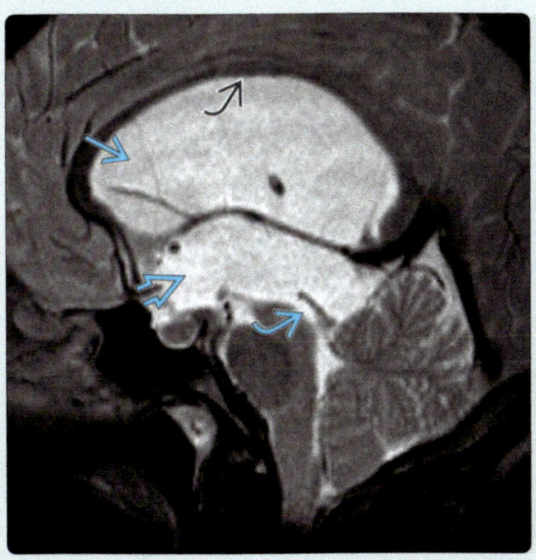

(Left) *Sagittal T2 SPACE MR demonstrates a normal aqueduct with a "flow void" due to cerebrospinal fluid flow from the 3rd ventricle into the 4th ventricle.* **(Right)** *Sagittal T2 SPACE MR demonstrates classic findings of aqueductal stenosis. There is an enlarged, funnel-shaped cerebral aqueduct and marked dilatation of the lateral and 3rd ventricles with thinning and upward bowing of the corpus callosum. Note the normal size of the 4th ventricle.*

Normal Pressure Hydrocephalus

KEY FACTS

TERMINOLOGY

- Normal pressure hydrocephalus (NPH)
- Ventriculomegaly with normal cerebrospinal fluid (CSF) pressure, altered CSF dynamics

IMAGING

- Enlarged lateral & 3rd ventricles, 4th ventricle relatively normal
- Disproportionately large ventricles compared with subarachnoid spaces (particularly sylvian fissures and basal cisterns)
  - Subarachnoid spaces over convexity may appear effaced
- Periventricular T2/FLAIR hyperintensity
- ↓ regional cerebral metabolism on F-18 FDG PET
- In-111 DTPA cisternography
  - Prominent ventricular reflux, with no flow over convexities at 24-48 hours

TOP DIFFERENTIAL DIAGNOSES

- Normal aging brain
- Other dementias (Alzheimer, multiinfarct, etc.)
- Subcortical arteriosclerotic encephalopathy

PATHOLOGY

- NPH pathogenesis poorly understood
- ↓ venous compliance in dural sinuses may impair CSF pulsations/absorption

CLINICAL ISSUES

- Heterogeneous syndrome
  - Classic triad = dementia, gait apraxia, urinary incontinence
- Test gait before/after removing CSF to check improvement

DIAGNOSTIC CHECKLIST

- Is ventricular dilation solely due to atrophy?
- Diagnostic challenge = identify shunt-responsive NPH

(Left) *Sagittal T1WI MR shows large lateral ventricles ➡, thinning of the corpus callosum ➡, and a relatively normal 4th ventricle ➡ in a patient with NPH.* **(Right)** *Axial CECT demonstrates typical findings suggestive of NPH. There is enlargement of the lateral ventricles and sylvian fissures ➡ out of proportion to the amount of general sulcal enlargement. The frontal horns show a characteristic rounded appearance. Periventricular hypodensities ➡ could reflect transependymal migration of cerebrospinal fluid.*

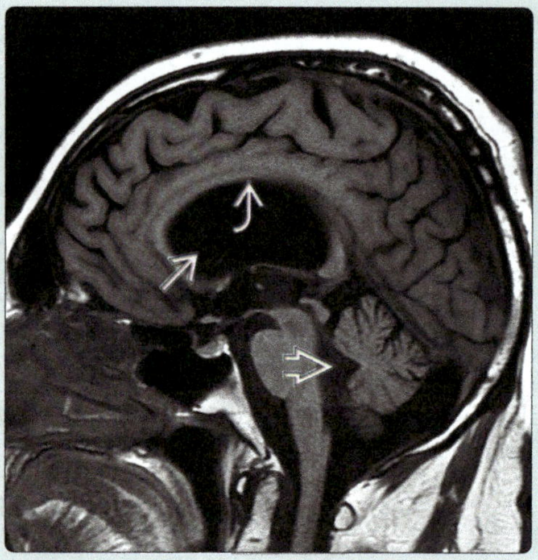

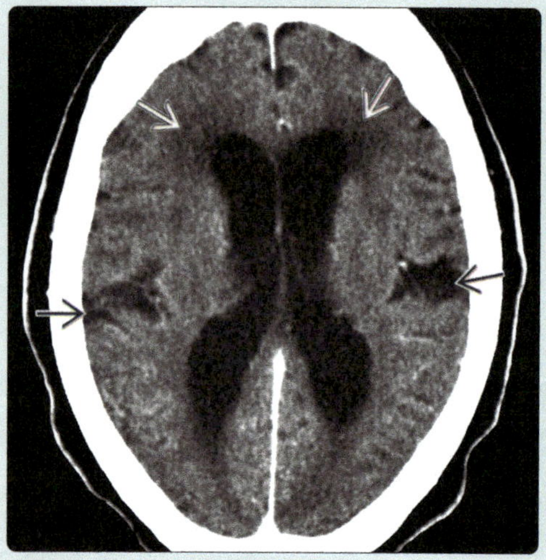

(Left) *Axial FLAIR MR shows enlarged ventricles out of proportion to the sulcal enlargement. Notice that periventricular hyperintensity is also present ➡.* **(Right)** *Axial T2WI MR in the same patient shows dilated ventricles. Normal pressure hydrocephalus accounts for ~ 5-6% of all dementias. The classic Hakim triad of dementia, gait apraxia, and urinary incontinence is present in a minority of patients.*

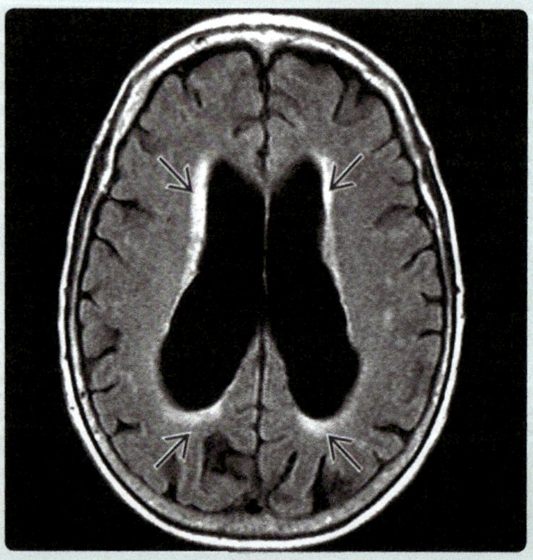

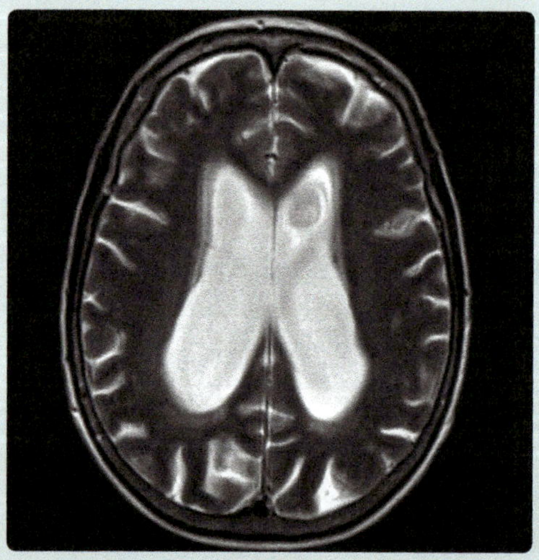

CSF Shunts and Complications

KEY FACTS

TERMINOLOGY

- Hydrocephalus
  - Enlargement of cerebral ventricles secondary to abnormal cerebrospinal fluid (CSF) formation, flow, or absorption resulting in ↑ CSF volume

IMAGING

- Shunt failure → dilated ventricles + edema around ventricles, along catheter and reservoir
- Use CT or MR to evaluate ventricle size, plain radiograph shunt series to identify mechanical shunt failure
- Baseline CT/MR following shunt insertion, follow-up at 1 year and as clinically needed
- Shunt radionuclide studies: Used to confirm distal obstruction

TOP DIFFERENTIAL DIAGNOSES

- Shunt failure with normal ventricle size or lack of interstitial edema
- Noncompliant ("slit") ventricle syndrome
- Intracranial hypotension, low pressure syndromes

PATHOLOGY

- Obstructive hydrocephalus: Secondary to physical blockage by tumor, adhesions, cyst
- Communicating hydrocephalus: Secondary to ↓ CSF absorption across arachnoid granulations

CLINICAL ISSUES

- Older children/adults: Headache, vomiting, lethargy, seizure, neurocognitive symptoms
- Infants: Bulging fontanelle, ↑ head circumference, irritability, lethargy

DIAGNOSTIC CHECKLIST

- Shunt + headache not always shunt failure
- Confirm programmable shunt valve setting after MR
- Compare current CT with prior studies to detect subtle changes in ventricle size

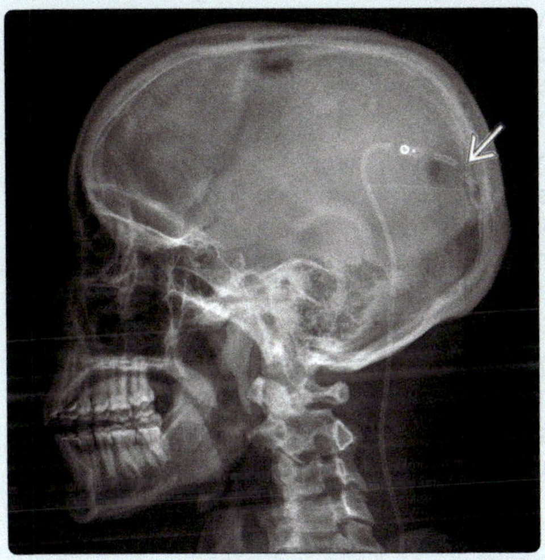
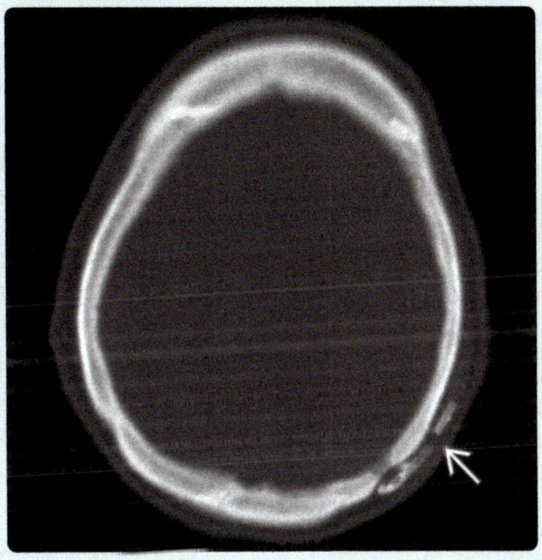

(Left) *Lateral skull radiograph of acute ventriculoperitoneal shunt failure from a plain radiograph shunt series demonstrates a mechanical shunt catheter disconnection → between the programmable valve and the reservoir.* **(Right)** *Axial bone CT in the same patient reveals the mechanical catheter disconnection → between the reservoir and the programmable shunt valve. This finding had not appeared on the most recent comparison CT scan (not shown).*

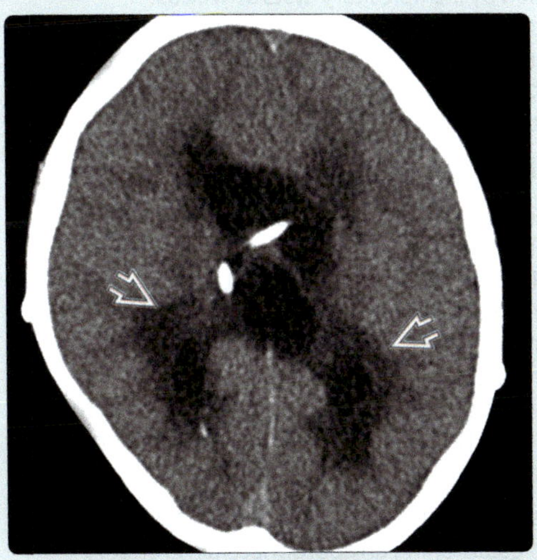
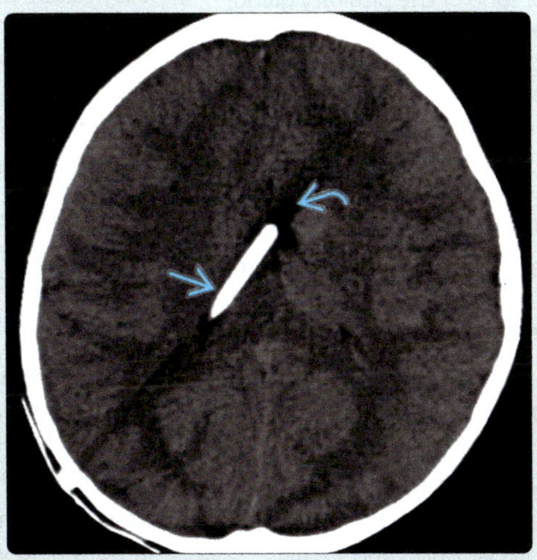

(Left) *Axial NECT in a patient with acute ventriculoperitoneal (VP) shunt failure shows symmetric periventricular interstitial edema → within the deep white matter. The ventricles were larger than on prior CTs (not shown).* **(Right)** *Axial NECT in a patient with VP shunt → who presented with severe headaches shows collapsed lateral ventricles →. Slit ventricle syndrome presents as severe headaches due to noncompliant ventricles and should not be confused with radiological slit ventricles.*

Gross Anatomy

Sella

Bony anatomy: The sella turcica ("Turkish saddle") is a concave, midline depression in the basisphenoid that contains the pituitary gland (also called the hypophysis). The anterior borders of the sella are formed by the anterior clinoid processes of the lesser sphenoid wing and the tuberculum sellae, whereas the posterior border is formed by the dorsum sellae. The top of the dorsum sellae expands to form the posterior clinoid processes, which in turn form the upper margin of the clivus. The floor of the sella is part of the sphenoid sinus roof, which is partially or completely aerated. The cavernous segments of the internal carotid artery lie in shallow grooves, called the carotid sulci, which are located inferolateral to the sella.

Meninges: The meninges in and around the sella turcica form important anatomic landmarks. Dura covers the bony floor of the sella itself. A thin dural reflection borders the pituitary fossa laterally and forms the medial cavernous sinus wall. A small circular dural shelf, the diaphragma sellae, forms a roof over the sella turcica that, in most cases, almost completely covers the pituitary gland. The diaphragma sella has a variably sized central opening that transmits the pituitary stalk. In some cases, this dural opening is large and gapes widely. In such cases, arachnoid with or without accompanying cerebrospinal fluid may protrude from the suprasellar cistern inferiorly through the diaphragma sellae opening into the sella turcica and cause the imaging appearance of an empty sella.

Pituitary Gland

Overview: The pituitary gland, also called the hypophysis cerebri, consists of 3 major parts: The adenohypophysis (AH), the neurohypophysis (NH), and the pars intermedia (PI) plus the infundibulum, which are generally considered together as a unit.

Adenohypophysis: The AH, also called the anterior lobe, wraps anterolaterally around the NH in a U-shaped configuration. The AH contains acidophil, basophil, and chromophobe cells, as well as other cells, such as tanycytes. Cells of the AH secrete trophic hormones (TSH, ACTH, LH, and FSH) as well as growth hormones. The AH forms 80% of the pituitary gland by volume.

Neurohypophysis: The NH, sometimes called the pars nervosa, consists of the posterior lobe of the pituitary gland, infundibular stem, and median eminence of the hypothalamus. The NH is formed from the embryonic diencephalon (forebrain) as a downward extension of the hypothalamus. Vasopressin and oxytocin are formed within the hypothalamus, pass inferiorly along the hypothalamohypophysial tract, and are stored in the NH. The NH comprises ~ 20% of the pituitary gland.

Pars intermedia: The PI is derived from the buccal ectoderm of the embryonic Rathke pouch. It is relatively small (< 5% of the pituitary volume). Axons from the hypothalamus carry granules of releasing hormones to the AH.

Imaging Recommendations

MR

MR is generally the imaging procedure of choice. Recommended sequences include precontrast thin-section, small field of view sagittal and coronal T1WIs and T2WIs followed by postcontrast sagittal and coronal T1WI C+ FS images. Whole-brain FLAIR is a useful sequence to add. T2*/SWI may be helpful in detecting pituitary hemorrhage. If microadenoma is suspected, dynamic imaging with coronal thin-section T1WIs obtained at 5-10-s intervals following rapid bolus injection of contrast is recommended. At least 3 sections (3 mm or less with no interslice gap), sorted by slice, are typically obtained. Some 20-30% of microadenomas are detected only on dynamic contrast-enhanced MR.

CT

Thin-section coronal CT with sagittal/coronal reconstruction may be a useful imaging adjunct when lesions affecting the sella &/or cavernous sinus arise in the basisphenoid.

Imaging Anatomy

Size: The overall height of the pituitary gland varies with both sex and age. In prepubescent children, 6 mm or less is considered normal. Physiologic hypertrophy, with a normal height of up to 10 mm, is common in young menstruating female patients. An upwardly convex gland is common in these patients. Pregnant and lactating female patients can have an even larger gland with a height of 12 mm. The upward limit of normal in men and postmenopausal women is 8 mm.

Signal intensity: Pituitary gland signal varies. With the exception of neonates (in whom the AH can be large and very hyperintense), the AH is typically isointense to gray matter on precontrast T1WIs. A dark or black pituitary gland seen on T2* is found in iron overload states (thalassemia, hemochromatosis). A uniformly white pituitary gland on T1WI is uncommon and can be seen in liver failure.

The NH usually has a short T1 (posterior pituitary "bright spot," PPBS) likely caused by vasopressin/oxytocin neurosecretory granules. The "bright spot" does not suppress with FS, as it does not contain fat. Although the absence of a PPBS is common in central diabetes insipidus, up to 20% of normally imaged patients lack a PPBS.

Enhancement: The pituitary gland does not have a blood-brain barrier, so it enhances rapidly and strongly following contrast administration. Enhancement is typically slightly less intense than that of venous blood in the adjacent cavernous sinuses.

Pituitary "incidentalomas" are common on T1WI C+ scans (found in 15-20% of cases). Seen as focal areas of hypointensity within the intensely enhancing pituitary gland, they can be caused by intrapituitary cysts as well as nonfunctioning microadenomas. Both are very common at autopsy. If a pituitary "incidentaloma" does not enhance at all, then a benign nonneoplastic cyst [such as a pars intermedia or Rathke cleft cyst (RCC)] is more likely than a microadenoma.

Differential Diagnosis Approach

Overview: Because the sellar region is anatomically very complex, at least 30 different lesions occur in and around the pituitary gland. They can arise from the pituitary gland or any adjacent structure (brain, 3rd ventricle, meninges, cavernous sinus, arteries, cranial nerves, etc.). At least 75-80% of all sellar/juxtasellar masses are in the "Big 5": Macroadenoma, meningioma, aneurysm, craniopharyngioma, and astrocytoma. All other lesions (e.g., RCC and arachnoid cysts, germinoma, lymphoma, metastasis, etc.) are each 1-2% or less.

Keys to diagnosis: Anatomic sublocation is the most important key to establishing an appropriate differential diagnosis. Initially dividing lesions into 3 categories, (1) intrasellar, (2) suprasellar, and (3) infundibular, is the 1st step.

The key to determining anatomic sublocation accurately is asking the question, "Can I find the pituitary gland separate from the mass?" If the gland **is** the mass, it is most likely a macroadenoma. Less likely pathologies that can enlarge the pituitary gland and sometimes appear indistinguishable from macroadenoma include infiltrating lesions, such as sarcoidosis, histiocytosis, hypophysitis, lymphoma, germinoma, and metastasis. If the mass can indeed be identified as separate from the pituitary gland, it is most likely not macroadenoma and arises from structures other than the hypophysis.

Clinical considerations: Patient age is an important consideration in differential diagnosis. Lesions that are common in children (craniopharyngioma and astrocytoma of the optic chiasm/hypothalamus) are less common in adults, in whom the most common masses are macroadenoma, meningioma, and aneurysm. Macroadenomas are very common in adults but, with the exception of adolescent girls, are quite rare in children. Beware: A lesion in a prepubescent boy that looks like a macroadenoma usually isn't; it is more often nonphysiologic nonneoplastic hyperplasia from end-organ failure.

Imaging appearance: Imaging appearance can be very helpful in evaluating a sellar/juxtasellar lesion. Is the lesion calcified? Does it appear cystic? Does it contain blood products? Is it focal or infiltrating? Does it enhance?

Intrasellar Lesions

Empty sella: Empty sella is seen in 5-10% of patients as an intrasellar CSF collection that flattens the pituitary gland against the sellar floor. Other than empty sella, most intrasellar masses are lesions of the pituitary gland itself.

Pituitary hyperplasia: Diffuse pituitary enlargement or hyperplasia is common and can be physiologic in young menstruating female patients and postpartum/lactating female patients. Less commonly, pituitary hyperplasia occurs as a result of end-organ failure, such as hypothyroidism. Rarely, intracranial hypotension and dural arteriovenous fistulas cause pituitary enlargement, probably due to passive venous congestion.

Macro- and microadenomas: The most common "real" intrasellar masses are pituitary microadenomas (defined as < 10 mm) and macroadenomas. Macroadenomas may extend superiorly through the diaphragma sella, opening into the suprasellar compartment. Occasionally macroadenomas can appear very aggressive and extremely invasive, extending into the cavernous sinus and eroding the skull base. Pituitary carcinoma is exceptionally rare, typically diagnosed at the time of metastatic spread.

Miscellaneous lesions: A number of neoplastic and nonneoplastic processes can infiltrate the pituitary gland and adjacent structures, such as neurosarcoid, lymphoma, and metastases.

Suprasellar Lesions

Children vs. adults: Once a lesion is defined as suprasellar, patient age is key to the differential diagnosis. Pediatric suprasellar masses are most often either craniopharyngiomas or pilocytic astrocytomas (hypothalamus, optic chiasm). All other lesions, such as germinoma and histiocytosis, are much less common.

At least 1/2 of all suprasellar masses in adults are upward extensions of macroadenomas through the diaphragma sella. Macroadenomas are typically heterogeneously enhancing masses that may contain cysts or blood products. Macroadenomas often enlarge or remodel the sella turcica. Meningioma and aneurysm are common in adults, accounting for ~ 10% each of all adult suprasellar masses. Both are rare in children. Meningiomas are homogeneously enhancing masses, separate from the pituitary gland. Aneurysms may be identified on MR by a flow void or pulsation artifact. If thrombosed, an aneurysm may have a laminated appearance. CTA or MRA may be helpful in further characterizing a sellar region aneurysm.

Imaging appearance: Cystic-appearing suprasellar masses are often nonneoplastic [enlarged 3rd ventricle, RCC, suprasellar arachnoid cyst, and inflammatory cysts, such as neurocysticercosis (NCC)]. RCCs may be intrasellar (40%) or suprasellar (60%). RCCs may be asymptomatic or present with pituitary dysfunction, visual changes, or headache. RCCs are noncalcified, nonenhancing, cystic lesions on CT and MR. A helpful clue on MR is the presence of an intracystic nodule. Craniopharyngioma is the most common suprasellar mass in a child and is often known as the 90% tumor; 90% are cystic, 90% are calcified, and 90% enhance. With the exception of craniopharyngioma, cystic-appearing neoplasms are rare in this location. Pilocytic astrocytoma is the overall most common pediatric glial neoplasm in this area. Pilocytic astrocytomas of the optic chiasm/hypothalamus are solid, not cystic (as they often are when they occur in the posterior fossa).

The presence of calcification is helpful. In older patients, atherosclerosis (cavernous and supraclinoid internal carotid arteries), saccular aneurysm, and meningioma are common lesions that calcify. In children, a calcified suprasellar mass is most often a craniopharyngioma. NCC can calcify and may be found in both children and adults, but the suprasellar cistern is a rare location for NCC cysts.

Hemorrhage into a sellar/suprasellar mass can be detected with T2* imaging or SWI. Hemorrhagic macroadenoma, pituitary apoplexy, and thrombosed aneurysm can show "blooming." The pilomyxoid variant of pilocytic astrocytoma is a rare but important cause of a hemorrhagic suprasellar mass in a child or young adult.

Infundibular Stalk Lesions

Infundibular stalk lesions are a distinct differential diagnosis. The normal infundibular stalk should be 2 mm or less in transverse diameter and taper gradually from top to bottom.

A "thick stalk" in a child is usually histiocytosis or germinoma. In an adult, neurosarcoid, lymphocytic hypophysitis, lymphoma, and metastasis are more common. Lesions of the infundibulum often present with diabetes insipidus. Enhancement is often unhelpful, as the normal infundibulum lacks a blood-brain barrier and enhances intensely following contrast administration. Neurosarcoid may affect the infundibulum only and appear as a thickened, enhancing stalk but more commonly presents with other CNS lesions. Hypophysitis may be related to an autoimmune inflammatory disorder, granulomatous disease, IgG4 related, or drug related. A recent cancer immunotherapy (ipilimumab) has been associated with lymphocytic hypophysitis, which may affect the gland &/or only the infundibulum.

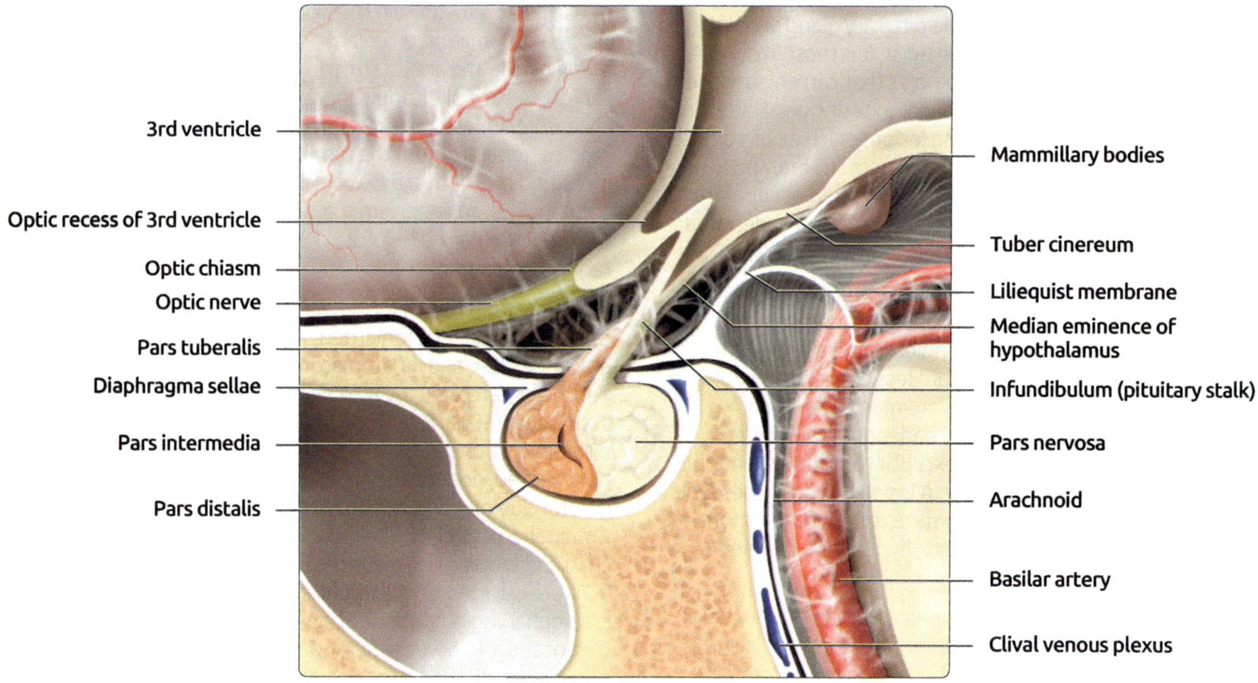

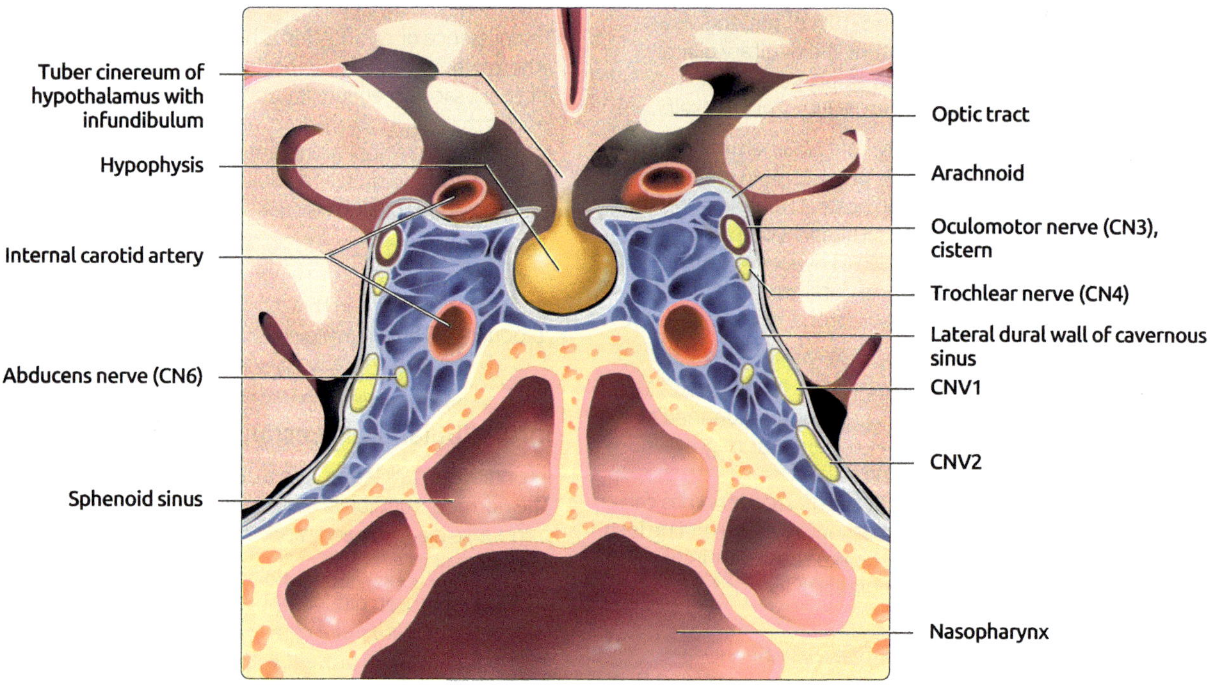

(Top) *Lateral graphic of a normal pituitary shows the adenohypophysis composed of the pars tuberalis, pars intermedia, and pars distalis. The neurohypophysis is composed of the median eminence of the hypothalamus, infundibulum, and pars nervosa. Periosteal dural layer covers the sellar floor.* **(Bottom)** *Coronal graphic depicts the cavernous sinus contents. The cranial nerves that traverse the cavernous sinus within the lateral wall, from superior to inferior, are oculomotor (CN3), trochlear (CN4), and the 1st (ophthalmic or V1) and 2nd (maxillary or V2) divisions of trigeminal (CN5) nerves. The only cranial nerve actually within the venous sinusoids of the cavernous sinus is the abducens nerve (CN6). The abducens nerve is often the 1st cranial nerve affected by a cavernous carotid artery aneurysm.*

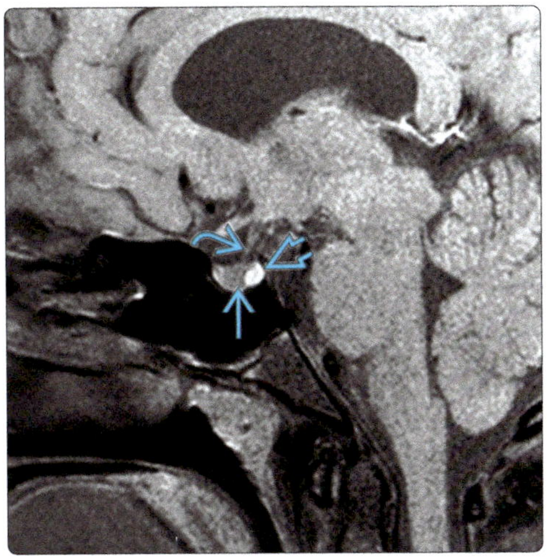

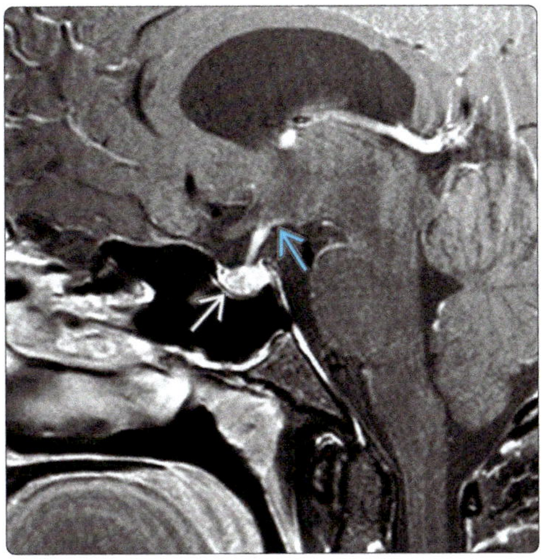

(Left) *Sagittal 3T T1WI with FS MR shows that the normal adenohypophysis is isointense with gray matter; the posterior pituitary is hyperintense. This posterior pituitary "bright spot" does not suppress on FS sequences. Note the gradual top-to-bottom tapering of the infundibulum.* **(Right)** *Sagittal T1 C+ FS MR in the same patient shows intense, slightly inhomogeneous enhancement of the pituitary gland. The stalk enhances, as does the tuber cinereum of the hypothalamus, anterior to the mammillary bodies.*

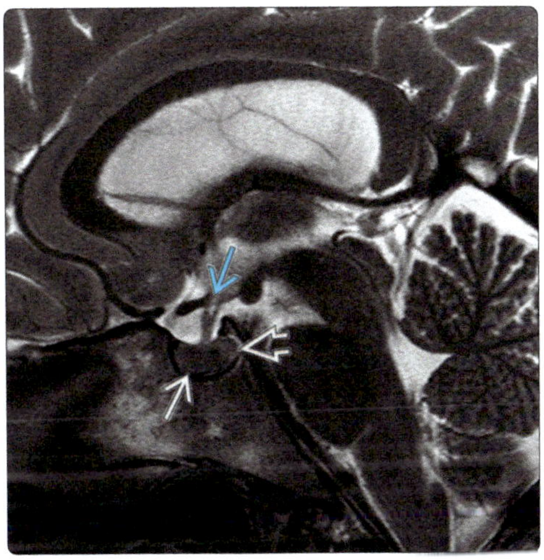

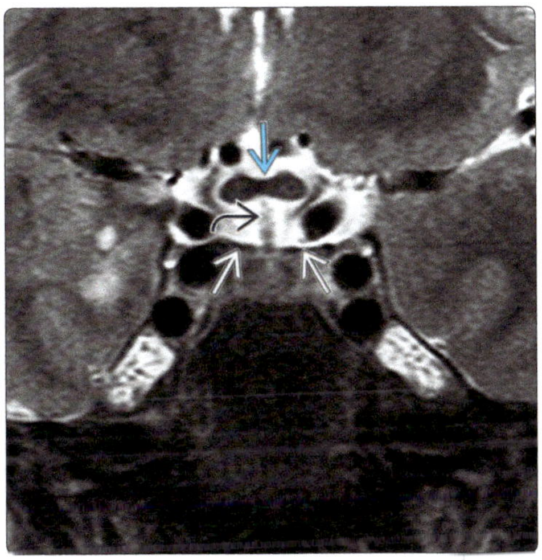

(Left) *Sagittal T2WI MR shows the adenohypophysis (AH) is isointense with brain. The neurohypophysis is slightly hyperintense compared with the AH. Note the infundibular recess of the 3rd ventricle.* **(Right)** *Coronal T2WI MR shows the infundibular stalk passing inferiorly through a small discontinuity in the thin shelf of dura, the diaphragma sellae, seen here as thin black lines forming the roof of the pituitary fossa. The optic chiasm is present superiorly within the suprasellar cistern and is often affected by suprasellar masses.*

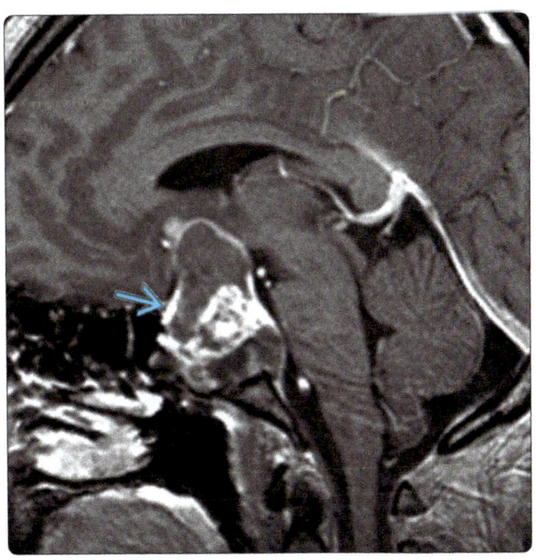

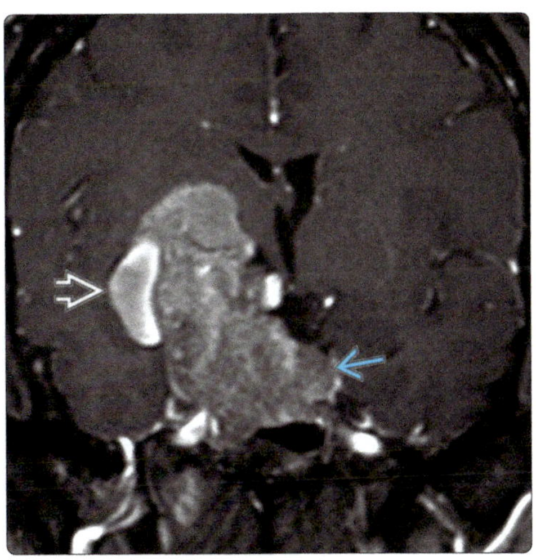

(Left) *Sagittal T1 C+ MR in a child shows a complex, cystic, and solid sellar and suprasellar mass related to an adamantinomatous craniopharyngioma. These masses represent > 50% of pediatric suprasellar neoplasms.* **(Right)** *Coronal T1 C+ MR in an adult with visual symptoms shows a complex sellar and suprasellar macroadenoma with regions of hemorrhage. Macroadenomas are among the most common of all CNS neoplasms, accounting for 10-15% of primary intracranial neoplasms.*

Pituitary Anomalies

KEY FACTS

TERMINOLOGY

- Congenital anomalies of pituitary stalk → potential hypothalamic/pituitary axis malfunction

IMAGING

- Posterior pituitary ectopia (PPE)
- Duplicated pituitary gland/stalk (DP)
- PPE: No (or tiny) pituitary stalk, ectopic posterior pituitary on midline sagittal T1WI MR
  - Look for associated anomalies: Heterotopia, optic nerve hypoplasia, corpus callosum anomalies
- DP: 2 pituitary stalks on coronal view, thick tuber cinereum on midline sagittal view

TOP DIFFERENTIAL DIAGNOSES

- PPE
  - Surgical or traumatic stalk transection
  - Central diabetes insipidus
  - Hypothalamic lipoma (in tuber cinereum)
- DP
  - Dilated infundibular recess of 3rd ventricle ("pseudoduplication")
  - Tuber cinereum hamartoma

PATHOLOGY

- PPE: Genetic mutation → defective neuronal migration during embryogenesis
- DP: Genetic mutation unknown; may constitute polytopic field defect due to splitting of notochord

CLINICAL ISSUES

- PPE: Short stature
- DP: Unsuspected finding on craniofacial imaging for other indications

DIAGNOSTIC CHECKLIST

- PPE: Assess optic and olfactory nerves, frontal cortex
- DP: Oral tumors compromise airway patency

(Left) *Sagittal graphic demonstrates ectopia of the posterior pituitary gland located at the distal end of a truncated pituitary stalk along the median eminence of the hypothalamus. The sella turcica and adenohypophysis are both small.* **(Right)** *Sagittal T1WI MR shows an ectopic posterior pituitary gland located at the median eminence. The pituitary infundibulum is absent, the anterior pituitary gland is small, and the normal bright posterior pituitary gland is not identified in its typical location.*

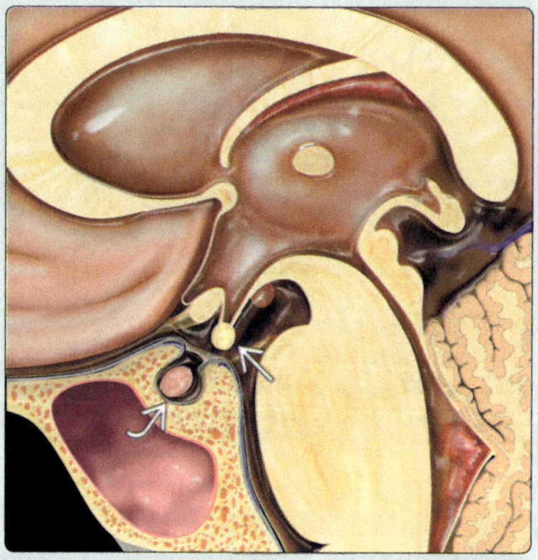

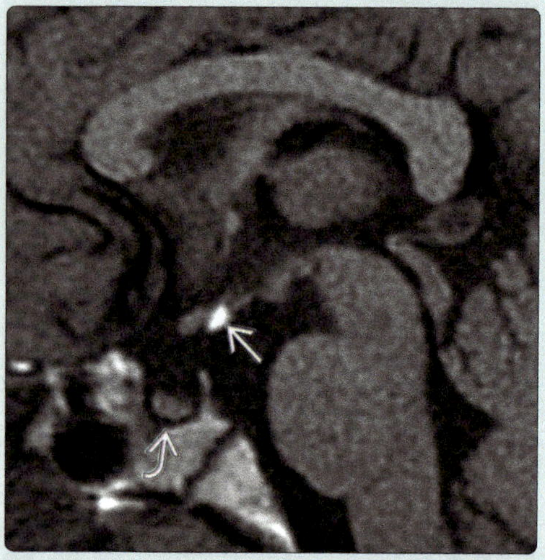

(Left) *Coronal T1WI MR depicts the ectopic posterior pituitary gland location at the median eminence. A pituitary stalk is not visualized below the ectopic posterior pituitary. The septum pellucidum is present, and the optic tracts are of normal size.* **(Right)** *Sagittal T2 MR in a patient with complete absence of the posterior pituitary bright spot shows a small sella turcica and pituitary gland. The optic apparatus is also hypoplastic. A clearly defined pituitary stalk is present.*

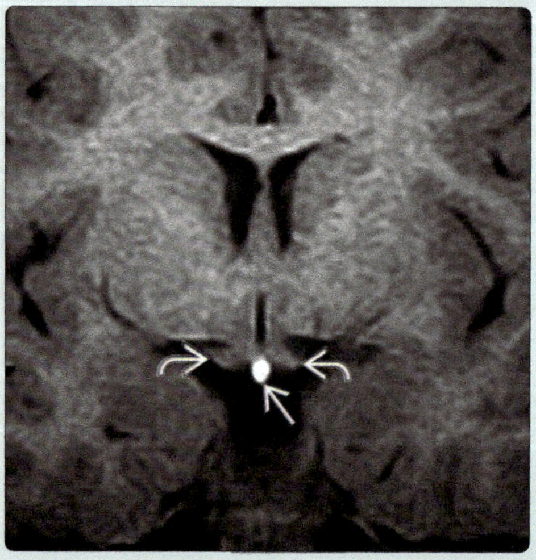

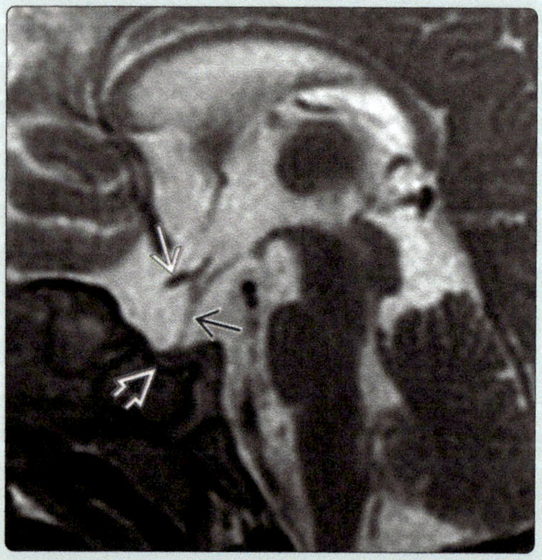

Pituitary Microadenoma

KEY FACTS

TERMINOLOGY

- Microadenoma: ≤ 10 mm in diameter

IMAGING

- Intrasellar mass is typical location
  - Rare: Ectopic origin outside pituitary fossa
- Best technique = dynamic contrast-enhanced thin-section T1-weighted MR
  - Generally enhance more slowly than adjacent normal pituitary
  - Beware: 10-30% can be seen only on dynamic contrast-enhanced scans
  - Occasionally, adenoma may be cystic or hemorrhagic
- Intrapituitary "filling defect" may be benign nonneoplastic cyst, as well as incidental microadenoma

TOP DIFFERENTIAL DIAGNOSES

- Rathke cleft cyst
- Craniopharyngioma
- Pituitary hyperplasia
- Other nonneoplastic cyst (e.g., pars intermedia cyst)

PATHOLOGY

- Adenomas are almost always WHO grade I
  - Pituitary carcinoma exceedingly rare (diagnosed when metastatic disease identified)
- Can occur as part of multiple endocrine neoplasia type 1, Carney complex, or McCune-Albright syndrome

CLINICAL ISSUES

- Symptoms of secreting tumors vary according to type
  - Prolactinoma is most common functional adenoma
  - Asymptomatic/nonfunctioning adenoma most common
- ~ 20-25% incidental finding at autopsy
- Medical therapy (bromocriptine, cabergoline) reduces prolactin secretion to normal in 80%
- Surgical (transsphenoidal) curative in 60-90%

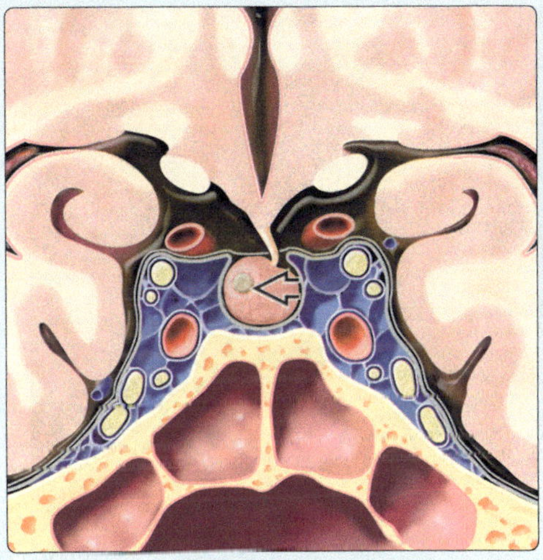

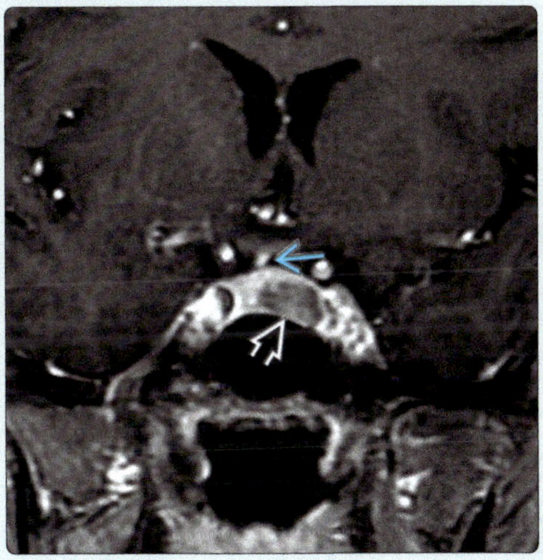

(Left) *Coronal graphic shows a small microadenoma that slightly enlarges the right side of the pituitary gland and deviates the infundibulum toward the left.* **(Right)** *Coronal T1 C+ MR in a 41-year-old woman with amenorrhea and elevated prolactin levels shows a mass in the left pituitary gland with displacement of the infundibulum to the right. Prolactin-secreting microadenoma was found at resection. The microadenoma enhances less than the normal pituitary gland.*

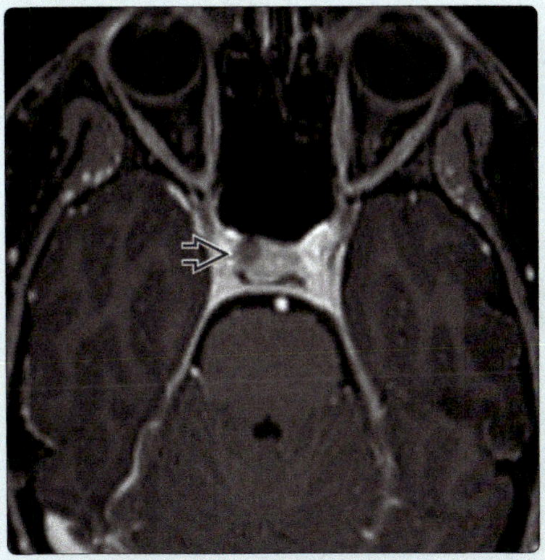

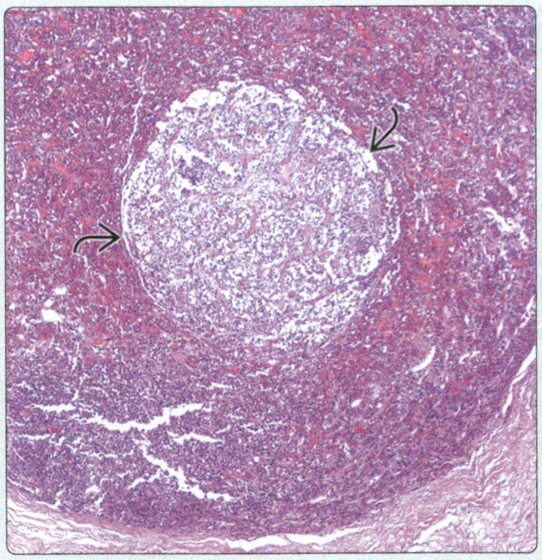

(Left) *Axial T1 C+ MR in a 31-year-old woman with elevated prolactin shows a discrete mass related to a microadenoma in the anterior right pituitary gland. Prolactinomas are typically located laterally within the adenohypophysis, as the prolactin secreting cells are present laterally within the normal gland.* **(Right)** *Coronal microscopic image shows a normal pituitary gland surrounding a small nonfunctioning microadenoma that was found incidentally at autopsy. (Courtesy J. Townsend, MD.)*

Pituitary Macroadenoma

KEY FACTS

TERMINOLOGY

- Benign neoplasm of adenohypophysis

IMAGING

- Upward extension of macroadenoma = most common suprasellar mass in adults
- Best imaging technique
  - MR with sagittal/coronal thin-section imaging through sella + T1 C+ with FS
- Sellar mass without separate identifiable pituitary gland = macroadenoma
- Mass **is** pituitary gland
- Usually isointense with gray matter
- Enhance strongly, often heterogeneously
- Cavernous sinus invasion difficult to determine

TOP DIFFERENTIAL DIAGNOSES

- Pituitary hyperplasia
- Saccular aneurysm
- Meningioma (diaphragma sellae)
- Metastasis
- Lymphocytic hypophysitis
- Craniopharyngioma

PATHOLOGY

- WHO grade I
- MIB-1 > 1% suggests early recurrence, rapid regrowth
- Invasive adenoma > > pituitary carcinoma (rare)

CLINICAL ISSUES

- Beware: Adenoma-like mass in adolescent/prepubescent boys may represent hyperplasia secondary to end-organ failure
- Prolactin-secreting adenoma is most common functional adenoma

DIAGNOSTIC CHECKLIST

- No matter how aggressive/invasive it looks, pituitary tumors are almost never malignant

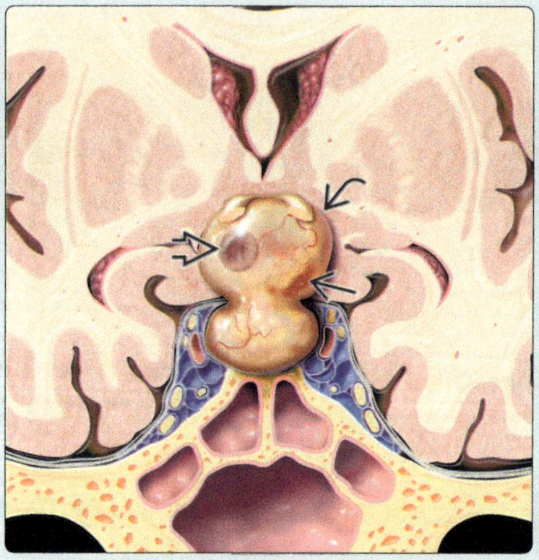
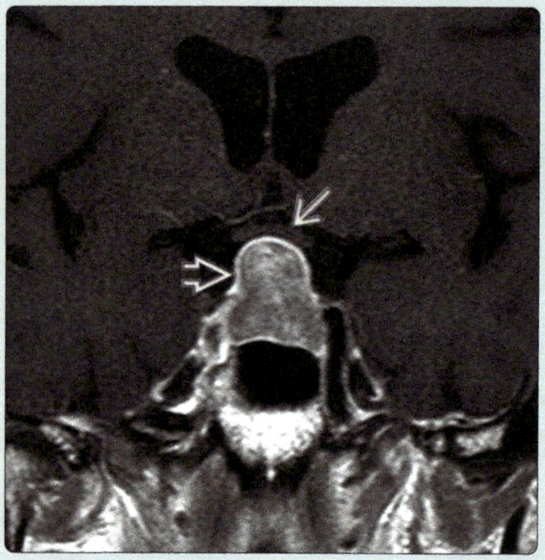

(Left) *Coronal graphic shows a snowman-shaped or "figure 8" sellar/suprasellar mass ➔. Small foci of hemorrhage ➔ and cystic change ➔ are present within the lesion. The pituitary gland cannot be identified separate from the mass; indeed, the gland is the mass.* **(Right)** *T1 C+ MR in a 68-year-old man with elevated prolactin shows a classic "figure 8" or "snowman" appearance of the pituitary macroadenoma ➔. There is mild displacement of the optic chiasm ➔. The pituitary gland cannot be separated from the mass.*

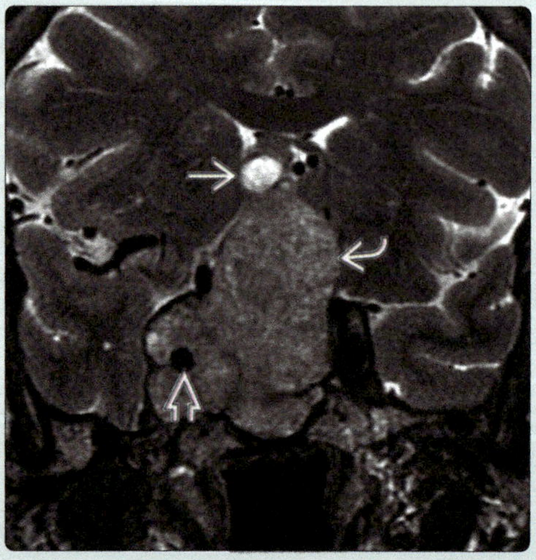
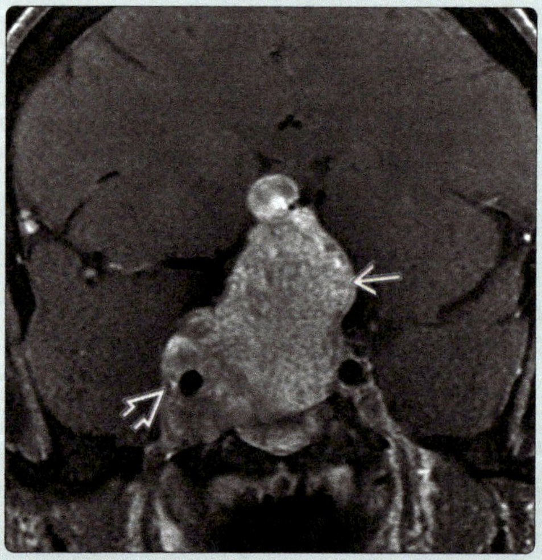

(Left) *Coronal T2 MR in a 64-year-old woman with visual changes shows a large adenoma ➔ with cystic change ➔ filling the sella and suprasellar region. Note the patent cavernous carotid artery ➔.* **(Right)** *Coronal T1 C+ MR in same patient shows heterogeneous enhancement ➔ of the macroadenoma. There is tumor lateral to the cavernous carotid artery representing cavernous sinus invasion ➔ and nonfunctional adenoma found at resection. The cavernous sinus disease was treated with radiation therapy.*

Pituitary Apoplexy

KEY FACTS

TERMINOLOGY

- Acute clinical syndrome with headache, visual defects/ophthalmoplegia, altered mental status, variable endocrine deficiencies
- Caused by either hemorrhage or infarction of pituitary gland
- Preexisting pituitary macroadenoma common

IMAGING

- CT
  - Sellar/suprasellar mass with patchy or confluent hyperdensity
  - Peripheral enhancement, ± hemorrhage
  - May be associated with subarachnoid hemorrhage
- MR
  - Enlarged, hypointense (hemorrhagic), or hyperintense (nonhemorrhagic) pituitary on T2WI
  - T2* (SWI/GRE) "blooming" (best sequence if blood products present)
  - Restricted diffusion within adenoma may be early sign of apoplexy
- Associated findings
  - Adjacent dural thickening, enhancement in 50%
  - Thickening of sphenoid sinus mucosa in 80%

TOP DIFFERENTIAL DIAGNOSES

- Pituitary macroadenoma (nonhemorrhagic)
- Craniopharyngioma
- Rathke cleft cyst
- Lymphocytic hypophysitis
- Giant thrombosed intrasellar aneurysm
- Pituitary abscess
- Primary intrapituitary hemorrhage

DIAGNOSTIC CHECKLIST

- Rim enhancement or fluid level in snowman-shaped sellar/suprasellar mass may represent pituitary apoplexy

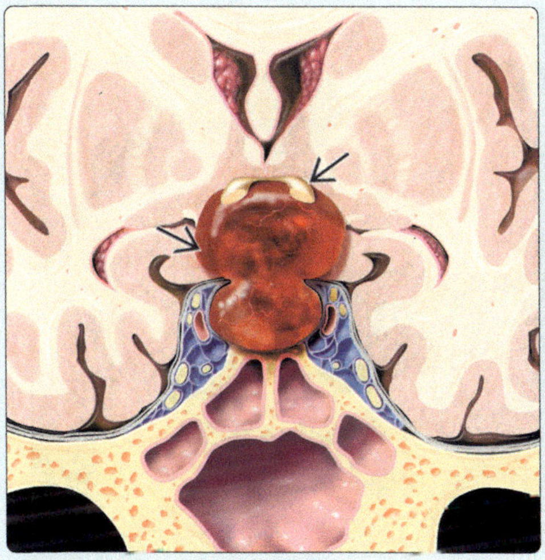

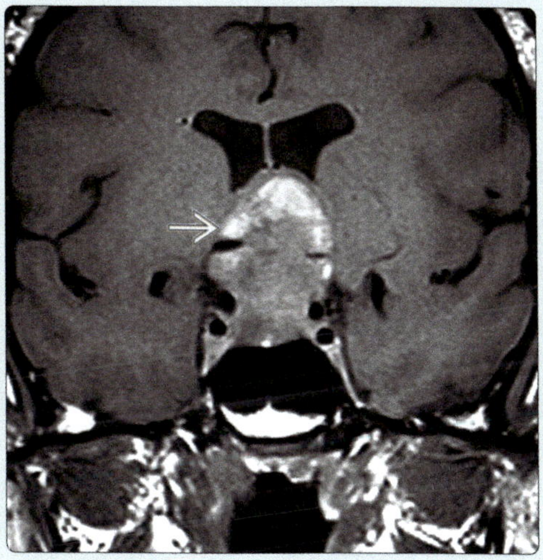

(Left) *Coronal graphic shows a macroadenoma with acute hemorrhage → causing pituitary apoplexy. Superior displacement of the optic chiasm is common.* **(Right)** *Coronal T1 MR shows a hemorrhagic sellar and suprasellar macroadenoma in a 58-year-old woman with acute onset of headache and ophthalmoplegia. Note the T1 shortening → in the superior aspect of the macroadenoma related to subacute blood products.*

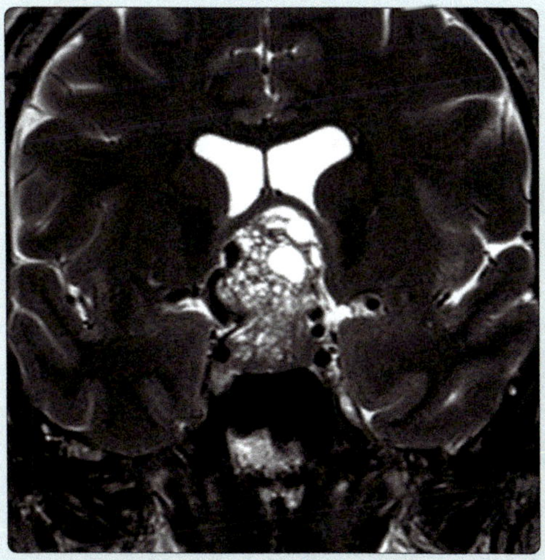

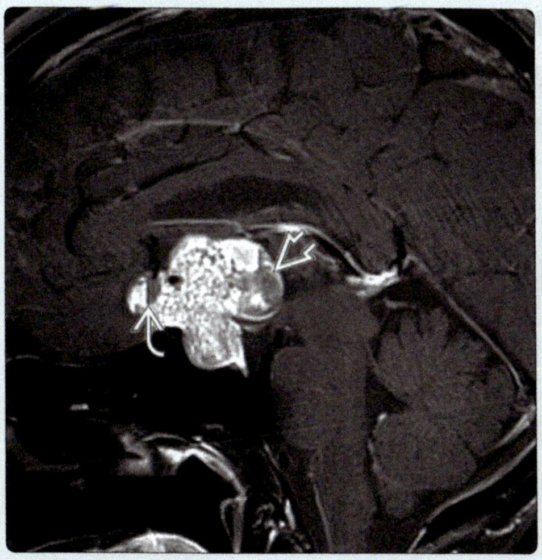

(Left) *Coronal T2 MR in the same patient shows heterogeneous signal throughout the sellar and suprasellar mass, typical of pituitary apoplexy.* **(Right)** *Sagittal T1 C+ FS MR in the same patient shows heterogeneous enhancement of the mass with a blood-fluid level → and regions of nonenhancement → related to necrotic adenoma. A necrotic, hemorrhagic, nonfunctional adenoma was found at surgery. A preexisting macroadenoma is present in the vast majority of patients with pituitary apoplexy.*

Rathke Cleft Cyst

KEY FACTS

TERMINOLOGY

- Nonneoplastic cyst arising from remnants of embryonic Rathke cleft
- Benign sellar region endodermal cyst lined by ciliated, mucus-producing epithelium

IMAGING

- Nonenhancing, noncalcified, intrasellar &/or suprasellar cyst with intracystic nodule
  - Completely intrasellar (40%), suprasellar extension (60%)
  - Density/signal intensity varies with cyst content (serous vs. mucoid)
- Most symptomatic Rathke cleft cysts (RCCs): 5-15 mm in diameter
- Occasionally, RCCs can become very large
- Claw sign = enhancing rim of compressed pituitary surrounding nonenhancing cyst
- No internal enhancement

TOP DIFFERENTIAL DIAGNOSES

- Craniopharyngioma
- Cystic pituitary adenoma
- Arachnoid cyst
- Other nonneoplastic cyst (pars intermedia, colloid cyst)

CLINICAL ISSUES

- Most are asymptomatic, found incidentally at imaging or autopsy
- Common presenting features when symptomatic: Headache, pituitary dysfunction, visual changes
- Rare but important: Apoplexy, cavernous sinus syndrome
  - Can be indistinguishable from pituitary apoplexy
- Conservative management if asymptomatic
  - Have been reported to resolve without therapy
- Surgical aspiration, partial excision, or resection if symptomatic
  - Recurrence rates in up to 18% of patients

(Left) *Coronal graphic shows a typical suprasellar Rathke cleft cyst interposed between the pituitary gland → and the optic chiasm →.* **(Right)** *Sagittal T1WI MR in a 32-year-old woman with amenorrhea shows a hyperintense mass within the pituitary gland → anterior to the normal T1-hyperintense neurohypophysis →. Imaging mimics a hemorrhagic pituitary microadenoma. Rathke cleft cyst was found at resection. Small Rathke cleft cysts are most commonly asymptomatic and may be managed conservatively.*

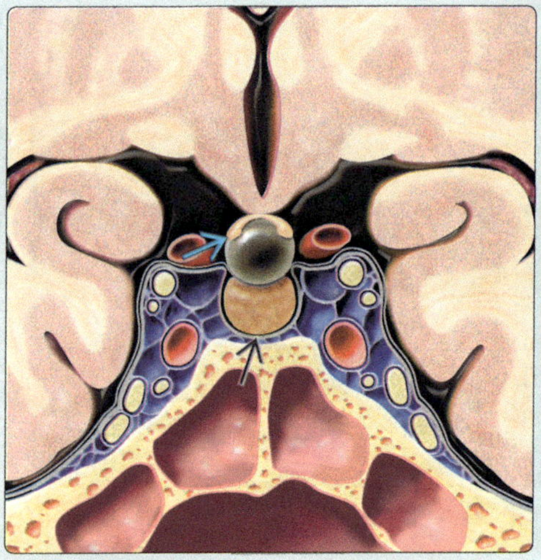

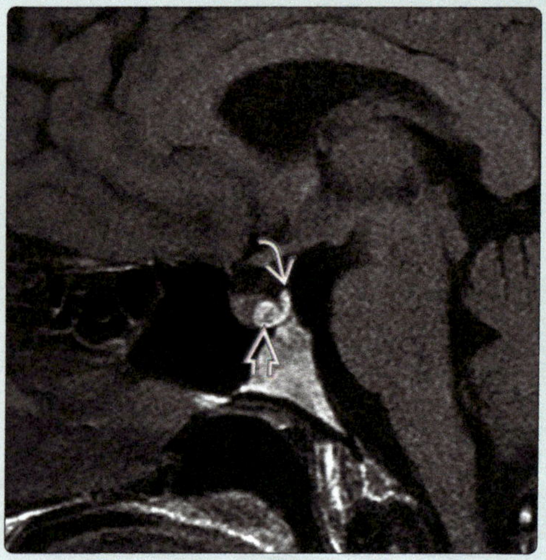

(Left) *Coronal T1WI C+ MR in a 62-year-old woman with headaches shows a cystic suprasellar mass → with mild peripheral enhancement, the so-called claw sign → related to compression of the adjacent residual pituitary gland by the Rathke cleft cyst. Note the lack of enhancement within the cyst.* **(Right)** *Coronal T2WI MR in the same patient shows a hyperintense cyst with a hypointense intracystic nodule →. An intracystic nodule may be seen in up to 75% of Rathke cleft cysts and is a helpful clue to the correct diagnosis.*

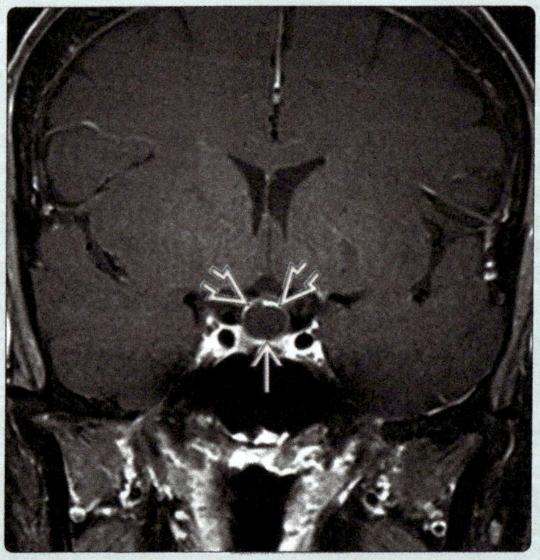

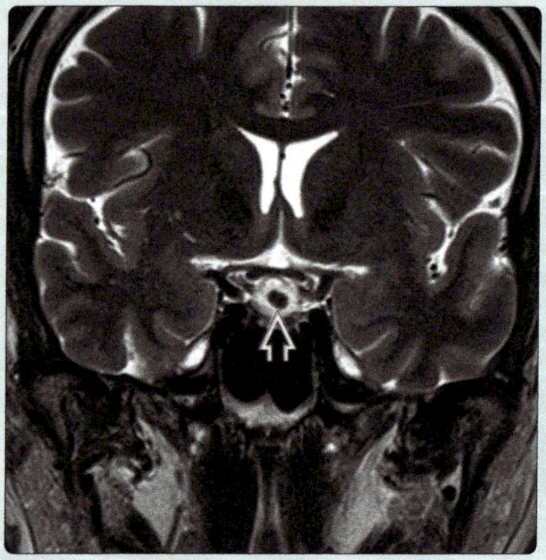

KEY FACTS

TERMINOLOGY

- Benign, often partially cystic sellar region tumor derived from Rathke pouch epithelium
- 2 types
  - Adamantinomatous (cystic mass in childhood)
  - Papillary (solid mass in older adults)

IMAGING

- General features
  - Multilobulated, often large (> 5 cm)
  - Occasionally giant, multicompartmental
- CT
  - Cystic (90%), Ca++ (90%), enhancing (90%)
- MR: Signal varies with cyst contents
  - Cysts variably hyperintense on T1WI and T2WI
  - Solid portions enhance heterogeneously; cyst walls enhance strongly
  - Cyst contents show broad lipid peak (0.9-1.5 ppm) on MR spectroscopy

PATHOLOGY

- Most common pediatric intracranial tumor of nonglial origin
- WHO grade I
- Craniopharyngiomas arise from remnants of craniopharyngeal duct

CLINICAL ISSUES

- Bimodal age distribution
  - Peak 5-15 years; papillary craniopharyngioma > 50 years
- Pediatric patient with morning headache, visual defect, short stature
  - Endocrine disturbances include growth hormone deficiency
  - Others = hypothyroidism > adrenal failure > diabetes insipidus
- Surgical resection is primary therapy
- Surgery, radiation therapy, or cyst aspiration for recurrent tumors

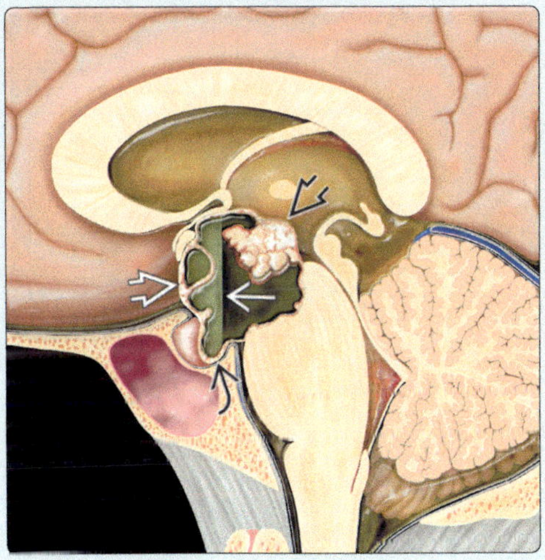
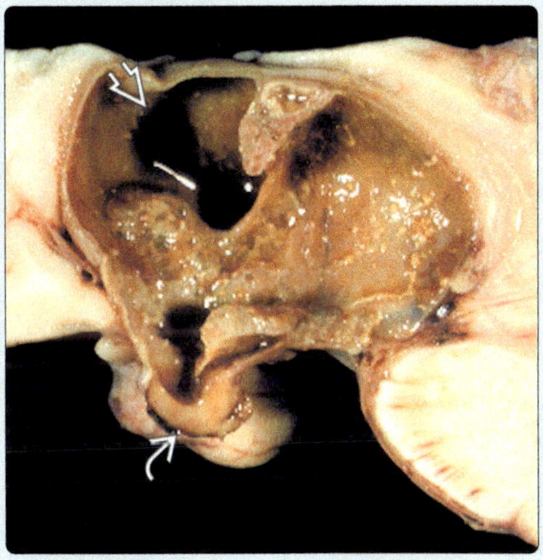

(Left) *Sagittal graphic shows a predominantly cystic, partially solid suprasellar mass with focal rim calcifications. Note the small intrasellar component and fluid-fluid level. Craniopharyngiomas are the 90% tumors (90% cystic, 90% calcified, and 90% enhancing).* **(Right)** *Sagittal gross pathology shows classic adamantinomatous craniopharyngioma with mixed solid, cystic components. The classic machine or "crank case oil" is present. Note the intrasellar extension. (Courtesy R. Hewlett, MD.)*

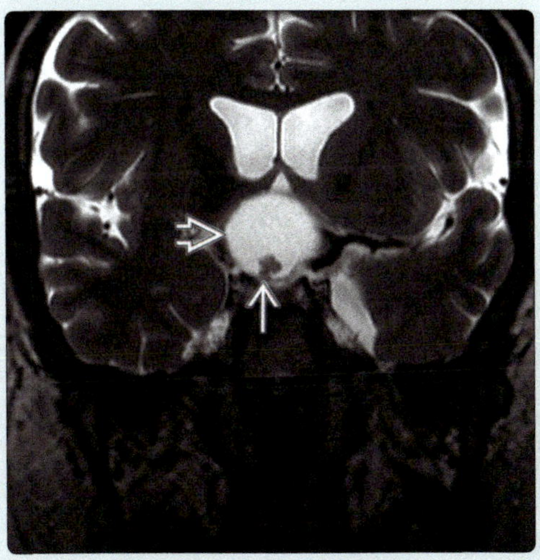
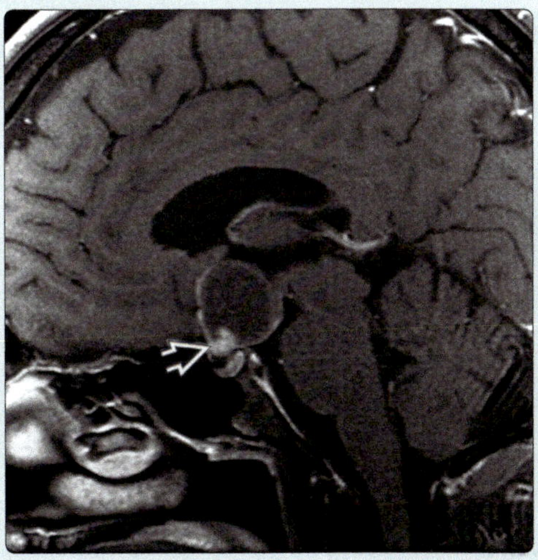

(Left) *T2 MR in a 48-year-old man who presented with visual changes shows a cystic suprasellar mass with a focal T2-hypointense nodule. The T2 imaging mimics a Rathke cleft cyst.* **(Right)** *Sagittal T1 C+ MR in the same patient shows the enhancing nodule, which distinguishes this cystic lesion as a craniopharyngioma, not a Rathke cleft cyst. Surgical resection is the primary therapy for this WHO grade I neoplasm. However, the recurrence rate at 10 years approaches 20%.*

KEY FACTS

TERMINOLOGY

- Sella partially filled with arachnoid-lined cerebrospinal fluid (CSF) collection
- Primary empty sella
    - Common normal, incidental finding (15% of brain MRs)
    - Can be normal variant
    - Normal or increased CSF pressure
    - Near normal volume of compressed pituitary tissue
- Secondary empty sella
    - Prior pituitary surgery, radiation, or injury

IMAGING

- Intrasellar CSF, pituitary flattened against sellar floor
    - Bony sella may be normal or moderately enlarged (secondary to pulsatile CSF)
    - Bony margins intact, not eroded/demineralized
    - Infundibular stalk, pituitary gland enhance normally
- Fluid exactly like CSF
    - Suppresses completely on FLAIR
    - Does not restrict on DWI

TOP DIFFERENTIAL DIAGNOSES

- Idiopathic intracranial hypertension
- Secondary intracranial hypertension
- Arachnoid cyst
- Pituitary apoplexy

PATHOLOGY

- "Deficient" diaphragma sellae
    - Dural covering of sella is incomplete (widened)
    - Leaves large opening for infundibular stalk
    - Allows intrasellar herniation of arachnoid with CSF from suprasellar subarachnoid cistern above

CLINICAL ISSUES

- Mostly incidental, asymptomatic (adults); F:M = 5:1
- Headache, visual disturbances if related to intracranial hypertension
- Frequent endocrine abnormalities in children

(Left) *Sagittal graphic shows an empty sella. The extension of arachnoid with cerebrospinal fluid (CSF) through the diaphragma sellae ➡ flattens and displaces the pituitary gland ⇨ posteroinferiorly against the sellar floor.* **(Right)** *Axial gross pathology shows a primary empty sella found incidentally at autopsy. Note the wide opening of the diaphragma sellae ⇨ and CSF ↷ largely filling the bony sella. (Courtesy M. Sage, MD.)*

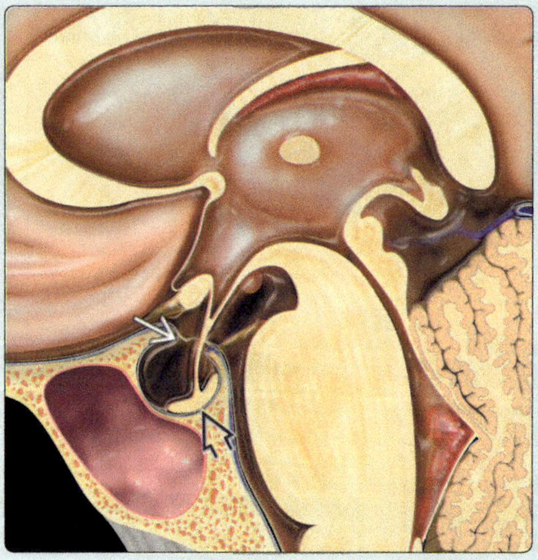

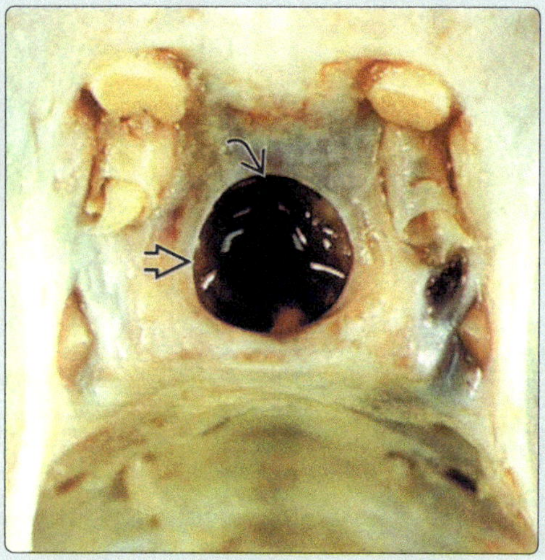

(Left) *Sagittal T1WI MR shows a 40-year-old man with incidentally found partially empty sella. No endocrine laboratory abnormalities are seen. Notice enlarged bony sella with thin rim of pituitary tissue ⇨.* **(Right)** *This T2WI MR was taken from the same patient with incidental partially empty sella. The bony sella is expanded and filled with CSF ➡. A normal pituitary infundibulum ↷ is present in the midline.*

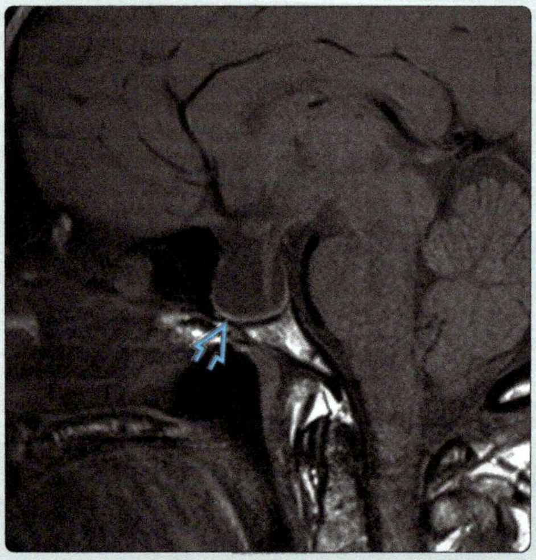

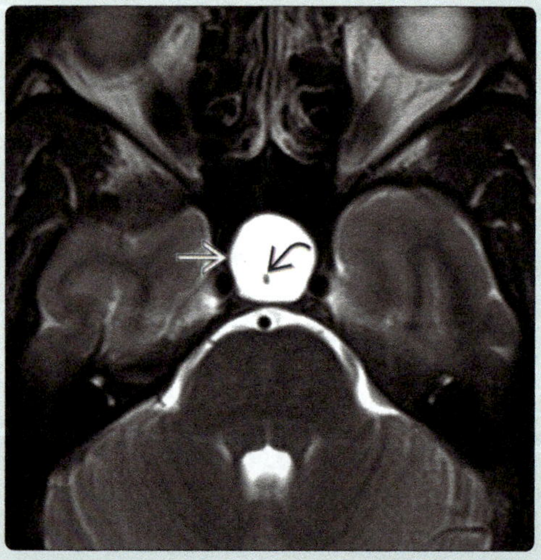

KEY FACTS

TERMINOLOGY

- Upper limit of normal pituitary height varies with age, sex
  - Pregnant/lactating female patients: 12 mm
  - Young menstruating female patients: 10 mm
  - Male patients, postmenopausal women: 8 mm
  - Infants, children: 6 mm
- Nonphysiologic hyperplasia seen with
  - Hypothyroidism, Addison disease, or other end-organ failure
  - Some neuroendocrine neoplasms

IMAGING

- Enlarged homogeneously enhancing pituitary gland with convex superior margin
- Best technique: High-resolution MR
  - Sagittal/coronal T1; coronal T2
  - Dynamic coronal T1WI
  - Postcontrast T1 FS sagittal/coronal T1
  - 3-4-mm slice thickness

TOP DIFFERENTIAL DIAGNOSES

- Pituitary macroadenoma
- Pituitary microadenoma
- Lymphocytic hypophysitis
- Venous congestion (intracranial hypotension, dural arteriovenous fistula)

PATHOLOGY

- Growth hormone cell hyperplasia usually diffuse, occurs with neuroendocrine tumors
- Prolactin cell hyperplasia: Diffuse > nodular
- Corticotroph hyperplasia: Nodular or diffuse
- Thyrotroph hyperplasia
  - Longstanding primary hypothyroidism, may have associated prolactin hyperplasia
- Gonadotroph hyperplasia (e.g., Turner, Klinefelter syndrome)

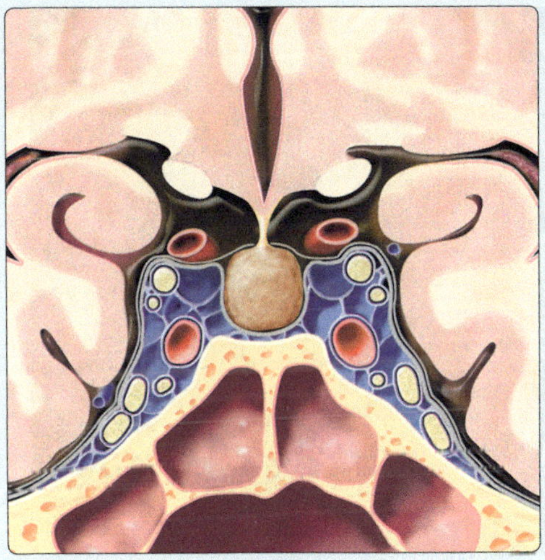

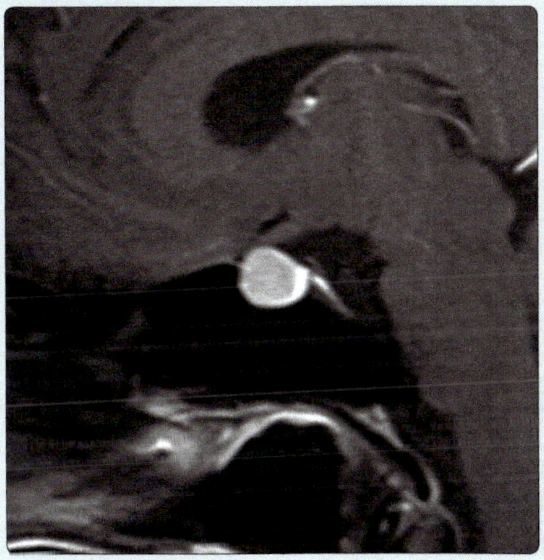

(Left) *Coronal graphic shows physiologic pituitary hyperplasia. The gland is uniformly enlarged and has a mildly convex superior margin.* **(Right)** *Sagittal T1W C+ MR in a 38-year-old woman undergoing infertility treatment imaged for headache shows a homogeneously enhancing pituitary measuring 12 mm.*

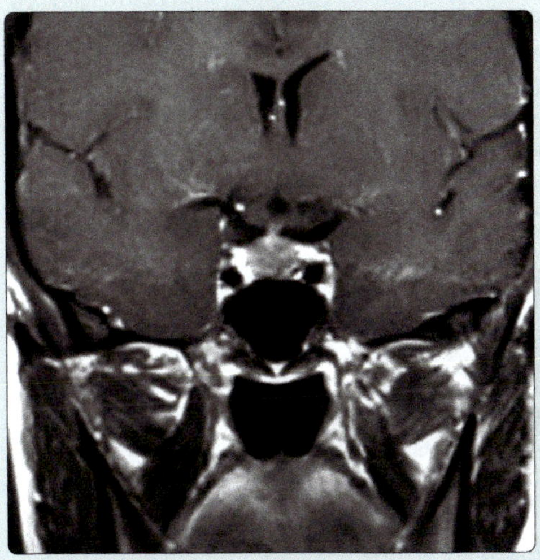

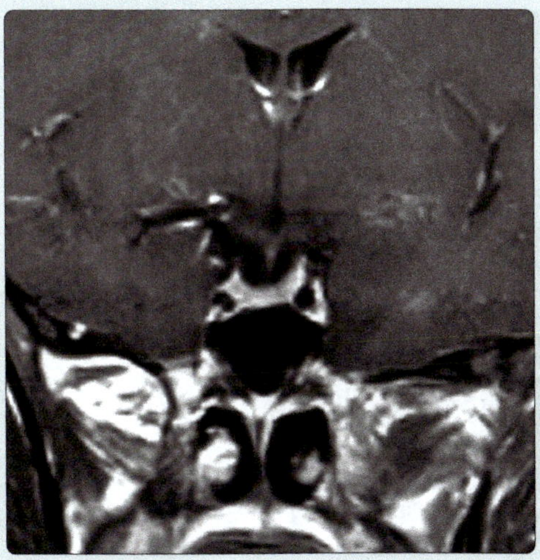

(Left) *Coronal T1WI C+ MR shows typical physiologic pituitary hyperplasia in a 28-year-old lactating woman. The gland has a mildly convex superior margin and measures nearly 14 mm in height.* **(Right)** *At follow-up 1 year later, coronal T1WI C+ MR reveals normal appearance to the pituitary gland with interval resolution of the postpartum physiologic enlargement.*

Lymphocytic Hypophysitis

KEY FACTS

TERMINOLOGY

- Lymphocytic hypophysitis (LH)
- Synonyms: Adenohypophysitis, primary hypophysitis, stalkitis
- Idiopathic inflammation of pituitary gland &/or stalk

IMAGING

- Thick stalk (> 2 mm + loss of normal "top to bottom" tapering)
- ± enlarged pituitary gland
- 75% show loss of posterior pituitary "bright spot"
- Enhances intensely, uniformly
- May have adjacent dural or sphenoid sinus mucosal thickening

TOP DIFFERENTIAL DIAGNOSES

- Macroadenoma
- Pituitary hyperplasia
- Adolescent pituitary gland
- Granulomatous disease
- Pituitary "dwarf"
- Ectopic posterior pituitary gland

CLINICAL ISSUES

- Peripartum woman with headache, multiple endocrine deficiencies
- Middle-aged man with diabetes insipidus (lymphocytic infundibuloneurohypophysitis)
- Mean in women = 35 years, men = 45 years
- M:F = 1:8-9
- Often self-limited
- Unrecognized, untreated LH can result in death from panhypopituitarism
- Conservative care (steroids, hormone replacement)

DIAGNOSTIC CHECKLIST

- LH can mimic pituitary adenoma

(Left) *Sagittal graphic shows lymphocytic hypophysitis. Note thickening of the infundibulum with loss of the normal "top to bottom" tapering as well as infiltration into the anterior lobe of the pituitary gland* ➔. **(Right)** *Coronal T2 MR in a pregnant woman with visual changes and endocrine abnormalities shows a hyperintense sellar/suprasellar mass with superior displacement of the optic chiasm* ➔. *Surgery for optic chiasm decompression disclosed lymphocytic hypophysitis. Imaging mimics pituitary macroadenoma.*

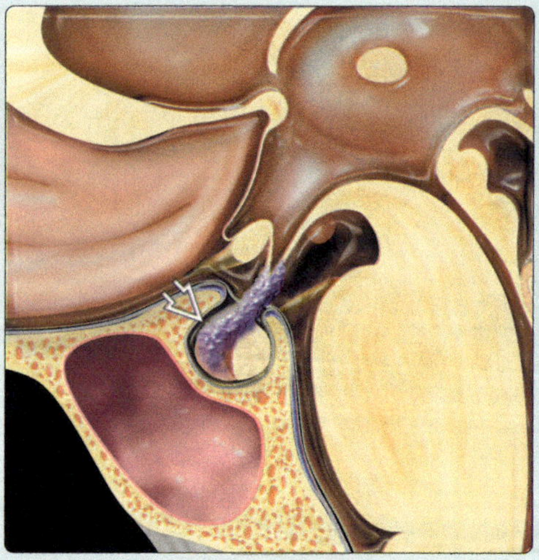

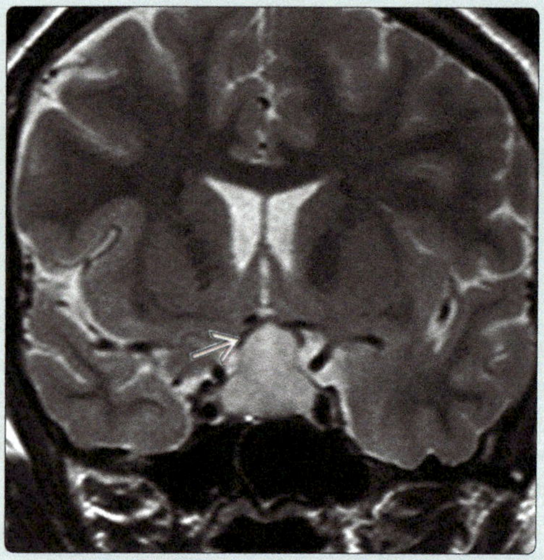

(Left) *Sagittal T1 C+ MR shows a prominent pituitary gland* ➔ *in a 37-year-old man with panhypopituitarism during treatment with ipilimumab for metastatic melanoma. The gland had doubled in size since MR 6 weeks prior. Findings are consistent with drug-induced hypophysitis.* **(Right)** *Sagittal T1 C+ MR in a 50-year-old patient with diabetes insipidus shows focal enlargement of the pituitary infundibulum* ➔ *related to lymphocytic infundibuloneurohypophysitis.*

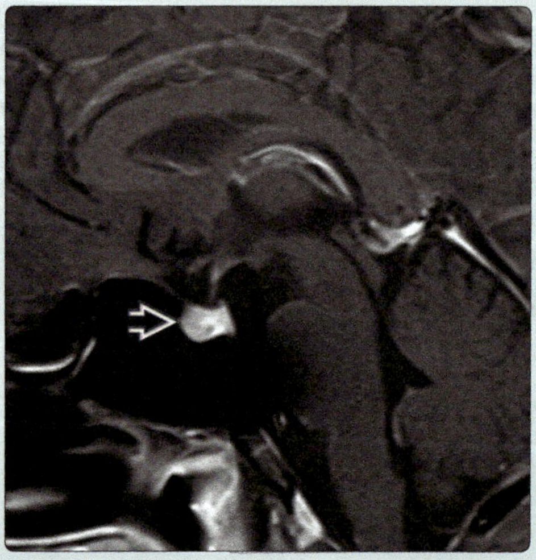

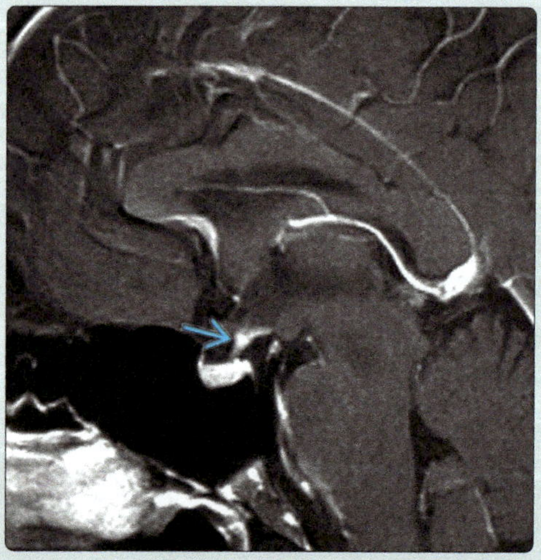

Terminology

The contents of the cerebellopontine angle (CPA) and internal auditory canal (IAC) cisterns include the facial nerve (CN7), the vestibulocochlear nerve (CN8), and the anterior inferior cerebellar artery (AICA) loop. The bony IAC, its fundal crests (vertical and horizontal), and its opening in the porus acusticus are also included as part of this discussion.

Embryology

The temporal bone forms as 3 distinct embryological events: (1) The external and middle ear, (2) the inner ear, and (3) the IAC. The practical implications of these 3 related but separate embryological events is that the presence or absence of the IAC is independent of the development of the inner, middle, or external ear.

The IAC develops in response to formation and migration of the facial and vestibulocochlear nerves through this area. IAC size depends on the number of migrating nerve bundles. The fewer the nerve bundles, the smaller the IAC. If the IAC is very small and only 1 nerve is seen, it is usually the facial nerve.

Imaging Anatomy of Cochlea, IAC, and CPA

The cochlear nerve portion of the vestibulocochlear nerve begins in the modiolus of the cochlea, where the bipolar **spiral ganglia** are found. Distally projecting axons reach the organ of Corti within the scala media. Proximally projecting axons coalesce to form the cochlear nerve itself within the fundus of the IAC.

CN8 in the IAC and CPA cisterns is made up of vestibular (balance) and cochlear (hearing) components. The cochlear nerve is located in the anteroinferior quadrant of the IAC. In the region of the porus acusticus, the cochlear nerve joins the superior and inferior vestibular nerve bundles to become the vestibulocochlear nerve in the CPA cistern.

The vestibulocochlear nerve crosses the CPA cistern as the posterior nerve bundle (CN7 is the anterior nerve bundle) to enter the brainstem at the junction of the medulla and pons. The entering cochlear nerve fibers pierce the brainstem and bifurcate to form synapses with both the **dorsal** and the **ventral cochlear nuclei**. These 2 nuclei are found on the lateral surface of the inferior cerebellar peduncle. Their location can be accurately determined by looking at high-resolution T2 axial images and identifying the contour of the inferior cerebellar peduncle. The entering vestibular nerve fibers divide into 4 branches to form synapses with the superior, inferior, medial, and lateral nuclei. The vestibular nuclei are clustered in the inferior cerebellar peduncle just anteromedial to the cochlear nuclei.

Remembering the normal orientation of nerves within the IAC cistern is assisted by the mnemonic "7-up, Coke down." CN7 is found in the anterosuperior quadrant, whereas the cochlear nerve is confined to the anteroinferior quadrant. Given this information, it is simple to remember that the superior vestibular nerve (SVN) is posterosuperior, whereas the inferior vestibular nerve (IVN) is posteroinferior.

Other normal structures to be aware of in the IAC include the **horizontal crest** (crista falciformis) and the **vertical crest** ("Bill's bar"). The horizontal crest is a medially projecting horizontal bony shelf in the IAC fundus that separates the CN7 and SVN above from the cochlear nerve and IVN below. The vertical crest is found between CN7 and the SVN along the superior fundal bony wall. The horizontal crest is easily seen on both bone CT and high-resolution MR. The vertical crest is more readily seen on bone CT.

Openings from the IAC fundus into the inner ear are numerous. The largest is the anteroinferior **cochlear nerve canal**, which conveys the cochlear nerve from the modiolus to the IAC fundus. Anterosuperiorly, the **meatal foramen** opens into the labyrinthine segment of CN7. The **macula cribrosa** is the multiply perforated bone that separates the vestibule of the inner ear from the IAC fundus.

Other nonneural normal anatomy of interest in the CPA cistern includes the AICA loop, flocculus, and choroid plexus. The **AICA** arises from the basilar artery, courses superolaterally into the CPA cistern, and then travels into the IAC cistern. Within the IAC, the AICA feeds the internal auditory artery of the cochlea. The AICA loop in the IAC or CPA cisterns may mimic a cranial nerve bundle on high-resolution T2WI MR. AICA vascular territory includes the cochlea, flocculus of the cerebellum, and anterolateral pons in the area of cranial nerve nuclei for CN5, CN7, and CN8 (AICA infarction is a rare cause of hearing loss). The **flocculus** is a lobule of the cerebellum that projects into the posterolateral CPA cistern. The 4th ventricle **choroid plexus** typically passes through the foramen of Luschka in the CPA cistern.

Imaging Techniques & Indications

The principal clinical indication requiring radiologists to examine the CPA-IAC is **sensorineural hearing loss (SNHL)**. Three principal parameters must be satisfied when completing the MR study in SNHL: (1) Use contrast-enhanced T1 fat-saturated thin-section sequences through the CPA-IAC to identify enhancing lesions in this location; (2) utilize high-resolution T2-weighted sequences to answer presurgical questions when a mass lesion is found; and (3) screen the brain for intraaxial causes, such as multiple sclerosis.

The gold standard for imaging patients with acquired SNHL is enhanced thin-section (≤ 3 mm) axial and coronal fat-saturated MR through the CPA-IAC. With these enhanced sequences, it is highly unlikely that a lesion causing SNHL will be missed. Be sure to obtain an axial or coronal precontrast T1 sequence and use fat saturation when contrast is applied to avoid the rare but troublesome mistake of calling a CPA-IAC lipoma a vestibular schwannoma. In the absence of fat saturation, the inherent high signal of lipoma will appear to enhance, leading to the misdiagnosis of vestibular schwannoma.

High-resolution T2-weighted thin-section (≤ 1 mm) MR sequences (CISS, FIESTA, T2 space) in the axial and coronal planes can be used as a screening exam without contrast to identify patients with mass lesions in the CPA-IAC area. However, these sequences are currently more commonly used as supplements when vestibular schwannoma is found on the enhanced T1 sequences to answer specific surgically relevant questions: What size is the fundal cap? What is the nerve of origin? Does the lesion enter the cochlear foramen?

Whenever MR is ordered for SNHL, remember to include whole-brain FLAIR, GRE, and DWI sequences. FLAIR will identify the rare multiple sclerosis patient presenting with SNHL as well as other intraaxial causes. GRE will demonstrate micro- or macrohemorrhage within a vestibular schwannoma and may help with aneurysm diagnosis when blooming of blood products or calcium in an aneurysm wall is seen. When

CPA Mass Differential Diagnosis

Pseudolesions	Vascular
Asymmetric cerebellar flocculus	Aneurysm (vertebrobasilar, PICA, AICA)
Asymmetric choroid plexus	Arteriovenous malformation
High jugular bulb	**Benign tumor**
Jugular bulb diverticulum	Choroid plexus papilloma
Marrow foci around IAC	Facial nerve schwannoma
Congenital	Hemangioblastoma, cerebellum
Arachnoid cyst	IAC hemangioma (venous malformation)
Epidermoid cyst	Meningioma
Lipoma	Vestibular schwannoma
Neurofibromatosis type 2	**Malignant tumor**
Infectious	Brainstem glioma, pedunculated
Cysticercosis	Ependymoma, pedunculated
Meningitis	Melanotic schwannoma
Inflammatory	Metastases, systemic or subarachnoid spread ("drop")
Idiopathic intracranial pseudotumor	
Sarcoidosis	

IAC = internal auditory canal; PICA = posterior inferior cerebellar artery; AICA = anterior inferior cerebellar artery.

DWI shows restricted diffusion in a CPA mass, the diagnosis of **epidermoid** is easily made.

Approaches to Imaging Issues of CPA-IAC

Approach to Sensorineural Hearing Loss in an Adult
Unilateral SNHL in an otherwise healthy adult is evaluated with MR (see prior section). Despite audiometric and brainstem-evoked response testing in the otolaryngology clinic, positive MR studies for lesions causing the SNHL are infrequent (< 5% even in highly screened patient groups). **Vestibular schwannoma** is by far the most common cause of unilateral SNHL (about 90% of lesions found with MR). It is important to become familiar with the wide range of appearances of vestibular schwannoma, including intramural cystic change, micro- and macroscopic hemorrhage, and associated arachnoid cyst.

Meningioma, epidermoid cyst, and CPA aneurysm are responsible for about 8% of lesions found in adult patients with SNHL. A long list of rare lesions, including otosclerosis, facial nerve, labyrinthine and jugular foramen schwannomas, IAC hemangioma, CPA metastases, labyrinthitis, sarcoidosis, lipoma, and superficial siderosis, make up < 2% of lesions causing unilateral SNHL in an adult that are found by MR.

Approach to Sensorineural Hearing Loss in a Child
When a child presents with unilateral or bilateral SNHL, the emphasis in the imaging work-up veers away from the typical adult tumor causes. Instead, congenital inner ear or CPA-IAC lesions are sought as the cause of the hearing loss. Complications of suppurative labyrinthitis (labyrinthine ossificans) are also included in the differential diagnosis.

When the child's presentation is bilateral profound SNHL, imaging is usually obtained as part of the work-up for possible **cochlear implantation**. High-resolution T2 MR is obtained in the axial and **oblique sagittal** planes to look for inner ear anomalies and labyrinthine ossificans as well as the presence or absence of a cochlear nerve in the IAC. If complex congenital inner ear disease is found, bone CT is often obtained to further define the inner ear fluid spaces and look for an absent cochlear nerve canal.

In reviewing the MR and CT in a child with SNHL, it is important to accurately describe any inner ear congenital anomaly, if present. If there is a history of meningitis, labyrinthine ossificans may be present. Look for bony encroachment on the fluid spaces of the inner ear. In particular, make sure the basal turn of the cochlea is open because occlusion by bony plaque may thwart successful cochlear implantation. Check the T2 oblique sagittal MRs for the presence of a normal cochlear nerve. If absent, cochlear implantation results may be negatively affected. Finally, look carefully at the IAC and CPA for signs of epidermoid cyst (restricted diffusion on DWI), lipoma (high signal on T1 precontrast sequences), and neurofibromatosis type 2 (bilateral CPA-IAC vestibular or facial schwannoma).

Selected References

1. Giesemann AM et al: The vestibulocochlear nerve: aplasia and hypoplasia in combination with inner ear malformations. Eur Radiol. 22(3):519-24, 2012
2. Burmeister HP et al: Identification of the nervus intermedius using 3T MR imaging. AJNR Am J Neuroradiol. 32(3):460-4, 2011
3. Sheth S et al: Appearance of normal cranial nerves on steady-state free precession MR images. Radiographics. 29(4):1045-55, 2009
4. Trimble K et al: Computed tomography and/or magnetic resonance imaging before pediatric cochlear implantation? Developing an investigative strategy. Otol Neurotol. 28(3):317-24, 2007
5. Rabinov JD et al: Virtual cisternoscopy: 3D MRI models of the cerebellopontine angle for lesions related to the cranial nerves. Skull Base. 14(2):93-9; discussion 99, 2004
6. Daniels RL et al: Causes of unilateral sensorineural hearing loss screened by high-resolution fast spin echo magnetic resonance imaging: review of 1,070 consecutive cases. Am J Otol. 21(2):173-80, 2000
7. Schmalbrock P et al: Assessment of internal auditory canal tumors: a comparison of contrast-enhanced T1-weighted and steady-state T2-weighted gradient-echo MR imaging. AJNR Am J Neuroradiol. 20(7):1207-13, 1999
8. Held P et al: MRI of inner ear and facial nerve pathology using 3D MP-RAGE and 3D CISS sequences. Br J Radiol. 70(834):558-66, 1997

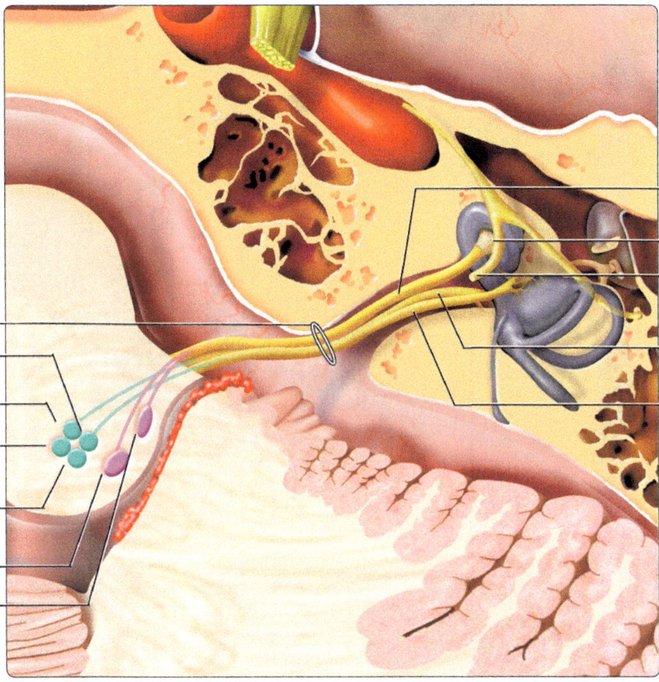

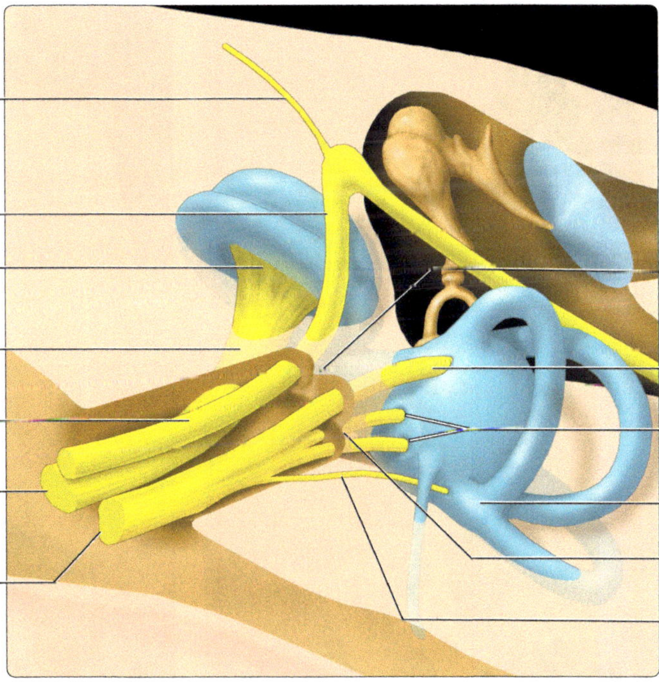

(Top) *Axial graphic depicts the vestibulocochlear nerve (CN8). The cochlear component of CN8 begins in bipolar cell bodies within the spiral ganglion in the modiolus. Central fibers run in the cochlear nerve to the dorsal and ventral cochlear nuclei on the lateral margin of the inferior cerebellar peduncle. Inferior and superior vestibular nerves begin in cell bodies in the vestibular ganglion; from there, they course centrally to 4 vestibular nuclei.* **(Bottom)** *Graphic shows the normal facial nerve and vestibulocochlear nerve in the internal auditory canal (IAC) and temporal bone. Notice that, by the mid-IAC, there are 4 main nerves present, including the facial, cochlear, superior vestibular, and inferior vestibular nerves. The singular nerve branches off the inferior vestibular nerve midway through the IAC on its way to the ampulla of the posterior semicircular canal. Multiple inferior vestibular nerve branches pierce the macular cribrosa, as does the superior vestibular nerve, on their way to the vestibule.*

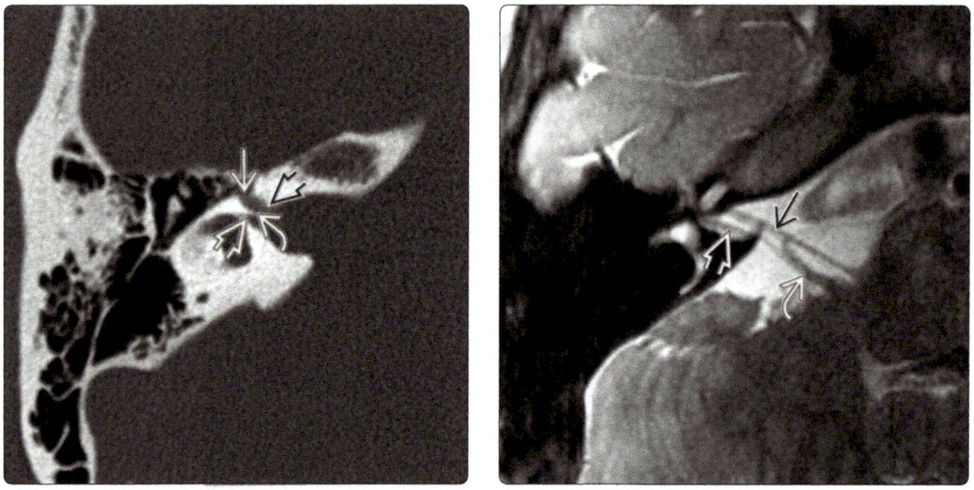

(Left) *Axial bone CT through the superior IAC reveals the labyrinthine segment of CN7 , the meatal foramen , the vertical crest , and the superior vestibular nerve connecting the IAC to the vestibule through the macula cribrosa.* **(Right)** *Axial T2WI MR through the superior IAC shows the anterosuperior CN7 , the superior vestibular nerve , and the vestibulocochlear nerve .*

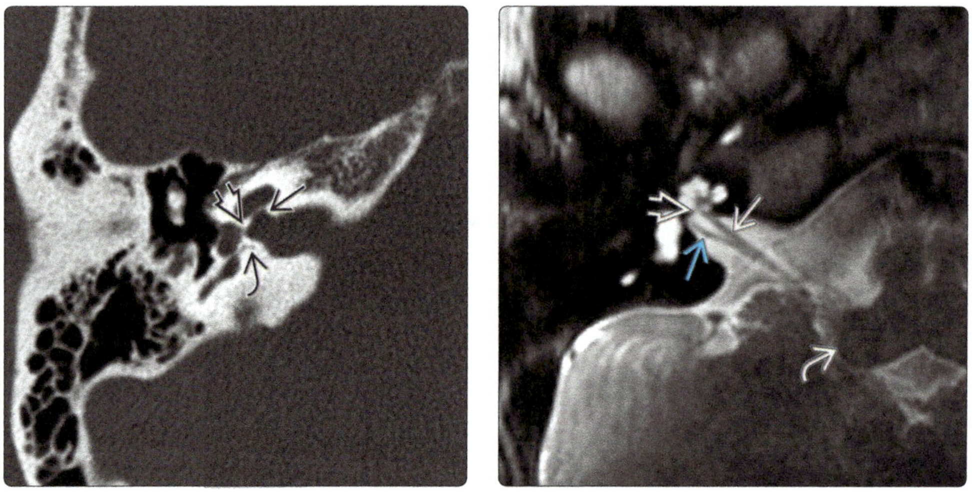

(Left) *Axial bone CT through the mid-IAC shows the cochlear nerve canal , inferior vestibular nerve leaving the fundus , and singular nerve canal containing the posterior branch of the inferior vestibular nerve .* **(Right)** *Axial T2WI MR through the inferior IAC reveals the cochlear nerve projecting into the cochlear nerve canal . Dorsal and ventral cochlear nuclei are not seen but are known to reside in the lateral inferior cerebellar peduncle margin . Note the inferior vestibular nerve .*

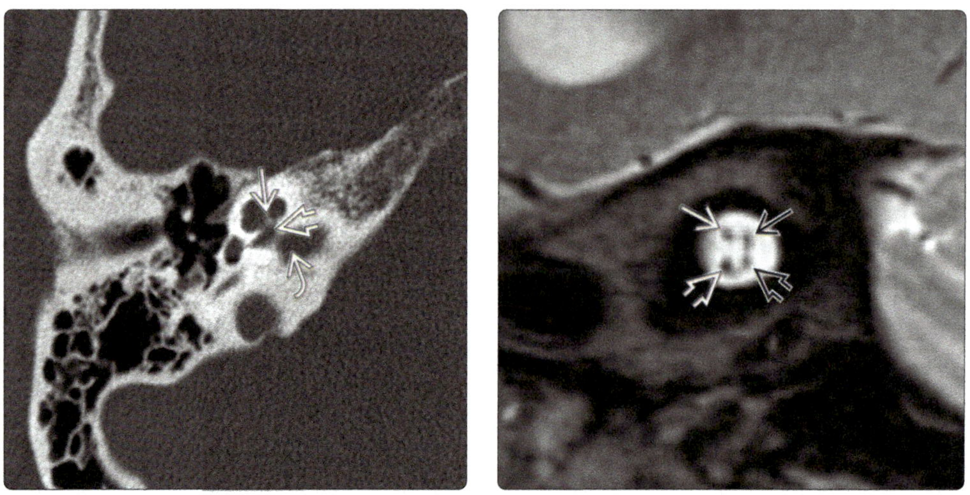

(Left) *Axial bone CT through the inferior IAC demonstrates the cochlear modiolus as a high-density structure at the cochlear base . The cochlear nerve canal and the fundus of the IAC are also labeled.* **(Right)** *Oblique sagittal T2WI MR shows the 4 nerve bundles of the mid-IAC cistern. CN7 is anterosuperior , the cochlear nerve is anteroinferior , and the superior and inferior vestibular nerves are posterosuperior and posteroinferior, respectively.*

KEY FACTS

TERMINOLOGY

- Definition: Congenital inclusion of ectodermal epithelial elements during neural tube closure

IMAGING

- CPA cisternal **insinuating** mass with high signal on DWI MR
  - 90% intradural, 10% extradural; margins usually scalloped or irregular; cauliflower-like margins with "fronds" possible
- T1 and T2: Isointense or slightly hyperintense to cerebrospinal fluid
- DWI: **Restricted diffusion** makes diagnosis

TOP DIFFERENTIAL DIAGNOSES

- Arachnoid cyst in CPA
- Cystic neoplasm in CPA
  - Cystic vestibular schwannoma
  - Cystic meningioma
  - Infratentorial ependymoma
  - Pilocytic astrocytoma
- Neurenteric cyst
- Neurocysticercosis, CPA

PATHOLOGY

- Surgical appearance: Pearly white CPA cistern mass
- Cyst wall: Internal layer of stratified squamous epithelium covered by fibrous capsule

CLINICAL ISSUES

- Clinical presentation
  - Principal presenting symptom: Dizziness and headache
    - Sensorineural hearing loss also common
  - If extends to lateral pons: Trigeminal neuralgia
  - Rarer symptoms: Facial palsy, seizure, hemifacial spasm
- Treatment: Complete surgical removal is goal
  - If adherent to neural structures, complete removal may not be possible; if recurs, takes many years to grow; DWI MR key to diagnosing recurrence

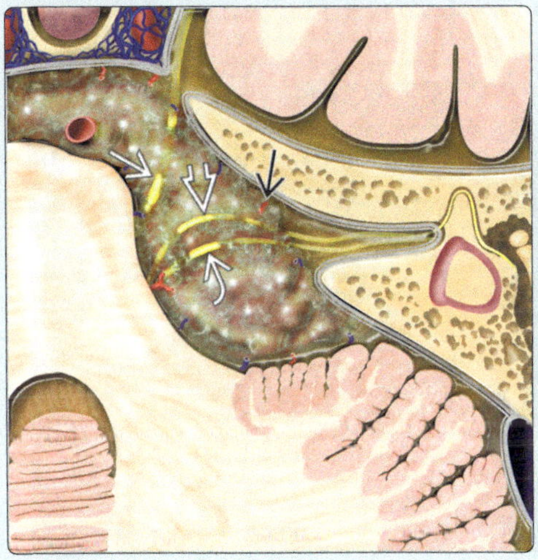

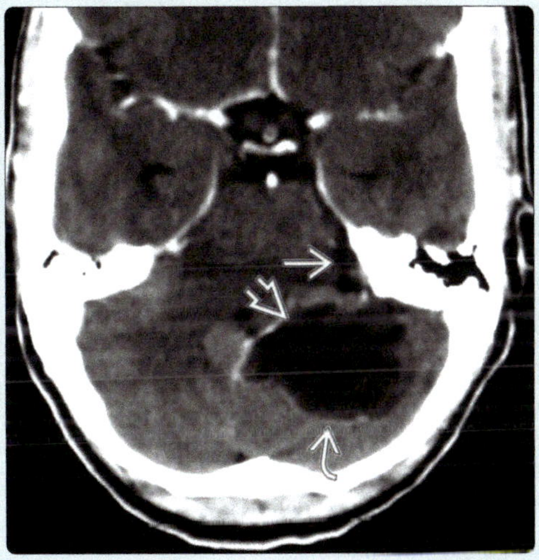

(Left) *Axial graphic shows a large cerebellopontine angle (CPA) epidermoid cyst within a typical "bed of pearls." Note that the 5th ➡, 7th ➡, and 8th ➡ cranial nerves along with the anterior inferior cerebellar artery loop ➡ are characteristically engulfed by this insinuating mass.* **(Right)** *Axial CECT shows a large CPA epidermoid cyst ➡. Note that this nonenhancing low-density lesion appears to invade the left cerebellar hemisphere ➡. Minimal rim enhancement is visible along the posterior margin of the cyst ➡.*

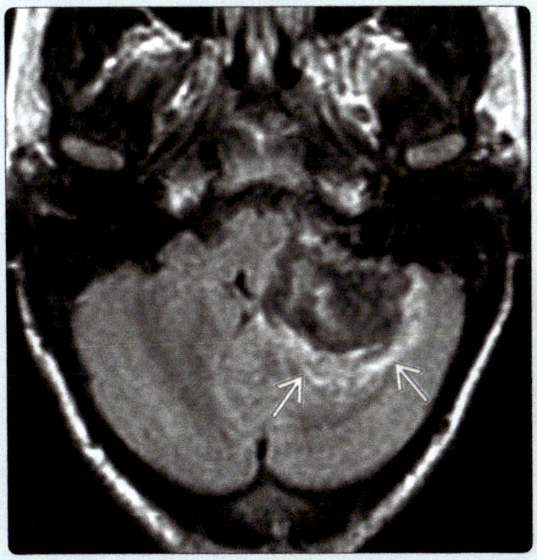

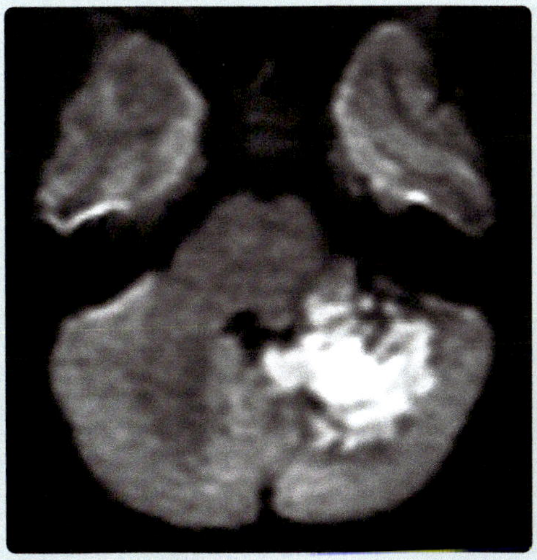

(Left) *Axial FLAIR MR of the same patient shows "incomplete" or partial nulling of the signal of this large epidermoid cyst. Associated high signal ➡ along the deep margins of the lesion is most likely due to gliosis of the cerebellar hemisphere.* **(Right)** *Axial DWI MR in the same patient reveals the expected high signal from epidermoid cyst diffusion restriction. DWI sequence allows straightforward differentiation of this epidermoid cyst from an arachnoid cyst.*

Arachnoid Cyst, CPA-IAC

KEY FACTS

TERMINOLOGY

- Arachnoid cyst (AC): Developmental arachnoid duplication anomaly creating cerebrospinal fluid (CSF)-filled sac

IMAGING

- Sharply demarcated ovoid extraaxial cisternal cyst with imperceptible walls with CSF density (CT) or intensity (MR)
- AC signal parallels (is isointense to) CSF on **all** MR sequences
- Complete fluid attenuation on FLAIR MR
- **No** diffusion restriction on DWI MR

TOP DIFFERENTIAL DIAGNOSES

- Epidermoid cyst in cerebellopontine angle (CPA)
- Cystic vestibular schwannoma
- Neurenteric cyst
- Cystic meningioma in CPA
- Cystic infratentorial ependymoma
- Cerebellar pilocytic astrocytoma

CLINICAL ISSUES

- Clinical presentation
  - Small AC
    - Asymptomatic, incidental finding (MR)
  - Large AC
    - Mostly asymptomatic
    - Symptoms may arise from direct compression ± ↑ intracranial pressure
- Natural history
  - Vast majority of ACs **do not** enlarge over time
- Treatment options
  - Most cases require **no** treatment
  - Treatment is highly selective process

DIAGNOSTIC CHECKLIST

- Differentiate AC from epidermoid cyst
  - AC: No restriction on DWI = best clue

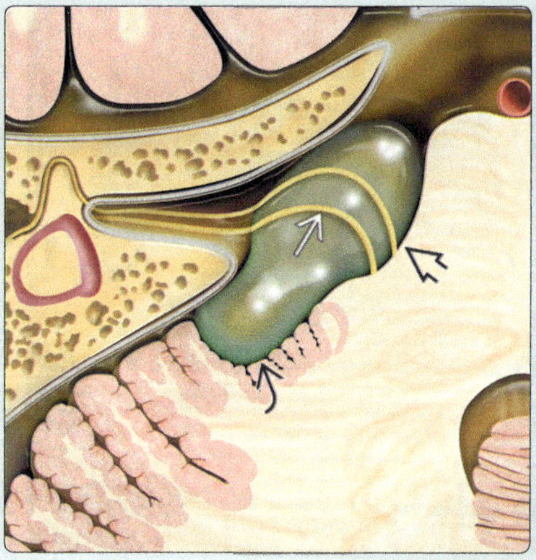
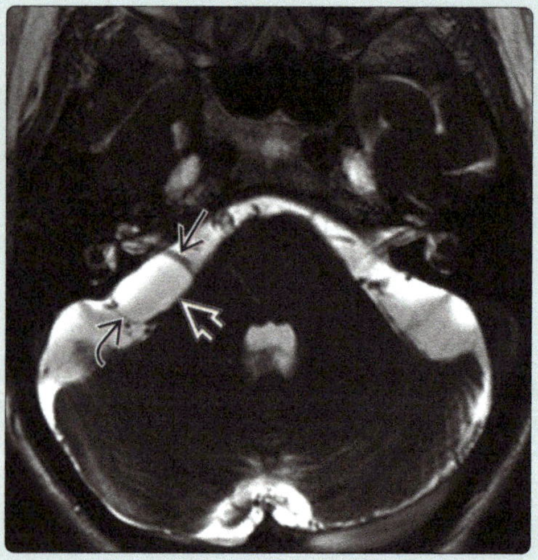

(Left) *Axial graphic of an arachnoid cyst (AC) in the cerebellopontine angle (CPA) shows a thin, translucent wall. Notice the cyst bowing the 7th and 8th cranial nerves anteriorly ➡ and effacing the brainstem ⇨ and cerebellum ⤳.* **(Right)** *Axial T2WI MR reveals a right CPA AC causing bowing of the facial and vestibulocochlear nerves anteriorly ➡, small bridging veins posteriorly ⤳, and flattening of the lateral margin of the brachium pontis ⇨.*

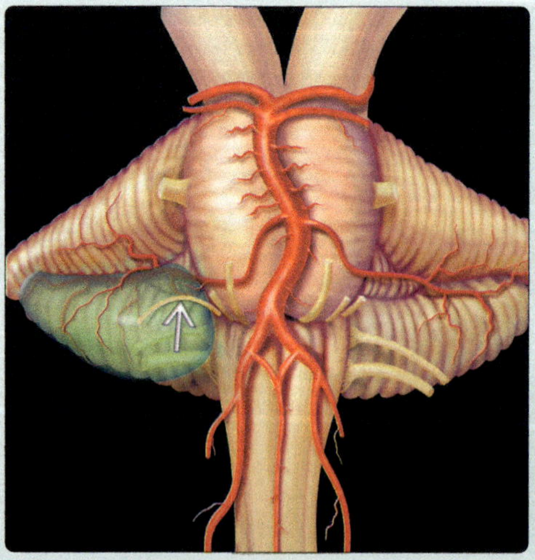
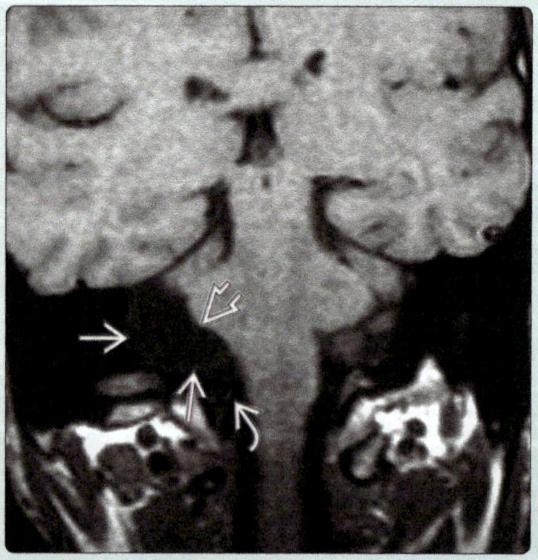

(Left) *Coronal graphic of a CPA AC depicts a typical translucent cyst wall. CN7 and CN8 are pushed by the cyst ➡ without being engulfed by it. In epidermoid cyst, cranial nerves are usually engulfed.* **(Right)** *Coronal T1WI MR demonstrates a small CPA AC ➡ that is almost identical with cerebrospinal fluid in the adjacent cistern ⤳. Note subtle mass effect on the adjacent brainstem ⇨. Complete fluid attenuation on FLAIR MR helps differentiate AC from an epidermoid cyst, which is the primary imaging differential diagnosis.*

Bell's Palsy

KEY FACTS

TERMINOLOGY

- Bell's palsy (BP): Herpetic peripheral facial nerve paralysis secondary to herpes simplex virus

IMAGING

- T1WI C+ fat-saturated MR: Fundal "tuft" and labyrinthine segment CN7 show intense asymmetric enhancement
  - Entire intratemporal CN7 may enhance
- Imaging note: Classic rapid-onset BP requires **no imaging** in initial stages
- If **atypical Bell's palsy**, search with imaging for underlying lesion

TOP DIFFERENTIAL DIAGNOSES

- Normal enhancement of intratemporal CN7
- Ramsay Hunt syndrome
- Lyme disease
- Facial nerve schwannoma
- Facial nerve venous malformation (hemangioma)
- Perineural tumor from parotid

PATHOLOGY

- Etiology-pathogenesis (current hypothesis)
  - Latent **herpes simplex** infection of geniculate ganglion with reactivation and spread of inflammatory process along proximal and distal intratemporal facial nerve fibers

CLINICAL ISSUES

- Classic clinical presentation
  - Acute-onset peripheral CN7 paralysis (36-hour onset)
- Medical therapy for BP
  - Tapering course of prednisone; begin within 3 days of symptoms for best result
  - Antiviral agents no longer used
- Surgical therapy for BP is controversial
  - Profound denervation (> 95%) treated with facial nerve decompression from internal auditory canal fundus to stylomastoid foramen

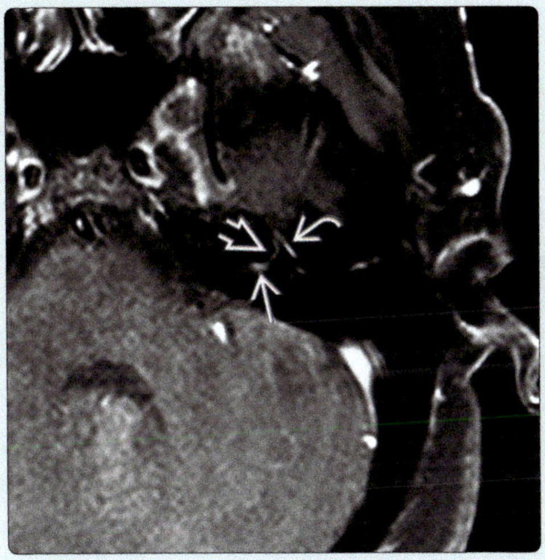
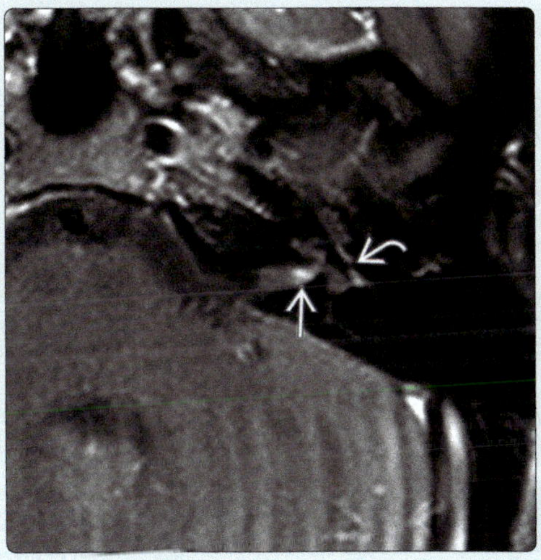

(Left) *Axial T1WI C+ FS MR shows classic findings of Bell's palsy with an internal auditory canal fundal "tuft" of enhancement ➔. The labyrinthine ➔ and tympanic ➔ facial nerve segments also enhance.* **(Right)** *Slightly lower axial T1WI C+ FS MR in the same patient again shows the internal auditory canal fundal "tuft" sign ➔ and tympanic segment of the facial nerve enhancement ➔. Remember that the geniculate ganglion and posterior genu/upper mastoid segment of the facial nerve may normally enhance.*

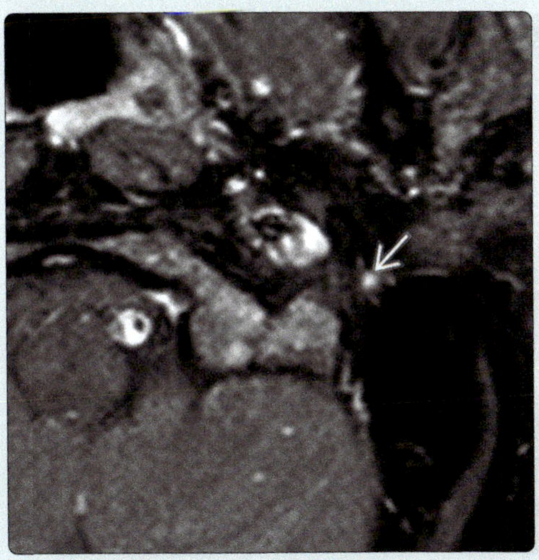
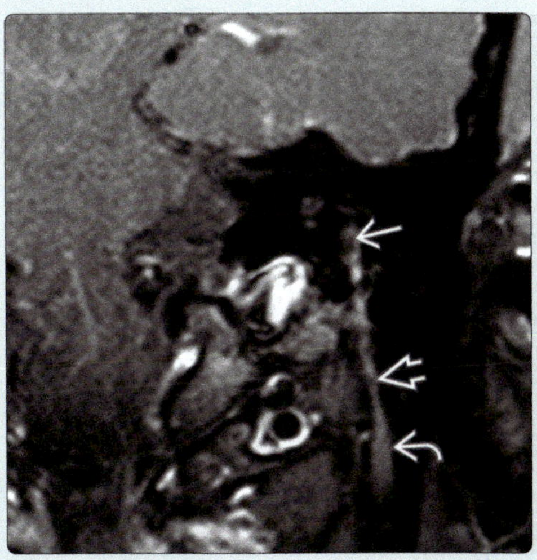

(Left) *Axial T1WI C+ FS MR in the same patient through the stylomastoid foramen demonstrates an enhancing, slightly enlarged facial nerve ➔. Swelling of the facial nerve is possible outside the bony facial nerve canal within the temporal bone.* **(Right)** *Coronal T1WI C+ FS MR in the same patient reveals avid enhancement in the mastoid ➔, stylomastoid ➔, and extracranial facial nerve ➔ in this patient with typical Bell's palsy.*

KEY FACTS

TERMINOLOGY

- Trigeminal neuralgia (TN) definition: Vascular loop compressing trigeminal nerve (CN5) at its root entry zone (REZ) or preganglionic segment (PGS)

IMAGING

- High-resolution MR: Serpiginous asymmetric signal void (vessel) in cerebellopontine angle (CPA) CN5 REZ or PGS
  - CN5 PGS atrophy: Severe, prolonged compression
  - Compressing vessel will bow PGS
- Offending vessels: **Superior cerebellar artery** (55%) > AICA (10%) > basal artery (5%) > variant vein (5%) > other

TOP DIFFERENTIAL DIAGNOSES

- Aneurysm in CPA-internal auditory canal
- Arteriovenous malformation in CPA
- Developmental venous anomaly in posterior fossa

PATHOLOGY

- CN5 REZ or PGS experiences "irritation" from vessel

CLINICAL ISSUES

- TN symptoms
  - Lancinating pain following V2 ± V3 distributions
  - May occur spontaneously or in response to "trigger" from tactile stimulation
- Treatment
  - Drug therapy (anticonvulsant) initially
  - Microvascular decompression or focused radiotherapy (~ 70% long-term success rate)

DIAGNOSTIC CHECKLIST

- 1st look for multiple sclerosis or developmental venous anomaly with draining vein along PGS
  - Also check for cisternal mass: Schwannoma, meningioma, epidermoid
- Next follow CN5 distally into cavernous sinus and face
  - Exclude perineural tumor, malignancies of face
- Last view high-resolution thin-section MR for causal vessel
  - Causal vessel will bow PGS or deform REZ

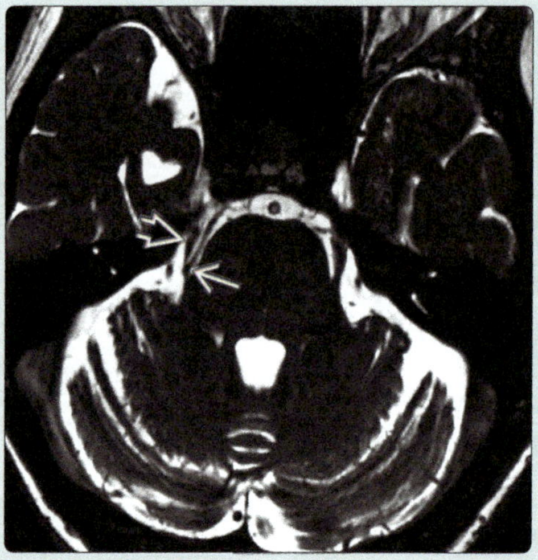
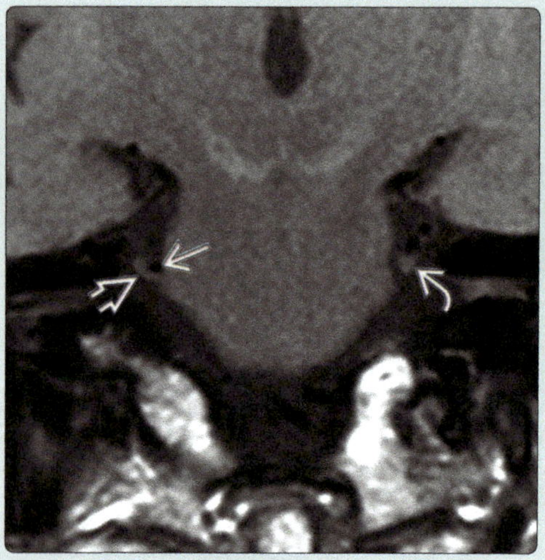

(Left) *Axial T2WI MR in this patient with right trigeminal neuralgia (TN) shows the low signal superior cerebellar artery impinging on the root entry zone of the preganglionic segment of the trigeminal nerve.* **(Right)** *Coronal T1WI MR in the same patient reveals the superior cerebellar artery compressing and deforming the right proximal preganglionic segment of CN5. Notice the larger, normal left preganglionic CN5, indicating that atrophy is a feature of the affected right side.*

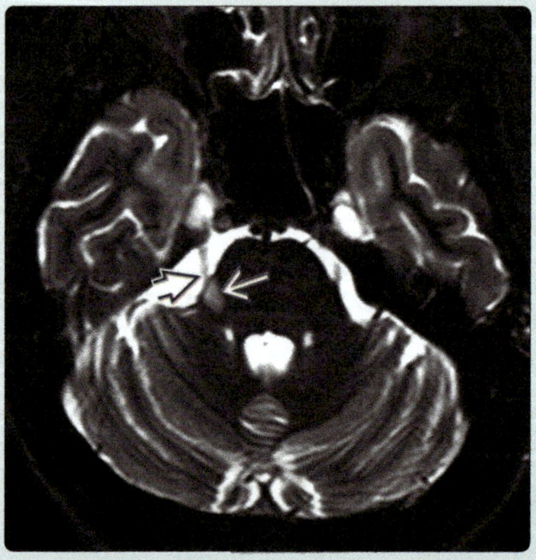
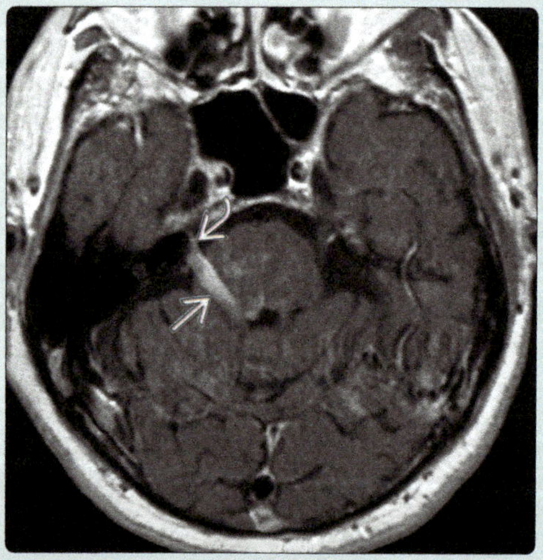

(Left) *Axial T2WI FS MR in a patient with right TN reveals a multiple sclerosis lesion involving the lateral pons at the root entry zone of the trigeminal nerve. Rarely, cisternal masses or MS may present with TN.* **(Right)** *Axial T1WI C+ MR in a patient with right TN shows a developmental venous anomaly of the cerebellum draining through the lateral pons and root entry zone of CN5. Less than 5% of patients with TN have a venous explanation for their symptoms.*

KEY FACTS

TERMINOLOGY

- Definition: Vascular loop compressing facial nerve at its root exit zone within cerebellopontine angle (CPA) cistern causing hemifacial spasm

IMAGING

- High-resolution T2WI MR or source MRA images show serpentine asymmetric signal void (vessel) in medial CPA
  - Anterior inferior cerebellar artery (50%) > posterior inferior cerebellar artery (30%) > vertebral artery (15%) > vein (5%)

TOP DIFFERENTIAL DIAGNOSES

- Aneurysm, CPA-IAC
- Arteriovenous malformation, CPA
- Developmental venous anomaly, posterior fossa

PATHOLOGY

- CN7 bundle experiences "irritation" from vessel
- Rare, nonvascular causes of hemifacial spasm (HFS)
  - Multiple sclerosis
  - Cisternal masses
    - Epidermoid, meningioma, schwannoma
  - T-bone and parotid lesions
    - Perineural CN7 malignancy

CLINICAL ISSUES

- Unilateral involuntary facial spasms (HFS)
- HFS begins with orbicularis oculi spasms
- Tonic-clonic bursts become constant over time

DIAGNOSTIC CHECKLIST

- Positive MR findings present in ~ 50% HFS patients
- 1st look for cisternal mass lesions, multiple sclerosis
- Then follow CN7 distally into T-bone and parotid
  - Exclude CN7 venous malformation, parotid malignancy
- Determine whether MRA source images or high-resolution T2WI identify causal vessel
  - Negative MR does not preclude surgical therapy

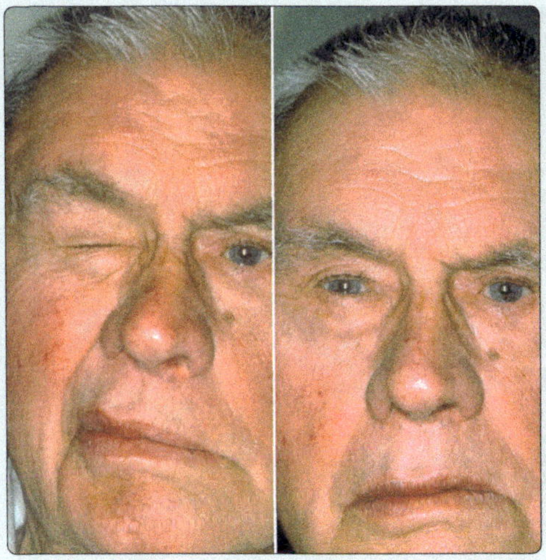

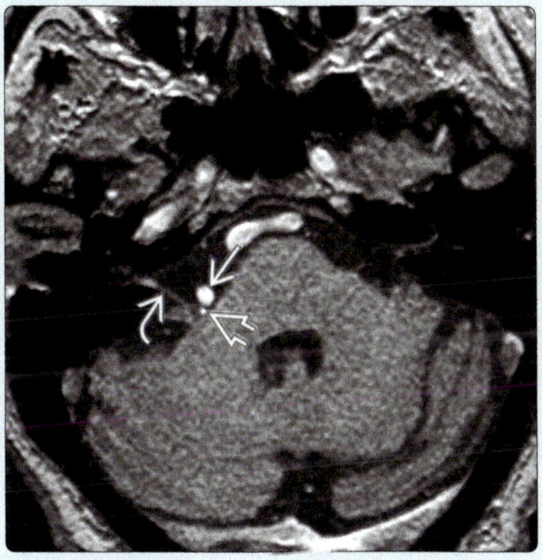

(Left) *(L) Clinical photograph shows a patient with severe right hemifacial spasm, which is synchronous right eyelid and face twitching. (R) In-between spasms, his face is normal.* **(Right)** *Axial MRA in a patient with right hemifacial spasm shows a tortuous right vertebral artery ➡ and associated posterior inferior cerebellar artery (PICA) ➡ pushing on the root exit zone of the facial nerve, visible in the cerebellopontine angle (CPA) cistern ➡.*

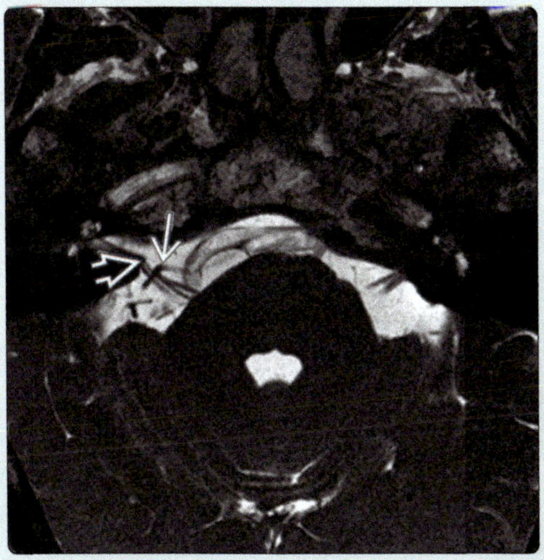

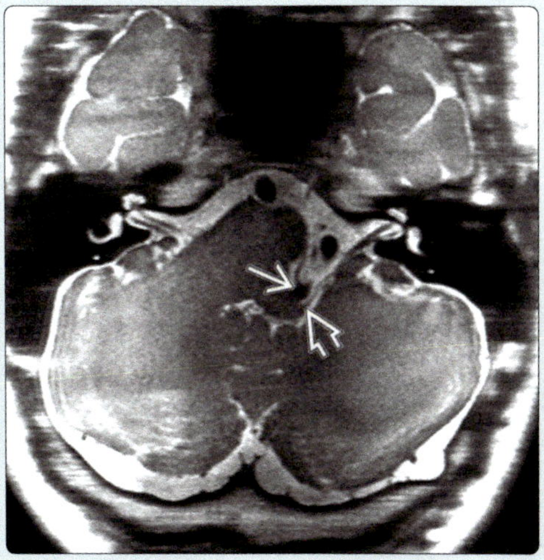

(Left) *Axial CISS MR through the CPA cisterns in a patient with right hemifacial spasm demonstrates a PICA loop ➡ pushing the cisternal CN7 and CN8 posteriorly, causing them to drape over the posterior margin of the porus acusticus ➡.* **(Right)** *Axial thin-section T2WI MR reveals a dolichoectatic vertebral artery ➡ impinging on the root exit zone ➡ of the facial nerve in the medial CPA cistern in this patient with hemifacial spasm.*

KEY FACTS

TERMINOLOGY

- Vestibular ("acoustic") schwannoma (VS): Benign tumor from Schwann cells that wrap vestibular CN8 branches in cerebellopontine angle-internal auditory canal (CPA-IAC)

IMAGING

- T1WI fat-saturated enhanced MR = gold standard
  - Focal, enhancing mass of CPA-IAC cistern centered on porus acusticus
  - Small VS: Ovoid-enhancing intracanalicular mass
  - Large VS: "Ice cream on cone" shape in CPA and IAC
  - 15% with intramural cysts (low signal foci)
  - 0.5% with associated arachnoid cyst/"trapped" CSF
- High-resolution T2 space, CISS, or FIESTA: "Filling defect" in hyperintense CSF of CPA-IAC cistern
- FLAIR: ↑ cochlear signal from ↑ protein
- T2* GRE: Microhemorrhages ↓ signal foci (common)
  - Characteristic VS finding when present
  - Not seen in meningioma

TOP DIFFERENTIAL DIAGNOSES

- Meningioma in CPA-IAC
- Epidermoid cyst in CPA
- Aneurysm in CPA
- Facial nerve schwannoma in CPA-IAC
- Metastases in CPA-IAC

PATHOLOGY

- Benign tumor arising from vestibular portion of CN8 at glial-Schwann cell junction

CLINICAL ISSUES

- Demographics and symptoms
  - Adults with unilateral sensorineural hearing loss
  - Other symptoms
    - Unsteady walking
    - Vertiginous sensation
    - Tinnitus
- Treatment: Surgery vs. radiosurgery

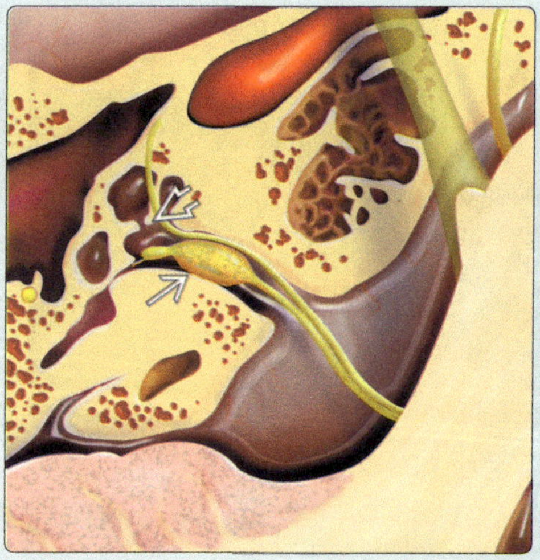

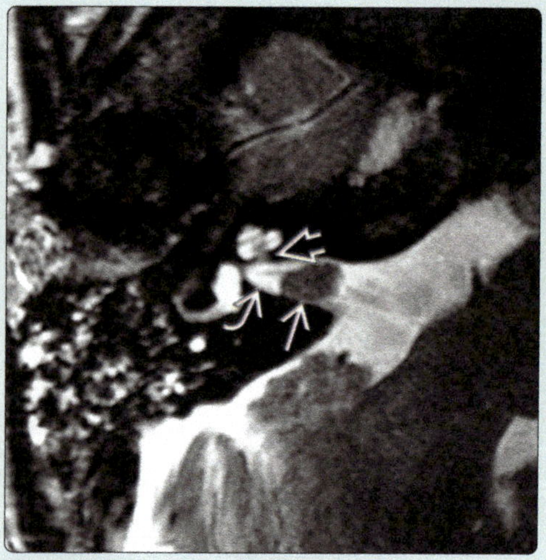

(Left) *Axial graphic shows small intracanalicular vestibular schwannoma arising from the superior vestibular nerve. Notice that the cochlear nerve canal is uninvolved.* **(Right)** *Axial T2WI MR reveals a small intracanalicular vestibular schwannoma visualized as a soft tissue intensity mass surrounded by high-intensity cerebrospinal fluid. The cochlear nerve canal is not involved, and an 8-mm fundal cap is present.*

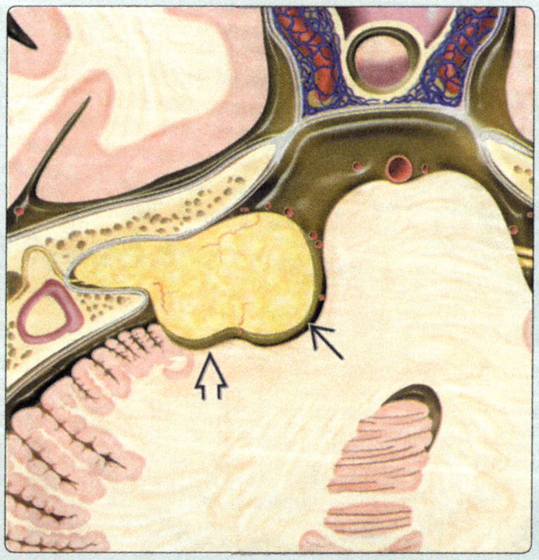

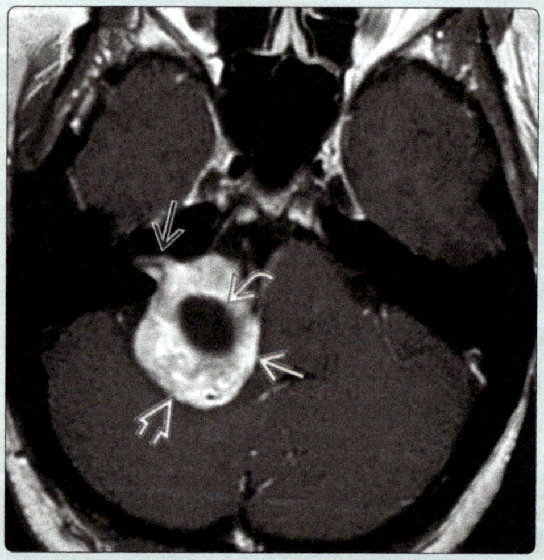

(Left) *Axial graphic of a large vestibular schwannoma reveals the typical "ice cream on cone" CPA-IAC morphology. Mass effect on the middle cerebellar peduncle and cerebellar hemisphere is evident.* **(Right)** *Axial T1WI C+ MR demonstrates a large CPA-IAC vestibular schwannoma compressing the middle cerebellar peduncle and cerebellar hemisphere. Enhancement within the IAC and the large intramural cyst makes the imaging diagnosis certain.*

KEY FACTS

TERMINOLOGY

- Benign encapsulated nerve sheath tumor composed of differentiated neoplastic Schwann cells
  - 99% of all schwannomas associated with cranial nerves
  - 95% involve CN8
  - < 1% of all intracranial schwannomas are intraparenchymal

IMAGING

- CT
  - Iso- to slightly hyperdense compared with brain
  - Adjacent bone, foramina may show smooth, scalloped enlargement
  - Avid, sometimes heterogeneous enhancement
- MR
  - Heterogeneously hyperintense on T2WI, FLAIR
  - 100% enhance (avid, heterogeneously)
  - Peritumoral arachnoid cyst common

TOP DIFFERENTIAL DIAGNOSES

- Cranial nerve schwannoma [enlarged, enhancing cranial nerve(s)]
  - Metastases
  - Lymphoma
  - Multiple sclerosis
  - Neurofibromatosis type 2
  - Schwannomatosis
- Parenchymal schwannoma (rare)
  - Ganglioglioma
  - Pleomorphic xanthoastrocytoma
  - Pilocytic astrocytoma

PATHOLOGY

- Spindle-shaped neoplastic Schwann cells
- Single cell type with 2 basic histologic patterns
  - High cellularity (Antoni A pattern)
  - Low cellularity ± lipidization ± cystic degeneration (Antoni B pattern)

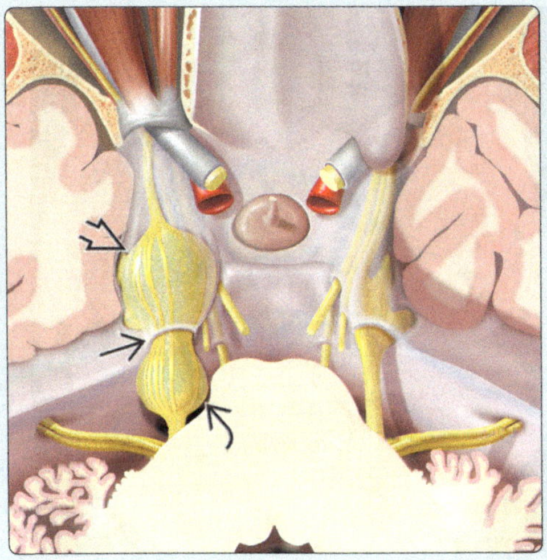

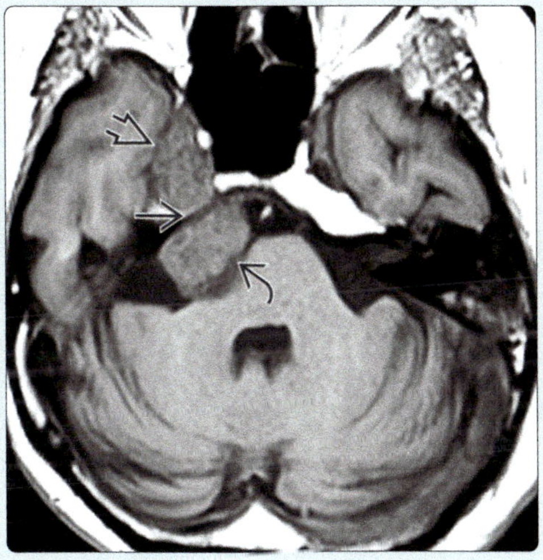

(Left) *Axial graphic depicts classic "dumbbell" trigeminal schwannoma. The dural ring of Meckel cave ➔ constricts the expansile lesion, with the cerebellopontine angle (CPA) segment ➔ and the Meckel cave segment ➔ forming the dumbbell.* **(Right)** *Axial T1WI shows a typical "dumbbell" trigeminal schwannoma with the Meckel cave segment ➔ and the large cerebellopontine angle segment ➔ constricted in the middle by the ring of dura ➔ at the entrance to Meckel cave.*

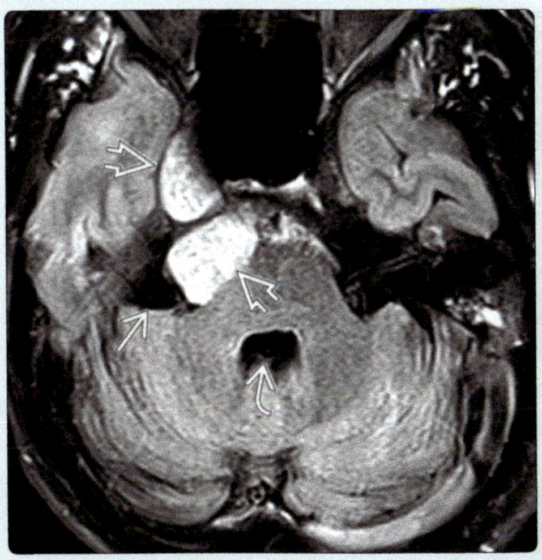

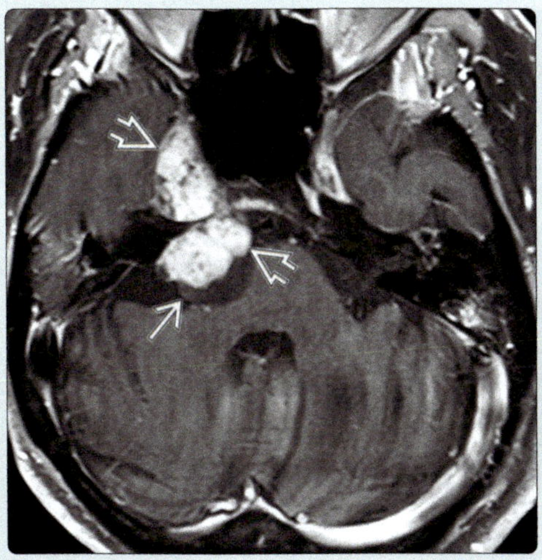

(Left) *Axial FLAIR in the same case shows that the lesion ➔ is heterogeneously hyperintense relative to the cerebrospinal fluid in the 4th ventricle ➔ and adjacent CPA cistern ➔.* **(Right)** *T1 C+ FS in the same case shows that the trigeminal schwannoma enhances intensely but somewhat heterogeneously ➔. There is a small arachnoid cyst ➔ adjacent to the tumor, a relatively common finding with cranial nerve schwannomas.*

KEY FACTS

TERMINOLOGY

- Definition: Benign, unencapsulated neoplasm arising from meningothelial arachnoid cells of CPA-IAC dura

IMAGING

- 10% occur in posterior fossa
- When in CPA, asymmetric to IAC porus acusticus
- NECT
    - Variable; often hyperdense
        - 25% calcified; 2 types seen
            - Homogeneous, sand-like (psammomatous)
            - Focal "sunburst," globular, or rim pattern
- Bone CT: Hyperostotic or permeative-sclerotic bone changes possible (en plaque type)
- T2WI MR: Pial blood vessels seen as surface flow voids between tumor and brain
    - High signal crescent from CSF ("CSF cleft")
- T1WI C+ MR: Enhancing dural-based mass with dural "tails" centered along posterior petrous wall
    - When IAC tail present, usually dural reaction, not tumor

TOP DIFFERENTIAL DIAGNOSES

- Vestibular schwannoma
- Epidermoid cyst, CPA-IAC
- Dural metastases, CPA-IAC
- Sarcoidosis, CPA-IAC
- Idiopathic inflammatory pseudotumor

CLINICAL ISSUES

- 2nd most common CPA tumor
- Slow-growing tumor, displacing adjacent structures
- Often found as incidental brain MR finding
- < 10% symptomatic; usually do not cause sensorineural hearing loss
- Treatment
    - Follow with imaging if smaller size and older patient
    - Surgical removal if medically safe
    - Adjunctive radiation therapy with incomplete surgery

(Left) *At level of the internal auditory canal (IAC), a large cerebellopontine angle (CPA) meningioma causes mass effect on the brainstem and cerebellum. Notice the broad dural base creating the shape of a mushroom cap. Dural "tails" ➡ are present in ~ 60% of cases, typically representing reactive rather than neoplastic change. CSF-vascular cleft is also visible ➡.* **(Right)** *Axial NECT scan in a 72-year-old woman shows a typical CPA meningioma as a hyperdense "mushroom cap-shaped" mass ➡ with its broad base toward the adjacent temporal bone.*

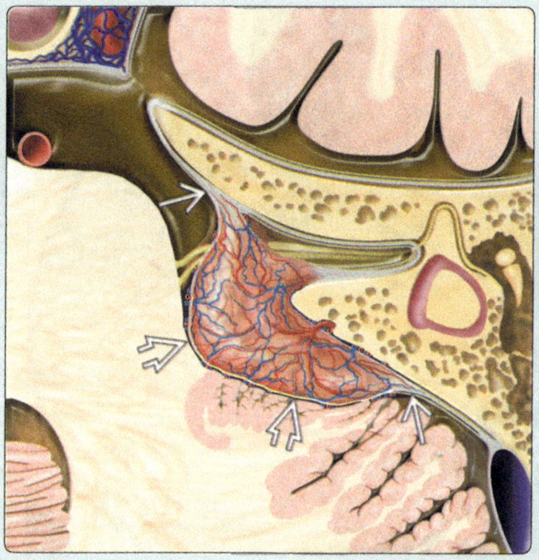

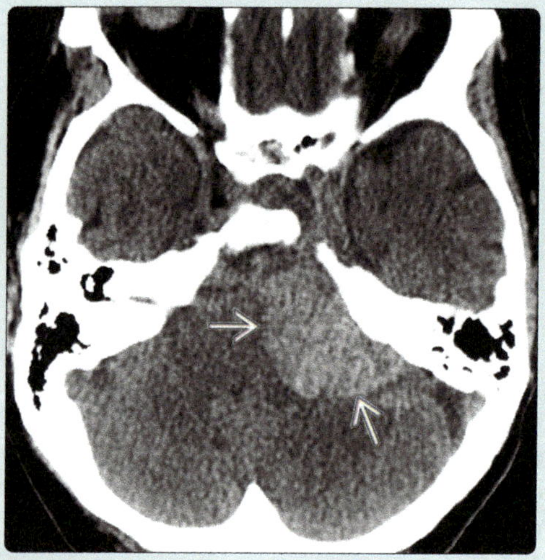

(Left) *Axial T1WI C+ FS MR through the IAC shows a meningioma overlying the porus acusticus. Note the dural "tail" ➡ extending along the temporal bone posterior wall. A dot of enhancement in the IAC fundus ➡ suggests that the low signal area in the IAC is a nonenhancing meningioma.* **(Right)** *Axial T2WI FS MR in the same patient reveals a high-velocity flow void ➡ representing a dural artery feeder penetrating the meningioma core. Low signal in the IAC ➡ is an intracanalicular meningioma.*

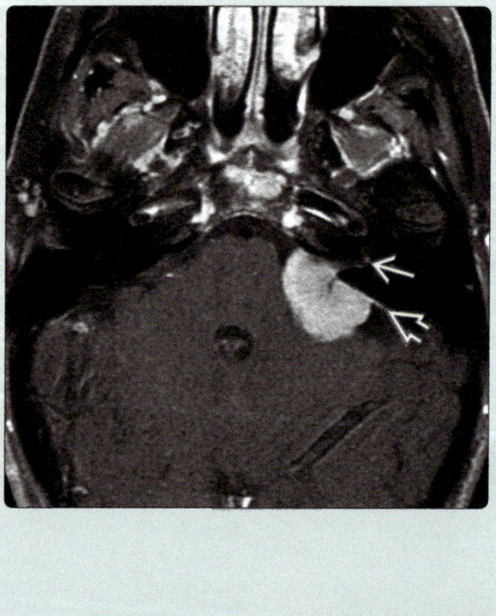

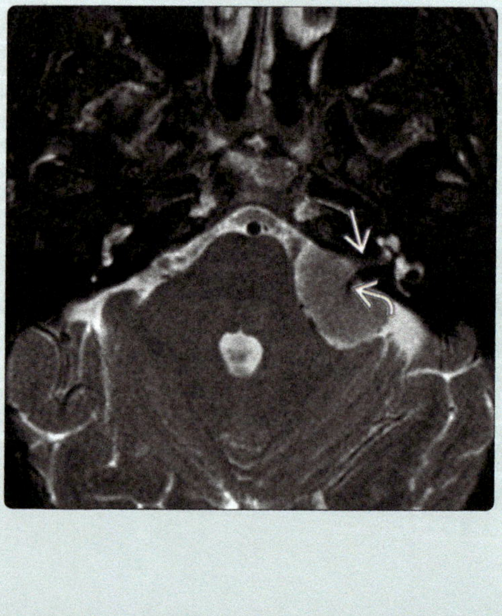

KEY FACTS

TERMINOLOGY

- Definition: Cerebellopontine angle-internal auditory canal (CPA-IAC) metastases refers to systemic or CNS neoplasia affecting area of CPA-IAC

IMAGING

- 4 major sites: Leptomeningeal (pia-arachnoid), dura, flocculus, and choroid plexus
- T1WI C+ MR
  - **Leptomeningeal metastases**: Diffuse thickening and enhancement of cranial nerves in IAC
  - **Dural metastases**: Thickened enhancing dura; may be diffuse or focal
  - **Floccular metastases**: Enhancing floccular mass extends into CPA cistern
  - **Choroid plexus metastases**: Enhancing nodular lesion along normal course of choroid plexus
  - Focal, enhancing brain metastases may be present
- FLAIR MR
  - Parenchymal brain metastases usually high signal

TOP DIFFERENTIAL DIAGNOSES

- Bilateral vestibular schwannoma (neurofibromatosis type 2, NF2)
- Sarcoidosis
- Meningitis
- Ramsay Hunt syndrome

CLINICAL ISSUES

- Rapidly progressive unilateral or bilateral facial nerve paralysis and sensorineural hearing loss
- Patient with past history of treated malignancy

DIAGNOSTIC CHECKLIST

- If trying to diagnose bilateral "vestibular schwannoma" in adult as NF2, probably CPA metastases instead
- Rapidly progressive 7th and 8th cranial nerve palsies + CPA mass suggest metastatic focus
  - Vestibular schwannoma rarely causes CN7 palsy

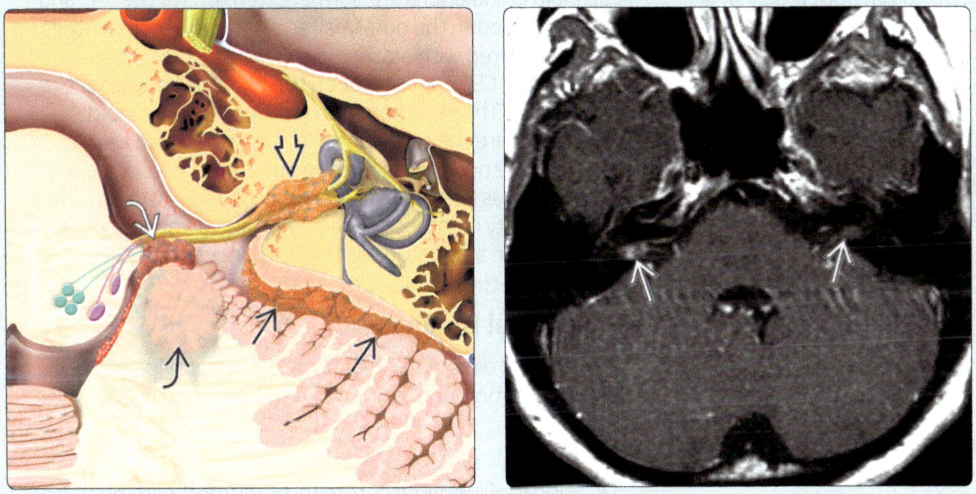

(Left) *In 4 major types of cerebellopontine angle-internal auditory canal (CPA-IAC) area metastases, along the posterolateral margin of the IAC, thickened dural metastases ➔ are visible. Within the IAC, metastatic leptomeningeal (pia-arachnoid) ➔ involvement is present. Choroid plexus ➔ and floccular ➔ metastases are also depicted.* **(Right)** *Axial T1WI C+ MR shows bilateral leptomeningeal breast carcinoma metastases ➔ within the IACs. Left-sided disease is more subtle than the right.*

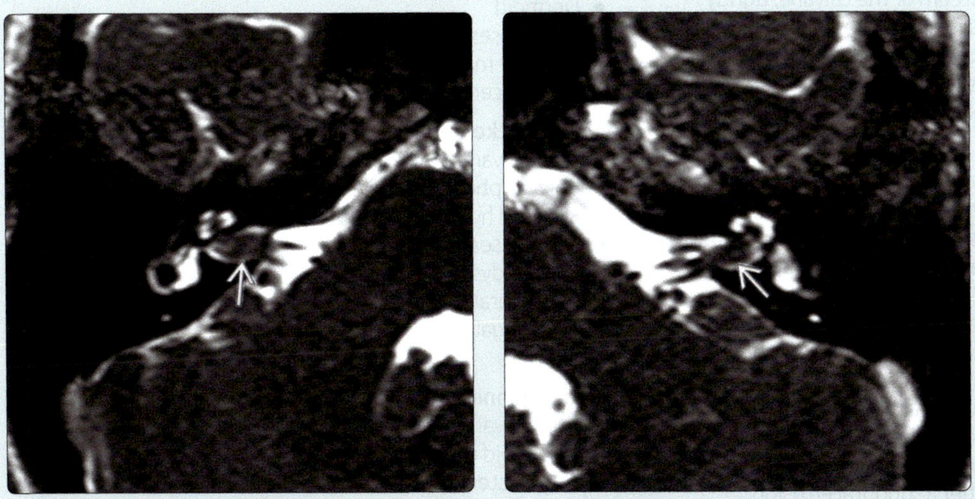

(Left) *Axial T2WI MR demonstrates right IAC leptomeningeal metastatic foci as thickening of the branches of CN7 and CN8 ➔ within the IAC.* **(Right)** *Axial T2WI MR reveals left IAC metastatic disease as subtle thickening of the branches of CN7 and CN8 ➔ within the IAC. In an adult patient with suspected bilateral vestibular schwannoma, consider metastatic disease rather than neurofibromatosis type 2.*

Overview

Understanding the anatomy of the skull, scalp, and meninges is key to formulating a correct imaging diagnosis. Several important differential diagnoses are based on location. However, each of these locations requires a different imaging approach.

For example, CT is often the best imaging modality for lesions of the skull and scalp. When faced with a complex skull base lesion, a combination of bone CT and contrast-enhanced MR is often required for optimal imaging. MR with contrast is the best imaging modality for meningeal processes.

Scalp

The scalp is made up of 5 layers including the dermis (skin), subcutaneous fibro-adipose tissue, epicranium and muscles, subaponeurotic areolar tissue, and pericranium. The first 3 layers are firmly connected and surgically act as a single layer.

The majority of scalp lesions are not imaged, as the area is easily accessible to both visual and manual inspection. Imaging becomes important when a scalp lesion is malignant or has a vascular component that could alter the surgical approach.

Skull Vault (Calvaria)

The calvaria is composed of 5 bones: Frontal, parietal, occipital, temporal, and sphenoid (greater wings) bones that are primarily connected by the major sutures, including the coronal, sagittal, and lambdoid sutures. The metopic suture is variably seen in adults.

There are many normal variants of the skull. These must be recognized to prevent misdiagnosis and unnecessary biopsy. Some of the most common skull normal variants include arachnoid granulations, vascular grooves from the meningeal arteries and veins, venous lakes, emissary veins, parietal thinning, asymmetric marrow (particularly in the petrous apex), aerated clinoid processes, and accessory sutures.

Meninges

Dura

The dura (or pachymeninges) is a thick, dense, fibrous connective tissue that is made up of 2 layers: An outer (peri- or endosteal) layer and an inner (meningeal) layer. These outer and inner layers are closely adherent and apposed except where they separate to enclose the venous sinuses.

The outer layer forms the periosteum of the calvaria, tightly attached to the inner table, particularly at the sutures. The inner layer folds to form the falx cerebri, tentorium, and diaphragma sellae. It also divides the cranial cavity into compartments. On imaging, the dura usually shows smooth, thin enhancement (< 2 mm).

The dura forms 2 important potential spaces. First, the epidural space is located between the dura and the inner table of the calvaria. Important lesions of the epidural space include hemorrhage related to trauma and infection causing an empyema, a rare but potentially lethal complication of sinusitis. Second, the subdural space is the potential space between the inner (meningeal) layer of the dura and the arachnoid. A traumatic subdural hematoma is the most common process to affect the subdural space (more accurately, it probably collects within the border cell layer along the inner margin of the dura). The subdural space may also be affected by infection, either a subdural effusion related to meningitis or a subdural empyema related to meningitis in a child or sinusitis in an adult.

Leptomeninges

The leptomeninges are formed by the arachnoid and pia. The arachnoid is loosely attached to the dural border cell layer. Pathologies often affect both the arachnoid and dura together, and the 2 areas cannot be easily differentiated on imaging.

The arachnoid is a thin, nearly transparent layer of meninges closely applied to the inner (meningeal) dura. It forms the outer margin of the subarachnoid space (SAS). It does not enter the sulci or fissures except along the falx, where it dips into the interhemispheric fissure. Trabeculae extend from the arachnoid across the SAS to the pia and are invested with a thin pia-like layer. The SAS is a cerebrospinal fluid (CSF)-filled space between the arachnoid and pia.

The pia is a thin, delicate membrane closely applied to the brain. It covers vessels and trabeculae in the SAS and lines the perivascular spaces.

Perivascular (Virchow-Robin) spaces are normal variants. They appear as interstitial fluid-filled, pial-lined spaces that accompany penetrating arteries and veins.

Arachnoid Granulations

Arachnoid granulations are normal extensions of the SAS and arachnoid through the dural wall and into the venous sinuses. They are covered with arachnoid cap cells and venous sinus endothelium. CSF drains through the endothelium into the venous sinus. The most common locations for arachnoid granulations are the superior sagittal sinus and transverse sinuses. These normal variants are important "pseudolesions" to recognize, as they may be misdiagnosed as pathology. They are CSF density or intensity on imaging and do not enhance. They are often associated with bone changes on CT, particularly in the occipital bone.

Differential Diagnosis

The following differential diagnosis lists are provided to help organize the most common scalp, skull, and meningeal lesions.

Scalp Masses

- Subgaleal hematoma, foreign body (most common)
- Trichilemmal ("sebaceous") cyst
- Lipoma
- Dermoid
- Metastases (extension from calvaria)
- Vascular malformation (sinus pericranii in a child)
- Skin cancer (basal cell or squamous cell)

Calvarial Thickening

- Normal variant (most common)
- Chronic phenytoin (Dilantin) therapy
- Shunted hydrocephalus
- Paget disease
- Fibrous dysplasia
- Hyperparathyroidism
- Acromegaly
- Anemias

Calvarial Thinning

- Normal variants (parietal thinning) (most common)
- Arachnoid cyst
- Mega cisterna magna

- Peripherally located tumors (oligodendroglioma, dysembryoplastic neuroepithelial tumors)

"Hair on End"
- Classic appearance of anemias: Thalassemia, sickle cell disease, hereditary spherocytosis
- Skull hemangioma
- Metastases (commonly neuroblastoma and prostate cancer)

Lytic Skull Lesion
- Normal variant or surgical defects (most common)
- Metastases
- Epidermoid cyst
- Eosinophilic granuloma
- Hemangioma
- Paget disease
- Plasmacytoma
- Osteomyelitis

Sclerotic Skull Lesion
- Metastasis (most common)
- Osteoma
- Fibrous dysplasia
- Meningioma-associated
- Paget disease

Diffuse Dura-Arachnoid Enhancement
- Post operative or post procedure (i.e., lumbar puncture)
- Chronic subdural hematoma
- Meningitis (leptomeningeal enhancement common)
- Neoplasm
- Neurosarcoid
- Intracranial hypotension (venous congestion)
- Hypertrophic pachymeningitis (may be IgG4 related)
- Dural sinus thrombosis

Pial Enhancement
- Meningitis (infectious or neoplastic); neurosarcoid

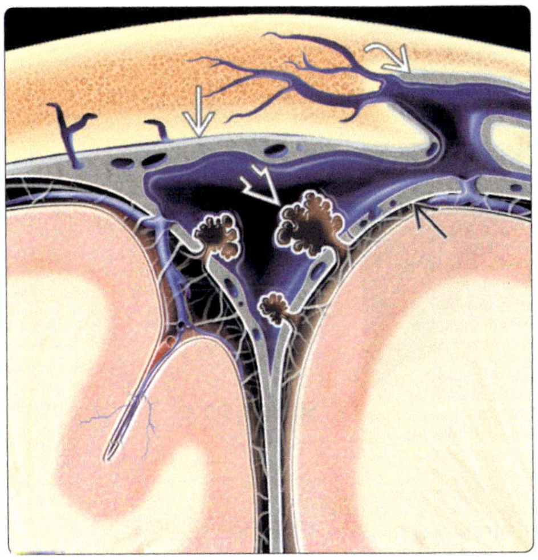

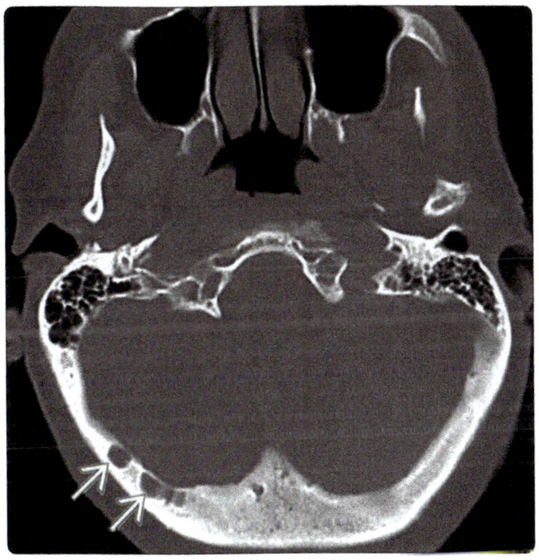

(Left) *Coronal graphic shows the calvarial apex with the superior sagittal sinus (SSS) and a venous lake ➡. The SSS is formed by 2 dural layers, an outer (periosteal) layer ➡ and inner (meningeal) layer. Arachnoid granulations ➡ extend from the arachnoid into the SSS. The arachnoid ➡ is closely applied to the inner layer of dura.* **(Right)** *Axial bone CT shows multiple sharply marginated, lucent, occipital bone lesions ➡ adjacent to the transverse sinus, characteristic of arachnoid granulations.*

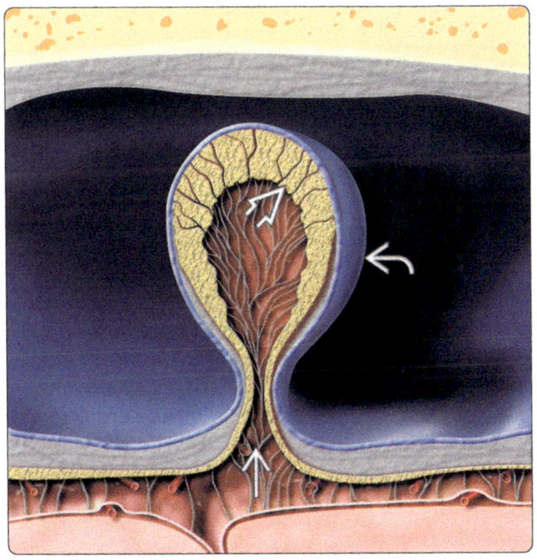

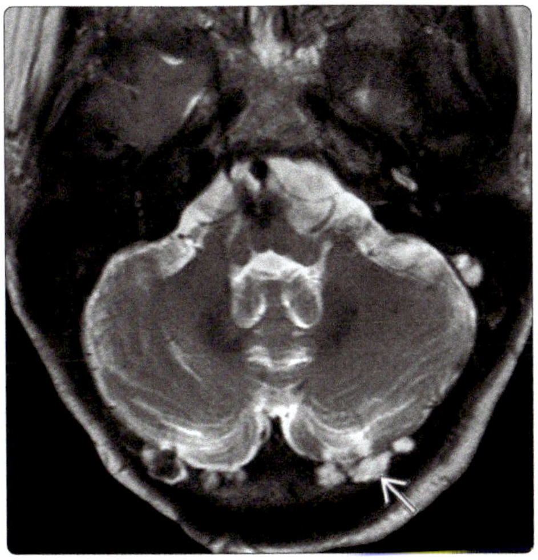

(Left) *Coronal graphic shows an arachnoid granulation projecting from the subarachnoid space (SAS) into the SSS. A cerebrospinal fluid (CSF) core ➡ extends into the arachnoid granulation and is separated by arachnoid cap cells ➡ from the venous sinus endothelium ➡. Arachnoid granulations allow drainage of CSF into the venous circulation.* **(Right)** *Axial T2WI FS MR shows multiple CSF signal intensity lesions representing arachnoid granulations ➡ in the occipital bone, a typical location.*

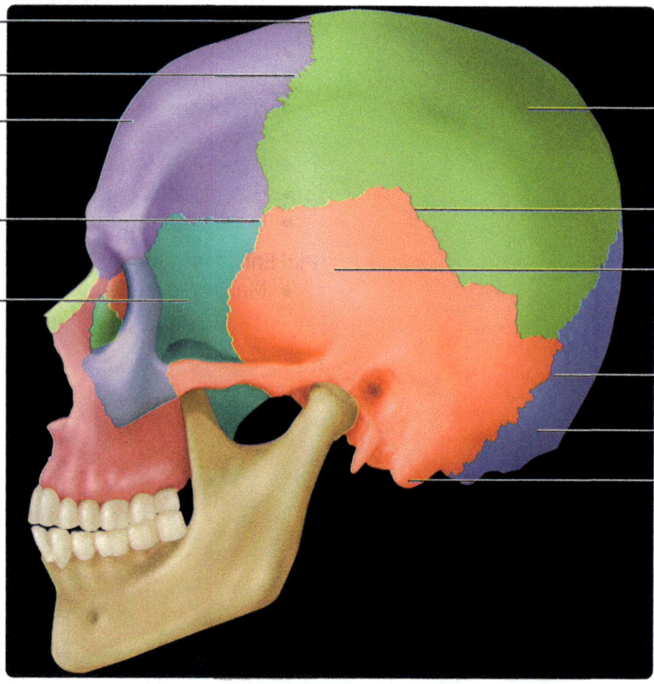

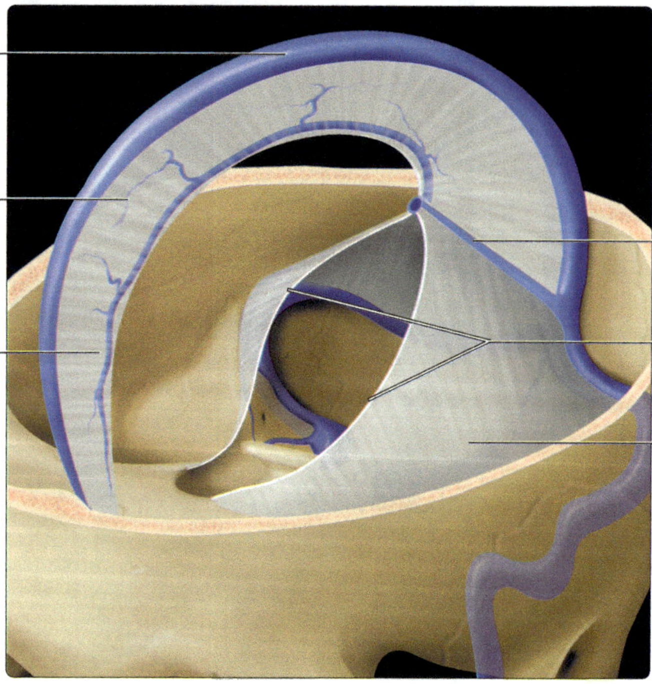

(Top) *Lateral view shows calvarial vault components. The pterion, an important surgical landmark, is a small area on the lateral skull at the intersection of the frontal, parietal, sphenoid, and squamosal temporal bones.* **(Bottom)** *Graphic shows the major dural sinuses as they relate to the falx cerebri and tentorium cerebelli. The falx inserts on the crista galli anteriorly and sweeps backward in the midline to the straight sinus, becoming taller as it passes posteriorly. The tentorium meets the falx at the tentorial apex and curves downward to contain the transverse sinuses. The leaves of the tentorium insert anteriorly on the petrous apex, and fibers extend forward to the anterior clinoid processes.*

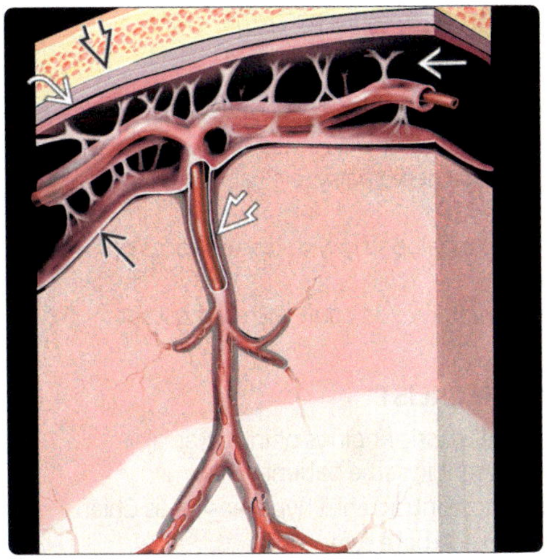

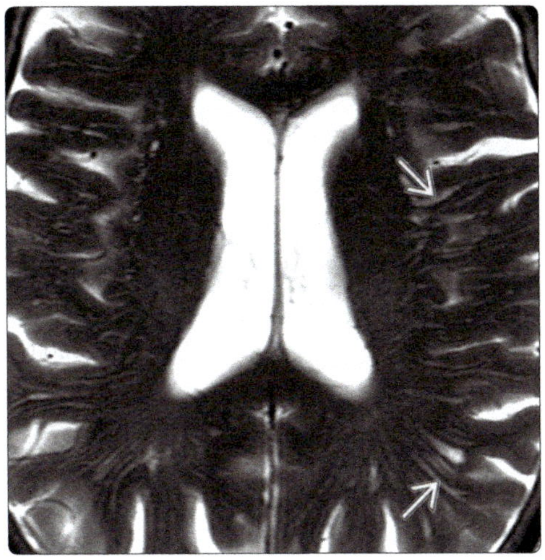

(Left) *Coronal graphic shows the cranial meninges and SAS ➡. The pia is a thin delicate membrane that covers the brain ⇨ as well as the vessels and trabeculae in the SAS. The pia also invaginates along a penetrating cortical artery to form a perivascular space ➡. The arachnoid ➡ forms the outer margin of the SAS and is loosely attached to the dura ⇨.* **(Right)** *Axial T2WI MR at 3T shows multiple normal perivascular spaces ➡ in the subcortical and deep white matter.*

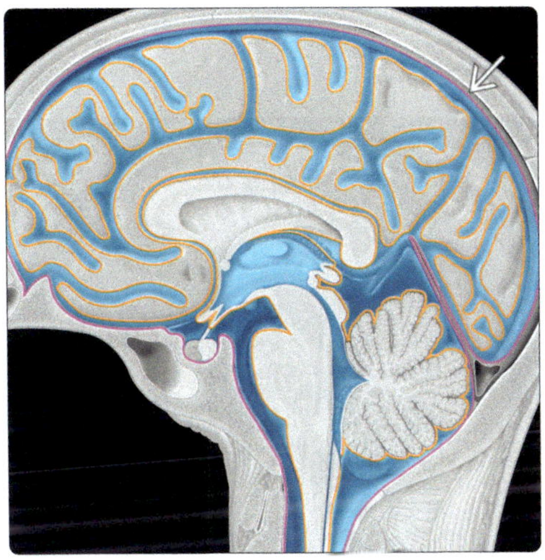

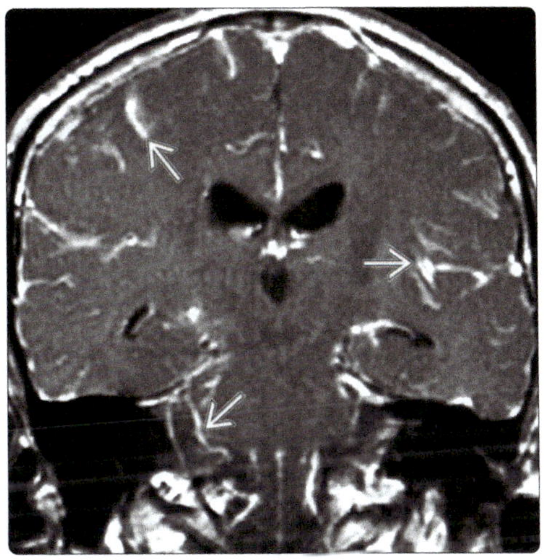

(Left) *Sagittal graphic depicts the cranial leptomeninges as they enclose the CSF cisterns, shown in blue. The arachnoid ➡ (purple) follows the dura around the inner calvaria but does not invaginate into the sulci. The pia (orange) is the innermost layer of leptomeninges and follows the brain surface and dips into the sulci. The SAS lies between the pia and arachnoid.* **(Right)** *Coronal T1 C+ MR shows extensive abnormal leptomeningeal enhancement ➡ related to infectious meningitis.*

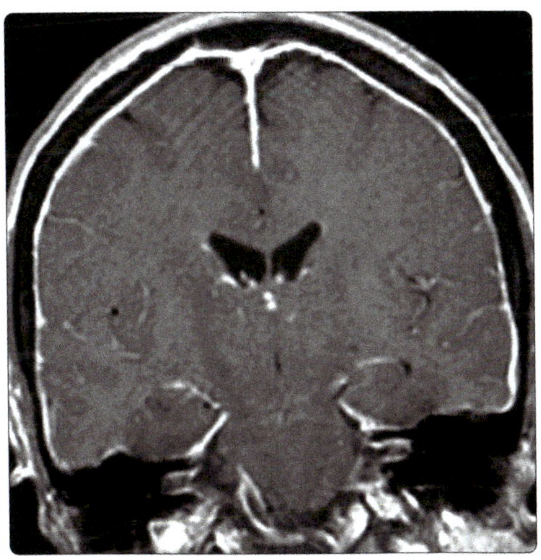

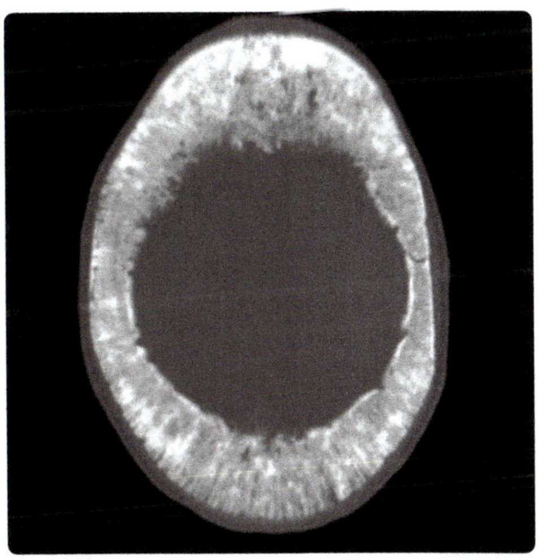

(Left) *Coronal T1 C+ MR shows diffuse dural enhancement related to intracranial hypotension in this patient with a CSF leak. Diffuse dural enhancement is commonly related to a prior procedure, infection, or inflammatory etiology. Venous congestion is the cause of the enhancement in intracranial hypotension.* **(Right)** *Axial bone CT shows diffuse calvarial thickening with widening of the diploic marrow resulting in a "hair on end" appearance. Thalassemia major is the most common cause of this classic imaging finding.*

KEY FACTS

TERMINOLOGY

- Headache caused by ↓ intracranial CSF pressure

IMAGING

- Classic imaging
  - Diffuse dural thickening/enhancement
    - Smooth, not nodular or "lumpy-bumpy"
  - Downward displacement of brain through incisura ("slumping" midbrain)
  - Veins, dural sinuses distended
  - ± subdural hygromas/hematomas
- Other: Midbrain elongated, ambient cisterns effaced on axial T2WI

TOP DIFFERENTIAL DIAGNOSES

- Meningitis
- Meningeal metastases
- Chronic subdural hematoma
- Dural sinus thrombosis
- Postsurgical dural thickening
- Idiopathic hypertrophic cranial pachymeningitis

CLINICAL ISSUES

- Severe headache (orthostatic, persistent, pulsatile, or even associated with nuchal rigidity)
- Uncommon: Cranial nerve palsy (e.g., abducens), visual disturbances
- Rare: Severe encephalopathy with disturbances of consciousness
- Profile: Young/middle-aged adult with orthostatic headache

DIAGNOSTIC CHECKLIST

- Only rarely are **all** classic findings of intracranial hypotension present in same patient
- Do not misdiagnose intracranial hypotension as Chiari 1
  - Surgery can exacerbate symptoms
  - In rare cases can be fatal

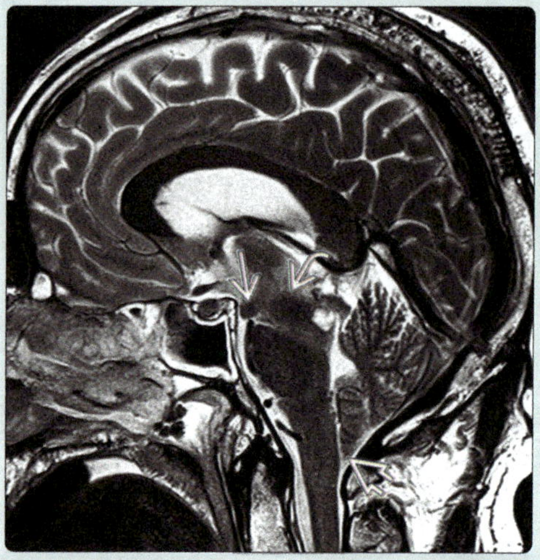
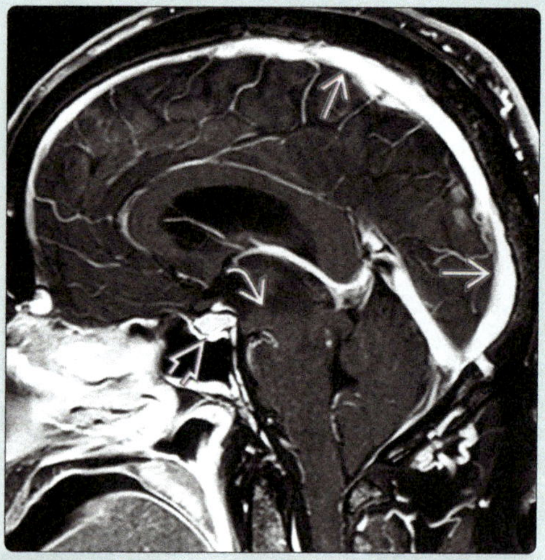

(Left) *Sagittal T2WI in a 57-year-old man treated for "migraine" headaches shows severe midbrain "slumping", downwardly displaced cerebellar tonsils, draping of hypothalamus over dorsum sellae with mammillary bodies below dorsum.* **(Right)** *Sagittal T1 C+ FS MR in the same case shows the severe midbrain "slumping" and inferiorly displaced tonsils. In addition, the pituitary gland appears "fat", and the dural venous sinuses are engorged.*

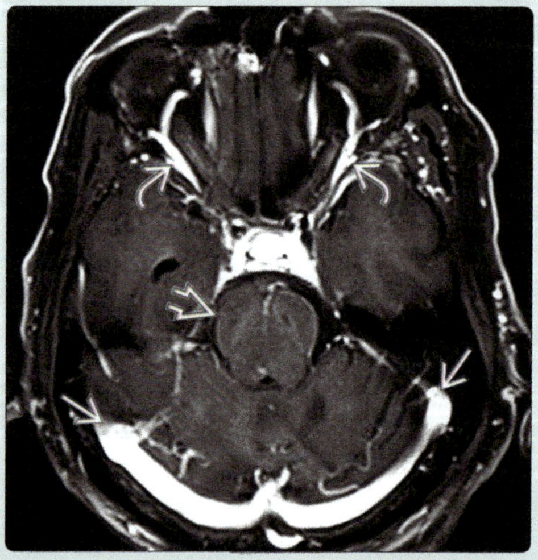
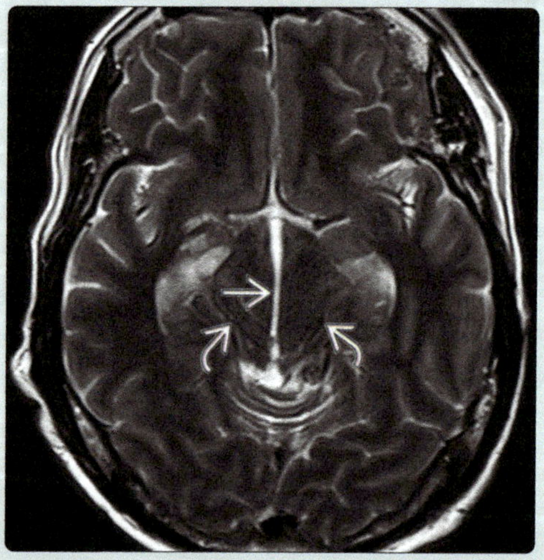

(Left) *Axial T1 C+ FS scan in the same case shows a "fat" midbrain/pons, prominent superior ophthalmic veins, and engorged, outwardly convex transverse/sigmoid sinuses. No subdural hematomas were identified. Severe intracranial hypotension was treated successfully with blood patch.* **(Right)** *Axial T2WI in the same case shows the inferiorly displaced 3rd ventricle superimposed on the compressed midbrain. The ambient cisterns are completely effaced.*

Skull Base CSF Leak

KEY FACTS

IMAGING

- Best clue
  - Anterior or central skull base (**SB**) **defect** on bone CT with **positive β2-transferrin** test on nasal secretions
- Anterior SB bone CT findings
  - Bone defect in cribriform plate, lateral lamella of middle turbinate or ethmoid roof
  - Other evidence for fracture, functional endoscopic sinus surgery (FESS), congenital cephalocele
- Central SB bone CT findings
  - Bone defect in sella floor (transnasal pituitary surgery, craniopharyngeal canal persistence), lateral wall sphenoid (arachnoid granulation)

TOP DIFFERENTIAL DIAGNOSES

- Vasomotor rhinitis
- SB defect without cerebrospinal fluid (CSF) leak

PATHOLOGY

- Can be congenital or acquired (post trauma, surgery)
- **Congenital** CSF leak
  - Cribriform plate defect, congenital cephalocele, persistent craniopharyngeal canal
- **Acquired** leak: From arachnoid granulation (pit, osteodural defect) or "spontaneous"
  - Lateral roof of sphenoid sinus
- **Posttraumatic** leak: Can occur with any sinonasal fracture
  - Roof or lateral wall of sphenoid sinus or cribriform plate/ethmoid roof
- **Postoperative** defect: Can occur after any sinonasal or anterior or central SB surgery

CLINICAL ISSUES

- Rhinorrhea with Valsalva or head-down maneuvers
- **β2-transferrin** is single best test to confirm fluid from nose is CSF
- Persistent CSF leaks endoscopically repaired

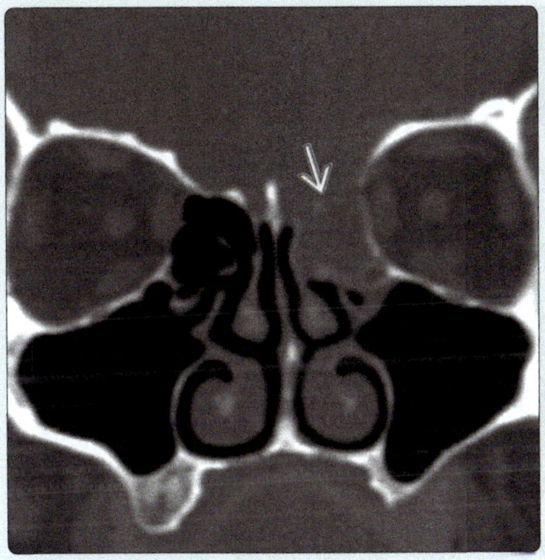

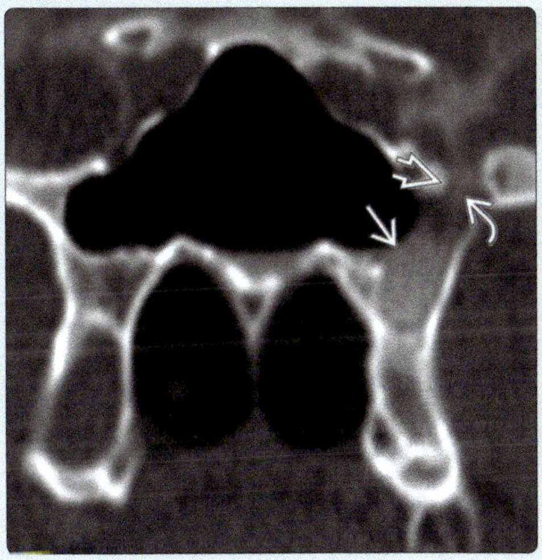

(Left) *Coronal bone CT shows large bony defect in left ethmoid roof, lateral to insertion of middle turbinate. Because there is complete opacification of the ethmoid cells, an MR was performed that showed meningoencephalocele.* **(Right)** *Coronal bone CT after intrathecal contrast placement shows CSF in left sphenoid chamber, bone defect, and contrast extending through defect. CT-cisternography is rarely necessary when high-resolution bone CT and MR are performed 1st for CSF leak.*

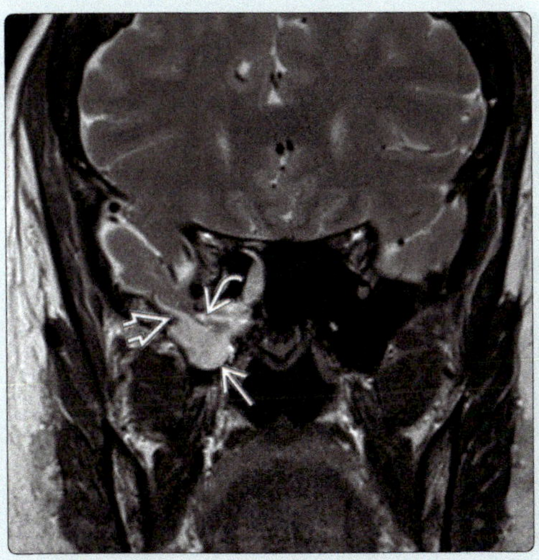

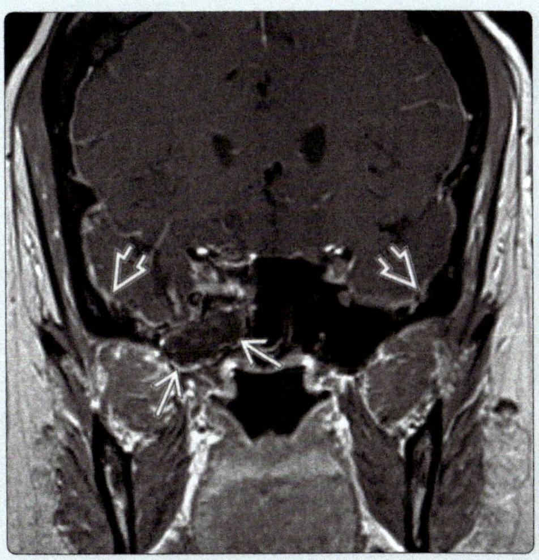

(Left) *Coronal T2WI MR reveals lateral wing of sphenoid sinus filled with CSF. Osseous defect is in roof of lateral sphenoid roof, and brain herniates through defect. This woman had a "spontaneous" CSF leak. Many such leaks are caused by large arachnoid granulations.* **(Right)** *Coronal T1WI C+ MR in the same patient shows peripheral enhancement on the margin of the sphenoid meningoencephalocele. Note diffuse thin dural enhancement, including at the defect site, secondary to leak.*

KEY FACTS

TERMINOLOGY

- Definition: Nonspecific, nonneoplastic benign inflammatory lesion without identifiable local or systemic causes characterized by polymorphous lymphoplasmacytic infiltrate
- Idiopathic orbital inflammation
  - May involve any part(s) of orbit
- Idiopathic extraorbital inflammation
  - **Intracranial involvement**: Spread through superior orbital fissure (SOF) or optic canal (OC)
    - Cavernous sinus, dura, Meckel cave
  - **Skull base-extracranial involvement**: Spreads from inferior orbital fissure (IOF) or through orbital wall
    - Anterior skull base, sinuses, nasopharyngeal spaces
- IgG4-related disease: Subgroup of idiopathic inflammation with systemic involvement
  - Intracranial noncontiguous sites: Pituitary, infundibulum
  - Extracranial noncontiguous H&N sites: Parotid, submandibular glands, thyroid

IMAGING

- T1WI C+ FS MR: Diffusely enhancing, infiltrating mass
  - Extends from orbit through SOF ± OC to cavernous sinus, dura, Meckel cave
  - Extends through IOF to pterygopalatine fossa, nose, deep nasopharyngeal spaces
- T2: Iso- to **hypointense** lesion; ↑ fibrosis, ↓ intensity

TOP DIFFERENTIAL DIAGNOSES

- En plaque meningioma
- Meningeal non-Hodgkin lymphoma
- Nasopharyngeal carcinoma
- Neurosarcoid

CLINICAL ISSUES

- Symptoms: Painful proptosis ± headaches ± cranial neuropathies (Tolosa Hunt syndrome)
- Diagnosis of exclusion (draw IgG4 levels; biopsy)
- Treatment: High-dose systemic **steroids**

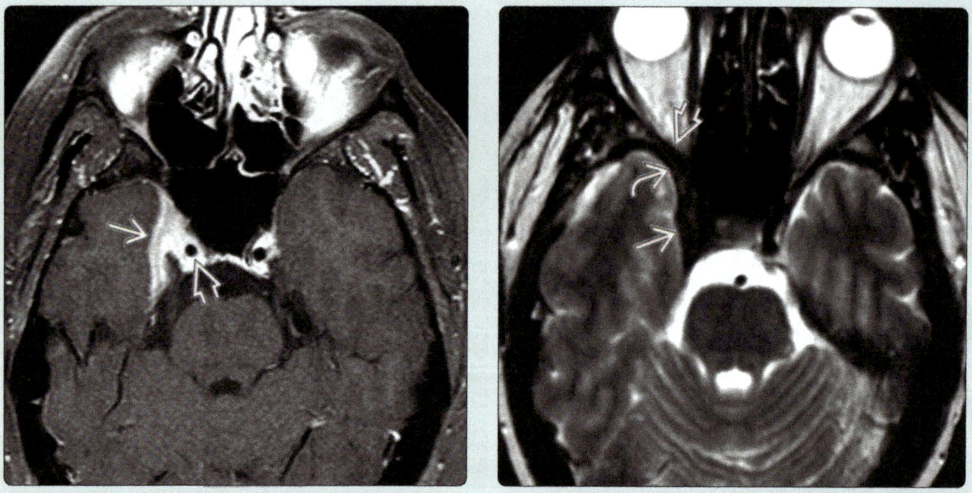

(Left) *Axial T1WI C+ FS MR shows a focus of enhancing idiopathic extraorbital inflammation (IEI) involving the right cavernous sinus with subtle narrowing of the intracavernous internal carotid artery.* **(Right)** *Axial T2WI MR in the same patient reveals that an idiopathic orbital inflammation lesion connects to the cavernous sinus IEI through the superior orbital fissure. Both areas of idiopathic inflammation are hypointense due to the fibrosis often found within this lesion.*

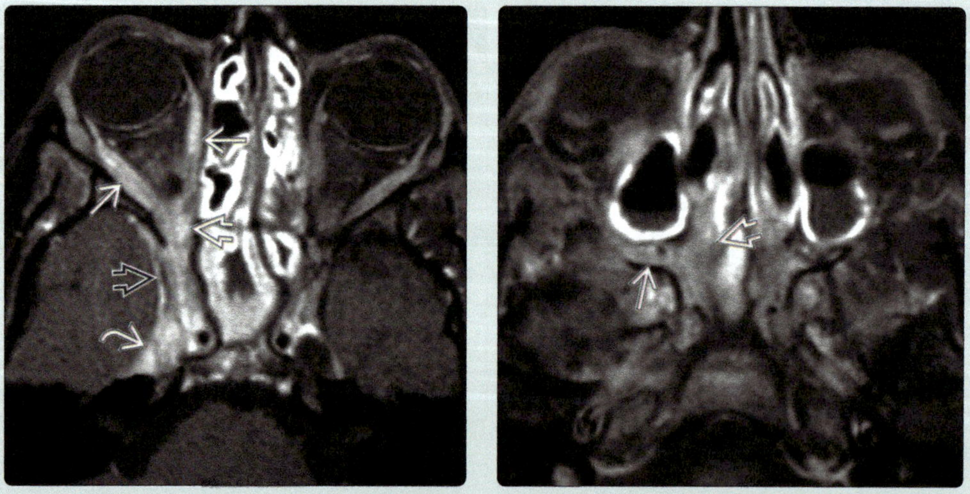

(Left) *Axial T1WI C+ FS MR through the orbits shows enlarged, enhancing orbital rectus muscles connecting through the superior orbital fissure with the cavernous sinus and Meckel cave. First impression of adenoid cystic carcinoma gave way to biopsy-proven idiopathic inflammation with both intraorbital and intracranial components.* **(Right)** *Axial T1WI C+ FS MR in the same patient shows the lesion invading inferiorly through the inferior orbital fissure into the pterygopalatine fossa and nose.*

KEY FACTS

TERMINOLOGY

- IgG4-related disease (IgG4-RD)
- Chronic fibroinflammatory disease characterized by IgG4(+) plasma cell infiltrates

IMAGING

- Diffusely infiltrating enhancing mass
  - Orbital adnexa (lacrimal gland most common)
  - Dura-arachnoid (IgG4-related hypertrophic pachymeningitis)
  - Pituitary gland, stalk (hypophysitis)
  - Other: Cranial nerves (especially infraorbital nerve), brain (autoimmune-like encephalopathy)
- MR
  - Isointense to brain on T1WI, hypointense on T2WI
  - Enhances strongly, uniformly

TOP DIFFERENTIAL DIAGNOSES

- Idiopathic inflammatory pseudotumor
- Meningioma
- Neurosarcoid
- Lymphoma

CLINICAL ISSUES

- All ages, but 6th-7th decades most common
  - Exophthalmos, headache
  - Cranial neuropathy
- Clinical course
  - Glucocorticosteroids → improvement/remission (relapses common if tapered/discontinued)
- Between 3-30% of IgG4-RD patients have normal serum IgG4 concentrations
- Elevated serum IgG4 is **not** diagnostic of IgG4-RD (neither sensitive nor specific)

DIAGNOSTIC CHECKLIST

- Best diagnostic clue is combination of clinical history, physical examination, laboratory, imaging

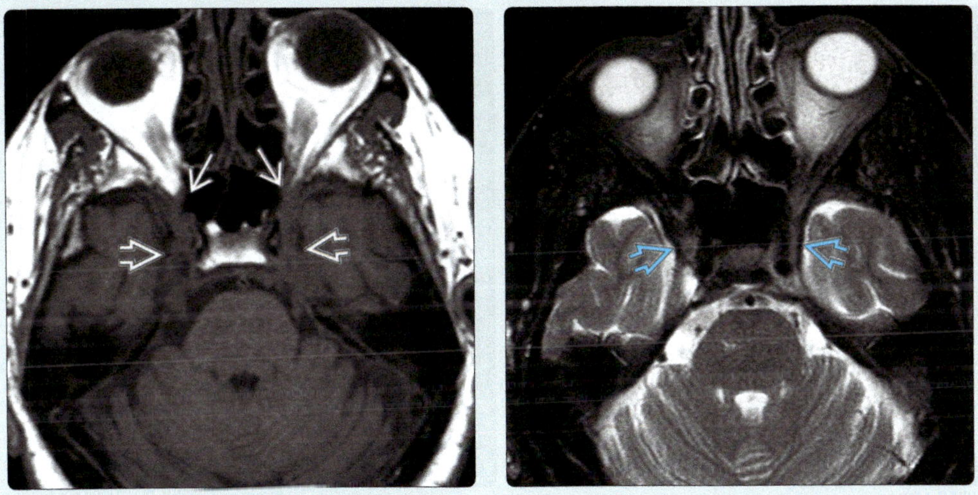

(Left) *Axial T1WI MR in an 81-year-old man with decreasing vision in his left eye shows diffuse infiltration of the cavernous sinus* ➡ *and orbital apices* ➡ *by soft tissue that is isointense relative to the brain. The lacrimal glands are not affected.* **(Right)** *Axial T2 FS MR in the same patient shows that the infiltrates* ➡ *are hypointense relative to the brain.*

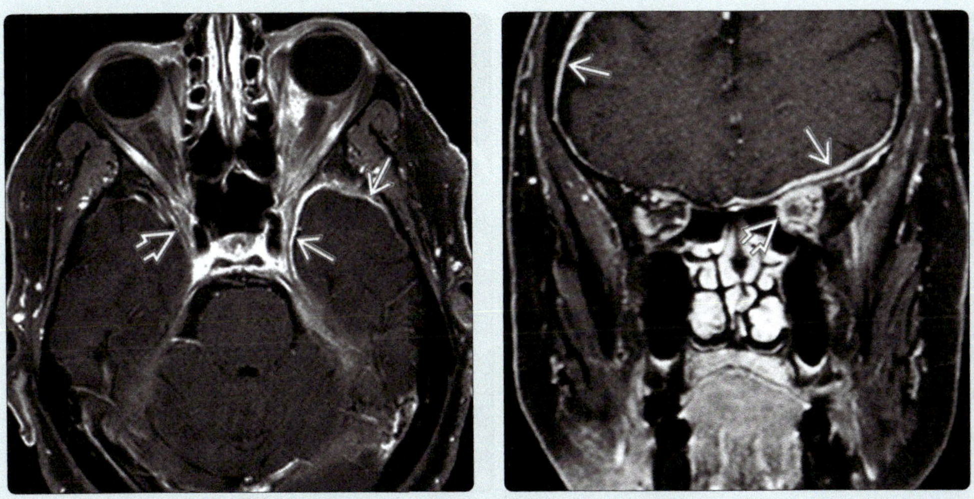

(Left) *T1 C+ FS MR in the same patient shows that the cavernous sinus* ➡ *and orbital apex infiltrates enhance strongly. In addition, note thickened, enhancing dura-arachnoid* ➡ *in the left middle cranial fossa.* **(Right)** *Coronal T1 C+ FS scan in the same case shows that the dura-arachnoid enhancement is bilateral* ➡*, and the posterior orbit is filled with enhancing soft tissue* ➡ *that surrounds and encases the left optic nerve. Biopsy disclosed IgG4-related disease is shown.*

Fibrous Dysplasia

KEY FACTS

TERMINOLOGY

- Fibrous dysplasia (FD)
  - Synonyms: Craniofacial fibrous dysplasia (CFD), osteitis fibrosa, osteodystrophy fibrosa
- McCune-Albright syndrome (MAS)
  - 1 of most common FD syndromes
- Congenital disorder characterized by expanding lesion(s)
  - Defect in osteoblastic differentiation, maturation
  - Contains mixture of fibrous tissue, woven bone

IMAGING

- Best diagnostic clue: Ground-glass matrix in bone lesion on CT
- CFD: Majority have > 1 bone involved
- MR: ↓ T2WI signal throughout (if solid) or in rim (if cystic)
  - Variable enhancement
  - Rim, diffuse, or none

TOP DIFFERENTIAL DIAGNOSES

- Paget disease
- Garré sclerosing osteomyelitis
- Meningioma

CLINICAL ISSUES

- Most common signs/symptoms: Painless swelling or deformity
- Demographics
  - < 6 years (39%), 6-10 years (27%), > 10 years (39%)
  - MAS usually (but not exclusively) female
  - Monostotic FD 6x more common than polyostotic FD
  - Monostotic FD (75%): 25% found in skull, face
  - Polyostotic FD (25%): 50% found in skull, face
  - Calvarial involvement differs: Polyostotic FD (50%) > monostotic FD (25%)
- RARE progression to fibro-, osteo-, chondro-, and mesenchymal sarcoma

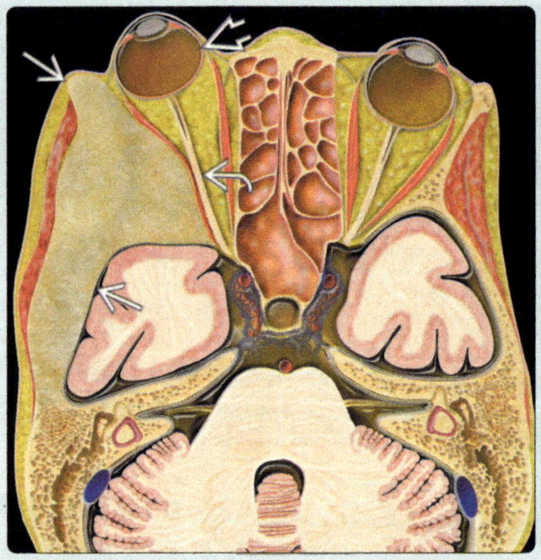

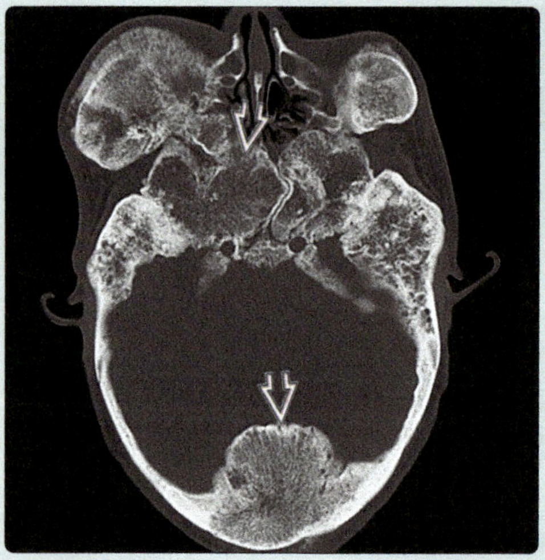

(Left) *Axial graphic shows expansion of the lateral orbital rim, sphenoid wing, and temporal squamosa by fibrous dysplasia (FD) ➡. Note the exophthalmos ➡ and stretching of the optic nerve ➡ on the ipsilateral side.* **(Right)** *Axial bone CT scan in a 19-year-old man with craniofacial dysplasia (polyostotic FD) shows gross overgrowth of facial bones, skull base with classic "ground glass" matrix in the affected bones ➡.*

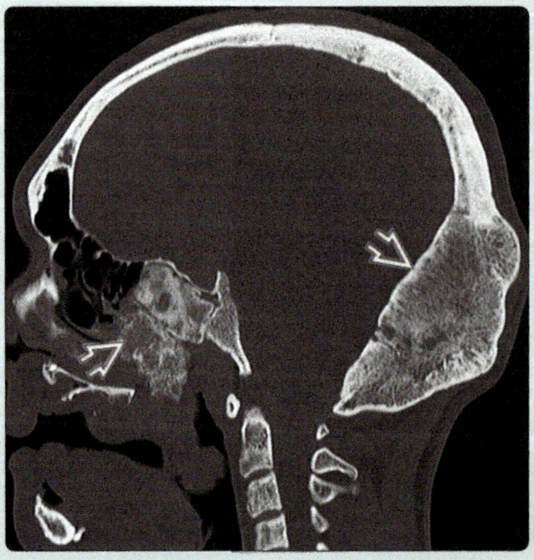

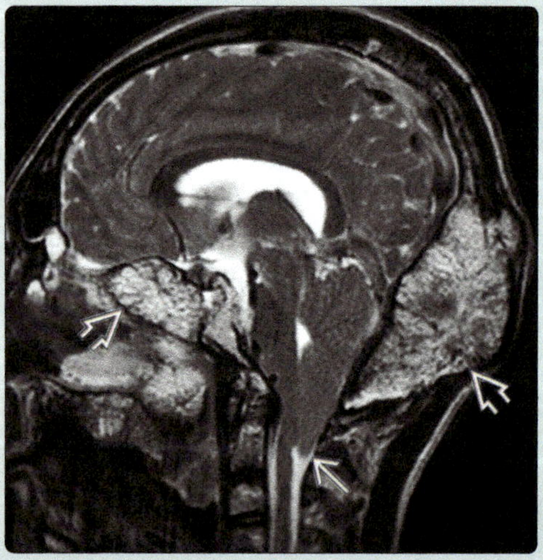

(Left) *Sagittal bone CT reformatted from the axial scan data in the same case demonstrates the "ground glass" ➡ in the expanded bones typical for FD.* **(Right)** *Sagittal T2WI in the same case shows that the expanded bones appear hyperintense ➡. Signal intensity in FD is quite variable. In older patients with "burned out" sclerotic FD, the signal intensity is often quite hypointense (dark). Note compression of brainstem and cerebellum, with inferiorly displaced tonsil ➡.*

KEY FACTS

TERMINOLOGY

- Chronic metabolic skeletal disorder
- Characterized by bony expansion with variable destruction ± sclerosis

IMAGING

- Well-circumscribed, sharply marginated defects &/or marked thickening + sclerosis
- Skull in 25-65% (may be isolated to skull base)
  - Diploic widening, coarse trabecula, thick cortices
  - "Tam-o'-shanter" skull: Marked ↑ diploic space, particularly inner table
  - "Cotton wool" skull: Focal sclerosis within previous areas of "osteoporosis circumscripta"
- Platybasia
- Typically "hot" throughout all bone scan acquisitions (blood flow, blood pool, static)
- Bone scans + radiographs abnormal in 56-86%

TOP DIFFERENTIAL DIAGNOSES

- Osteosclerotic metastases
- Osteolytic metastases
- Fibrous dysplasia
- Other causes of calvarial thickening

PATHOLOGY

- Excessive and abnormal remodeling of bone, with both active and quiescent phases
  - Localized areas of ↑ bone resorption + exuberant but aberrant new bone formation
- Individual sites progress at variable rates
  - PD of differing phases may be seen within same patient

CLINICAL ISSUES

- 20% asymptomatic; pain, tenderness, ↑ hat size
- New pain/swelling → malignant transformation

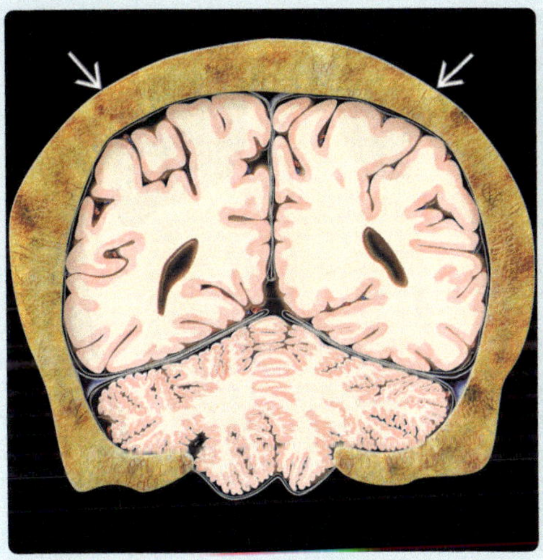

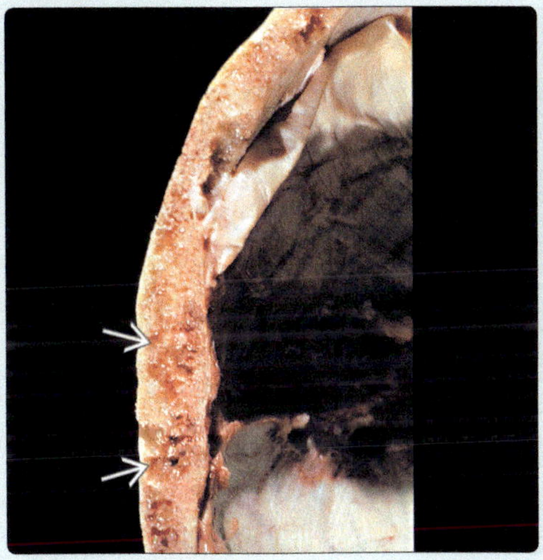

(Left) *Coronal graphic illustrates diffuse Paget disease of the skull with severe diploic widening ➡.* **(Right)** *Autopsy specimen shows pagetoid changes in the calvaria with diffuse thickening, replacement of fatty marrow with fibrovascular tissue ➡. (Courtesy E.T. Hedley-Whyte, MD.)*

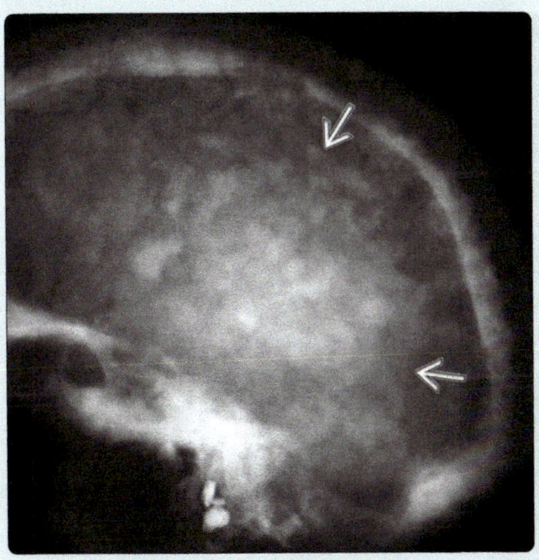

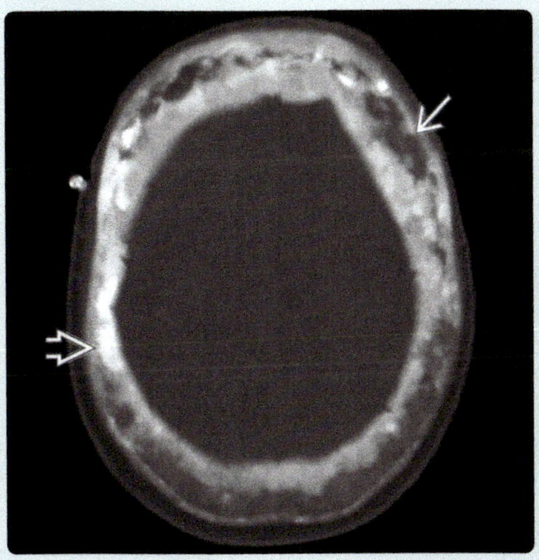

(Left) *Lateral radiograph shows classic cotton wool appearance ➡ of mixed active stage Paget disease, with enlarged bone (thickened calvaria), mixed lytic and sclerotic foci, and confluent nodular calcifications.* **(Right)** *Axial bone CT shows the mixed areas of bony lysis ➡ and sclerosis ➡ that produces the cotton wool appearance seen on digital radiographs of mixed active stage Paget disease.*

KEY FACTS

TERMINOLOGY

- Skull thickening (ST)
  - Diploic space expanded ± thickened cortex

IMAGING

- Widened calvaria (skull width)
  - Can be diffuse or focal
- NECT best for most causes of ST
  - Thin-section bone CT for detailed skull base evaluation
- MR C+ contrast: Look for adjacent dural involvement

TOP DIFFERENTIAL DIAGNOSES

- Normal variation (most common cause)
- Shunted hydrocephalus or infantile brain injury
  - Neonatal meningitis or cerebritis
  - Hypoxia/ischemia/hypoglycemia in neonatal period
  - Metabolic/genetic disease with infantile brain atrophy
  - ± phenytoin
- Metastases (diffuse sclerotic)
- Microcephaly
- Chronic anemias

CLINICAL ISSUES

- Often asymptomatic
- Patients with skull base ST
  - Look for foraminal/canal overgrowth/encroachment
  - May cause cranial neuropathy
- In many cases, evaluation of underlying brain can help to establish diagnosis
- Many tests can help discriminate among etiologies
- Skull findings often harbinger of underlying disease
- Therapy aimed at treating underlying etiology

DIAGNOSTIC CHECKLIST

- What could be underlying clinical cause of ST?
  - Normal variant (most common)
  - Other: Metastases, anemia, parathyroid disorder, etc.

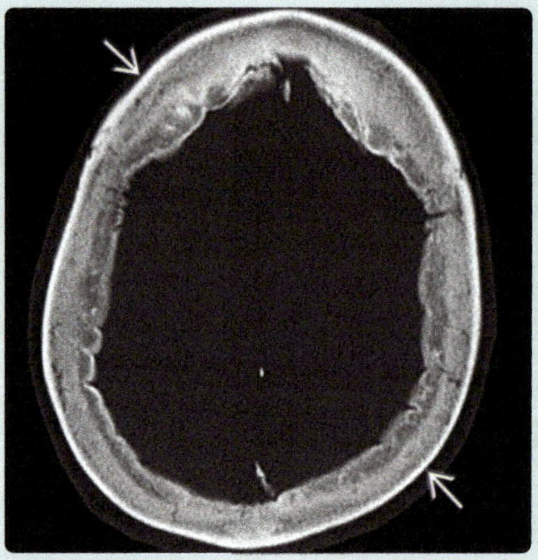

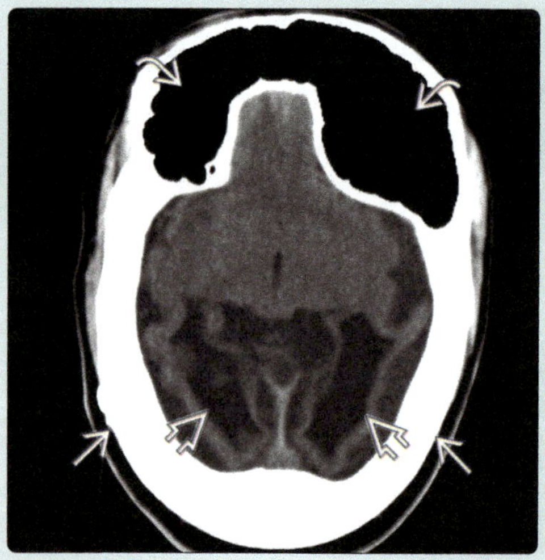

(Left) *Bone CT in a 64-year-old woman with nonspecific headaches, normal neurologic examination, shows a diffuse, circumferentially thickened calvaria ➔. The most common cause of diffusely thickened skull is a normal variant.* **(Right)** *The skull may thicken if the underlying brain is abnormally small. Due to the severe perinatal brain injury in this child, the brain is atrophic with ventriculomegaly ➔, the calvaria is massively thickened ➔, and the frontal sinuses ➔ are massively enlarged.*

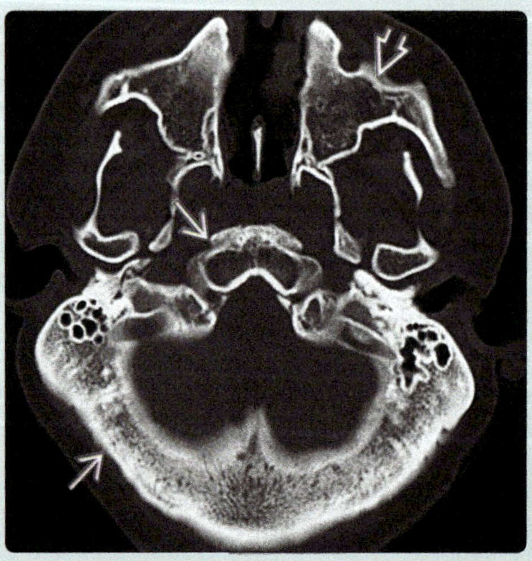

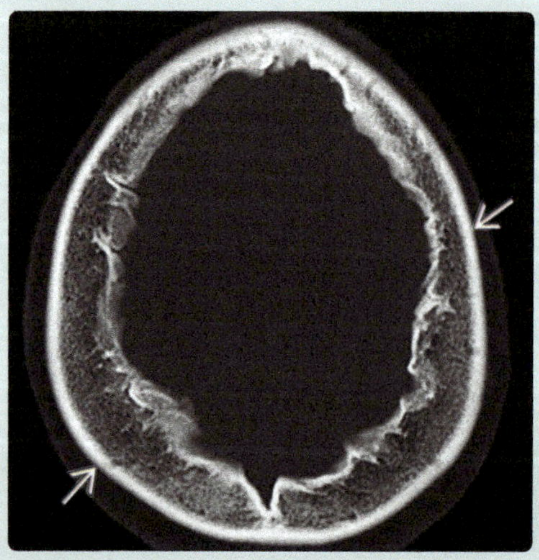

(Left) *The calvaria can be thickened in a spectrum of inherited disorders. In this 19-year-old man with known craniometaphyseal dysplasia, the occipital bone (including the clivus) is markedly thickened ➔, as are the maxillary sinuses ➔.* **(Right)** *More cephalad image in the same patient shows that the calvarial vault is also diffusely and symmetrically thickened ➔, most strikingly in the parietal bones.*

KEY FACTS

TERMINOLOGY

- Langerhans cell histiocytosis (LCH)
- LCH now best understood as neoplastic disease
  - Activating somatic *BRAF* mutations, LCH cell clonality

IMAGING

- NECT
  - Sharply marginated lytic skull defect
    - Beveled edges
  - Mastoid: Geographic destruction, soft tissue mass
- MR
  - Absent posterior pituitary "bright spot" on T1WI
  - Thick enhancing infundibulum
  - Enhancing masses in choroid plexus, leptomeninges, basal ganglia
  - Sometimes cerebellar white matter disease

TOP DIFFERENTIAL DIAGNOSES

- Lytic calvarial lesions
  - Surgical (burr hole, shunt, surgical defect)
  - Epidermoid
  - Dermoid
- Pituitary infundibular/hypothalamic thickening, enhancement
  - Germinoma; metastasis; pituicytoma; neurosarcoid

CLINICAL ISSUES

- Can be confined only to skull (often asymptomatic) but can involve other tissues also (skin, lymph glands, lungs, CNS); if > 1 organ involved, may have symptoms

DIAGNOSTIC CHECKLIST

- Calvaria is most frequent bony site involved by LCH
- Thick enhancing pituitary stalk is most common CNS manifestation of LCH
  - If initially "normal" MR in patient with diabetes insipidus, repeat in 2-3 months
- Consider LCH for ataxic patient with choroid plexus masses, cerebellar white matter demyelination

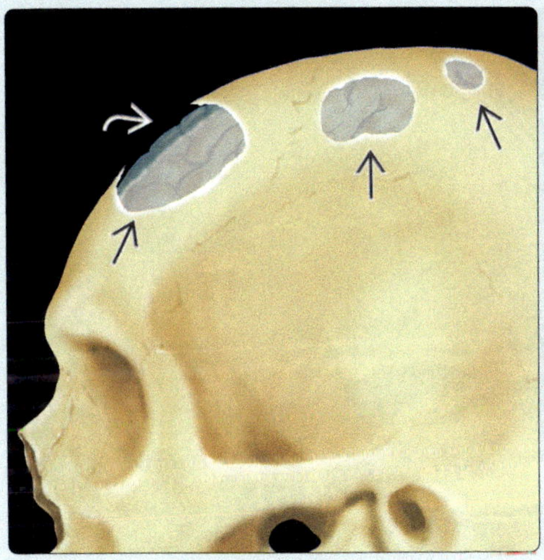

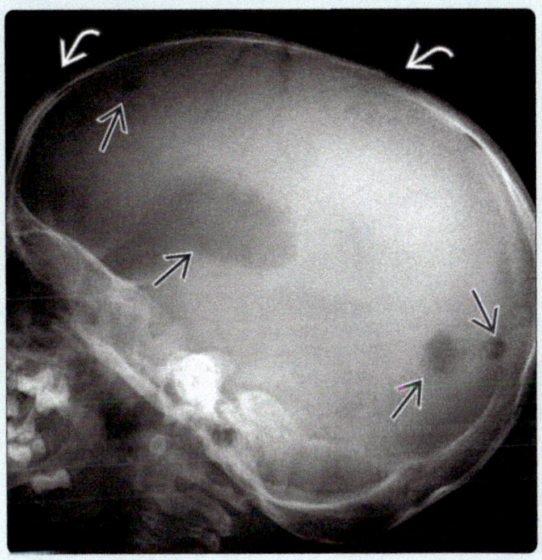

(Left) *Lateral graphic demonstrates 3 sharply defined lytic lesions* → *of the membranous calvaria with geographic destruction. Note the beveled margins of the bony lysis* ➡. **(Right)** *Lateral radiograph in a 3-year-old boy with several subcutaneous masses and central diabetes insipidus demonstrates multiple lytic lesions of the skull* →. *Note the "cookie cutter" sharp pattern of bony lysis and the beveled edge pattern* ➡ *of differential inner and outer table calvarial involvement.*

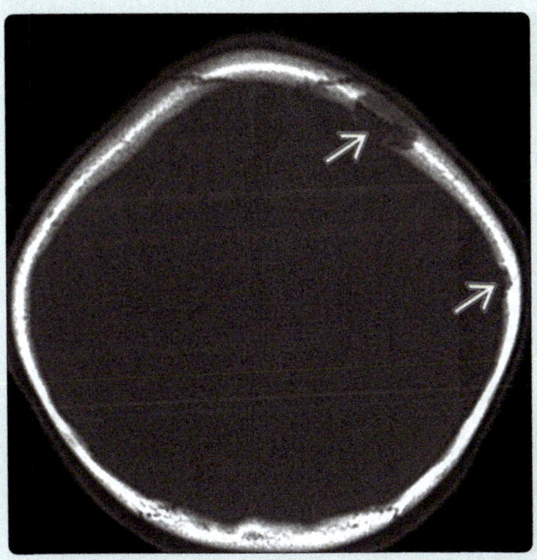

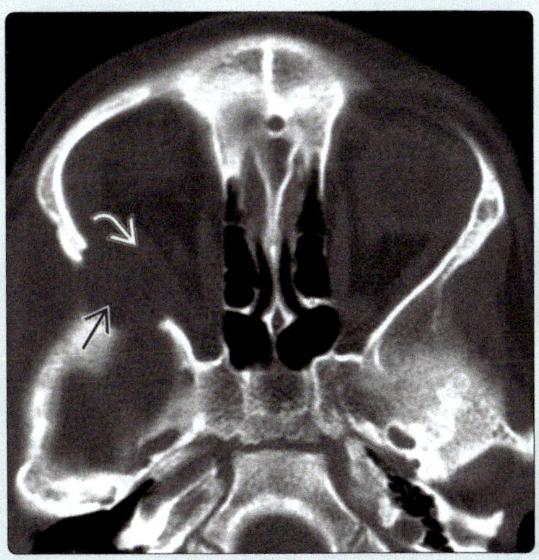

(Left) *Axial NECT in a 5-year-old girl with multiple scalp masses demonstrates 2 lytic lesions* ➡ *of the left frontal bone. Both lesions show the characteristic pattern of sharply defined geographic bony lysis. Note the unequal inner and outer table involvement creating a beveled edge appearance.* **(Right)** *Axial NECT in a proptotic 10-year-old boy shows a sharply defined lytic lesion of the lateral orbital wall* →. *Note the soft tissue mass displacing the lateral rectus muscle* ➡.

KEY FACTS

TERMINOLOGY

- Multisystem inflammatory disease characterized by noncaseating epithelioid-cell granulomas

IMAGING

- Solitary or multifocal CNS mass(es) ± abnormal CXR
  - CXR abnormal in > 90% with neurosarcoid (NS)
- Wide spectrum of MR manifestations
  - Dura-arachnoid thickening (diffuse or focal))
  - May coat pia, cranial nerves, fill internal auditory canals
  - Pituitary stalk/hypothalamus thickening
  - Can thicken, infiltrate choroid plexi
  - Can infiltrate orbital adnexa, optic nerve
  - Rare
    - Small vessel vasculitis/angiitis in white matter
    - Focal parenchymal mass

TOP DIFFERENTIAL DIAGNOSES

- Meningitis
- Meningioma
- Metastases
- Lymphocytic hypophysitis

PATHOLOGY

- Etiology remains unknown
- May infiltrate along perivascular spaces into brain

CLINICAL ISSUES

- Often indolent disease (up to 50% asymptomatic)
- CNS involved in 5% (clinical) to 27% (autopsy)
  - Most common CNS symptom: Cranial nerve deficit(s), most often facial nerve palsy
- Natural history
  - 2/3 of NS self-limited monophasic illness; remainder have chronic remitting-relapsing course

DIAGNOSTIC CHECKLIST

- Protean manifestations make NS "great mimicker"

(Left) *Sagittal graphic illustrates common neurosarcoid locations: (1) enveloping the infundibulum and extending into the parasellar region ➡; (2) contiguous disease wrapping the inferior frontal lobes ➡; and (3) synchronous lesions of the superior vermis ➡ and 4th ventricle choroid plexus ➡.* **(Right)** *Sagittal T1 C+ FS MR in a patient with neurosarcoidosis and diabetes insipidus demonstrates thickening of the infundibulum and hypothalamus ➡.*

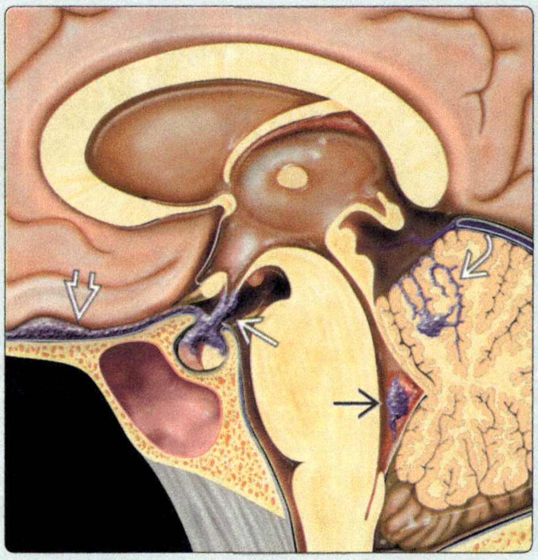

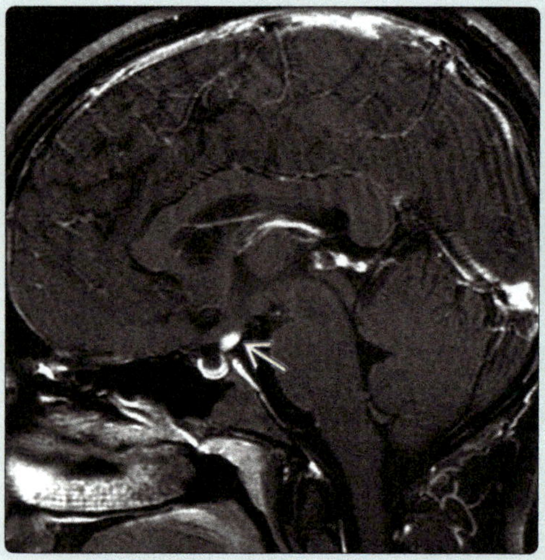

(Left) *Axial T1 C+ MR in a 44-year-old woman with worsening headaches and diplopia shows diffuse dura-arachnoid thickening over the left hemisphere ➡. Extension into the sulci ➡ and underlying brain ➡ is present. Biopsy disclosed neurosarcoid with brain invasion.* **(Right)** *Axial T1 C+ MR in a case of proven neurosarcoid demonstrates diffuse pial enhancement over the surface of the upper pons ➡ and cerebellum ➡.*

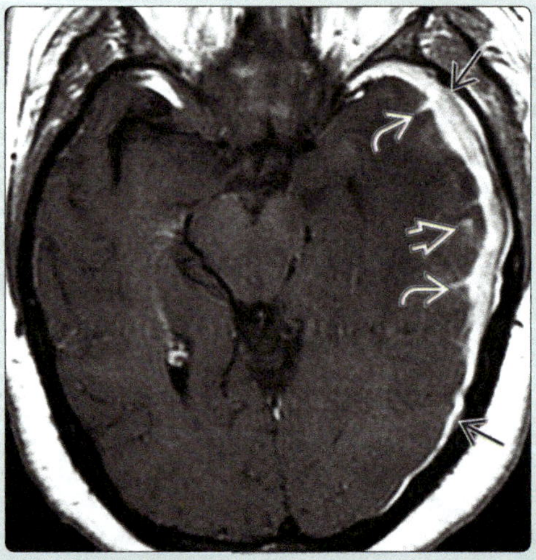

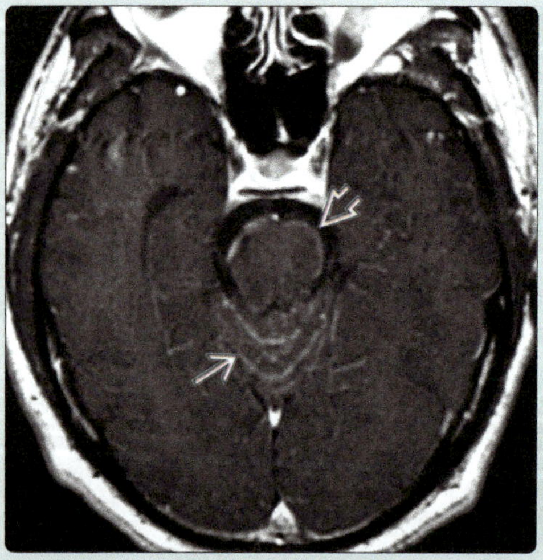

KEY FACTS

TERMINOLOGY

- Trichilemmal cyst (TC) is preferred term
  - Sebaceous cyst commonly used but incorrect
  - Variant = proliferating trichilemmal tumor
- Keratin-containing cyst
  - Lined by stratified squamous epithelium
  - Pathology looks like root sheath of hair follicle

IMAGING

- General features
  - Most within dermis or subcutaneous tissue
  - Size varies (few millimeters to several centimeters)
  - Can be single or multiple
- CT
  - Round/ovoid, well-delineated scalp mass
  - Multifocal punctate/curvilinear/coarse Ca++
- MR
  - Isointense with brain, muscle on T1WI
  - Inhomogeneously hypointense on T2WI
  - Does not suppress on FLAIR
  - Multifocal "blooming" foci common on T2*
  - Simple sebaceous cysts usually do not enhance

TOP DIFFERENTIAL DIAGNOSES

- Basal cell, squamous cell carcinoma
- Dermoid cyst
- Epidermoid cyst
- Metastasis
- Cephalocele

CLINICAL ISSUES

- Classic presentation
  - Subepidermal scalp mass in women > 60 years of age
  - Hairless, rubbery, nontender, mobile subcutaneous scalp mass(es)
  - Usually nonpainful

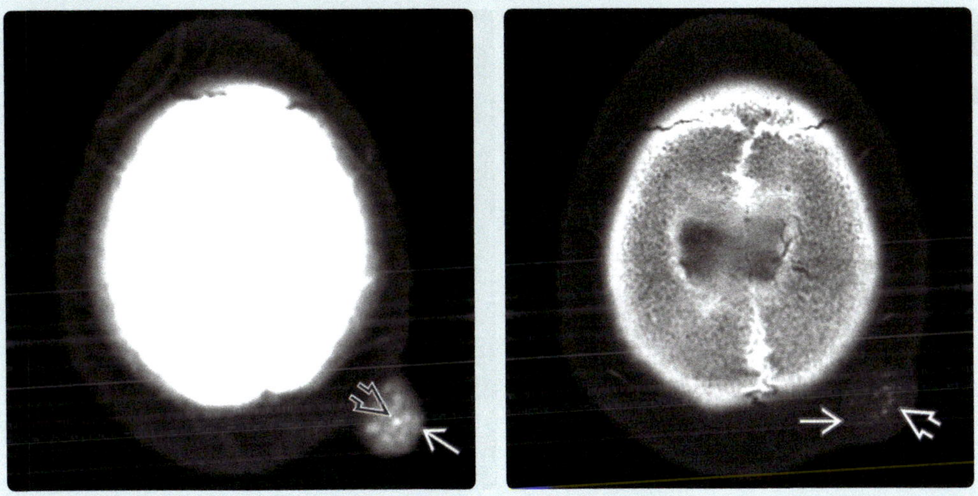

(Left) *Axial NECT in a 63-year-old man was obtained for trauma evaluation. A superficial scalp mass ➡ that contained several hyperintense foci suggesting calcifications ⇨ was incidentally noted.* **(Right)** *Axial bone CT in the same patient shows that the scalp mass ➡ is sharply delineated. Multiple punctate and curvilinear calcifications ⇨ within the mass can be seen. Note the lack of bone erosion or invasion. The remainder of the scalp appears normal. This was presumed to be a sebaceous cyst.*

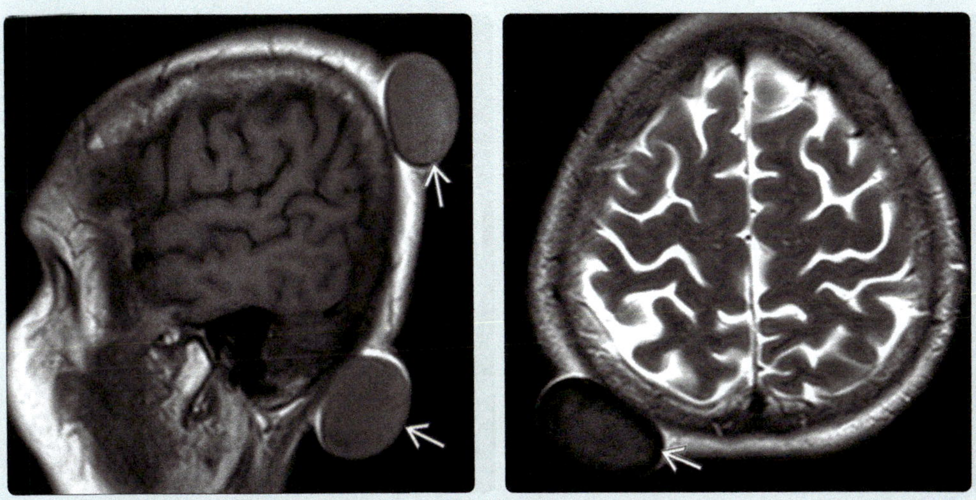

(Left) *Sagittal T1WI MR in a 68-year-old woman with headaches shows 2 large but very well-circumscribed scalp masses ➡. The masses are incompletely surrounded by fat and isointense with brain and muscle.* **(Right)** *Axial T2WI MR in the same patient shows the mass ➡ to be inhomogeneously hypointense. Both lesions demonstrated some internal "blooming" on T2* that suggested calcifications. These lesions had been slowly enlarging over many years and are benign proliferating trichilemmal cysts.*

KEY FACTS

TERMINOLOGY

- Typical ("benign") meningioma = WHO grade I

IMAGING

- Location
  - Supratentorial (90%)
    - Parasagittal/convexity (45%), sphenoid (15-20%)
    - Olfactory groove (5-10%), parasellar (5-10%)
  - Infratentorial (8-10%) (CPA most common site)
  - Multiple meningiomas in 1-9% of cases
- General features
  - Extraaxial mass with broad-based dural attachment
  - > 90% enhance homogeneously, intensely
- CT
  - Hyper- (70-75%), iso- (25%), hypodense (1-5%)
  - Hyperostosis, irregular cortex, ↑ vascular markings
  - Ca++ (20-25%) (diffuse, focal, sand-like, "sunburst," globular, rim)
  - Necrosis, cysts common; hemorrhage rare
- MR
  - Look for CSF/vascular "cleft" between tumor, brain; dural "tail" (35-80% but nonspecific)
- Correlation between imaging, ↑ tumor grade
  - Indistinct tumor-brain interface
  - Capsular enhancement
  - Heterogeneous tumor enhancement

TOP DIFFERENTIAL DIAGNOSES

- Dural metastasis
- Granuloma (TB, sarcoid)
- Idiopathic hypertrophic pachymeningitis
- Extramedullary hematopoiesis
- Hemangioma, dura/venous sinuses

CLINICAL ISSUES

- Most common adult primary intracranial neoplasm (20-35%); peak age = 40-60 years (rare in children unless NF2); often asymptomatic, incidentally found, grow slowly

(Left) *Coronal graphic depicts classic meningioma with broad base toward dura with reactive dural tail ⇨. Note the CSF-vascular cleft ⇨ between invaginating tumor and brain. Typical "sunburst" of dural vessels ⇨ (in this case, the middle meningeal artery) supplies center of lesion, whereas pial vessels supply periphery.* **(Right)** *Axial T2 FS MR in a 59-year-old man with headaches shows a moderately hyperintense extraaxial mass ⇨ with "sunburst" of vessels (flow voids) supplying center of tumor ⇨.*

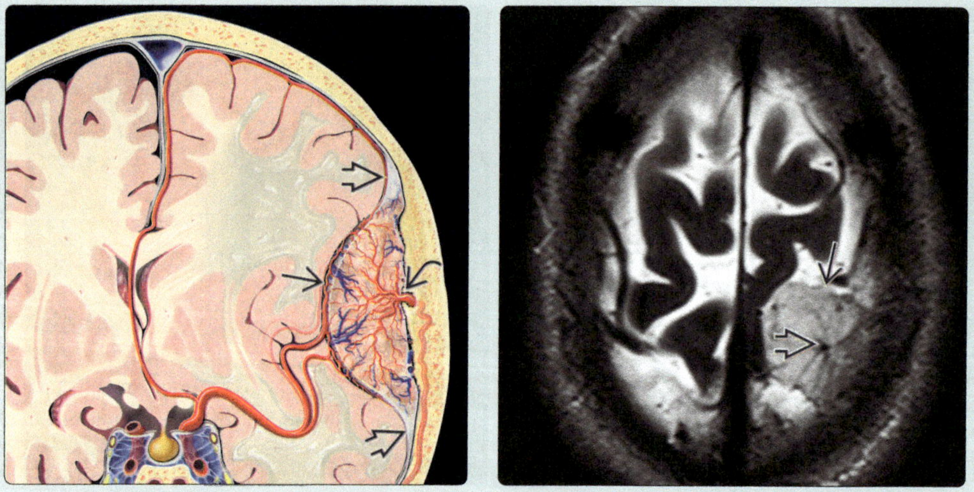

(Left) *Axial T1 C+ MR in the same patient shows that the mass ➡ enhances strongly and uniformly.* **(Right)** *Coronal T1 C+ MR shows the enhancing mass ➡ with slightly more intensely enhancing dural tail ➡. A WHO grade I meningioma was removed at surgery. The dural tail was not involved by tumor.*

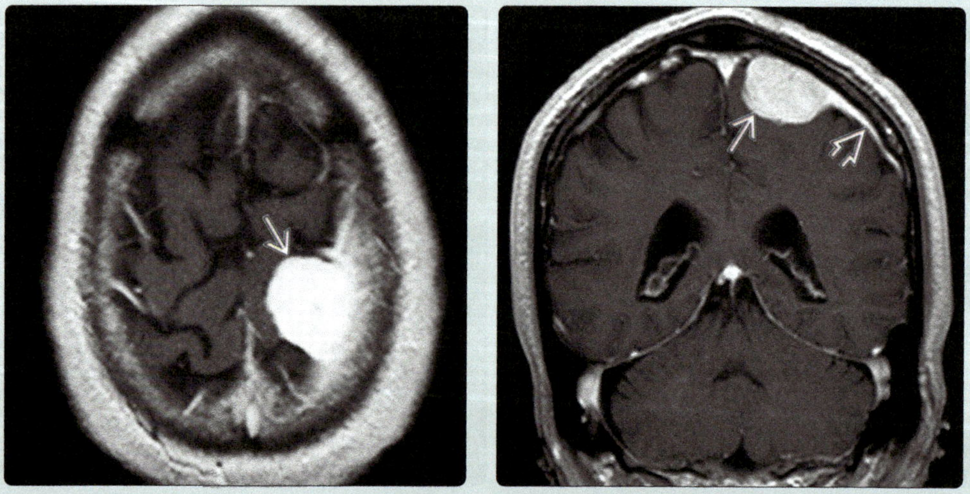

Atypical and Malignant Meningioma

KEY FACTS

TERMINOLOGY

- Typical (benign) meningioma = WHO grade I
- Atypical meningioma (AM) = WHO grade II
- Malignant meningioma (MM) = WHO grade III

IMAGING

- CT triad of MM: Extracranial mass, osteolysis, intracranial tumor
- MR
  - Dural-based locally invasive lesion with areas of necrosis, marked brain edema
  - Indistinct tumor margins (tumor invades, interdigitates with brain)
  - Prominent tumor pannus extending away from mass = "mushrooming"
  - Marked peritumoral edema
  - DWI, ADC correlate with hypercellular histopathology (high signal on DWI, low ADC)

TOP DIFFERENTIAL DIAGNOSES

- Meningioma (typical)
- Dural metastasis
- Lymphoma
- Sarcoma (osteosarcoma, Ewing, gliosarcoma, etc.)

PATHOLOGY

- AM: High mitotic activity
- MM: AM features + findings of frank malignancy

CLINICAL ISSUES

- AM 29% recurrence (26% become MM)
- MM 50% recurrence

DIAGNOSTIC CHECKLIST

- Difficult to predict meningioma tumor grade on imaging
- Imaging findings of typical meningioma do not exclude atypical, malignant variants

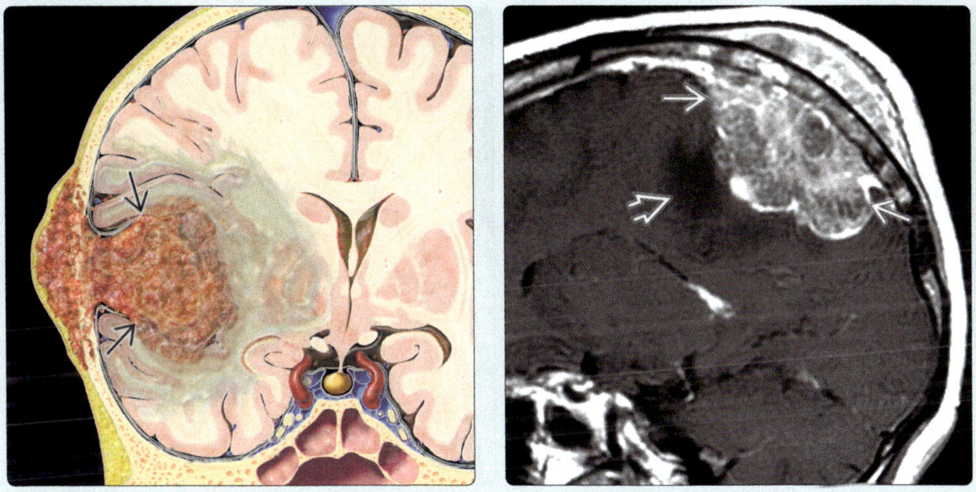

(Left) *Coronal graphic illustrates a malignant meningioma infiltrating the scalp, skull, and underlying brain. Extensive vasogenic edema (in gray) is present. Note osteolysis, invasion through dura/arachnoid, tumor "mushrooming" ➡, and interdigitation with the brain.* **(Right)** *Sagittal T1WI C+ MR of malignant meningioma shows enhancing tumor involving the scalp, skull, and underlying brain. Note "mushrooming" of tumor through the dura ➡, prominent hypointense brain edema ➡.*

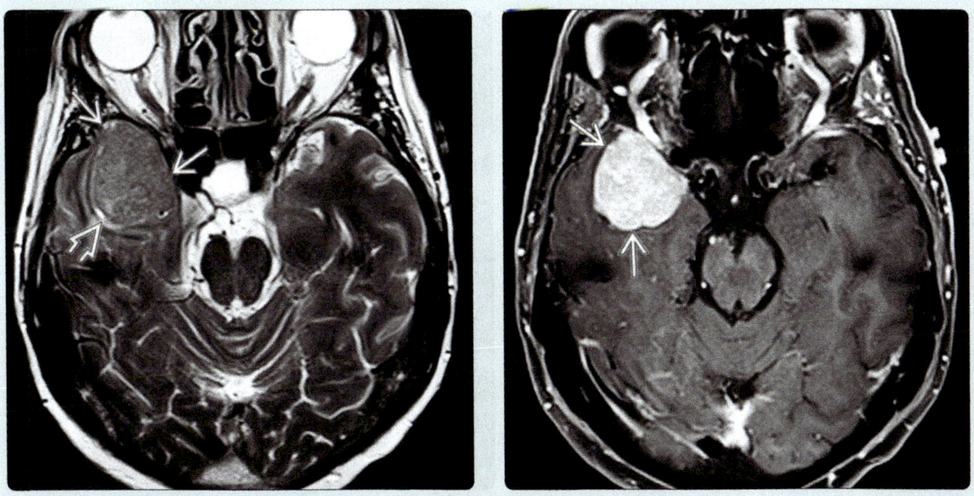

(Left) *Axial T2WI MR in a 71-year-old man shows well-demarcated dural-based mass along right greater sphenoid wing ➡. Mass is isointense with cortex & distinct cerebrospinal fluid-vascular cleft ➡ with no evidence for focal brain invasion.* **(Right)** *Axial T1 C+ FS MR scan shows intense, uniform enhancement ➡. At surgery there was no evidence for invasion of adjacent parenchymal. Pathology disclosed WHO grade II meningioma. This case illustrates the difficulty of predicting meningioma tumor grade on imaging.*

Calvarial Hemangioma

KEY FACTS

TERMINOLOGY

- Benign intraosseous skull lesion with predominantly vascular and some avascular components

IMAGING

- Best clue
  - Sharply marginated expansile skull lesion
- Frontal, temporal, parietal bone in decreasing order
- Most often solitary, but multiple in 15%
- Best imaging tool: Bone CT
  - Sharply marginated expansile lesion
  - Thin peripheral sclerotic rim in 1/3
  - Intact inner and outer table
  - Outer table often more expanded than inner table
  - Trabecular thickening with radiating spicules
- MR signal characteristics dependent on
  - Quantity of slow-moving venous blood
  - Ratio of red marrow to converted fatty marrow
  - Hypointense trabeculae
- T1WI
  - Hypo- to isointense
- T2WI
  - Usually heterogeneously hyperintense ("light bulb bright")
- T1 C+
  - Enhances diffusely and heterogeneously
  - "Fills in" with delayed imaging
  - May have dural tail

PATHOLOGY

- Classified on basis of dominant vessels: Capillary, cavernous, or mixed

CLINICAL ISSUES

- Most often asymptomatic
- Calvarial hemangiomas rare: 0.2% of bone tumors
- Rarely requires treatment

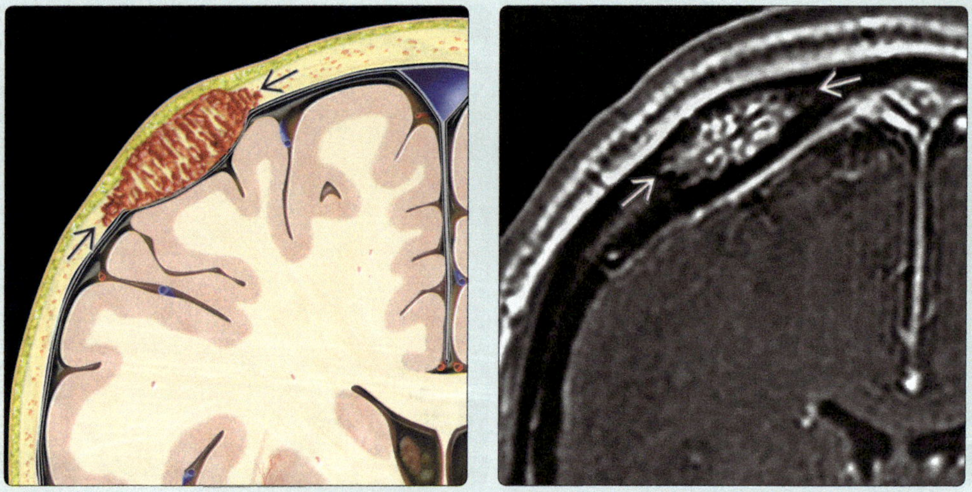

(Left) *Coronal graphic illustrates a sharply marginated expansile skull lesion ➡ with a slight honeycomb-appearing pattern from intradiploic trabecular thickening.* **(Right)** *Coronal T1WI C+ MR shows diffuse yet heterogeneous enhancement of an expansile calvarial hemangioma ➡. Heterogeneity is a result of vascular enhancement combined with hypointense bony trabeculae.*

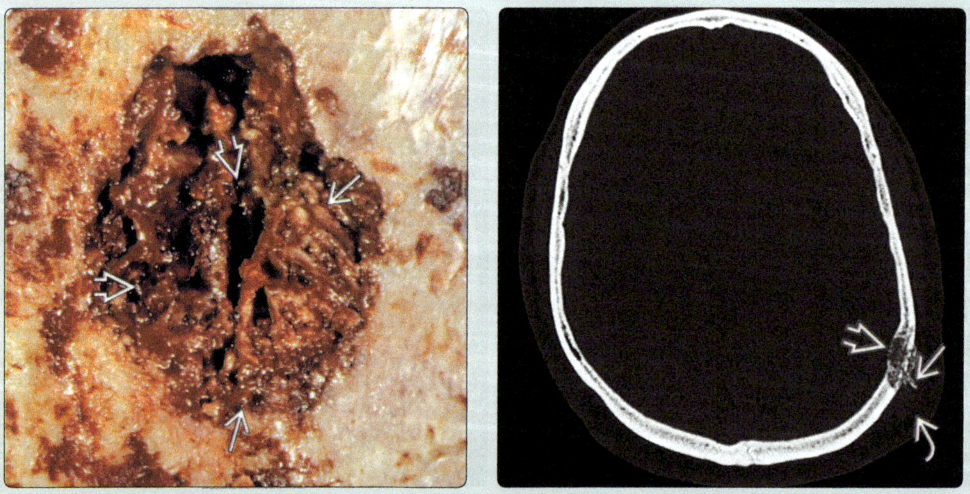

(Left) *Image shows a close-up view of resected calvarial hemangioma. Note the radiating spicules of lamellar bone ➡ interspersed with vascular channels of varying sizes ➡.* **(Right)** *Axial bone CT shows a scalp mass ➡ with the spiculated bone ➡ of an underlying calvarial hemangioma ➡.*

Myeloma

KEY FACTS

TERMINOLOGY

- Clonal B-lymphocyte neoplasm of terminally differentiated plasma cells
  - Solitary = plasmacytoma
    - Brain/CNS is extramedullary plasmacytoma
  - Multifocal = multiple myeloma (MM)

IMAGING

- Intracranial MM rare (1% of MM)
- Can occur as solitary (primary) plasmacytoma or manifestation of systemic MM (secondary)
  - **Secondary**
    - Extension from osteolytic skull lesion > hematogenous spread
  - **Primary** CNS myeloma rare
    - Extraaxial dural-based nonosseous lesions
    - CNS "myelomatosis" involving leptomeninges &/or cranial nerves
    - Parenchymal masses (discrete nodules)
- Best overall imaging tool: Radiography (skeletal survey)
  - Detects 80% of sites in 90% of patients
  - Up to 20% of radiographs and MR may be "normal"
- CNS disease
  - Bone CT for calvaria, skull base
  - MR ± T1 C+ FS for nonosseous intracranial lesions

TOP DIFFERENTIAL DIAGNOSES

- Surgical defect
- Lytic metastasis
- Hemangioma
- Hyperparathyroidism

CLINICAL ISSUES

- Peak onset = 65-70 years
  - Most common symptom: Bone pain (68%)
- Prognosis
  - 70% of plasmacytomas progress to MM

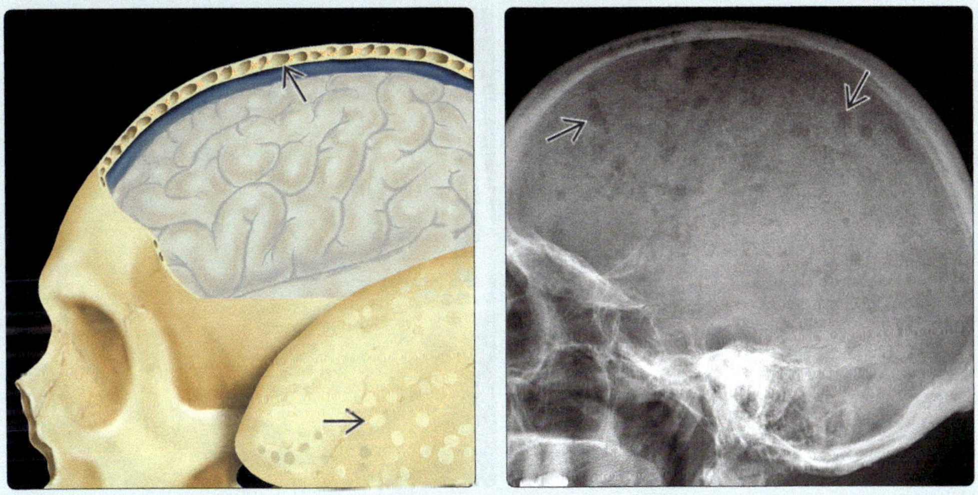

(Left) *Sagittal graphic depicts the multiple "punched-out" lesions ➡ of multiple myeloma in the calvaria.* **(Right)** *Lateral digital radiograph in a patient with multiple myeloma shows the classic salt and pepper appearance of the skull caused by innumerable "punched-out" lesions ➡.*

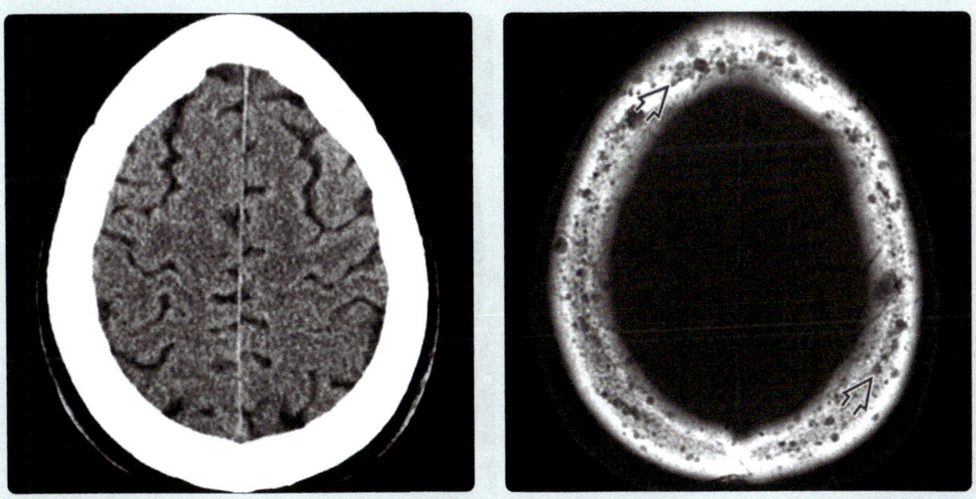

(Left) *Axial NECT in a 50-year-old man with altered mental status, "possible TIA," shows no abnormalities.* **(Right)** *Axial bone CT with bone algorithm reconstruction in the same patient shows innumerable well-defined lytic lesions ➡ in the calvaria. Further evaluation disclosed metastatic multiple myeloma.*

KEY FACTS

IMAGING

- Enhancing lesion(s) with skull/meningeal destruction/infiltration
- Skull, dura, leptomeninges, arachnoid/subarachnoid, pia, and subgaleal
- Many manifestations: Smooth thickening, nodularity, loculation, lobulation, fungating masses

TOP DIFFERENTIAL DIAGNOSES

- Skull metastases: Surgical defect (burr hole, craniectomy), myeloma
- Dural metastases: Epidural/subdural hematoma, meningioma
- Leptomeningeal metastases: Subarachnoid hemorrhage, sarcoidosis, infectious meningitis

CLINICAL ISSUES

- 18% of patients with extracranial and intracranial malignancies
- Primary tumor never identified in 2-4%
- All metastases: May be asymptomatic and unsuspected clinically
- Headache is most common symptom (50%)
- CSF cytology often falsely negative
- Accuracy of single lumbar puncture (LP) is 50-60% but 90% after 3 attempts
- Bimodal → children (medulloblastoma & leukemia); adults (breast, lung, melanoma, prostate)
- Average age ~ 50 years (relatively young secondary pediatric cancer and young women with breast cancer)
- Entire neuraxis must be treated, as tumor cells are often widely disseminated throughout CSF

DIAGNOSTIC CHECKLIST

- Both enhanced MR and LP should be performed, especially if initial test is negative

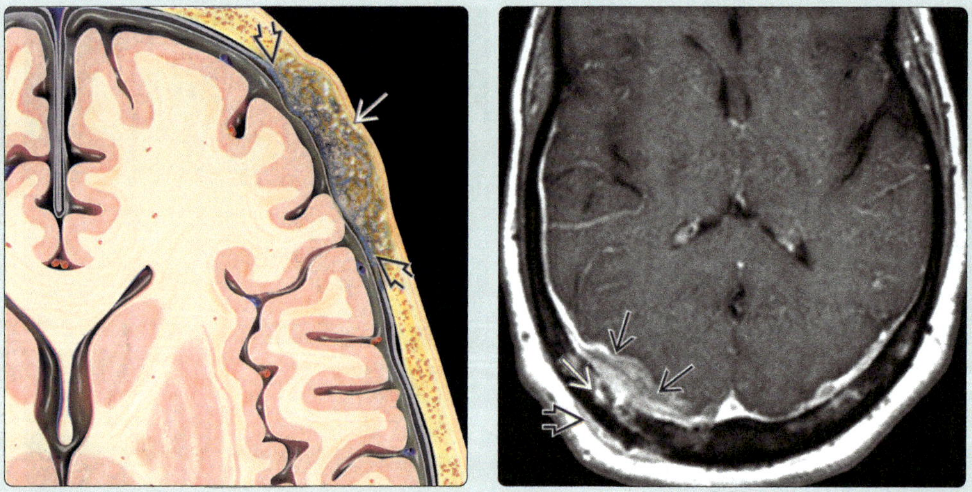

(Left) *Axial graphic illustrates a destructive skull metastasis ➔ expanding the diploic space and invading/thickening the underlying dura (light blue linear structure) ⇒.* **(Right)** *Axial T1WI C+ MR shows skull metastasis with enhancement of the diploic space ➔. There is associated small subgaleal soft tissue ⇒ and extensive nodular dural thickening →.*

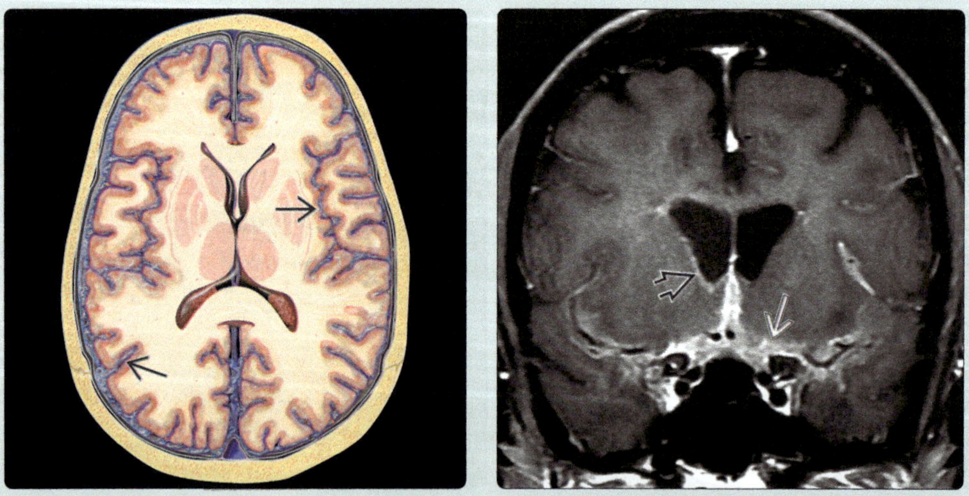

(Left) *Axial graphic illustrates diffuse leptomeningeal metastases, shown here as abnormal blue material → coating the pial surface of the brain and filling the subarachnoid spaces between interdigitating sulci.* **(Right)** *Carcinomatous "meningitis" can be indistinguishable on imaging from pyogenic meningitis. In this case of diffuse cerebrospinal fluid spread from glioblastoma, there is both sulcal-cisternal ➔ and ependymal ⇒ spread of tumor.*

Imaging Approach & Indications

General Approach

Imaging of the orbit encompasses 2 clinically distinct areas of ophthalmology: (1) The eye or globe and (2) the bony orbit, soft tissues, and periorbita.

Lesions in these 2 areas result in specific clinical profiles that affect different patient groups. When a patient is referred for imaging, it is usually clear to the clinician whether the problem involves the eye proper versus some other structure of the orbit.

The term "orbital" refers to those bony structures and soft tissues that are extrinsic to the eye, as opposed to the term "ocular," which refers to the globe itself. Most imaging referrals come from oculoplastic surgeons, neurologists, neuroophthalmologists, neurosurgeons, and otolaryngologists who need help characterizing orbital processes extrinsic to the globe. However, in some instances imaging of the globe provides complementary information to the physical and ophthalmoscopic examination.

Ultrasound

Ultrasound of the eye is a readily available complement to funduscopic examination and is traditionally performed in the ophthalmology clinic. In addition to providing imaging of the globe, transocular ultrasound provides a limited, high-resolution assessment of other soft tissue orbital structures.

Because of the availability of ultrasound, many simple diagnoses can be made without the need of further imaging. In this regard, imaging of the orbit is a function that is shared between the ophthalmologist and the neuroradiologist.

CT

Because of its superior bony characterization, CT has advantages over MR for orbital lesions that arise from or directly affect the bones, such as epithelial inclusions, osteocartilaginous tumors with matrix, osteodystrophic processes, benign masses that cause bony scalloping, and aggressive malignancies that cause bony destruction.

The presence of calcification is a specific differentiating feature in some lesions, and, therefore, CT can provide essential diagnostic information, even after an MR has been obtained. Examples include retinoblastoma, perioptic meningioma, and end-stage ocular disease (phthisis bulbi). It is worth noting that orbital cavernous hemangioma, a common intraconal orbital mass in the adult, rarely shows phleboliths or calcification.

In many instances, CT can provide enough information to allow for a definitive diagnosis and guide therapy without the need for MR. Examples include thyroid ophthalmopathy, clinically benign lacrimal mass, and orbital cavernous hemangioma.

When the diagnosis is clinically apparent, CT is often adequate to identify associated findings or complications that directly impact treatment decisions. For example, in a patient with orbital cellulitis, enhanced CT can identify the presence of sinus disease &/or abscess, thus guiding surgical therapy.

In children, CT has the particular advantage of rapid acquisition that obviates the need for sedation. However, the risk of radiation exposure is a mitigating factor that must also be considered.

MR

For evaluating complex orbital disease, MR is the preferred modality. Superior soft tissue differentiation and enhancement make MR ideal for characterizing the extent of complicated lesions, including extraocular tumors, vascular malformations, and complex inflammatory processes.

In particular, MR is the optimal modality for delineating the extent of malignant orbital disease. Important features visible on MR include perineural tumor spread, optic nerve invasion, hematogenous or cerebrospinal fluid (CSF) disseminated metastases, and intracranial extension.

Although ultrasound is usually the 1st line for imaging the globe, MR can provide a more accurate visualization of retrobulbar extension of intraocular malignancy, including retinoblastoma, ocular melanoma, and ocular metastases. Additionally, MR provides exquisite characterization of the globe itself, which is particularly useful in circumstances in which funduscopic evaluation is obscured, such as swollen or injured eye, retinal detachment, large intraocular mass, vitreal hemorrhage, or opaque media from any cause.

Imaging Anatomy

Bony Orbit

Major portions of the bony orbital walls are contributed by the frontal bone superiorly, zygomatic bone laterally and inferiorly, maxillary bone inferiorly and medially, and ethmoid bone medially. Smaller contributions medially include the lacrimal bone, nasal bone, and a tiny portion of the palatine bone. The sphenoid bone makes up a large portion of the orbit posteriorly and laterally, forming the complex foramina at the orbital apex.

Globe

The aqueous-filled anterior segment includes anterior and posterior chambers, both anterior to the lens. The vitreous-filled posterior segment occupies the bulk of the globe posteriorly. There is limited visualization of other normal anatomical substructures on routine imaging.

Orbital Septum

Fascia arising from the orbital periosteum inserts onto the aponeurosis of the tarsal plates of the lids, providing a barrier between the anterior periorbita and the intraorbital contents. Although the septum itself is often not discernible, its presence is readily evident when a disease process is contained on 1 side of the barrier.

Lacrimal Apparatus

The lacrimal gland lies in a bony fossa at the anterior aspect of the superolateral orbit. Lacrimal drainage is via canaliculi and sac at the inferomedial orbit, and from there through the nasolacrimal duct, which drains via the inferior meatus.

Extraocular Muscles (EOM)

The 4 rectus muscles originate from the annulus of Zinn at the apex and insert on the corneoscleral surface. The superior oblique has similar origin and insertion but courses through the trochlea ("pulley") at the superomedial orbital rim. The inferior oblique has a short, more direct course originating from the anteroinferior orbital rim. The levator palpebrae superioris originates at the annulus, coursing just above the superior rectus to insert at the upper eyelid.

Optic Nerve-Sheath Complex

Actually a central tract, the optic nerve (CN2), traverses the optic canal to insert at the optic nerve head. The surrounding

Differential Diagnosis: Orbit

Congenital Lesions	Infectious Lesions	Benign Tumors
Coloboma	Ocular toxocariasis	Orbital infantile hemangioma
Persistent hyperplastic primary vitreous	Orbital subperiosteal abscess	Optic pathway glioma
Coats disease	Orbital cellulitis	Optic nerve sheath meningioma
Orbital dermoid and epidermoid	**Inflammatory Lesions**	Lacrimal gland benign mixed tumor
Orbital neurofibromatosis, type 1	Orbital idiopathic pseudotumor	**Malignant Tumors**
Vascular Lesions	Orbital sarcoidosis	Retinoblastoma
Orbital lymphatic malformation	Thyroid ophthalmopathy	Ocular melanoma
Orbital varix	Optic neuritis	Orbital lymphoproliferative lesions
Orbital cavernous hemangioma	**Tumor-Like Lesions**	Lacrimal gland carcinoma
Orbital infantile hemangioma*	Orbital Langerhans histiocytosis	

**Infantile hemangioma is classified as a benign neoplasm but is also listed alongside the vascular malformations for comparison.*

dural sheath is contiguous with the intracranial dura and the sclera. A thin layer of CSF surrounding the nerve is typically visible on MR and is contiguous with CSF in the suprasellar cistern.

Peripheral Cranial Nerves

CN3, CN4, and CN6 supply motor innervation to the EOMs and parasympathetics to the iris via CN3. These nerves are not reliably identifiable within the orbit. However, knowledge of their course via the cavernous sinus and superior orbital fissure (SOF) allows localization of pathology that involves these nerves.

Two of the branches of CN5 course through the orbit. V1 passes with other nerves in through the SOF, and V1 exits through the supraorbital foramen. V2 passes through foramen rotundum and inferior orbital fissure and exits through the infraorbital foramen.

Vascular Structures

The ophthalmic artery enters the orbit within the optic nerve; it is frequently visible in the orbit as it exits the nerve near the apex. The superior ophthalmic vein is found between the superior rectus muscle and the optic nerve.

Orbital Fat

In addition to providing volume "filler" for the orbital cavity, orbital fat provides intrinsic imaging contrast, making other structures and disease processes more conspicuous.

Anatomy-Based Imaging Issues

In approaching orbital lesions, it is useful to localize the process to a subregion of the orbit and ascertain the relationship of the lesion to critical structures.

- Globe: Is the lesion entirely intraocular, or is there transscleral extension?
- Optic nerve: Does the lesion arise within the nerve proper or involve primarily the dural sheath?
- EOM: Is the lesion intraconal, extraconal, or does it arise from the muscles themselves? Is muscle involvement symmetric?
- Lacrimal gland: Is the lesion unilateral or is it bilateral, indicating a systemic process?
- Bone: Does the bone show benign scalloped remodeling or aggressive destruction?
- Focality: Is the lesion isolated or multiple? Does the lesion extend beyond the orbit?

Imaging Protocols

CT

Routine imaging of the orbit with CT does not require special discussion, but 1 circumstance is worth noting: Intermittent proptosis due to orbital varix. This dynamic lesion enlarges with increases in venous pressures and is best demonstrated with provocation. After routine enhanced CT is performed, the scan is repeated with the breath held in Valsalva maneuver, increasing venous pressures and enlarging the varix.

MR

Routine imaging of the orbit with MR is usually adequate for the vast majority of ophthalmologic indications. The protocol includes 3 sequence types: precontrast T1WI; T2WI with fat suppression, or STIR; and postcontrast T1WI with fat suppression. Each of these is performed in axial and coronal planes at 3.0-mm slice thickness and 18-cm field of view. Whole-brain imaging is added when indicated.

Pathologic Issues: Vascular Malformations

Vascular malformations are congenital, nonneoplastic lesions in which classification reflects their histologic and hemodynamic features.

Lymphatic/venolymphatic malformation: Lesions may have no flow (type 1), venous flow (type 2), or may be mixed. There may be a distensible component, resulting in varix. Outdated terminology includes "lymphangioma" and "cystic hygroma."

Venous malformation: Purely venous malformations occur elsewhere in the head and neck but are relatively uncommon in the orbit unless part of a larger transspatial lesion. The misnomer "hemangioma" should be avoided.

Orbital cavernous hemangioma (OCH): This common mass is actually a malformation that is unique to the orbit. It is encapsulated, with low-flow arterial (type 3) hemodynamics but also some venous features. The term "OCH" is a misnomer but is widely used.

Arteriovenous malformations (AVM): True orbital AVMs are rare lesions, with high-flow arterial (type 3) hemodynamics.

Selected References

1. Rootman J. Diseases of the Orbit: A Multidisciplinary Approach. Philadelphia: Lippincott, 2003

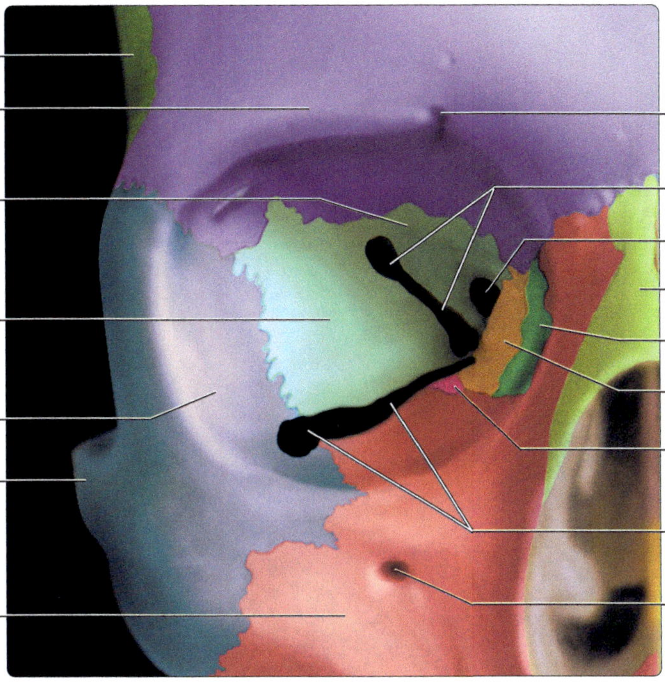

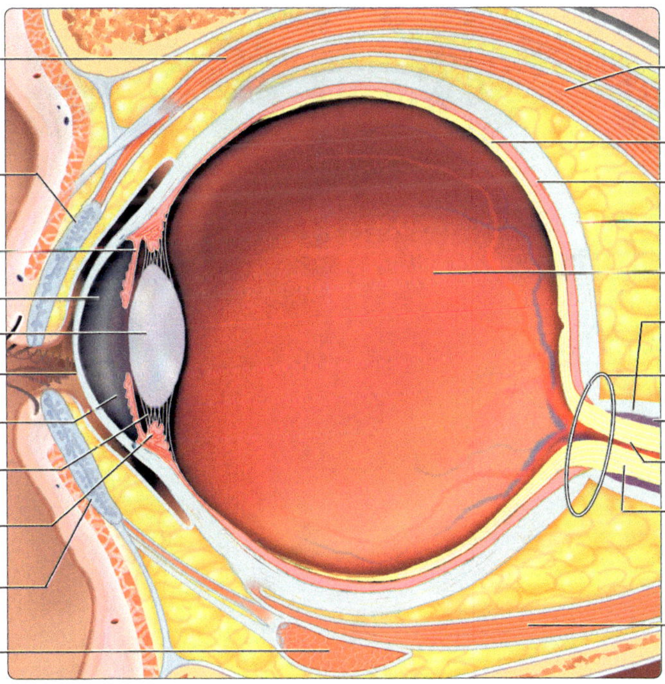

(Top) *Frontal graphic demonstrates the complex anatomy of the bony orbit. The walls of the orbital cavity receive contributions from 8 different bones of the skull. The complex foramina and fissures at the apex are located primarily within the greater and lesser wings of the sphenoid bone and its junctions with adjacent bones.* **(Bottom)** *Sagittal graphic demonstrates the anterior and posterior segments of the globe. The aqueous anterior segment is comprised of the anterior chamber and very small posterior chamber. The much larger posterior segment is filled by the vitreous chamber. The layered tunicae of the retina, choroid, and sclera are demonstrated as well as the components of the optic nerve at its insertion. Some of the extraocular muscles and eyelid structures are also demonstrated.*

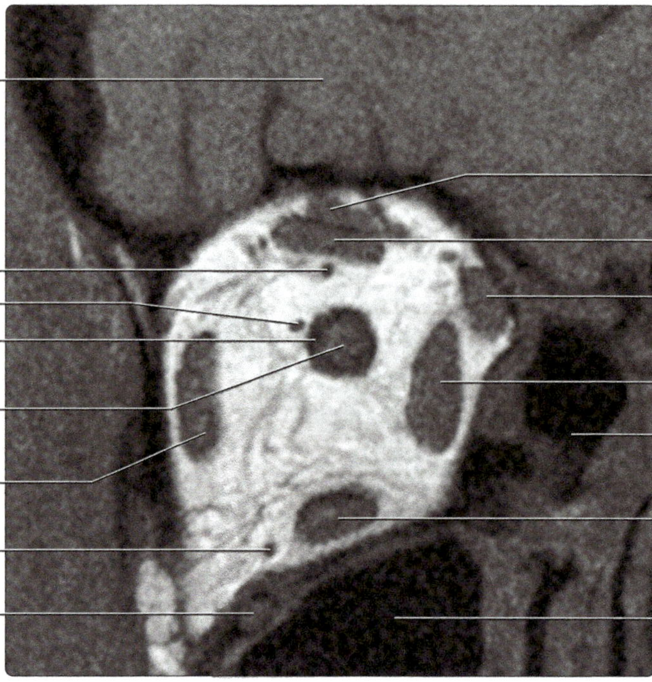

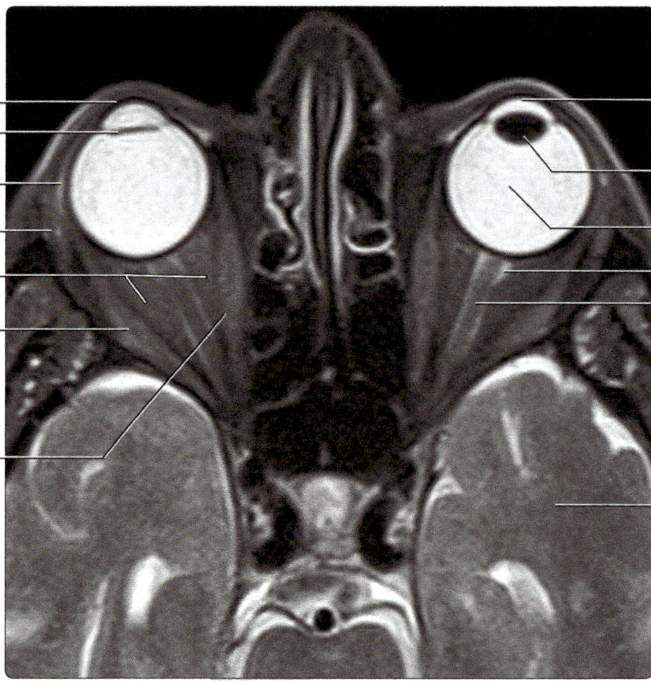

(Top) *Coronal T1WI MR demonstrates the peripherally located extraocular muscles, the central optic nerve sheath complex, and the vascular structures of the orbit. The intrinsic T1 signal of the orbital fat provides excellent contrast for visualizing the intraorbital contents.* **(Bottom)** *Axial T2WI MR with fat suppression nearly eliminates signal from orbital fat, allowing for conspicuity of fluid signal structures. A small amount of cerebrospinal fluid surrounding the optic nerve is usually visible on T2WI. The normal extraocular muscles show intermediate to low signal. A small portion of the lacrimal gland is seen, but the majority of the gland is located further superiorly. The anterior segment of the eye shows water signal, primarily representing the anterior chamber; the posterior chamber is not discernible on routine MR. The posterior segment also shows water signal, comprised of the vitreous chamber. Note that this patient has a prosthetic lens on the right.*

Optic Neuritis

KEY FACTS

IMAGING

- Focal or segmental T2 hyperintensity of optic nerve
  - Nerve normal in size or minimally enlarged
- Central or diffuse nerve enhancement
  - ± peripheral sheath enhancement

TOP DIFFERENTIAL DIAGNOSES

- Neuromyelitis optica
- Ischemic optic neuropathy
- Infectious optic neuritis (ON)
- Idiopathic perineuritis (pseudotumor)
- Granulomatous optic neuropathy (sarcoid)
- Optic nerve sheath meningioma
- Optic nerve glioma

CLINICAL ISSUES

- Symptoms and signs
  - Acute loss of visual acuity
  - Relative afferent pupillary defect if unilateral
  - Impaired color vision
  - Eye pain
- Optic disc acutely looks normal
  - About 1/3 demonstrate mild swelling
- Distinct clinical profiles
  - Acute ON
  - Neuromyelitis optica (Devic syndrome)
  - Acute demyelinating encephalomyelitis
  - Pediatric ON
- Spontaneous recovery of vision is characteristic
  - Corticosteroids accelerate acute recovery
  - Early interferon therapy mitigates risk of MS

DIAGNOSTIC CHECKLIST

- Identification of demyelinating lesions in CNS is most important neuroimaging task in setting of ON
  - High incidence of MS in patients with ON
  - Findings on MR strongly predictive of MS
- Recommend brain and spinal cord imaging

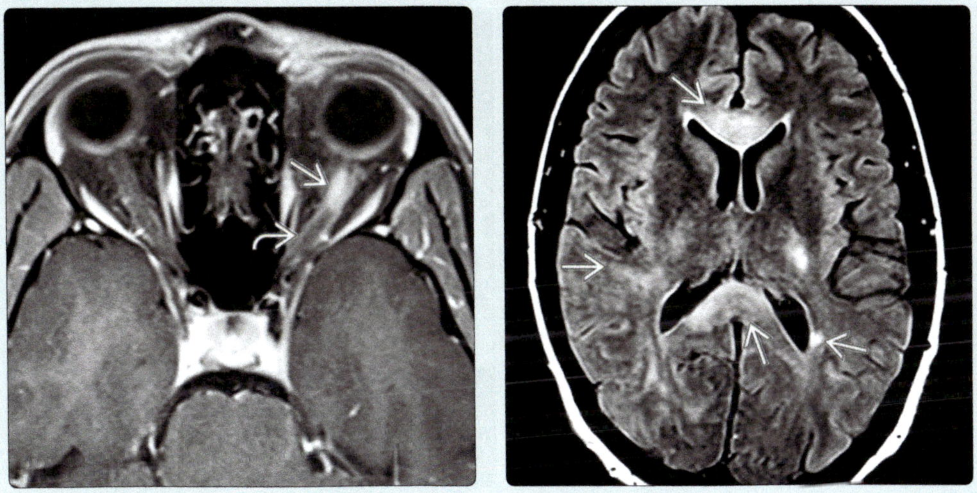

(Left) *Axial T1WI C+ FS MR in a woman with left eye pain and decreased color vision shows intense segmental enhancement of the left intraorbital optic nerve ➔. A component of peripheral nerve sheath enhancement is seen extending posteriorly ➔.* **(Right)** *Axial FLAIR MR of the brain in the same patient shows multiple periatrial, capsular, callosal, and subcortical white matter lesions ➔. Cerebrospinal fluid (CSF) analysis yielded oligoclonal bands, and the patient was diagnosed with multiple sclerosis.*

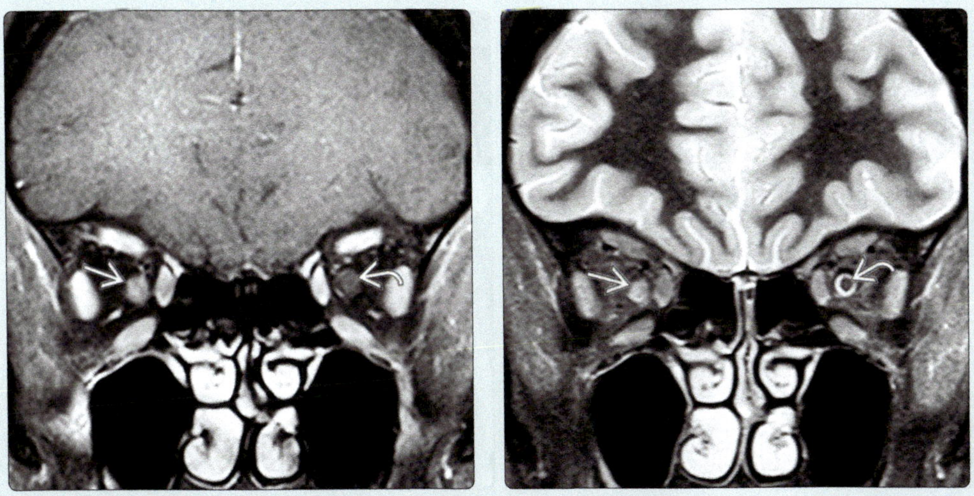

(Left) *Coronal T1WI C+ FS MR in 22-year-old woman with right eye vision loss, pain, afferent pupillary defect shows enhancement of the intraorbital optic nerve ➔ (compared with normal nonenhancing left nerve ➔).* **(Right)** *Coronal STIR MR in the same patient shows increased signal in the right optic nerve ➔. Note that the hyperintense signal of the right nerve is similar to CSF in the optic nerve sheath, whereas the normal left nerve ➔ is distinct from the surrounding CSF.*

KEY FACTS

TERMINOLOGY

- Synonyms: **Graves ophthalmopathy,** thyroid orbitopathy
- Autoimmune orbital inflammatory condition associated with thyroid dysfunction

IMAGING

- CT
  - For uncomplicated disease and surgical planning
  - Nonuniform, symmetric, or asymmetric extraocular muscle involvement
  - Enlargement of muscle bellies, sparing tendinous insertions
  - **"I'M SLO"** mnemonic for sites of predilection
    - **I**nferior > **m**edial > **s**uperior > **l**ateral > **o**blique
  - Increased volume of orbital fat
    - Caution: Extraocular muscles may look normal
- MR
  - Assess disease activity
  - ↑ T2WI MR signal acutely due to edema
  - ↓ T2WI MR signal chronically due to fibrosis
- US: Effective for bedside diagnosis

TOP DIFFERENTIAL DIAGNOSES

- Idiopathic orbital inflammatory pseudotumor
- Sarcoidosis
- Lymphoproliferative lesions

PATHOLOGY

- Autoantibodies target thyrotropin receptors found in both thyroid gland and orbit
- Cellular infiltrate with hyaluron deposition acutely
- Fibrosis and muscle degeneration in chronic phase

CLINICAL ISSUES

- Typical patient is middle-aged woman with periorbital edema, proptosis, and restricted gaze
- Corticosteroids 1st line of therapy in acute disease
- Surgery for decompression in severe cases

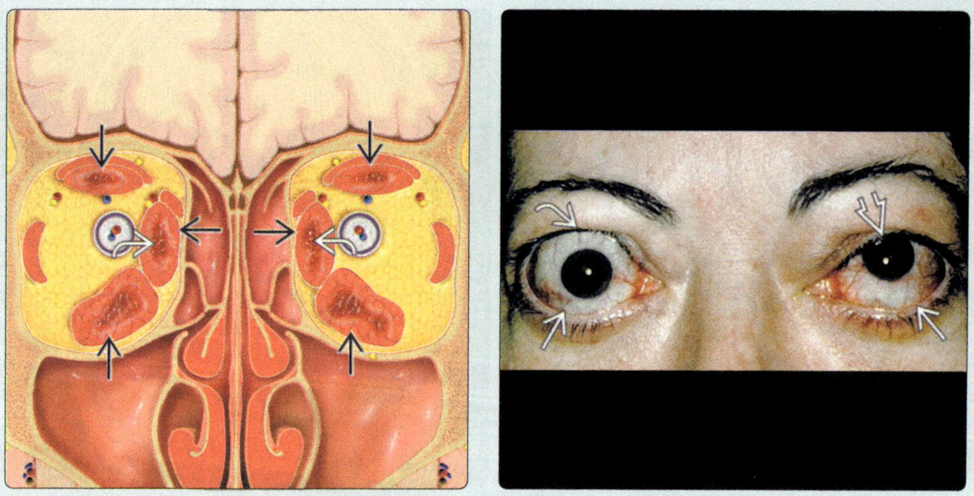

(Left) *Coronal graphic shows bilateral symmetric enlargement of extraocular muscles. Irregularity within the muscles represents accumulation of lymphocytes and mucopolysaccharide deposition.* **(Right)** *Clinical photograph of a patient with severe thyroid ophthalmopathy shows bilateral proptosis, lid retraction, and disconjugate gaze.*

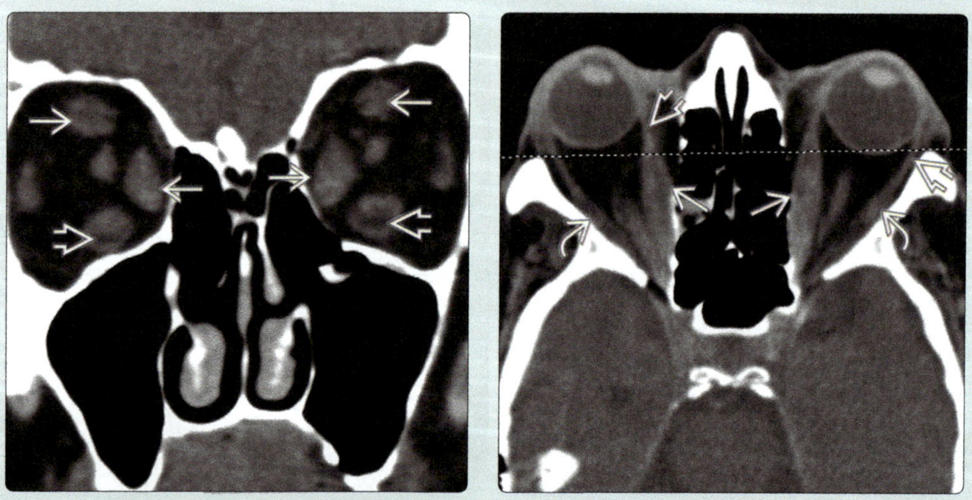

(Left) *Coronal NECT shows enlargement of the bilateral inferior, medial, and superior rectus muscles in a patient with thyroid ophthalmopathy. Mucopolysaccharide deposition manifests as areas of low density within the muscles, particularly inferior recti.* **(Right)** *Axial NECT in another case with thyroid ophthalmopathy demonstrates proptosis (globes displaced anteriorly beyond the lateral orbital walls/dotted line), fusiform enlargement of medial and lateral recti with striking sparing of tendon sheaths.*

Orbital Idiopathic Inflammatory Pseudotumor

KEY FACTS

TERMINOLOGY

- Nonspecific orbital inflammation, not due to any known etiology or systemic illness

IMAGING

- Best imaging tool: Contrast-enhanced MR with fat suppression
- Poorly marginated mass-like enhancing soft tissue involving any area of orbit
- Categorized by area(s) of involvement
  - Myositic, lacrimal, anterior, diffuse, apical
- Moderate diffuse enlargement, irregularity, and enhancement of involved structures
- Isointense or slightly hyperintense on T2WI or STIR
  - ↓ signal compared with many orbital lesions due to cellular infiltrate and fibrosis
  - ↓ signal in chronic disease suggests sclerosing variant and portends worse prognosis

TOP DIFFERENTIAL DIAGNOSES

- Lymphoproliferative lesions
- IgG4-related disease
- Thyroid ophthalmopathy
- Sarcoidosis
- Wegener granulomatosis
- Orbital cellulitis

PATHOLOGY

- Polymorphous chronic inflammation and fibrosis

CLINICAL ISSUES

- Symptoms: Pain and swelling, restricted eye motion, diplopia, proptosis, and impaired vision
- 3rd most common orbital disorder
- Steroid treatment effective in most patients

DIAGNOSTIC CHECKLIST

- Pseudotumor is diagnosis of exclusion

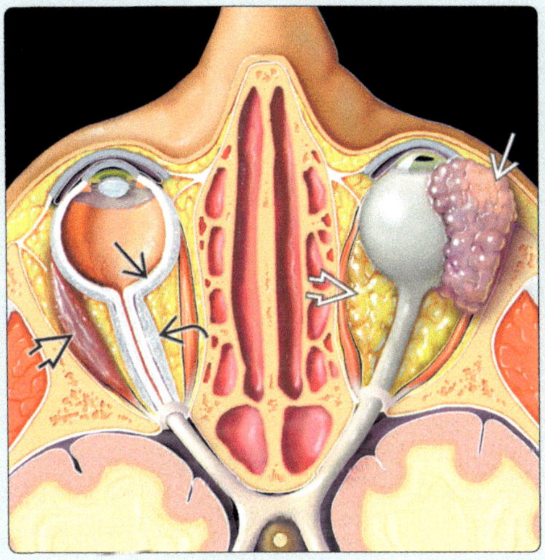

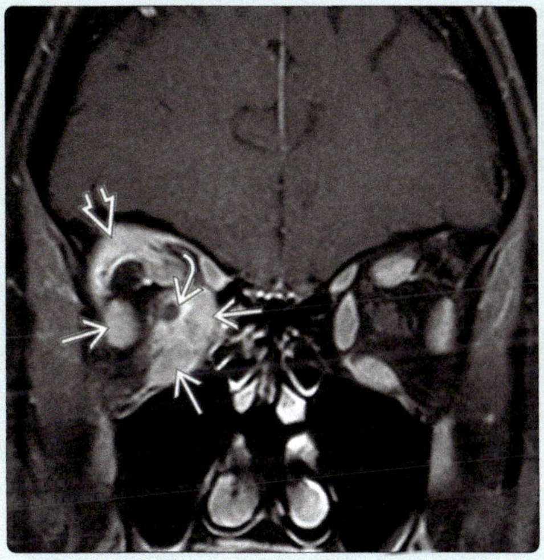

(Left) *Axial graphic depicts multifocal orbital idiopathic inflammation, including involvement of the extraocular muscles ⇨, orbital fat ➡, lacrimal gland ➡, sclera ⇨, and optic sheath ⇨.* **(Right)** *Coronal T1WI C+ FS MR demonstrates extensive orbital inflammation, with ill-defined enlargement and enhancement of the rectus muscles ➡, extraconal infiltration extending to the lacrimal gland ➡, and intraconal enhancement partially surrounding the optic nerve ➡.*

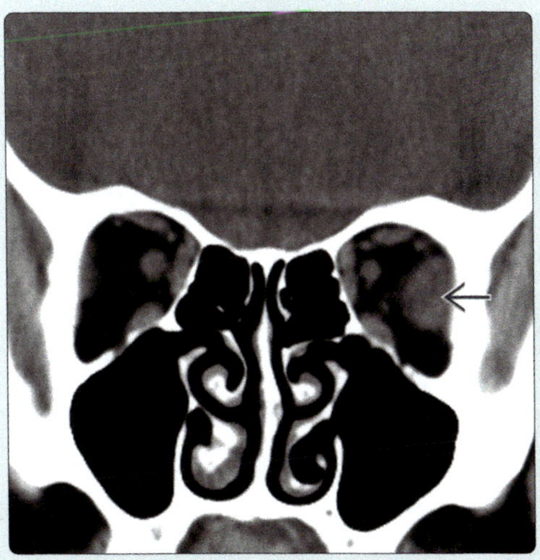

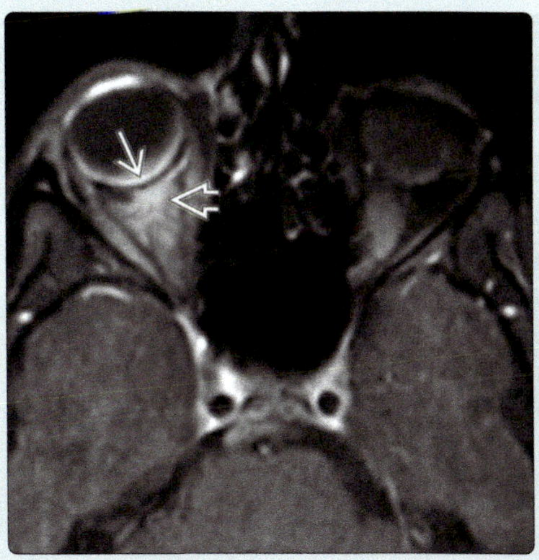

(Left) *Coronal NECT in a middle-aged woman with left eye pain and diplopia shows enlargement and mild hypodensity of the left lateral rectus ⇨. Isolated lateral rectus myositis is a typical manifestation of orbital pseudotumor, rare in thyroid orbitopathy.* **(Right)** *Axial T1WI C+ FS MR in a patient with symptoms of uveitis shows orbital inflammatory changes of the anterior right orbit. Marked right uveoscleral "shaggy" enhancement is evident ➡, as well as ill-defined enhancement of the retrobulbar fat ➡.*

KEY FACTS

TERMINOLOGY

- Optic pathway glioma (OPG)
- Primary neuroglial tumor of optic pathway
- 3 broad clinical subtypes
  - Childhood syndromic [neurofibromatosis type 1 (NF1)], childhood sporadic, adult

IMAGING

- Fusiform optic nerve (ON) mass with variable posterior pathway involvement
- MR is preferred imaging modality
  - Isointense to mildly hypointense on T1WI
  - Variably hyperintense on T2WI
  - Enhancement varies from none/minimal to intense
- Associated neuroimaging findings in NF1: ↑ T2 foci in brain, other CNS tumors, sphenoid dysplasia, buphthalmos

TOP DIFFERENTIAL DIAGNOSES

- Optic neuritis
- ON sheath meningioma
- Idiopathic orbital inflammatory pseudotumor
- Sarcoidosis

PATHOLOGY

- Childhood OPG: Low-grade glioma
- Adult OPG: Anaplastic astrocytoma or glioblastoma multiforme

CLINICAL ISSUES

- Decreased vision, proptosis; often asymptomatic
- Childhood OPG: Onset 0.5-15 years
- 30-40% of patients with OPG have NF1
- 11-30% of patients with NF1 have OPG
- Natural history highly variable
  - Generally indolent in childhood OPG
  - Much more aggressive in adults
    - Poor prognosis; often rapidly fatal

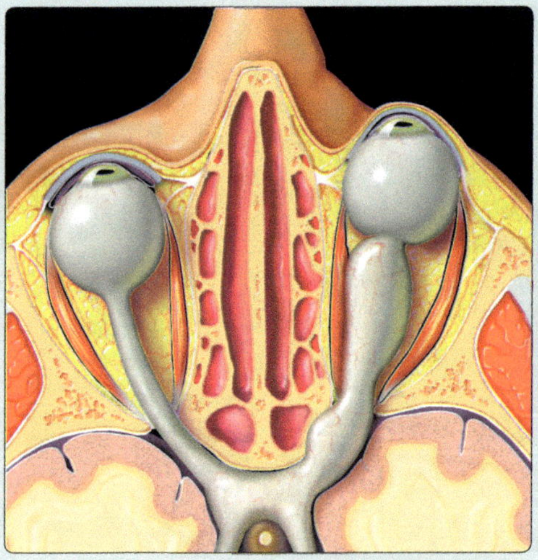

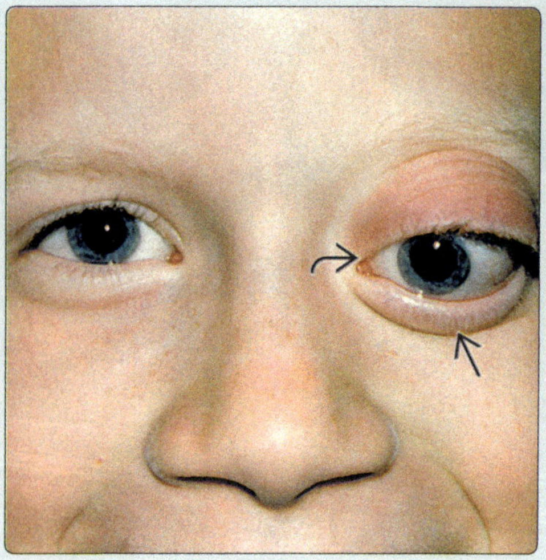

(Left) *Axial graphic depicts a left optic pathway glioma extending along the length of the intraorbital nerve, through the enlarged optic canal, and into the prechiasmatic segment. The fusiform pattern of enlargement is typical.* **(Right)** *Clinical photograph of a child with a large optic nerve glioma shows striking proptosis with bulging orbital contents, diplopia.*

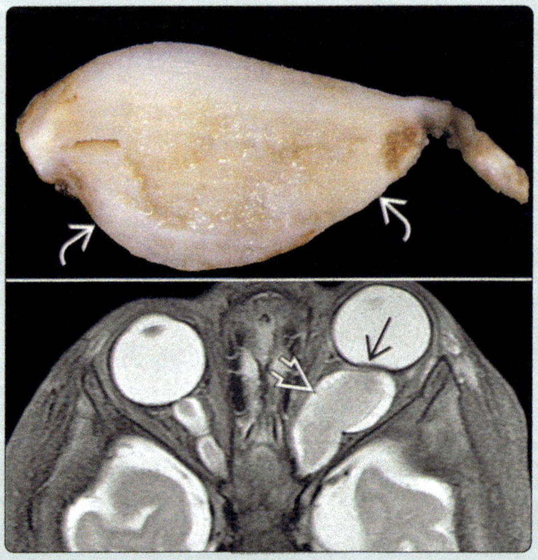

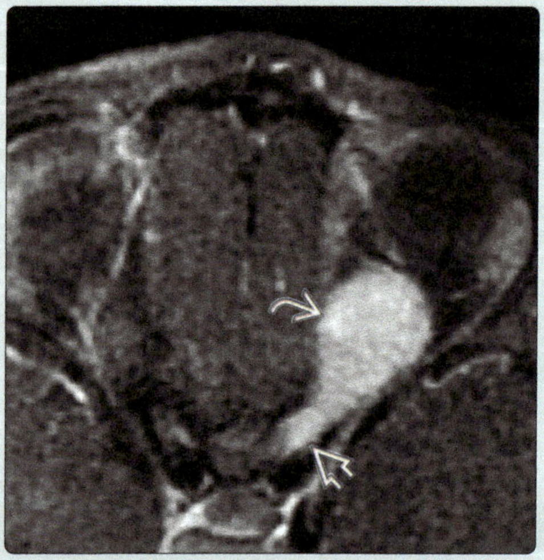

(Left) *(Top) Gross pathology of optic nerve glioma shows fusiform enlargement of the optic nerve. (Bottom) Axial T2WI shows optic nerve glioma with anterior displacement, compression of the globe.* **(Right)** *Axial T1C+ FS in another case of optic pathway glioma shows fusiform enlargement, enhancement of the prechiasmatic segment of the left optic nerve, in addition to the marked enlargement and enhancement of the intraorbital optic nerve.*

KEY FACTS

TERMINOLOGY

- Optic nerve sheath meningioma
  - Also known as perioptic meningioma
- Benign, slow-growing tumor of optic nerve sheath
- Distinct entity from intracranial (spheno-orbital) meningioma that extends through orbital apex into orbit

IMAGING

- NECT
  - "Tram-track" Ca++ on either side of optic nerve
    - Seen in 1/3 to 1/2 of cases
- CECT
  - Tubular enhancing mass surrounding intraorbital optic nerve
- MR
  - Variably hyperintense to hypointense on T2WI
  - Uniform, moderately intense enhancement

TOP DIFFERENTIAL DIAGNOSES

- Optic nerve glioma
- Orbital pseudotumor
- Orbital sarcoidosis
- Metastasis
- Orbit lymphoproliferative lesions

PATHOLOGY

- Benign tumor arising from arachnoid "cap" cells within optic nerve sheath
- May be associated with neurofibromatosis type 2

CLINICAL ISSUES

- Classic: Visual loss, optic atrophy, optociliary venous shunting, choroidal fold

DIAGNOSTIC CHECKLIST

- MR is preferred imaging modality for tumor assessment, but look for Ca++ on CT when diagnosis in doubt

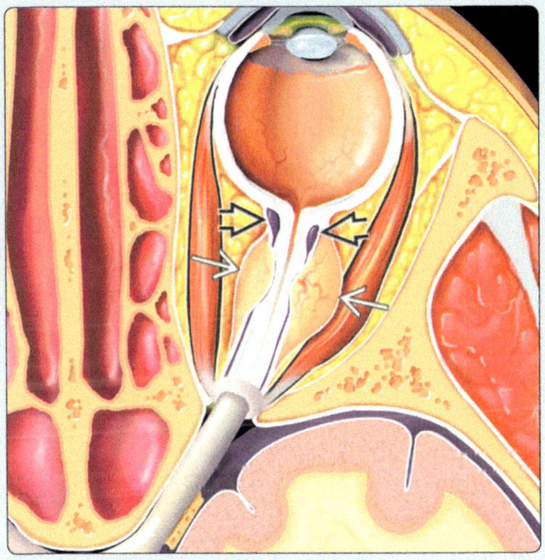
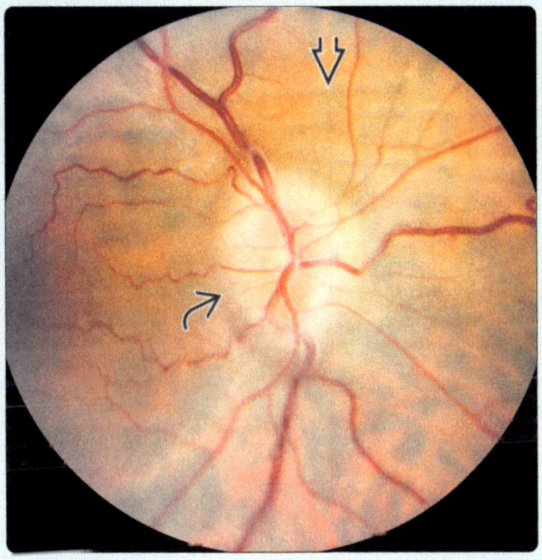

(Left) *Axial graphic depicts a fusiform meningioma ➡ arising from the optic nerve sheath. Characteristic "perioptic cyst" evident behind the globe ⇨ represents trapped cerebrospinal fluid within the nerve sheath.* **(Right)** *Funduscopic examination in a patient with optic nerve sheath meningioma shows optic disc edema and pallor ⇨ together with prominent choroidal folds ⇨.*

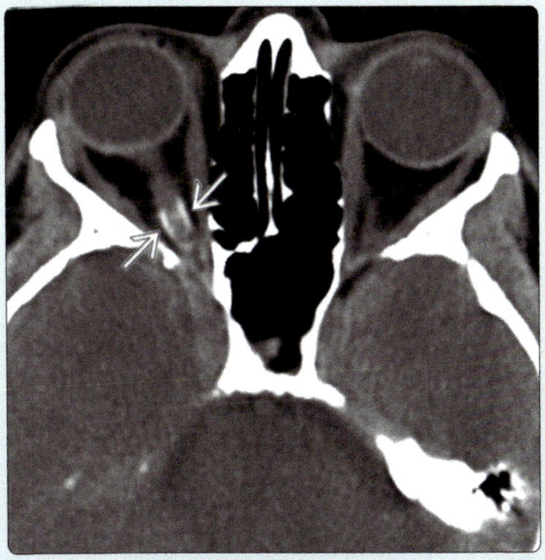
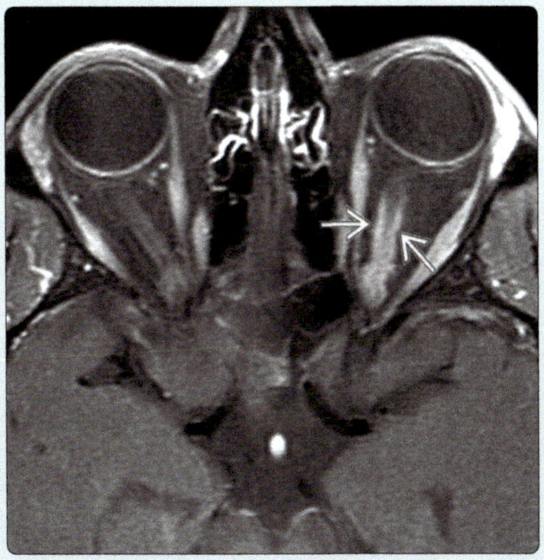

(Left) *NECT scan shows typical "tram track" calcifications ➡ of optic nerve sheath meningioma. No obvious soft tissue abnormality is seen on this noncontrast CT study.* **(Right)** *Axial T1WI C+ FS MR in another case shows a symmetric en plaque thickening/enhancement of the left nerve sheath characteristic of meningioma ➡. Enhancing tumor outlining the nerve results in the "tram-tracks" mimicking calcification described on CT.*

PART II: SPINE
SECTION 1

Normal Anatomy and Congenital Disorders

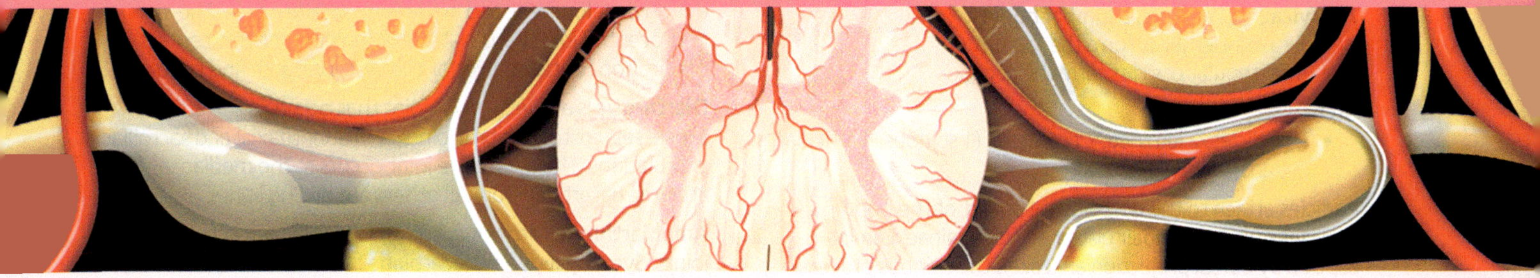

Anatomy

Malformations, Congenital Disorders, and Scoliosis

Imaging Anatomy

There are **33** spinal vertebrae, which comprise 2 components: A cylindrical ventral bone mass, which is the vertebral **body**, and the dorsal **arch**.

7 cervical, 12 thoracic, 5 lumbar bodies

- 5 fused elements form the sacrum
- 4-5 irregular ossicles form the coccyx

Arch

- 2 pedicles, 2 laminae, 7 processes (1 spinous, 4 articular, 2 transverse)

Pedicles attach to the dorsolateral aspect of the body. Pedicles unite with a pair of arched flat laminae. Lamina capped by dorsal projection are called the spinous process. Transverse processes arise from the sides of the arches.

The 2 articular processes (zygapophyses) are diarthrodial joints. The 1st is a superior process bearing a facet with the surface directed dorsally. The 2nd is an inferior process bearing a facet with the surface directed ventrally.

Pars interarticularis is the part of the arch that lies between the superior and inferior articular facets of all subatlantal movable elements. The pars are positioned to receive biomechanical stresses of translational forces displacing superior facets ventrally, whereas inferior facets remain attached to dorsal arch (spondylolysis). C2 exhibits a unique anterior relation between the superior facet and the posteriorly placed inferior facet. This relationship leads to an elongated C2 pars interarticularis, which is the site of the hangman's fracture.

Cervical

The cervical bodies are small and thin relative to the size of the arch and foramen, with the transverse diameter greater than the AP diameter. The lateral edges of the superior surface of the body are turned upward into the uncinate processes. The transverse foramen perforates the transverse processes. The vertebral artery resides within the transverse foramen, most commonly starting at the C6 level.

C1 has no body and forms a circular bony mass. The superior facets of C1 are large ovals that face upward, and the inferior facets are circular in shape. Large transverse processes are present on C1 with fused anterior and posterior tubercles.

The C2 complex consists of the axis body with dens/odontoid process. The odontoid embryologically arises from the centrum of the first cervical vertebrae.

The C7 vertebral body shows a transitional morphology with a prominent spinous process.

Thoracic

Thoracic bodies are heart-shaped and increase in size from superior to inferior. Facets are present for rib articulation, and the laminae are broad and thick. Spinous processes are long and are directed obliquely caudally. Superior facets are thin and directed posteriorly. The T1 vertebral body shows a complete facet for the capitulum of the first rib and an inferior demifacet for capitulum of second rib.

Lumbar

The lumbar vertebral bodies are large, wide, and thick and lack a transverse foramen or costal articular facets. The pedicles are strong and directed posteriorly. The superior articular processes are directed dorsomedially and almost face each other. The inferior articular processes are directed anteriorly and laterally.

Joints

Synarthrosis is an immovable joint of cartilage and occurs during development and in the first decade of life. The neurocentral joint occurs at the union point of two centers of ossification for two halves of the vertebral arch and centrum.

Diarthrosis is a true synovial joint that occurs in the articular processes, costovertebral joints, and atlantoaxial and sacroiliac articulations. The pivot-type joint occurs at the median atlantoaxial articulation. All others are gliding joints.

Amphiarthroses are nonsynovial, movable connective tissue joints. **Symphysis** is a fibrocartilage fusion between 2 bones, as in the intervertebral disc. **Syndesmosis** is a ligamentous connection common in the spine, such as the paired ligamenta flava, intertransverse ligaments, and interspinous ligaments. An unpaired syndesmosis is present in the supraspinous ligament.

Atlantooccipital articulation is composed of a diarthrosis between the lateral mass of atlas and occipital condyles and the syndesmoses of the atlantooccipital membranes. Anterior atlantooccipital membrane is the extension of the anterior longitudinal ligament (ALL). The posterior atlantooccipital membrane is homologous to the ligamenta flava.

Atlantoaxial articulation is a pivot joint. The transverse ligament maintains the relationship of the odontoid to the anterior arch of atlas. Synovial cavities are present between the transverse ligament/odontoid and the atlas/odontoid junctions.

Disc

The intervertebral disc is composed of 3 parts: The **cartilaginous endplate**, the **anulus fibrosis**, and the **nucleus pulposus**. The height of the lumbar disc space generally increases as one progresses caudally. The anulus consists of concentrically oriented collagenous fibers, which serve to contain the central nucleus pulposus. These fibers insert into the vertebral cortex via Sharpey fibers and also attach to the ALL and posterior longitudinal ligament (PLL). Type I collagen predominates at the periphery of the anulus, whereas type II collagen predominates in the inner anulus. The normal contour of the posterior aspect of the anulus is dependent on the contour of its adjacent endplate. Typically, this is slightly concave in the axial plane; although commonly at L4-L5 and L5-S1, these posterior margins will be flat or even convex. A convex shape on the axial images alone should not be interpreted as degenerative bulging.

The nucleus pulposus is a remnant of the embryonal notochord and consists of a well-hydrated, noncompressible proteoglycan matrix with scattered chondrocytes. Proteoglycans form a major macromolecular component, including chondroitin 6-sulfate, keratan sulfate, and hyaluronic acid. Proteoglycans consist of protein core with multiple attached glycosaminoglycan chains. The nucleus occupies an eccentric position within the confines of anulus and is more dorsal with respect to the center of the vertebral body. At birth, ~ 85-90% of the nucleus is water. This water content gradually decreases with advancing age. Within the nucleus pulposus on T2-weighted sagittal images, there is often a linear hypointensity coursing in an anteroposterior direction, the intranuclear cleft. This region of more prominent fibrous tissue should not be interpreted as intradiscal air or calcification.

Anterior Longitudinal Ligament (ALL)

The ALL runs along the **ventral** surface of the vertebral bodies from the skull to the sacrum. The ALL is narrowest in the cervical spine and is firmly attached at the ends of each vertebral body. It is loosely attached at the midsection of the disc.

Posterior Longitudinal Ligament (PLL)

The PLL runs on the **dorsal** surface of the vertebral bodies from the skull to the sacrum. The PLL has a segmental denticulate configuration and is wider at the disc space but narrows and becomes thicker at the vertebral body level.

Craniocervical Ligaments

The craniocervical ligaments are located anteriorly to spinal cord and occur in 3 layers: Anterior, middle, and posterior. Anterior ligaments consist of the odontoid ligaments (apical and alar). The apical ligament is a small fibrous band extending from dens tip to basion. Alar ligaments are thick, horizontally directed ligaments extending from the lateral surface of dens tip to anteromedial occipital condyles. The middle layer consists of the cruciate ligament. The **transverse ligament** is a strong horizontal component of the cruciate ligament extending from behind the dens to the medial aspect of C1 lateral masses. The craniocaudal component consists of a fibrous band running from the transverse ligament superiorly to the foramen magnum and inferiorly to C2. Posteriorly, the tectorial membrane is the continuation of PLL and attaches to anterior rim of the foramen magnum.

Vertebral Artery

The vertebral artery arises as the 1st branch of the subclavian artery on both sides. The vertebral artery travels cephalad within the foramen transversarium (transverse foramen) within the transverse processes. The 1st segment of the vertebral artery extends from its origin to the entrance into the foramen of the transverse process of the cervical vertebrae, usually the 6th. The most common variation is the origin of the left vertebral from the arch, between the left common carotid and the left subclavian arteries (2-6%). The vertebral artery in these variant cases almost always enters the foramen of the transverse process of C5. The second segment runs within the transverse foramen to the C2 level. Nerve roots pass posterior to the vertebral artery. The 3rd segment starts at the C2 level where the artery loops and turns lateral to ascend in the C1 transverse foramen. It then turns medial crossing on top of C1 in a groove. The 4th segment starts where the artery perforates the dura and arachnoid at lateral edge of posterior occipitoatlantal membrane, coursing ventrally on the medulla to join with the other vertebral to make the basilar artery.

Vertebral Column Blood Supply

Paired segmental arteries (intercostals, lumbar arteries) arise from the aorta and extend dorsolaterally around the middle of the vertebral body. Near the transverse process, the segmental artery divides into lateral and dorsal branches. The lateral branch supplies dorsal musculature, and the dorsal branch passes lateral to the foramen, giving off branch(es) and providing major vascular supply to bone and vertebral canal contents. The posterior central branch supplies disc and vertebral body, whereas the prelaminal branch supplies the inner surface of the arch, ligamenta flava, and regional epidural tissue. The neural branch entering the neural foramen supplies pia, arachnoid, and cord. The postlaminar branch supplies musculature overlying lamina and branches to bone.

Spinal Cord Vascular Supply

The spinal cord vasculature is derived from the vertebral arteries as well as segmental vessels at multiple levels. A single anterior spinal artery supplies the anterior 2/3 of the cord; paired posterior spinal arteries supply the posterior 1/3. Both are augmented by numerous segmental feeders from radicular branches. Penetrating medullary branches to the central cord arise from multiple radicular branches that have few collaterals.

The artery of Adamkiewicz is the dominant anterior radicular feeding vessel to the thoracic cord, typically arising from one of the left T9-12 branches. It courses cephalad along the anterior cord, then makes a characteristic "hairpin" turn, and courses inferiorly to the conus.

Venous drainage occurs through a network of interconnected veins that form a tortuous venous plexus over the pial surface of the cord. The plexus consists of median and lateral longitudinal veins, which drain the cord and terminate in anterior and posterior internal vertebral venous plexi (of Batson) within the epidural space. The plexi are a series of irregular, thin-walled, valveless sinuses arranged in a continuous ladder-like series of cross-connected expansions extending throughout the epidural fat. The anterior plexus also receives basivertebral veins from the vertebral bodies. The internal vertebral venous plexi drain into external plexi that surround the vertebral column and interconnect with the inferior and superior vena cavae as well as the azygous/hemiazygos systems and the intracranial dural sinuses.

Nerves

Spinal nerves are arranged in 31 pairs and grouped regionally: 8 cervical, 12 thoracic, 5 lumbar, 5 sacral, 1 coccygeal. Ascensus spinalis is the apparent developmental rising of the cord related to differential spinal growth. The course of nerve roots becomes longer and more oblique at lower segments.

Meninges are divided into dura, arachnoid, and pia.

Dura is a dense, tough covering corresponding to the meningeal layer of the cranial dura. The epidural space is filled with fat, loose connective tissue, and veins. The dura continues with spinal nerves through the foramen to fuse with the epineurium. Cephalic attachment of the dura is at the foramen magnum and the caudal attachment at the back of the coccyx.

Arachnoid is the middle covering, which is thin, delicate, and continuous with cranial arachnoid. The arachnoid is separated from the dura by the potential subdural space.

Pia is the inner covering of delicate connective tissue closely applied to the cord. Longitudinal fibers are laterally concentrated as denticulate ligaments lying between posterior and anterior roots and attach at 21 points to dura. Longitudinal fibers are concentrated dorsally as the septum posticum attaching the dorsal cord to the dorsal midline dura.

(Left) *Sagittal view of CVJ shows: 1) Ant. atlantooccipital membrane, 2) apical lig., 3) ant. longitudinal lig., 4) cruciate lig., 5) tectorial membrane, 6) transverse lig., 7) post. longitudinal lig., and 8) post. atlantooccipital membrane. Red star is basion; blue star is opisthion.* **(Right)** *Posterior view of CVJ shows: 1) Sup. cruciate ligament, 2) cruciate lig., 3) odontoid ant. to cruciate lig., 4) atlantoaxial jt., 5) accessory atlantoaxial lig., 6) inf. cruciate lig., 7) transverse lig., 8) alar lig., and 9) atlantooccipital jt. Red star is basion.*

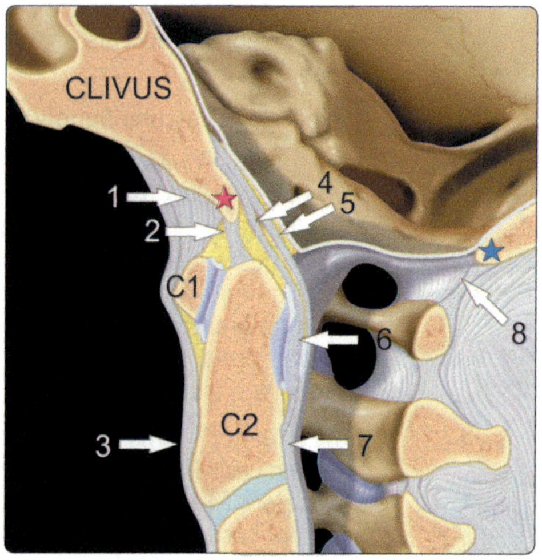

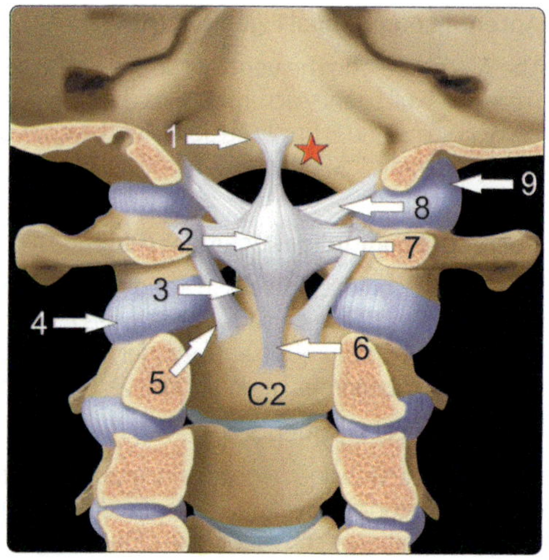

(Left) *Graphic shows cervical vertebra from above. Vertebral body is broad transversely, central canal is large and triangular in shape, pedicles are directed posterolaterally, and laminae are delicate. Lateral masses contain the transverse foramen for passage of vertebral artery and veins.* **(Right)** *Mid-C5 body at the pedicle level: Transverse foramina are prominent, encompassing the vertical course of vertebral artery. The anterior and posterior tubercles give rise to muscle attachments in neck.*

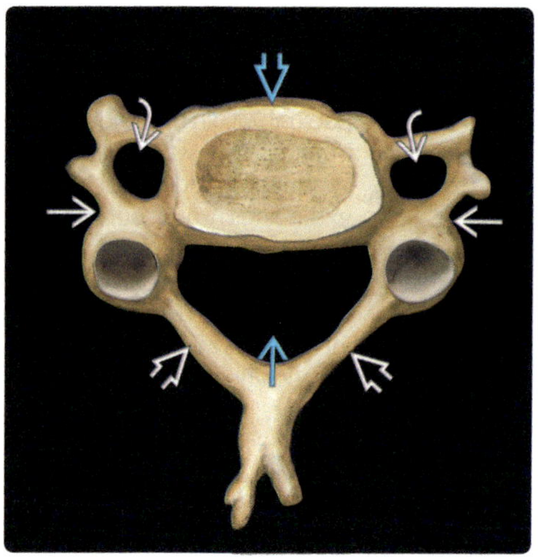

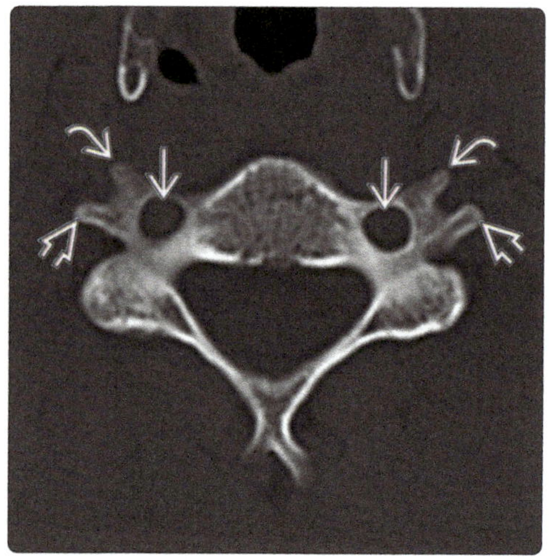

(Left) *Graphic shows a thoracic vertebral body from above. Thoracic bodies are characterized by long, spinous and transverse processes. Complex rib articulation includes both costotransverse joints and costovertebral joints. Facet joints are oriented in the coronal plane.* **(Right)** *Image through the pedicle level of the thoracic spine shows that the coronal orientation of the facet joints is well identified in this section. The pedicles are thin and gracile, with adjacent rib articulations.*

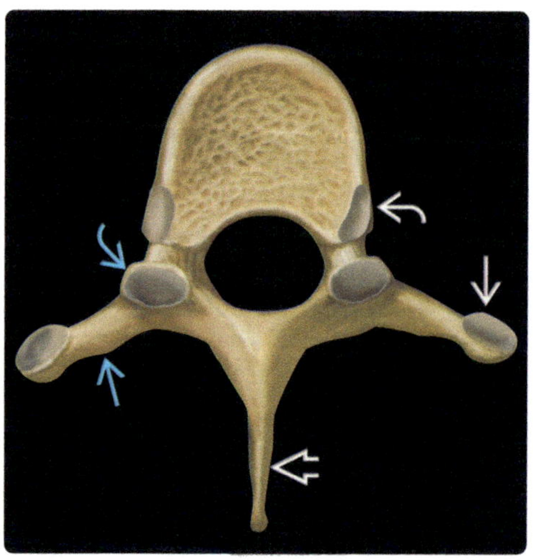

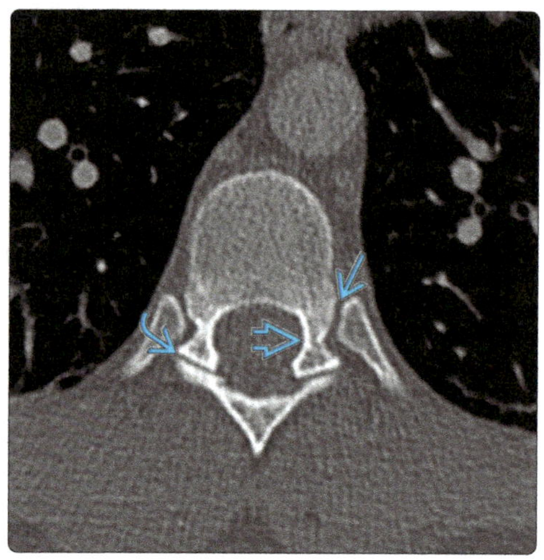

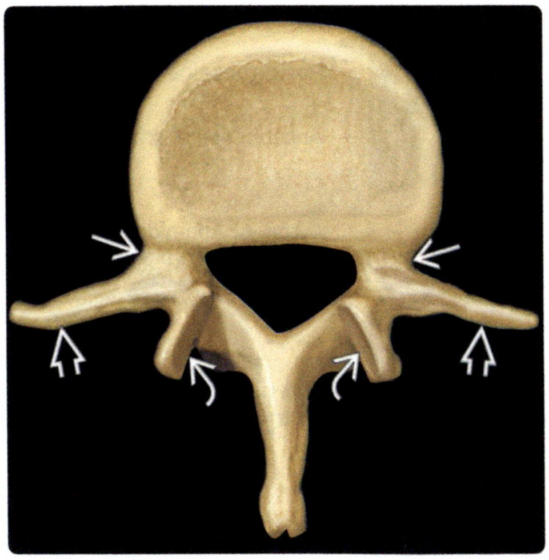

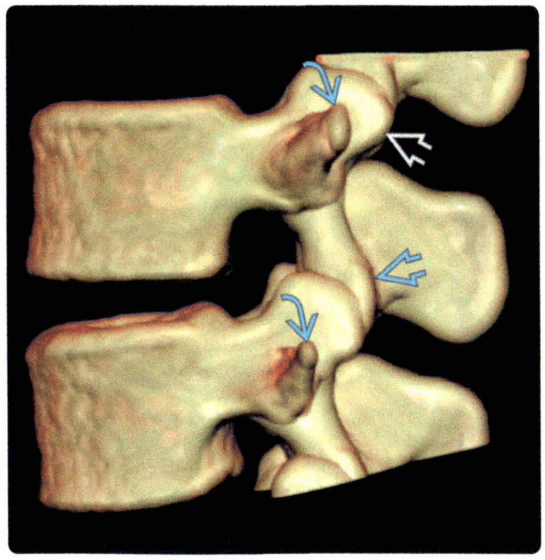

(Left) *Graphic shows lumbar body from above. Large, sturdy lumbar bodies connect to thick pedicles and transversely directed transverse processes. Facets maintain oblique orientation favoring flexion/extension.* **(Right)** *Lateral 3D scan of the lumbar spine shows large bodies joined by thick posterior elements with the superior and inferior articular processes angled in lateral plane. Transverse processes jut out laterally for muscle attachments.*

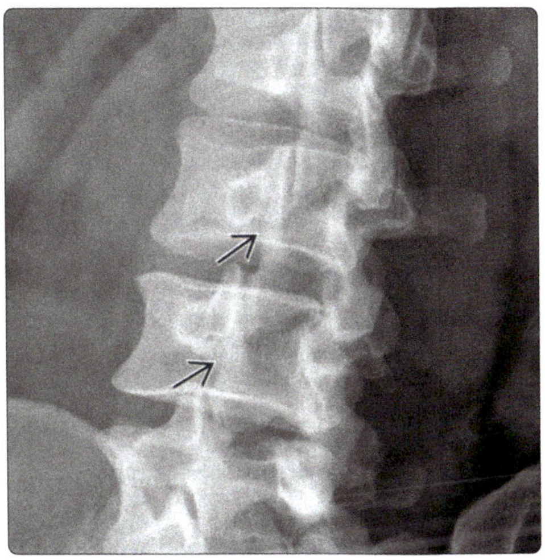

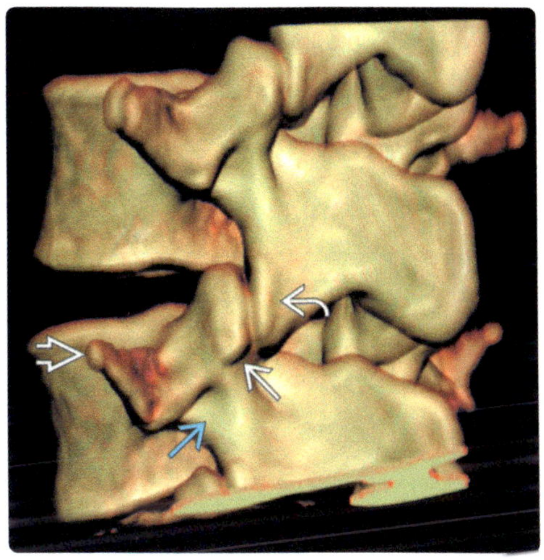

(Left) *Coronal oblique view of the lumbar spine shows the typical "Scotty dog" appearance of the posterior elements. The neck of the "dog" is the pars interarticularis.* **(Right)** *Oblique 3D exam of lumbar spine shows surface anatomy of "scotty dog": Transverse process (nose), superior articular process (ear), inferior articular process (front leg), and intervening pars interarticularis (neck). Pedicle that forms "eye" on CT reconstructions is obscured.*

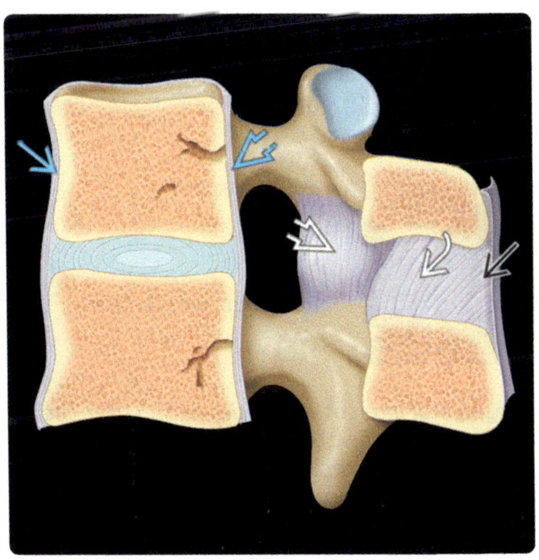

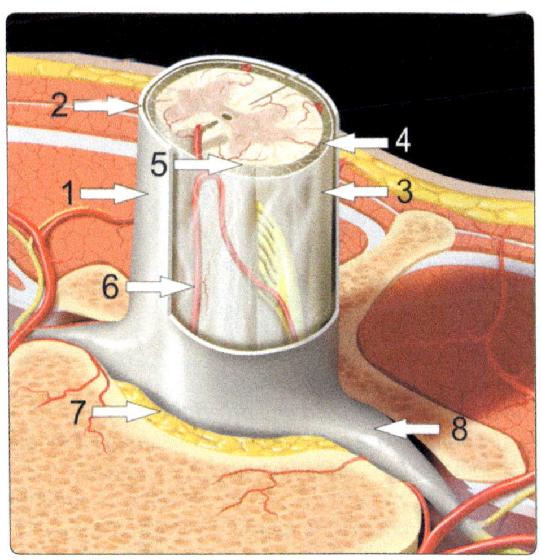

(Left) *Cut-away graphic shows lumbar vertebral bodies joined by disc & anterior & posterior longitudinal ligaments. Paired ligamentum flavum & interspinous ligament join posterior elements, with midline supraspinous ligament.* **(Right)** *Graphic shows spinal cord and coverings: (1) dura mater, (2) subdural space, (3) arachnoid mater, (4) subarachnoid space, (5) pia mater, (6) ant. spinal artery, (7) epidural space, and (8) root sleeve.*

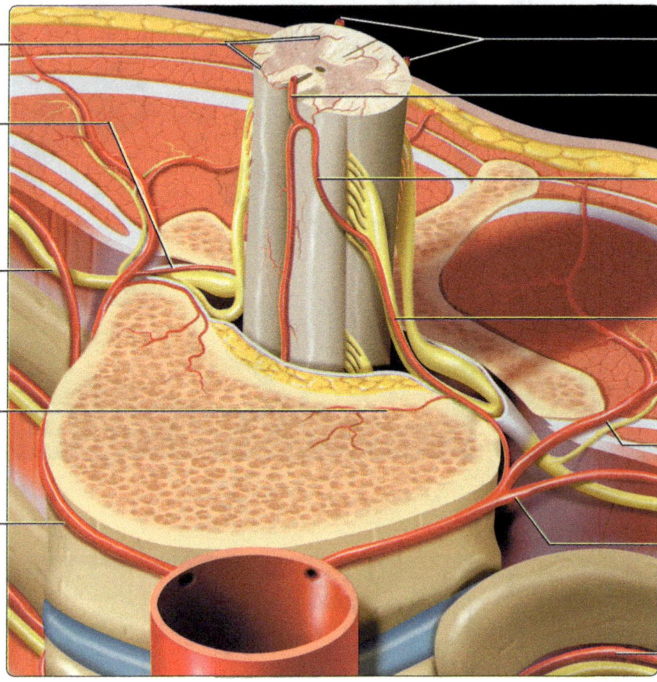

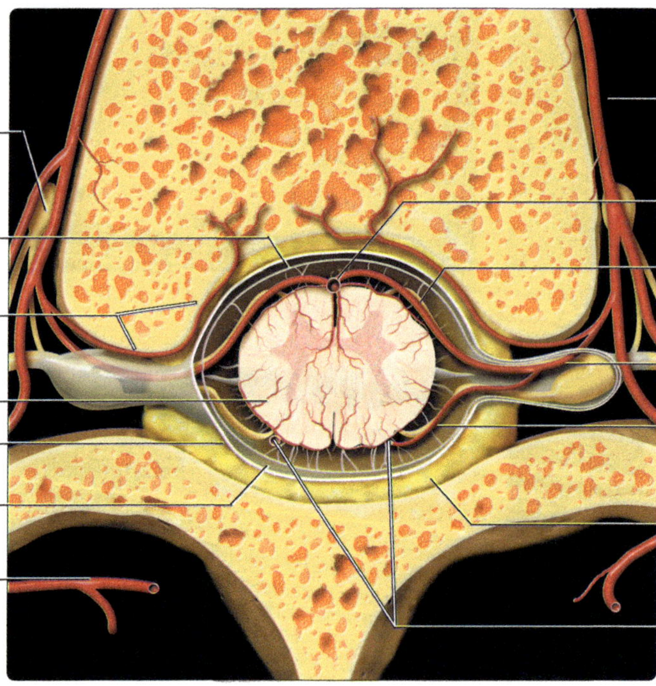

(Top) *Oblique axial graphic of the thoracic spinal cord and arterial supply at T10 shows segmental intercostal arteries arising from the lower thoracic aorta. The artery of Adamkiewicz is the dominant segmental feeding vessel to the thoracic cord, supplying the anterior aspect of the cord via the anterior spinal artery. Adamkiewicz has a characteristic "hairpin" turn on the cord surface as it first courses superiorly, then turns inferiorly.* **(Bottom)** *Axial graphic shows the anterior and posterior radiculomedullary arteries anastomosing with the anterior and posterior spinal arteries. Penetrating medullary arteries in the cord are largely end-arteries with few collaterals. The cord "watershed" zone is at the central gray matter.*

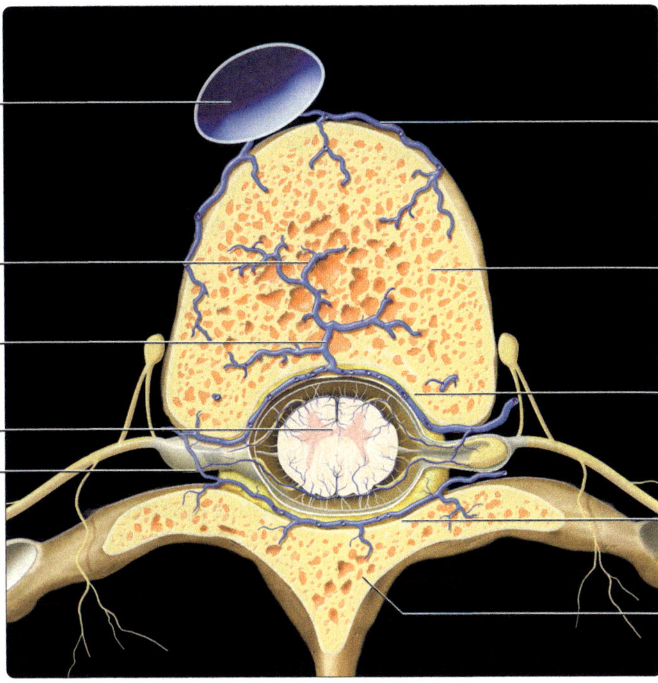

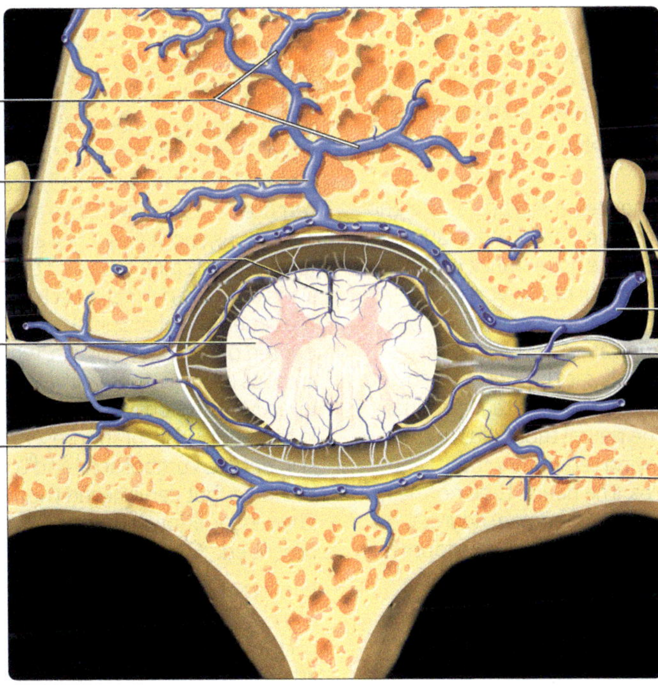

(Top) *Axial graphic shows thoracic vertebral bodies and venous anatomy. The vertebral bodies are drained by anterior perforating veins, as well as via the basivertebral venous plexus. The anterior perforating veins are part of the anterior external plexus, whereas the basivertebral veins are part of the anterior internal plexus. The spinal central canal contains the anterior and posterior internal vertebral venous plexi.* **(Bottom)** *Magnified graphic shows the internal vertebral venous plexus. The radicular veins course along the dorsal and ventral rami, eventually draining into components of the anterior or posterior internal plexus, and subsequently the segmental veins, which will drain into the superior or inferior vena cava.*

Terminology

Definitions

Morphogenetic fields
- Embryological cellular regions with potential for development into discrete anatomic structures

Gradient fields
- Describe gradually varying potential to form specific individual bones and organs within morphogenetic field

Homeobox genes
- Gene family complexes that regulate early embryologic differentiation
- Located on separate chromosomes
- Arranged linearly in same order as expression along craniocaudal axis

Imaging Protocols

Multiplanar magnetic resonance imaging best evaluates soft tissues, neural structures, and ligaments. Multidetector axial CT with sagittal and coronal reconstruction optimally defines bone anatomy.

Embryology

The spinal axis develops following a (mostly) orderly progression of steps, with the vertebral axis and spinal cord developing synchronously. Embryological spine formation begins in the occipital region, then subsequently commences at multiple other sites simultaneously. These sites progress at different rates and thus will be at different developmental stages at any given point in time. The cephalic spine (to about the conus level) forms by the process of primary neurulation, whereas the caudal spine forms separately by secondary neurulation (also called canalization and retrogressive differentiation). Most spinal anomalies may be explained by 1 or more events going awry during these steps.

Primary Neurulation

Embryonic spinal formation commences at the end of the 2nd gestational week with formation of the Hensen node and at the beginning of the 3rd week with the appearance of the neural plate during gastrulation (2-germ cell layer embryo → 3-germ cell layer embryo). The notochordal process forms at days 16-17, with transient communication of the amnion through notochordal canal to the yolk sac through neurenteric canal of Kovalevsky. Abnormalities during this stage produce the neurenteric cyst spectrum. The neural tube folds and closes at the end of 3rd week, leaving temporary cranial and caudal openings called neuropores. The neural tube normally closes by days 25-27, signaling the end of primary neurulation. A closed neural tube is a prerequisite for normal development of the posterior neural arch.

During primary neurulation, the neural tube separates from the overlying ectoderm during the process of dysjunction. If dysjunction occurs prematurely (premature dysjunction), perineural mesenchyme is permitted access to the neural groove and ependymal lining, differentiates into fat, and prevents complete neural tube closure, leading to the lipomatous malformation spectrum. Conversely, if dysjunction fails to occur (nondysjunction), an ectodermal-neuroectodermal tract forms that prevents mesenchymal migration, leading to focal or widespread dysraphism and the open neural tube defect spectrum, including myelomeningocele (MMC), dorsal dermal sinus, and myelocystocele. It is important to note that nondysjunction and premature dysjunction anomalies can coexist in combination simultaneously.

Premature Dysjunction

Premature dysjunction of the neural tube from the overlying ectoderm allows the perineural mesenchyme to access the neural groove and differentiate into fat, physically preventing completion of neural tube closure and resulting in a spinal lipoma, with or without closed posterior spinal dysraphism. The most commonly premature dysjunction anomalies are lipomyelomeningocele (LMMC) and intradural (juxtamedullary) lipoma. LMMC is a skin-covered, closed dysraphism anomaly in which the neural placode is complexed with a lipoma contiguous with the subcutaneous fat through a posterior dysraphic defect. In all cases, the lipoma attaches to and tethers the spinal cord. LMMC accounts for 20-56% of occult spinal dysraphism and 20% of skin-covered lumbosacral masses. Spinal lipoma is subdivided into intradural (juxtamedullary, subpial) and terminal lipomas. Intradural lipomas most commonly occur near the conus. Conversely, terminal lipoma is variably considered within both the premature dysjunction and abnormal caudal cell mass differentiation spectra, with findings overlapping both mechanisms. Some authorities ("lumpers") combine all of the premature dysjunction disorders featuring lipomas into a lipomatous malformation spectrum for simplicity, recognizing that there is considerable overlap between the LMMC and lipoma malformations.

Nondysjunction

In contrast, anomalies resulting from nondysjunction related to teratogens or faulty notochord induction occur when the neural tube fails to dissociate from adjacent cutaneous ectoderm over either a focal or long interval. The least extensive variation is the dorsal dermal sinus, which occurs when a single connection remains, forming a fibrous cord from skin to conus or central spinal cord canal. The dermal sinus tract usually has an atypical dimple at the ostium that is remote (> 2.5 cm) from the anus, often combined with other cutaneous anomalies. They are most common in the lumbosacral spine followed by the occipital region, and the sinus opening dermatomal level correlates with the metameric level of spinal cord attachment. All have some degree of focal dysraphism, which may be as subtle as a bifid spinous process. More extensive nondysjunction produces the open MMC lesion associated with maternal folate deficiency. In this entity, the infant presents with an open, red, weeping skin defect. Lumbosacral and thoracolumbar MMC are most common, but cervical and thoracic MMC are observed rarely. Their association with the Chiari 2 malformation is well described.

Important mimics of the dorsal dermal sinus are the low sacral (coccygeal) dimple and pilonidal sinus. The low sacral or coccygeal dimple is common and features a low skin dimple affixed to the coccyx by a "spot weld." These are found within the intergluteal cleft, never communicate with the spinal canal, and require no treatment. A pilonidal sinus has a low ostium, does not communicate with the spinal canal, and may present later with cutaneous infection.

Secondary Neurulation (Canalization and Retrogressive Differentiation)

By day 30, neural tube development below the caudal neuropore has commenced within the undifferentiated caudal cell mass of the primitive streak, which subsequently regresses. This process is inherently less precise than primary neurulation, which leads to more bizarre anomalies, and is characterized by the development of cysts in the caudal cell mass that coalesce into an ependymal-lined tubular structure that subsequently unites with the rostral neural tube. At day 48, a transient ventriculus terminalis appears in the future conus. If this persists after birth, it is noted incidentally as a persistent ventriculus terminalis or 5th ventricle, usually of no clinical significance. Failure of proper canalization and retrogressive differentiation leads to caudal regression spectrum, terminal myelocystocele, anterior sacral meningocele, tethered cord spectrum, or sacrococcygeal teratoma. By the 3rd gestational month, the spinal cord extends the entire length of the developing spinal column. It is the more rapid elongation of the vertebral column and dura relative to the spinal cord that produces the apparent cord ascent during gestation. The conus should be at adult level soon after birth, and conus persistence below L2 after the 1st month of life in a full-term infant is probably abnormal.

Caudal cell mass anomalies are a diverse group of anomalies with a significant range of severity resulting from aberrant differentiation and retrogressive differentiation of the caudal cell mass. The etiology is postulated to be a metabolic or toxic insult to the caudal cell mass prior to the 4th gestational week. Most cases are sporadic, although a dominantly inherited defect in *HLBX9* has been recently described. 15-20% are infants of diabetic mothers, whereas 1% of diabetic mother offspring are afflicted. There is an association with vertebral, anal, cardiac, tracheal, esophageal, renal, and limb (VACTERL) anomalies, omphalocele, bladder extrophy, imperforate anus, and Currarino triad.

Hypogenesis or agenesis of the caudal cell mass produces the caudal regression syndrome (CRS). Two types are described; the more severe type 1 CRS shows a foreshortened terminal vertebral column with high-lying, wedge-shaped conus termination and severe associated anomalies, whereas the less severe type 2 CRS demonstrates a low-lying, tethered cord with milder associated malformations. In general, the higher the cord termination, the more severe the sacral anomalies. The most severe CRS presentations are lumbosacral agenesis, where the spine terminates at the lower thoracic level, and severe sacral dysgenesis with fused lower extremities in a so-called "mermaid" configuration (sirenomelia). In contrast, the mildest CRS cases manifest only a missing terminal sacral segment and are clinically asymptomatic. CRS is associated with myriad other congenital abnormalities, including renal/pulmonary hypoplasia and anorectal malformations. Other congenital spinal malformations, such as open dysraphism, segmentation and fusion anomalies, and split cord malformations, are also commonly associated, and imaging should include a search to exclude those entities as well.

A rarer presentation of caudal cell mass dysplasia than CRS is the anterior sacral meningocele, which is a large meningocele traversing an enlarged sacral foramen producing a presacral cystic mass. Most are sporadic, with a minority showing an inherited predisposition within the Currarino triad or in syndromes featuring dural dysplasia (neurofibromatosis type 1, Marfan syndrome). As with other caudal cell mass dysplasias, anorectal malformations, caudal dysgenesis, and dermoid/epidermoid tumors may be found as well.

Terminal myelocystocele is very rare and manifests as a hydromyelic spinal cord traversing a meningocele terminating in a skin-covered myelocystocele. Associated anorectal and other visceral anomalies are common and drive the early management while producing much of the morbidity and mortality.

Perhaps the most common lesion in the caudal cell mass dysplasia spectrum is tethered cord syndrome (TCS). Semantically speaking, TCS refers only to patients with a low-lying cord and thickened filum and not patients with other spinal anomalies and cord abnormalities, although those patients may look "tethered" and clinically present similarly. It is important to consider TCS as a clinical diagnosis, with imaging relegated to the role of preoperative planning rather than for establishing the primary diagnosis. On imaging, TCS manifests either as a taut spinal cord without definitive conus or low-lying conus with thickened, shortened filum and variably an associated lipomatous malformation.

Finally, if the primitive streak incompletely regresses and leaves a caudal remnant, a sacrococcygeal teratoma (SCT) may arise from the residual totipotential cell rests (Hensen node). SCTs demonstrate tissue derived from all 3 cell layers and contain varying proportions of mature and immature elements.

Vertebral Formation and Segmentation

Vertebral body formation occurs simultaneously with spinal cord development. During neurulation, the notochord induces the surrounding paraxial mesoderm derived from primitive streak to form paired somite blocks (myotomes, sclerotomes). The myotomes form the paraspinal muscles and skin cover, whereas the sclerotomes divide into medial and lateral formations to produce the vertebral body, intervertebral disc, meninges, spinal ligaments (medial), and posterior spinal elements (lateral). Failure of correct notochordal induction leads to incomplete splitting of the neural plate from the notochord and produces the split notochord syndromes [neurenteric cyst and diastematomyelia (DSM)]. At day 24, a remarkable process known as sclerotomal resegmentation commences and continues until the 5th week. During sclerotomal resegmentation, a horizontal sclerotomal cleft appears in the vertebra, and the caudal half of 1 vertebra combines with the rostral half of the vertebra below to form a "new" vertebral body. The notochord within the vertebral body subsequently degenerates, and the intervertebral notochordal remnant becomes the intervertebral disc nucleus pulposus. Between days 40-60, the vertebral body and neural arches undergo chondrification and then subsequent ossification continuing past birth and into young adulthood. Ossification begins in the lower thoracic and upper lumbar regions and diverges cranially and caudally. In the cervical region, the vertebral primary ossification centers appear after the neural arch centers, beginning in lower cervical spine (C6, C7) and commencing rostrally. Cells of sclerotomal origin migrate dorsally to form the neural arch and condense to produce the spinous processes. The neural arches are situated intersegmentally with respect to the myotomes, so that each neural arch is associated with 2 successive myotomal segments. Absence of a ganglion at a vertebral level is postulated to allow unilateral arch fusion (congenital osseus bar).

Anomalies of vertebral formation and segmentation arise from aberrancies in vertebral column formation. These are generally divided into anomalies resulting from failure (partial or total) of vertebral formation (FVF) and failure to correctly segment after vertebral formation (vertebral segmentation failure). The abnormal vertebra may be supernumerary or replace a normal vertebral body. As a rule of thumb, the more severe the segmentation and fusion anomalies, the higher the incidence of concurrent visceral organ or other neuraxis anomalies. Abnormal *PAX1* expression is postulated to be etiological in the development of the segmentation anomalies, and other visceral and neuraxis anomalies are commonly identified as well. With FVF, the degree and location of vertebral formation failure predict morphology; unilateral chondral center deficiency and failure of ossification produce a hemivertebra, whereas central failure of ossification centers to unite produces a "butterfly" vertebra. Conversely, vertebral segmentation failure presents with composite or "block" vertebra and posterior element fusions. Not surprisingly, block vertebra frequently coexist with FVF hemivertebra and butterfly vertebra, leading many to lump them together into the working term "segmentation and fusion anomalies" (SFAs). Many clinical syndromes prominently feature SFAs, including Klippel-Feil and Jarcho-Levin (spondylothoracic dysplasia). Therefore, SFAs are not a finding that implicates a specific disorder but rather function more as an imaging marker for a possible syndromic process.

Spinal Cord

Spinal cord formation occurs in conjunction with vertebral formation. Within the spinal cord, the neuroepithelial cells (neuroblasts) around the central tube form the mantle layer, which produces the spinal cord gray matter. The outermost layer forms the marginal layer, which myelinates to produce the spinal cord white matter. The central neuroepithelial cells differentiate into ependymal cells along the central canal. Neural crest cells along each side of the neural groove form the dorsal root ganglia, autonomic ganglia, Schwann cells, leptomeninges, and adrenal medulla.

Notochordal Anomalies

Notochordal anomalies, primarily neurenteric cyst and DSM, produce some of the most bizarre congenital spinal anomalies. Neurenteric cysts, consisting of an intraspinal cyst lined by enteric mucosa, are most common in the thoracic spine followed by the cervical spine. They arise from a putative abnormal persistent connection between the primitive endoderm and ectoderm during the 3rd embryonic week. Whereas normally the notochord separates the ventral endoderm (foregut) and dorsal ectoderm (skin, spinal cord) during embryogenesis, in a neurenteric cyst there is failure of separation that "splits" the notochord and hinders development of mesoderm, trapping a small piece of the primitive gut within the developing spinal canal. This gut remnant may become isolated, forming a cyst, or maintain connections with the gut, skin, or both, producing the spectrum of fistulae and sinuses comprising the dorsal-enteric spinal anomalies spectrum. The most severe cases maintain communication through a primitive vertebral canal of Kovalevsky, but even mild cases usually show some kind of vertebral segmentation anomalies on close inspection.

DSM arises from a similar aberrant process to neurenteric cyst, resulting in a splitting of the spinal cord into two hemicords, each with one ventral and one dorsal root. The hemicords may be symmetric or asymmetric (partial DSM), and 1 or both may feature hydromyelia or tethering. Because the notochord influences vertebral development, vertebral segmentation anomalies are very commonly associated with DSM. The presence (type 1) or absence (type 2) of an osseous or fibrous spur and whether the cords reside in separate or a single dural tube are important for preoperative planning. Occasionally, the nerve root(s) will become adherent to the dura and tether the spinal cord, producing the so-called "meningocele manqué." DSM may be isolated or found in conjunction with other spinal anomalies, particularly MMC, and it is thus critical to search for DSM prior to operative repair of a spinal anomaly or scoliosis correction.

Congenital and Developmental Anomalies of Unknown Etiology

Other uncommon but important anomalies in which the etiology is not definitively known include the simple dorsal meningocele and the lateral meningocele. Dorsal meningocele by definition occurs dorsally, often in the lumbosacral spine, and strictly defined features a skin-covered meningocele devoid of neural elements protruding through a posterior dysraphic defect. In practice, however, it is not uncommon to find pieces of dysplastic nerve root or other neural tissue within the meningocele. Lateral meningoceles present as cerebrospinal fluid-filled paraspinal masses contiguous with the thecal sac extending through a neural foramen with adjacent pedicular and foraminal osseous remodeling.

Selected References

1. Babu R et al: Concurrent split cord malformation and teratoma: dysembryology, presentation, and treatment. J Clin Neurosci. 21(2):212-6, 2014
2. Gupta P et al: Congenital spinal cord anomalies: a pictorial review. Curr Probl Diagn Radiol. 42(2):57-66, 2013
3. Rufener S et al: Imaging of congenital spine and spinal cord malformations. Neuroimaging Clin N Am. 21(3):659-76, viii, 2011
4. Rossi A et al: Current classification and imaging of congenital spinal abnormalities. Semin Roentgenol. 41(4):250-73, 2006
5. Tortori-Donati P et al: Magnetic resonance imaging of spinal dysraphism. Top Magn Reson Imaging. 12(6):375-409, 2001
6. Tortori-Donati P et al: Spinal dysraphism: a review of neuroradiological features with embryological correlations and proposal for a new classification. Neuroradiology. 42(7):471-91, 2000
7. Pang D: Sacral agenesis and caudal spinal cord malformations. Neurosurgery. 32(5):755-78; discussion 778-9, 1993
8. Pang D et al: Split cord malformation: Part I: A unified theory of embryogenesis for double spinal cord malformations. Neurosurgery. 31(3):451-80, 1992

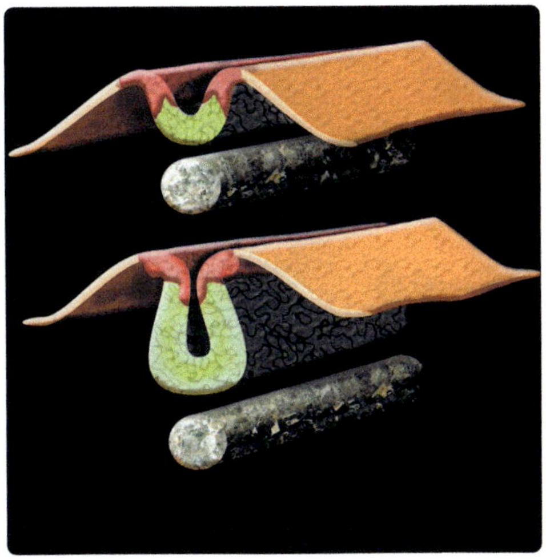

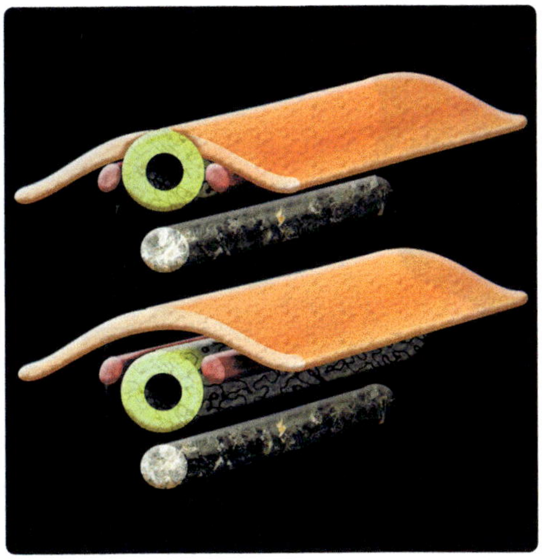

(Left) *3D graphic of neural tube embryology demonstrates normal formation of neural plate (top) and neural groove (bottom). Note the cutaneous epithelium (orange), neural crest (red), neural ectoderm (green), and notochord (gray).* **(Right)** *3D graphic of neural tube formation depicts normal neural tube closure (top) and subsequent dysjunction (bottom). Note the cutaneous epithelium (orange), neural crest (red), neural ectoderm (green), and notochord (gray).*

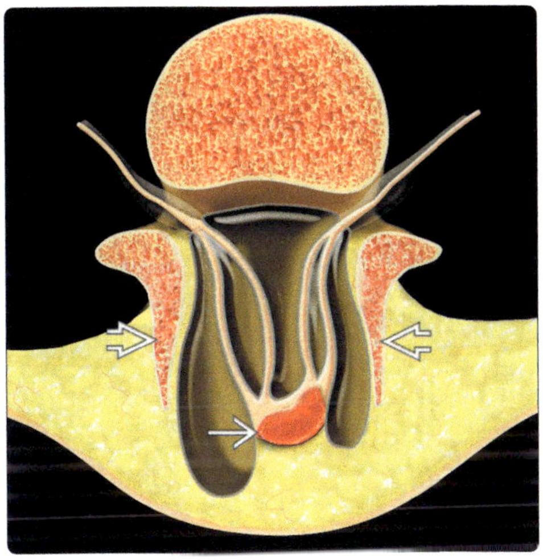

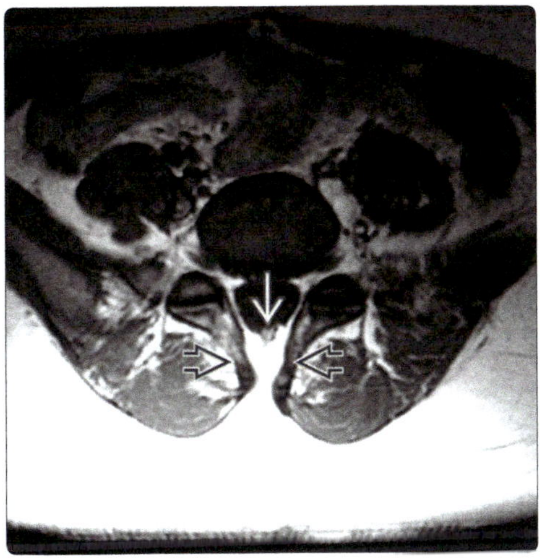

(Left) *Axial graphic illustrates premature dysjunction with a classic lipomyelomeningocele. The neural placode ➡ is displaced through the dysraphic unfused posterior elements ➡ into a meningocele sac.* **(Right)** *Axial T1WI MR (lipomyelomeningocele) shows the distal spinal cord ➡ inserting into a lipoma merging imperceptibly with lumbosacral subcutaneous fat through dysraphic posterior elements ⇨.*

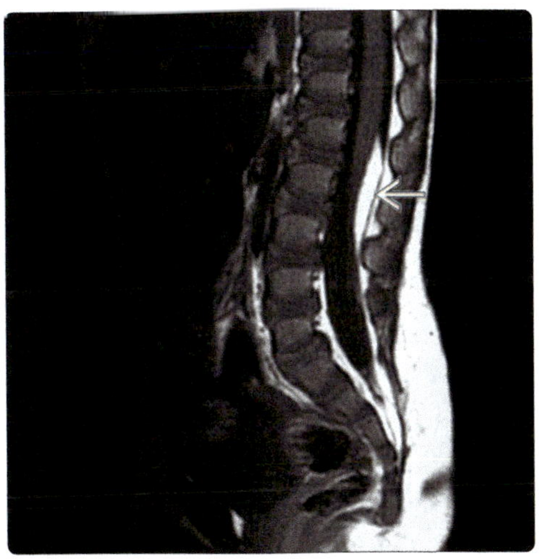

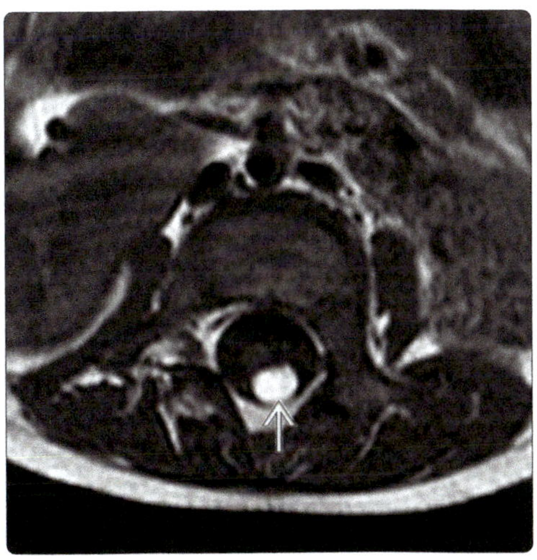

(Left) *Sagittal T1WI MR demonstrates the typical hyperintense appearance of a juxtamedullary or subpial conus lipoma ➡. The conus is low lying at L2/L3. These lipomas classically arise from premature dysjunction.* **(Right)** *Axial T1WI MR confirms the intradural location and close relationship of the lipoma ➡ with the dorsal conus surface. Additionally, the misshapen right kidney and empty left renal fossa were proven to represent crossed fused renal ectopia.*

(Left) *Axial graphic (nondysjunction) shows a classic myelomeningocele, with the nerve roots traversing a large meningocele sac from the exposed neural placode →, which merges into adjacent cutaneous fat and skin.* **(Right)** *Axial T1WI MR (unrepaired lumbar myelomeningocele) demonstrates nondysjunction, characterized by open dysraphism with lack of skin covering over the neural placode →. The neural elements are in direct contact with the outside environment.*

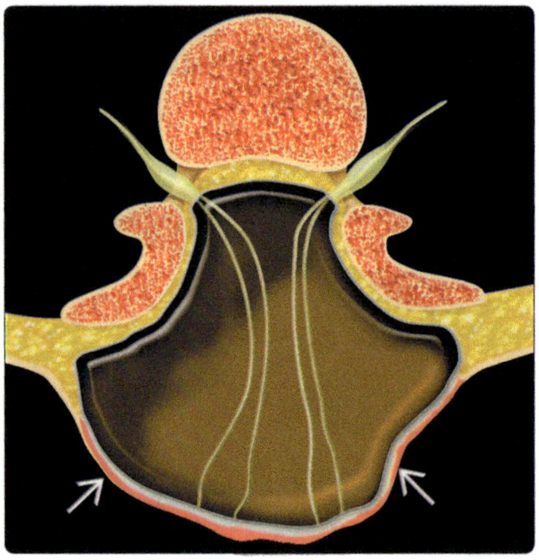

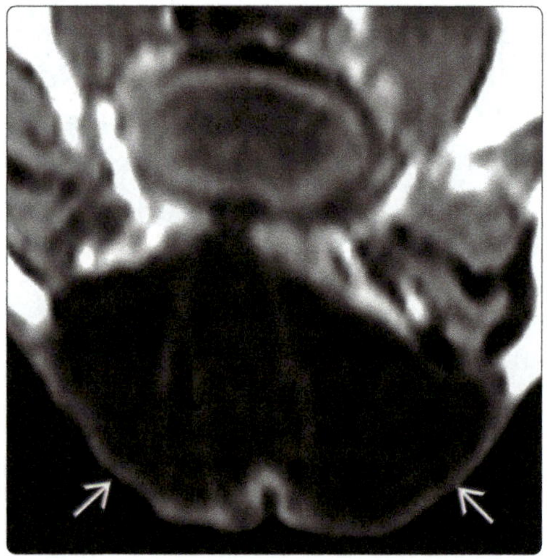

(Left) *Sagittal graphic illustrates focal nondisjunction, with a dorsal dermal cutaneous sinus tract → extending from skin surface to conus. A hairy vascular cutaneous lesion marks the sinus ostium. Note the epidermoid deposits ↪ along the sinus tract.* **(Right)** *Sagittal T1WI MR reveals a hypointense dermal sinus → extending through the L5 posterior elements and coursing intradural to tether the low-lying conus at L2/L3. A vitamin E capsule has been placed to mark the skin opening of the sinus ⇨.*

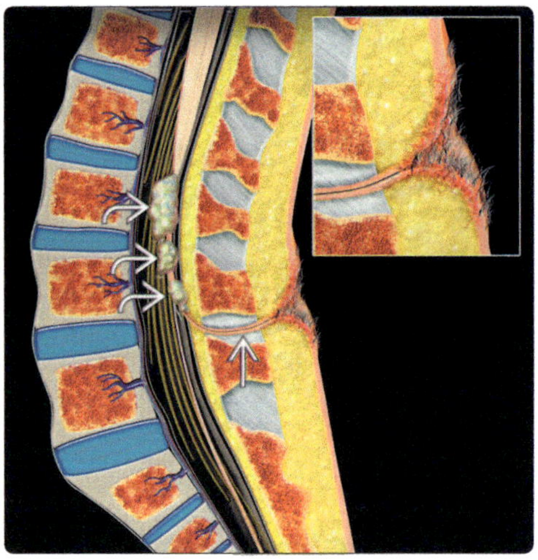

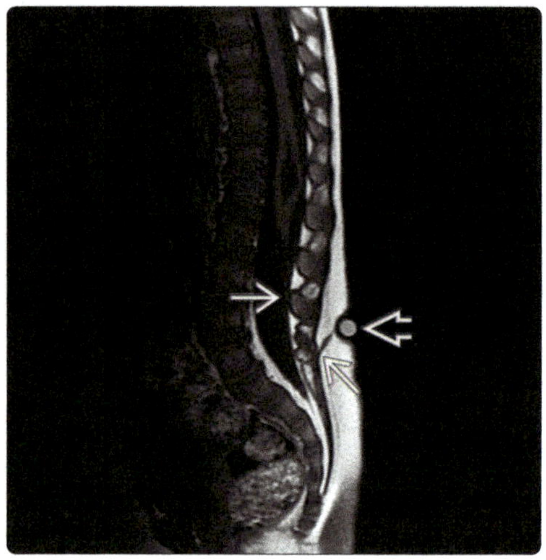

(Left) *Sagittal graphic depicts aberrant secondary neurulation resulting in severe caudal regression and vertebral column termination at the lower lumbar spine. The blunt, abnormally high conus → is characteristic of type 1 caudal regression syndrome.* **(Right)** *Sagittal T1WI MR (caudal regression) reveals abnormal vertebral column termination at the low lumbar level. The abnormal conus → shows a characteristic blunt wedge shape. Sacral absence permits medial migration of the iliac wings ⇨.*

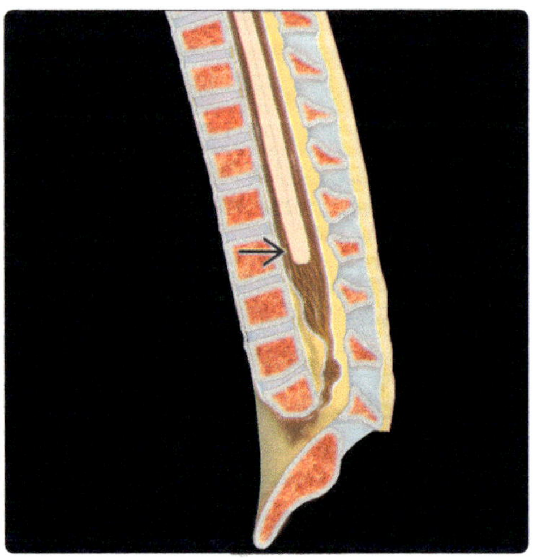

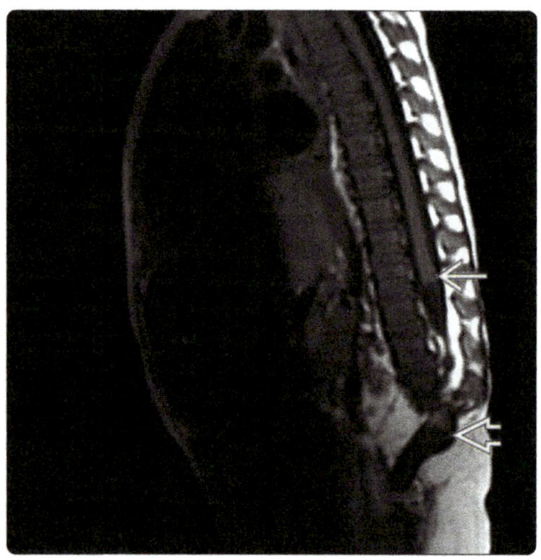

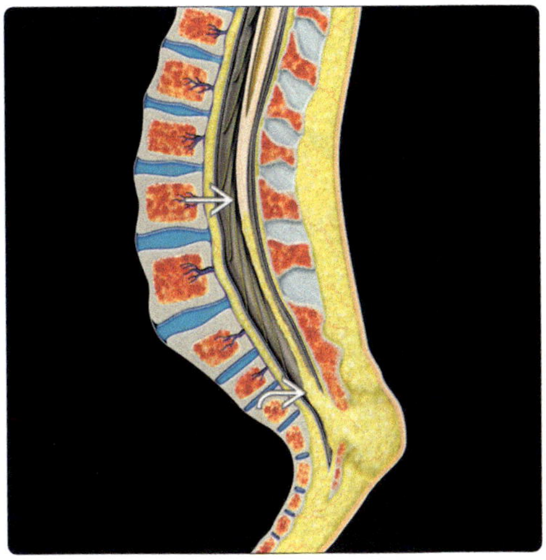

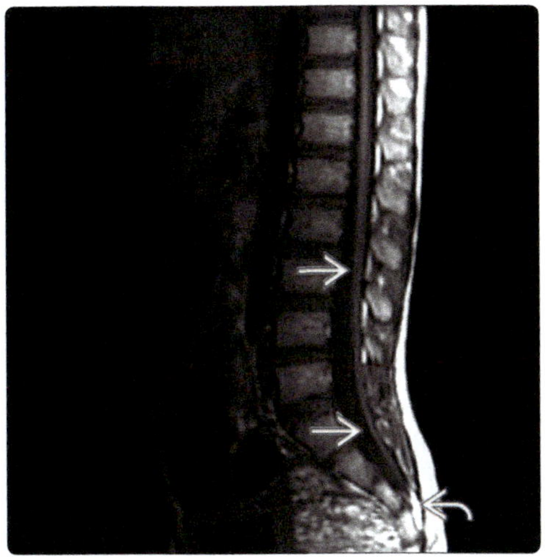

(Left) *Sagittal graphic (tethered spinal cord) demonstrates abnormal elongation of the low-lying spinal cord ➔, which inserts into a terminal lipoma ↪ at the end of a thick, shortened fatty filum.* **(Right)** *Sagittal T1WI MR (tethered spinal cord) reveals an abnormally elongated spinal cord ➔ extending to at least L5, subtly transitioning into a thickened filum terminale that terminates in a small terminal lipoma ↪. No syrinx or hydromyelia is present.*

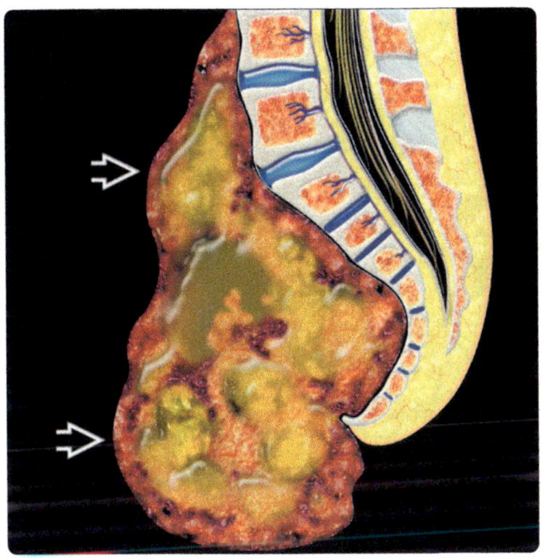

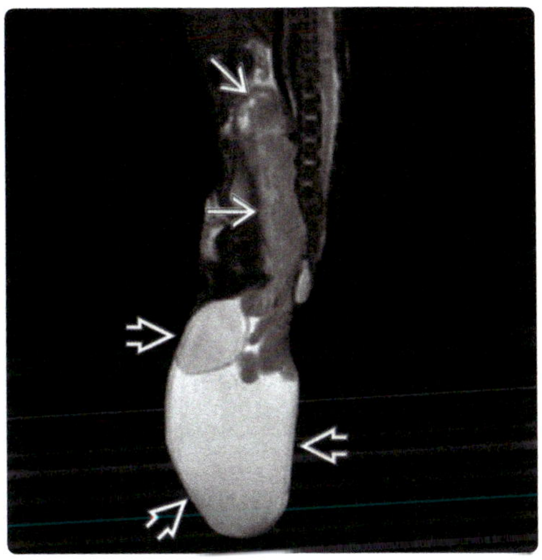

(Left) *Sagittal graphic (AAP II sacrococcygeal teratoma) shows a heterogeneous necrotic neoplasm ⇨ located ventral to the sacrum. Approximately equal external and internal components classify the tumor as AAP type II. Absence of sacral invasion is characteristic.* **(Right)** *Sagittal T2WI MR (AAP II sacrococcygeal teratoma) depicts a mixed cystic and solid pelvic mass. The internal portion ➔ is predominately solid, whereas the external portion ⇨ is more cystic.*

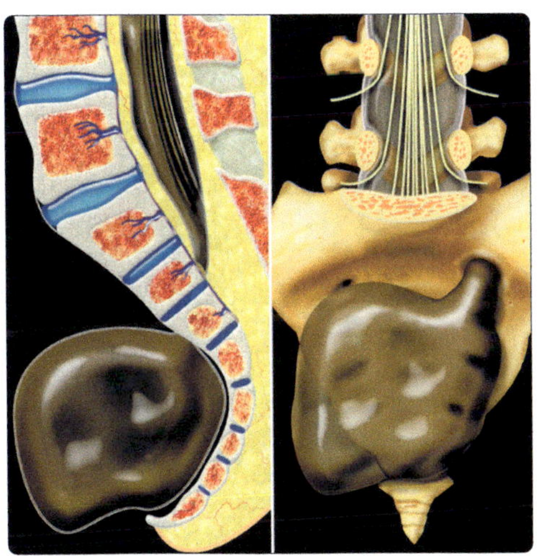

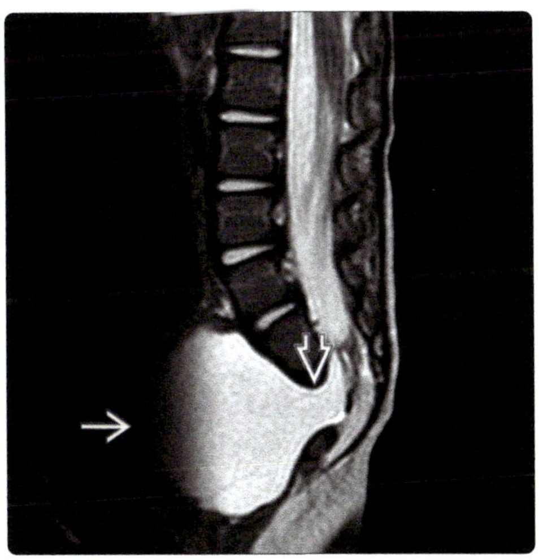

(Left) *Sagittal and coronal graphics demonstrate a classic anterior sacral meningocele. The sac enters the presacral space through an enlarged sacral neural foramina.* **(Right)** *Sagittal T2WI MR (anterior sacral meningocele) imaged parasagittal off-midline demonstrates continuity of the ventral meningocele sac ➔ with the thecal sac through an abnormally enlarged sacral foramen ⇨.*

(Left) *Sagittal graphic demonstrates a typical terminal myelocystocele, with posterior spinal dysraphism and classic "cyst within a cyst" configuration.* **(Right)** *Sagittal T1WI MR shows the classic appearance of terminal myelocystocele, with a low-lying tethered spinal cord with distal hydromyelia ➔ traversing a meningocele ⇨ produced by obstruction of the subarachnoid space. Also note the hypoplastic sacrum.*

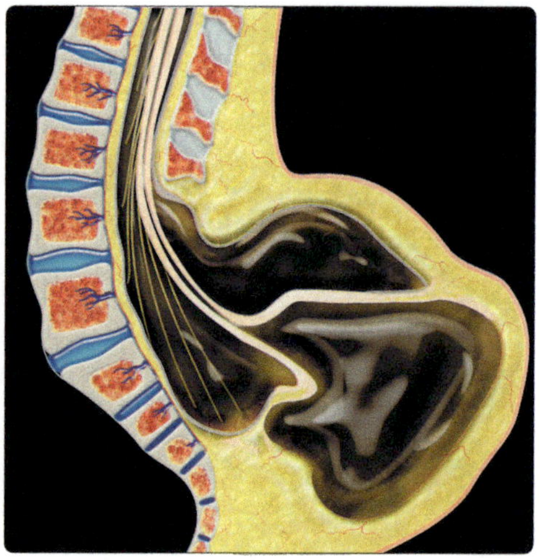

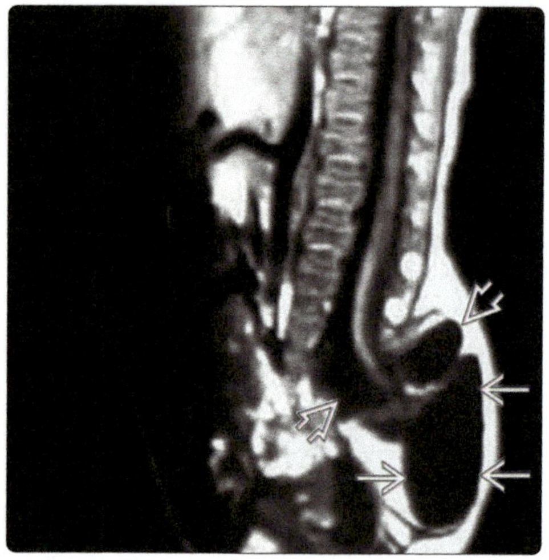

(Left) *Sagittal bone CT of the sacrum and coccyx in a 24-month-old child demonstrates normal ossification of the 5 sacral vertebra and first 3 coccygeal vertebra. The underlying cartilaginous model is faintly visible as soft tissue density containing the ossified centra.* **(Right)** *Axial bone CT in a 3-day-old infant demonstrates normal CT imaging appearance of the vertebral centrum ➔ and neural arch ⇨, primary ossification centers separated by cartilaginous synchondroses ↷.*

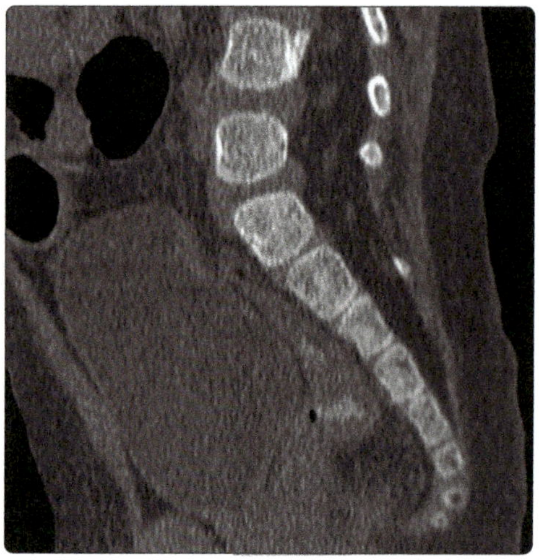

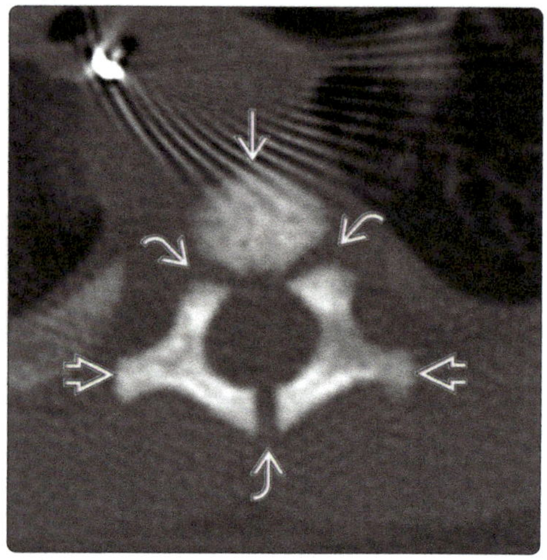

(Left) *Anteroposterior radiograph demonstrates 2 thoracic hemivertebra ➔. These hemivertebra are on opposite sides and "cancel" to limit spinal curvature. This "balanced" configuration is less likely to show progressive curvature than "unbalanced" hemivertebra.* **(Right)** *Coronal T1WI MR shows thoracic dextroscoliosis with extensive vertebral segmentation failure. Low signal intensity between the dysplastic vertebral elements represents nonossified cartilage in this young, skeletally immature patient.*

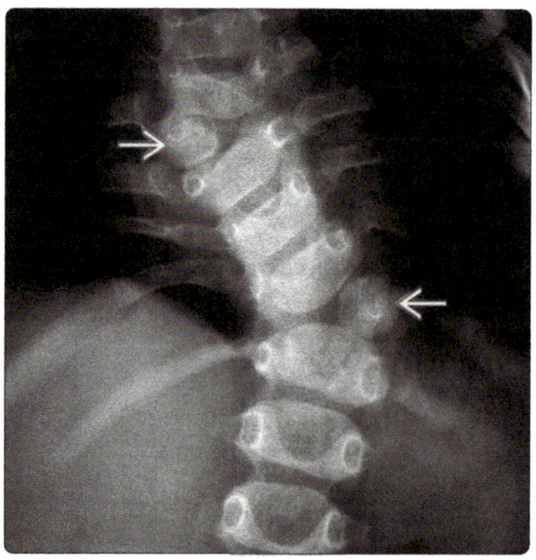

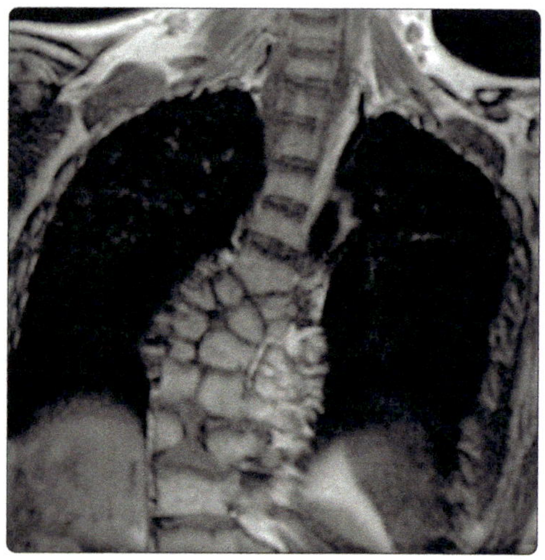

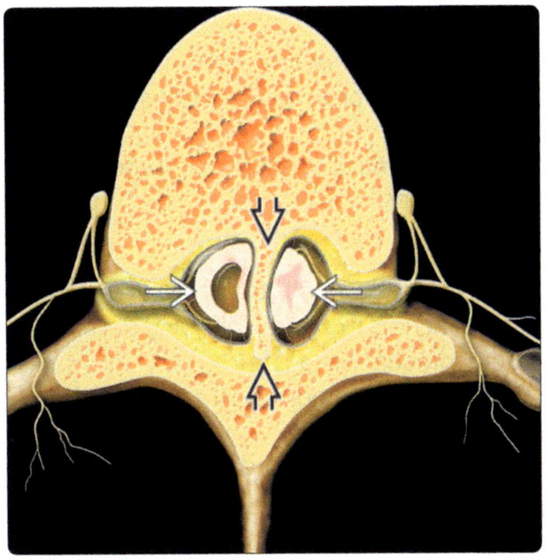

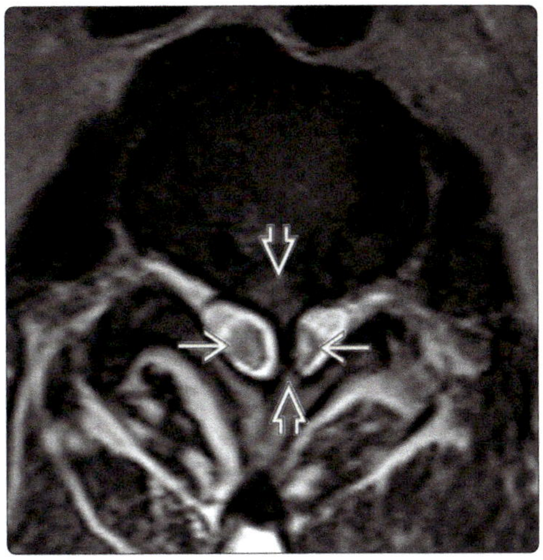

(Left) *Axial graphic demonstrates type 1 diastematomyelia, with a large osseous spur connecting the vertebral body to posterior elements, dividing the spinal cord into 2 hemicords, each within a separate dural tube. The right hemicord has a syrinx.* **(Right)** *Axial T1WI MR (split notochord syndrome) depicts classic type 1 diastematomyelia, with an ossified spur dividing the dural sac and spinal cord into 2 separate hemicords, each within their own dural tube.*

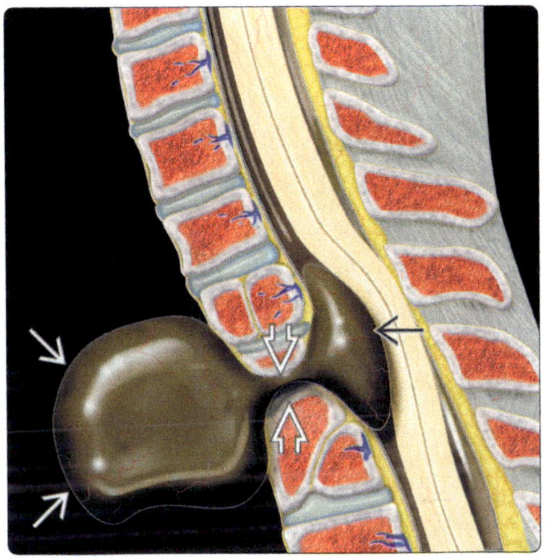

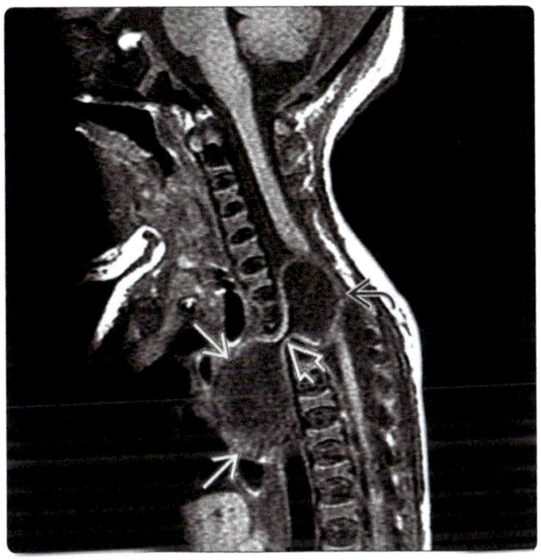

(Left) *Sagittal graphic (split notochord syndrome) shows upper thoracic vertebral segmentation anomalies with a persistent canal of Kovalevsky, permitting communication of the mediastinal enteric cyst with the extradural neurenteric cyst.* **(Right)** *Sagittal T1WI MR demonstrates a large, dumbbell-shaped neurenteric cyst. The mediastinal enteric cyst extends into the ventral spinal canal through the canal of Kovalevsky to produce an intracanalicular neurenteric cyst.*

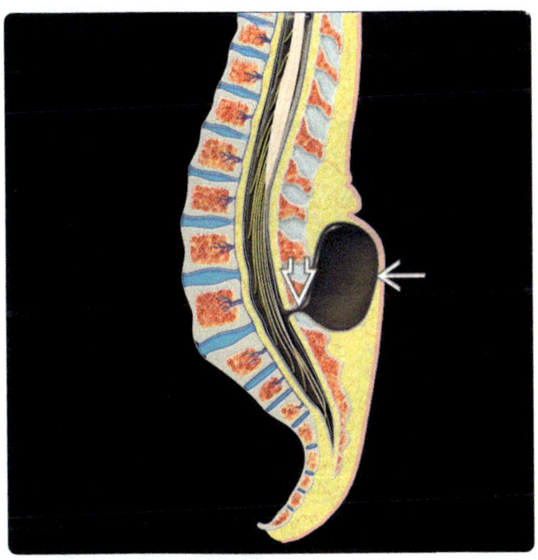

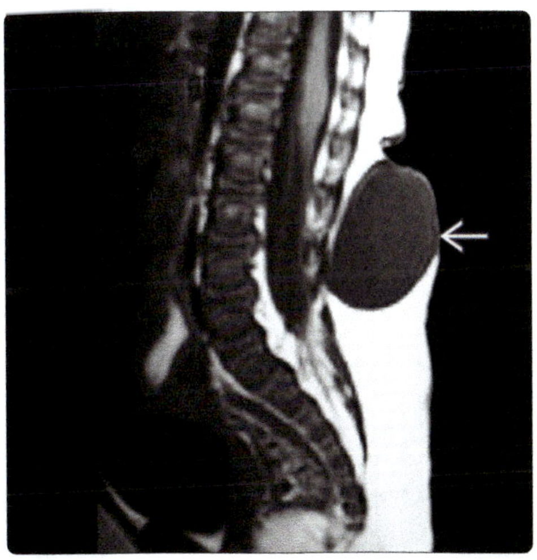

(Left) *Sagittal graphic demonstrates a dorsal spinal meningocele, a malformation of unknown etiology. The meningocele sac communicates with the dural sac by a thin isthmus. There are no neural elements within the meningocele sac.* **(Right)** *Sagittal T1WI MR shows the classic appearance of a dorsal spinal meningocele. The meningocele sac extends through the posterior elements via a thin isthmus, representing mild focal closed spinal dysraphism.*

Myelomeningocele

KEY FACTS

TERMINOLOGY

- Posterior spinal defect lacking skin covering → neural tissue, cerebrospinal fluid (CSF), and meninges exposed to air
- Synonyms: Meningomyelocele, open spinal dysraphism, spina bifida aperta, spina bifida cystica

IMAGING

- Lumbosacral (44%) > thoracolumbar (32%) > lumbar (22%) > thoracic (2%)
- Preoperative: Posterior spinal defect lacking skin covering → neural tissue, CSF, and meninges exposed to air
- Postoperative: Dysraphism, low-lying cord/roots, postoperative skin closure changes

TOP DIFFERENTIAL DIAGNOSES

- Dorsal meningocele
- Closed (occult) spinal dysraphism
- Postoperative pseudomeningocele

PATHOLOGY

- Failure of neural tube closure at 3-4 weeks
  - Placode may be segmental or terminal
- Association with maternal folate deficiency or abnormal folate metabolism
- Usually accompanied by multiple neurological and orthopedic complications

CLINICAL ISSUES

- Can be diagnosed (MR, ultrasound), treated in utero
- Stable neurological deficits expected following closure
- Neurological deterioration → imaging
  - Cord retethering most common spinal cause of delayed deterioration
  - Other = dural ring constriction, cord ischemia, syrinx

DIAGNOSTIC CHECKLIST

- Low-lying cord on MR does not always equate to clinical tethering

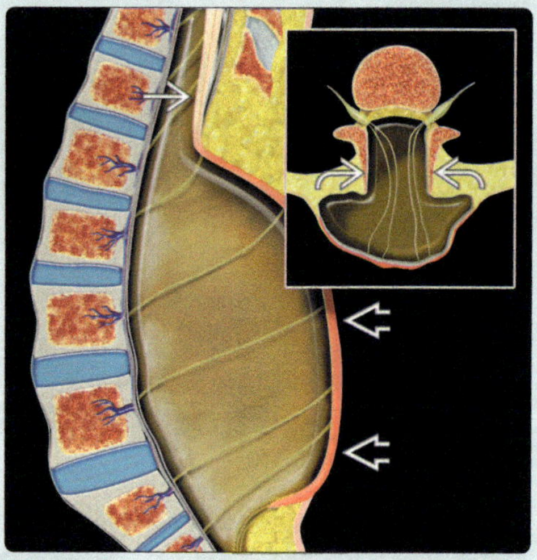

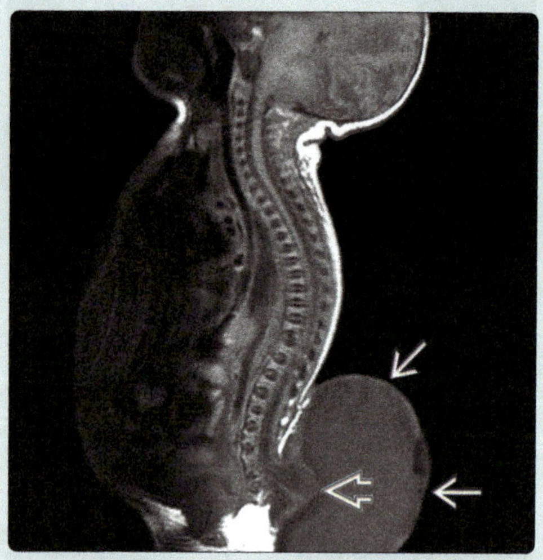

(Left) *Sagittal graphic shows ballooning of meninges through dysraphic spinal defect, with low-lying cord ➡ terminating in the red neural placode ➡. Axial insert shows origin of spinal roots from ventral placode and protrusion of meninges and placode through dysraphic posterior elements ➡.* **(Right)** *Sagittal T1WI MR shows a large unrepaired lumbosacral myelomeningocele sac ➡ protruding through a posterior dysraphic defect. Neural elements are seen protruding into the sac ➡.*

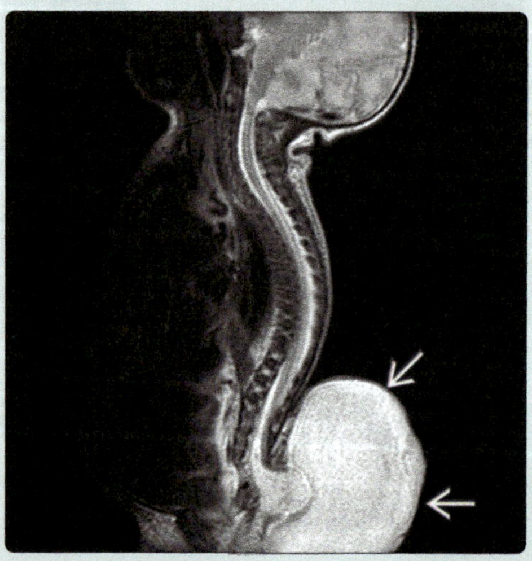

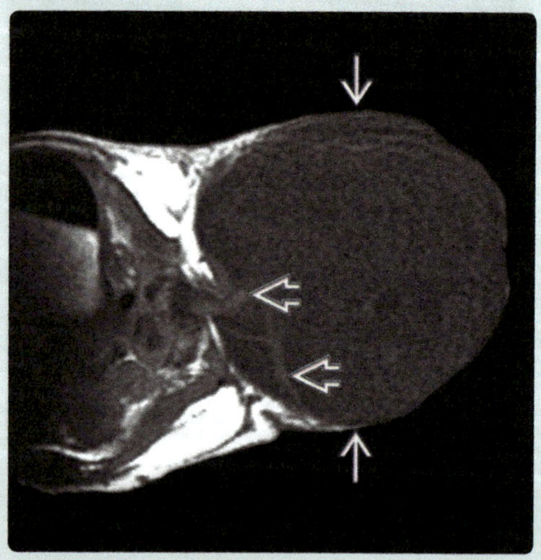

(Left) *Sagittal T2WI MR shows typical posterior fossa Chiari 2 malformation changes. The large myelomeningocele lumbosacral sac ➡ has not been surgically repaired, and it protrudes dorsally through a large posterior dysraphic defect.* **(Right)** *Axial T1WI MR of unrepaired lumbosacral myelomeningocele confirms an exophytic meningeal sac ➡ and extension of dysplastic neural elements ➡ through the osseous spinal dysraphic defect into the myelomeningocele.*

KEY FACTS

TERMINOLOGY

- Synonyms: Dermal sinus tract (DST)
- Midline/paramedian stratified squamous epithelial-lined sinus tract
- Extends inward from skin surface for variable distance

IMAGING

- Sinus tract easily identified superimposed on background of cutaneous fat
- Terminus usually conus medullaris (lumbosacral) or central spinal canal (cervical, thoracic)

TOP DIFFERENTIAL DIAGNOSES

- Low coccygeal midline dimple
- Pilonidal sinus
- (Epi)dermoid tumor without dermal sinus

PATHOLOGY

- Focal incorporation of cutaneous ectoderm into neural ectoderm during disjunction at circumscribed point only → focal segmental adhesion
- Spinal cord ascends relative to spinal canal, stretches adhesion into long, tubular tract

CLINICAL ISSUES

- Infancy → 3rd decade
- Presentation either asymptomatic (incidentally noted skin dimple) or infection, neurological deficits secondary to cord tethering or compression

DIAGNOSTIC CHECKLIST

- Must differentiate DST from simple sacral dimple or pilonidal sinus
- Identify sinus course, termination for surgical planning

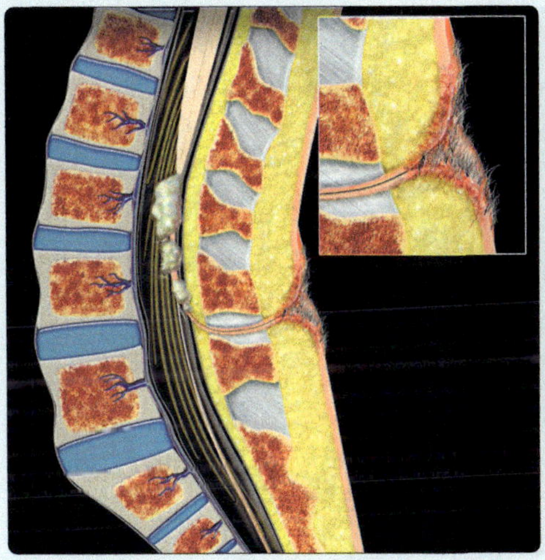

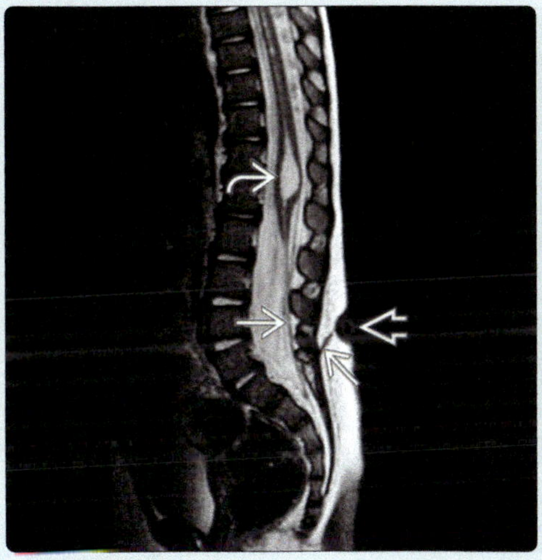

(Left) *Sagittal graphic shows a dermal sinus extending from the skin surface into the spinal canal to terminate at conus with epidermoid cysts. A skin dimple with capillary angioma and hairy tuft (cutaneous marker) indicates sinus opening.* **(Right)** *Sagittal T2WI MR shows hypointense dermal sinus ➡ extending through L5 posterior elements and coursing intradural to tether the low-lying hydromyelic conus ↪ at L2-L3. A vitamin E capsule has been placed to mark the skin opening of the sinus ⇨.*

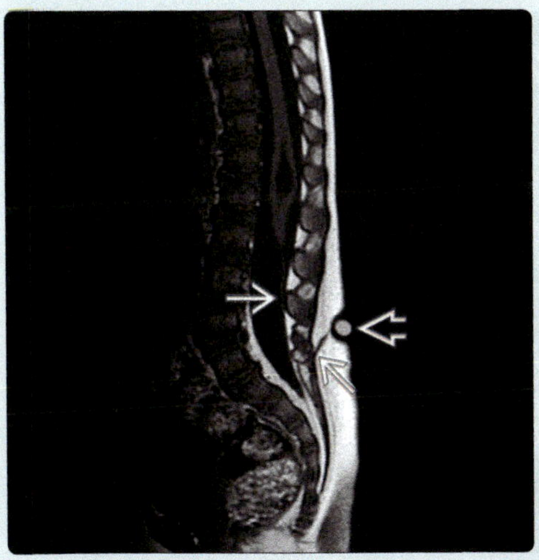

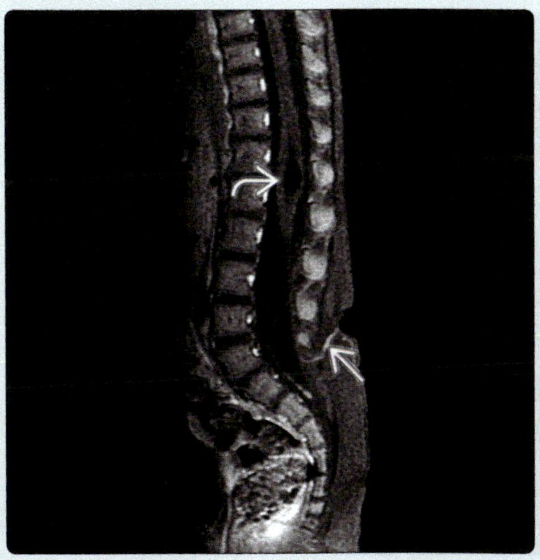

(Left) *Sagittal T1WI MR reveals hypointense dermal sinus ➡ extending through L5 posterior elements and coursing intradural to tether the low-lying conus at L2-L3. A vitamin E capsule marks skin opening of the sinus ⇨.* **(Right)** *Sagittal T1WI C+ FS MR confirms mild dermal sinus tract enhancement ➡ without abscess. Note that the terminal cord central canal is dilated ↪, probably representing syringohydromyelia rather than ventriculus terminalis because of low-lying cord and presence of dermal sinus.*

KEY FACTS

TERMINOLOGY

- Synonym: Sacral dimple

IMAGING

- Low sacral dimple connecting to coccyx by fibrous tract
  - Usually resides within intergluteal cleft
  - No intradural extension by definition
- Variable size; deeper dimples usually evoke more physician and parental concern

TOP DIFFERENTIAL DIAGNOSES

- Dorsal dermal sinus
- Pilonidal sinus

PATHOLOGY

- Congenital
- Tract usually atretic; may occasionally be patent with fluid in lumen

CLINICAL ISSUES

- Often asymptomatic discovery by parents during diaper change or bathing
  - Dimple becomes less conspicuous as patient grows
  - No specific treatment indicated; reassure parents
- Occasionally presents with acute inflammation or purulent discharge

DIAGNOSTIC CHECKLIST

- Important to distinguish from dorsal dermal sinus, which requires surgical excision
  - Low dimple opening within intergluteal cleft usually but not always coccygeal dimple
  - High dimple position, leaking of fluid more likely dorsal dermal sinus
- Look for hypointense tract surrounded by bright fat on MR
- Always mark skin dimple ostium with MR visible marker

(Left) *Sagittal graphic of the lumbosacral spine demonstrates a low sacral dimple (marked by vitamin E capsule ⇨), which is connected to the coccyx tip by a fibrous tract ⇨. There is no intradural extension, and the conus/intradural structures are normal.* **(Right)** *Sagittal T2WI MR demonstrates a deep low sacral dimple with vitamin E marker capsule ⇨ placed. The conus terminates at normal L1 level. The dimple and tract → connect directly to the coccyx ↪ with no intradural extension.*

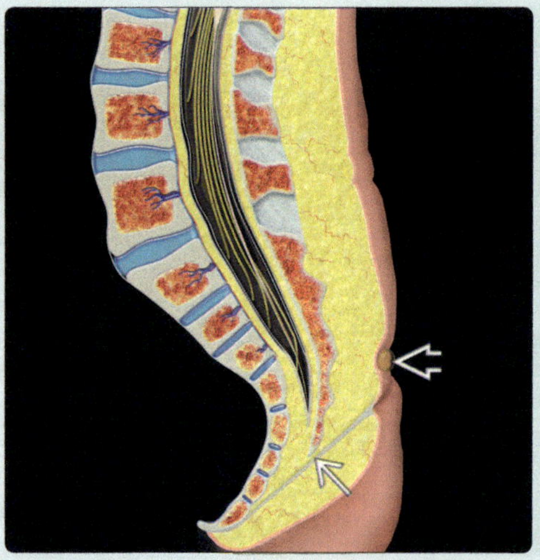

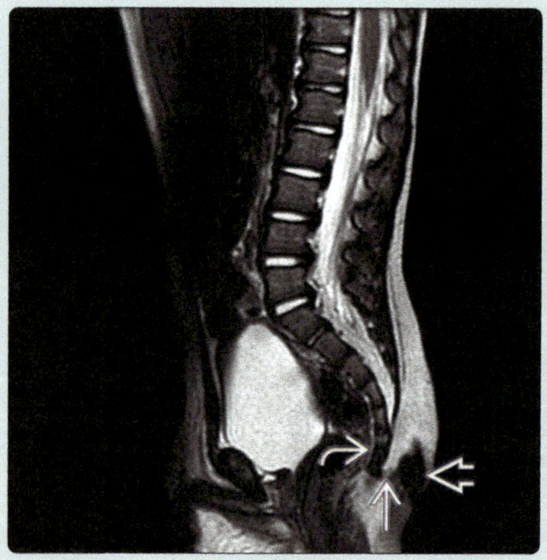

(Left) *Sagittal T1WI MR reveals a deep sacral dimple marked for imaging with a vitamin E capsule ⇨. The conus terminates at normal L1 level. The dimple shows typical "spot-welded" proximity to the coccyx via a short fibrous tract →.* **(Right)** *Axial T1WI MR confirms that the sacral dimple, marked with vitamin E capsule ⇨, and tract → connect directly to the coccyx ↪ without intradural extension.*

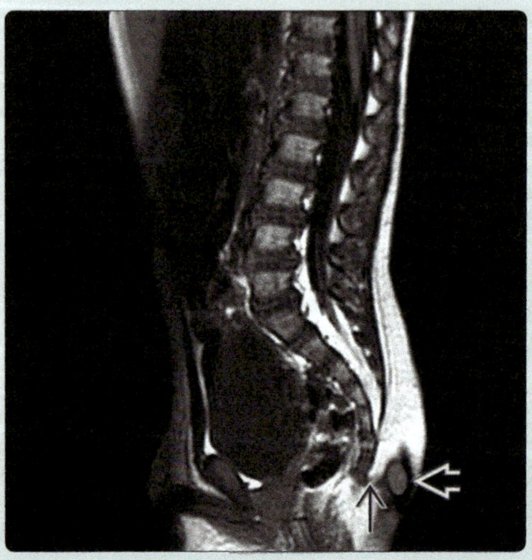

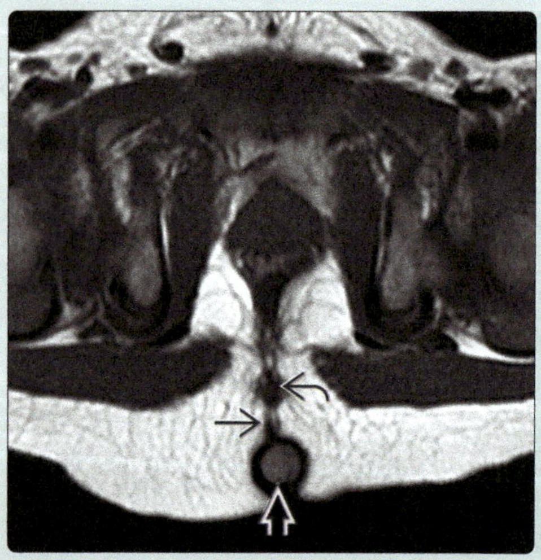

KEY FACTS

TERMINOLOGY

- Synonyms: Tethered cord syndrome (TCS), tight filum terminale syndrome

IMAGING

- Stretched, thinned cord with low-lying conus, thickened filum
- ± fibrolipoma/terminal lipoma, dysraphism, vertebral segmentation anomalies
- ↓ spinal cord motion

TOP DIFFERENTIAL DIAGNOSES

- Normal variant low-lying conus
- Open or closed spinal dysraphism
- Postsurgical low-lying conus

PATHOLOGY

- Tethering stretches nerve fibers, arterioles, and venules → impaired oxidative metabolism of conus and nerve roots → syringohydromyelia, myelomalacia
- Tethered filum histologically abnormal, even if conus terminates at normal level

CLINICAL ISSUES

- Low back and leg pain, gait and sensory abnormalities, urinary bladder dysfunction
- Symptomatic presentation most common during rapid somatic growth (adolescent growth spurt, school age 4-8 years), or secondary to kyphosis (elderly)

DIAGNOSTIC CHECKLIST

- TCS is clinical diagnosis; imaging role is detection of low-lying conus/thick filum, associated anatomic abnormalities for surgical decision making
- Clinical tethering may be present despite normal conus level
- Measure filum thickness at L5/S1; stretching at more rostral levels may erroneously thin filum into "normal" size range

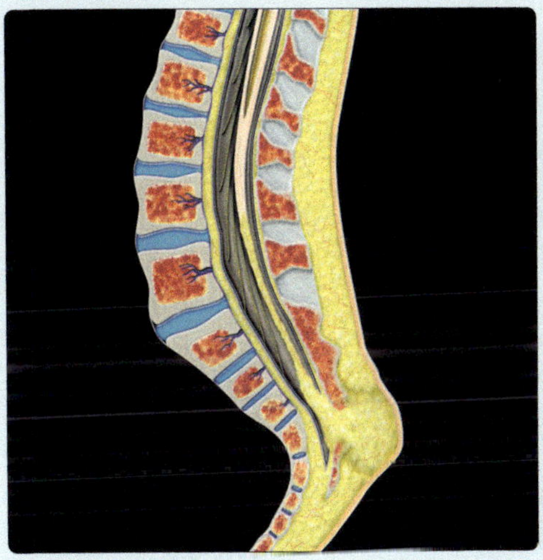

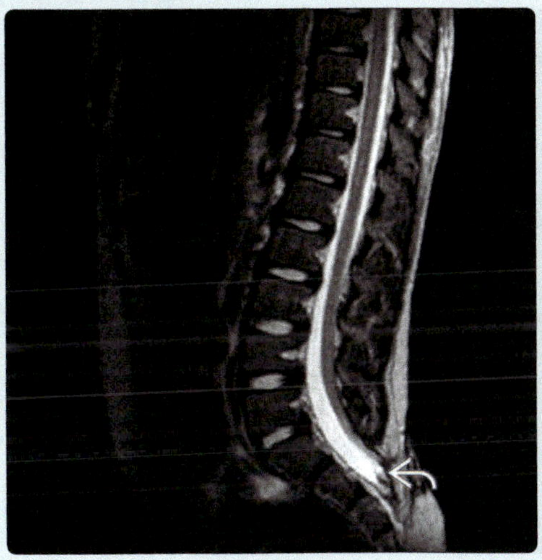

(Left) *Sagittal graphic of the lumbosacral spine depicts composite tethered cord syndrome (TCS) findings of low-lying, hydromyelic tethered cord with thickened filum and fibrolipoma inserting into a terminal lipoma that is contiguous with subcutaneous fat through dorsal dysraphism.* **(Right)** *Sagittal T2WI MR (clinical TCS) demonstrates an elongated low-lying spinal cord extending to the S2 level, where it ends in a small terminal lipoma. Focal sacral posterior dysraphism is also present.*

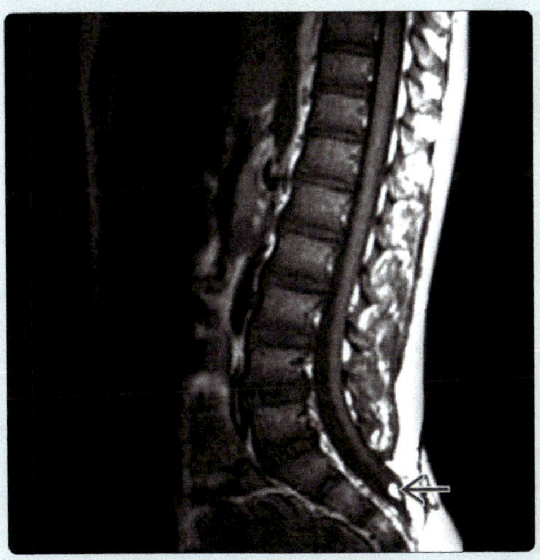

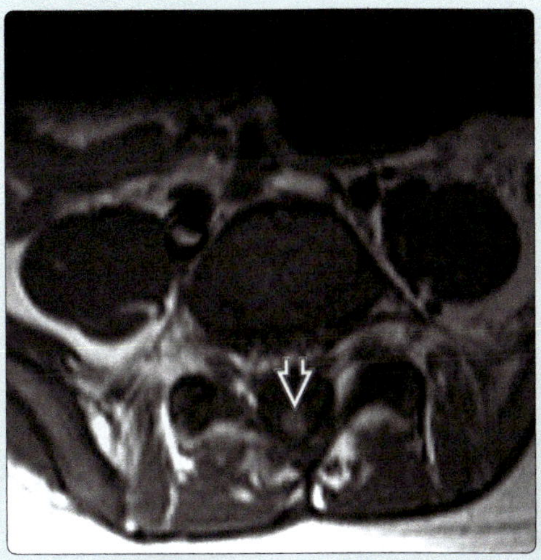

(Left) *Sagittal T1WI MR (clinical TCS symptoms) confirms an elongated low-lying spinal cord extending to the S2 level and ending in a small terminal lipoma. Focal sacral posterior dysraphism is also conspicuous. In general, lipomas are considerably more conspicuous on T1WI than T2WI.* **(Right)** *Axial T1WI MR at the lumbosacral transition reveals that the abnormal elongated, low-lying spinal cord continues to the sacral level.*

KEY FACTS

TERMINOLOGY

- Synonyms: Klippel-Feil syndrome (KFS)
- Congenital spinal malformation characterized by segmentation failure of ≥ 2 cervical vertebrae ± thoracic, lumbar segmentation failure

IMAGING

- Single- or multiple-level congenital cervical segmentation and fusion anomalies
- C2-3 (50%) > C5-6 (33%) > craniovertebral junction, upper thoracic spine
- Vertebral bodies usually smaller than normal
- Vertebral body narrowing ("wasp waist") at fused rudimentary disc space ± fusion of posterior elements

TOP DIFFERENTIAL DIAGNOSES

- Juvenile idiopathic arthritis
- Surgical fusion
- Chronic sequelae of discitis
- Ankylosing spondylitis

PATHOLOGY

- No universally accepted etiology; embryonic insult postulated between 4th and 8th weeks
- Sporadic; familial genetic component with variable expression identified in many patients

CLINICAL ISSUES

- Classic triad (33-50%): Short neck, low posterior hairline, and limited cervical motion
- In practice, however, wide variation in clinical, anatomical expression

DIAGNOSTIC CHECKLIST

- Much KFS morbidity and nearly all mortality related to visceral system dysfunction
- Look for instability, progressive degenerative changes, cord/brainstem compression

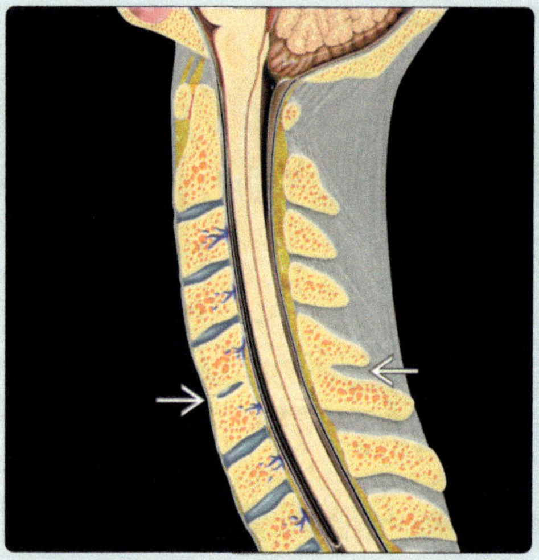

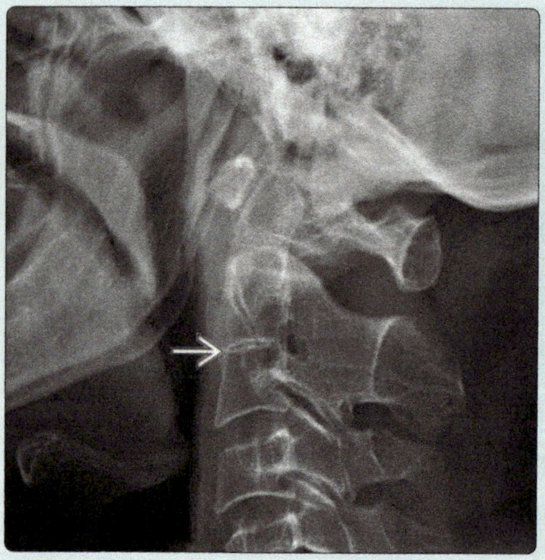

(Left) *Sagittal graphic (KFS 2) shows congenital fusion ➡ of the C5-C6 vertebrae and spinous processes, with characteristic rudimentary disc space and distinctive "waist" typical of congenital fusion.* **(Right)** *Lateral radiograph (KFS type 2) demonstrates typical C2/3 congenital segmentation failure ("fusion") with characteristic rudimentary disc space ➡ and fusion of the facets and spinous processes. The disc space appearance helps distinguish from postcervical fusion.*

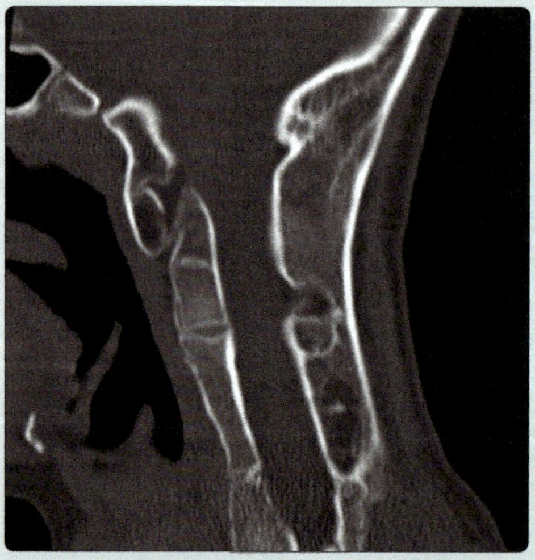

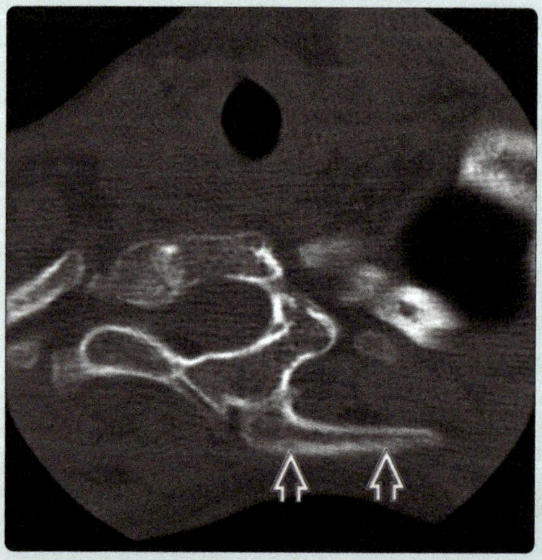

(Left) *Sagittal bone CT (KFS 1) reveals extensive fusion of all cervical vertebrae and posterior elements, with the characteristic hypoplastic appearance of the vertebrae and intervertebral disc spaces. In this patient, there is additionally incorporation of C1 into the skull base ("occipitalization of the atlas").* **(Right)** *Axial bone CT (KFS 1, severe segmentation anomalies) demonstrates the vertebral articulation of a unilateral left omovertebral bone ➡.*

Dural Dysplasia

KEY FACTS

TERMINOLOGY

- Synonym: Dural ectasia

IMAGING

- Smooth remodeling of posterior vertebral body, expansion of osseous spinal canal, ± kyphoscoliosis
  - Pedicular attenuation, widened interpediculate distance, erosion of anterior and posterior elements
- Patulous, expansile dural sac enlargement
- Easiest to appreciate on sagittal images

TOP DIFFERENTIAL DIAGNOSES

- Congenital vertebral dysplasia
- Spinal tumor or syrinx
- Cauda equina syndrome of ankylosing spondylitis

PATHOLOGY

- Etiologies include NF1, connective tissue disorders (Marfan syndrome, Ehlers-Danlos syndrome, Loey-Dietz syndrome, homocystinuria), idiopathic
- Association with lateral thoracic or lumbar meningocele, anterior sacral meningocele, kyphoscoliosis, joint hypermobility, lens abnormalities, aneurysm, arterial dissection, and peripheral or central neoplasms
- Dura in ectatic areas is extremely thin, fragile

CLINICAL ISSUES

- Most commonly presents with back pain ± radiculopathy
- Other complaints include headache, incontinence, pelvic symptoms
- May present at any age depending on severity, underlying etiology

DIAGNOSTIC CHECKLIST

- Recognition of specific imaging clues and integration of available clinical data permit more specific diagnosis
- Important to determine underlying disorder for treatment planning, genetic counseling, and determining prognosis

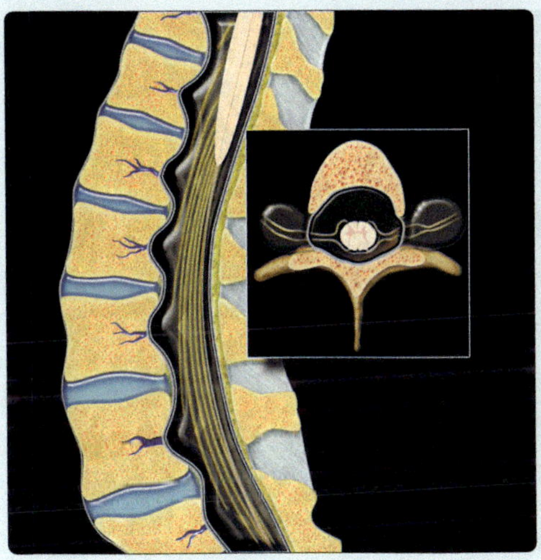

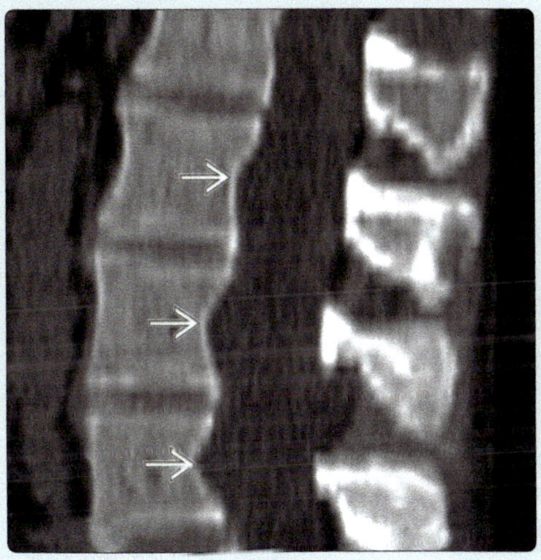

(Left) *Sagittal graphic of the lumbosacral spine demonstrates scalloping of the posterior vertebral bodies and central spinal canal enlargement. Note that the dural sac generally fills the concavity produced in the posterior vertebral body. Also conspicuous (inset) are bilateral lumbar lateral meningoceles.* **(Right)** *Sagittal bone CT (neurofibromatosis type 1, NF1) reveals characteristic posterior vertebral remodeling and scalloping ➡ with resultant widening of the central spinal canal.*

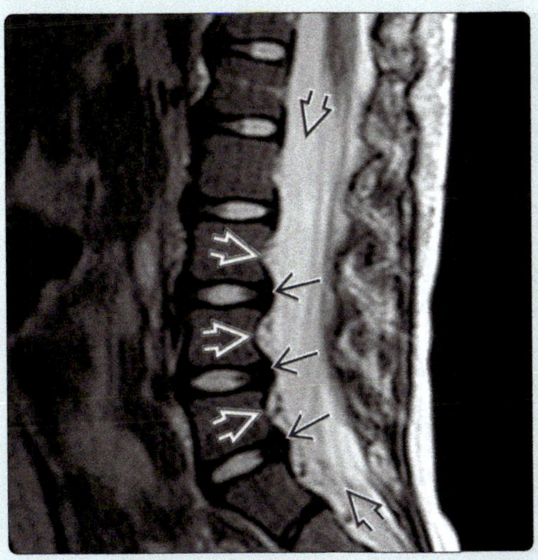

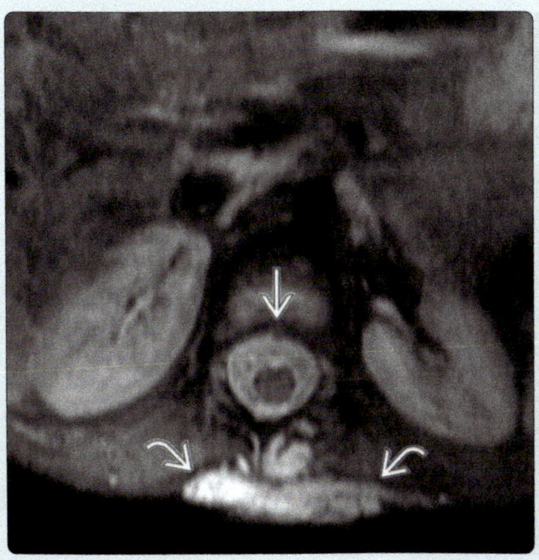

(Left) *Sagittal T2WI MR (NF1) shows posterior vertebral body scalloping ➡ and patulous thecal sac ➡. The discs ➡ are normal; the vertebral abnormalities make them appear bulging.* **(Right)** *Axial STIR MR (neurofibromatosis type 1) demonstrates posterior vertebral body remodeling ➡ related to dural dysplasia. Note also the typical appearance of a hyperintense dorsal lumbar subcutaneous infiltrative plexiform neurofibroma ➡, the clinical indication for imaging.*

KEY FACTS

TERMINOLOGY

- Synonyms: von Recklinghausen disease, peripheral neurofibromatosis
- Mesodermal dysplasia with neurofibromas (NFs), spinal deformity, neoplastic and nonneoplastic brain lesions, and cutaneous stigmata

IMAGING

- Kyphoscoliosis ± multiple nerve root tumors, plexiform neurofibroma, dural ectasia/lateral meningocele
- Tumors range from tiny to very large

TOP DIFFERENTIAL DIAGNOSES

- Neurofibromatosis type 2 (NF2) (central neurofibromatosis)
- Chronic inflammatory demyelinating polyneuropathy
- Congenital hypertrophic polyradiculoneuropathies

PATHOLOGY

- Autosomal dominant
  - *NF1* gene mutation on chromosome 17q11.2
- Characteristic lesion is plexiform neurofibroma, although 3 types of spinal NF seen in NF1
  - Localized NF (90% of all NF)
  - Diffuse NF
  - Plexiform NF (pathognomonic for NF1)

CLINICAL ISSUES

- Prominent pigmentation anomalies (café au lait, axillary freckling, Lisch nodules)
- Focal or acute angle kyphoscoliosis ± myelopathy
- Palpable spinal or cutaneous masses

DIAGNOSTIC CHECKLIST

- Multiple nerve sheath tumors, ≥ 1 NF, bizarre kyphoscoliosis with deformed vertebra → consider NF1
- Absence of visible stigmata does not exclude NF1
- Characteristic plexiform NF imaging appearance best displayed using FS T2WI or STIR MR

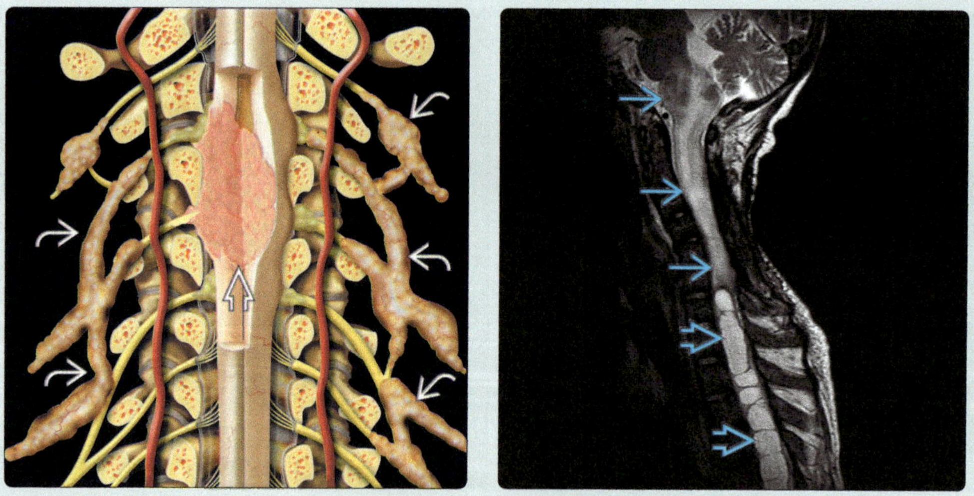

(Left) *Coronal graphic of the cervical spine demonstrates multiple manifestations of neurofibromatosis type 1, including a large intramedullary spinal cord tumor and bilateral brachial plexus plexiform neurofibromas.* **(Right)** *Sagittal T2WI MR demonstrates a large expansile intramedullary primary spinal cord neoplasm expanding into the brainstem. A large neoplastic syrinx is present. Note also cervical lordosis reversal, probably secondary to laminectomy for cord biopsy.*

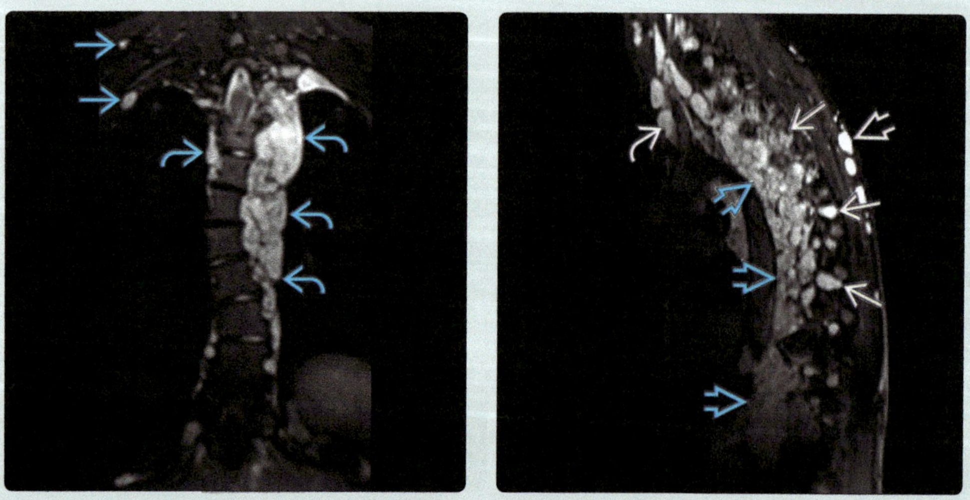

(Left) *Coronal STIR MR reveals extensive plexiform neurofibromas involving the bilateral paraspinal sympathetic chains, as well as involvement of multiple intercostal nerves.* **(Right)** *Sagittal STIR MR obtained off midline demonstrates innumerable T2 hyperintense plexiform neurofibromas involving the spinal nerves, sympathetic chains, bilateral brachial plexus, as well as multiple cutaneous nerves.*

KEY FACTS

TERMINOLOGY

- Rare autosomal dominant disease from chromosomal 22 defect in which all patients develop CNS tumors
- Mnemonic for NF2 tumors: **M**ultiple **i**nherited **s**chwannomas, **m**eningiomas, and **e**pendymomas (MISME)

TOP DIFFERENTIAL DIAGNOSES

- Metastases
- Hemangioblastomas
- Nonsyndromic schwannoma
- Nonsyndromic meningioma
- Nonsyndromic ependymoma
- Lymphoma

PATHOLOGY

- 22q12 deletion correlates with loss of *NF2* gene product "merlin" (a.k.a. schwannomin)
- Definite diagnosis of NF2
  - Bilateral CN8 (vestibular) schwannomas
  - 1st-degree relative with NF2 and either unilateral early-onset vestibular schwannoma (age < 30 years) or any 2: Meningioma, glioma, schwannoma, juvenile posterior subcapsular lenticular opacity
- Presumptive diagnosis of NF2
  - Early-onset unilateral CN8 schwannomas (age < 30 years) and 1 of the following
    - Meningioma, glioma, schwannoma, juvenile posterior subcapsular lenticular opacity
    - Multiple meningiomas (> 2) and unilateral vestibular schwannoma
  - Or 1 of these: Glioma, schwannoma, juvenile posterior subcapsular lenticular opacity

CLINICAL ISSUES

- Minimal to no cutaneous stigmata

DIAGNOSTIC CHECKLIST

- Screen using MR C+ of brain and entire spine

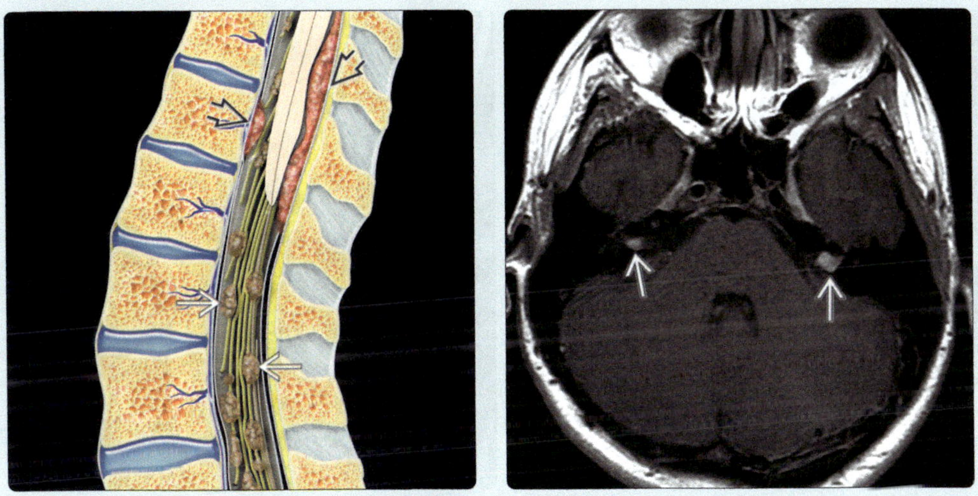

(Left) *Sagittal graphic illustrates multiple rounded schwannomas (brown) ➡ along the cauda equina, as well as flat dural-based meningiomas (red) ➡ impinging the conus.* **(Right)** *Axial T1WI C+ MR shows bilateral enhancing cerebellopontine angle masses ➡ due to vestibular schwannomas in this patient with neurofibromatosis type 2.*

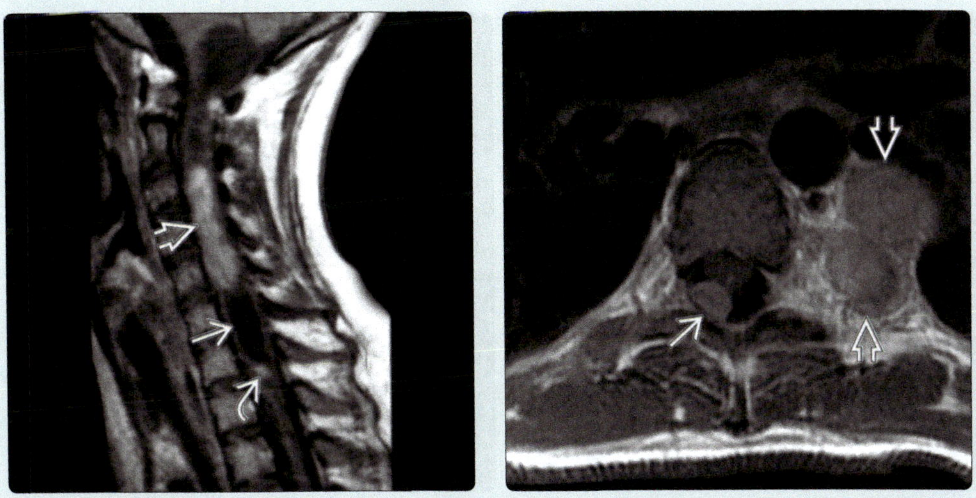

(Left) *Sagittal T1WI C+ MR demonstrates multiple intramedullary enhancing ependymomas. The largest is at the C3-C5 level ➡, with an associated inferior cyst ➡, with a smaller 2nd tumor at C7-T1 level ➡.* **(Right)** *Axial T1 C+ MR shows heterogeneous enhancement of paraspinal schwannomas ➡, as well as an intradural extramedullary tumor with a broad dural base consistent with meningioma ➡.*

KEY FACTS

TERMINOLOGY

- Autosomal-dominant dwarfism affecting spine and extremities
- a.k.a. achondroplastic dwarfism

IMAGING

- Shortened vertebral pedicles
  - Decreasing interpediculate distance toward lower levels of lumbar spine
- Mildly flattened &/or anteriorly wedged vertebral bodies
- Thoracolumbar kyphosis
- Lumbar hyperlordosis
- Small foramen magnum
- Other
  - Growth disturbance more obvious in proximal limbs (rhizomelic dwarfism)
  - "Champagne glass" pelvis: Pelvic inlet is flat and broad
  - Squared iliac wings
  - Short ribs
  - Enlarged skull with constricted skull base

TOP DIFFERENTIAL DIAGNOSES

- Pseudoachondroplasia
- Hypochondroplasia
- Diastrophic dysplasia
- Spondyloepiphyseal dysplasia
- Thanatophoric dysplasia
- Osteogenesis imperfecta

PATHOLOGY

- Defect in *FGFR3*, responsible gene mapped to 4p16.3
- Usually spontaneous mutation (80%)
- Results in defective enchondral bone formation
- Autosomal dominant transmission

CLINICAL ISSUES

- Surgical correction of progressive/unresolving kyphosis
- Surgical decompression of foramen magnum in severe cases

(Left) *Graphic shows progressive narrowing of interpediculate distance in caudad direction. Axial insert image shows spinal stenosis related to short pedicles and decreased interpediculate distance.* **(Right)** *Sagittal T2WI MR shows constricted skull base relative to the visualized cranial vault. Stenosis of the foramen magnum ➔ compresses the cervicomedullary junction, with mildly increased signal in the upper cervical cord due to myelopathic changes.*

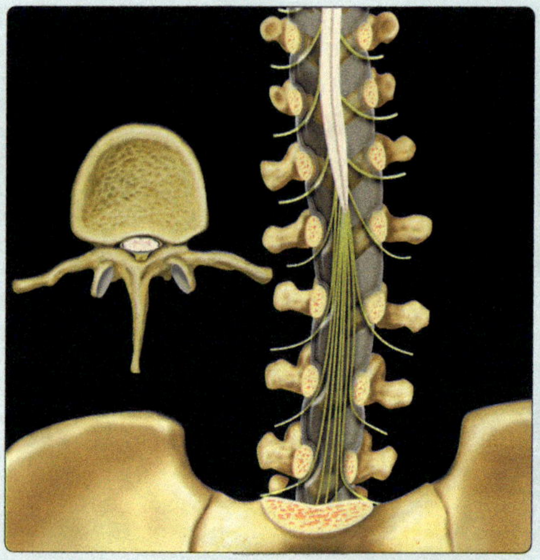

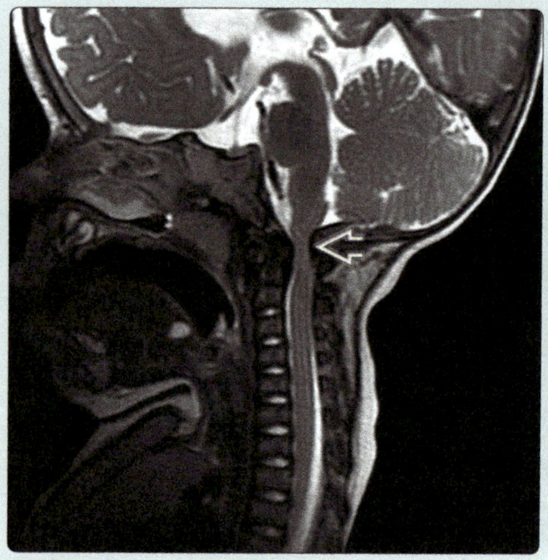

(Left) *AP radiograph of the lumbar spine shows narrowing of the interpediculate distance and progressive interpedicular narrowing between L1 ⇨ and L4 ➔, causing narrowing of the lumbar canal in the transverse dimension.* **(Right)** *Sagittal T2WI MR shows a diffusely narrowed AP dimension of the lumbar spinal canal, reflecting shortened vertebral pedicles. Congenital canal stenosis is further narrowed by a small disc protrusion ➔ at L2-L3.*

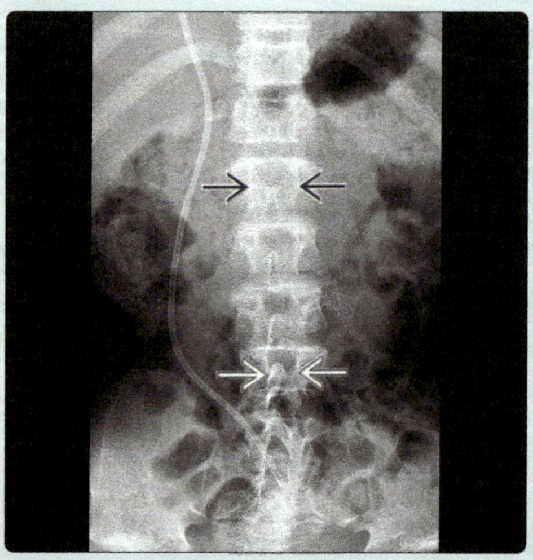

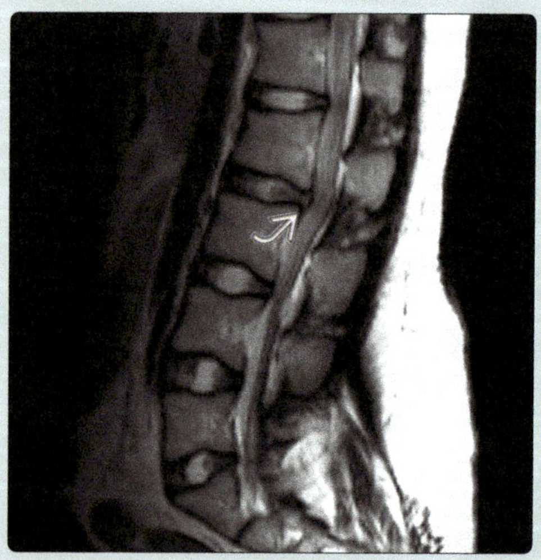

KEY FACTS

TERMINOLOGY

- Spinal curvature secondary to vertebral anomalies
- Hemivertebra: Unilateral or anterior vertebral hypoplasia
- "Butterfly" vertebra: Central vertebral cleft due to failure of central vertebral body development
- "Fused" vertebrae: Embryological failure of segmentation rather than fusion
- Klippel-Feil syndrome: Multiple cervical segmentation anomalies

IMAGING

- Accentuated dorsal thoracic spine curvature on lateral image
- Look for vertebral anomalies in patient with scoliosis or kyphosis
- May have multiple kyphotic and scoliotic curves if multiple anomalies present

TOP DIFFERENTIAL DIAGNOSES

- Scheuermann kyphosis
- Idiopathic kyphosis
- Kyphosis or scoliosis due to syndromes
- Traumatic kyphosis
- Osteomyelitis, granulomatous

PATHOLOGY

- May be congenital or acquired
- Congenital abnormalities due either to failure of development &/or failure of segmentation

CLINICAL ISSUES

- May be isolated anomaly or associated with multisystem anomalies (VACTERL)

DIAGNOSTIC CHECKLIST

- Image entire spine (particularly in children) to exclude additional bone or cord abnormalities, Chiari 1 malformation

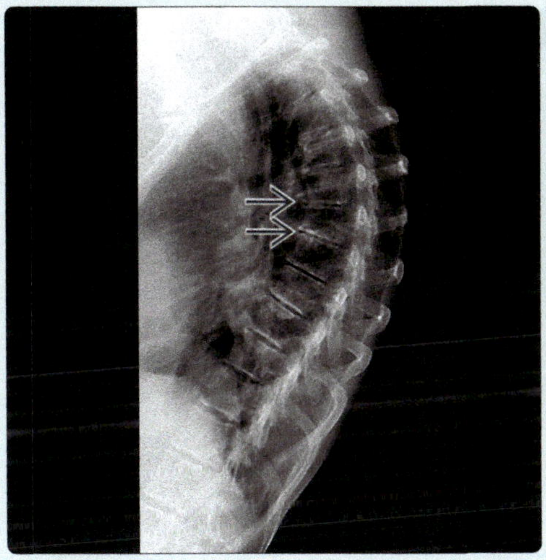
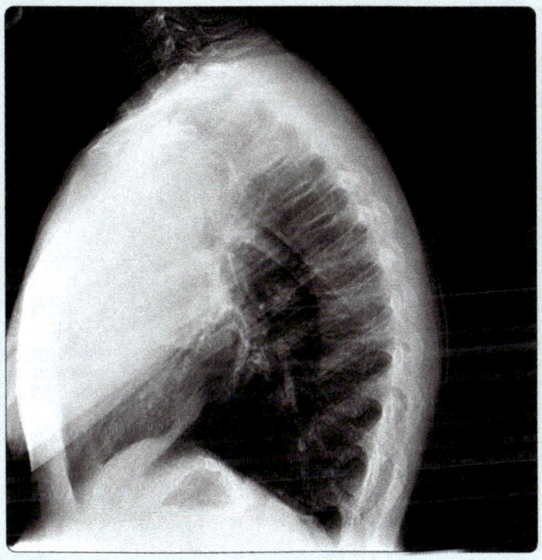

(Left) *Lateral radiograph demonstrates smoothly curved thoracic kyphosis, with premature upper thoracic degenerative disc disease ➙, in this patient with degenerative kyphosis.* **(Right)** *Lateral chest radiograph (idiopathic kyphosis) reveals diffuse upper thoracic kyphosis with a round-back deformity. There is no underlying cause of kyphosis (e.g., Scheuermann disease, prior trauma, congenital anomaly, or infection).*

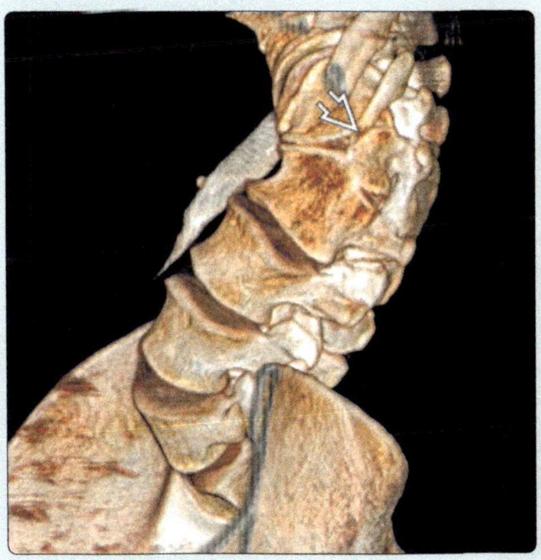
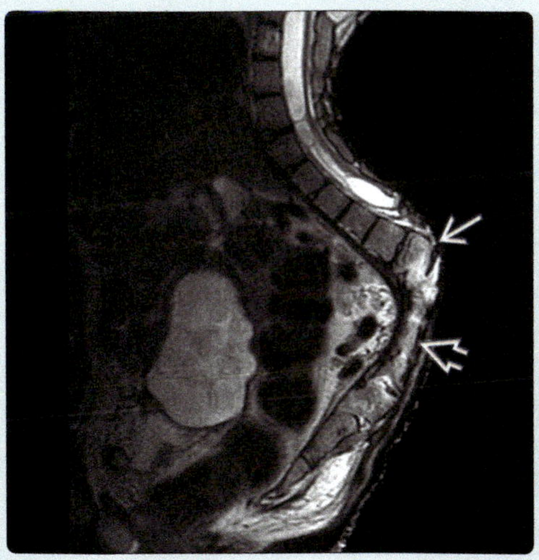

(Left) *Lateral 3D reformation CT shows a posterior hemivertebra ➙ fused to the vertebra below and causing kyphoscoliosis. Congenital scoliosis is often complex in morphology and most easily appreciated on 3D reformations.* **(Right)** *Sagittal T2WI MR of a child with a repaired high myelomeningocele and congenital vertebral segmentation failure ➙ shows severe focal lumbosacral kyphotic curvature ➙.*

Scoliosis

KEY FACTS

TERMINOLOGY

- General term for any lateral curvature of spine

IMAGING

- Lateral curvature of spine
  - Returns to midline at ends of curve
  - Rotational component common
- Most commonly thoracic or thoracolumbar
- Imaging approach
  - Radiography for initial diagnosis
  - Multiplanar MR to screen for bone, cord abnormalities
  - CT for surgical planning, complications

TOP DIFFERENTIAL DIAGNOSES

- Idiopathic scoliosis
- Neuromuscular scoliosis
- Congenital scoliosis
- Scoliosis due to congenital syndromes without vertebral anomalies
- Degenerative scoliosis
- Scoliosis due to infection
- Scoliosis due to tumor
- Scoliosis due to trauma
- Curvature related to limb length inequality
- Positional scoliosis

CLINICAL ISSUES

- Usually presents in childhood or adolescence
- Idiopathic scoliosis usually asymptomatic
  - Painful scoliosis indicates underlying abnormality
- Surgical fusion for rapidly progressive curves, curves > 40°

DIAGNOSTIC CHECKLIST

- Short-curve or painful scoliosis usually has underlying abnormalities
- Curve may progress rapidly, especially during growth spurts

(Left) *Anteroposterior radiograph in an idiopathic scoliosis patient shows the typical curve of idiopathic scoliosis that is convex to the right in the thoracic spine and convex to the left in the lumbar spine. No vertebral anomalies are present, excluding congenital scoliosis.* **(Right)** *Coronal 3D reformatted bone CT reveals a right L3 hemivertebra resulting in convex right congenital scoliosis. There are rudimentary left L3 pedicle and posterior elements.*

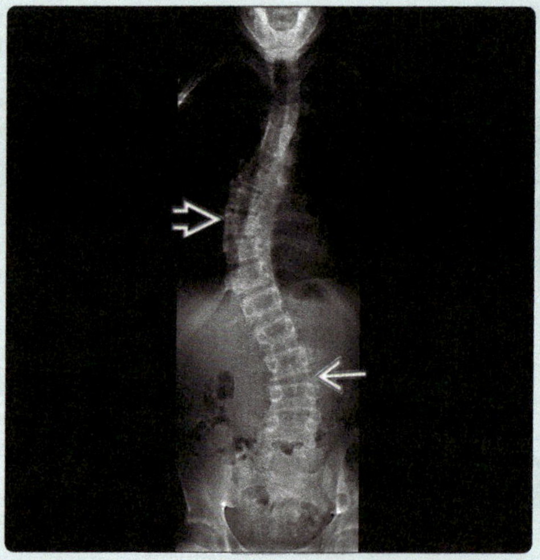

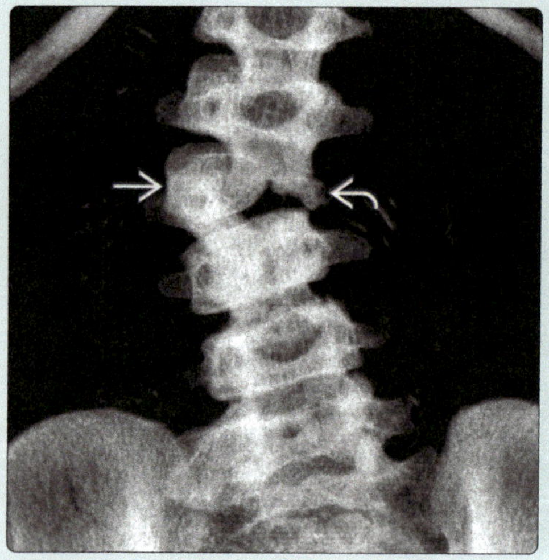

(Left) *Anteroposterior 3D reformatted bone CT of idiopathic scoliosis shows rotation as well as scoliosis to be present on the apical vertebra and terminal vertebrae.* **(Right)** *Axial bone CT 3D reformation demonstrates the rotation of the apical vertebra compared with the terminal vertebrae. 3D CT is valuable in surgical planning to evaluate severity of rotation.*

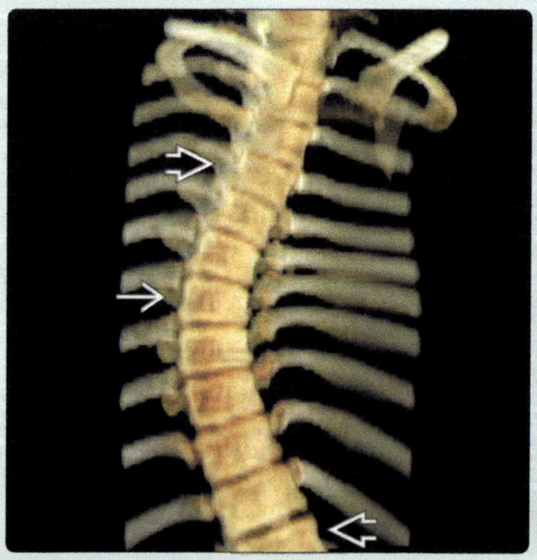

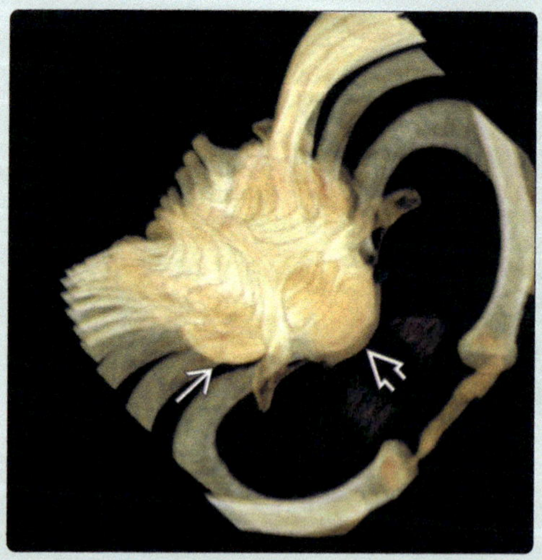

KEY FACTS

TERMINOLOGY

- Lateral curvature in spine due to degenerative disc and facet disease in older patients
- Deformity in skeletally mature patient with Cobb angle of > 10° in coronal plane
- Predominance of lower lumbar curves

IMAGING

- Conventional standing full-length PA and lateral radiographs for monitoring curve progression
- Most common from L1 to L4
  - Lateral listhesis, vertebral rotation
  - Disc space loss, endplate sclerosis
  - Circumferential endplate spurring
  - Facet arthropathy
  - Spondylolisthesis, loss of lordosis

TOP DIFFERENTIAL DIAGNOSES

- Adult idiopathic scoliosis
- Neuromuscular
- Congenital scoliosis
- Post-traumatic, inflammatory, or neoplastic
- Dysplasias (neurofibromatosis type 1, Marfan)

PATHOLOGY

- Asymmetric degenerative change at multiple levels
  - Asymmetric loading of spinal segments gives 3-dimensional deformity
  - Spondylolisthesis &/or rotatory listhesis

CLINICAL ISSUES

- Low back pain, radiculopathy
  - Pain worse with prolonged spinal extension
  - Radiculopathy not reliably relieved by flexion
    - In contrast to spinal stenosis without scoliosis
- Deformity and waist asymmetry
- Gait disturbance

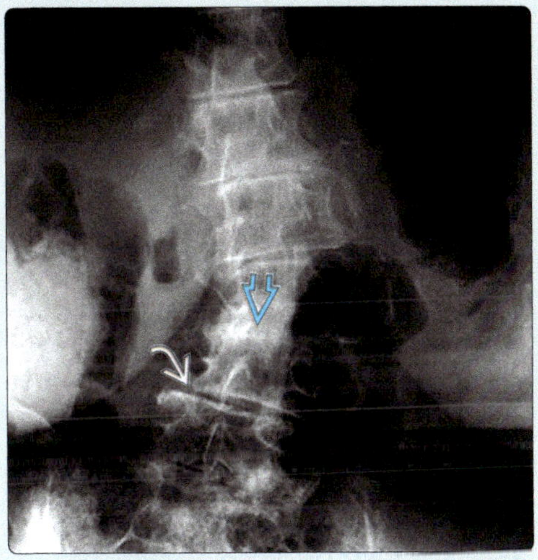
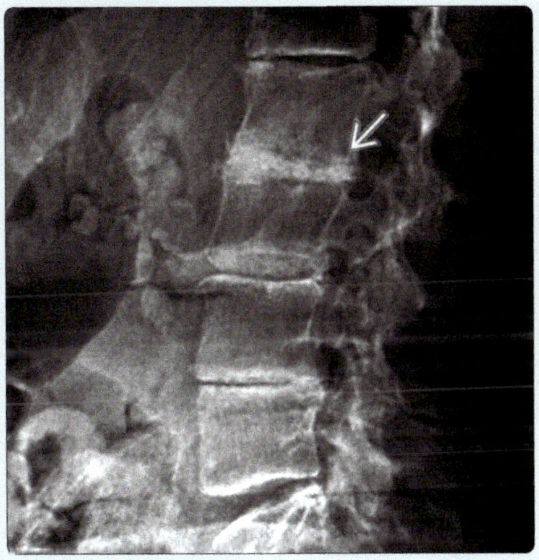

(Left) *Anteroposterior radiography shows lumbar rotatory levoscoliosis (convex left) with associated multilevel marked disc height loss and endplate sclerosis . There is left lateral listhesis of L4 on L5 .* **(Right)** *Lateral radiography shows loss of lumbar lordosis with multilevel disc space height loss and degenerative endplate bony eburnation (sclerosis), worst at L2-L3 .*

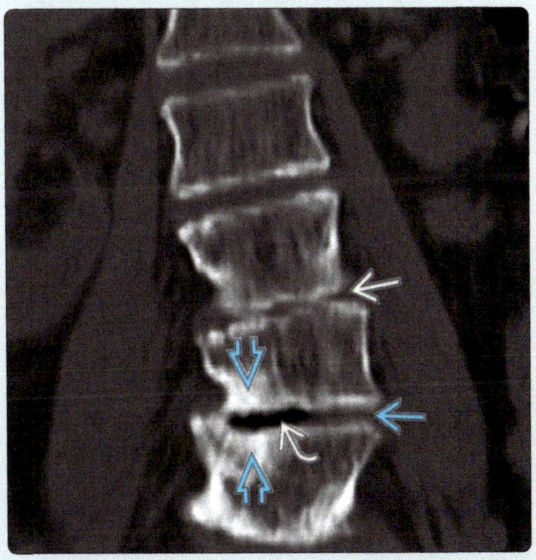
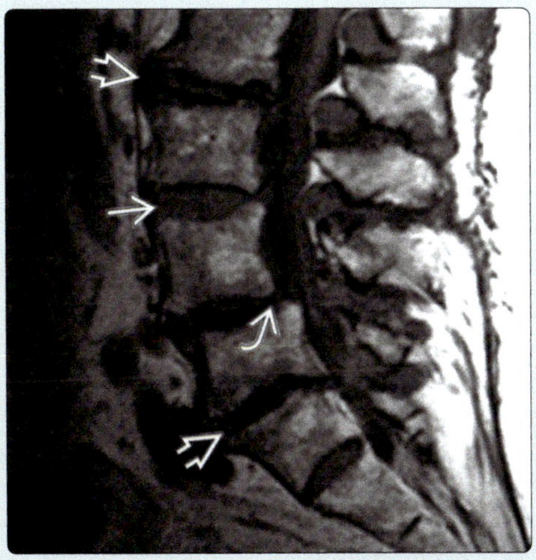

(Left) *Coronal reformation of nonenhanced lumbar spine CT shows mild levoscoliosis at L4-L5 with vacuum disc phenomenon and right-sided endplate sclerosis . There is disc height loss at L3-L4 and L4-L5 .* **(Right)** *Sagittal T1WI MR shows grade 1 anterolisthesis of L4 on L5 with severe disc degeneration. Degenerative discs are also present at L2-L3 and L5-S1. Compare this to a more normal disc at L3-L4 .*

PART II: SPINE
SECTION 2

Trauma and Hemorrhage

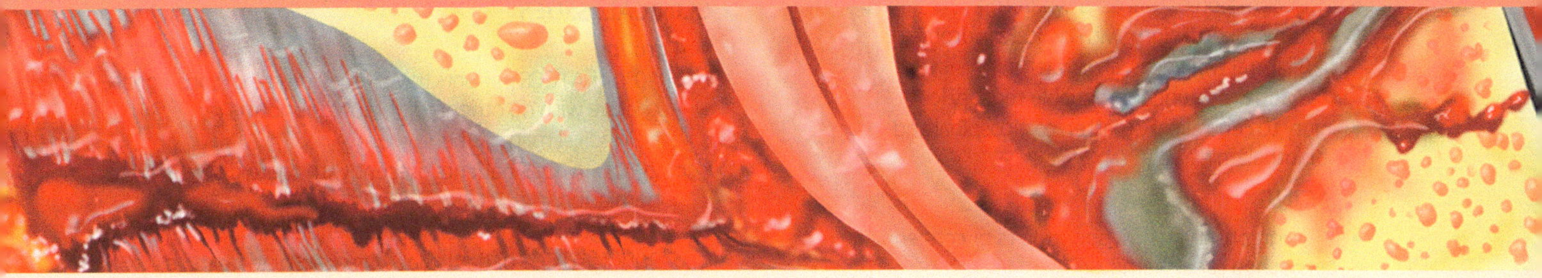

Central Spinal Cord Syndrome

KEY FACTS

TERMINOLOGY

- Central cord syndrome (CCS), acute traumatic central cord syndrome (ATCCS)
- Most common partial cord syndrome
- Traumatic cord injury, with clinical syndrome of
  - Bilateral weakness, arms > legs
  - Bladder dysfunction, variable sensory loss
- Injury to central gray matter, corticospinal and spinothalamic tracts

IMAGING

- Radiographs may show spondylosis or congenitally diminished canal diameter
- MR shows hyperintense signal in central spinal cord on T2WI
- Significant percentage shows fracture/dislocations

PATHOLOGY

- Often with preexisting canal stenosis
  - Congenital canal stenosis
  - Disc herniation, osteophyte
  - Facet/ligamentous hypertrophy

CLINICAL ISSUES

- **4 groups**
  - 10% of ATCCS patients have MR evidence of cord signal change with no other radiographic abnormality
    - Medical management
  - 20% of ATCCS patients present with acute disc herniation
    - Surgical intervention recommended
  - 30% of ATCCS patients have cervical spine fracture subluxation injuries
    - Early realignment of spinal column with spinal cord decompression is recommended
  - 40% of ATCCS patients have spinal stenosis without evidence of bony or ligamentous injury
    - Management remains controversial

(Left) *Sagittal reformatted spine CT shows focal flexion deformity at C5-C6 ➡ with splaying of the posterior elements ➡, demonstrating a hyperflexion injury in this trauma patient with marked upper extremity weakness.* **(Right)** *Sagittal T2WI of the same patient again shows the focal flexion deformity at C5-C6. There is extensive moderately hyperintense signal in the cord from C2-C3 through C6-C7 ➡, demonstrating contusion within the spinal cord. Also note edema within prevertebral soft tissues ➡.*

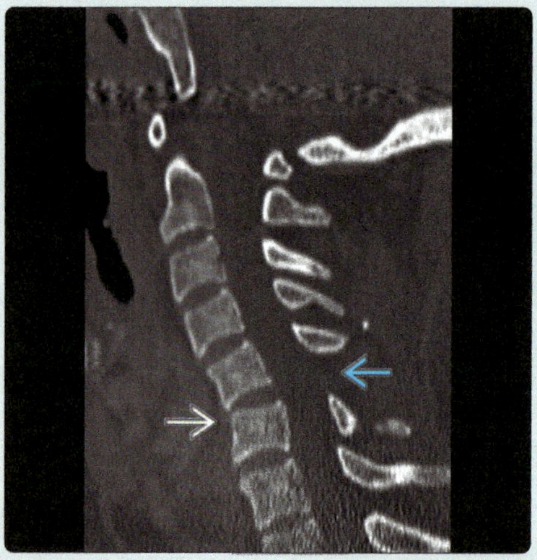

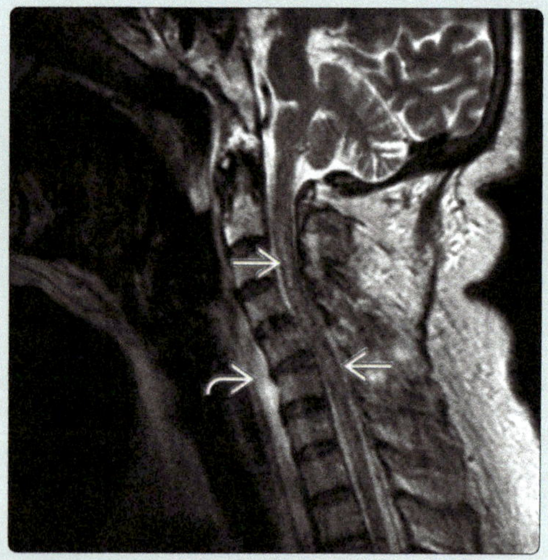

(Left) *Lateral radiograph in this injured child presenting with central cord syndrome shows borderline thickening of the prevertebral soft tissues ➡ but is otherwise unremarkable.* **(Right)** *Sagittal T2WI MR in the same child shows a normal vertebral column and prevertebral soft tissues (seen better on other sequences). There is extensive hyperintense signal within the cord from the cervicomedullary junction ➡ through T4-T5 ➡ demonstrating spinal cord contusion.*

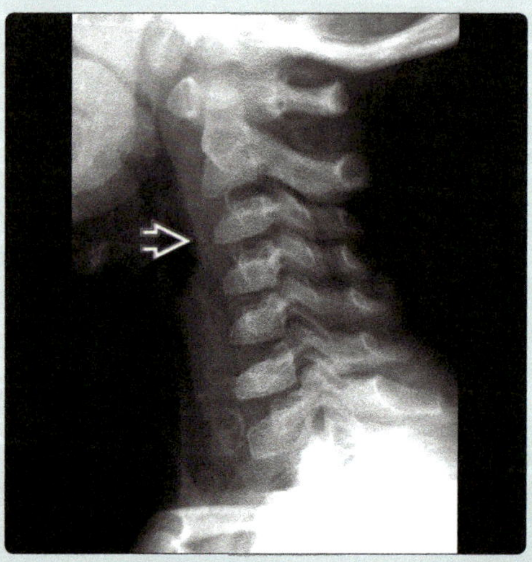

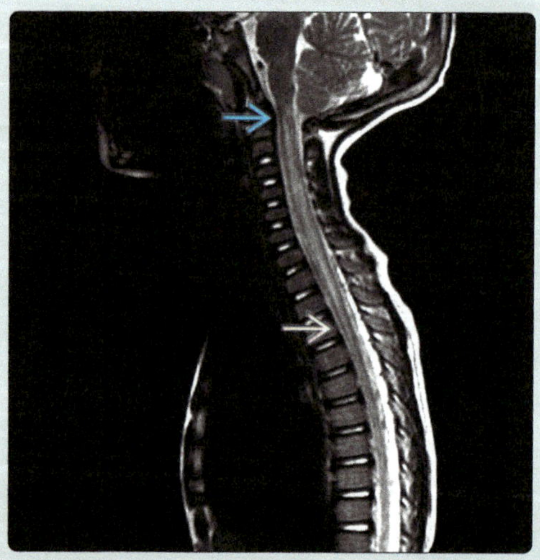

KEY FACTS

IMAGING

- Fusiform intramedullary hyperintensity tracking cerebrospinal fluid (CSF) signal
  - Myelomalacia precedes overt syrinx formation = "presyrinx state"
- Cystic expansile cord lesion
  - May appear to be "expansile" lesion, relative finding in presence of cord atrophy
- Consider cine ("dynamic") PC CSF flow study if suspected obstruction to CSF flow (e.g., arachnoid adhesions)

TOP DIFFERENTIAL DIAGNOSES

- Gibbs artifact
- Nontraumatic syrinx
- Myelitis
- Myelomalacia

PATHOLOGY

- Current treatment assumes syrinx is related to posttraumatic arachnoid scarring and CSF flow obstruction at trauma level

CLINICAL ISSUES

- Symptoms include spasticity, hyperhidrosis, pain, sensory loss, automotive hyperreflexia
- Classic presentation: Severe pain unrelieved by analgesics; ascending disassociated sensory loss
- Surgery reserved from patients with progressive neurological symptoms
  - First-line treatment has moved away from shunting of syrinx to restoring normal CSF flow patterns at traumatic site
    - Untethering of cord
    - Duraplasty
    - Spine realignment or fusion may be added if angulation or stability is problematic

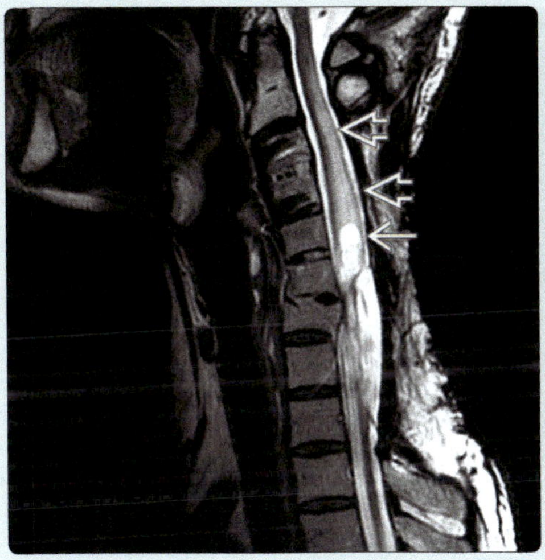
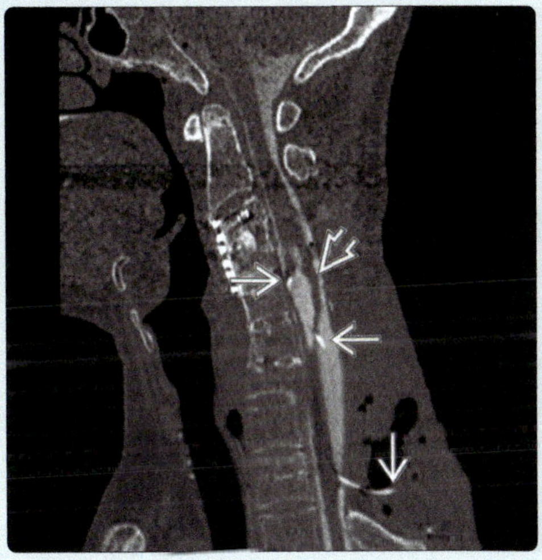

(Left) *Sagittal images showing extension of syrinx over time into regions of "presyrinx" edema are presented. Initial T2 MR after C3-C4 fusion and prior flexion injury at C5-C6 shows the well-defined syrinx cavity at the C5-C6 level with cord expansion ➡. T2 hyperintense signal within the cord extends cephalad from the syrinx to the C2 level due to cord edema ➡.* **(Right)** *Sagittal CT myelogram following placement of a syringoperitoneal shunt shows the shunt catheter ➡ within the syrinx cavity, which is decreased in size ➡.*

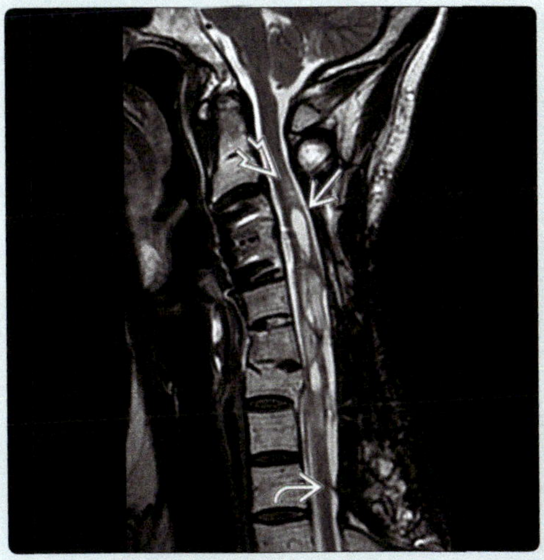
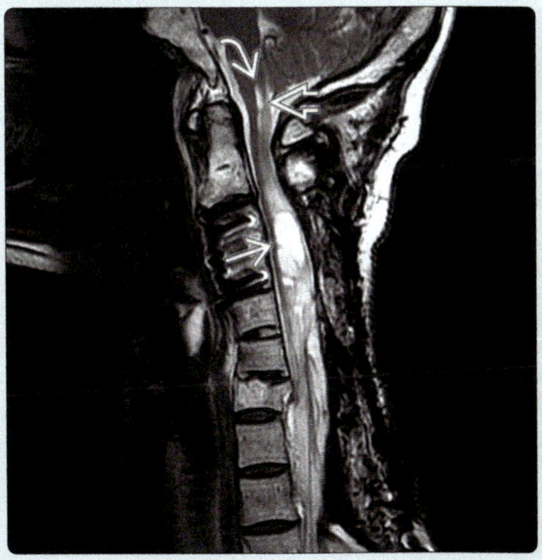

(Left) *Follow-up sagittal T2 MR 3 months later shows extension of the syrinx to the C3 level ➡ with slight edema ➡ cephalad to this site. Note the presence of a shunt catheter ➡, which has not stopped the syrinx progression.* **(Right)** *Sagittal T2 MR 6 months later shows expansion of the syrinx at the C3 level ➡ and marked, increased "presyrinx" edema extending cephalad to the medulla ➡ with a small focus of syringobulbia ➡.*

Spinal Cord Contusion-Hematoma

KEY FACTS

TERMINOLOGY

- Spinal cord injury (SCI)
- Traumatic axonal injury, cord edema, &/or hemorrhage

IMAGING

- Abnormal cord signal on MR in setting of trauma
- Most common level of adult SCI is C4-C6
- Commonly associated fracture or subluxation in younger adults (16-45 years)
- Underlying degenerative change (canal stenosis) predisposes to cord injury in older population
- SCI without radiographic abnormality is common in pediatric population (< 8 years)
- Cord injury typically occult on CT

PATHOLOGY

- Overall incidence of SCI in trauma estimated at 3.7%
- High-velocity mechanisms more common in youth and young adults
- If > 45 years, more likely due to fall; short falls (< 1 m) may result in significant injury in elderly patients

CLINICAL ISSUES

- Edema without hemorrhage: Good prognosis for recovery
- Hematoma: Poor prognosis, often without recovery
  - Extent of intramedullary hemorrhage and cord swelling are key predictors of neurologic recovery after traumatic cervical cord injury
- 30-60 new cases per million per year in USA

DIAGNOSTIC CHECKLIST

- Sagittal STIR is key sequence
  - Sensitive to cord edema
  - Ligamentous/muscular injury
  - Marrow edema
- Sagittal and axial gradient-echo images for cord hemorrhage

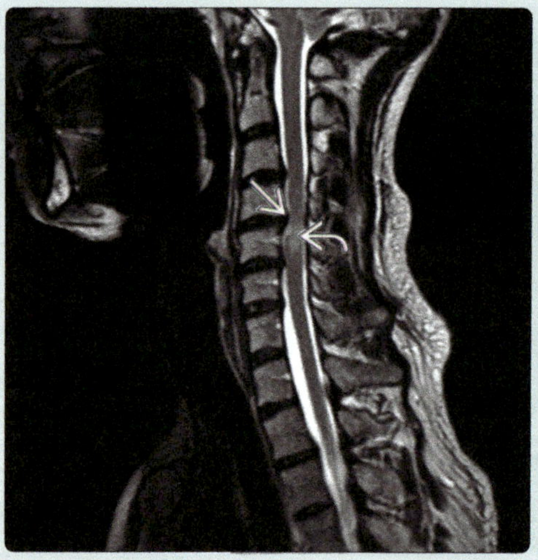

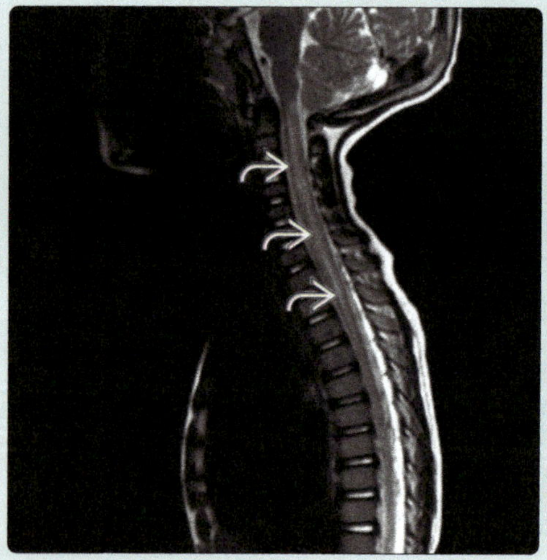

***(Left)** Sagittal T2WI MR of a patient presenting days after an MVA with upper > lower extremity weakness shows congenital narrowing of the canal with multiple disc bulges and levels of canal stenosis, worst at C4-C5. Caudally, mild, patchy T2 hyperintensity shows nonhemorrhagic cord contusion. **(Right)** Sagittal T2WI MR in a child shows diffuse contusion in the cord from C1 through the upper thoracic cord. The patient presented with 4 extremity neurologic deficits after fall. Plain films would be normal.*

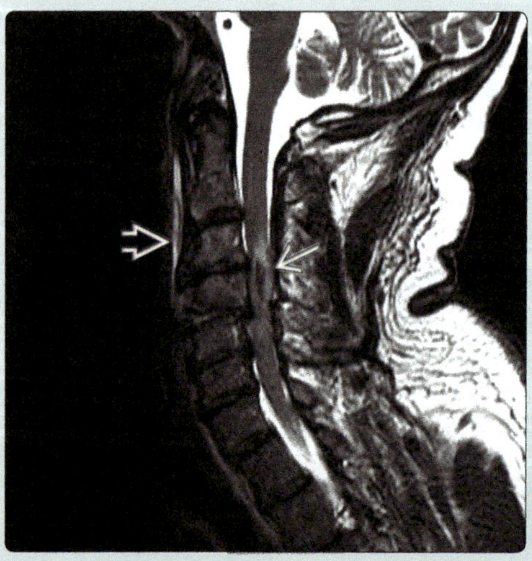

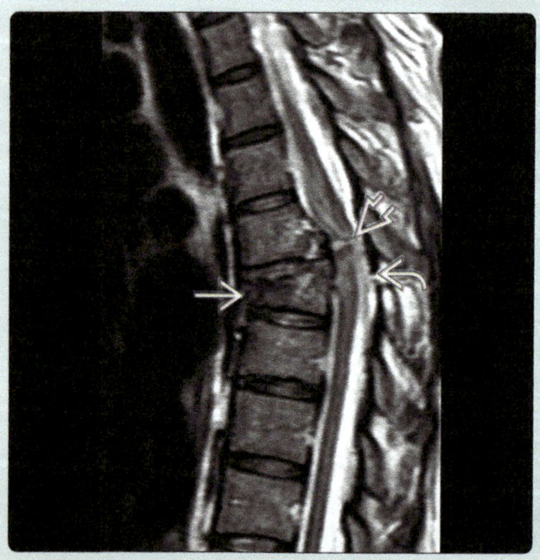

***(Left)** Sagittal T2 MR in this trauma patient shows low signal intensity cord hemorrhage at C4 with surrounding edema in the setting of severe cervical canal stenosis. Prevertebral edema is present. **(Right)** Sagittal T2WI shows a midthoracic burst fracture and disruption of ligamentum flavum. There is complete transection of the spinal cord, demonstrated by a cerebrospinal fluid-filled cleft, with adjacent edema.*

KEY FACTS

TERMINOLOGY

- Hemorrhage build-up between dura and spine not caused by significant trauma or iatrogenic procedures

IMAGING

- Extradural multisegmental T1 hyperintense fluid collection
- Thoracic, lumbar > cervical
  - Lentiform or biconvex
  - Outlined by dorsal epidural fat cranially and rostrally
- T1WI acute: < 48 hours
  - Isointense > hypo-/hyperintense
- T1WI subacute and chronic
  - Hyperintense > isointense
- T2WI heterogeneously hyperintense

TOP DIFFERENTIAL DIAGNOSES

- Epidural metastasis
- Lymphoma
- Disc extrusion, migration
- Epidural abscess
- Subdural hematoma
- Epidural fat lipomatosis

PATHOLOGY

- Idiopathic: 40-50%
- Minor trauma
- Anticoagulation
- Coagulopathy
- Disc herniation
- Vascular anomaly

CLINICAL ISSUES

- Acute onset of neck, back pain
- Progressive paraparesis
- Bladder or bowel dysfunction

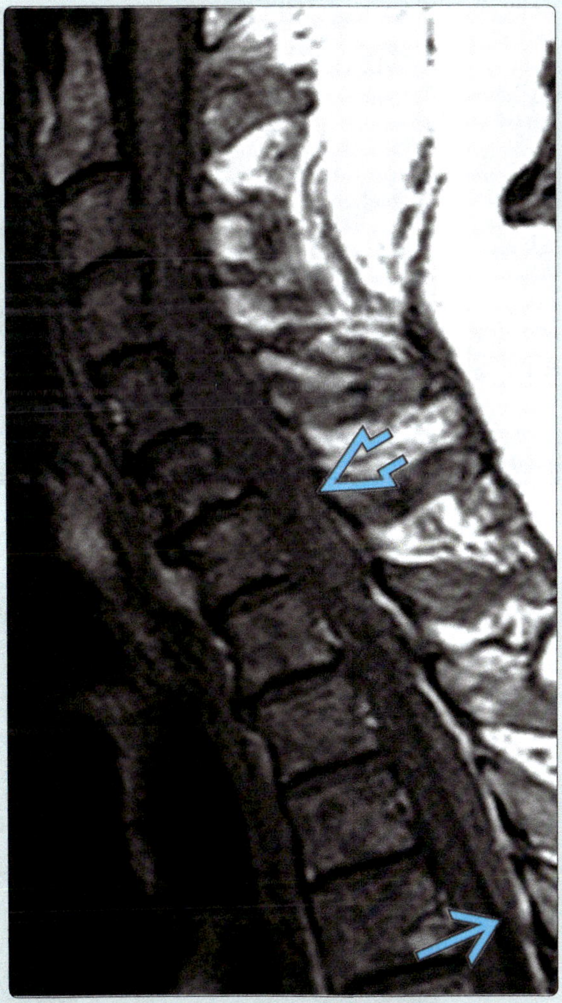

Sagittal T1WI MR shows an indistinct margin of the cervical cord due to an isointense mass within the dorsal epidural space ⇨. The location of the mass is best identified at the inferior margin as extradural ⇨.

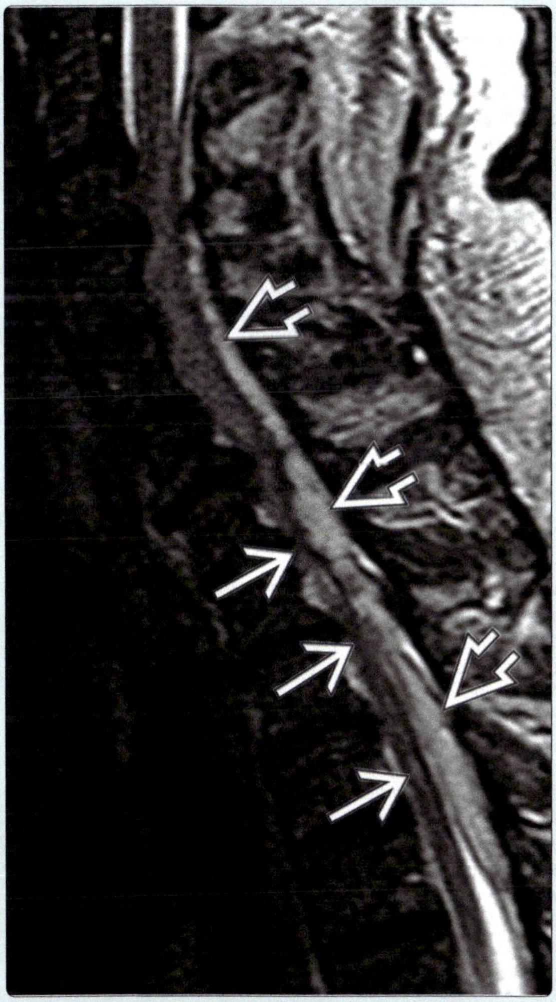

Sagittal T2WI MR of the same patient shows a slightly heterogeneous, long-segment hyperintense mass ➡ within the posterior epidural space spanning the C2-T4 level. The cord ➡ is severely compressed and displaced anteriorly.

KEY FACTS

TERMINOLOGY

- Accumulation of blood between dura, arachnoid

IMAGING

- Intradural collection hyperintense on T1WI, predominantly hypointense on T2WI or gradient-echo imaging
- Thoracolumbar > lumbar or lumbosacral > cervical
- Clumped, loculated masses of hemorrhagic density/intensity

TOP DIFFERENTIAL DIAGNOSES

- Epidural hematoma
- Subdural abscess
- Cerebrospinal fluid leakage syndrome
- Spinal meningitis
- Idiopathic hypertrophic spinal pachymeningitis

PATHOLOGY

- Trauma
- Bleeding diathesis: 54% of reported cases
- Iatrogenic cause is factor in 2/3 of those with abnormal coagulation parameters
- Neoplasm
- Arteriovenous malformation
- Postoperative complication
- Spontaneous: 15%

CLINICAL ISSUES

- Acute onset of neck or back pain
- Radicular pain, bladder/bowel dysfunction
- Much less common than spinal epidural hematoma
- Treatment
  - May resolve spontaneously
  - Decompressive laminectomy with clot evacuation
    - Indicated with severe and progressive deterioration of neurologic symptoms

(Left) *Sagittal T1WI MR without fat saturation shows prominent hyperintense linear collections both ventral* → *and dorsal* → *within the bony spinal canal, with narrowing of the thecal cerebrospinal fluid (CSF) space.* **(Right)** *Sagittal T1WI MR with fat saturation shows the hyperintense linear subdural blood collection to better advantage. There is marked narrowing of thecal CSF space* →*. Iatrogenic cause is a factor in 2/3 of those with abnormal coagulation parameters.*

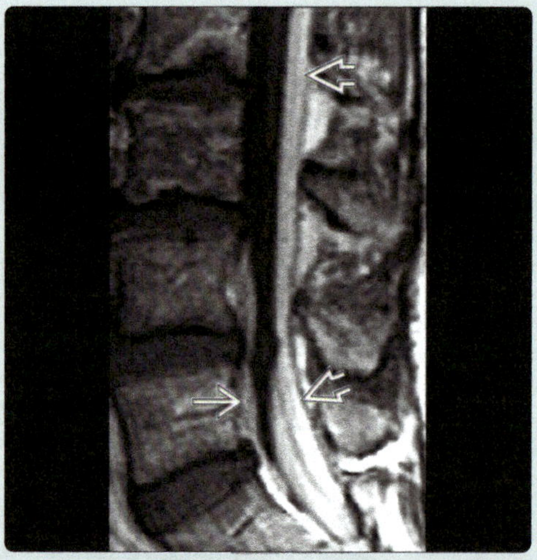

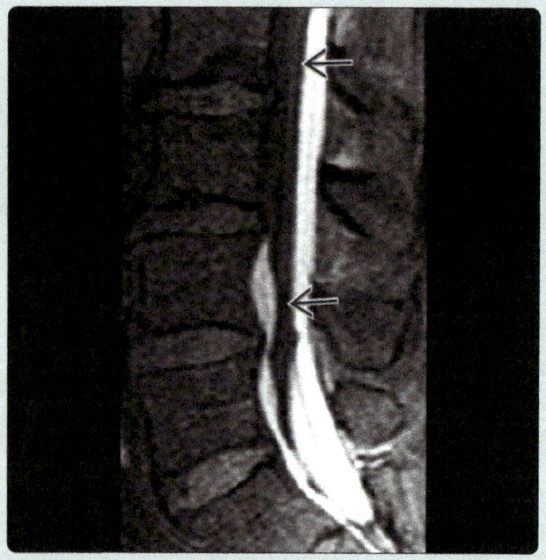

(Left) *Axial T1WI FS MR in the same patient shows the typical appearance of a subdural hemorrhage, with a well-defined outer margin bounded by the dura* →*, and an inner lobulated margin, giving a Mercedes Benz sign* →*.* **(Right)** *Sagittal T1WI MR in a patient with a subdural hematoma shows diffuse ventral* → *and dorsal* → *intraspinal hyperintense collections, with intracranial extension* →*.*

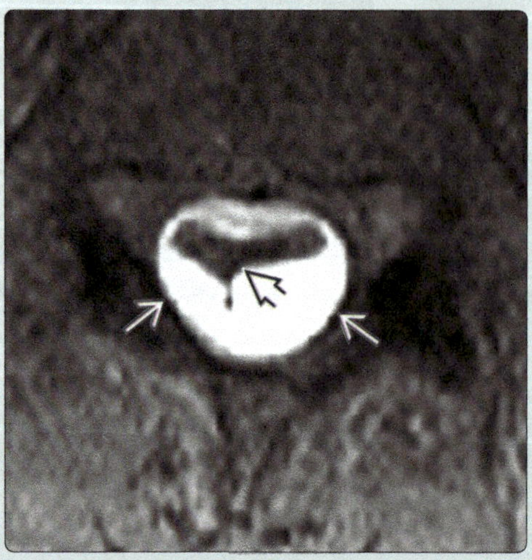

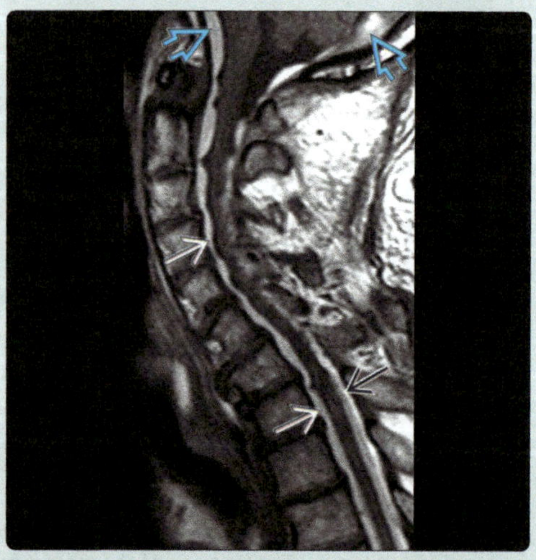

KEY FACTS

TERMINOLOGY

- Hemorrhage into spinal subarachnoid space from variety of etiologies
  - Trauma (> 50%)
  - Aneurysmal subarachnoid hemorrhage (SAH) with spinal extension
  - Spinal arteriovenous malformations
    - Mainly types II, III, IVc, conus malformations
  - Tumor
  - Anticoagulant therapy
  - Infection (pneumococcal meningitis, herpes)
  - Systemic disease
  - Spinal artery aneurysm (rare)

IMAGING

- Fluid-fluid level within thecal sac
- Variable depending on stage of blood breakdown and byproducts
- Dynamic enhanced MRA useful as screen for spinal vascular malformation

TOP DIFFERENTIAL DIAGNOSES

- Epidural hemorrhage
- Subdural hemorrhage
- Intramedullary hemorrhage

PATHOLOGY

- Rare reports of cervical/thoracic arachnoiditis developing following spinal SAH

CLINICAL ISSUES

- Acute back or radicular pain ± signs of cord compression (numbness, weakness)
- Massive spinal SAH may give acute cord compression, paraplegia, fecal and urinary incontinence

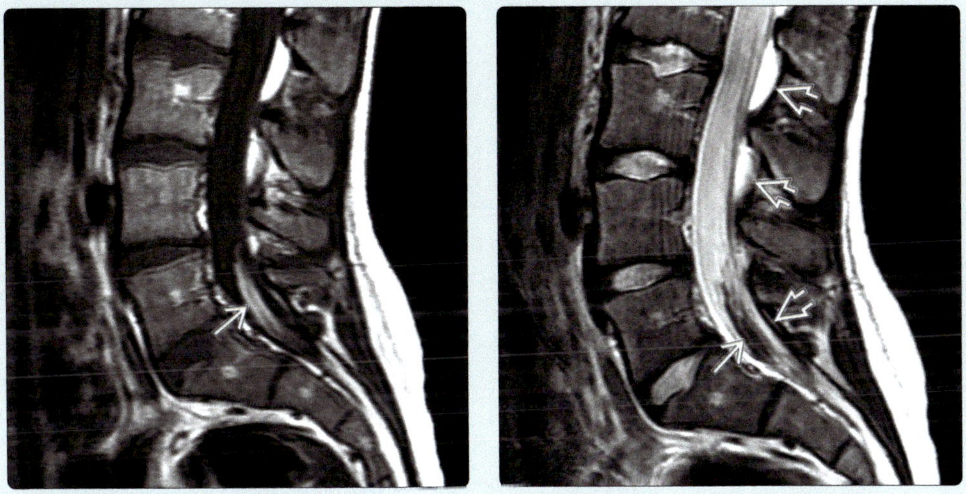

(Left) *Sagittal T1WI MR of subarachnoid blood following epidural blood patch, presumably related to incorrect needle position, shows oblong focus of T1 hyperintensity within distal thecal sac at the L5-S1 level due to methemoglobin ➡. No epidural lesion is present.* **(Right)** *Sagittal T2WI MR in the same patient shows the blood is low signal intensity ➡. The epidural space is normal ⇨.*

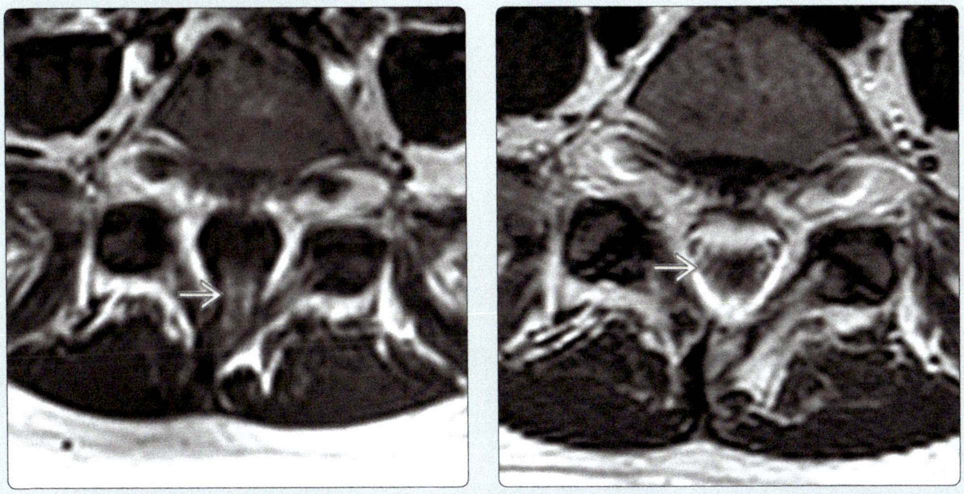

(Left) *Axial T1WI MR (same patient) of subarachnoid blood following epidural blood patch shows focus of T1 hyperintensity ➡ within distal thecal sac at the L5-S1 level.* **(Right)** *Axial T2WI MR shows diffuse subarachnoid blood in the distal thecal sac as hypointensity ➡.*

PART II: SPINE
SECTION 3

Degenerative Diseases and Arthritides

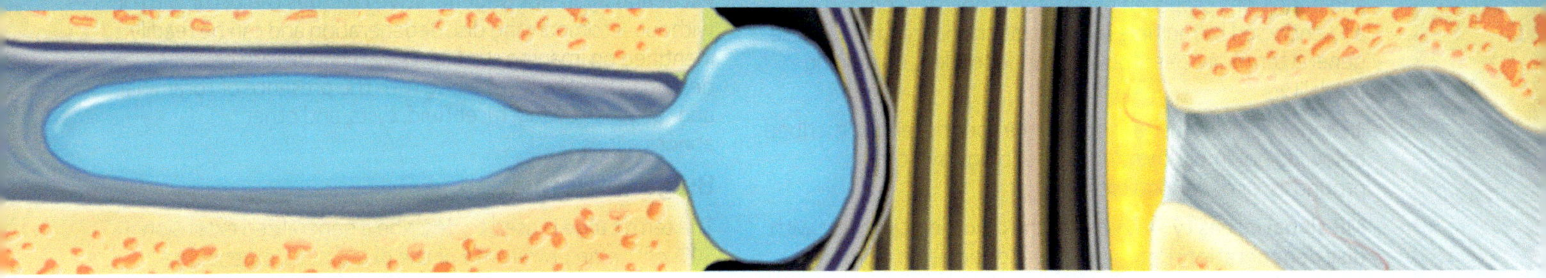

Spine Degenerations

Spondylolisthesis and Spondylolysis

Inflammatory, Crystalline, and Miscellaneous Arthritides

Disc Degeneration

Overview. Describing morphology alterations seen in degenerative disc disease requires common terminology to standardize communication. A series of pathoanatomic terms and definitions proposed by an interdisciplinary committee and endorsed by multiple societies is summarized here. These general terms are descriptive and independent of imaging modality.

It cannot be overemphasized that the specific terms described below do not imply knowledge of etiology, symptoms, prognosis, or need for treatment.

MR signal intensity. Any or all of the following can occur with **disc degeneration**: Real or apparent desiccation, fibrosis, narrowed intervertebral disc space, bulging, fissuring/mucinous degeneration of the anulus, osteophytes of the vertebral apophyses, and endplate/adjacent marrow changes.

Severely degenerated discs with markedly decreased signal intensity may demonstrate linear areas of high signal intensity on T2-weighted images that may represent free fluid within cracks or fissures of the degenerated complex. Signal intensity changes in the intervertebral disc on T1-weighted images, while much less common than the loss of signal noted on T2-weighted images, can also be seen with degeneration.

Regions of decreased or absent signal within **heavily calcified discs** may occur. Signal loss has been attributed to a low mobile proton density as well as, in the case of gradient echo imaging, its sensitivity to the heterogeneous magnetic susceptibility found in calcified tissue.

Focal or diffuse areas of hyperintensity on T1-weighted spin-echo sequences may also be encountered in densely calcified intervertebral discs. These changes are related to T1 relaxation times secondary to a surface relaxation mechanism. These regions of high signal intensity on T1 are unaffected by fat suppression, suggesting that it is a T1 shortening effect rather than the presence of lipid. Hyperintensities within severely degenerated intervertebral discs that suppress on fat-saturation techniques presumably relate to areas of fatty marrow.

Separation between, or avulsion of, anular fibers from their vertebral body insertions, or breaks through fibers that extend transversely in a radial fashion, or concentrically through layers of the anular lamellae, are referred to as **anular fissures**. On MR, these changes are seen on T2-weighted images as high signal intensity within the outer anulus/posterior longitudinal ligament complex (the so-called "high-intensity zone"). These regions will also sometimes enhance following the administration of paramagnetic contrast, an effect thought to be secondary to reactive reparative tissue. The term "anular tear" should be avoided.

The role of anular disruption as the principle causal agent of disc degeneration has not been proven. In light of the continuing controversy surrounding the concept of "internal disc disruption," it is probably unwarranted to imply that radial tears are more than a manifestation of advanced degeneration. While no data clearly support an unequivocal causal relationship between these degeneration changes and symptoms, anular disruption is important to consider because of a controversial concept of "discogenic pain" and its implications concerning the usefulness of discography for diagnosis. Back pain is thought to occur in some patients without morphological abnormalities, such as herniation or stenosis, which are thought to be related to leakage of nuclear material through the disrupted anulus into the epidural space.

Facet and ligament degenerative changes can occur with or without accompanying disc degeneration and can be readily identified on imaging studies. These changes are best described level by level, along with the presence of foraminal and canal narrowing, facet fluid, cysts, and other abnormalities.

Bulge vs. Herniation

The term **bulge** is used to describe a generalized extension > 50% of the circumference of the disc tissues, extending a short distance (< 3 mm) beyond the edges of the adjacent apophyses. A bulge is not a herniation, although 1 portion of the disc may be bulging and another portion of the disc may herniate.

A bulge is often a normal variant, particularly in children in whom all normal discs appear to extend slightly beyond the vertebral body margin. Bulge may also be associated with disc degeneration or may occur as a response to axial loading or angular motion with ligamentous laxity. Occasionally, a bulge in 1 plane is really a central subligamentous disc herniation in another plane. Asymmetric bulging of disc tissue > 25% of the disc circumference may be seen as an adaptation to adjacent deformity and is not considered a form of herniation.

Herniations are a localized displacement of disc material beyond the limits of the intervertebral disc space in any direction. The disc space is defined in the cranio-caudad direction by the vertebral body endplates and peripherally by the outer edges of the vertebral ring apophyses, exclusive of any osteophytes. If the herniation is < 25% of the disc circumference, it is referred to as **focal or localized**. If it is between 25% and 50%, it has been referred to as **broad based**. This term has been eliminated in the latest version of the nomenclature.

Protrusions are herniations in which the greatest distance in any plane between the edges of disc material beyond the disc space is less than the distance between the edges of the base in the same plane. In practical terms, this looks like a triangle on sagittal images, with the base of the triangle at the disc margin and the apex of the triangle within the epidural space.

Extrusions are herniations in which, in at least 1 plane, any 1 distance between the edges of the disc material beyond the disc space, is greater than the distance between the edges of the base in the same plane, or when no continuity exists between the disc material beyond the disc space and that material within the disc space. In practical terms, this looks like the toothpaste sign on the sagittal image, with the larger component of the herniation within the epidural space and a smaller pedicle connecting to the intervertebral disc.

If extruded disc material is not contiguous to the disc space, it is referred to as a **sequestration** (or **"free fragment"**). The extrusion is referred to as "migrated" if it has been displaced from the site of extrusion, regardless of whether or not it is sequestrated. The signal intensity of the extruded portion may be increased or decreased on T2-weighted images. All disc herniations, small or large, can be associated with enhancement, and this enhancement may constitute a large portion of the extradural mass. Acute disc herniations may also cause focal epidural hemorrhage.

Sequestrated fragments can lie anterior to the posterior longitudinal ligament, especially if they have migrated behind the vertebral bodies where the posterior longitudinal ligament is not in direct opposition. Fragments may also lie posterior to the ligament. Sequestrated fragments within the lateral recess and the neural foramen have been shown to produce eroded cortical bone and expansion of those spaces and, thus, should be considered in the differential diagnosis of a mass arising and expanding the neural foramen and lateral recess.

In rare instances, disc herniation may extend through the dura and arachnoid. The mechanism of **intradural disc herniation** is thought to be the development of chronic inflammation leading to adhesions between the dura and the posterior longitudinal ligament. Nevertheless, there is almost invariably penetration through the posterior longitudinal ligament posteriorly, where it is fused with the anulus, or superiorly or inferiorly, where it fuses with the vertebral body margin. Intradural disc herniations may enhance and mimic neoplasm.

The characterization of a disc herniation is not always clear cut, and it may appear as a protrusion in 1 plane and an extrusion in another. If there is displacement away from the disc space in any plane, it should be referred to as an extrusion. Containment refers to the integrity of the outer anulus covering the disc herniation.

One may view the continuum of herniated disc disease as starting with anular disruption, proceeding on to small focal herniation (which is not broken completely through the anulus-ligamentous complex) to frank herniation (extrusion). The extrusion has dissected through the anulus and posterior ligamentous complex completely. These extrusions may show variable degrees of containment, and a line of decreased signal intensity has been reported around sequestrated fragments and large extruded discs, where there has clearly been disruption of the anulus and ligament. This is thought to be secondary to anular and ligamentous fibers that are carried away with the disc herniation.

The anulus fibrosus and posterior longitudinal ligament are so intertwined at the level of the disc that a distinction between the 2 structures may be impossible or, for that matter, irrelevant. Technical limitations of CT and MR usually preclude the distinction of a contained from an uncontained disc herniation. In the transverse plane, the disc abnormality is usually described as **central**, **right** or **left central**, **subarticular**, **foraminal**, or **extraforaminal** (far lateral). In the sagittal plane, **discal**, **infrapedicular**, **suprapedicular**, and **pedicular** are most commonly employed.

Several nonstandard terms should be avoided. These include "disc material beyond the interspace" (DEBIT), which has been superseded by protrusion and extrusion categorization. "Herniated nucleus pulposus" is an old favorite but is not accurate because much of what herniates is not nucleus pulposus (cartilage, fibrous tissue). "Ruptured" disc has no role in a report because this implies a specific knowledge of a traumatic etiology, which is nearly always lacking. Finally, "prolapse" is synonymous with the standard term "protrusion."

Degenerative Endplate Changes

The relationship among the vertebral body, endplate, and disc has been studied by using both degenerated and chymopapain-treated discs as models. A common observation in MR is signal intensity changes in the vertebral body marrow adjacent to endplates of a degenerative disc. These changes appear to take 3 main forms.

Type I changes demonstrate a decreased signal intensity on T1-weighted images and an increased signal intensity on T2-weighted images, and these changes have been identified in ~ 4% of patients scanned for lumbar disease. Type I changes are also seen in ~ 30% of chymopapain-treated discs, which may be viewed as a model of acute disc degeneration.

Type II changes are represented by increased signal intensity on T1-weighted images and an isointense or slightly hyperintense signal on T2-weighted images. These changes are seen in ~ 16% of cases. In both types I and II, there is evidence of associated degenerative disc disease at the level of involvement. Mild enhancement of type I vertebral body marrow changes is seen with Gd-DTPA, which at times can extend to involve the disc itself. This enhancement is presumably related to vascularized fibrous tissue within adjacent marrow.

Histopathological sections of a disc with type I changes demonstrate disruption and fissuring of the endplate and vascularized fibrous tissues within the adjacent marrow, producing prolongation of T1 and T2. Discs with type II changes also show evidence of endplate disruption with yellow marrow replacement in the adjacent vertebral body, resulting in a shorter T1. There appears to be a relationship between the different endplate types, as type I changes have been observed to convert to type II with time, and type II changes seem to remain stable.

Type III changes are represented by decreased signal intensity on both T1- and T2-weighted images. These findings seem to correlate with the presence of extensive bony sclerosis.

While the signal intensity changes of type I may be similar to those seen in vertebral osteomyelitis, the distinguishing factor (at least in the adult population) is the involvement of the intervertebral disc, which shows an abnormal high signal intensity and abnormal configuration on T2-weighted images with infection. Increased signal from the disc may suggest an active inflammatory process. Disc narrowing, sclerosis, and vertebral endplate irregularity suggestive of osteomyelitis has also been demonstrated in long-term hemodialysis and calcium pyrophosphate disease. Classically, in the patient with hemodialysis spondyloarthropathy, the intervertebral disc maintains low signal intensity on both T1- and T2-weighted sequences. Crystal disorders should show increased signal intensity on long TE/TR sequences.

Selected References

1. Fardon DF et al: Lumbar disc nomenclature: version 2.0: Recommendations of the combined task forces of the North American Spine Society, the American Society of Spine Radiology and the American Society of Neuroradiology. Spine J. 14(11):2525-45, 2014
2. Fardon DF et al: Nomenclature and classification of lumbar disc pathology. Recommendations of the Combined task Forces of the North American Spine Society, American Society of Spine Radiology, and American Society of Neuroradiology. Spine (Phila Pa 1976). 26(5):E93-E113, 2001
3. Milette PC: The proper terminology for reporting lumbar intervertebral disk disorders. AJNR Am J Neuroradiol. 18(10):1859-66, 1997

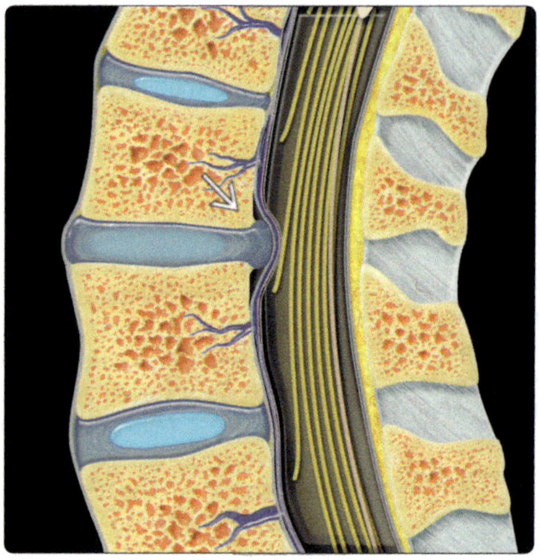

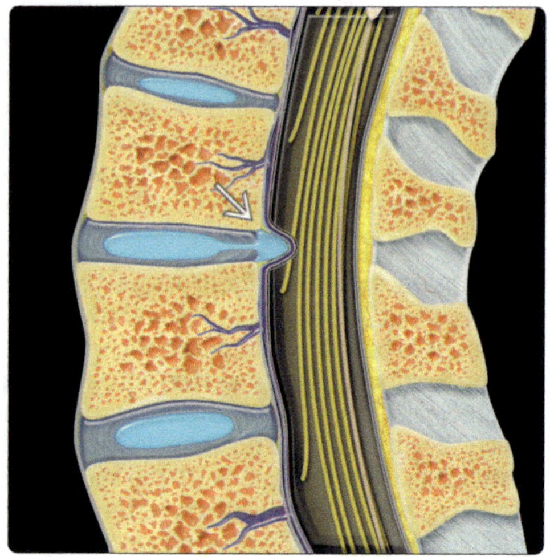

(Left) *Sagittal graphic of a disc bulge shows generalized extension of the disc margin beyond the vertebral body.* *An axial view must show generalized extension > 90° of the disc margin to be a bulge; < 90° would be a protrusion.* **(Right)** *Sagittal graphic of a disc protrusion shows extension of disc material beyond the interspace margin, where the base of the herniation is wider than the portion in the epidural space.*

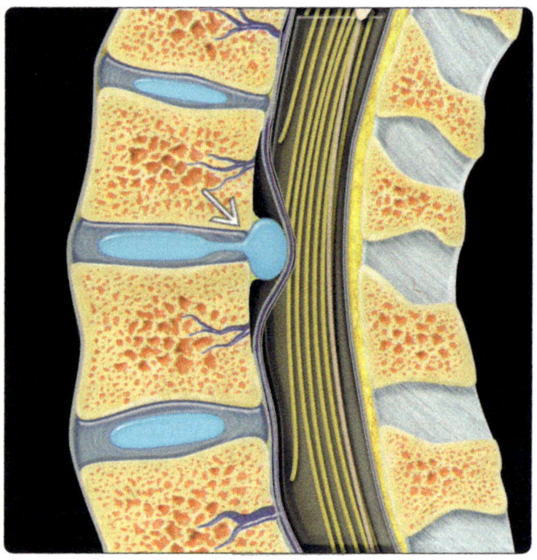

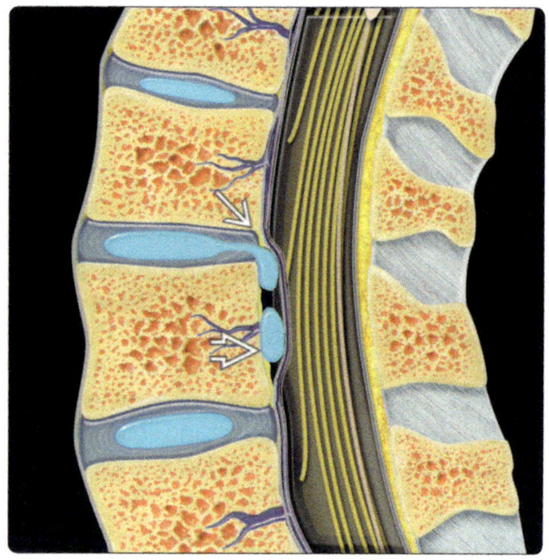

(Left) *Sagittal graphic of a disc extrusion shows extension of disc material beyond the interspace, where the base of the herniated material is smaller than the component in the epidural space.* **(Right)** *Sagittal graphic shows a disc extrusion with free fragment. Extruded disc demonstrates extension of disc material beyond the interspace with the base narrower than the portion in the epidural space. A 2nd component has separated from the parent disc and is a free fragment or sequestered disc.*

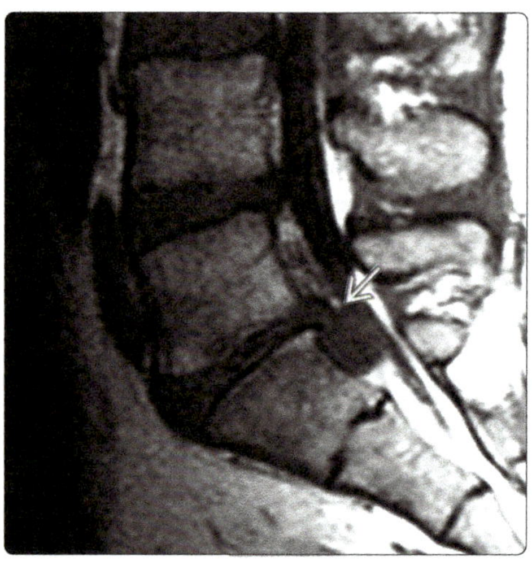

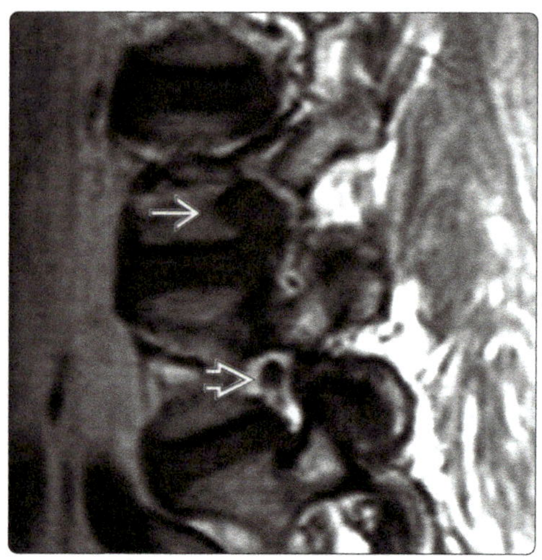

(Left) *Sagittal T1WI MR shows severe disc degeneration at L5-S1 with disc extrusion, where the base of herniation is narrower than the portion extending into epidural space. There is inferior migration of herniation consistent with free fragment.* **(Right)** *Sagittal T1WI MR shows a large L3-L4 far lateral disc extrusion, which is located within the neural foramen (foraminal herniation) and obscures the exiting L3 nerve root. Note the normal exiting root at the level below for comparison.*

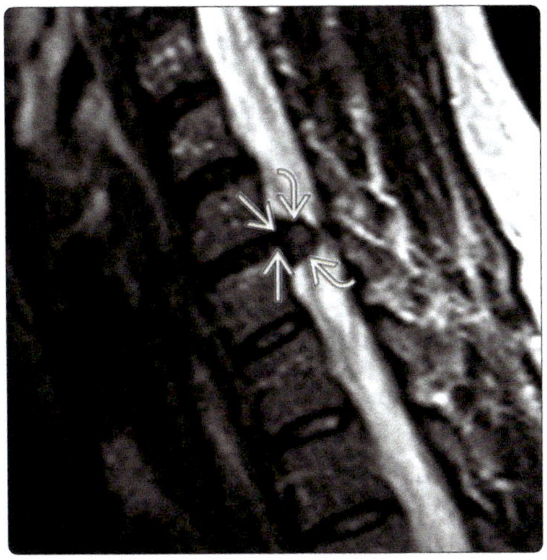

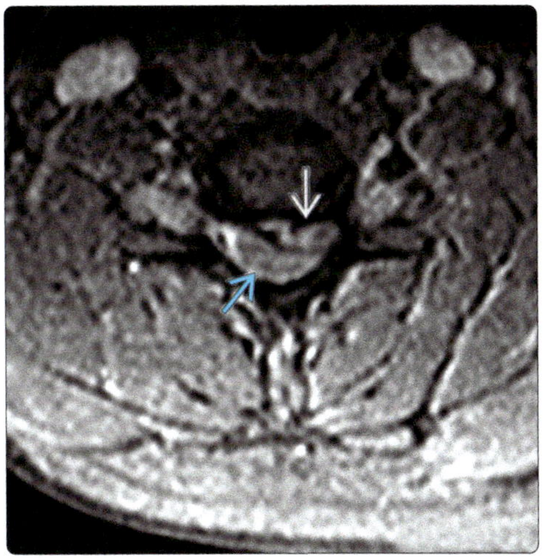

(Left) *Sagittal T2WI MR shows C5-C6 disc extrusion, where the base of the herniation is smaller than the rest of the epidural component.* **(Right)** *Axial T2* GRE MR in a different patient shows a large left central disc extrusion with moderate compression of the thecal sac and cord.*

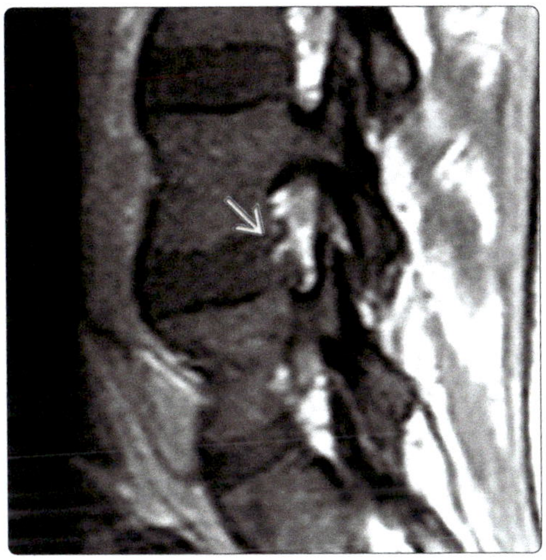

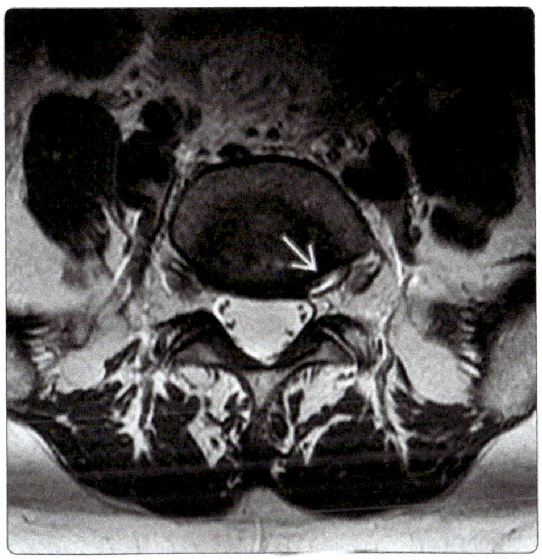

(Left) *Sagittal T1 C+ MR shows an anular fissure as focal enhancement within the posterolateral anulus fibrosus. There is no disc herniation, and the foramen is normal in size. The term anular tear is to be avoided.* **(Right)** *Axial T2WI shows an anular fissure along the posterior lateral margin of the disc, defined as linear hyperintensity without focal contour abnormality.*

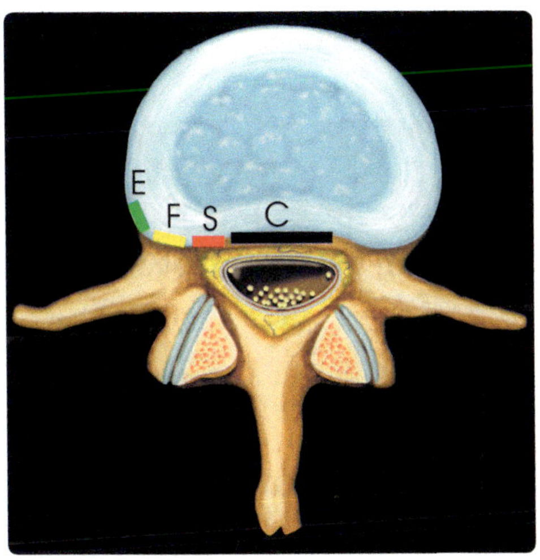

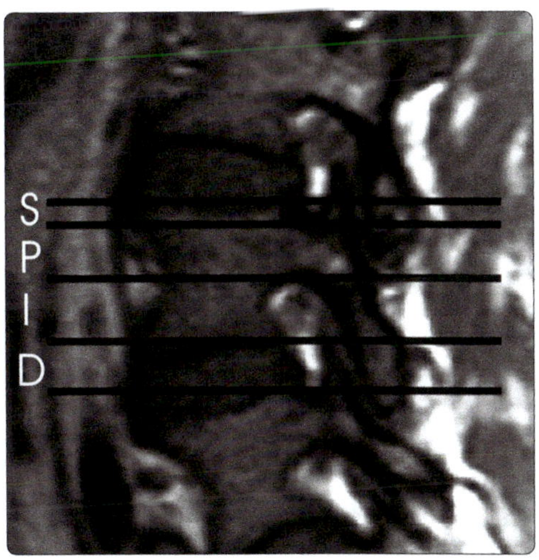

(Left) *Axial graphic of a lumbar intervertebral disc shows right-left location nomenclature classification for disc disease: C (central), S (subarticular), F (foraminal), and E (extraforaminal or far-lateral).* **(Right)** *Sagittal T1W1 MR through the neural foramen of the lumbar spine shows the level classification and nomenclature. The space between the 2 lines is classified as: S (suprapedicular), P (pedicular), I (infrapedicular), and D (disc).*

Degenerative Disc Disease

KEY FACTS

TERMINOLOGY

- Generalized and multifactorial process affecting discovertebral unit leading to biomechanical/morphologic alterations

IMAGING

- Loss of disc space height, vacuum phenomenon seen as low signal within disc
- Degenerative endplate changes I → III
  - Type I: Replacement with fibrovascular marrow
  - Type II: Replacement by fatty marrow
  - Type III: Bony sclerosis with little residual marrow
- T2 shows loss of signal from nucleus, loss of horizontal nuclear cleft
- Disc may show linear enhancement with degenerative disc disease, enhancement within Schmorl nodes

TOP DIFFERENTIAL DIAGNOSES

- Disc space infection
- Hemodialysis spondyloarthropathy
- Seronegative spondyloarthropathy

PATHOLOGY

- Etiology of disc degeneration multifactorial
- Individuals involved in manual materials handling, with repeated heavy lifting, at increased risk
- Some studies show strong familial predisposition to discogenic back pain

CLINICAL ISSUES

- Asymptomatic or associated with back/neck pain ± radiculopathy
- Lifetime incidence of back pain (all causes) in United States 50-80%
- Prevalence among adults ranges from 15-30%
- Back pain most common cause of disability in persons younger than 45 years
- Of patients complaining of chronic pain (> 3 months), 1/3 have disabling symptoms

(Left) *Sagittal graphic shows degeneration of L4-5 and L5-S1 intervertebral discs with loss of disc height, associated type II fatty endplate change, and osteophyte formation.* **(Right)** *Sagittal NECT reformat shows multilevel severe loss of disc height and vacuum phenomenon, which appears as black pockets of gas in the disc. Endplate eburnation (sclerosis) is most obvious at L3-4. Osteophytes are present at several levels.*

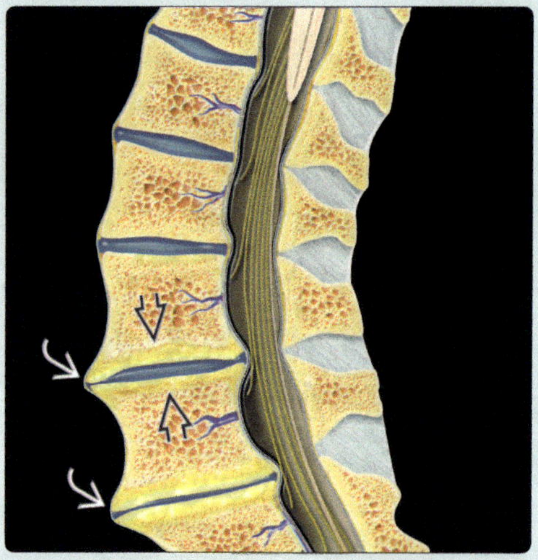

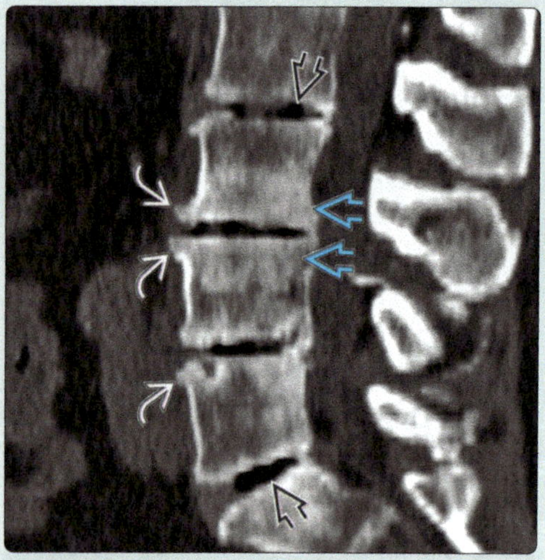

(Left) *Sagittal T2WI MR shows degenerated disc as low signal at L4-5, L5-S1 compared to normal disc signal intensity at L3-4. Degenerative disc disease is also seen as loss of disc height at L4-5, disc herniation at L5-S1, and anular tear at L4-5.* **(Right)** *Axial T2WI MR shows protrusion compressing the exiting root. Degenerated disc shows low signal centrally with disrupted internal disc contents pointing toward the herniation.*

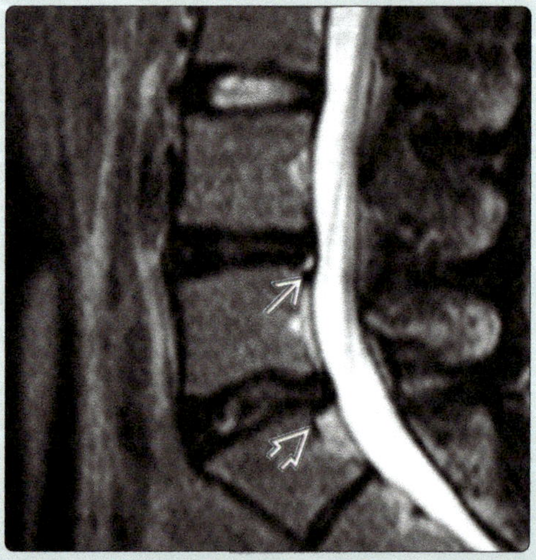

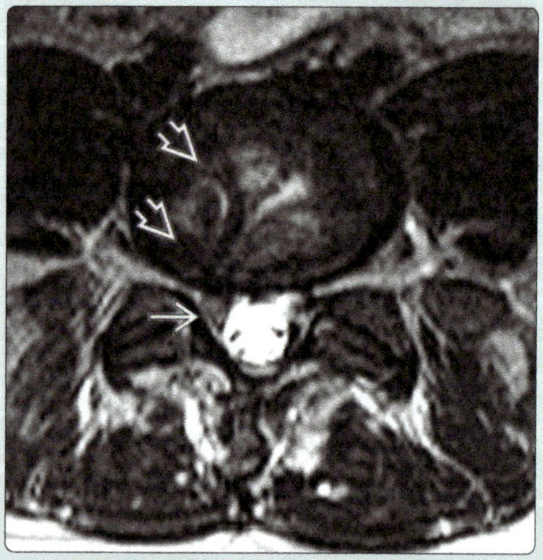

KEY FACTS

TERMINOLOGY

- Anular bulge
- Generalized extension of disc beyond edges of vertebral ring apophyses

IMAGING

- Circumferential disc "expansion" beyond confines of vertebral endplates
  - Short radius of extension: ≤ 3 mm
  - > 25% of disc circumference
  - If morphologic abnormality is < 25% of disc circumference, then it is herniation and not bulge
- Smooth ventral extradural defect in contrast column, with indentation on anterior thecal sac
  - Central canal and subarticular recesses usually not compromised unless associated with ligamentous hypertrophy
- T1WI and T2WI MR with sagittal and axial planes
- Discography may help identify symptomatic disc

TOP DIFFERENTIAL DIAGNOSES

- Disc protrusion (< 25% of disc circumference)
- Ossification of posterior longitudinal ligament
  - Most common in cervical spine (70%)
- Vertebral endplate bony spur
  - Continuous with vertebral endplate

PATHOLOGY

- Bulge less important as separate entity but associated with disc degeneration and anular fissures → "discogenic" pain

CLINICAL ISSUES

- Low back pain
- Up to 39% of asymptomatic adults have bulging discs
- > 80-90% success rate with conservative treatment

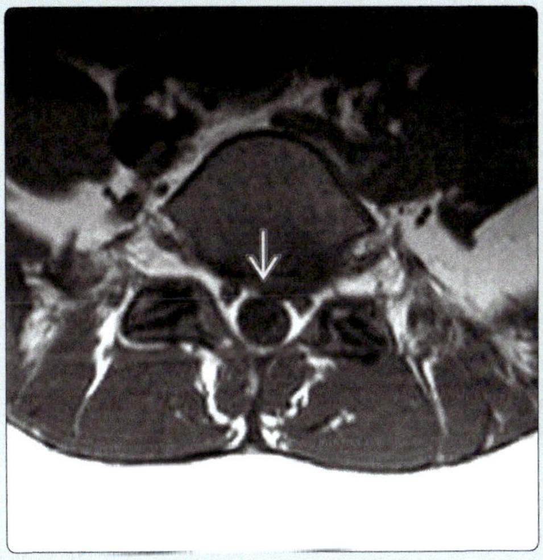

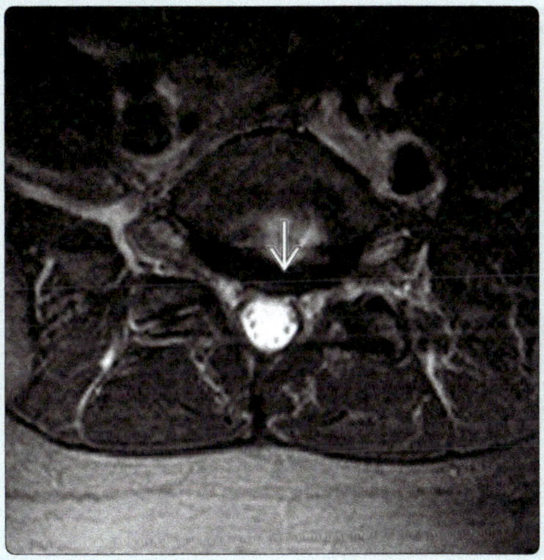

(Left) *Axial T1WI MR shows the typical pattern of a lumbar broad-based vertebral disc bulge ➡ at L5-S1. The disc extension beyond the vertebral body margin is diffuse, with no focal protrusion.* **(Right)** *Axial T2WI FS MR in the same patient demonstrates the broad-based appearance of the bulging disc ➡ with predominately low signal intensity. Associated anular fissure would show focal high signal.*

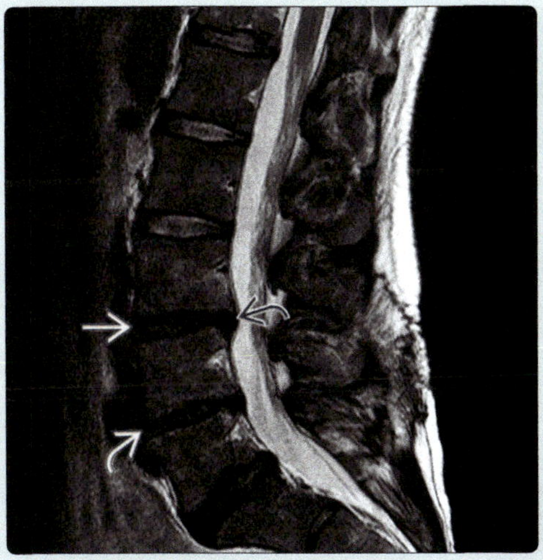

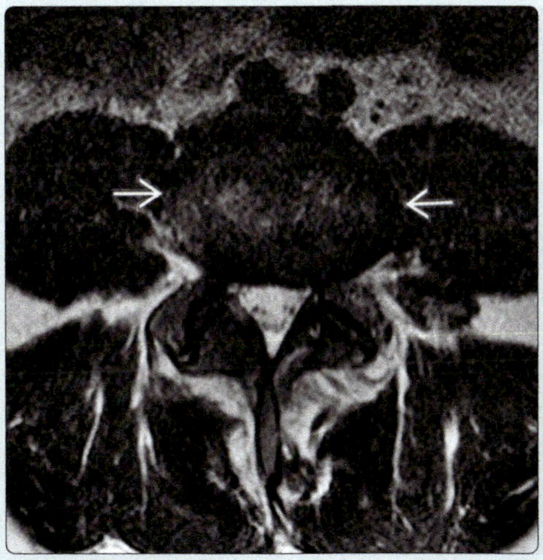

(Left) *Sagittal T2WI in a 39-year-old man with low back pain shows desiccation, loss of height of both L3-4 ➡ and 4-5 ➡. Note indentation on the anterior aspect of the thecal sac at L3-4 ⇨ caused by mild diffuse disc bulge at this level.* **(Right)** *Axial T2WI through the L3-4 disc in the same case shows mild circumferential bulging of the disc ➡, seen here as smoothly rounded contour without any focal protrusion of disc material.*

KEY FACTS

TERMINOLOGY

- Protruded disc, extruded disc, free fragment, sequestered disc
- Localized (< 50% of disc circumference) displacement of disc material beyond edges of vertebral ring apophyses

IMAGING

- Small mass in ventral spinal canal, contiguous with intervertebral disc
- Protrusion is herniated disc with broad base at parent disc
- Extrusion is herniated disc with narrow or no base at parent disc
- Sequestered or free fragment: Extruded disc without contiguity to parent disc
- Migrated: Disc material displaced away from site of herniation, regardless of continuity to parent disc

TOP DIFFERENTIAL DIAGNOSES

- Ossification posterior longitudinal ligament
- Osteophyte
- Tumor
- Hemorrhage
- Abscess

CLINICAL ISSUES

- 10% of people under age 40 have cervical herniation
- Acute radiculopathy usually self-limited disorder with full recovery expected
  - Neck pain (90%)
  - Radicular pain (65%)
  - Paresthesia (89%)
- Treatment
  - Conservative treatment
  - Multiple surgical approaches without clear consensus

DIAGNOSTIC CHECKLIST

- Use fast STIR for cord disease
- Axial GRE, T2* GRE for disc definition

(Left) *Sagittal graphic shows disc extrusion ➡, with the base of the herniation smaller than the epidural component, effacing the thecal sac and causing cord compression.* **(Right)** *Sagittal T2WI MR shows C5-C6 disc extrusion with the base of herniation smaller than the component extending into the epidural space.*

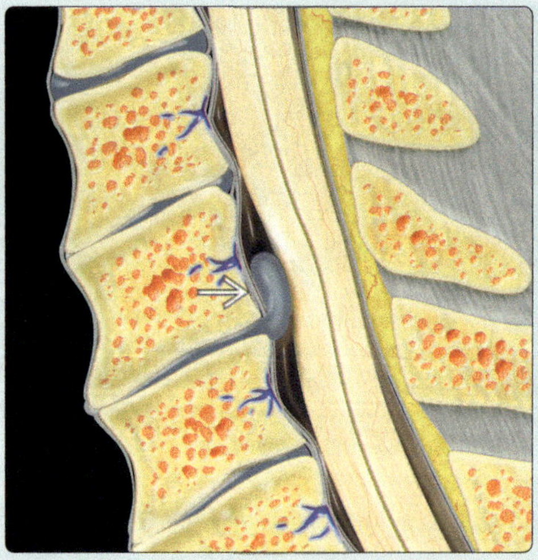

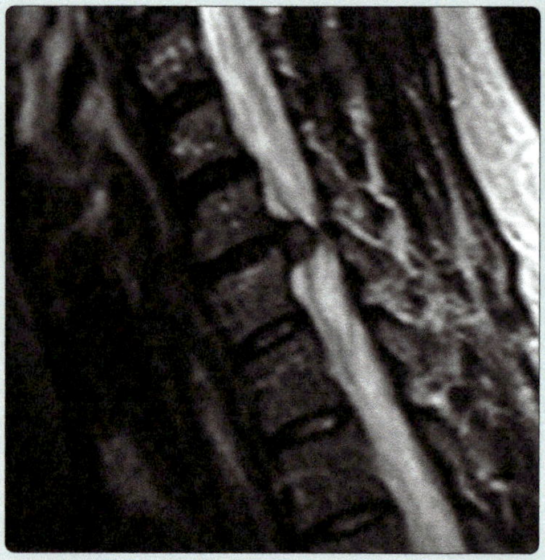

(Left) *Sagittal T1WI C+ MR shows C4-5 extrusion ➡ impinging on the cord. Smaller C5-C6 protrusion also compresses the ventral cord ➡. Peripheral enhancement ➡ is related to epidural plexus and granulation tissue.* **(Right)** *Axial T2* GRE MR shows left-sided extrusion ➡ effacing the left side of the thecal sac and extending toward the left neural foramen ➡. Note the compression of the spinal cord ➡.*

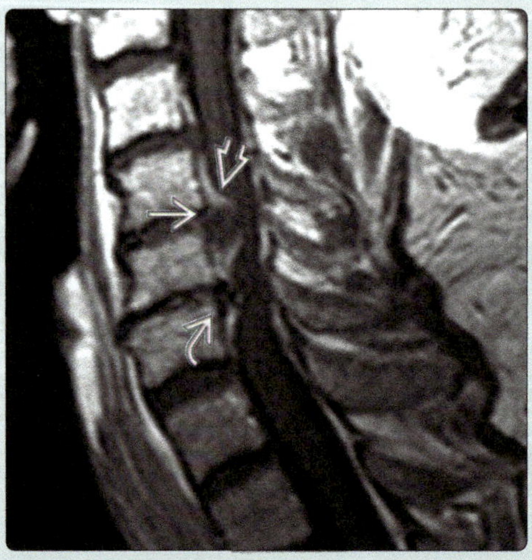

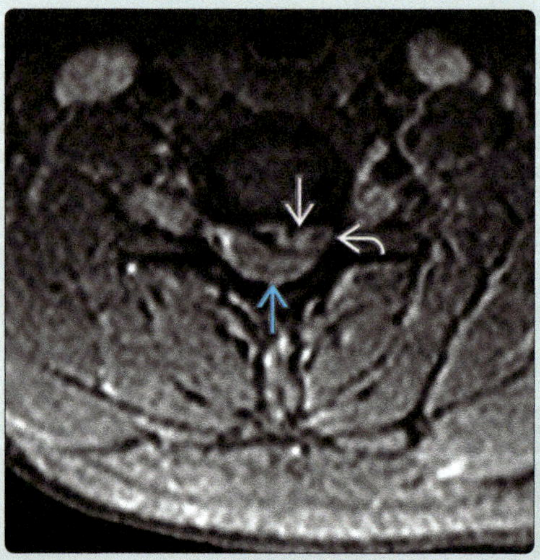

KEY FACTS

IMAGING

- Small mass in spinal canal contiguous with intervertebral disc
  - Ventral epidural
  - Rare in upper thoracic spine (T1-T3)
- May enhance peripherally after intravenous contrast material due to granulation tissue or dilated epidural plexus
  - Peripheral enhancement may give "lifted band" or "tent" configuration

TOP DIFFERENTIAL DIAGNOSES

- Osteophyte
  - Sharp margins not arising directly from intervertebral disc level
- Tumor
  - Homogeneous enhancement
- Hemorrhage
  - Elongated within epidural space, tends to be posterior
- Abscess
  - May mimic large herniation with peripheral enhancement

CLINICAL ISSUES

- 5th decade
- Uncommon entity
- Thoracic disc surgery uncommon, represents 1-2% of all disc surgery
- History of Scheuermann disease (kyphosis secondary to multiple Schmorl nodes → vertebral body wedging)

DIAGNOSTIC CHECKLIST

- Calcification (65%)
- Multiple herniation (14%)
- T2WI critical because herniation may not be visible on T1WI due to calcification
- **Check and recheck herniation level, counting from C2 and L5 levels**

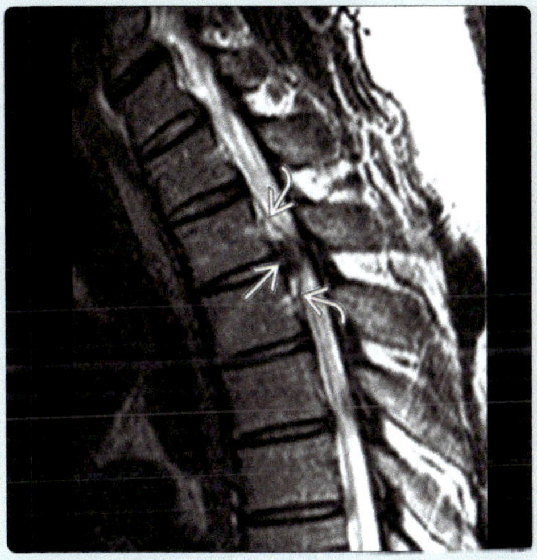

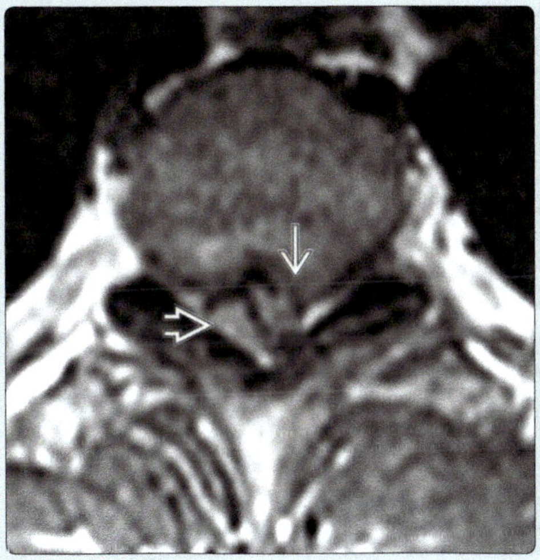

(Left) *Sagittal T2WI MR shows a large low signal disc extrusion at T2-T3 effacing the thecal sac and tenting the ventral dura.* **(Right)** *Axial T1WI MR demonstrates the large left-sided extrusion severely compressing the left side of the cord.*

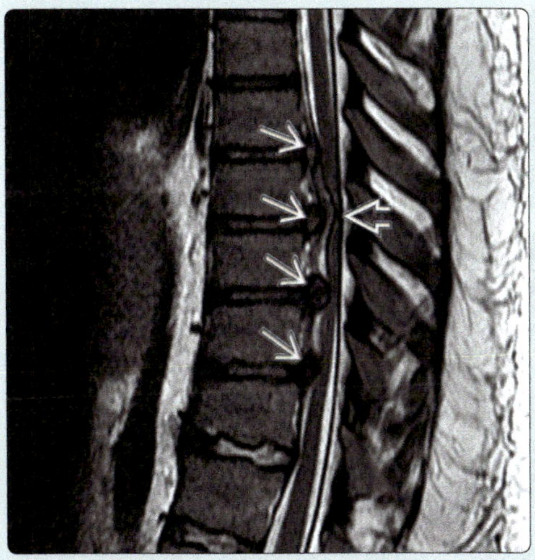

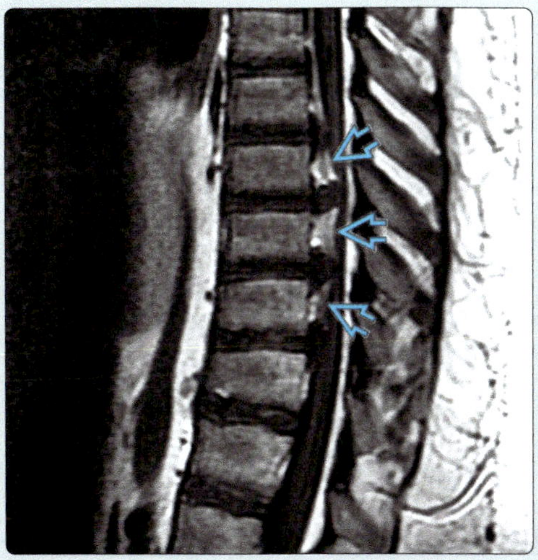

(Left) *Sagittal T2WI MR shows multiple large, lower thoracic disc herniations, which severely compress the cord at multiple levels. Thoracic herniations are most common from T7-T12.* **(Right)** *Sagittal T1WI C+ MR in the same patient shows pronounced peripheral enhancement surrounding the herniations related to tented and distended epidural plexus and herniation-associated granulation tissue.*

Lumbar Intervertebral Disc Herniation

KEY FACTS

TERMINOLOGY

- Localized (< 25% of disc circumference) displacement of disc material beyond confines of disc space
- Protrusion
  - Herniated disc with broad base at parent disc
- Extrusion
  - Herniated disc with narrow or no base at parent disc
- Sequestered: Free fragment

IMAGING

- Anterior extradural mass contiguous with disc space extending into spinal canal
- Axial: Central, subarticular (lateral recess), foraminal, or extraforaminal (far lateral)
- Sagittal: Disc level, infrapedicle, pedicle, suprapedicle

TOP DIFFERENTIAL DIAGNOSES

- Peridural/epidural fibrosis
- Epidural metastasis
- Nerve sheath tumor

CLINICAL ISSUES

- Low back pain
- Radiculopathy
  - Most common: Posterolateral radiating pain down lower extremity
    - Can be anterior (e.g., anterior thigh pain if foraminal/far lateral L3-4 herniation)
    - Positive straight-leg raising test (Lasègue sign)
  - Cauda equina syndrome
    - Saddle anesthesia, bowel/bladder dysfunction, etc.
    - Occasionally caused by massive disc herniation
- Back pain ± radiculopathy usually resolves in 6-8 weeks
- Treatment options
  - Conservative
  - Minimally invasive techniques (many variations)
  - Standard open techniques, such as laminotomy/discectomy

(Left) *Graphic of large recurrent disc herniation shows displacement of the nuclear material ➡ through a large defect in the posterior annular fibers ➡, with effacement of the ventral thecal sac and displacement of the intrathecal nerve roots.* **(Right)** *Sagittal T1 MR shows a very large disc extrusion at L5-S1 level ➡ with superior migration of a large component to L4-L5 level ➡. The thecal sac is nearly completely effaced by the large herniation.*

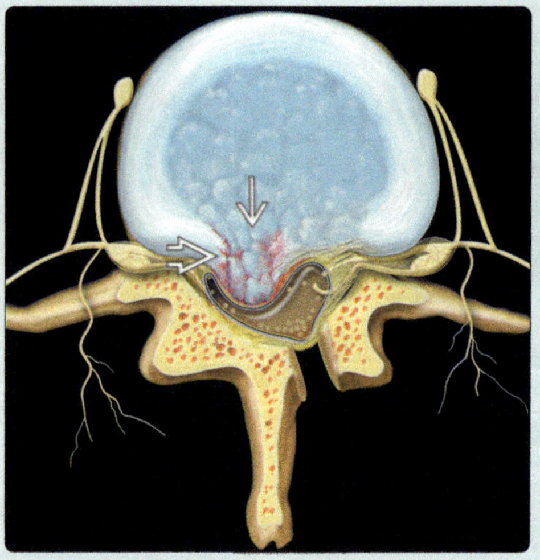

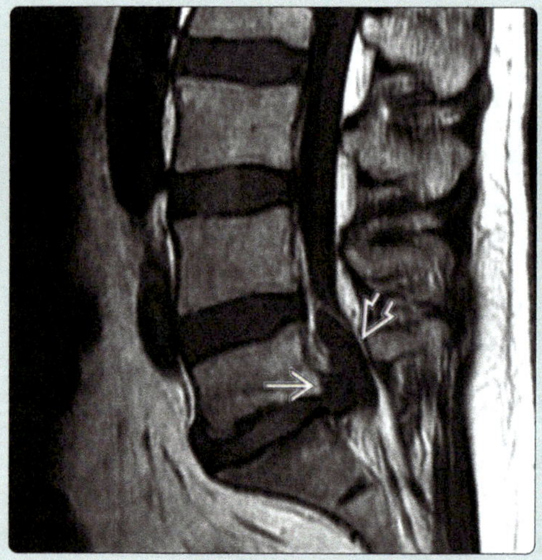

(Left) *Sagittal T2 TSE shows a large extrusion of the intervertebral disc at the L5-S1 level with a sequestered component (free fragment) ➡ that is migrated superiorly.* **(Right)** *Axial T2WI MR shows a large central and left extrusion of the intervertebral disc ➡ with severe effacement of the thecal sac ➡. The herniation extends into the left neural foramen ➡.*

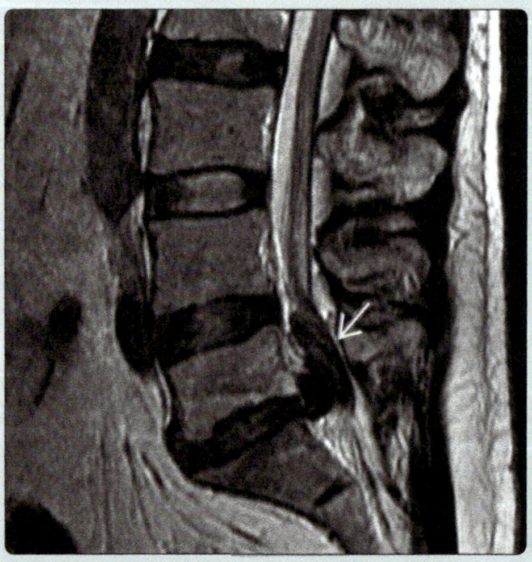

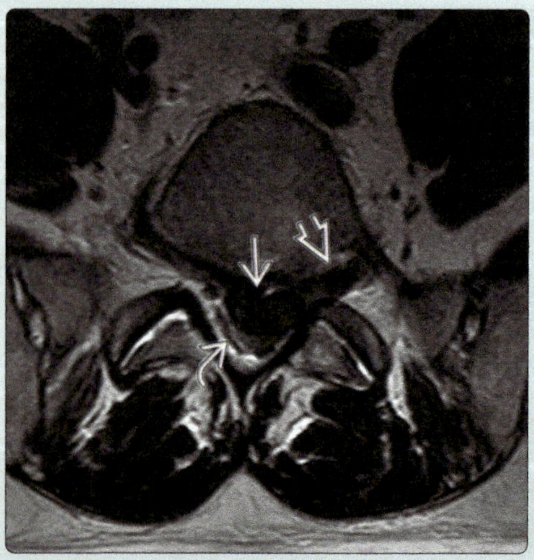

KEY FACTS

TERMINOLOGY

- Extruded disc material within neural foramen
- Far lateral is disc material lateral to neural foramen

IMAGING

- Obliterated perineural fat in neural foramen on sagittal images
- Soft tissue mass contiguous with parent disc
- T1WI isointense to parent disc
- T2WI iso-, hypo-, or hyperintense to parent disc
- May enhance peripherally
- Often missed on myelography

TOP DIFFERENTIAL DIAGNOSES

- Schwannoma
- Spinal nerve root diverticulum
- Large facet osteophyte

CLINICAL ISSUES

- 5-10% of all disc herniations
- Severe radicular pain
  - Mass effect on exiting nerve root in narrow confines of neural foramen
  - More symptomatic compared with central disc herniations
  - Lumbar: 25% sciatic and 75% femoral distribution
- Lateral bending, sitting, and increased intraabdominal pressure worsen pain
- Pain relieved by rest with hip and knee in flexion
- May stabilize or resolve spontaneously
- Surgery
  - Failed conservative therapy after 6-8 weeks; progressive deficits
  - Interlaminal approach with partial medial facetectomy
  - Endoscopic lateral approaches more commonly used, but no change in outcome relative to open procedures

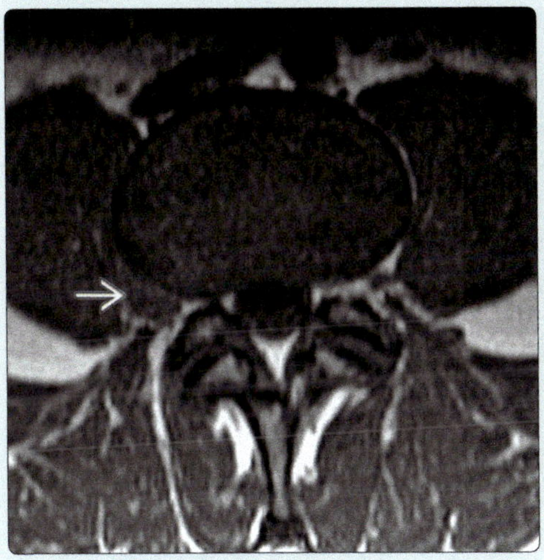

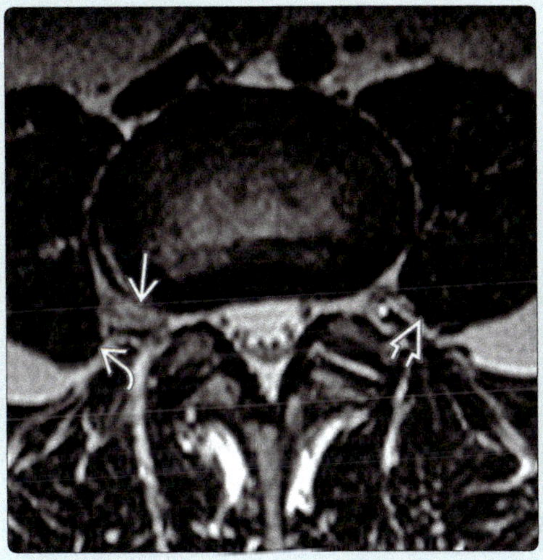

(Left) *Axial T1WI MR shows large right lateral and intraforaminal disc herniation ➡ at L4-L5. The disc herniation involves the lateral aspect of the neural foramen.* **(Right)** *Axial T2WI MR in the same patient shows that the large right lateral and intraforaminal disc herniation ➡ is almost isointense in signal to the adjacent paravertebral soft tissue. There is slight lateral displacement of the psoas muscle ➡ (compared with the opposite side ➡).*

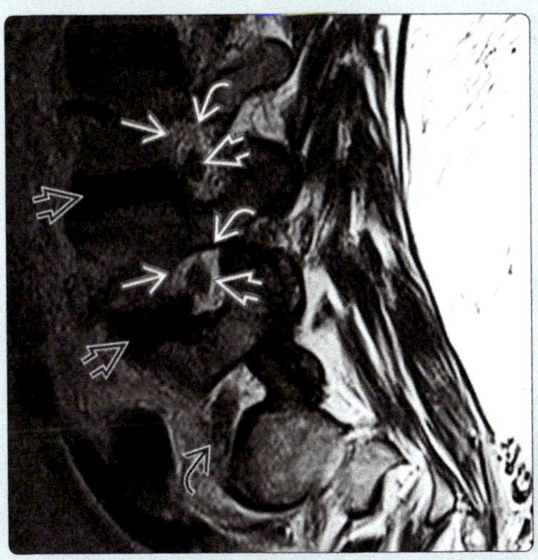

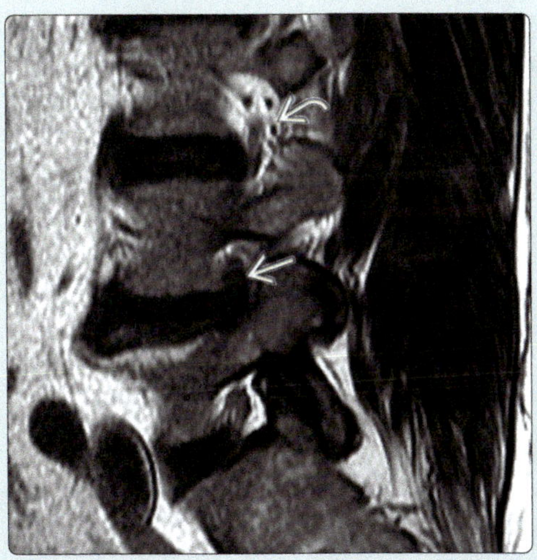

(Left) *Sagittal T2WI through a normal lower lumbosacral spine shows the "keyhole-shaped" neural foramina ➡ at L3-4 and L4-5. Bright fat ➡ surrounds the dorsal root ganglia (DRG) ➡ and fills the neural foramina. Note that the exiting DRGs lie slightly above the level of the intervertebral discs ➡. The L5 nerve root ➡ is seen exiting the L5-S1 neural foramen.* **(Right)** *Sagittal T2WI shows an L4-5 foraminal/far lateral disc herniation ➡ filling the neural foramen. Contrast with the normal "keyhole-shaped" L3-4 neural foramen above ➡.*

KEY FACTS

TERMINOLOGY

- Facet arthrosis, degenerative facet disease, degenerative joint disease

IMAGING

- Osseous facet overgrowth impinging on neural foramina in conjunction with articular joint space narrowing
- Facet joint osteophytes producing foraminal narrowing
- Mushroom-cap facet appearance
- Joint space narrowing with sclerosis and bone eburnation
- Intraarticular gas ("vacuum phenomenon")
- Enhancing inflammatory soft tissue changes surrounding facet joint are common
- Joint space narrowing, thinning of articular cartilage
- Facet effusions as linear hyperintensity

TOP DIFFERENTIAL DIAGNOSES

- Septic facet
- Healing facet fracture
- Inflammatory arthritides
- Paget disease
- Myositis ossificans
- Metastasis

CLINICAL ISSUES

- Mechanical neck pain (facet arthrosis syndrome)
  - Related to irritation of innervation of joint from medial branch(es) of dorsal primary ramus
  - Capsular distension, inflammatory synovitis, entrapment of synovial villi between 2 articular processes, or nerve impingement by osteophytes
- Pain aggravated by rest and alleviated by gentle movement
  - Worse in morning
- Poor correlation between duration/severity of pain and extent of facet degeneration

DIAGNOSTIC CHECKLIST

- Best detail with thin-section CT

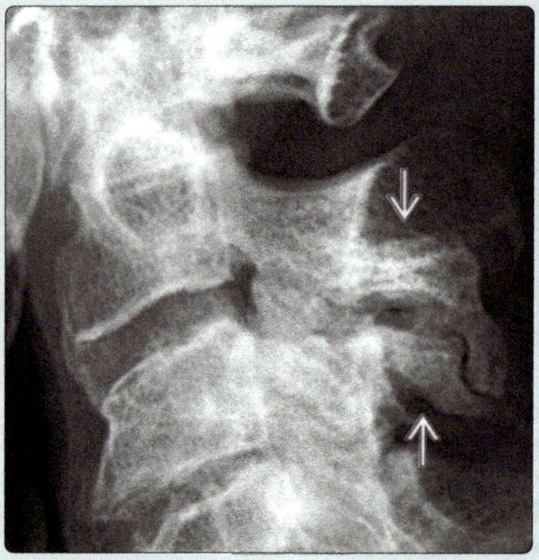

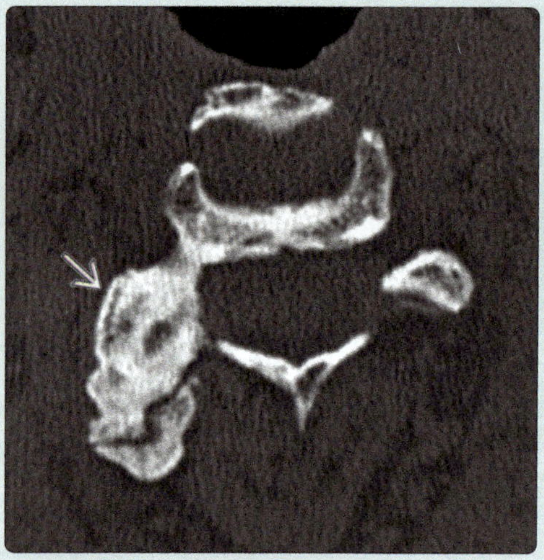

(Left) *Lateral radiograph shows severe facet hypertrophic degenerative arthropathy at C2-C3* ➡ *with marked hypertrophy of the facets.* **(Right)** *Axial NECT shows severe, exuberant right facet degenerative arthropathy* ➡. *This has been described as a mushroom-cap appearance.*

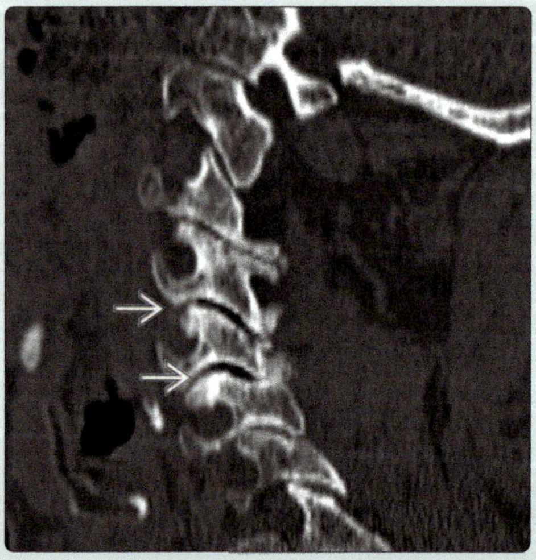

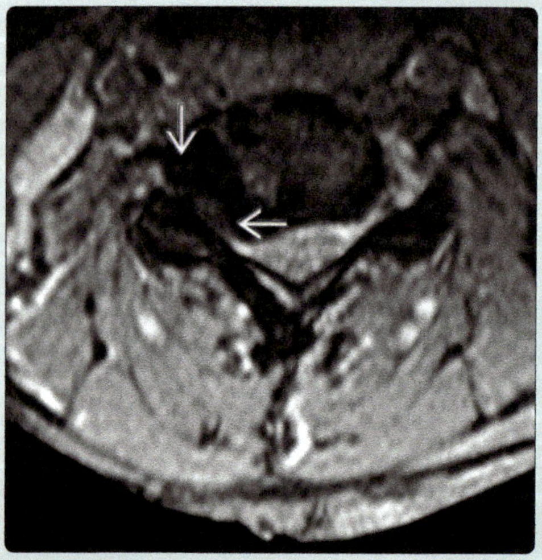

(Left) *Sagittal NECT shows multilevel hypertrophic facet degenerative arthropathy with "vacuum phenomenon"* ➡, *bony eburnation, and osteophyte formation.* **(Right)** *Axial T2* GRE MR shows severe right uncovertebral hypertrophic degenerative arthropathy with severe foraminal stenosis* ➡ *with facet degenerative change.*

KEY FACTS

TERMINOLOGY

- Facet arthrosis, degenerative facet disease, degenerative joint disease, facet hypertrophy
- Osteoarthritis of synovially lined lumbar apophyseal joints

IMAGING

- Osseous overgrowth impinging on foramina in conjunction with articular joint space narrowing
  - Mushroom cap facet appearance
  - Joint space narrowing with sclerosis/bone eburnation, ligamentum flavum hypertrophy
  - Intraarticular gas, effusion
  - Spondylolisthesis not uncommon
- CT more sensitive than plain films for detecting presence and degree of arthrosis
  - Facet hypertrophic degenerative arthropathy, particularly superior articular facet extending into lumbar foramen
- MR best demonstrates degenerative facet compression of thecal sac and fat-filled neural foramina
  - Enhancing inflammatory soft tissue changes surrounding facet joint not uncommon
- Consider CT myelography if MR contraindications or MR does not demonstrate facet relationship to neural foramina

TOP DIFFERENTIAL DIAGNOSES

- Septic facet
- Inflammatory arthritides
- Paget disease
- Tumor
  - Metastasis
  - Lymphoma

DIAGNOSTIC CHECKLIST

- Look for associated **synovial cysts**

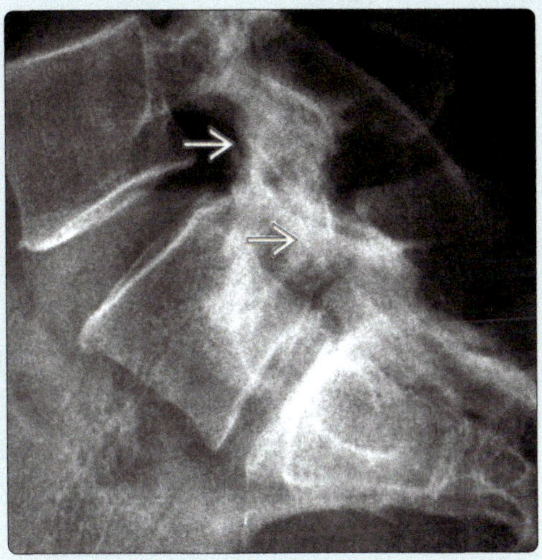
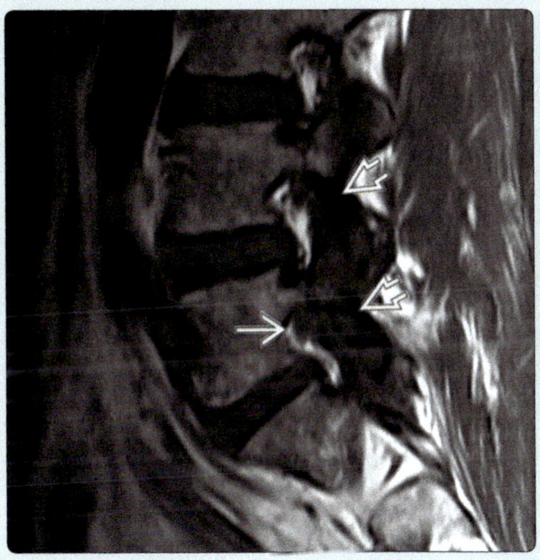

(Left) *Lateral radiograph shows facet hypertrophy and bony eburnation of the L4-L5 and L5-S1 facets.* **(Right)** *Sagittal T1WI MR shows L4-L5, L5-S1 facet degenerative arthropathy with bony hypertrophy and low signal involving the facets from bony sclerosis. There is narrowing of the L5-S1 foramen primarily by the hypertrophied superior articular facet of S1.*

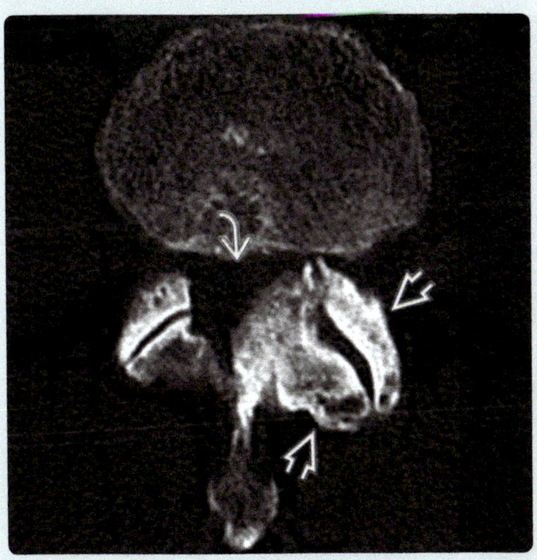
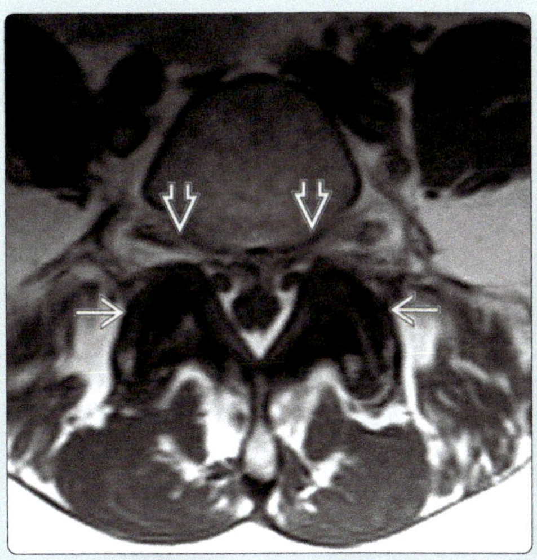

(Left) *Axial bone CT shows severe left unilateral facet overgrowth, causing moderately severe central stenosis. The facet overgrowth has been described as having a mushroom cap appearance.* **(Right)** *Axial T1WI MR shows marked facet hypertrophic degenerative arthropathy with enlarged facets, producing moderately severe foraminal stenosis.*

KEY FACTS

TERMINOLOGY

- Definition: Node within vertebral body due to vertical disc extension (intravertebral disc herniation) through vertebral endplate
    - Any level, although thoracic, thoracolumbar > cervical

IMAGING

- Focal invagination of endplate by disc material surrounded by sclerotic (old) or edematous (acute) bone
- Plain films
    - Contour defect within endplate, extending from disc space into vertebral body spongiosa with well-corticated margins
- CT
    - Island of low density surrounded by condensed bone on axial slice through vertebral body
- MR
    - Focal defect in endplate filled by disc ± adjacent marrow edema, fatty marrow conversion

TOP DIFFERENTIAL DIAGNOSES

- Acute compression fracture
- Degenerative endplate change
- Discitis
    - Both endplates show defect
- Limbus vertebrae
    - Seen at vertebral body corners
- Bone island (sclerotic nodule)
- Focal metastasis
    - No contiguity with parent disc
- Scheuermann disease
    - Thoracic, with anterior wedging

CLINICAL ISSUES

- Seen in up to 75% of all normal spines
- Conservative management

DIAGNOSTIC CHECKLIST

- Schmorl node is always contiguous with parent disc

(Left) *Sagittal CT shows multiple Schmorl nodes (SN) of varying size ➡. There is variable sclerosis adjacent to nodes. Wedging at T12 ➡ is a normal anatomic variant often seen at T11-L1. It is distinguished from compression fracture by normal contour and equal involvement of both endplates.* **(Right)** *Lateral fluoroscopy image (different patient) during discography reveals a superior endplate SN ➡. Contrast injected into the contiguous intervertebral disc fills the herniated disc within the vertebral SN defect.*

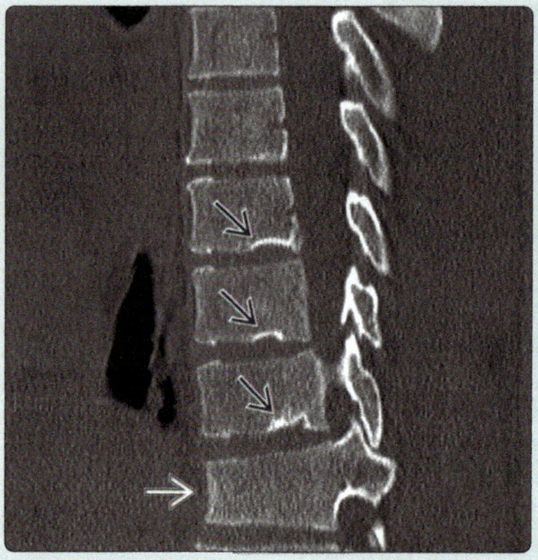

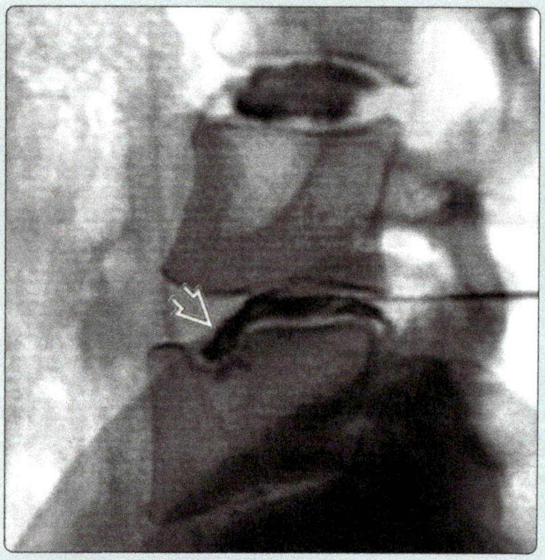

(Left) *Sagittal T2WI MR demonstrates the typical pattern of fatty marrow ➡ outlining chronic endplate herniation (SN) ➡.* **(Right)** *Axial T2WI MR (same patient) shows a well-defined focus of low signal ➡ in the superior S1 endplate representing an SN. There is a thin concentric rind of fatty marrow conversion ➡ surrounding the SN.*

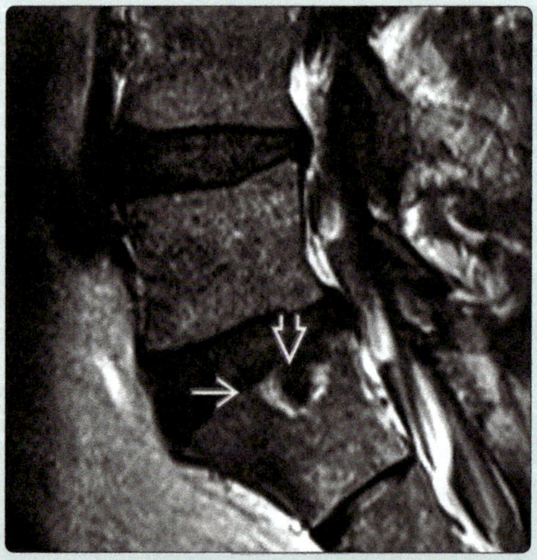

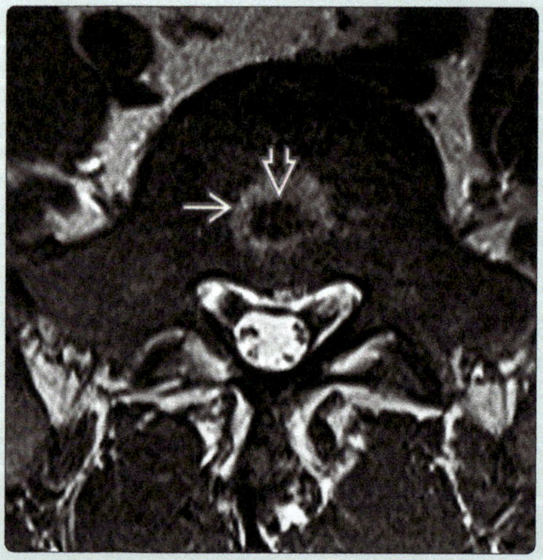

KEY FACTS

TERMINOLOGY

- Juvenile kyphosis, Scheuermann kyphosis
- Kyphosis secondary to multiple Schmorl nodes → vertebral body wedging

IMAGING

- Wedged-shaped **thoracic** vertebrae with irregular endplates
  - ≥ 3 contiguous vertebrae, each showing ≥ 5° of kyphosis
  - Undulation of endplates secondary to extensive disc invaginations
  - Disc spaces narrowed, with greatest narrowing anteriorly
  - Well-defined Schmorl nodes often present

TOP DIFFERENTIAL DIAGNOSES

- Postural kyphosis
- Wedge compression fractures
- Congenital kyphosis
- Tuberculosis
- Osteogenesis imperfecta
- Neuromuscular disease (clinical)

PATHOLOGY

- Disc extrusions through weakened regions of vertebral endplates
- Weightlifting, gymnastics, and other spine-loading sports may contribute

CLINICAL ISSUES

- Thoracic spine pain worsened by activity
- Kyphosis develops in adolescence, may present later in life
- Peak incidence: 13-17 years
- Initial treatment includes observation, bracing
- Surgical treatment for > 75° kyphosis in skeletally immature person

DIAGNOSTIC CHECKLIST

- Schmorl nodes without anterior wedging are not indicative of Scheuermann disease

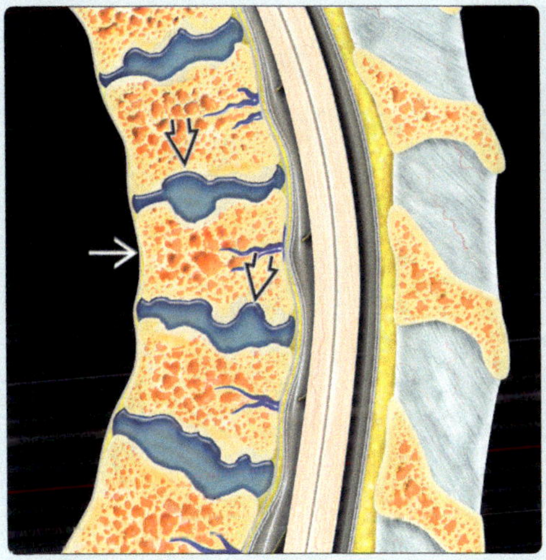

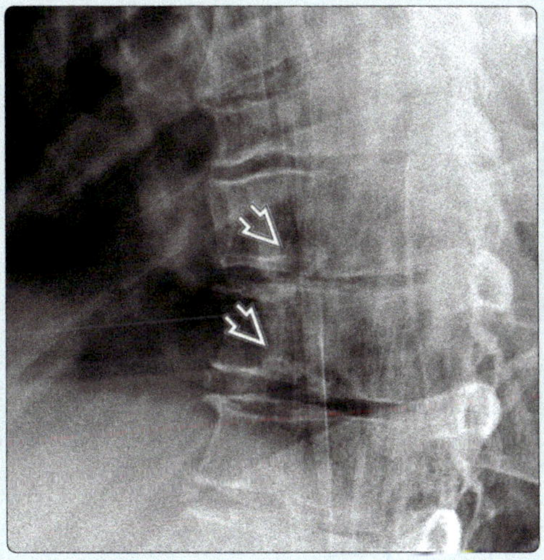

(Left) *Sagittal graphic demonstrates anterior vertebral wedging ➡ and herniation of disc material through the vertebral endplates ⇨, creating focal subcortical bone defects in conjunction with thoracic kyphotic deformity. Undulation of endplates reflects sequelae of the osseous reparative process.* **(Right)** *Lateral radiography reveals anterior wedging deformity and undulation of vertebral endplates with multiple Schmorl nodes at each level ⇨.*

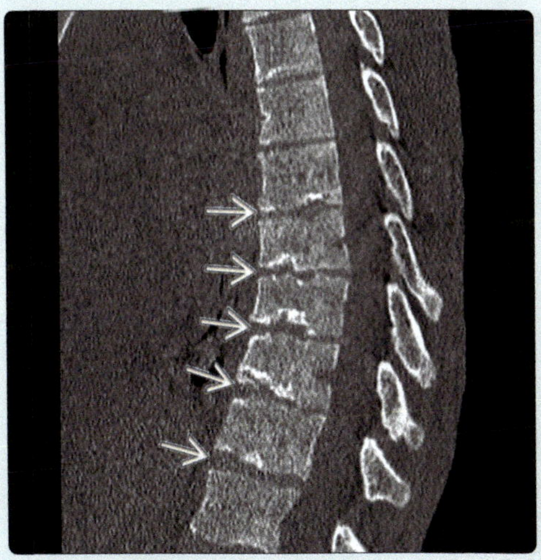

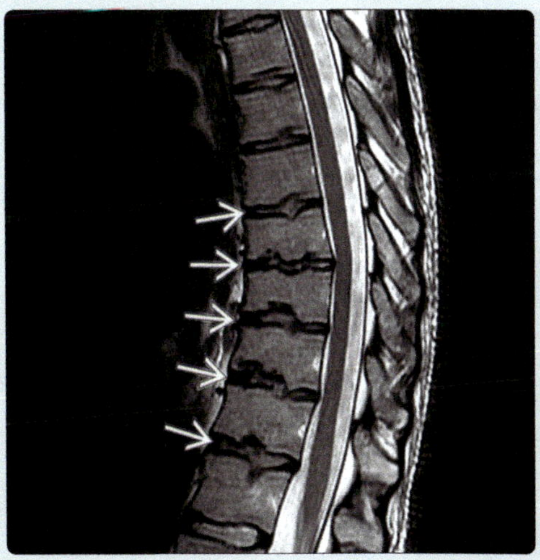

(Left) *Sagittal bone CT shows loss of anterior vertebral height and endplate irregularity involving multiple thoracic discs ➡. There are multiple (> 3) contiguous levels of endplate irregularities (Schmorl node) and increased thoracic kyphosis.* **(Right)** *Sagittal T2WI MR (same patient) confirms loss of disc height and signal intensity at multiple thoracic levels ➡. The thoracic spinal cord is normal, and there are no associated thoracic disc herniations into the spinal canal.*

Acquired Lumbar Central Stenosis

KEY FACTS

TERMINOLOGY

- Spinal canal narrowing in lumbar spine
  - Secondary to multifactorial degenerative changes, being progressive and dynamic process

IMAGING

- Trefoil appearance of lumbar spinal canal on axial imaging
- Sagittal diameter of bony lumbar canal < 10 mm

TOP DIFFERENTIAL DIAGNOSES

- Disc herniation
- Metastatic disease
- Paget disease
- Epidural hemorrhage

CLINICAL ISSUES

- Chronic low back pain
- Neurogenic claudication
  - Leg pain (80%)
  - Bilateral lower extremity pain, paresthesia, and weakness
  - Relief of pain by squatting or sitting (flexion) in 80%
- Bladder dysfunction and sexual difficulty (10%)
- Radicular pain (10%)
- Rare but important presentation: Legs suddenly "giving out"
- Operative treatment includes surgical decompression or X-Stop interspinous implant-like devices
- Natural history: Majority of symptomatic patients stable over months to years (40-70%)
  - 1/3 improve with nonoperative treatment
  - 1/3 deteriorate

DIAGNOSTIC CHECKLIST

- Axial T2WI mandatory for stenosis identification

(Left) *Axial T2WI MR demonstrates severe central canal stenosis with marked facet degenerative arthropathy. The thecal sac has assumed a trefoil appearance.* **(Right)** *Axial T1WI MR in another case shows central canal stenosis primarily related to facet and ligamentous hypertrophy/thickening with little ventral epidural disease.*

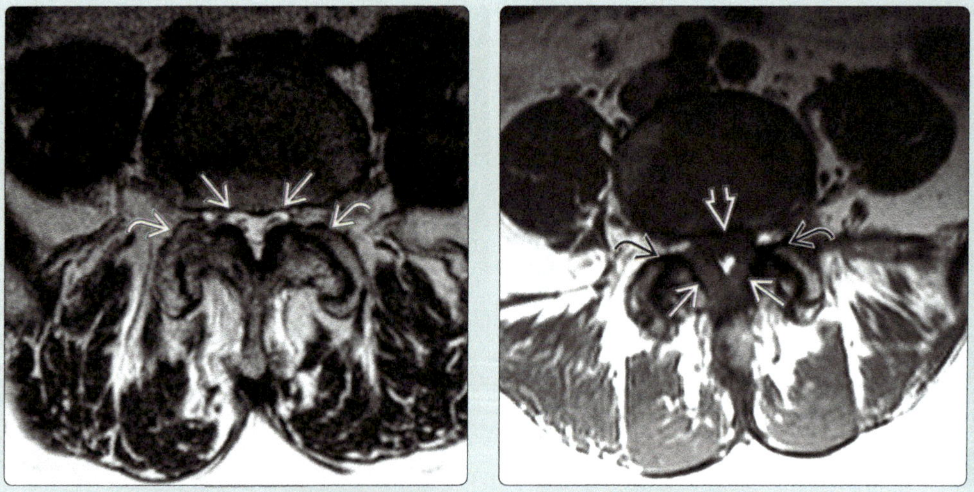

(Left) *Sagittal T2WI MR shows severe central stenosis at L4-L5 due to marked posterior ligamentum flavum thickening. Hyperintensity within the interspinous ligament denotes degeneration, which is also called Baastrup disease or interspinous bursitis.* **(Right)** *Sagittal T2WI MR shows canal stenosis at L3-L4 with a bulging disc and ligamentous thickening. Note serpentine areas of low signal within the cephalad thecal sac due to redundant nerve roots.*

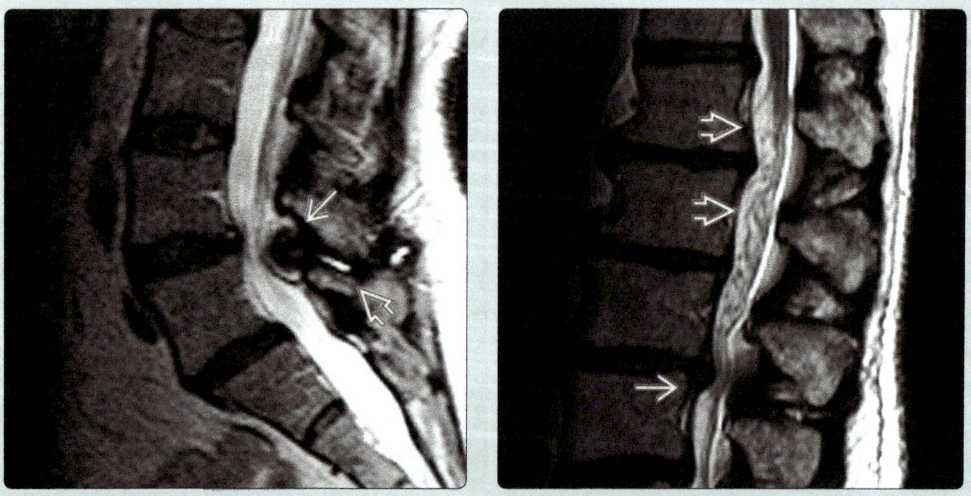

Congenital Spinal Stenosis

KEY FACTS

TERMINOLOGY

- Reduced AP canal diameter secondary to short, squat pedicles and laterally directed laminae

IMAGING

- Central canal diameter is smaller than normal
  - Cervical spine: Absolute AP diameter < 14 mm
  - Spinal stenosis present if AP canal diameter at L1 < 20 mm, L2 < 19 mm, L3 < 19 mm, L4 < 17 mm, L5 < 16 mm, S1 < 16 mm
    - Lumbar spine: Critical stenosis at L4 < 14 mm, L5 < 14 mm, S1 < 12 mm
- Short, thick pedicles
- Trefoil-shaped lateral recesses
- Laterally directed laminae

TOP DIFFERENTIAL DIAGNOSES

- Acquired spinal stenosis
- Inherited spinal stenosis
  - Achondroplasia
  - Mucopolysaccharidoses

PATHOLOGY

- Torg ratio (AP canal diameter/AP vertebral body diameter) < 0.8
- Idiopathic

CLINICAL ISSUES

- Symptomatic cervical or lumbar stenosis symptoms at younger age than typical of degenerative stenosis
  - These patients typically lack complicating medical problems (diabetes or vascular insufficiency)
- Athletes present with temporary neurological deficit following physical contact that subsequently resolves
- Lumbar: Decompressive laminectomy, posterior foraminotomy at involved levels
- Cervical: Posterior cervical laminectomy or laminoplasty

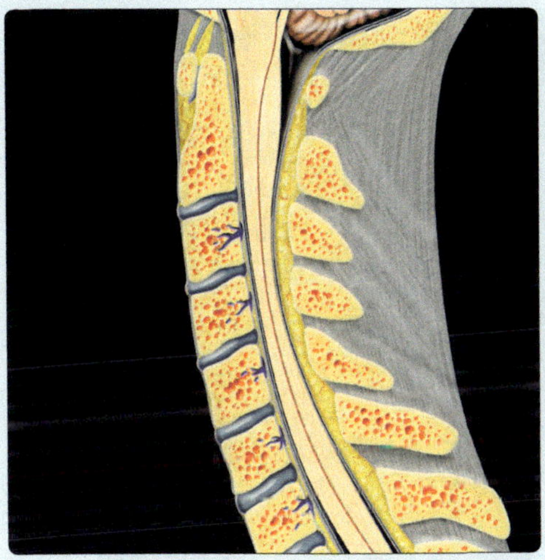
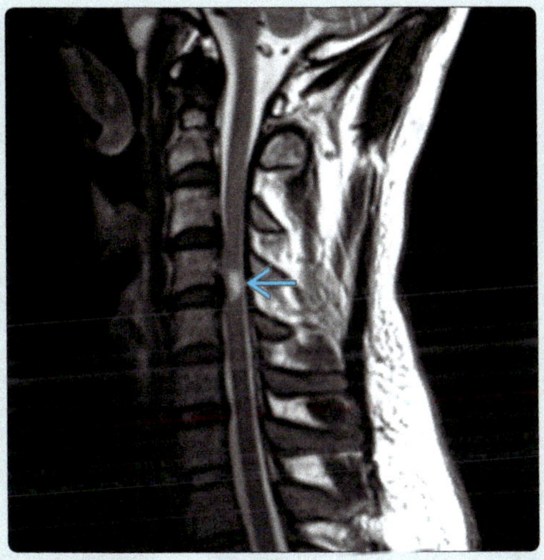

(Left) *Sagittal graphic shows marked congenital anteroposterior narrowing of the central spinal canal.* **(Right)** *Sagittal T2WI MR reveals moderate congenital AP canal narrowing exacerbated by C4-C5 disc herniation. The protrusion produces spinal cord T2 hyperintensity → corresponding to clinical myelopathy.*

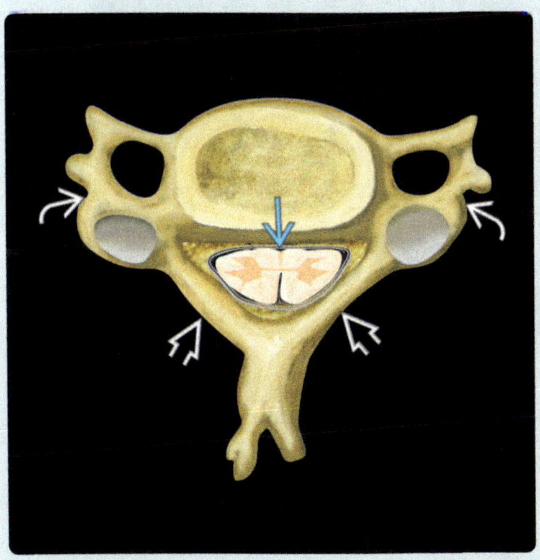
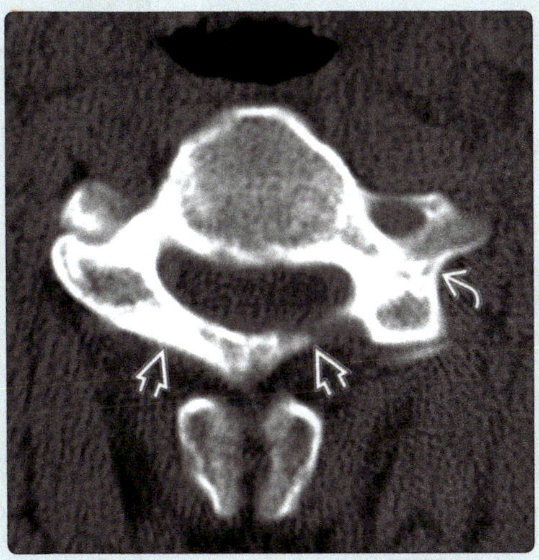

(Left) *Axial graphic depicts congenital cervical AP spinal narrowing with generalized narrowing of the subarachnoid space. The pedicles ➡ are short, thick, and laterally directed with resultant flattening of laminae ➡ and compression of the spinal cord →.* **(Right)** *Axial bone CT demonstrates marked AP canal reduction attributable to developmentally short pedicles ➡ and laterally oriented laminae ➡.*

KEY FACTS

TERMINOLOGY

- Spinal canal and neural foraminal narrowing in cervical spine secondary to multifactorial degenerative changes

IMAGING

- Cervical spine, ventral epidural, centered at disc levels
- Sagittal diameter of cervical canal < 13 mm
- Disc osteophyte complex protruding into canal and compressing thecal sac and cord
- Completely effaced subarachnoid space at disc levels in cervical spine → "washboard spine"
- Variable degrees of cord compression

TOP DIFFERENTIAL DIAGNOSES

- Ossification of posterior longitudinal ligament
- DDx of abnormal cord signal
  - Cord tumor
  - Syrinx
  - Multiple sclerosis
  - Motor neuron disease

PATHOLOGY

- Multilevel disc degeneration with decreased disc hydration and fissures
- Disc herniation, bulge with associated broad osteophytes
- Uncovertebral joint osteoarthritic change with foraminal stenosis

CLINICAL ISSUES

- Acquired spinal stenosis (cervical) has no pathognomic symptoms or signs
  - Can exhibit both central AND peripheral findings
- Spastic paraparesis commonly seen
- Upper extremity numbness, weakness ("myelopathic hand")
- Natural history of insidious onset, periods of static disability, and episodic worsening

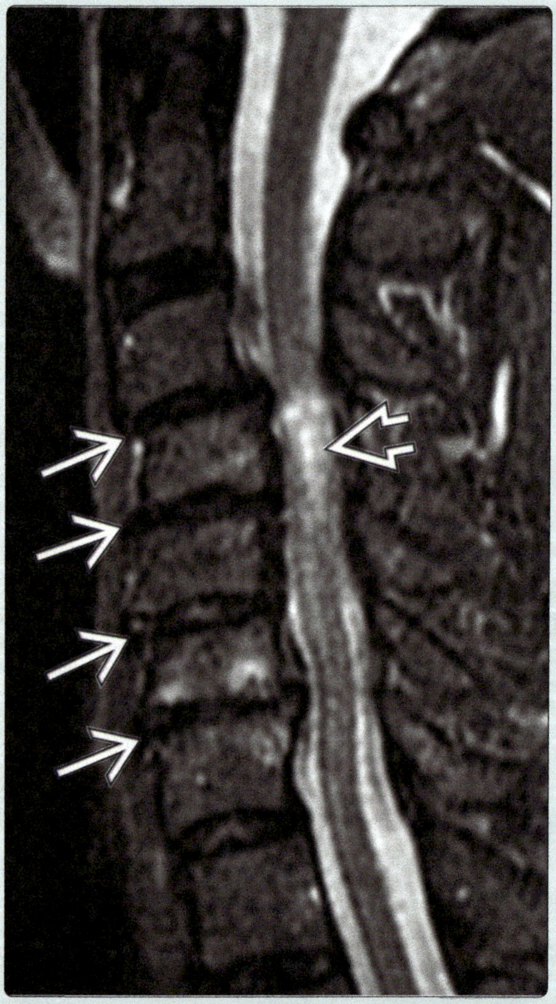

Sagittal T2WI MR shows multilevel degenerative disc disease and disc osteophyte complexes with canal stenosis spanning C3-C4 through C6-C7. T2 hyperintensity present within the cord centered at C3-C4 reflects myelomalacia.

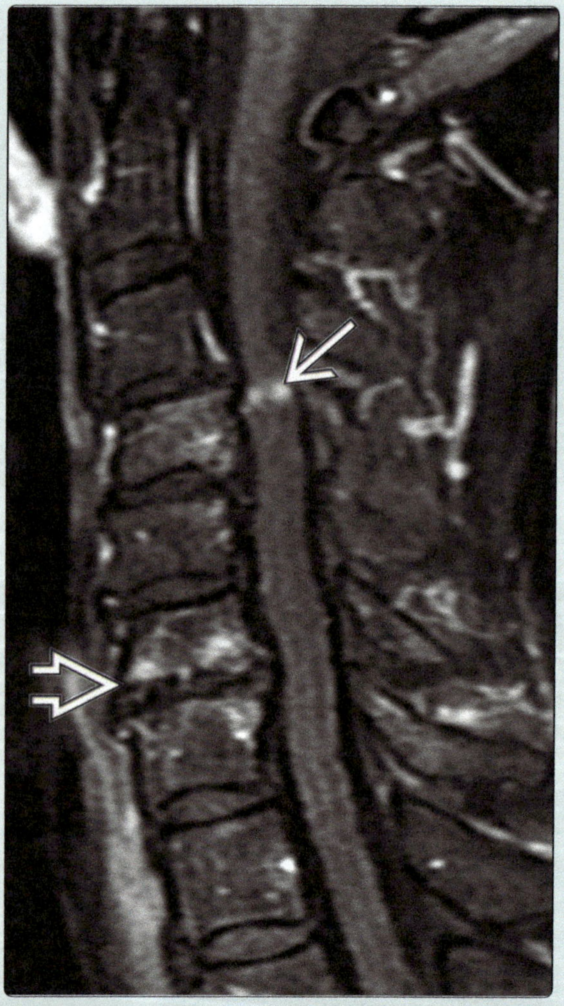

Sagittal T1WI C+ FS MR in the same case shows horizontal linear enhancement within the cervical cord at C3-C4 due to chronic myelomalacia. There is also enhancement of type I degenerative endplate changes at C6-C7.

Diffuse Idiopathic Skeletal Hyperostosis (DISH)

KEY FACTS

TERMINOLOGY

- Diffuse idiopathic skeletal hyperostosis (DISH)
- Forestier disease, senile ankylosing hyperostosis, asymmetrical skeletal hyperostosis

IMAGING

- Flowing anterior vertebral ossification with minimal degenerative disc disease, facet arthropathy, absent facet ankylosis
- Thoracic spine (100%) > cervical (65-80%), lumbar spine (68-90%); R > L
- Lateral radiography inexpensive, reliable
- Reserve MR to evaluate for coexistent OPLL or spondylosis-related cord compression

TOP DIFFERENTIAL DIAGNOSES

- Spondylosis
- Ankylosing spondylitis
- Psoriatic or reactive (Reiter) arthritis

PATHOLOGY

- Exact cause for exaggerated new bone formation stimuli unknown
  - Exuberant entheseal reaction at tendon, ligament, and joint capsule insertions
  - Associated with OPLL
  - Dysphagia related to DISH multifactorial
- Primary diagnostic criteria for DISH
  - Flowing anterior ossification extending over at least 4 contiguous vertebral bodies
  - No apophyseal or SI joint ankylosis
  - Mild degenerative disc changes, no facet ankylosis

CLINICAL ISSUES

- Majority of cases incidental
- Osteophyte resection if severe symptoms
- Increased risk of extension-type fractures with high morbidity

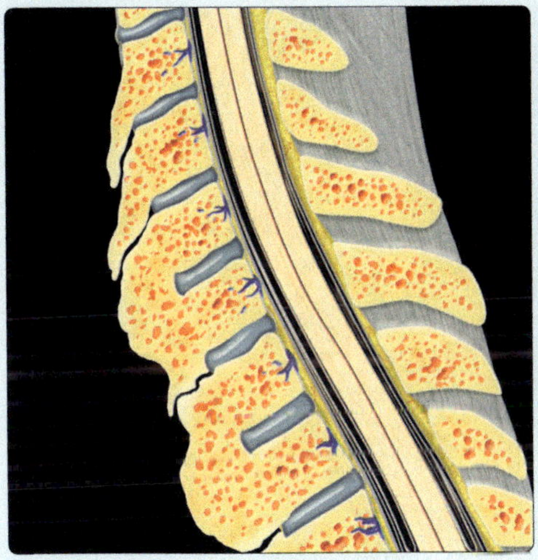

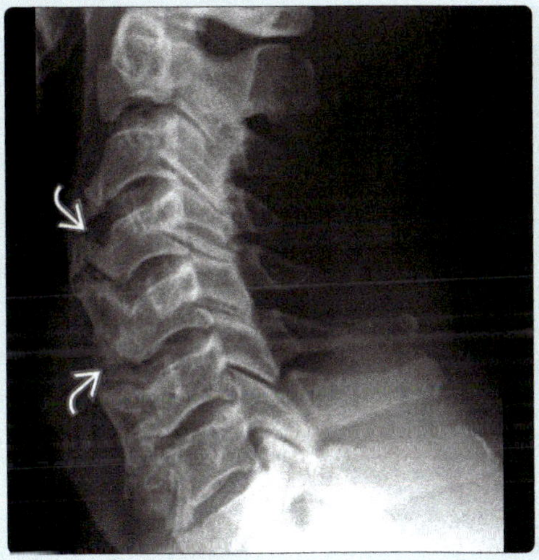

(Left) *Sagittal graphic shows bulky flowing ossification of the anterior longitudinal ligament extending over > 4 contiguous vertebra. Disc spaces are relatively preserved.* **(Right)** *Lateral radiograph shows a large anterior ossified mass ➡ that is discontinuous at several disc spaces, a variation implying some degree of continued cervical spine mobility.*

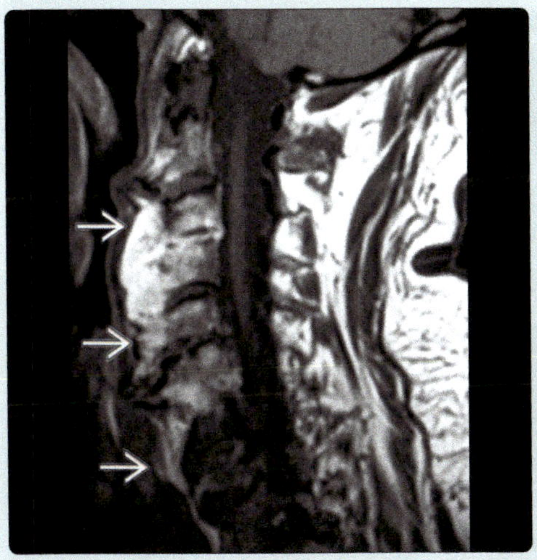

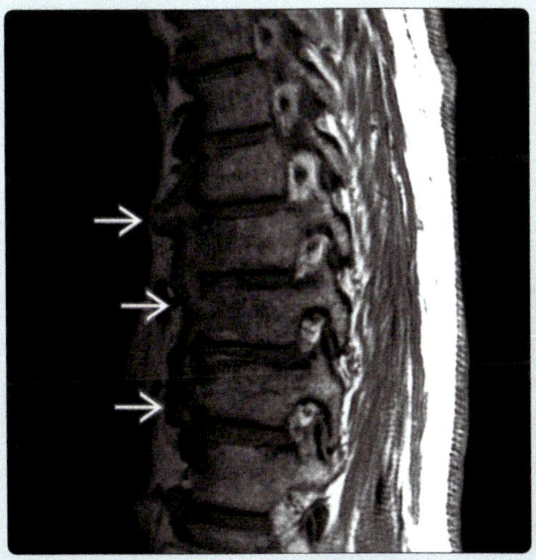

(Left) *Sagittal T1WI MR shows bulky anterior flowing ossification ➡ consistent with DISH. Fatty marrow is responsible for high T1 signal intensity within the anterior ossification.* **(Right)** *Sagittal T1WI MR right parasagittal slice shows bulky flowing ALL ossification ➡ spanning more than 4 vertebral levels but minimal disc abnormality that is typical of DISH.*

Ossification of Posterior Longitudinal Ligament (OPLL)

KEY FACTS

TERMINOLOGY

- Ossification of posterior longitudinal ligament (OPLL)

IMAGING

- Flowing multilevel ossification posterior to vertebral bodies
  - Relatively minimal degenerative disc disease, absent facet ankylosis
  - Midcervical (C3-C5) > midthoracic (T4-T7)
  - PLL ossification narrows AP spinal canal dimension → spinal stenosis, cord compression
- Characteristic "upside-down T" or "bowtie" PLL configuration on axial images
  - CT with sagittal reformats to confirm MR diagnosis, clarify extent of ossification for surgical planning
  - Sagittal T1WI, T2WI to evaluate spinal cord compression, extent of ligamentous ossification

TOP DIFFERENTIAL DIAGNOSES

- Spondylosis
- Calcified herniated disc
- Meningioma

PATHOLOGY

- Variable extent
  - Continuous
    - Ossified mass over several vertebral segments
  - Segmental
    - Fragmented ossified lesions behind each vertebral body
  - Mixed
    - Combination of continuous and segmental
  - Focal
    - Ossification confined to disc level

CLINICAL ISSUES

- Spastic paresis → paralysis (17-22%)
- ↑ risk for developing progressive myelopathy if > 60% canal stenosis, ↑ cervical range of motion

(Left) *Sagittal graphic shows flowing multilevel ossification of the posterior longitudinal ligament (OPLL), producing canal narrowing and cord compression.* **(Right)** *Axial postmyelogram bone CT shows the classic "upside-down T" configuration of OPLL. This is causing mild compression of the contrast-filled thecal sac but does not deform the spinal cord.*

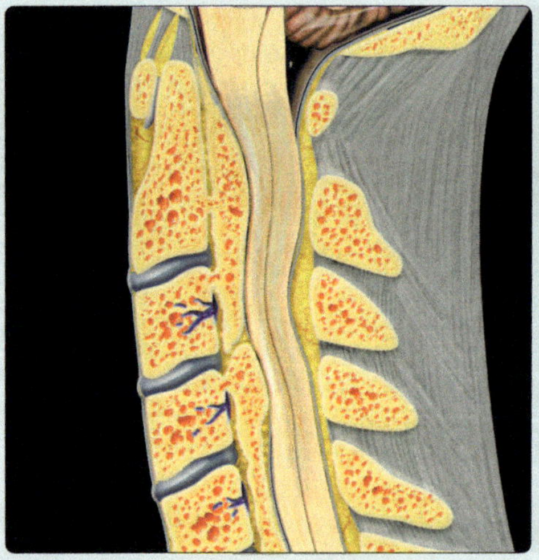

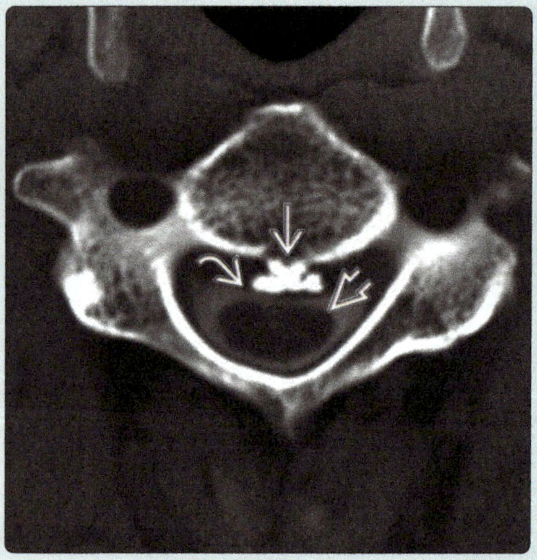

(Left) *Sagittal STIR MR shows the typical pattern of continuous-type OPLL seen as low signal ventral to the cord with severe cord compression. Note the associated diffuse idiopathic skeletal hyperostosis with multilevel fusion.* **(Right)** *Sagittal T1 C+ MR in the same case shows a slightly heterogeneous mass ventral to the cervical cord, with severe cord compression at the C4 level. OPLL may show low or heterogeneous increased signal on T1WI due to marrow content with fat elements.*

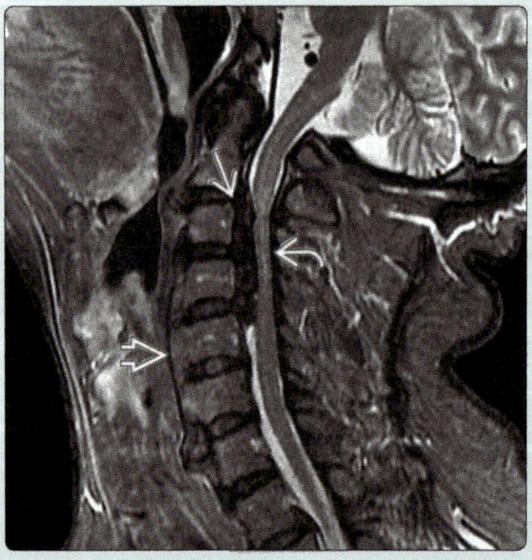

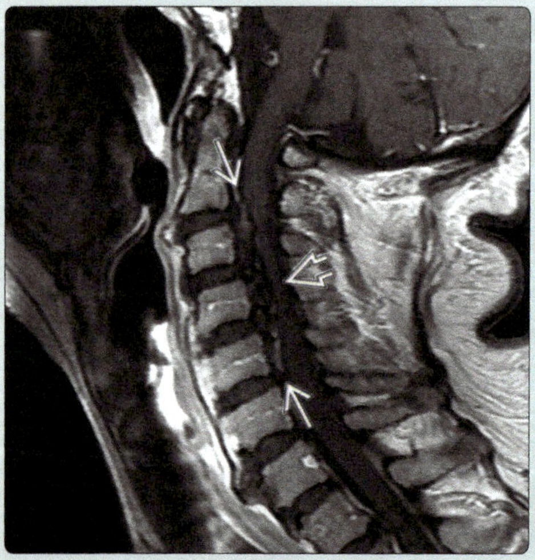

KEY FACTS

TERMINOLOGY

- Anterolisthesis: Anterior displacement of vertebral body relative to 1 below
- Retrolisthesis: Posterior displacement of vertebral body relative to 1 below

IMAGING

- Lateral flexion and extension to evaluate for instability
  - Napoleon's-hat sign on AP plain film
  - Instability uncommon in degenerative listhesis
    - 90% of normal volunteers show 1-3-mm translation on flexion-extension radiographs
- Spondylolysis may be difficult to identify on MR
  - T1-weighted sagittal images critical
  - CT for definitive diagnosis of subtle fracture

PATHOLOGY

- Degenerative spondylolisthesis (DS)
  - Degenerative retrolisthesis associated with disc degeneration
  - Sagittal oriented facets more likely to have DS
- Spondylolysis (isthmic)
  - Bilateral in 80%
- Postsurgical: Loss of posterior element stability
- Dysplastic: Small L5 body leading to pars lysis
- Trauma: Severe to produce vertebral body displacement
- Pathologic: Underlying tumor with instability

CLINICAL ISSUES

- **9.2% overall complication rate for treatment of spondylolisthesis**
  - Complications related to higher-grade spondylolisthesis, DS > isthmic, older age (> 65)
- DS + stenosis treated surgically show greater improvement in pain and function over 4 years compared with nonsurgical treatment

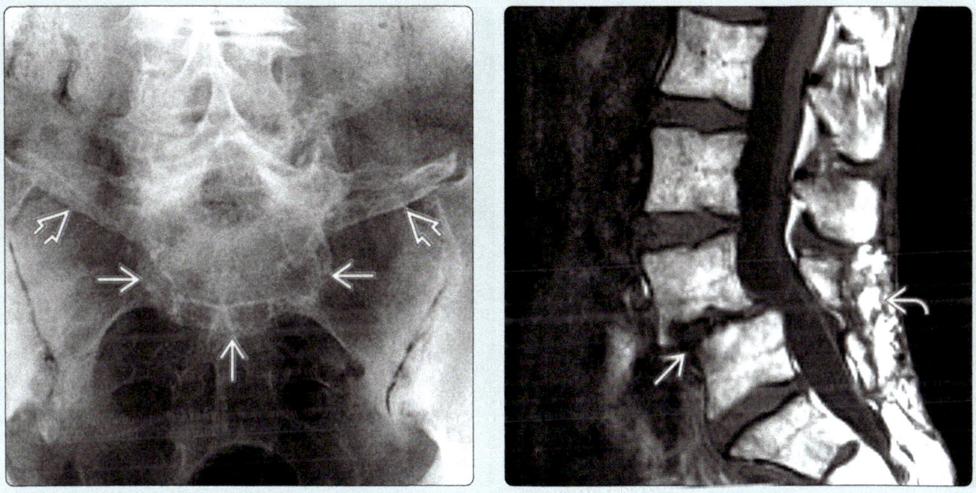

(Left) *Anteroposterior radiograph shows Napoleon's-hat sign. The hat is inverted, with the crown ➡ representing the anterior cortex of vertebral body and the brim ➡ representing the transverse processes.* **(Right)** *Sagittal T1WI MR shows postoperative spondylolisthesis following lumbar laminectomy ➡. There are advanced degenerative changes of the L4-L5 intervertebral disc space ➡ with anterior subluxation of L4 on L5.*

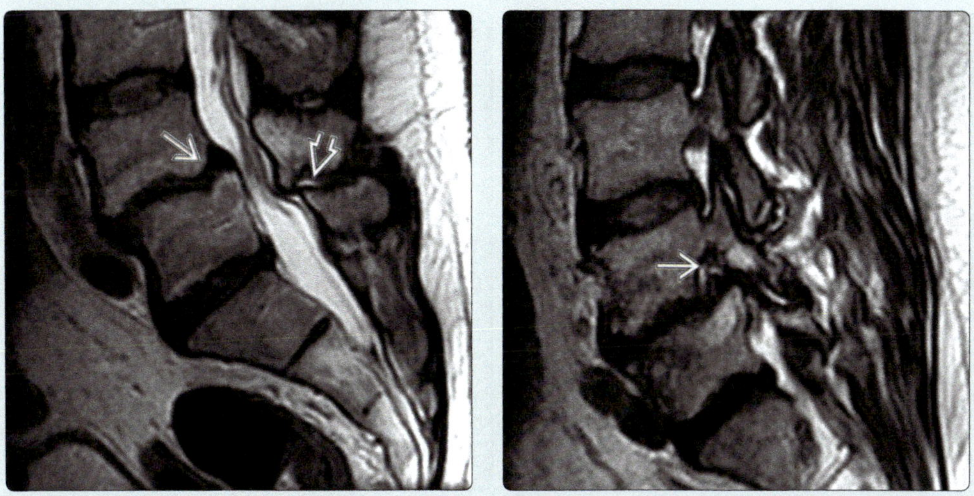

(Left) *Sagittal T2WI MR shows grade I spondylolisthesis of L4 on L5 ➡, with intervertebral disc degeneration and associated fatty endplate change. There is also degeneration of the interspinous ligament ➡.* **(Right)** *Sagittal T2WI MR shows a grade I spondylolisthesis of L4 on L5 with resultant severe foraminal stenosis ➡.*

KEY FACTS

TERMINOLOGY

- Defects in pars interarticularis (PI) thought to result from repetitive stress injury
  - Pars is junction of pedicle, lamina, and facet

IMAGING

- Most common at L5: 80-90%
- Discontinuity in neck of "Scotty dog" on oblique plain films
- Elongation of spinal canal at level of pars defects on axial imaging
- Incomplete-ring sign on axial imaging

TOP DIFFERENTIAL DIAGNOSES

- Acute traumatic fracture of posterior elements
- Facet arthropathy with marrow edema
- Septic facet with marrow edema
- Bone tumor with marrow edema
- Pedicle stress fracture
- Congenital defect with pars cleft

PATHOLOGY

- Repeated microfractures of PI lead to fatigue fracture

CLINICAL ISSUES

- 6-8% in general population
- 10-20 years old is typical age range
- Symptoms of chronic low back pain
- Conservative measures in grade 1-2 spondylolisthesis
- Wide variety of practice patterns for treatment
  - 50% of surgeons agreed on surgical treatment
  - No consensus on optimum surgical strategy

DIAGNOSTIC CHECKLIST

- Look for integrity of PI on sagittal MR and pars/pedicle marrow edema

(Left) *Lateral graphic shows chronic L5 spondylolisthesis ➡ and spondylolysis ➡ with defect in the pars interarticularis (PI) and resultant foraminal stenosis.* **(Right)** *Coronal oblique radiograph shows a thin lucency ➡ in the right L5 PI with adjacent bony sclerosis.*

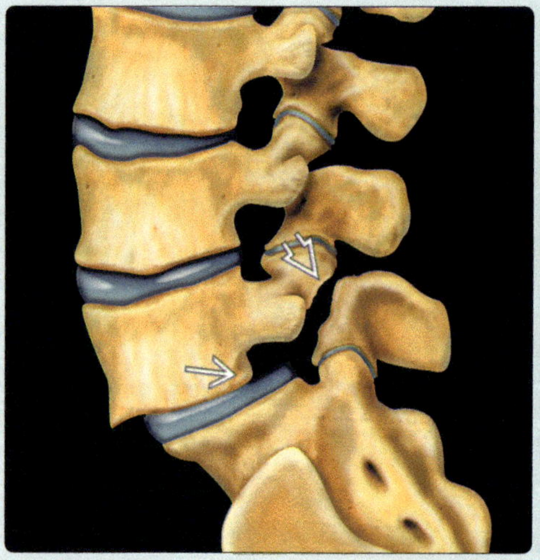

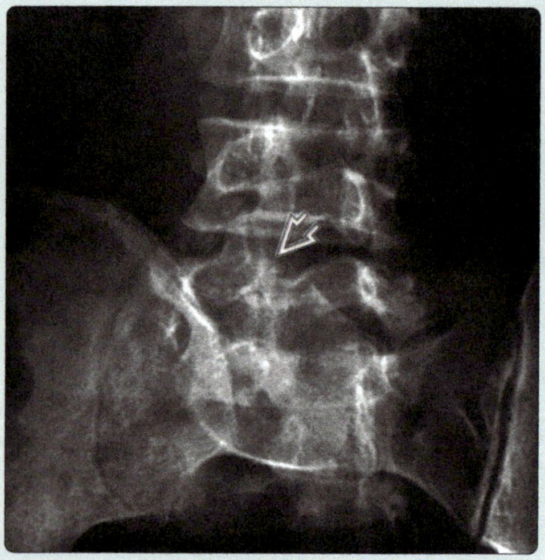

(Left) *Lateral radiography shows a defect and mild angulation in L5 PI ➡ with anterolisthesis of L5 on S1. There is disc height loss at L5-S1 with associated sclerotic endplate changes ➡.* **(Right)** *Sagittal bone CT reformation shows L5 pars defect ➡ without anterolisthesis.*

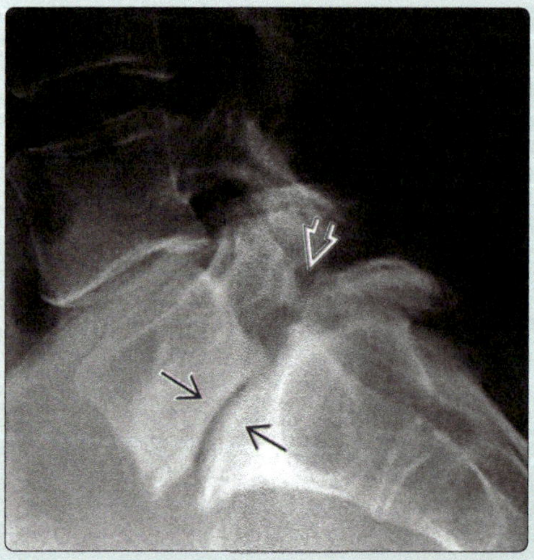

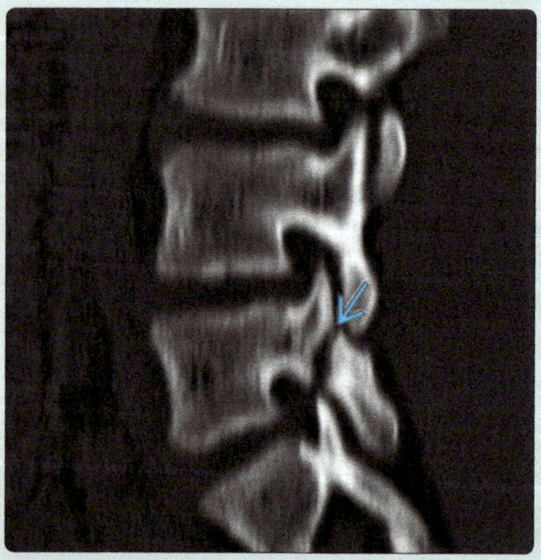

KEY FACTS

IMAGING

- Erosions of dens, uncovertebral joints, facet joints
- Atlantoaxial instability in 20-86% patients with RA
- Cranial settling occurs in 5-8% of RA patients
- Lower cervical spine: Facet and uncovertebral joint erosions, instability
- Neutral, flexion, and extension lateral radiographs performed for evaluation of instability
    - Normal = 2 mm between inner margin anterior ring of C1 and dens
    - If distance ≥ 9 mm, high correlation with neurologic symptoms
- Pannus is mass-like and surrounds and erodes dens, facet joints, uncovertebral joints
    - Low signal on T1WI
    - Heterogeneous signal on T2WI, STIR
    - Enhances avidly with gadolinium

TOP DIFFERENTIAL DIAGNOSES

- Seronegative spondyloarthropathy
- Calcium pyrophosphate dihydrate deposition (CPPD) disease
- Juvenile chronic arthritis
- Osteoarthritis

CLINICAL ISSUES

- 50-60% of RA patients have involvement of cervical spine
- Never involves spine before hands &/or feet
- May develop radiculopathy, myelopathy
- Instability → significant morbidity, mortality

DIAGNOSTIC CHECKLIST

- Calcifying mass with odontoid erosions is **not** RA
    - Indicates crystalline arthropathy, usually CPPD

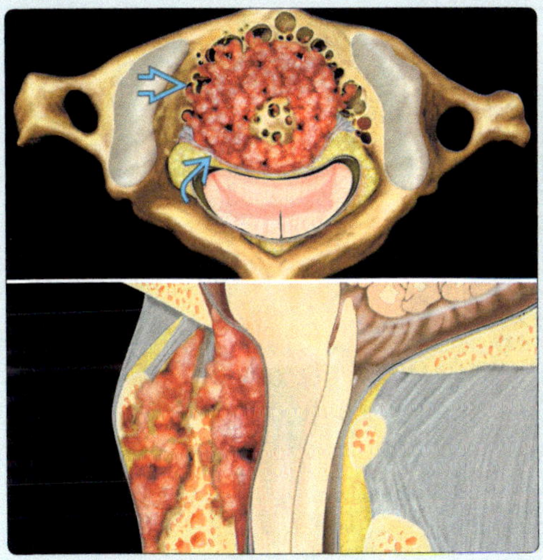

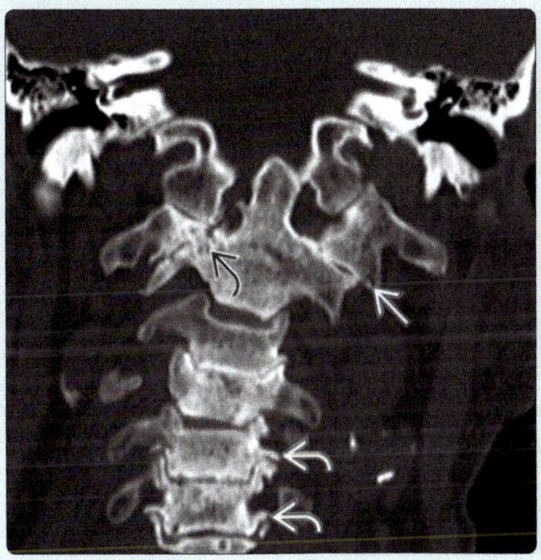

(Left) *Axial and sagittal graphics show erosion of dens by hypertrophied synovial tissue (pannus). Pannus has eroded the transverse ligament of the dens, resulting in instability. The spinal cord is compressed.* **(Right)** *Coronal CT reconstruction illustrates erosive changes at the right C1-2 joint and lateral subluxation of C1 with respect to C2. Inflammatory synovial proliferation and destruction of surrounding bone also affect the uncovertebral joints in the subaxial spine.*

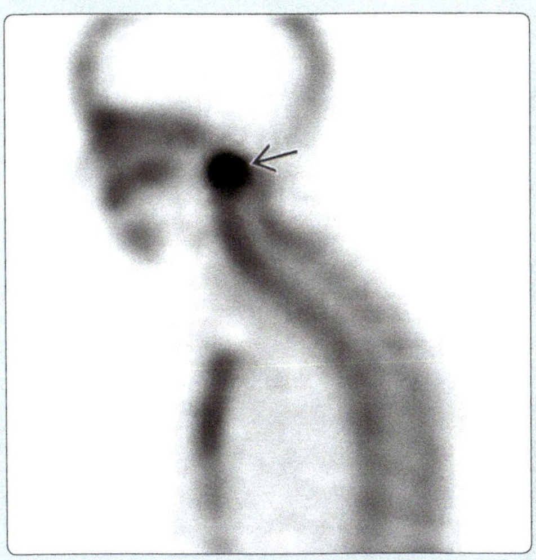

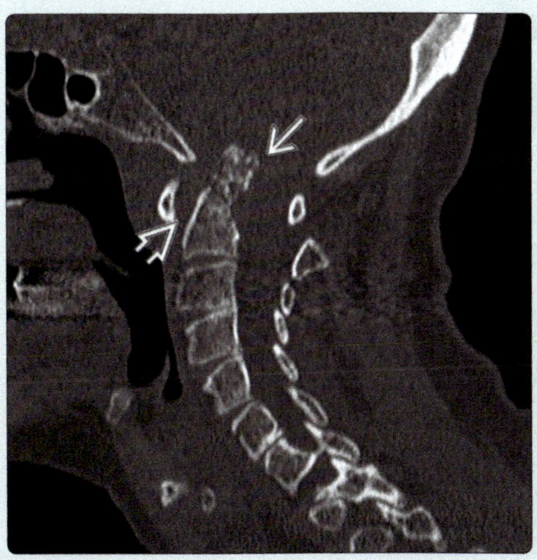

(Left) *Lateral view from a bone scan shows focal marked uptake at the C1-2 junction in this patient with RA.* **(Right)** *Sagittal NECT scan shows upward translocation of the odontoid and widened atlantodental interval. The skull and C1 have remained together, with the ligamentous laxity and disruption at C1-2 (coupled with the C1 lateral mass collapse), allowing C2 to migrate cephalad into the foramen magnum with brainstem compression (not shown).*

Calcium Pyrophosphate Dihydrate Deposition (CPPD)

KEY FACTS

TERMINOLOGY

- Metabolic arthropathy
- Crowned dens syndrome: Pain due to calcium pyrophosphate dihydrate deposition around dens

IMAGING

- Soft tissue calcifications
  - Usually linear, occasionally globular
  - Seen in ligaments, discs, facet joint capsules, hyaline cartilage
  - Horseshoe-shaped calcification around dens
- Erosions of odontoid process, vertebral endplates
  - Usually sharply demarcated, often corticated
- MR findings nonspecific
  - Calcium usually not visible, low signal intensity on all sequences
  - Soft tissue mass surrounding dens
  - Erosions of dens, vertebral endplates

TOP DIFFERENTIAL DIAGNOSES

- Degenerative disc disease
- Rheumatoid arthritis, adult
- Osteomyelitis, pyogenic
- Seronegative spondyloarthropathy
- Hemodialysis arthropathy
- Hyperparathyroidism
- Gout

CLINICAL ISSUES

- Acute attack of pain ± fever ± radiculopathy
  - Almost any joint may be involved
- Other
  - Chronic back pain common
  - Myelopathy due to cord compression

DIAGNOSTIC CHECKLIST

- CT useful in distinguishing from rheumatoid arthritis, which does not calcify

(Left) *Sagittal T1WI MR shows a large pseudopannus posterior to the odontoid process ➡ with moderately severe effacement of the ventral thecal sac and mild mass effect upon the cervicomedullary junction. A large degenerative cyst is present in the odontoid process ➡.* **(Right)** *Axial bone CT shows marked thickening of the retroodontoid soft tissues ➡ with scattered calcifications ➡ that are consistent with a diagnosis of calcium pyrophosphate dihydrate deposition (CPPD).*

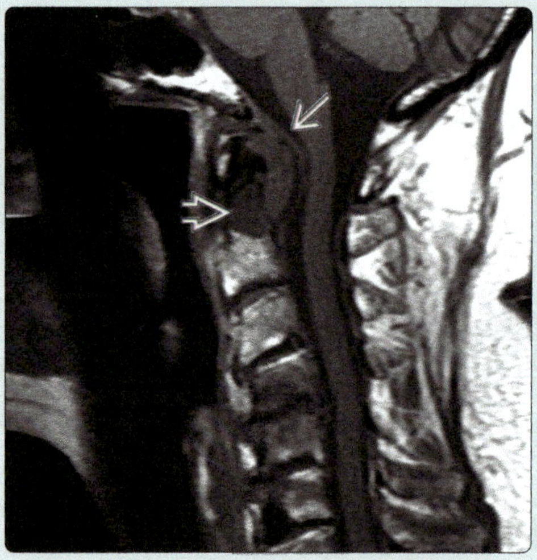

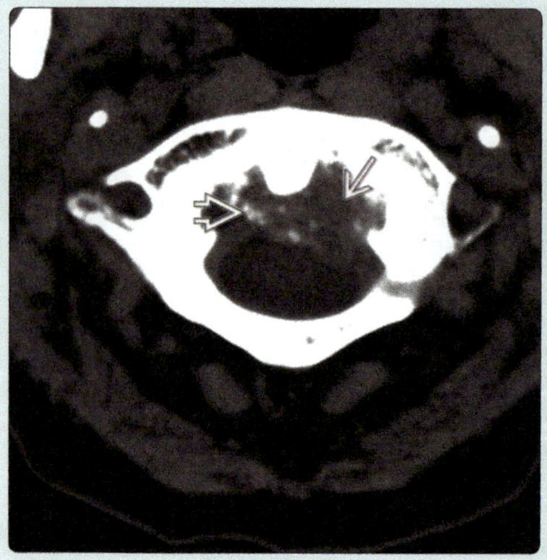

(Left) *Sagittal bone CT shows severe CPPD at the craniocervical junction. There is a large calcified mass posterior to the dens ➡ and severe odontoid erosion. Calcification is seen in the ligamentum flavum ➡ and intervertebral discs ➡.* **(Right)** *Axial CTA study shows multiple punctate foci of calcification ➡ within a large soft tissue mass posterior to the odontoid process, which causes cord compression ➡.*

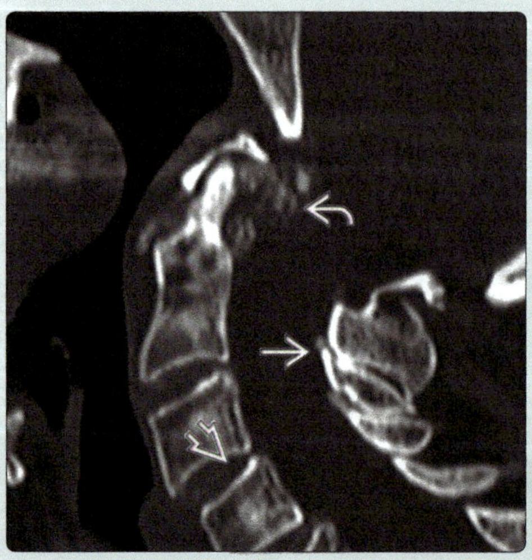

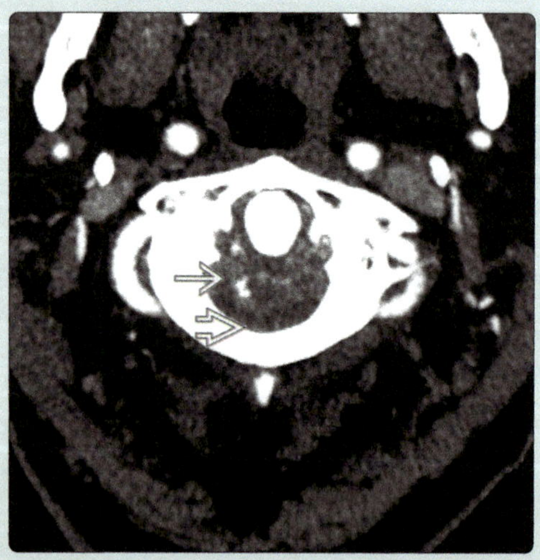

Ankylosing Spondylitis

KEY FACTS

IMAGING

- Location
    - Discs and synovial joints of spine
    - Joints of axial skeleton, less commonly peripheral joints
    - Tendon and ligament attachments (entheses)
- Sacroiliac joints (SIJs): Bilaterally symmetric erosive arthropathy → fusion
- Facet, uncovertebral joints: Erosions → fusion
- Squaring of vertebral bodies → corner erosions → "shiny corner" (corner sclerosis) → ankylosis
- Erosions, new bone formation at tendon and ligament attachments
- Trauma
    - Often hyperextension injury, involving all 3 columns of spine
    - Fracture may occur through fused regions
    - MR should be considered to exclude occult fracture, as these may be subtle secondary to osteopenia

TOP DIFFERENTIAL DIAGNOSES

- Diffuse idiopathic skeletal hyperostosis
- Psoriatic arthritis and reactive arthropathy
- Rheumatoid arthritis
- Osteitis condensans ilii

PATHOLOGY

- Associated findings
    - Pulmonary interstitial fibrosis, decreased chest excursion, uveitis, aortitis, aortic valve insufficiency
- 90% of patients HLA-B27 positive

CLINICAL ISSUES

- Complications: Kyphotic deformity, fractures of fused spine
- Pain centered over SIJs, back stiffness

DIAGNOSTIC CHECKLIST

- Normal SIJs preclude imaging diagnosis of ankylosing spondylitis

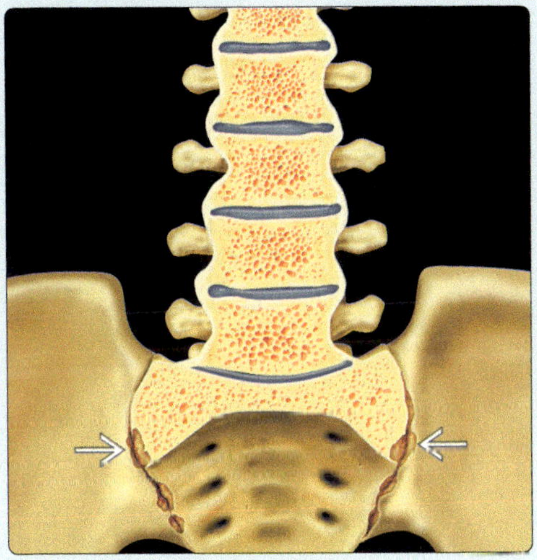

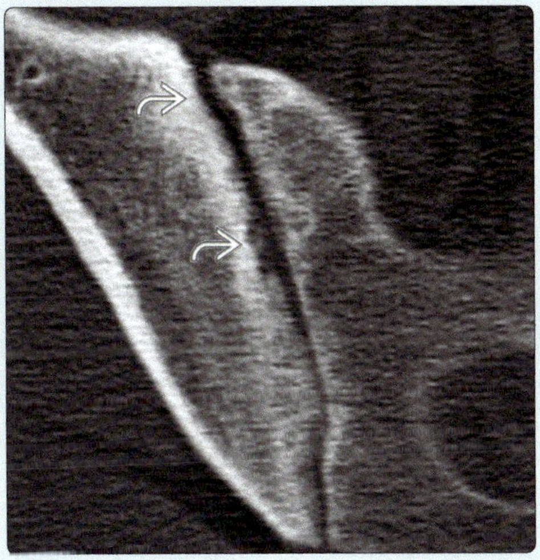

(Left) *Graphic shows sacroiliac joint (SIJ) erosions. Erosions are best seen in the inferior 1/3 of the joint, which is primarily synovial. More superiorly, the articulation is primarily ligamentous, with only a small synovial portion, and erosions are difficult to see.* **(Right)** *Axial bone CT shows classic appearance of SIJ inflammatory arthropathy, including small erosions, blurring of the subchondral bone plate, and adjacent sclerosis. Findings are more severe on the iliac side of joint.*

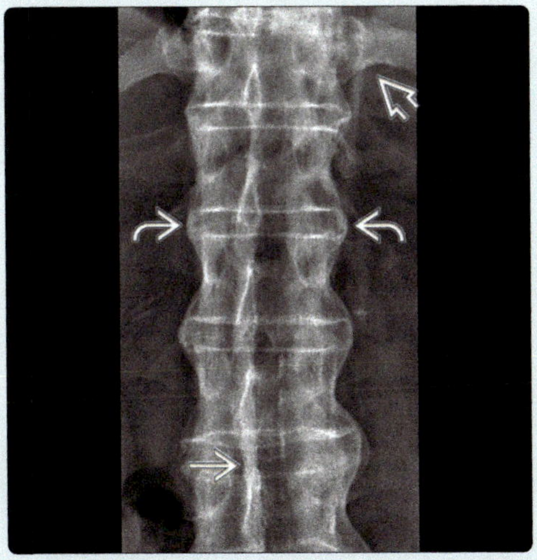

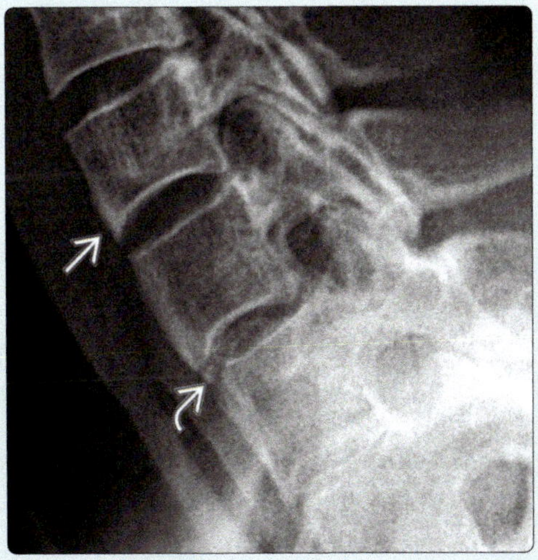

(Left) *Anteroposterior radiograph shows the "bamboo spine" typical of advanced ankylosing spondylitis, where ossification of the outer fibers of the annulus fibrosus mimics the joints of the bamboo plant. Fusion of the costotransverse joints and between the spinous processes is also visible.* **(Right)** *Lateral radiograph shows the shiny-corner sign. Bone resorption beneath the anterior longitudinal ligament creates a squared vertebral body contour. A single, thin syndesmophyte is visible.*

PART II: SPINE
SECTION 4

Infection and Inflammatory Disorders

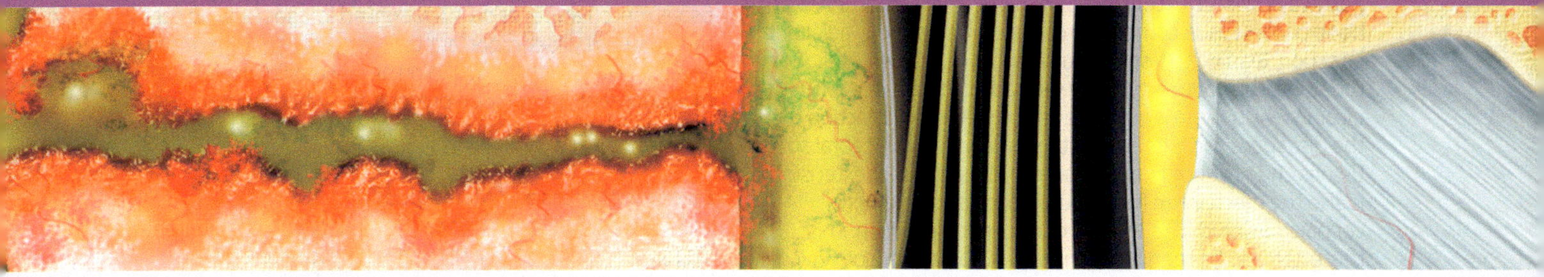

Infections

Inflammatory and Autoimmune Disorders

Anatomy-Based Imaging Issues

Spread of infection may occur along 1 of many different tracts, including **direct extension**, **lymphatic spread**, **hematogenous spread**, and along the **cerebrospinal fluid pathways**. **Direct extension**, as its name implies, occurs when bone or soft tissue comes into contact with a directly adjacent infection, leading to a soft tissue abscess or osteomyelitis. For the spine, this route is typically seen adjacent to a decubitus ulcer in which there is adjacent osteomyelitis. An infection of the disc space can extend into the adjacent paravertebral soft tissues and produce psoas muscle abscesses. Direct extension is also the mechanism for epidural abscess involvement cephalad or caudad to the site of disc space infection. This route can also be seen for an intramedullary spinal cord abscess in which the infection occurs through congenital dysraphism or a dermal sinus tract. Lymphatic spread is of limited importance in the spine relative to the much more commonly seen direct extension and hematogenous spread. **Lymphatic spread** may be seen in cases of retroperitoneal node enlargement from pelvic or abdominal primary neoplasms.

Hematogenous Spread

Hematogenous spread is the major pathway of infection spread to the axial skeleton. Vertebral bodies have areas that function physiologically in a similar manner to long bone metaphyses. The metaphyseal equivalent bone occurs near the anterior longitudinal ligament and has an end-arteriole network, making it susceptible to bacterial seeding. These areas have distal nonanastomosing vessels that have slow flow, and occlusion of these vessels will lead to avascular necrosis. In the vertebral bodies, segmental arteries usually supply 2 adjacent vertebral bodies and the intervening disc, giving the typical disc space infection patterns. The venous route is classically through Batson plexus, which is a longitudinal network of valveless veins running parallel to the spinal column. These veins lie outside of the thoracoabdominal cavity. These veins communicate with multiple aspects of the venous system, including the vena cava, portal venous system, azygos system, intercostal veins, and pulmonary and renal veins. Flow direction within the plexus is variable due to the variable intrathoracic and intraabdominal pressures. The pharyngovertebral plexus serves the same physiologic purpose. The contiguity of the cerebrospinal fluid spaces between the intracranial vault and the thecal sac allows for direct communication of neoplasm and infection. Intracranial neoplasms may seed throughout the cervical, thoracic, or lumbar thecal sac. Likewise, even distal neoplasms involving the caudal thecal sac may propagate cephalad and extend into the intracranial cerebrospinal fluid space.

Pathologic Issues

Types of spinal infection can be divided into disc space infection/vertebral osteomyelitis, subdural empyema, meningitis, intramedullary cord abscess, and septic arthritis/facet joint involvement. Disc space infection shows the typical pattern of low signal intensity on T1-weighted images involving the disc space proper and extending to the adjacent endplates. Endplate irregularity is a typical feature. T2 hyperintensity is generally present within the intervertebral disc in a nonanatomic pattern, with adjacent T2 hyperintensity extending to the vertebral bodies. Contrast enhancement tends to be irregular when it involves the intervertebral disc, with diffuse enhancement extending to the involved vertebral bodies. Extension into the paravertebral soft tissues is an important aspect of disc space infections and should be evaluated via either fat-suppressed, postcontrast T1-weighted images looking for enhancement of the paravertebral and psoas musculature, or on T2-weighted images looking for T2 hyperintensity. It is important to comment, not only on the level of involvement, but also on any instability or malalignment that may be present and whether there is extension into the paravertebral regions, epidural space, and psoas musculature.

Epidural Abscess and Meningitis

Isolated epidural abscesses can occur without concomitant disc space infections, but they can be associated with indwelling spinal catheters or prior spinal instrumentation. Uncommonly, these may occur as a result of hematogenous spread. Meningitis typically manifests on postcontrast T1-weighted images as linear enhancement along the pial surface of the cord or the roots of the cauda equina. With fungal infection, a more nodular enhancement pattern can be seen, which mimics the appearance of neoplastic spread. Spinal subdural empyemas are an uncommon manifestation of infection but may be seen in the setting of a severe disc space infection with adjacent extension into the epidural space. Presumably this is the result of direct extension through the dura and infection of the subdural space.

Intramedullary spinal cord abscesses are uncommon but can occur via both the hematogenous route and by direct extension. In adults, direct extension is the more typical mechanism. In children, the typical mechanism is direct extension through a dermal sinus. Septic arthritis/facet joint involvement may occur via hematogenous extension or by direct extension. Early infection may only be identified by slight T2 hyperintensity involving the bone of the facets, associated with facet effusion.

Adult vs. Pediatric

The routes of pyogenic infection will differ between adults and children due to developmental differences. In adults, the vertebral endplates become infected first, spreading to adjacent disc space and subsequently to the adjacent vertebral body, paravertebral tissues, and epidural space. In children, vascular channels are present across the growth plate, allowing primary infection of the intervertebral disc with subsequent secondary infection of the vertebral body. Disc space infections occur most commonly in the lumbar spine, followed by thoracic and cervical regions. Risk factors are many but include age over 50 years, intravenous drug abuse, diabetes, rheumatoid arthritis, AIDS, steroid administration, urinary tract instrumentation, prior spinal fracture, and paraplegia. *Staphylococcus aureus* is the most common organism. Pseudomonas may occur in the setting of drug abuse. *Salmonella* is the classic infection seen in sickle cell patients; however, *S. aureus* is still the most common overall in this population.

Classification

The Cierny and Mader classification of bone infection divides the pathology into 4 anatomic disease types and 3 host categories, yielding 12 clinical stages. The 4 anatomic disease types are: (1) Early hematogenous or medullary osteomyelitis, (2) superficial osteomyelitis (contiguous spread), (3) localized or full-thickness sequestration, and (4) diffuse osteomyelitis. The 3 host classifications are: (A) Normal physiologic response, (B) locally or systemically compromised response, and (C) treatment of the osteomyelitis would be worse than infection itself.

The spinal tuberculosis classification of Mehta (2001) divides the disease into 4 groups: (1) Stable anterior lesions without kyphotic deformity are treated with anterior debridement and strut grafting; (2) global lesions with kyphosis and instability are treated with posterior instrumentation and anterior strut grafting; (3) patients who are at high risk if treated by transthoracic surgery are treated with posterior decompression and instrumentation; and (4) isolated posterior lesions can be treated with posterior decompression.

Clinical Implications

Spinal involvement with infection represents 2-5% of all osteomyelitis sites. Axial spine pain is the most common presentation. This is progressive although it can have a fairly insidious onset, producing pain without relief from rest. Fever is variable and may be present in < 50% of cases. High-grade fever is present in < 5%, and motor and sensory deficits occur in 10-15% of patients. Rarely, intramedullary abscess can present with motor or sensory neurological deficits. Delay in diagnosing spinal infection is common. Intramedullary abscesses are fatal in 8%, with persistent neurological deficits in over 70%. Erythrocyte sedimentation rate is positive in more than 90%. C-reactive protein is also elevated. Blood cultures are positive with spinal osteomyelitis in 25-60% of cases.

Operative debridement with fusion may be necessary for a variety of reasons, including necessity to obtain a specific microorganism, abscess drainage, persistent neurological deficit, presence of spine instability and deformity, and failure of medical treatment. Long-term intravenous antibiotics remain the 1st line of therapy if there is no acute or evolving neurological deficit. A 6-week course of intravenous antibiotics is typical, which may also include an additional oral antibiotic regimen at the completion of the intravenous phase. External spine immobilization and bracing may be used. Recurrent bacteremia, paravertebral abscesses, and chronically draining sinuses are associated with relapse. Chronic autofusion of the infected level with successful nonoperative treatment is a common outcome.

Differential Diagnosis

The primary diagnostic modality in the evaluation of epidural abscess is MR, which is as sensitive as CT myelography for epidural infection but also allows the exclusion of other diagnostic choices, such as herniation, syrinx, tumor, and cord infarction. MR of epidural abscess demonstrates a soft tissue mass in the epidural space with tapered edges and an associated mass effect on the thecal sac and cord. The epidural masses are usually isointense to the cord on T1-weighted images and of increased signal on T2-weighted images. Contrast-enhanced MR is necessary for full elucidation of the abscess. The patterns of MR contrast enhancement of epidural abscess include: (1) Diffuse and homogeneous, (2) heterogeneous, and (3) thin peripheral. Enhancement is a very useful adjunct for identifying the extent of a lesion when the plain MR scan is equivocal, demonstrating activity of an infection and directing needle biopsy and follow-up treatment. Successful therapy should cause a progressive decrease in enhancement of the paraspinal soft tissues, disc, and vertebral bodies. In the initial stages of vertebral osteomyelitis, when the disc space is not yet involved, it may be difficult to exclude neoplastic disease, type I degenerative endplate changes, or compression fracture from the differential diagnosis using only MR. Follow-up studies are usually necessary to further define the nature of the lesion.

Boden et al. (1992) suggested that, in the postoperative spine, the triad of intervertebral disc space enhancement, annular enhancement, and vertebral body enhancement leads to the diagnosis of disc space infection, with the appropriate laboratory findings, such as an elevated sedimentation rate. However, there is a group of normal postoperative patients with annulus enhancement (at the surgical curette site), intervertebral disc enhancement, and vertebral endplate enhancement without evidence of disc space infection. In postoperative normal enhancement, the intervertebral disc enhancement is typically seen as thin bands paralleling the adjacent endplates, and the vertebral body enhancement is enhancement associated with type I degenerative endplate changes. This pattern should be distinguished from the amorphous enhancement seen within the intervertebral disc with disc space infection.

Selected References

1. Duarte RM et al: Spinal infection: state of the art and management algorithm. Eur Spine J. 22(12):2787-99, 2013
2. Malghem J et al: Necrotizing fasciitis: contribution and limitations of diagnostic imaging. Joint Bone Spine. 80(2):146-54, 2013
3. Go JL et al: Spine infections. Neuroimaging Clin N Am. 22(4):755-72, 2012
4. DeSanto J et al: Spine infection/inflammation. Radiol Clin North Am. 49(1):105-27, 2011
5. Celik AD et al: Spondylodiscitis due to an emergent fungal pathogen: Blastoschizomyces capitatus, a case report and review of the literature. Rheumatol Int. 29(10):1237-41, 2009
6. Hong SH et al: MR imaging assessment of the spine: infection or an imitation? Radiographics. 29(2):599-612, 2009
7. Karikari IO et al: Management of a spontaneous spinal epidural abscess: a single-center 10-year experience. Neurosurgery. 65(5):919-23; discussion 923-4, 2009
8. Mylona E et al: Pyogenic vertebral osteomyelitis: a systematic review of clinical characteristics. Semin Arthritis Rheum. 39(1):10-7, 2009
9. Petruzzi N et al: Recent trends in soft-tissue infection imaging. Semin Nucl Med. 39(2):115-23, 2009
10. Posacioglu H et al: Rupture of a nonaneurysmal abdominal aorta due to spondylitis. Tex Heart Inst J. 36(1):65-8, 2009
11. Sobottke R et al: Treatment of spondylodiscitis in human immunodeficiency virus-infected patients: a comparison of conservative and operative therapy. Spine (Phila Pa 1976). 34(13):E452-8, 2009
12. Thwaites G et al: British Infection Society guidelines for the diagnosis and treatment of tuberculosis of the central nervous system in adults and children. J Infect. 59(3):167-87, 2009
13. Dai LY et al: Anterior instrumentation for the treatment of pyogenic vertebral osteomyelitis of thoracic and lumbar spine. Eur Spine J. 17(8):1027-34, 2008
14. Mehta JS et al: Tuberculosis of the thoracic spine. A classification based on the selection of surgical strategies. J Bone Joint Surg Br. 83(6):859-63, 2001
15. Mader JT et al: Staging and staging application in osteomyelitis. Clin Infect Dis. 25(6):1303-9, 1997
16. Boden SD et al: Postoperative diskitis: distinguishing early MR imaging findings from normal postoperative disk space changes. Radiology. 184(3):765-71, 1992

(Left) *Sagittal graphic shows lumbar disc space infection with vertebral body osteomyelitis with endplate destruction. There are ventral and dorsal abscess collections.* **(Right)** *Sagittal T1WI C+ FS MR in this case of disc space infection shows enhancement of L5 and S1 bodies and intervertebral disc, with prevertebral and epidural phlegmon extension.*

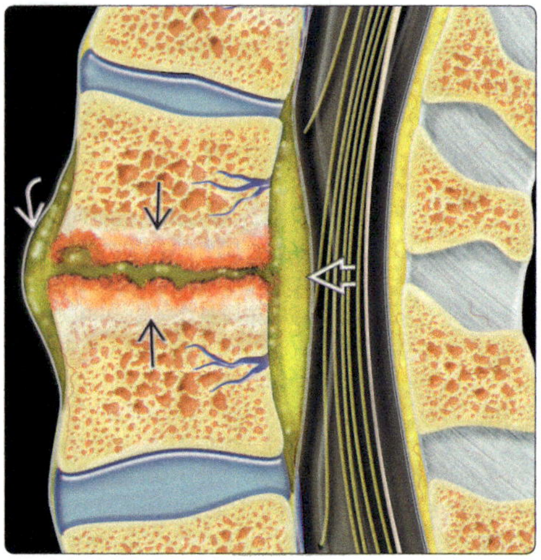

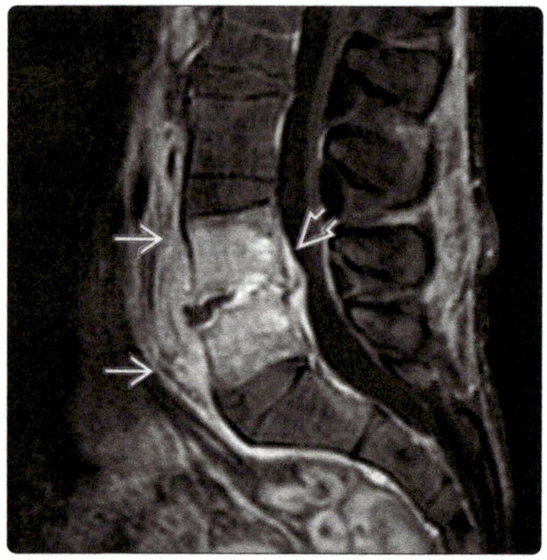

(Left) *Axial T1WI C+ MR of a disc space infection shows inflammatory extension into the prevertebral space, psoas muscles, and dorsal spinal muscles. Phlegmon extends into the ventral epidural space with thecal sac compression.* **(Right)** *Axial T2WI FS MR shows inflammatory extension into the prevertebral space, psoas muscles, and dorsal spinal muscles.*

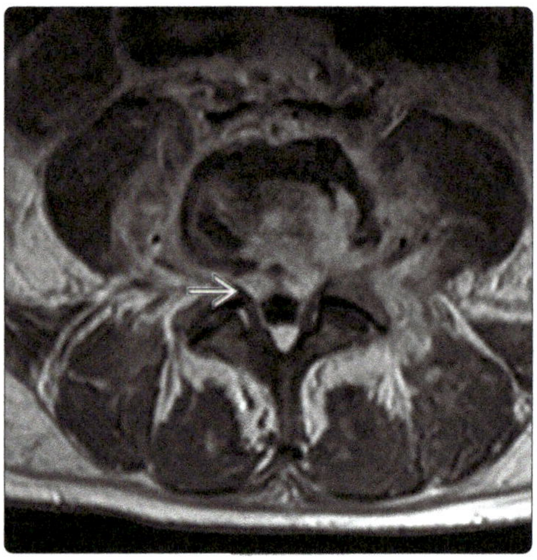

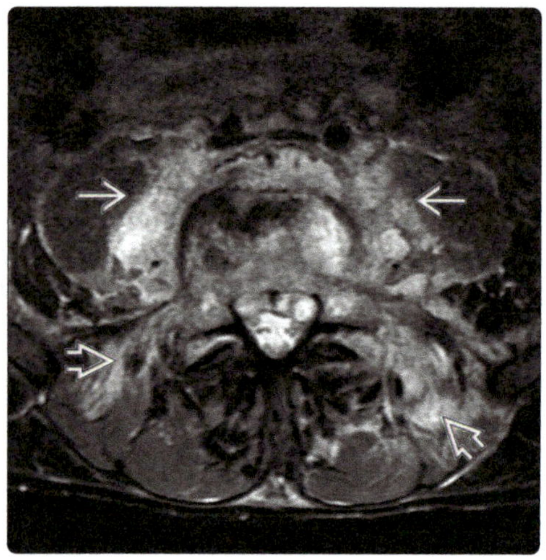

(Left) *Axial T1WI C+ MR shows disseminated coccidioidomycosis with diffuse bone and soft tissue involvement and adjacent paraspinal extension and extension into lung.* **(Right)** *Axial T2WI MR in another case of coccidioidomycosis shows huge paraspinal abscesses. There is effacement of the normal thecal sac within the spinal canal due to disc space infection and osteomyelitis.*

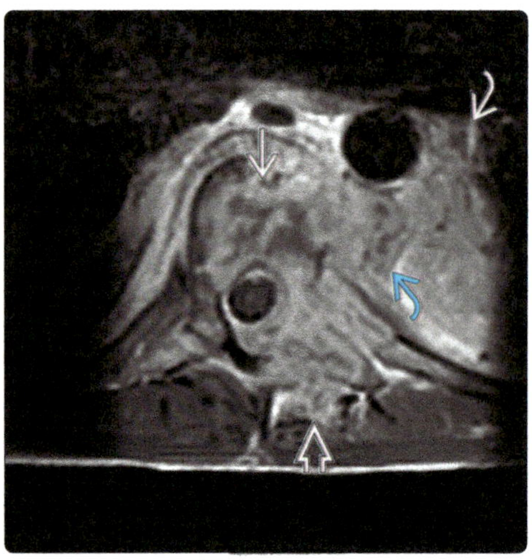

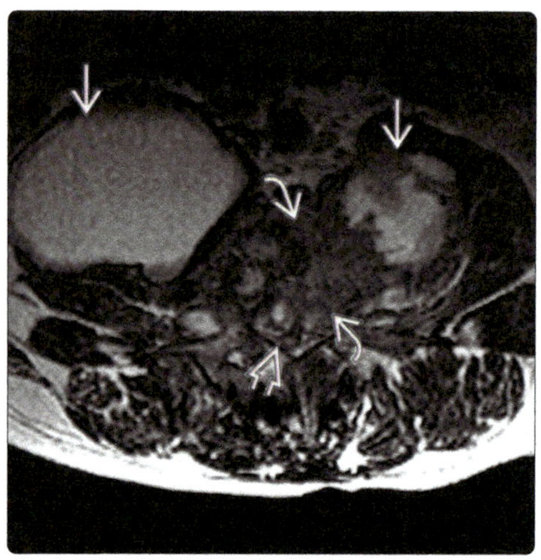

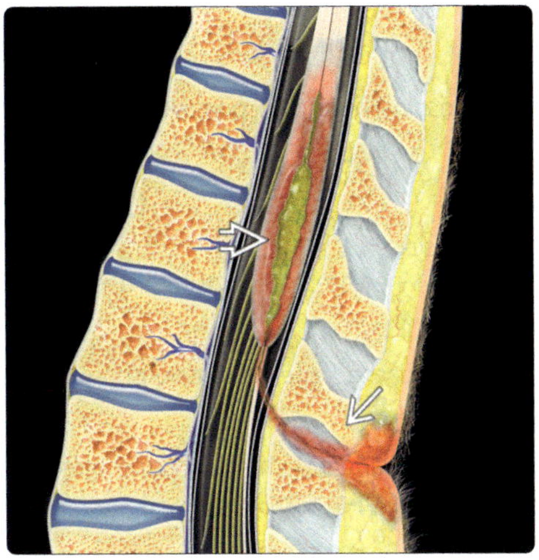

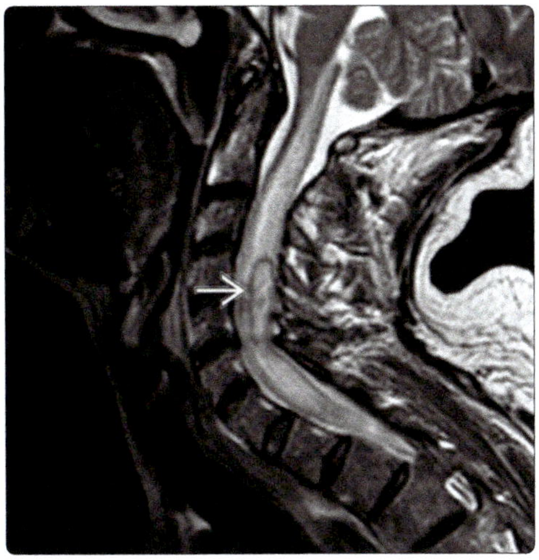

(Left) *Sagittal graphic shows dermal sinus extending from skin surface to conus, with conus abscess and extensive cord edema.* **(Right)** *Sagittal T2WI MR in a patient with a cervical cord abscess and streptococcal endocarditis shows diffuse cord expansion, with a ring-shaped area of low T2 signal (abscess capsule) within the cord from C4 to C5-C6.*

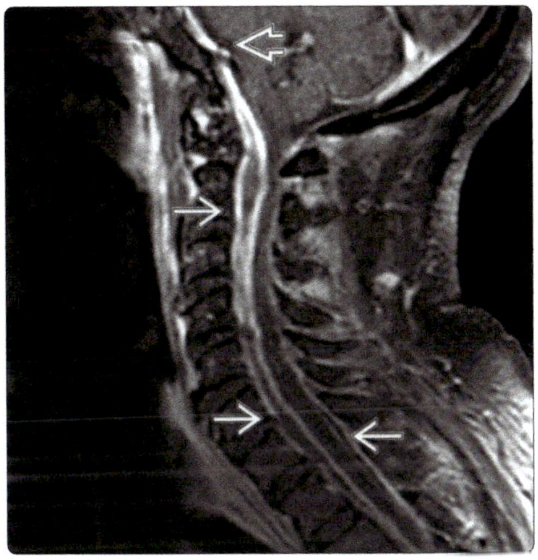

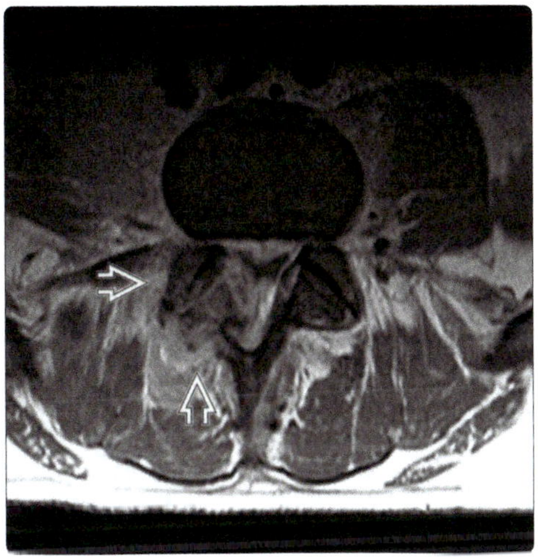

(Left) *Sagittal T1WI C+ MR with fat suppression shows extensive subdural empyema with peripheral enhancement throughout the cervical spine and extending along clivus.* **(Right)** *A septic facet joint is shown. Axial T1WI C+ MR at L4-L5 shows extension of the infection to the right facet joint with diffuse facet bone enhancement and juxta facet soft tissue involvement.*

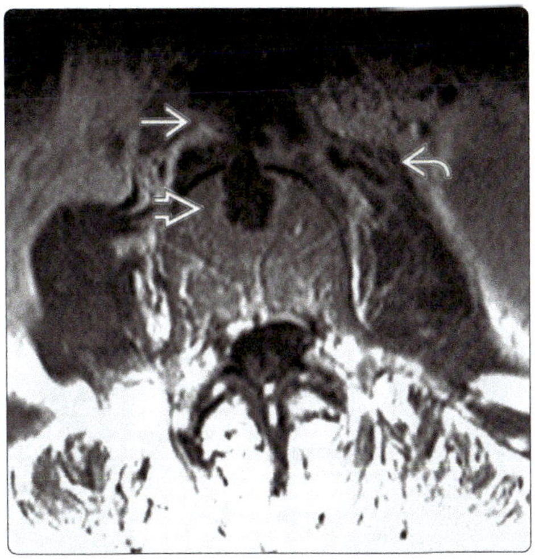

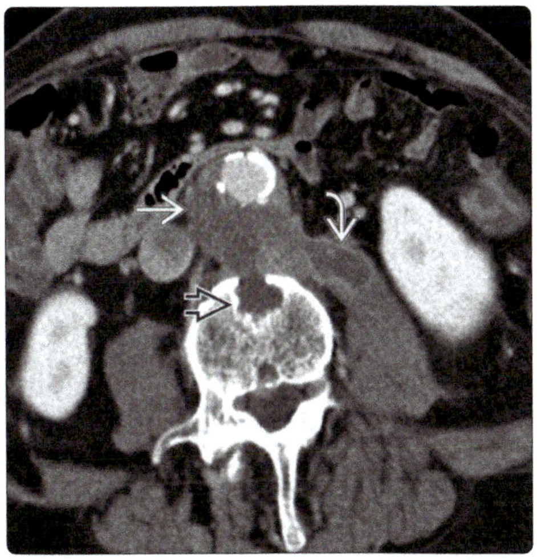

(Left) *Axial T1WI C+ MR shows direct extension of infection from mycotic aortic aneurysm into the ventral vertebral body, producing bone destruction and osteomyelitis. There is also direct extension of infection into psoas muscle.* **(Right)** *Axial CECT shows direct extension of infection from mycotic aortic aneurysm into vertebral body and left psoas muscle.*

Spinal Meningitis

KEY FACTS

IMAGING

- MR
  - Diffuse, extensive subarachnoid enhancement
  - Smooth or irregular meningeal enhancement

TOP DIFFERENTIAL DIAGNOSES

- Carcinomatous meningitis
  - Focal or diffuse, sheet-like or nodular enhancement along cord or nerve roots
- Sarcoidosis
  - Leptomeningeal + nerve root enhancement mimics spinal meningitis
- Lumbar arachnoiditis
  - Empty-sac sign (nerve roots stuck to inside of thecal sac)
- Guillain-Barré syndrome
  - Inflammatory demyelination typically following recent viral illness
- Intracranial hypotension (spontaneous or iatrogenic)
  - Engorged epidural venous plexi, not dura/arachnoid or pia

PATHOLOGY

- Infection of cerebrospinal fluid (CSF), pia covering spinal cord/roots
- Associated findings
  - Spondylodiscitis
  - Spinal epidural abscess
  - Blocked CSF flow → increased pressure in cord → syrinx

CLINICAL ISSUES

- Acute fever, chills, headache ± altered consciousness

DIAGNOSTIC CHECKLIST

- Imaging often negative early, so lumbar puncture necessary
  - Positive in advanced bacterial meningitis or granulomatous infection
- Intravenous gadolinium increases sensitivity in detecting meningeal disease

(Left) *Sagittal T1WI C+ MR shows diffuse mildly irregular leptomeningeal enhancement. No extradural or vertebral inflammatory changes are apparent. Abnormal contrast agent enhancement is noted in only 55-70% of patients with proven infectious meningitis on contrast-enhanced MR. Contrast-enhanced MR is particularly insensitive to viral meningitis.* **(Right)** *Axial T1WI C+ MR in the same patient shows marked thickening and enhancement of the nerve roots.*

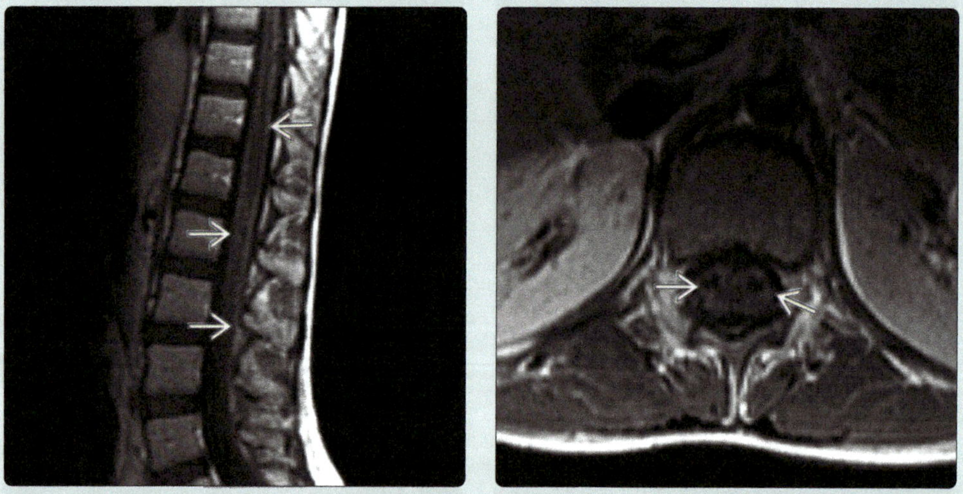

(Left) *Sagittal T1 C+ MR exhibits diffuse leptomeningeal enhancement extending into the posterior fossa.* **(Right)** *Sagittal T2 MR reveals diffuse intramedullary hyperintensity consistent with spinal cord ischemia complicating meningitis. Inflammatory vasculitis acutely produces vascular compromise. Vascular insufficiency secondary to arachnoiditis gives delayed complications, such as paraparesis, sensory loss, and urinary incontinence.*

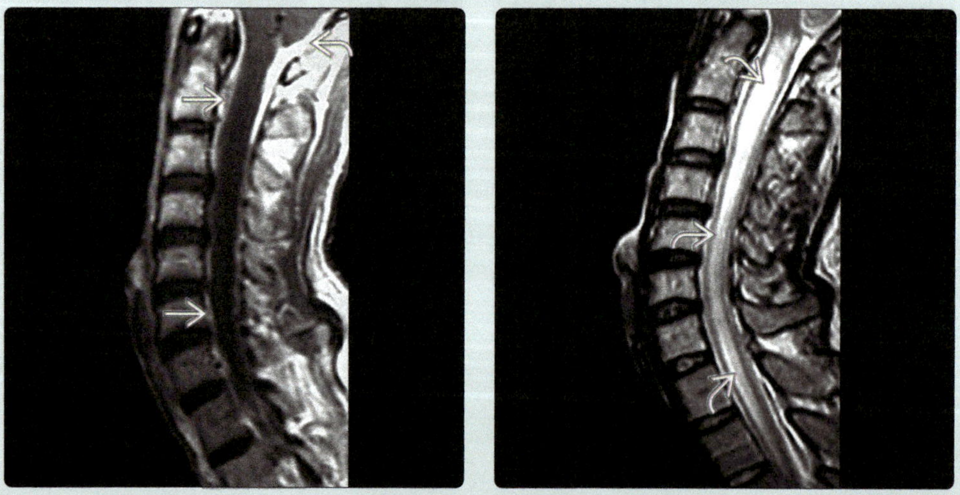

KEY FACTS

TERMINOLOGY

- Tuberculosis (TB); TB spondylitis (TS)
  - Extrapulmonary granulomatous infection of spine/adjacent tissues
  - Also known as Pott (Pott's) disease

IMAGING

- Gibbus vertebrae with relatively intact intervertebral discs, large paraspinal abscesses
- Midthoracic or thoracolumbar > lumbar, cervical
- Isolated posterior element involvement possible
- MR best modality to evaluate extent of disease, assess response to treatment
  - Sagittal STIR or FSE T2 with fat saturation most sensitive for bone marrow edema, epidural involvement
  - T1 C+
    - Marrow, subligamentous, discal, dural enhancement
    - Diffusely enhancing soft tissue = phlegmon
    - Ring-enhancing = abscess

TOP DIFFERENTIAL DIAGNOSES

- Pyogenic spondylitis
  - Initial infection in subchondral bone
  - Intervertebral discs typically affected
- Fungal spondylitis
- Spinal metastases
  - Extraosseous epidural or paraspinal extension
  - Disc space preserved
- Brucellar spondylitis

PATHOLOGY

- Hematogenous or lymphatic spread
- Initially in anterior vertebral body
  - Spread under longitudinal ligaments → other (often noncontiguous) vertebrae

CLINICAL ISSUES

- Chronic back pain, focal tenderness, fever
- Neurologic deficits common in TS

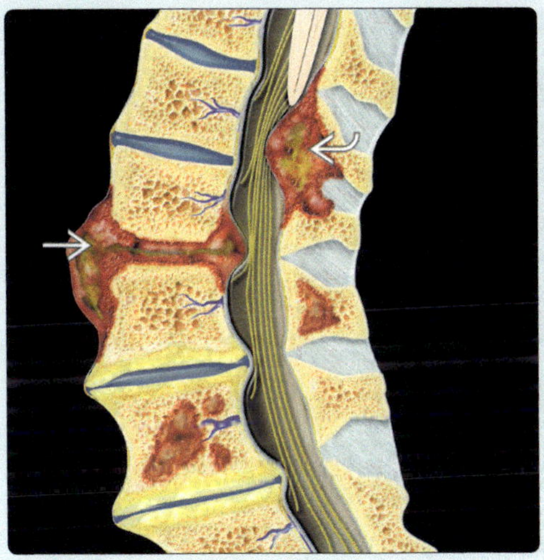

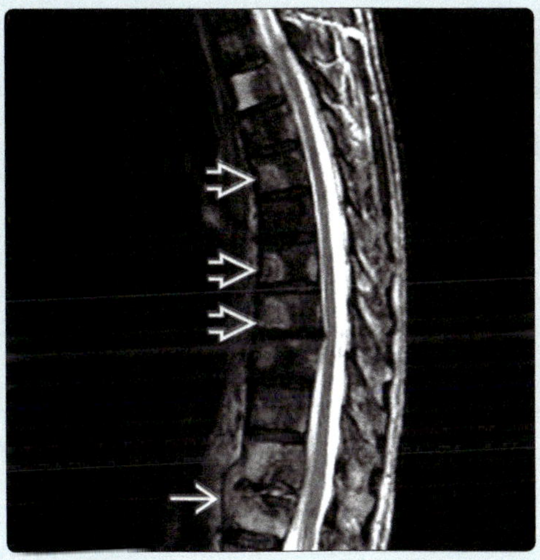

(Left) *Sagittal graphic through lumbar spine depicts multifocal granulomatous osteomyelitis. Frank abscesses are present at L3-L4 disc space → and between spinous process of L2 and L3 →.* **(Right)** *Sagittal STIR MR in a patient with TB infection shows involvement of contiguous vertebral bodies, with subligamentous abscess spread and partial disc involvement →. Multiple focal bone lesions are present without adjacent disc involvement →.*

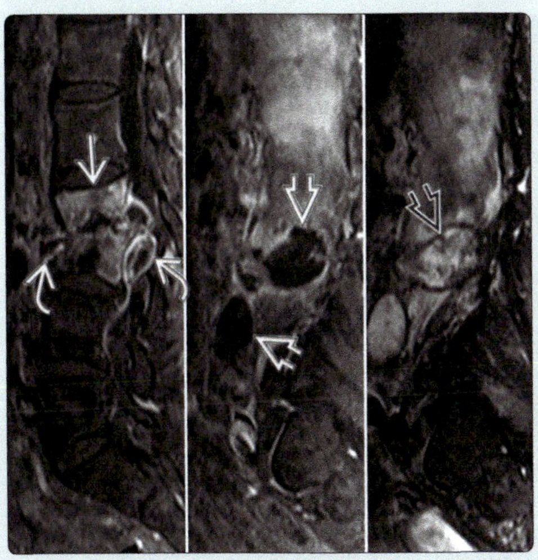

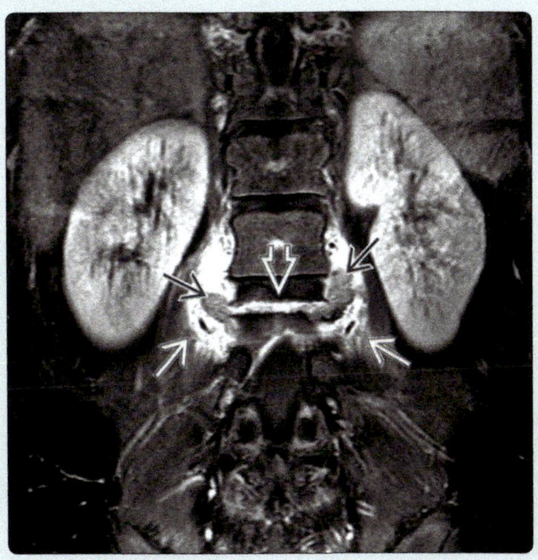

(Left) *Sagittal T1WI C+ FS MR demonstrates focal kyphosis at L2-L3, collapse of the disc space, avid vertebral body enhancement →, and ventral and dorsal paravertebral abscesses →. There are peripherally enhancing abscesses in the paraspinal soft tissues →, which exhibit hypointense rims →.* **(Right)** *Coronal T1WI C+ FS MR shows TB osteomyelitis with L2 vertebra plana →. Psoas involvement with swelling and marked enhancement → is present. Inflammatory soft tissue surrounds the disc →.*

KEY FACTS

TERMINOLOGY

- Paraspinal phlegmon surrounding peripherally enhancing fluid collections

IMAGING

- **Pre**vertebral/**para**vertebral space
- Multiple or multiloculated collections along muscle plane
- NECT
    - Amorphous low-density intramuscular collection
    - Calcified psoas abscesses characteristic of tuberculous paraspinal abscess
    - Endplate destruction
- MR
    - Iso- to hypointense on T1WI
    - Hyperintense fluid collection and surrounding muscle on T2WI and STIR
    - Diffuse enhancement: Phlegmon
    - Peripherally enhancing fluid collection(s): Abscess

TOP DIFFERENTIAL DIAGNOSES

- Neoplasm, primary or metastatic
- Retroperitoneal hematoma
- Extramedullary hematopoiesis

PATHOLOGY

- Most common pathogens: *Staphylococcus aureus, Mycobacterium tuberculosis, Escherichia coli*

CLINICAL ISSUES

- Fever (50%) at presentation
- Back pain and tenderness
- ↑ erythrocyte sedimentation rate, ↑ white blood cell count

DIAGNOSTIC CHECKLIST

- Peripherally enhancing collection in paravertebral soft tissue with associated spondylitis characteristic of paraspinal abscess

(Left) *Axial graphic through a lumbar disc space demonstrates an extensive abscess infiltrating bilateral psoas muscles ➔ and epidural space ➔. Abnormal retroperitoneal lymph nodes are also present ➔.* **(Right)** *Axial NECT depicts bilateral calcified paraspinal masses ➔ in a patient with tuberculosis spondylodiscitis. Anterior aspect of the vertebral body adjacent to the subchondral plate is affected with spread to adjacent discs. Abscesses may descend down the sheath of the psoas and are typically calcified.*

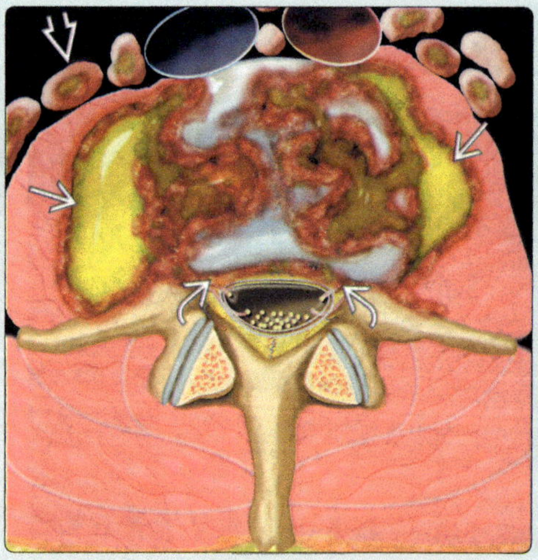

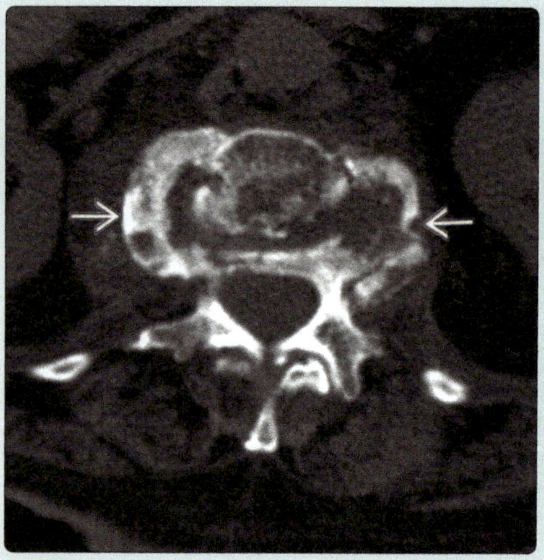

(Left) *Sagittal CT (L) illustrates a low-density collection in the operative bed status post schwannoma resection. The collection has faint peripheral enhancement ➔. Sagittal T1WI C+ MR (R) in the same patient better delineates irregular peripheral enhancement ➔ of the postoperative collection and enhancement in the neural foramen ➔. The patient presented with fever and leukocytosis.* **(Right)** *Axial T1WI C+ MR shows a peripherally enhancing collection ➔ in the left neural foramen operative site.*

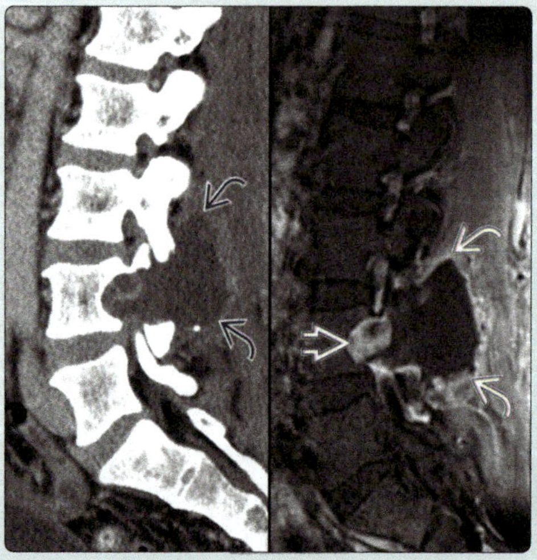

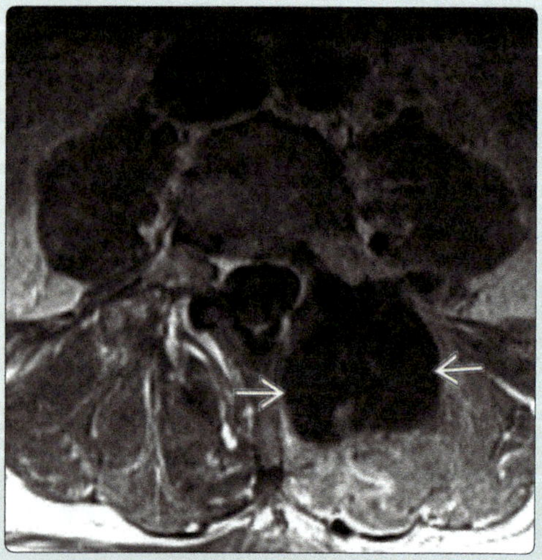

KEY FACTS

TERMINOLOGY

- Spinal epidural abscess
- Extradural spinal infection with abscess formation

IMAGING

- Lower thoracic and lumbar > upper thoracic and cervical
- CT
  - Enhancing epidural mass narrowing central canal
- MR
  - T1WI: Iso- to hypointense to cord
  - T2WI/STIR: Hyperintense
  - T1WI C+: Homogeneously or heterogeneously enhancing **phlegmon**
  - Peripherally enhancing necrotic **abscess**
- Fat saturation: STIR, T2WI FS, T1WI C+ FS
  - Increases lesion conspicuity by suppressing signal from epidural fat and vertebral marrow
- Signal alteration in spinal cord secondary to compression, ischemia, or direct infection
- Persistent epidural enhancement without mass effect on follow-up MR imaging
  - Probable sterile granulation tissue or fibrosis
  - Correlate with ESR and CRP for disease activity

TOP DIFFERENTIAL DIAGNOSES

- Extradural metastasis
  - Often contiguous with vertebral lesion
- Epidural hematoma
  - ± mild peripheral enhancement

PATHOLOGY

- *Staphylococcus aureus* most common cause; *Mycobacterium tuberculosis* next most frequent

CLINICAL ISSUES

- Fever, acute or subacute spinal pain, and tenderness
- Neurosurgical emergency if cord complications (bowel, bladder dysfunction)
  - Decompression + 4-6 weeks of IV antibiotics

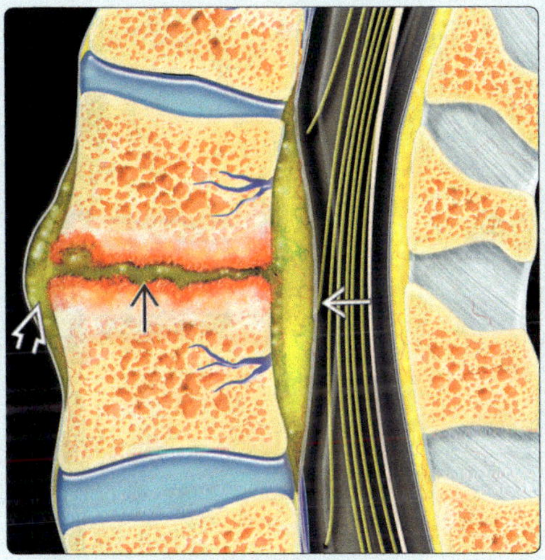

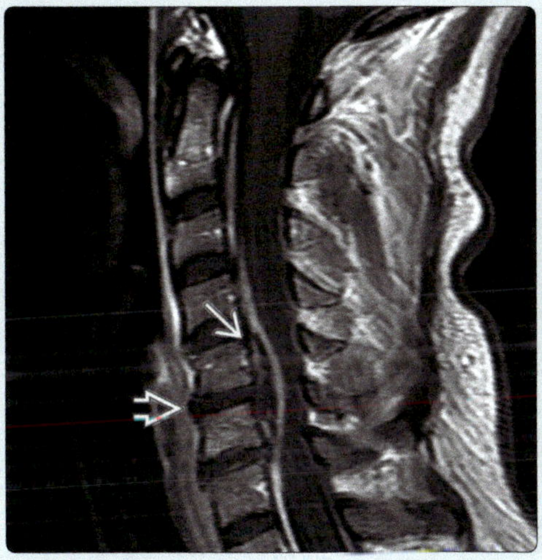

(Left) *Sagittal graphic through the lumbar spine demonstrates vertebral osteomyelitis with an intervertebral abscess extending ventrally and dorsally into the epidural space, where it is narrowing the central canal.* **(Right)** *Sagittal T1WI C+ MR in an intravenous drug abuser shows a large ventral epidural abscess collection with peripheral enhancement causing a severe mass effect upon the cervical cord. There is relative preservation of the C5-C6 endplates with no disc enhancement.*

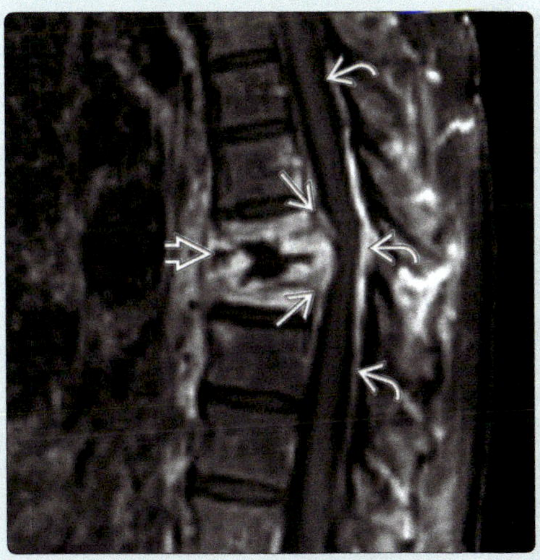

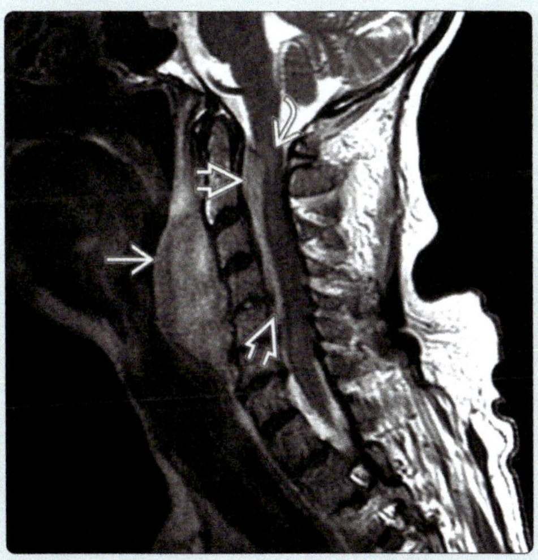

(Left) *Sagittal T1WI C+ FS MR shows homogeneously enhancing epidural phlegmon in the ventral epidural space adjacent to the osteomyelitis/discitis. Dorsal epidural phlegmon contributes to the mass effect on the cord.* **(Right)** *Sagittal T2WI MR shows a large prevertebral abscess as increased signal. Note the extensive ventral epidural abscess with posterior displacement of the cord. A small amount of cord edema is present.*

KEY FACTS

TERMINOLOGY

- Spinal subdural abscess (SSA)
- Intradural extramedullary ring-enhancing fluid collection of pus in "potential" space between dura and arachnoid

IMAGING

- Thoracolumbar region most common
- Presence suggested by mass effect on cord and obliterated subarachnoid space
- Cord displacement: ± impingement and edema
- Increased subdural density on NECT
- MR
  - T2 hyperintense/T1 hypointense
  - Heterogeneous, diffuse subdural enhancement
  - Rim-enhancing fluid collection
- Best imaging modality
  - MR with contrast → ↑ sensitivity in detecting SSA
  - Axial sequences confirm subdural location (inside dural margin)

TOP DIFFERENTIAL DIAGNOSES

- Abscess: Epidural, paravertebral
  - Typically associated with spondylodiscitis
- Subdural hematoma
  - Predominantly hypointense on T2WI or gradient-echo

PATHOLOGY

- Predisposing factors
  - Intravenous drug abuse, immunocompromised state, diabetes, cirrhosis, renal failure

CLINICAL ISSUES

- Fever
- Neck or back pain and tenderness

DIAGNOSTIC CHECKLIST

- Ring-enhancing intradural extramedullary collection outlined by epidural fat and cerebrospinal fluid on axial imaging

(Left) *Sagittal T2WI MR shows a heterogeneously hyperintense collection ➡ in the dorsal intradural extramedullary space, with hypointense rim causing marked mass effect on cervical cord ➡.* **(Right)** *Sagittal CT shows a hyperdense spinal subdural abscess (SSA) ⇨ in the dorsal spinal canal. Osseous destruction of the L4 & L5 endplates ⇨ & intradiscal hypodense fluid ➡ at this level are seen. This extensive SSA began as a lumbar spinal epidural abscess caused by Serratia marcescens.*

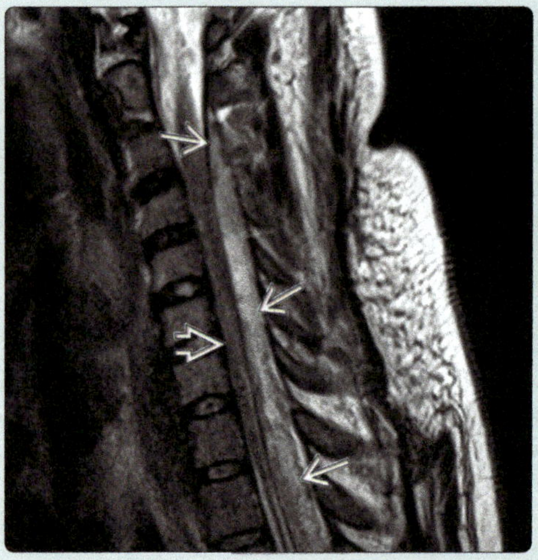

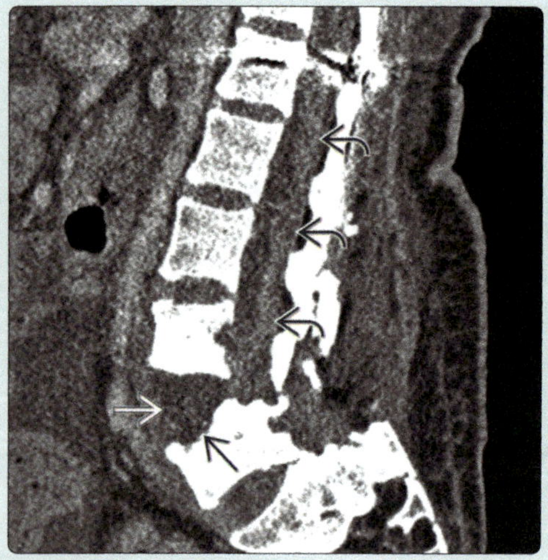

(Left) *Axial T1WI C+ MR depicts a rim-enhancing fluid collection ➡ in the dorsal spinal canal, causing mass effect upon and anteriorly displacing the cervical cord ➡.* **(Right)** *Sagittal T1 C+ MR exhibits a low-intensity collection with thick peripheral enhancement ⇨ spanning the cervical and thoracic dorsal spinal canal. The SSA causes severe impingement of the cord ➡. Initially, CT-guided drainage was attempted but with limited success. Subsequently, surgical decompression was performed.*

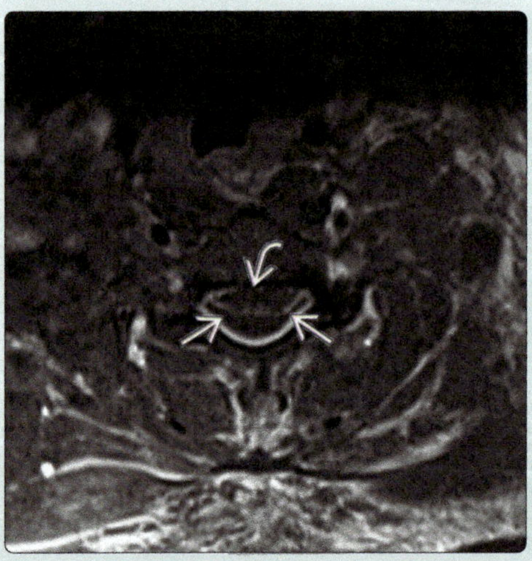

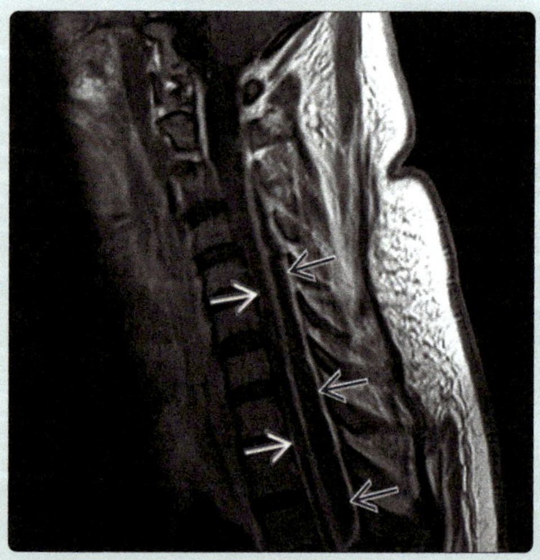

KEY FACTS

TERMINOLOGY

- Acute inflammatory insult of spinal cord due to direct viral infection or postviral immunologic attack

IMAGING

- Swollen, edematous spinal cord with segmental contiguous involvement
  - From 1 segment to extensive cord involvement
- Fusiform expansion of spinal cord
- Diffuse increase in T2 signal intensity through involved segment
- Variable, patchy enhancement of involved cord segment

TOP DIFFERENTIAL DIAGNOSES

- "Idiopathic" transverse myelitis
- Multiple sclerosis
- Acute cord infarct
- Neuromyelitis optica

PATHOLOGY

- Since near complete eradication of polio, other enteroviruses most common etiology
- Edematous, boggy cord ± necrosis

CLINICAL ISSUES

- Acute onset of weakness following febrile illness or upper respiratory tract infection
- Cerebrospinal fluid shows elevated mononuclear counts and protein level
- Principal treatment supportive with antiviral drugs ± steroids, variable efficacy

DIAGNOSTIC CHECKLIST

- Strong diagnostic clue in patients with acute onset of myelopathy: Long, segmental cord enlargement and edema without focal lesions

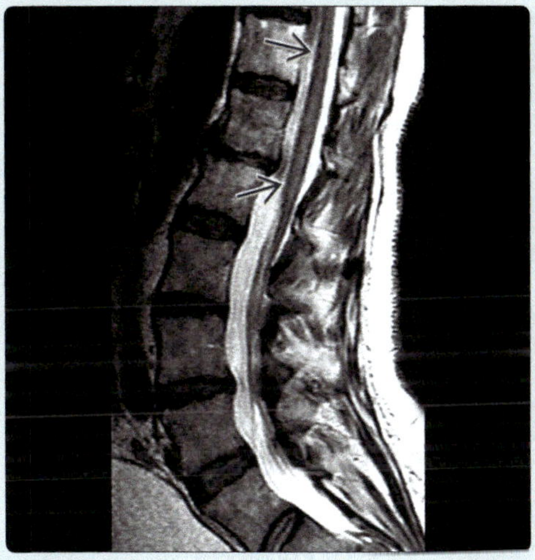

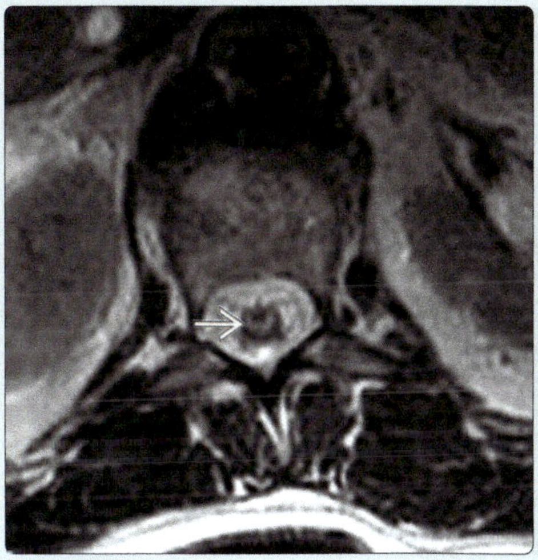

(Left) *Sagittal T2WI MR shows hyperintensity in the distal thoracic cord and conus ➡ in this patient with West Nile virus (WNV), confirmed with positive IgM serology. WNV can cause meningitis, encephalitis, ± an irreversible acute flaccid paralysis. WNV shows a predilection for the deep gray nuclei in the brain and the spinal cord.* **(Right)** *Axial T2WI MR in the same patient with WNV demonstrates hyperintensity in the distal thoracic cord central gray matter ➡.*

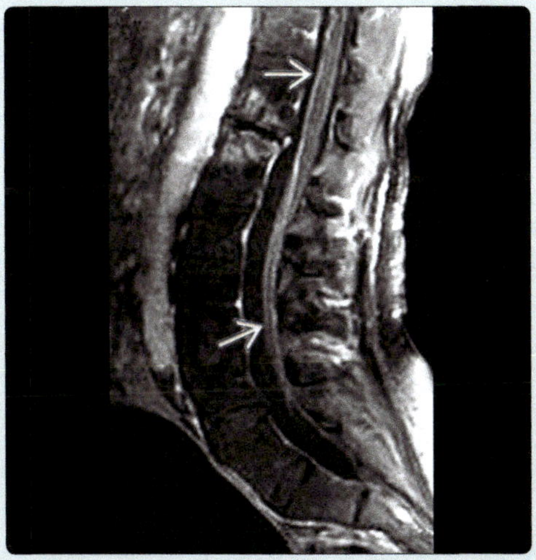

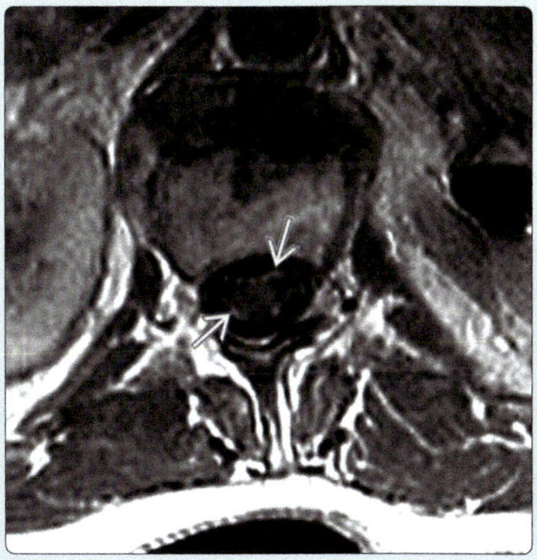

(Left) *Sagittal T1WI C+ FS MR displays enhancement along the distal cord and cauda equina ➡ due to WNV. This patient had a poliomyelitis-like syndrome.* **(Right)** *Axial T1WI C+ MR of the same patient illustrates linear enhancement of the cauda equina ➡. Most WNV-associated acute flaccid paralysis is due to spinal motor neuron involvement producing an anterior myelitis.*

KEY FACTS

TERMINOLOGY

- Myelopathy resulting from primary HIV infection

IMAGING

- Most common: Atrophy
- Spinal cord T2 hyperintensity ± patchy enhancement
  - Thoracic > cervical; ↑ rostral as disease progresses

TOP DIFFERENTIAL DIAGNOSES

- B12 deficiency
- Infection (varicella-zoster virus, human T-cell leukemia/lymphoma virus)
- Multiple sclerosis
- Transverse myelitis
- Delayed radiation myelopathy

PATHOLOGY

- DNA lentivirus/retrovirus attacks spine monocytes, macrophages
  - Disease of cord and brain often occurs separately, suggesting different pathogenetic mechanisms
- Opportunistic CNS and PNS infections and malignancies

CLINICAL ISSUES

- Insidious progressive spastic paraparesis with ataxia, urinary problems, and sensory loss
  - May have acute myelitic syndrome shortly after seroconversion
- Immune reconstitution inflammatory syndrome → myelopathy
- Diagnosis of exclusion based on clinical, laboratory, and radiologic findings
  - MR excludes other extrinsic or intrinsic processes

DIAGNOSTIC CHECKLIST

- Important to exclude other treatable causes of myelopathy
- Spinal cord atrophy is most common MR abnormality, typically involving thoracic spinal cord ± cervical cord involvement

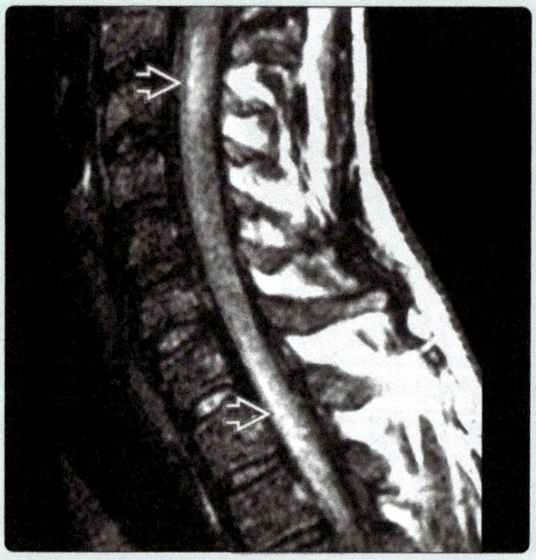
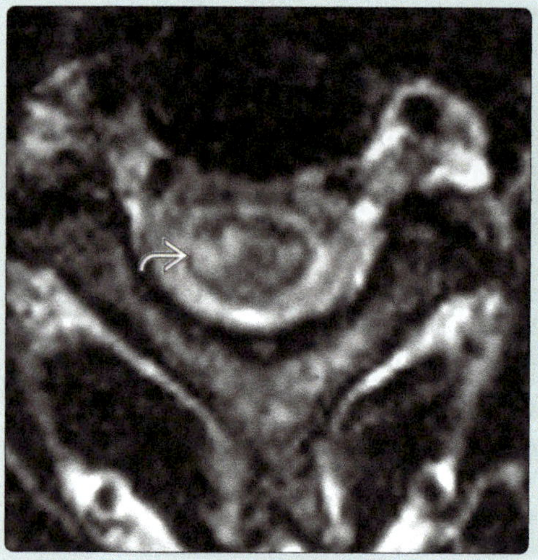

(Left) *High signal intensity abnormalities are seen in the cervical spinal cord on sagittal FLAIR MR. The cord is not swollen. The findings are consistent with HIV-related changes in the spinal cord.* **(Right)** *Axial T2WI MR demonstrates hyperintense signal in the right hemicord. The cord is not swollen. No enhancement was observed on postcontrast T1WI (not shown). The findings are consistent with HIV-related changes in the spinal cord.*

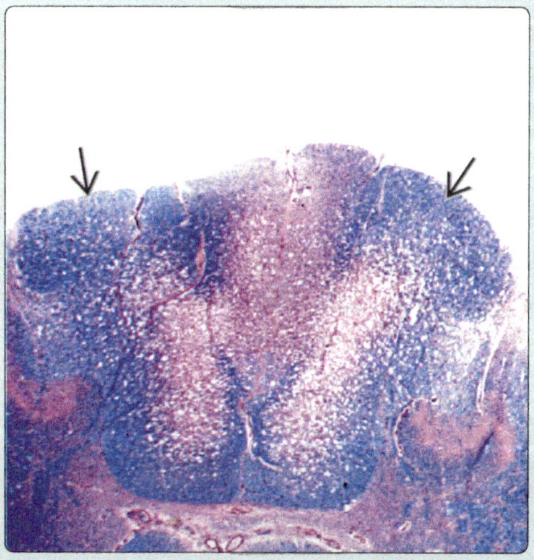
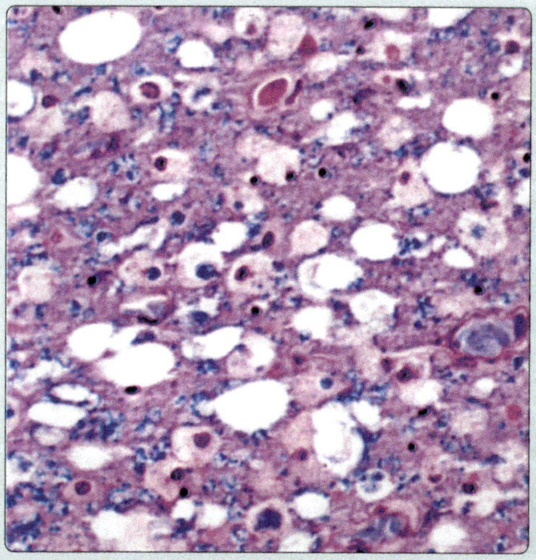

(Left) *Micropathology, low power with Luxol fast blue stain, shows extensive spongiform changes within white matter from vacuolar myelopathy. Disease of cord and brain often occur separately, suggesting different pathogenetic mechanisms. (Courtesy R. Schmidt, MD.)* **(Right)** *Micropathology, high power with Luxol fast blue stain, shows marked vacuolation within white matter from HIV myelopathy. (Courtesy R. Schmidt, MD.)*

KEY FACTS

TERMINOLOGY

- Infection in setting of immunocompromised state
  - HIV(+)
  - Chronic/systemic illness
  - Steroid therapy
  - Cancer ± chemotherapy

IMAGING

- Discitis/osteomyelitis → loss of disc height, bony endplate erosive changes
  - Enhancement of irregular adjacent endplates, blurring of dark cortical margin of endplates
- Epidural abscess/phlegmon → soft tissue in ventral/dorsal extradural space
  - Homogeneous enhancement of phlegmon
  - Rim enhancement of abscess
- Paraspinal abscess/phlegmon
- Infectious arachnoiditis → thickening, clumping of nerve roots
- Intramedullary abscess → peripherally enhancing intramedullary lesion

TOP DIFFERENTIAL DIAGNOSES

- Osteomyelitis, pyogenic
- Meningitis, spinal
- Acute disseminated encephalomyelitis, spinal cord
- Acute transverse myelitis, idiopathic

CLINICAL ISSUES

- Fever
- Back/neck pain
- Paraparesis
- Treatment targeted to pathogen

DIAGNOSTIC CHECKLIST

- Consider complete neuraxis imaging if immunocompromised patients develop neurologic symptoms

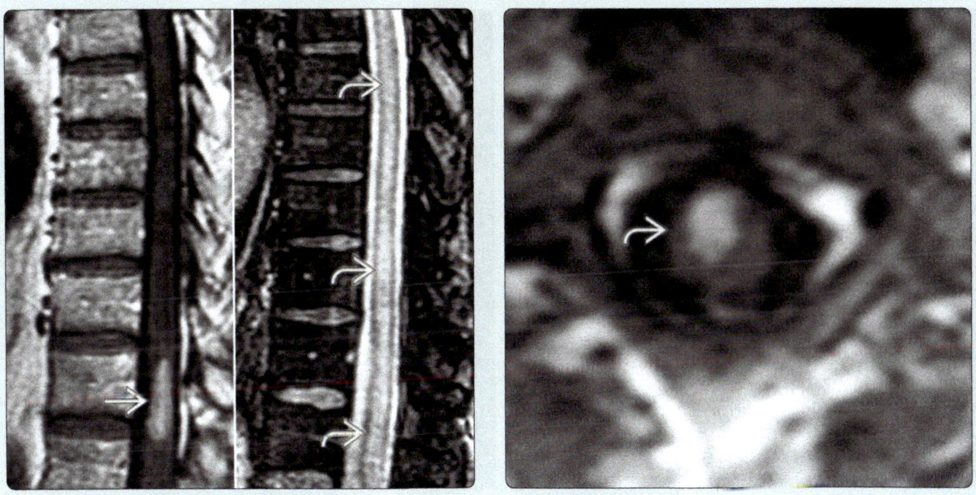

(Left) *Sagittal T1WI C+ MR (L) shows an intramedullary enhancement ➡ in the lower thoracic cord representing toxoplasma lesion. On the sagittal T2WI MR (R), abnormal hyperintense signal extends across multiple segments ⮫.* **(Right)** *Axial T1WI C+ MR demonstrates a nodular enhancing intramedullary lesion ⮫, which represents toxoplasma abscess of the spinal cord. The cord is slightly swollen. Spinal toxoplasmosis has only been described in HIV patients with simultaneously present cerebral toxoplasmosis.*

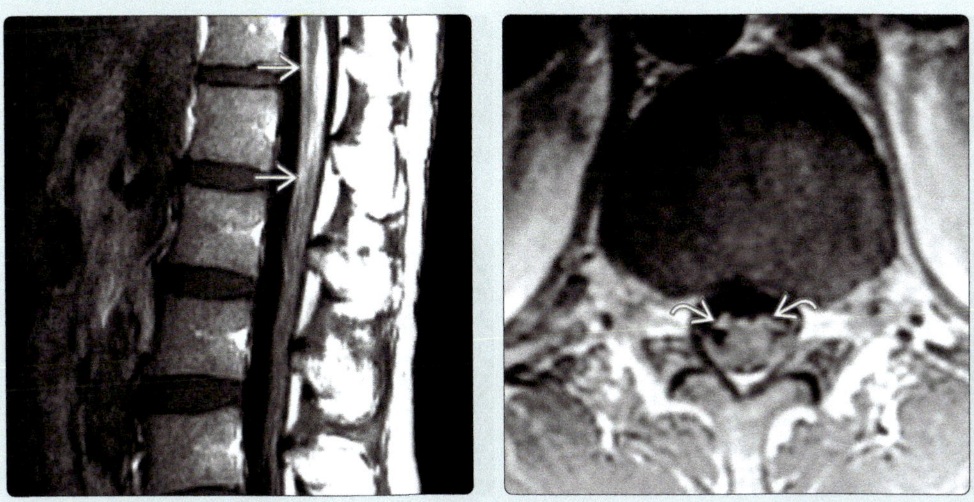

(Left) *Sagittal T1WI C+ MR in this case of CMV polyradiculopathy illustrates mild thickening of the proximal cauda equina and avid pial and cauda equina enhancement ➡.* **(Right)** *Axial T1WI C+ MR depicts diffuse cauda enhancement due to CMV radiculitis ⮫. The multiple root involvement with relatively smooth enhancement suggests CMV infection. Cerebrospinal fluid spread of tumor, lymphoma, and pyogenic meningitis can give a similar pattern but tends to be more nodular.*

Acute Transverse Myelopathy

KEY FACTS

TERMINOLOGY

- Noncompressive myelopathy
- Acute transverse myelopathy (ATM) is broad generic term encompassing heterogeneous group of disorders causing cord dysfunction
  - Etiologies include inflammatory causes (ATM) + vascular disease + radiation + paraneoplastic + idiopathic (unknown)
  - ATM is more specific term for cord dysfunction that is inflammatory in etiology
    - Inflammation defined by cerebrospinal fluid findings and MR enhancement

IMAGING

- Hyperintense lesion on T2WI with mild cord expansion ± enhancement
- Longitudinally extensive (3+ segments) = neuromyelitis optica (NMO), acute disseminated encephalomyelitis (ADEM), viral infection

TOP DIFFERENTIAL DIAGNOSES

- Inflammatory etiologies
  - Acquired demyelinating
    - Multiple sclerosis
    - NMO
    - ADEM
  - Parainfectious
  - Systemic autoimmune
  - Paraneoplastic (antineuronal immune disorder associated with cancer)
- Noninflammatory mimics
  - Radiation
  - Metabolic
  - Tumor and cysts
  - Vascular
    - Cord infarction
    - Dural fistula (type I arteriovenous fistula)
- Idiopathic ATM

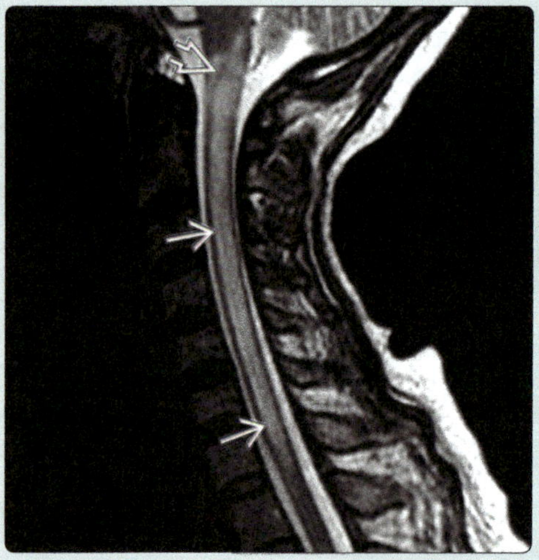
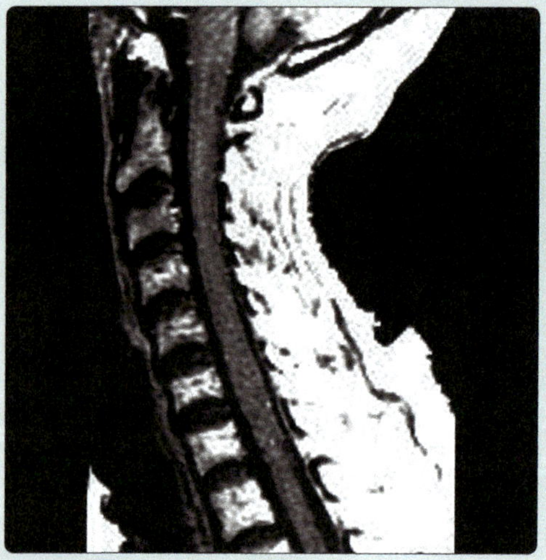

(Left) *Sagittal T2WI MR shows longitudinally extensive T2 hyperintensity throughout the cervical cord ➡ and lower medulla ➡. Differential diagnoses include neuromyelitis optica, acute disseminated encephalomyelitis, and parainfectious and systemic autoimmune disorders.* **(Right)** *Sagittal T1 C+ MR in the same patient does not demonstrate significant postgadolinium enhancement. The presence of longitudinally extensive abnormality in this patient suggests that MS is not the underlying abnormality.*

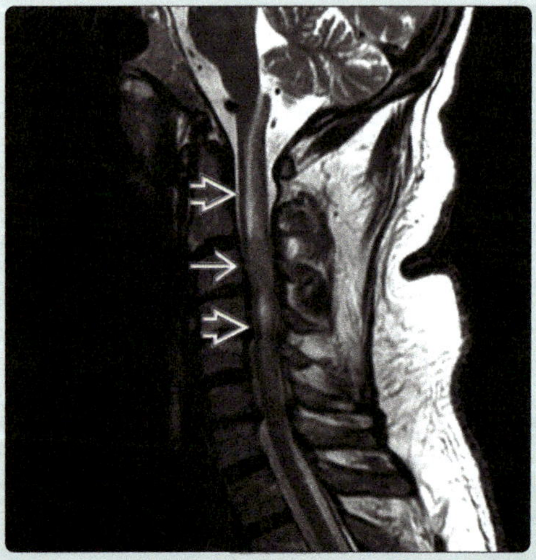
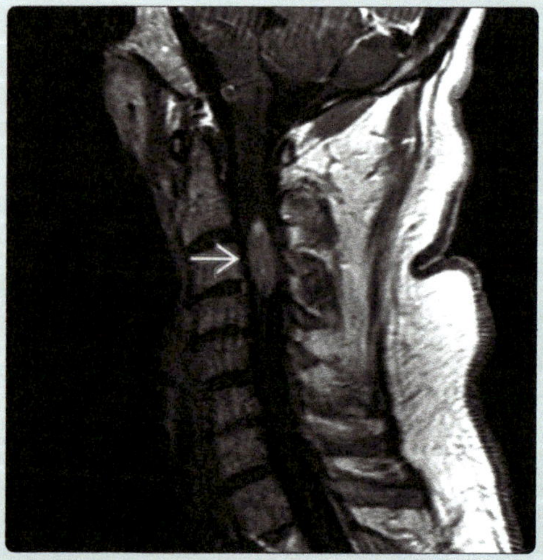

(Left) *Sagittal T2 TSE MR in this patient with lung cancer shows a focal mass at the C3 level ➡ with adjacent cord edema ➡ from a focal cord parenchymal metastasis.* **(Right)** *Sagittal T1 C+ MR shows enhancement of focal cord metastasis ➡ in this patient with lung carcinoma and worsening myelopathy.*

KEY FACTS

TERMINOLOGY

- Inflammatory disorder involving both halves of spinal cord, resulting in bilateral motor, sensory, and autonomic dysfunction

IMAGING

- Central cord expansile lesion > 2 vertebral segments in length ± variable eccentric enhancement

TOP DIFFERENTIAL DIAGNOSES

- Multiple sclerosis
- Neuromyelitis optica
- Spinal cord neoplasm
- Spinal cord infarction

PATHOLOGY

- Autoimmune phenomenon with formation of antigen-antibody complexes
- Small vessel vasculopathy → cord ischemia
- Associated demyelinating process

CLINICAL ISSUES

- Inclusion criteria
  - Sensory, motor, or autonomic dysfunction (including bowel/bladder involvement) attributable to spinal cord
  - Bilateral signs/symptoms with well-defined sensory level
  - Compressive etiology excluded by neuroimaging
  - Cord inflammation confirmed by cerebrospinal fluid pleocytosis, elevated IgG index, or gadolinium enhancement
- Exclusion criteria
  - History of spinal radiation within past 10 years
  - Cord ischemia/infarction, arteriovenous malformation
  - Connective tissue diseases
  - CNS infections, sarcoidosis, SLE, or Sjögren syndrome

DIAGNOSTIC CHECKLIST

- Central cord lesion > 2 vertebra in length, eccentric enhancement → consider acute transverse myelitis

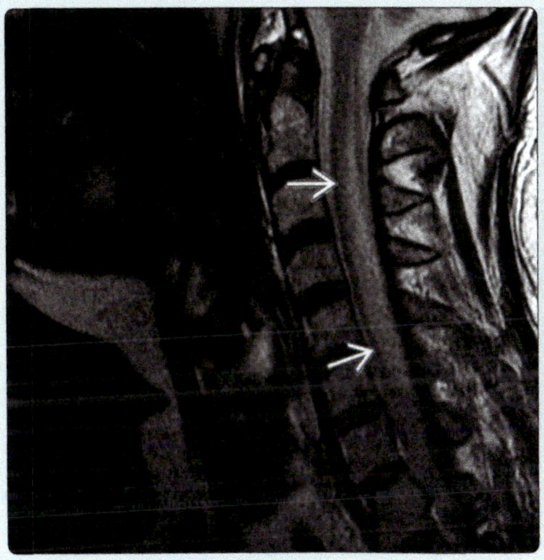

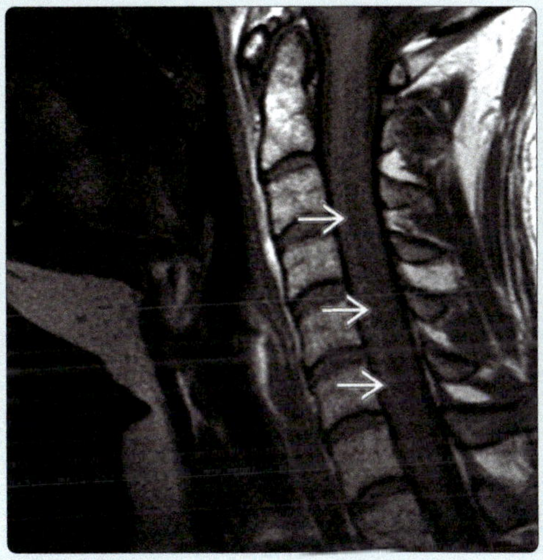

(Left) *Sagittal T2WI MR demonstrates mild, multilevel cervical cord expansion with confluent intramedullary T2 hyperintensity ➡ extending over 5 levels.* **(Right)** *Sagittal T1WI MR (same patient) reveals mild cervical cord expansion with subtle central intramedullary hypointensity ➡. Lesion extent on T1 MR is usually less conspicuous than on T2 MR.*

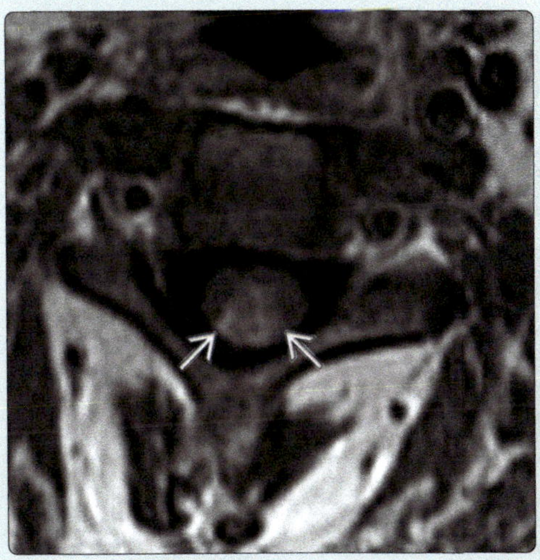

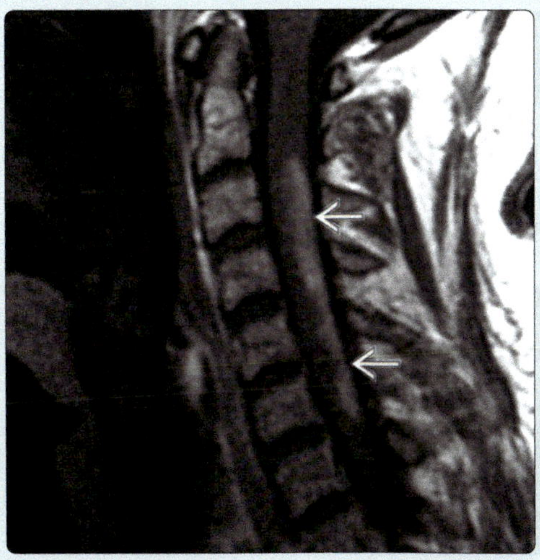

(Left) *Axial T1WI C+ MR (same patient) illustrates patchy, bilateral, central heterogeneous cervical spinal cord enhancement ➡ involving both gray and white matter.* **(Right)** *Sagittal T1WI C+ MR (same patient) confirms extensive parenchymal enhancement within the abnormal dorsal cervical spinal cord ➡.*

KEY FACTS

TERMINOLOGY

- Primary demyelinating disease of central nervous system with multiple lesions disseminated over time and space
  - Concomitant intracranial lesions in periventricular, subcallosal, brain stem, or cerebellar white matter

IMAGING

- Isolated spinal cord disease (10-20%)
- Cervical segment is most commonly affected
  - Dorsolateral aspect of cord
  - < 1/2 of cross-sectional area of spinal cord
  - < 2 vertebral segments in length
- Sagittal and axial T1WI & T2WI sequences with gadolinium
  - Lesions typically oval, peripheral, and asymmetric
  - Discrete vs. vague hyperintense lesions
  - Enhancement considered marker for active disease
    - Lasts 1-2 months (does not reflect disease progression)

TOP DIFFERENTIAL DIAGNOSES

- Intramedullary neoplasm
- Idiopathic transverse myelitis
- Neuromyelitis optica

PATHOLOGY

- Autoimmune, cell-mediated inflammatory process focused on CNS myelin

CLINICAL ISSUES

- Peak onset: 20-40 years
- Clinical types
  - Relapsing remitting (most common)
    - Can present with focal sensory or motor deficits, imbalance, vision changes, other neurologic impairment
  - Secondary progressive
  - Primary progressive
  - Progressive relapsing

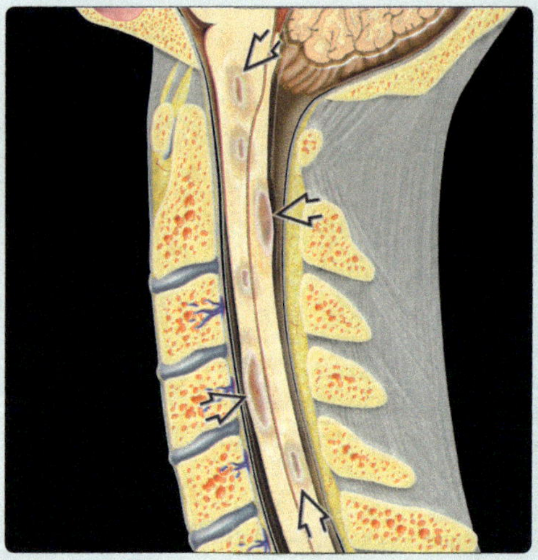

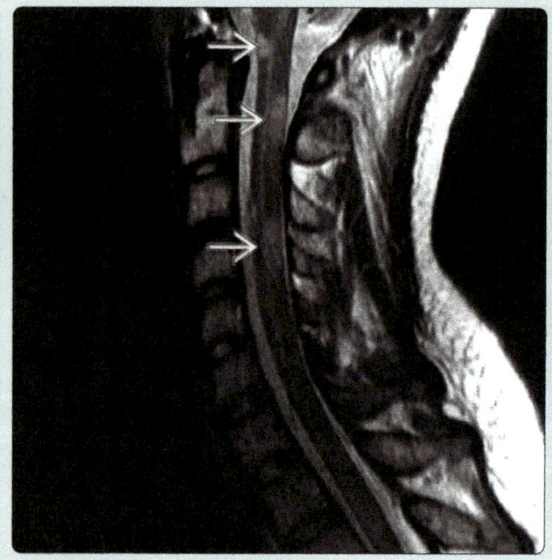

(Left) *Sagittal graphic depicts multiple demyelinating plaques ⇨ within the cervical spinal cord.* **(Right)** *Sagittal T2WI MR of the cervical spinal cord demonstrates multiple T2 hyperintense foci ➡, some well defined and others ill defined. The multiplicity of lesions and lack of edema or significant cord expansion is typical for demyelinating disease.*

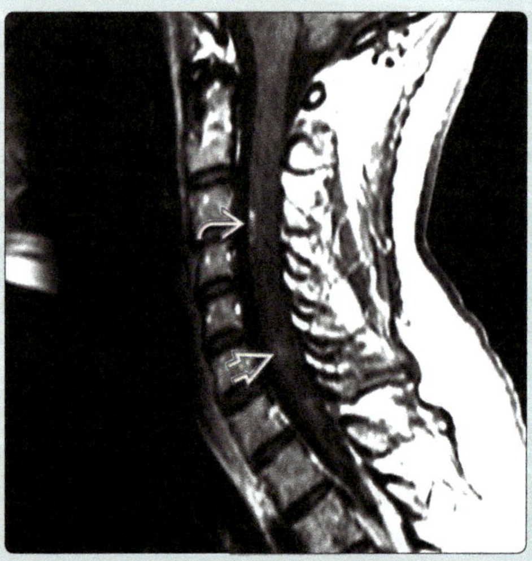

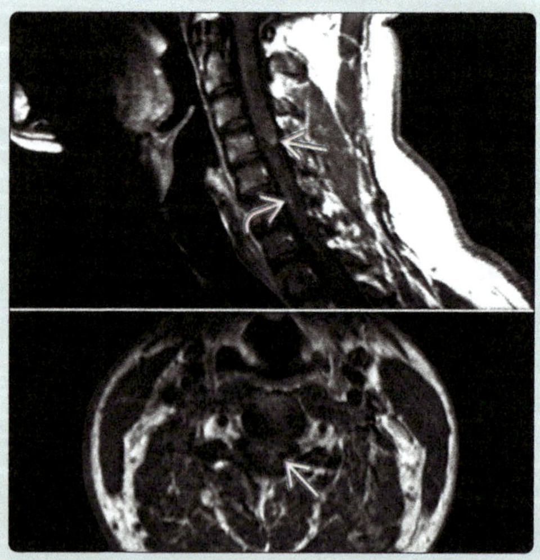

(Left) *Sagittal T1WI C+ MR shows multiple enhancing demyelinating lesions within the cervical spinal cord. Enhancement varies from focal ↪ to ill defined ⇨. The enhancement pattern changes with evolution of inflammation.* **(Right)** *T1WI C+ MR (sagittal on top, axial on bottom) illustrates an incomplete rim-enhancing lesion ➡ in the dorsal cervical cord at the C3-C4 level. A 2nd small enhancing focus is noted in the ventral cord at the C6 level ↪.*

KEY FACTS

TERMINOLOGY

- Synonyms: Devic disease, optic-spinal multiple sclerosis
- Definition: Autoimmune inflammatory disorder involving myelin of neurons of optic nerves and spinal cord, with limited brain parenchymal involvement

IMAGING

- Longitudinally extensive (> 3 vertebral segments) T2 hyperintensity within cord + enhancement of optic nerves (85% of cases)
- T2 abnormality tends to involve entire cross section of cord, unlike more focal involvement of MS

TOP DIFFERENTIAL DIAGNOSES

- Inflammatory etiologies
    - Multiple sclerosis
    - Acute disseminated encephalomyelitis (ADEM)
    - Parainfectious myelitis (viral, bacterial)
- Systemic autoimmune disease
- Noninflammatory mimics (dural arteriovenous fistula, neoplasm)
- Idiopathic acute transverse myelitis (diagnosis of exclusion)

PATHOLOGY

- Autoimmune disease targeting water channel proteins (aquaporin-4)

CLINICAL ISSUES

- **Revised diagnostic criteria (2006)**
    - Optic neuritis (ON), myelitis, and at least 2 of 3 supportive criteria
        - Contiguous cord lesion 3 or more segments in length, initial brain MR nondiagnostic for MS, or neuromyelitis optica (NMO)-IgG seropositivity

DIAGNOSTIC CHECKLIST

- Simultaneous ON and myelitis → NMO cannot be distinguished from ADEM at 1st attack

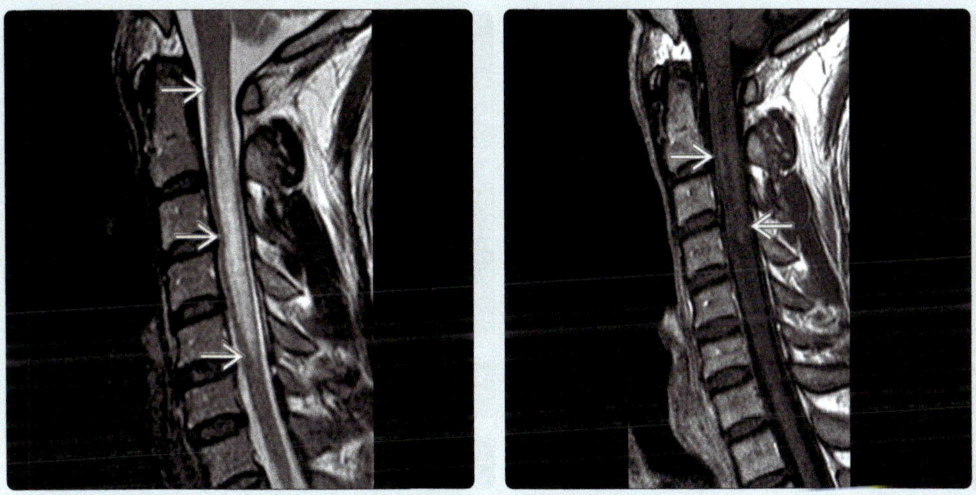

(Left) *Sagittal T2WI MR shows a long segment of cord enlargement with T2 hyperintensity* ➡. **(Right)** *Sagittal T1WI C+ MR shows cord enlargement and ill-defined enhancement* ➡. *Neuromyelitis optica (NMO) is an autoimmune disease possibly targeting the aquaporin-4 transmembrane water channel. The vasculocentric distribution of antigen of NMO-IgG correlates with the sites of immunoglobulin and complements deposition seen in spinal cord lesions of patients with NMO.*

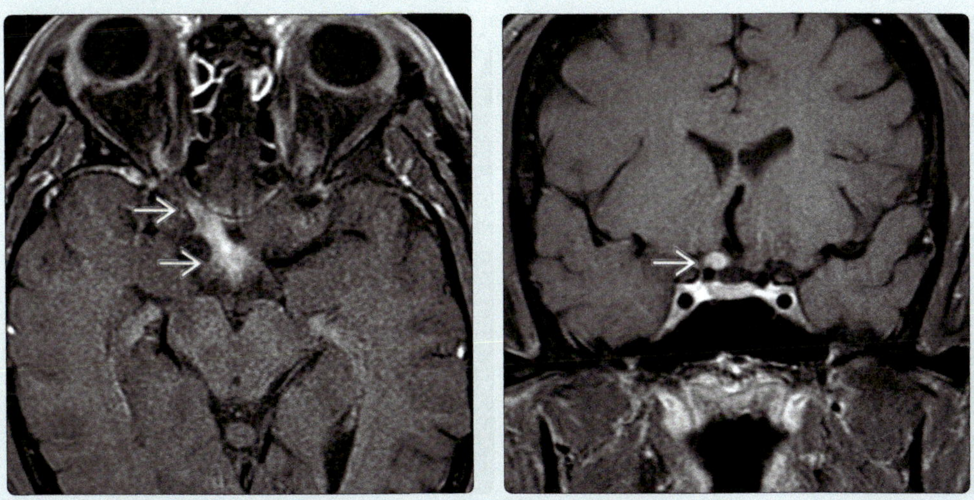

(Left) *Axial T1WI C+ FS MR reveals intense enhancement and mild enlargement of the intracanalicular and prechiasmatic segments of the right optic nerve* ➡. **(Right)** *Coronal T1WI C+ FS MR reveals intense enhancement and mild enlargement of the intracanalicular and prechiasmatic segments of the right optic nerve* ➡. *This is the classic appearance of Devic disease involving the optic nerves and spinal cord, with no brain parenchymal abnormalities.*

KEY FACTS

TERMINOLOGY

- Para-/postinfectious immune-mediated inflammatory disorder of white matter (WM)
  - Antibodies to pathogens exhibit cross-immunoreactivity with myelin basic protein

IMAGING

- Multifocal short-segment WM lesions with relatively little mass effect or vasogenic edema
  - Flame-shaped lesions with slight cord swelling
  - Dorsal white matter more voluminous
  - May see gray matter involvement
  - Variable enhancement, depending on stage of disease
  - May see nerve enhancement
- Brain almost always involved

TOP DIFFERENTIAL DIAGNOSES

- Inflammatory etiologies
  - Acquired demyelinating
    - Multiple sclerosis
    - Neuromyelitis optica
  - Parainfectious myelitis
  - Systemic autoimmune (vasculitis)
- Noninflammatory mimics
  - Vascular malformation
  - Infarction, spinal cord
  - Tumor and cysts
- Idiopathic acute transverse myelitis

CLINICAL ISSUES

- Typically monophasic illness lasting from 2-4 weeks
  - Encephalopathy, paresis
- Typically childhood or young adult
- Rx: High-dose corticosteroids (acute)

DIAGNOSTIC CHECKLIST

- Delay between clinical onset, appearance of imaging findings common, so rescan if initial study is negative

(Left) *Sagittal T1WI C+ MR shows linear enhancement along the dorsal surface of the midcervical cord* ➡*. Acutely, there is perivenous edema, demyelination, and infiltration with macrophages and lymphocytes, with relative axonal sparing. The late course of the disease is characterized by perivascular gliosis.* **(Right)** *Axial T2WI MR depicts a hyperintense focus in the right hemicord* ➡ *with minimal cord enlargement. ADEM is a postinfectious disease mediated by autoreactive cells or molecules.*

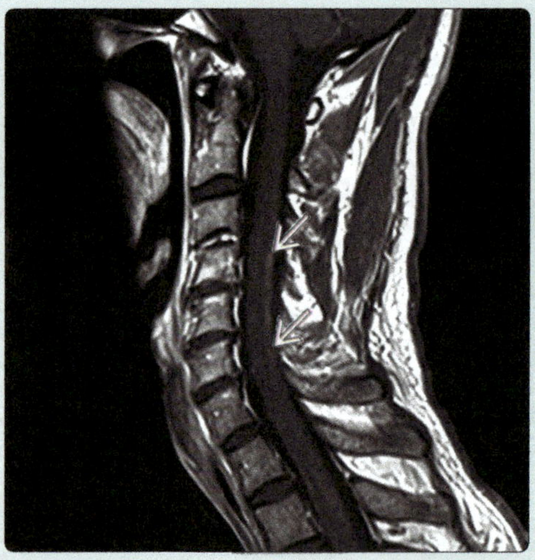

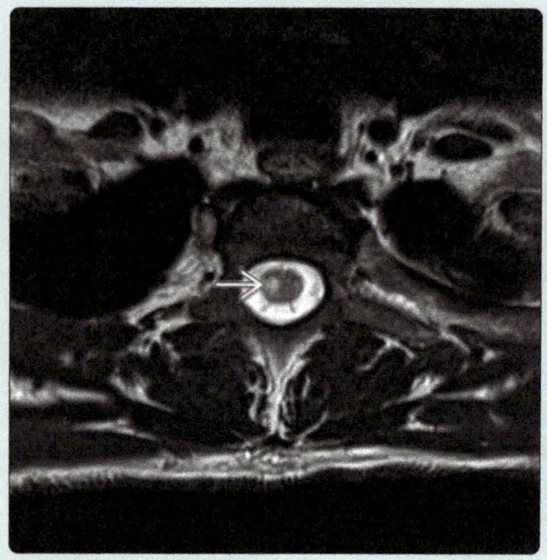

(Left) *Sagittal T2WI MR demonstrates a vague intramedullary focus of hyperintensity* ➡*. There is mild cord expansion.* **(Right)** *Sagittal T1WI C+ MR illustrates an ovoid intramedullary focus of enhancement in the upper thoracic cord* ➡*.*

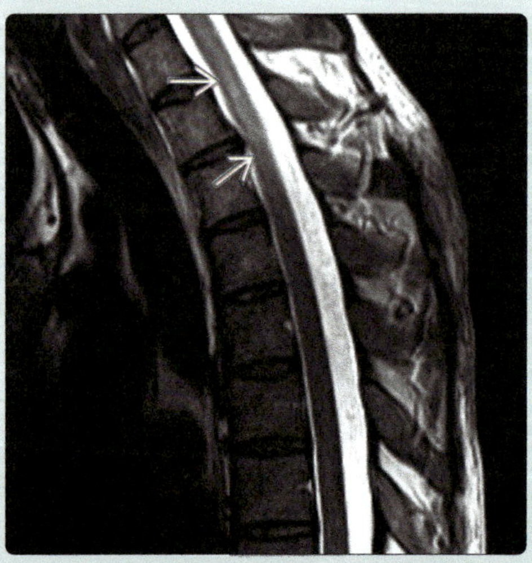

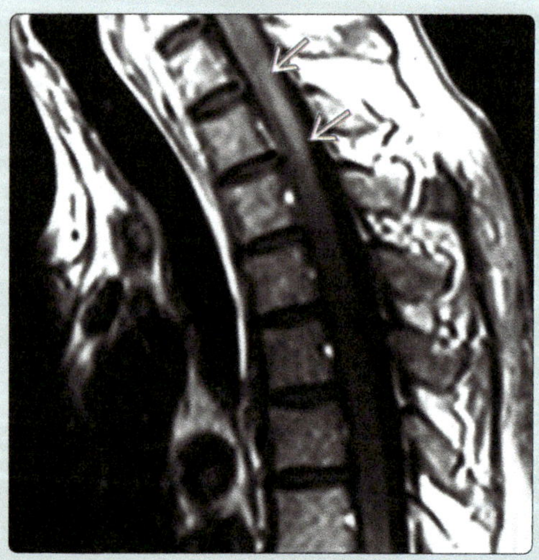

Acute Inflammatory Demyelinating Polyradiculoneuropathy (AIDP)

KEY FACTS

TERMINOLOGY

- Acute inflammatory demyelinating polyradiculoneuropathy (AIDP)
  - a.k.a. Guillain-Barré syndrome (GBS)
- Autoimmune postinfectious or postvaccinial acute inflammatory demyelination of peripheral nerves, nerve roots, cranial nerves

IMAGING

- Smooth pial enhancement of cauda equina and conus medullaris
  - Nerve roots often slightly enlarged
  - Conus not enlarged
- Axial T1WI C+ MR shows preferential contrast accentuation of ventral roots in cauda

TOP DIFFERENTIAL DIAGNOSES

- Miller-Fischer syndrome
- Chronic polyneuropathies
  - Subacute inflammatory demyelinating polyradiculoneuropathy
  - Chronic inflammatory demyelinating polyradiculoneuropathy
  - Hereditary polyneuropathies
- Carcinomatous or lymphomatous meningitis
- Anterior lumbar radiculopathy

PATHOLOGY

- Antecedent event or "trigger" in 70% of GBS cases
  - Usually follows recent viral illness

CLINICAL ISSUES

- Classically presents with "ascending paralysis"
  - If ascends to brainstem, may involve cranial nerves, require ventilator
  - Sensory loss common but less severe
- Cerebrospinal fluid shows albuminocytologic dissociation (↑ protein in absence of elevated WBCs)

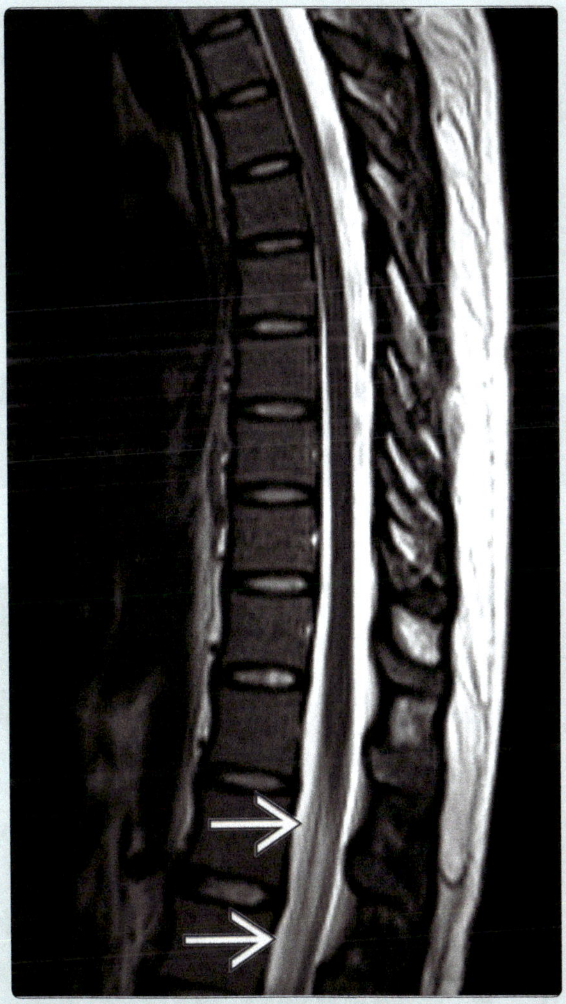

Sagittal T2WI MR in a Guillain-Barré syndrome patient reveals thickened cauda equina ➡. The conus has a normal morphology and exhibits normal signal intensities. Elevated antiganglioside antibody titer confirmed Guillain-Barré syndrome.

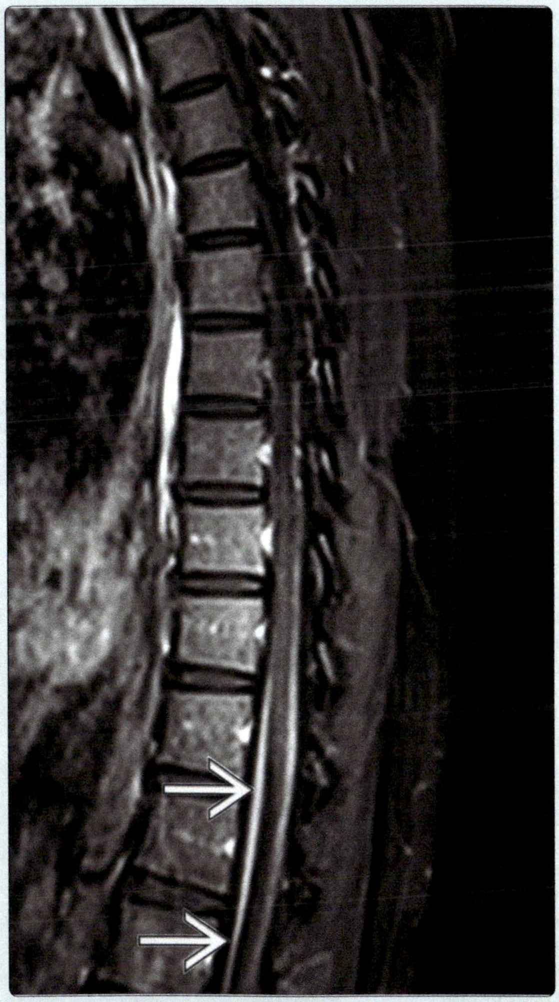

Sagittal T1WI C+ FS MR demonstrates smooth linear cauda equina thickening and enhancement ➡. This patient presented with typical acute onset of weakness and areflexia of the distal extremities.

Chronic Inflammatory Demyelinating Polyneuropathy (CIDP)

KEY FACTS

TERMINOLOGY

- Clinically heterogeneous, grossly symmetric, sensory and motor neuropathy evolving as monophasic, relapsing, or progressive disorder
  - Develops over > 8 weeks

IMAGING

- Enlargement and abnormal T2 hyperintensity of nerve roots, plexi, or peripheral nerves
- Spinal nerve roots and peripheral nerves (extraforaminal > intradural)
- Lumbar > cervical, brachial plexus, thoracic/intercostal > cranial nerve

TOP DIFFERENTIAL DIAGNOSES

- Guillain-Barré (acute inflammatory demyelinating polyneuropathy)
- Inherited demyelinating neuropathy
- Neurofibromatosis type 1

PATHOLOGY

- Autoimmune disease involving cellular and humoral immunity
- Hallmarks of chronic inflammatory demyelinating polyneuropathy (CIDP): Enlarged nerves with "onion bulb" formations, demyelination

CLINICAL ISSUES

- Diagnosis relies primarily on clinical, electrophysiologic examination supplemented by nerve biopsy
- Typical presentation
  - Progressive weakness/sensory loss in distal and proximal segments of 4 limbs with areflexia
  - Evolves over > 8 weeks
  - ↑ cerebrospinal fluid protein, heterogeneous slowing of nerve conduction
  - Responds to corticosteroids and/or IV immunoglobulin therapy

(Left) *Axial T1WI C+ FS MR demonstrates symmetric enlargement, mild enhancement of lumbar nerve roots ➡.* **(Right)** *Axial T2WI MR in same patient shows mild enlargement & iso- to hyperintensity of bilateral lumbar nerves ➡.*

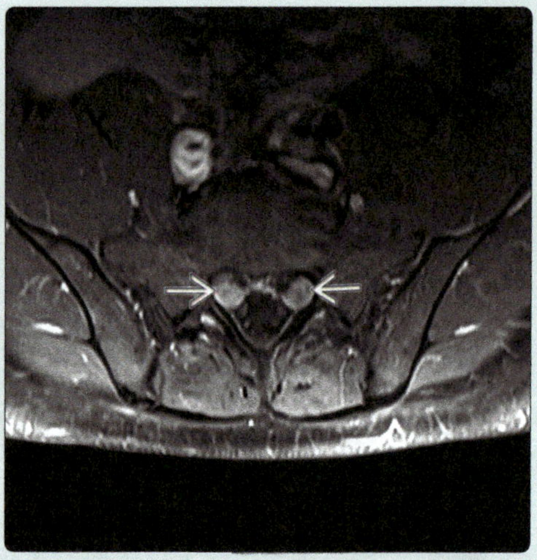

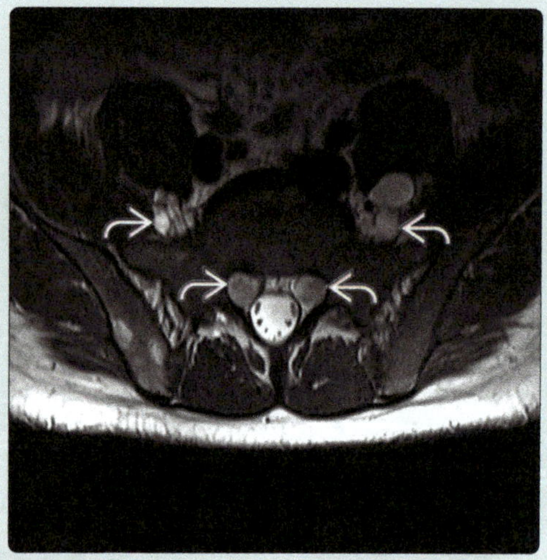

(Left) *Sagittal T2WI in the same case reveals enlargement, abnormal T2 hyperintensity of the exiting extradural lumbosacral nerves ➡.* **(Right)** *Axial T2WI in the same case shows enlargement, abnormal T2 hyperintensity of the exiting extradural lumbosacral nerves ➡. Imaging and associated progressive motor and sensory deficits with increased CSF protein content, electrophysiological features of demyelination, are characteristic of CIDP.*

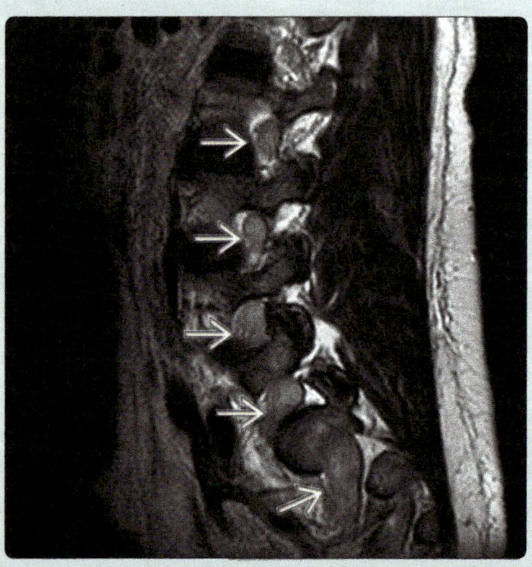

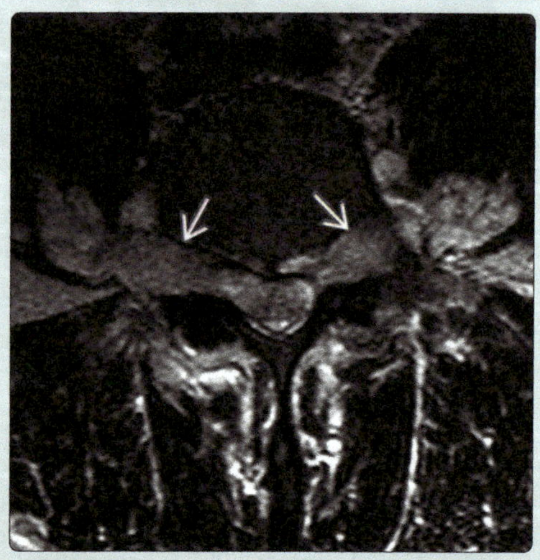

KEY FACTS

TERMINOLOGY

- Neurosarcoidosis
- Noncaseating granulomatous disease of spine and spinal cord

IMAGING

- Combination of leptomeningeal and peripheral intramedullary mass-like enhancement suggestive of spinal sarcoidosis
- Intramedullary
  - Fusiform cord enlargement
  - Enhancing intramedullary masses
  - Focal or diffuse T2-hyperintense lesions
- Intradural extramedullary
  - Leptomeningeal enhancement
  - Dural masses
- Extradural
  - CT/radiographs: Sclerotic or mixed lytic and sclerotic lesions
- Intracranial (look at brain on sagittal cervical spine scans!)
  - Frequently affects meninges, especially near base of brain
  - Cranial nerves often involved

TOP DIFFERENTIAL DIAGNOSES

- Intramedullary neoplasm
- Idiopathic transverse myelitis
- Lymphoma
- Intradural metastases
- Multiple sclerosis

CLINICAL ISSUES

- Clinical CNS involvement in patients with sarcoidosis (5%)
  - Spinal intramedullary sarcoidosis (< 1%)
- Lower extremity weakness, paresthesia
- Bladder and bowel dysfunction
- Treatment: Intravenous ± oral corticosteroids
  - Immunosuppressive therapy

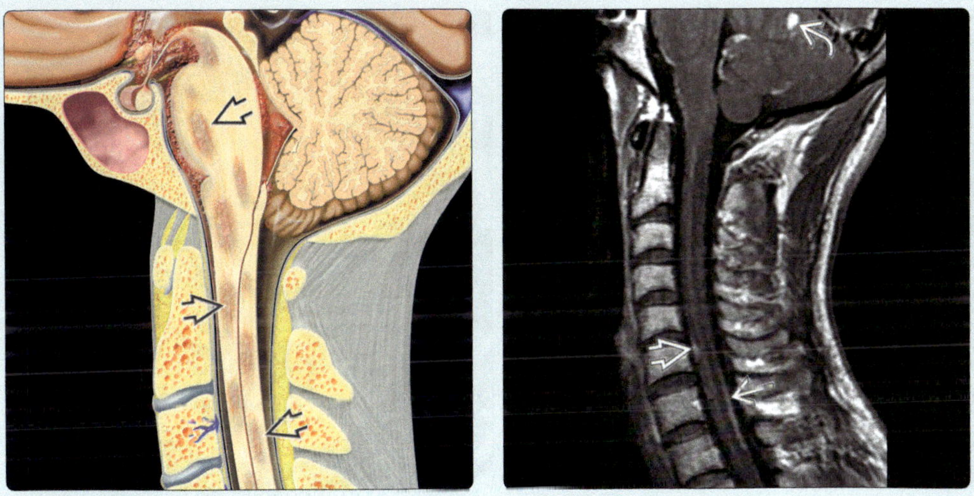

(Left) *Graphic depicts multiple intramedullary sarcoid granulomas ⇨ in brainstem and upper cervical cord. The intramedullary, intradural extramedullary, and extradural regions can be involved. Rare findings, such as calcifications and cyst formation, have also been described.* **(Right)** *Sagittal T1WI C+ MR demonstrates diffuse linear leptomeningeal enhancement ➔ with areas of more focal nodularity ⇨. Note the intracranial involvement ➔. Bulky leptomeningeal disease is unusual with neurosarcoidosis.*

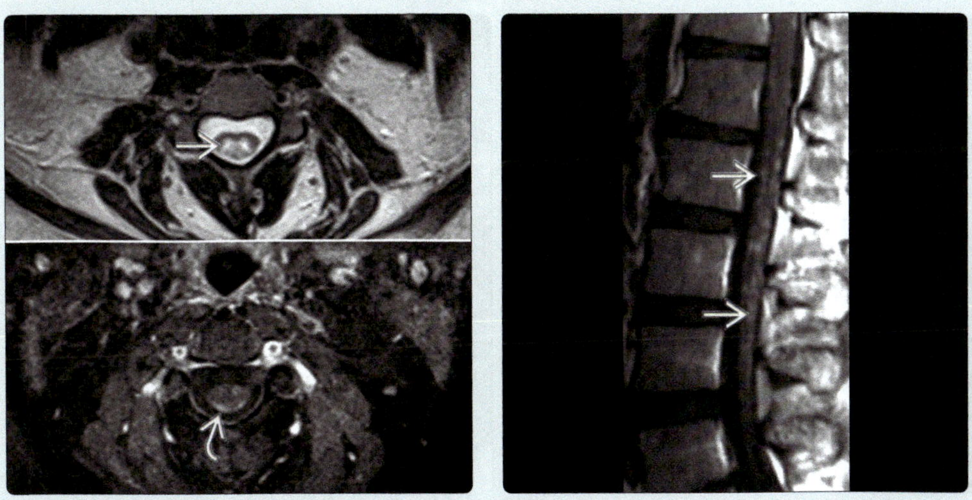

(Left) *Axial T2WI MR (top) shows intramedullary hyperintensity ➔. Axial T2WI MR (bottom) reveals irregular leptomeningeal enhancement along the cord ➔.* **(Right)** *Sagittal T1WI C+ MR of the lumbar spine exhibits multiple enhancing subarachnoid nodules ➔ interspersed among the cauda equina. Intradural extramedullary lesions are usually represented by leptomeningeal sarcoidosis infiltration, present in up to 60% of spinal cord lesions.*

Subacute Combined Degeneration

KEY FACTS

TERMINOLOGY

- Vitamin B12 deficiency produces selective degeneration of dorsal ± lateral spinal cord columns

IMAGING

- Longitudinal dorsal cord T2 signal abnormality
- Axial image → "inverted V" or "inverted rabbit ears" within dorsal spinal cord
- ± mild dorsal column enhancement

TOP DIFFERENTIAL DIAGNOSES

- Infectious myelitis
  - HIV vacuolar myelopathy
  - Varicella-Zoster/herpes
- Inflammatory demyelination
  - Multiple sclerosis
  - Acute disseminated encephalomyelitis
- Acute transverse myelitis
  - Acute presentation → diffuse multisegmental cord hyperintensity, swelling
- Infarction, spinal cord
  - Hyperacute presentation
- Copper deficiency, zinc toxicity (may look identical)

PATHOLOGY

- Malabsorption (most common)
  - Metabolic conditions: Copper deficiency, nitrous oxide anesthesia susceptibility, transcobalamin II deficiency

CLINICAL ISSUES

- Paraesthesia, stiffness, mild sensory ataxia, loss of position and vibration sense, spasticity, hyperreflexia
- Degree of resolution of clinical symptoms is inversely proportional to their duration and severity

DIAGNOSTIC CHECKLIST

- Neurologic findings may precede anemia and may not completely resolve following treatment

(Left) *Graphic shows dorsal column demyelination secondary to vitamin B12 deficiency. Major clinical findings of dysesthesia, gait disturbance, and impairment of position and vibration sense in the lower ± upper limbs are secondary to dorsal column, lateral corticospinal tract, and sometimes lateral spinothalamic tract dysfunction.* **(Right)** *Axial T2WI MR reveals T2 hyperintensity confined to the dorsal columns in an "inverted V" configuration, characteristic of B12 deficiency.*

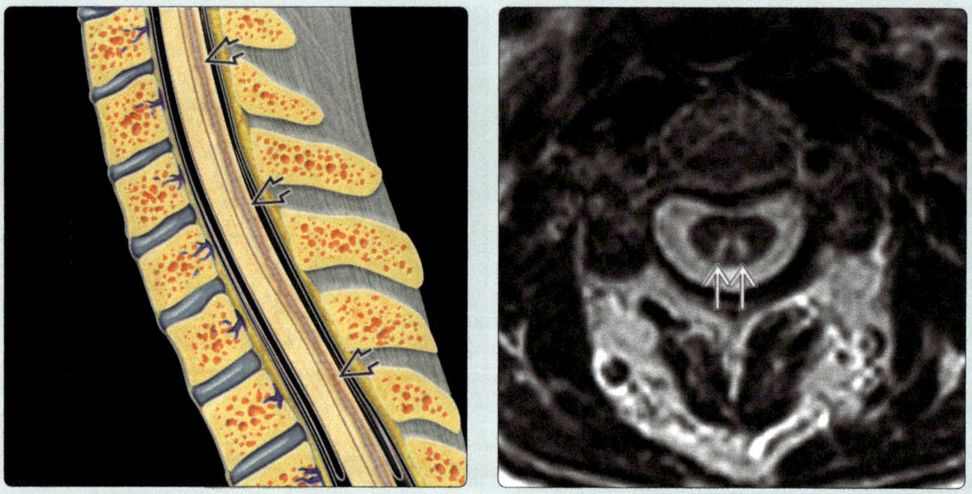

(Left) *Sagittal T1WI C+ MR reveals vague dorsal intramedullary enhancement. Lack of cobalamin (required as a cofactor for conversion of methylmalonyl-CoA to succinyl-CoA) leads to accumulation of methylmalonyl-CoA, causing ↓ in normal myelin synthesis and incorporation of abnormal fatty acids into neuronal lipids.* **(Right)** *Axial MR reveals patchy enhancement in bilateral dorsal columns, which reflects breakdown of the blood-cord barrier caused by perivascular demyelination and inflammation.*

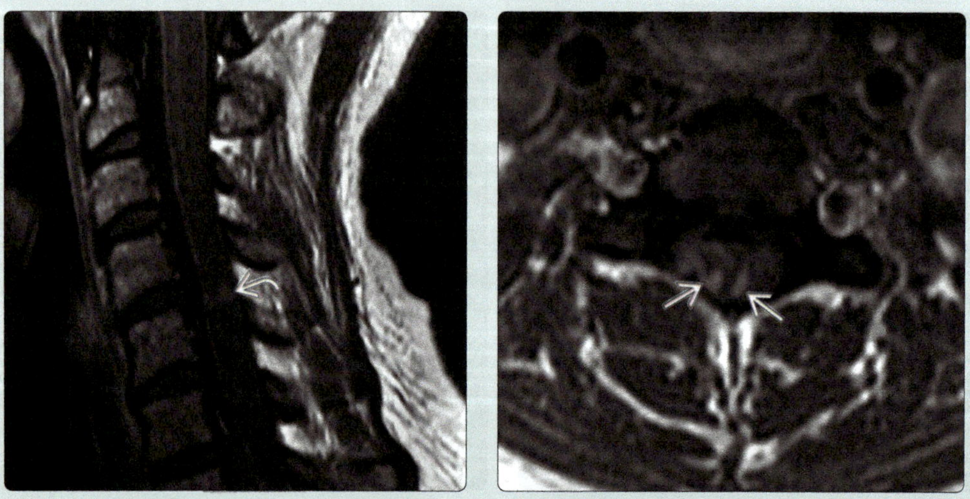

KEY FACTS

TERMINOLOGY

- Paraneoplastic neurologic disorder
- Antineuronal immune mechanism targeting CNS, occurring in conjunction with cancer

IMAGING

- Longitudinally extensive, symmetric, tract-specific signal changes within spinal cord that often enhance after gadolinium administration in patient with cancer
- Signal abnormality in ~ 70% of cases
- Lateral, dorsal columns
- Central gray matter

TOP DIFFERENTIAL DIAGNOSES

- Cord infarction
- Neuromyelitis optica
- B12 deficiency (subacute combined degeneration)
- Metastatic disease
- Neurosarcoidosis

PATHOLOGY

- Paraneoplastic disease usually
  - Antibodies against intracellular antigens
  - Older individuals, resistant to treatment
  - Mediated by T-cell mechanisms
- Most common with **lung** and **breast** cancer
- Most common antibodies causing myelopathy
  - Amphiphysin-IgG
  - Collapsin response-mediator protein-5

CLINICAL ISSUES

- Insidiously progressive myelopathy
- Often manifesting before detection of underlying cancer (2/3 of patients)
  - Median of 12 months from myelopathy onset to cancer detection
- Poor prognosis, often becoming wheelchair dependent

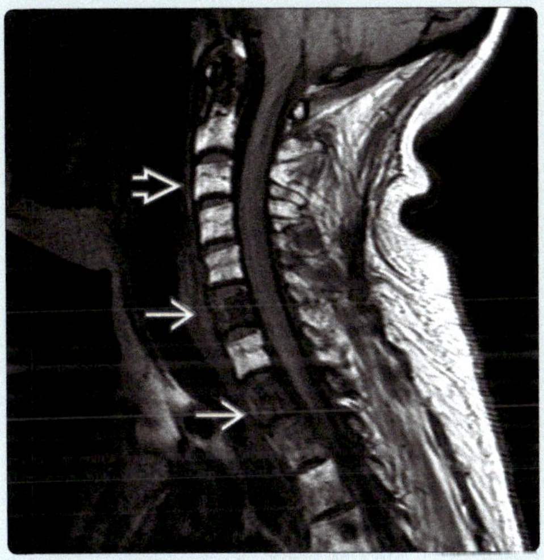
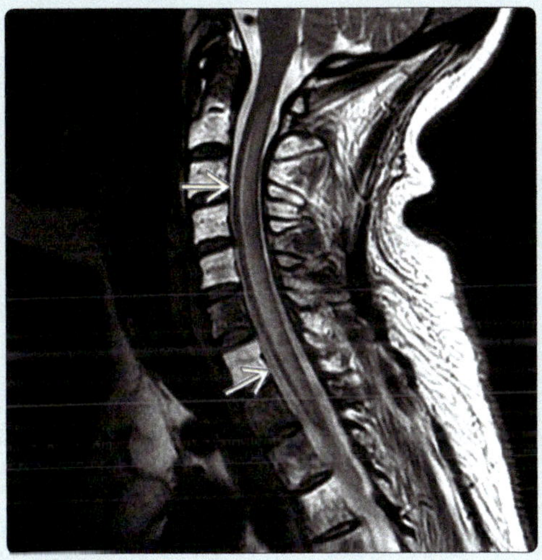

(Left) *Sagittal T1 MR shows multiple metastatic lesions ➡ involving the cervical and upper thoracic vertebral bodies, with marrow conversion from prior radiation therapy ➡. The cord is mildly expanded.* **(Right)** *Sagittal T2 MR in the same patient shows longitudinally extensive high signal within the cervical cord, with mild cord expansion ➡. This edema pattern is nonspecific, and cord metastases and radiation change should also be considered.*

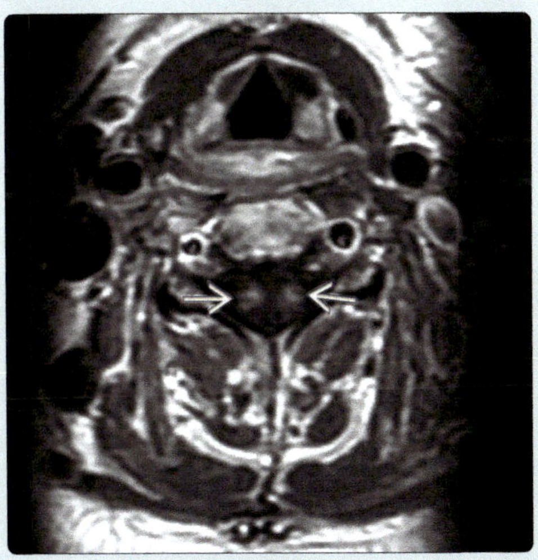
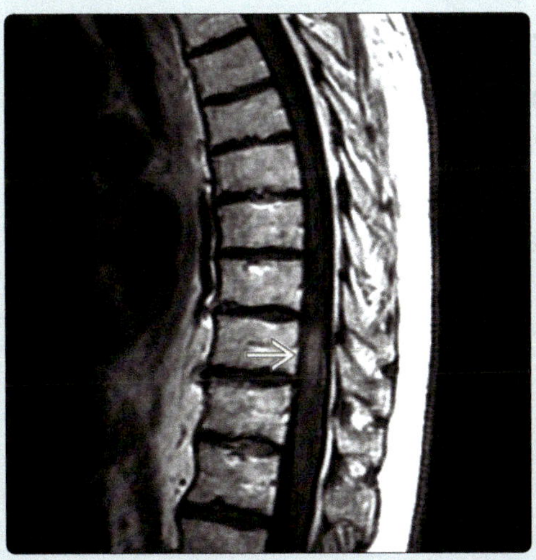

(Left) *Axial T1 C+ MR in the same patient shows the typical pattern of paraneoplastic myelopathy with focal central tract enhancement ➡ in a symmetrical fashion. This symmetrical tract involvement would not be seen with metastases or radiation change.* **(Right)** *Sagittal T1 C+ MR in a patient with a focal cord metastasis ➡ shows the very localized nature of the tumor to be contrasted, with the longitudinally extensive abnormality with paraneoplastic disease of the cord.*

PART II: SPINE
SECTION 5

Neoplasms, Cysts, and Other Masses

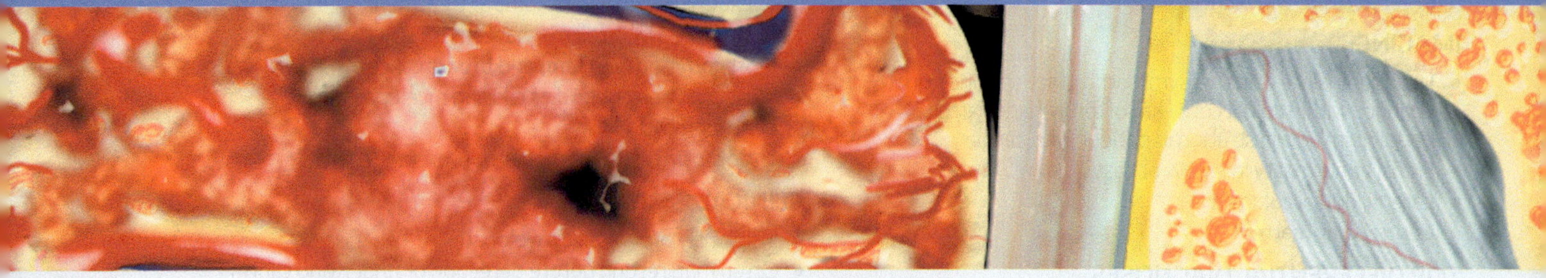

Neoplasms

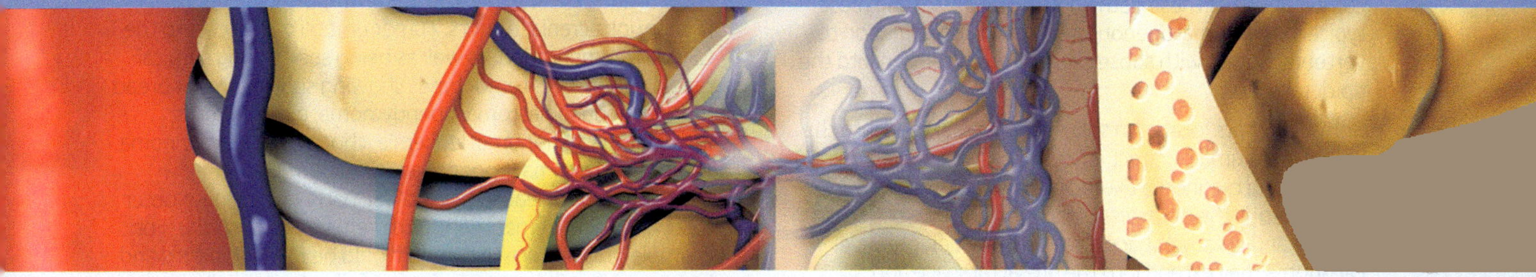

Nonneoplastic Cysts and Tumor Mimics

Vascular and Systemic Disorders

Anatomy-Based Imaging Issues

Neoplasms affecting the spine may spread by direct extension via the lymphatic system, the hematogenous route, or along the cerebrospinal fluid (CSF) pathways. There can also be combinations of these pathways involved, with the most typical being hematogenous metastatic dissemination to vertebral bodies with subsequent direct extension into the epidural space.

Primary tumors located in soft tissues may extend into the vertebral column by direct extension. An example would include lung carcinoma extending into the chest wall and subsequently the paravertebral region and into the spinal column and epidural space. Prostate, bladder, or bowel carcinoma may extend into the presacral space and subsequently into the vertebral column and epidural space. Nasopharyngeal carcinoma extends into the clivus and skull base and may track along the cranial nerves. In rare cases, there may be direct extension of a CNS tumor along the biopsy or surgical tract. There are also rare cases of CNS tumors extending through access via indwelling shunt tubing to give systemic metastases. Findings of direct extension of neoplasm in the spine consist of a soft tissue mass with adjacent bone destruction and variable neural compromise. Direct extension of neoplasm into the epidural space is more likely from vertebral body through the posterior longitudinal ligament. The anterior longitudinal ligament and disc are relatively resistant to tumor invasion. The anterior longitudinal ligament is stronger than the posterior longitudinal ligament and has fewer perforating vessels. Once the tumor has access into the epidural space, it comes against the tough dura, which is an effective barrier to tumor penetration. These barriers result in the distinguishing features between a disc space infection with adjacent vertebral osteomyelitis (with the epicenter at the level of the disc space) and neoplastic involvement (with the epicenter involving the vertebral bodies with sparing of the disc space). Direct extension of tumor may also be seen with a primary cord tumor within the cervical spine, with extension into the infratentorial space. Rarely, brainstem or cerebellar neoplasms may extend into the upper cervical cord.

Lymphatic spread is of limited importance in spine imaging relative to the more ubiquitous hematogenous spread. Local spread of pelvic tumors within the lumbar spine without pulmonary metastases would suggest venous or lymphatic route of extension.

Hematogenous spread is the major pathway of extension of malignant tumors to the axial skeleton. Batson plexus is a longitudinal network of valveless veins running parallel to the spinal column. These veins lie outside of the thoracoabdominal cavity and communicate with multiple aspects of the venous system, including vena cava, spinal, portal, azygos, intercostal, pulmonary, and renal veins. Flow direction in Batson plexus is variable due to the variable intrathoracic and intraabdominal pressures. Tumors in multiple anatomic sites could cause metastatic lesions along the course of the venous plexus without lung or liver involvement. Prostate carcinoma cells could seed vertebral bodies via Batson plexus and not necessarily extend into the vena cava. Breast carcinoma might also seed the vertebral bodies via the azygos system into Batson plexus. There is only 5-10% of portal blood flow that might shunt to Batson plexus, explaining the relatively low frequency of spinal metastatic lesions with GI and GU primaries. For the vast majority of spinal metastases, there may be no clear answer to the precise route to the end target. Homing properties of the tumor cells and receptive properties of the implantation site may be more important than any particular vascular route.

Spread along the CSF pathways is an important route for primary intracranial tumors. Tumor emboli gain access to the CSF via fragmentation, as well as being shed during surgical manipulation. CNS tumor types showing subarachnoid spread include medulloblastoma, ependymoma, pineal tumors, astrocytoma, lymphoma, leukemia, choroid plexus carcinoma, and retinoblastoma (poor prognosis with *MYCN* gene amplification). Spread along the CSF pathways can also occur following initial hematogenous dissemination of tumor. For example, this pattern of spread would be present in cord and leptomeningeal metastatic disease following the initial hematogenous dissemination in lung and breast metastatic disease.

Pathologic Issues

Forty percent of patients with cancer will develop visceral or bony metastases during their illness. The spinal column is the most common site of osseous metastases. Men are more frequently affected with vertebral metastases, with a male to female ratio of 3:2. Prostate, lung, and breast carcinomas account for the vast majority of spinal metastases. Locations are primarily thoracic (70%) > lumbar (20%) > cervical.

Primary tumors are generally composed of a variety of biologically different cells in regard to ultimate metastatic potential. Cells continually shed from the primary tumor and gain access to the circulatory system. Fewer than 0.01-0.10% of tumor cells survive to reach a distant site. Successful tumor spread requires completion of a complex pathway, including tumor separation from the primary source, access to blood, CSF, or lymphatic system, survival within the transport process, attachment to the endothelium of a distant vessel, exiting that vessel into the interstitial space, and finally developing the vascular supply at a distant site. The distant host environment site is a complex milieu. Multiple anatomic pathways may be involved with varying flow patterns within the veins and arteries.

Mechanisms of Tumorigenesis

Tumorigenesis in humans appears to be a multistep process. These steps reflect genetic alterations that drive progressive transformation of normal human cells into highly malignant versions. Cancers in humans have been shown to have an age-dependent incidence that implicates 4-7 rate-limiting, stochastic events. Tumor development proceeds via a succession of genetic changes, each conferring one or another type of growth advantage, which leads to the progressive conversion of normal human cells into cancer cells. By definition, cancer cells will have defects in regulatory circuits that govern cell proliferation and homeostasis. These defects have been categorized into 6 types of alterations in cell physiology: (1) Self-sufficiency in growth signals, (2) insensitivity to growth inhibitory signals, (3) evasion of programmed cell death (apoptosis), (4) limitless replicative potential, (5) sustained angiogenesis, and (6) tissue invasion and metastasis. Each of these 6 physiologic changes reflects the successful breaching of an anticancer defense mechanism that is hardwired into cells and tissues.

Normal cells require growth signals before they can move into an active proliferative state. The signals are transmitted to the cell via transmembrane receptors that bind a variety of signaling molecules, such as diffusible growth factors, extracellular matrix components, and cell-to-cell adhesion molecules (CAMs). Many cancer cells acquire the ability to synthesize growth factors to which they are responsive, which creates an abnormal positive feedback loop. Examples would be the production of platelet-derived growth factor by glioblastoma and tumor growth factor-α (TGF-α) by sarcomas. Epidermal growth factor receptor is upregulated in brain tumors.

Normal tissues have a variety of mechanisms that limit proliferation. The signals include both growth inhibitors and inhibitors within the extracellular matrix on the surface of adjacent cells. Many antiproliferative signals are channeled through the retinoblastoma tumor suppressor protein and its variations. Disruption of the retinoblastoma protein pathway will allow cell proliferation by rendering the cells insensitive to antigrowth factors by repressing the E2F transcription factors.

Evasion of programmed cell death (apoptosis) commonly occurs through mutations involving the *TP53* tumor suppressor gene. The inactivation of this *TP53* protein is seen in > 50% of human cancers.

Limitless replicative potential of cancer tumors is seen in cultures of tumor cells that have become immortalized. Normal human cell types in culture have a capacity for no more than 60-70 doublings. The ends of the chromosomes, telomeres, appear to be involved in this process. The erosion of the telomeres occurs through successive cycles of normal cell replication, causing them to lose their ability to protect the ends of the chromosome DNA. This leads to eventual cell crisis and cell death. In contrast, telomere maintenance is evident in all types of malignant cells. In cancer, telomeres are maintained at a length above some critical thresholds, which allows unlimited cell multiplication.

Abnormal angiogenesis is perhaps 1 of the more recognized aspects of abnormal cell physiology in cancer. Angiogenesis-promoting signals are classically seen with vascular endothelial growth factor and fibroblast growth factors. More than 2 dozen angiogenic-inducing factors are known, with a similar number of inhibiting-type proteins.

Metastatic Disease and Cell Motion

Tumor metastases are the cause of 90% of human cancer deaths. Tumor invasion and tumor metastases are very complex processes, with multiple genetic and biochemical factors. These can be described as tumor invasion, tumor cell dissemination through the blood stream or lymphatic system, colonization of distant organs, and outgrowth of the metastasis. Several classes of proteins are involved in tethering cells to their surroundings and are altered in invasion and metastases. CAMs and integrins are involved in this cell-to-cell regulatory signaling. The basement membrane is the first barrier tumor cells must breech. Receptors on the surface of cells recognize the glycoprotein of the basement membrane to which they attach. Attachment is followed by proteolysis of type IV collagen of the basement membrane by tumor-specific collagenase. Locomotion follows basement membrane lysis, with cells crossing that defective basement membrane with access to the interstitial space, lymphatics, and blood vessels. Chemoattractants can activate cell migration and invasion through activation of specific receptors and downstream intracellular signaling pathways. This appears to ultimately reorganize the actin cytoskeleton. Rho/Rac GTPases are well-known regulators of cytoskeletal organization. Rac activation induces membrane ruffles, adhesion complexes, and lamellipodia formation.

Tumor dissemination and cell motility occur along 3 different pathways including epithelial-to-mesenchymal transition (EMT), amoeboid transcription, and collective migration. In EMT, the cell elongates and degrades the local matrix by enzymes and migrates with pseudopodia-like projections. In amoeboid transcription, the cells become spherical and pass through gaps in the extracellular matrix. In collective migration, sheets or clusters of tumor cells migrate. EMT includes the downregulation of epithelial markers in tight junctions and cytokeratin filament network and upregulation of mesenchymal markers, like N-cadherin, vimentin, integrins, tenascin C, fibronectin, and fibroblast-specific protein 1. N-cadherin seems to be the most important of this group of markers. EMT can be controlled by intrinsic oncogenic activation like K-Ras mutation or HER2 overexpression. In some cancers, such as lung, the central role of EMT regulator belongs to TGF-β. TGF-β ultimately promotes EMT by regulating genes that control cell proliferation, apoptosis, differentiation, motility and migration.

Clinical Implications

Spine metastatic involvement presents with unrelenting back pain. Objective signs are uncommon or occur late in the disease (such as palpable mass and deformity). Back pain and weakness are a sign of epidural tumor extension. Due to spinothalamic tract crossing pattern, sensory levels may be 1-2 segments below the site of compression. Sensory abnormalities are an uncommon presenting sign of metastatic disease in the spine.

Selected References

1. Balic M et al: Circulating tumor cells: from bench to bedside. Annu Rev Med. 64:31-44, 2013
2. Perlikos F et al: Key molecular mechanisms in lung cancer invasion and metastasis: a comprehensive review. Crit Rev Oncol Hematol. 87(1):1-11, 2013
3. Ianari A et al: Cell death or survival: The complex choice of the retinoblastoma tumor suppressor protein. Cell Cycle. 9(1):23-4, 2010
4. Chen HZ et al. Emerging roles of E2Fs in cancer: an exit from cell cycle control. Nat Rev Cancer. 9(11):785-97, 2009
5. Fiorentino FP et al: Senescence and p130/Rbl2: a new beginning to the end. Cell Res. 19(9):1044-51, 2009
6. Mazel C et al. Cervical and thoracic spine tumor management: surgical indications, techniques, and outcomes. Orthop Clin North Am. 40(1):75-92, vi-vii, 2009
7. Sciubba DM et al: Solitary vertebral metastasis. Orthop Clin North Am. 40(1):145-54, viii, 2009
8. Fokas E et al: Metastasis: the seed and soil theory gains identity. Cancer Metastasis Rev. 26(3-4):705-15, 2007
9. Guillevin R et al: Spine metastasis imaging: review of the literature. J Neuroradiol. 34(5):311-21, 2007
10. Christofori G: New signals from the invasive front. Nature. 441(7092):444-50, 2006
11. Demopoulos A: Leptomeningeal metastases. Curr Neurol Neurosci Rep. 4(3):196-204, 2004
12. Batson OV: The function of the vertebral veins and their role in the spread of metastases. Ann Surg. 112(1):138-49, 1940

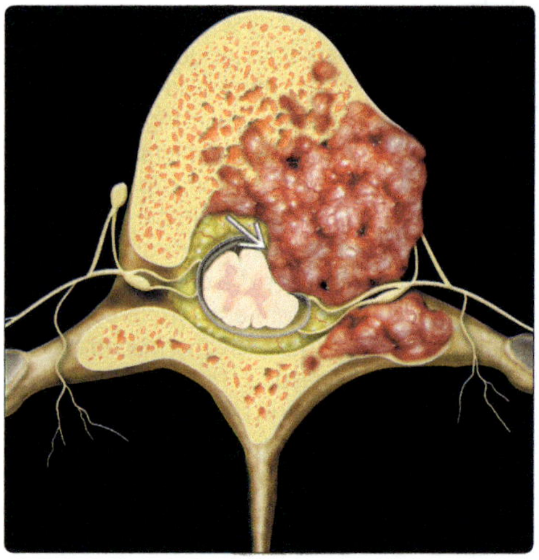

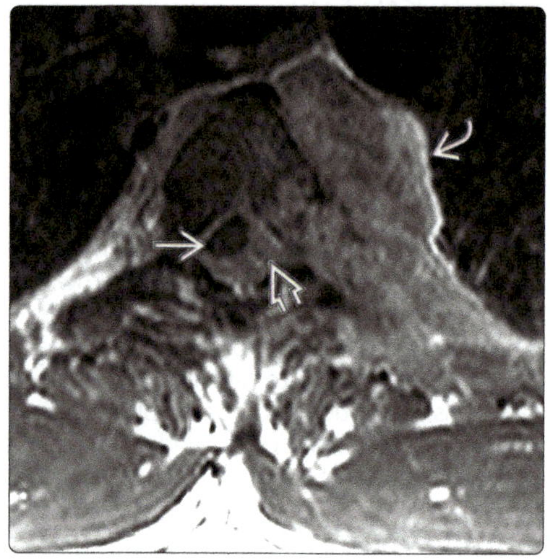

(Left) *Axial graphic shows hematogenously disseminated lytic metastatic lesion to thoracic vertebral body and pedicle, with subsequent direct epidural tumor extension and cord compression.* **(Right)** *Axial T1WI C+ MR shows a large hematogenously disseminated metastatic paravertebral mass lesion with direct tumor extension of tumor into the epidural space. Note the mass is causing cord compression.*

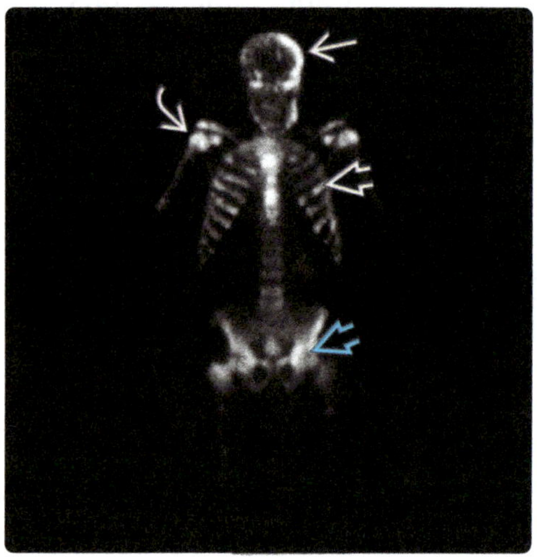

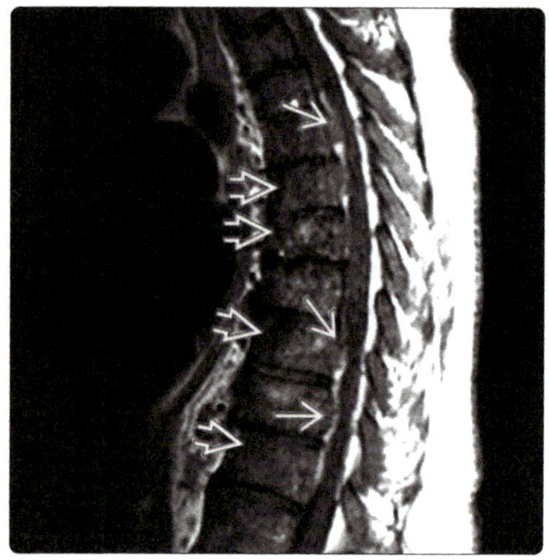

(Left) *Bone scan in a case of extensive blastic prostate carcinoma shows multiple foci of increased radiotracer uptake consistent with diffuse bone metastasis. This is particularly obvious in the pelvis, ribs, humeri, and skull.* **(Right)** *Sagittal T1WI C+ MR in a patient with extensive blastic prostate carcinoma shows diffuse abnormal decreased signal from all vertebral bodies with multiple foci of ventral epidural tumor extension, causing mild cord compression.*

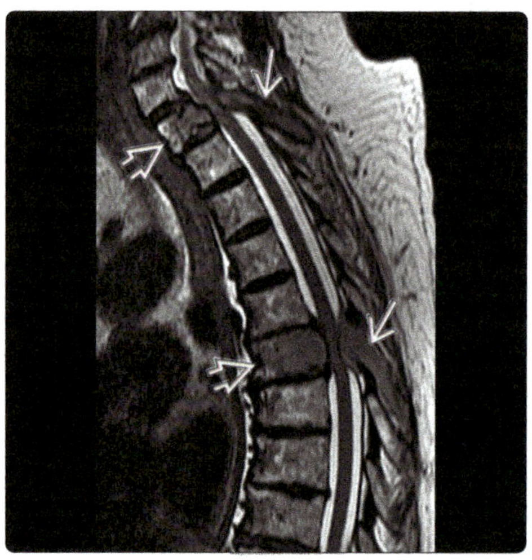

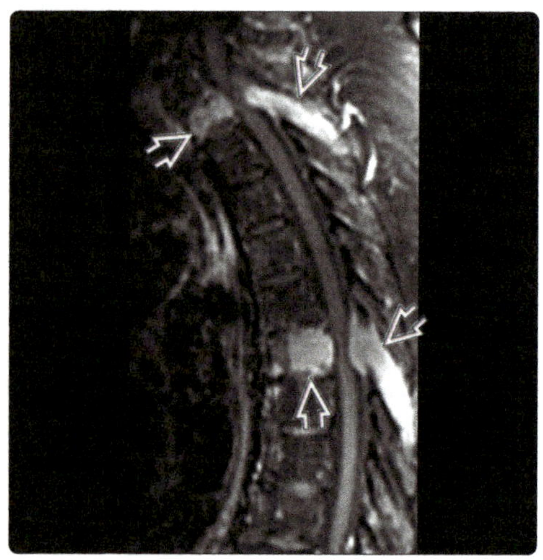

(Left) *Sagittal T2WI MR in a patient with multiple myeloma shows 2 vertebral levels of bony tumor involvement and slight spinous process expansion. There is severe cord compression at both levels.* **(Right)** *Sagittal T1 C+ FS MR of the same patient shows enhancement of the involved areas.*

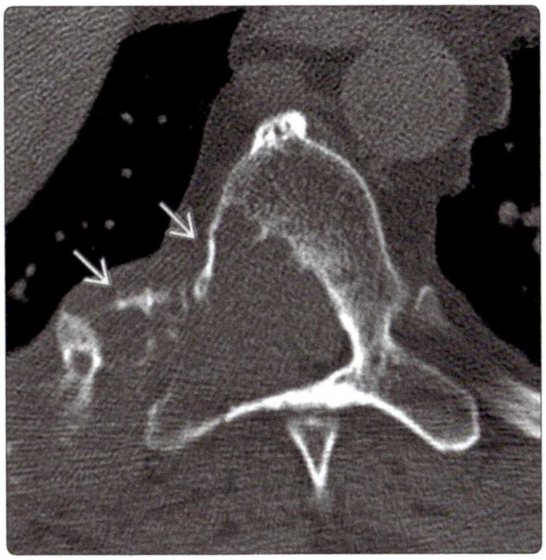

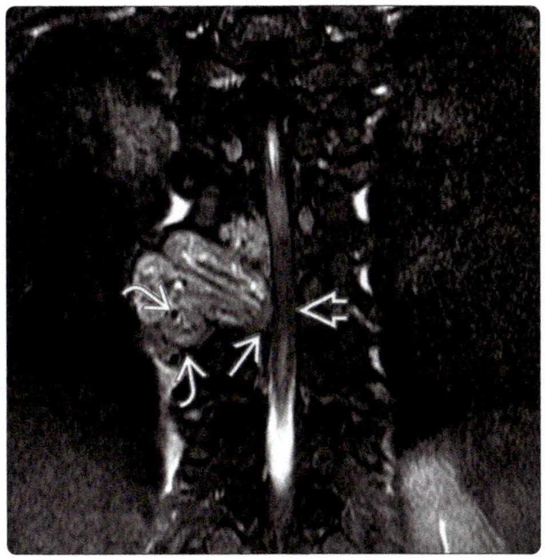

(Left) *Axial NECT in a patient with renal cell metastasis shows mass destroying the right side of T7-T8 bodies, extending into posterior elements, and crossing to involve right ribs and costovertebral joint. There is bony expansion with a thin rim soap-bubble pattern* ➔. **(Right)** *Coronal T2WI FS MR in the same patient with renal cell metastasis shows epidural extension of the mass* ➔ *and compression of the cord* ➔. *Multiple flow voids* ➔ *are present, indicating a very vascular tumor.*

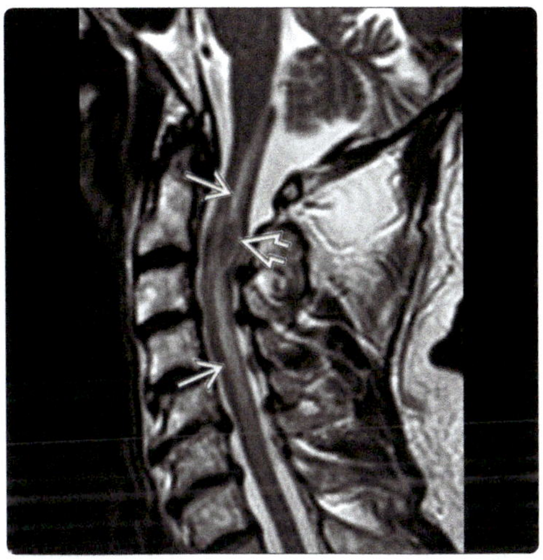

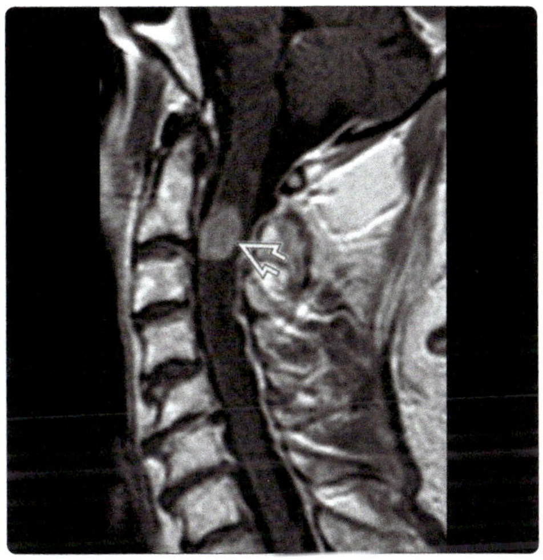

(Left) *Unenhanced T2WI MR in a patient with a large cervical cord metastatic lesion shows diffuse cord edema* ➔ *from cervicomedullary junction inferiorly to C5. A more focal signal abnormality is present at the C2-C3 level* ➔. **(Right)** *Sagittal T1WI C+ MR in the same patient shows enhancement of the large intramedullary metastatic lesion* ➔. *This was hematogenous dissemination from lung cancer.*

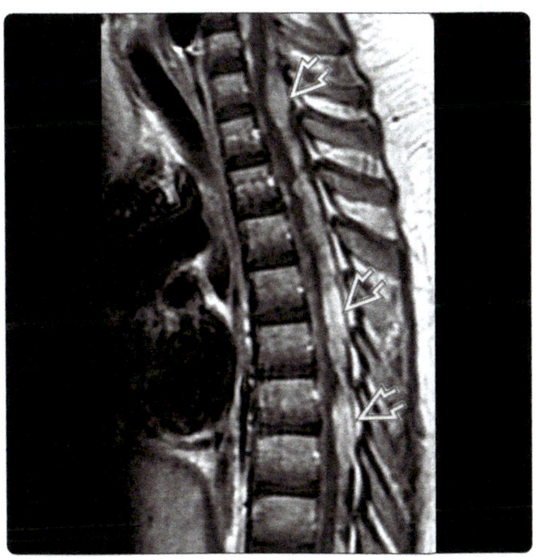

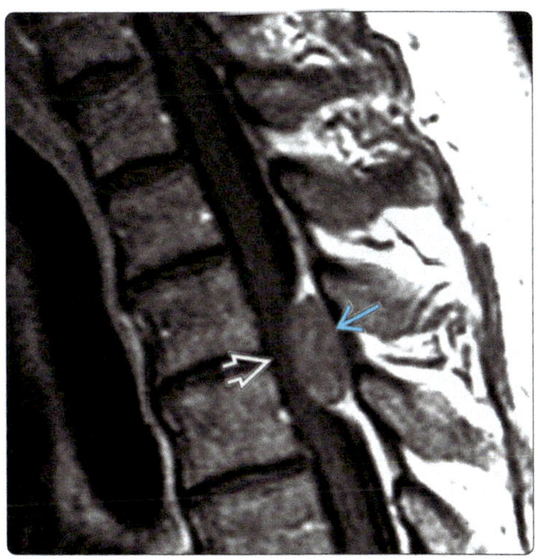

(Left) *Sagittal T1 C+ MR in a patient with extensive nodular leptomeningeal metastatic disease from high-grade brain oligodendroglioma shows massive nodular-enhancing leptomeningeal tumor following contrast administration* ➔. *This child had rapid onset of flaccid paraplegia, suggesting cord infarction from tumor compression.* **(Right)** *Sagittal T1 C+ MR shows focal epidural mass* ➔ *with cord compression* ➔ *from metastatic melanoma. Route of dissemination is presumed hematogenous.*

KEY FACTS

TERMINOLOGY

- Extension of primary tumor to spine where bone production exceeds bone destruction

IMAGING

- Multiple osteoblastic lesions in spine
  - May coexist with areas of osteolytic tumor, soft tissue mass
- Lesion distribution proportional to red marrow (lumbar > thoracic > cervical)
- MR signal typically diminished on T1, T2WI in areas of osteoblastic metastases
- Sclerotic metastases usually tracer avid on bone scan

TOP DIFFERENTIAL DIAGNOSES

- Treated metastases
- Discogenic sclerosis
- Hemangioma
- Paget disease
- Osteosarcoma

PATHOLOGY

- Marrow infiltration, tumor stimulates osteoblastic response
  - New bone deposition on trabeculae, within intertrabecular spaces
- Primary tumor, adults: Prostate, breast, carcinoid, lung, GI, bladder, nasopharynx, pancreas
- Primary tumor, children: Medulloblastoma, neuroblastoma, Ewing sarcoma

CLINICAL ISSUES

- Pain: Progressive axial, referred, or radicular
- Epidural tumor, if present, may cause neurologic dysfunction
- 90% of prostate metastases involve spine, with lumbar 3x more often than cervical

(Left) *Anteroposterior plain film shows diffuse extensive bone sclerosis of the spine, with all the vertebral bodies appearing whiter than normal, and pelvis due to diffuse osseous metastases from breast carcinoma.* **(Right)** *Anteroposterior bone scan shows diffuse, patchy tracer uptake in the thoracolumbar spine, pelvis, sternum, and multiple ribs due to diffuse osseous metastases from breast carcinoma.*

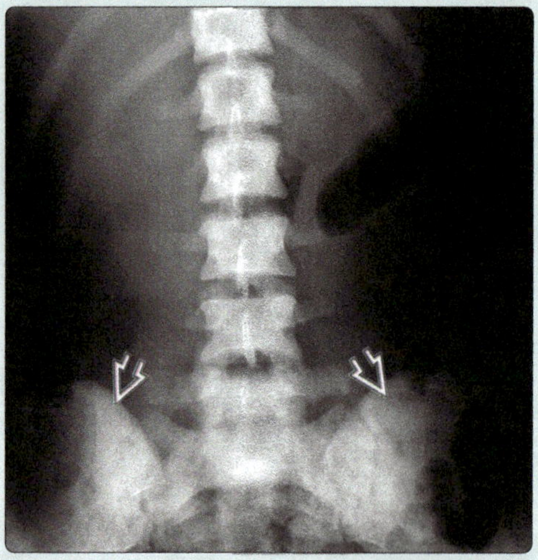

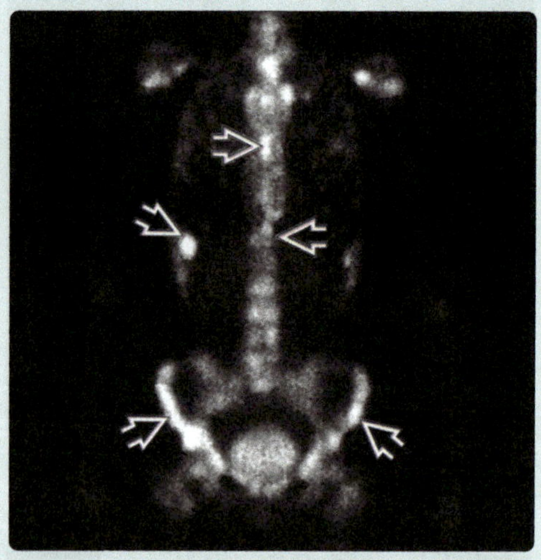

(Left) *Axial NECT shows diffuse sclerosis involving the left half of the vertebral body due to blastic metastasis in this patient with metastatic prostate carcinoma. A smaller abnormal area is present on the right.* **(Right)** *Sagittal T1-weighted MR shows low signal involving the L3 body and sacrum, reflecting diffuse metastatic disease. Extraosseous extension into the epidural space is seen at L3. There is no specific signal change on the MR to define the blastic nature of these metastatic lesions.*

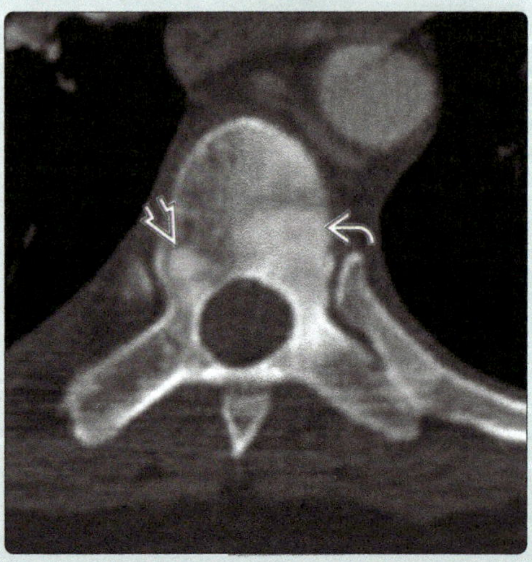

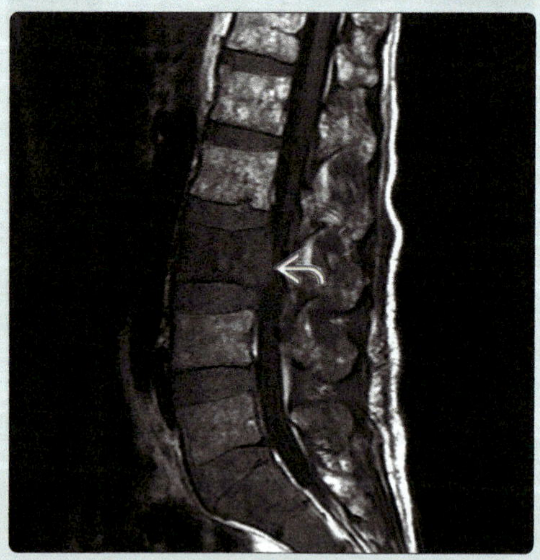

KEY FACTS

TERMINOLOGY

- Spread of primary tumor to spine, where bone destruction exceeds bone production

IMAGING

- Multiple osteolytic lesions in spine
- Compression fracture with bowing of posterior cortex, osteolysis extending into neural arch, extraosseous soft tissue
- Lesion distribution proportional to red marrow (lumbar > thoracic > cervical)
- Radiography requires 50-70% bone destruction and tumor size > 1 cm for detection
- Bone scan can give false-negatives with aggressively lytic tumor or with very small lesions

TOP DIFFERENTIAL DIAGNOSES

- Hematopoietic malignancy
- Benign (osteoporotic) compression fracture
- Schmorl node
- Normal heterogeneous marrow
- Spondylodiscitis

PATHOLOGY

- Spine is most common site of osseous metastases
  - Spine metastases found in 5-10% of cancer patients
- Common primaries causing osteolytic metastases
  - Breast, lung, renal most common
  - Other: Thyroid, GI tract, ovarian, melanoma

CLINICAL ISSUES

- Pain: Progressive axial, referred, or radicular
  - Compression fractures common
- Epidural tumor extension may cause neurologic dysfunction
  - Cord compression in 5% of adults with systemic cancers (70% solitary, 30% multiple sites)

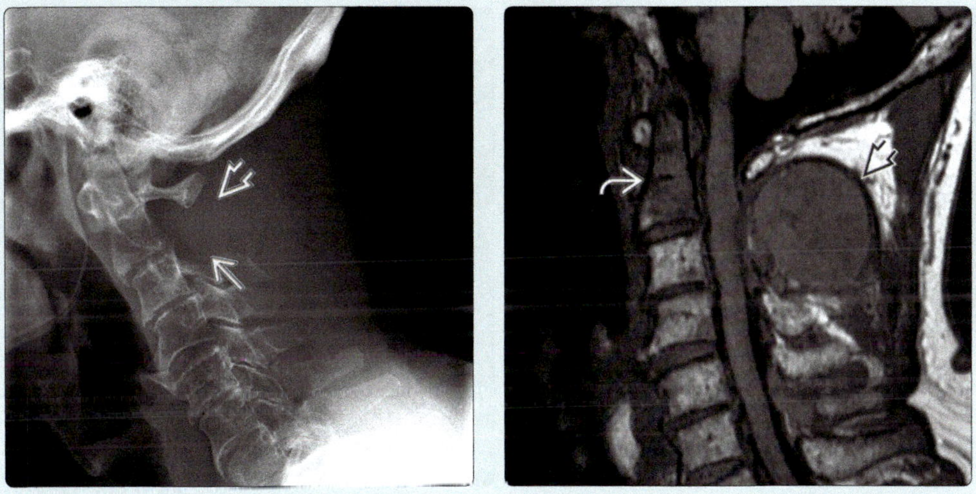

(Left) *Lateral radiograph shows osteolysis of the C2 neural arch ➡ and superior margin of the C3 arch ➡.* **(Right)** *Sagittal T1WI MR in the same patient shows a large soft tissue mass replacing the C2 arch ➡. There is also replacement of marrow in the C2 body and dens ➡. Subsequent work-up disclosed nonsmall cell lung carcinoma in the right upper lobe.*

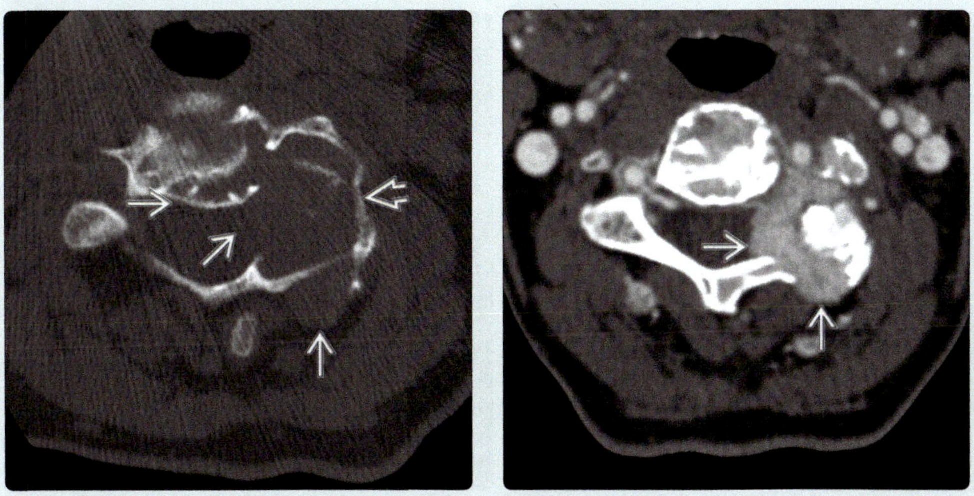

(Left) *Axial NECT shows large thyroid carcinoma metastasis to the vertebral body and left facet/lamina of C3. There is a thin rim of expanded bone ➡ partially surrounding the lesion. The extraosseous soft tissue mass is not clearly seen ➡ on bone windows.* **(Right)** *Axial contrast-enhanced CT at a slightly lower level shows enhancement of the mass ➡, typical of hypervascular tumors like thyroid carcinoma. The medial margin of the mass is in the spinal canal, effacing the thecal sac and likely contacting the cervical cord.*

Hemangioma

KEY FACTS

TERMINOLOGY

- Most common benign neoplasm of spine
    - Vascular/fatty marrow with fewer but thicker trabeculae

IMAGING

- CT: Well-circumscribed, hypodense lesion with coarse vertical trabeculae (corduroy appearance on sagittal, "white polka dots" on axial CT)
- MR: Circumscribed lesion, hyperintense on both T1 and T2WI, with hypointense vertical striations
    - Usually intraosseous, may have epidural component
    - Atypical hemangiomas may have reduced T1 signal due to paucity of fat
    - Strong, heterogeneous enhancement
- Often multiple (20-30%)
- Bone CT may supplement MR evaluation of suspected hemangioma with atypical imaging features concerning for neoplasm

PATHOLOGY

- Histology
    - Thin-walled sinusoidal channels lined by vascular endothelium
    - Interspersed thickened bony trabeculae
    - Fatty tissue

CLINICAL ISSUES

- Found in 10% of imaged adults
- Usually incidental finding
- Complications in < 1%
    - Pathologic compression fracture
    - Epidural hemangioma component with cord compression
- No follow-up typically necessary with pathognomonic imaging with small lesions and no extraosseous extension

(Left) *Sagittal graphic of the thoracolumbar junction shows the typical striated pattern of hemangioma, with thickened bony trabeculae. It fills the entire vertebral body, but there is neither extraosseous extension nor thecal sac compromise.* **(Right)** *Sagittal bone CT reformatted from the axial source data in a 43-year-old woman with low back pain shows the coarse, thickened vertical trabeculae and alternating fatty hypodense areas characteristic for vertebral hemangioma. The posterior cortex is indistinct.*

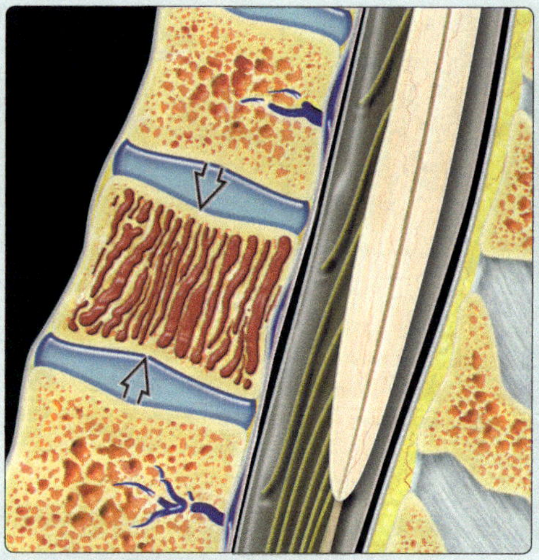

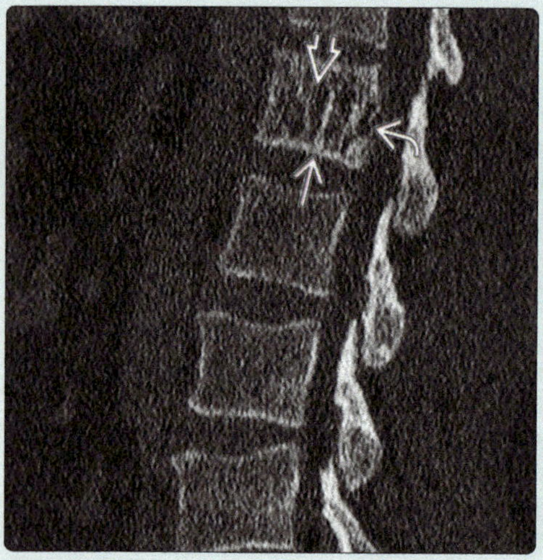

(Left) *Sagittal T1WI in the same case shows the "speckled" hyperintense marrow of the L1 vertebral body (compare with normal T12 and L1 vertebrae). Some transcortical extension into the epidural space is present. Contrast the appearance of this hemangioma with focal fatty marrow replacement in L5. Foci of fatty marrow are common normal findings in middle-aged and older patients.* **(Right)** *Sagittal T2WI in the same case shows the "speckled" fatty marrow or a classic vertebral hemangioma.*

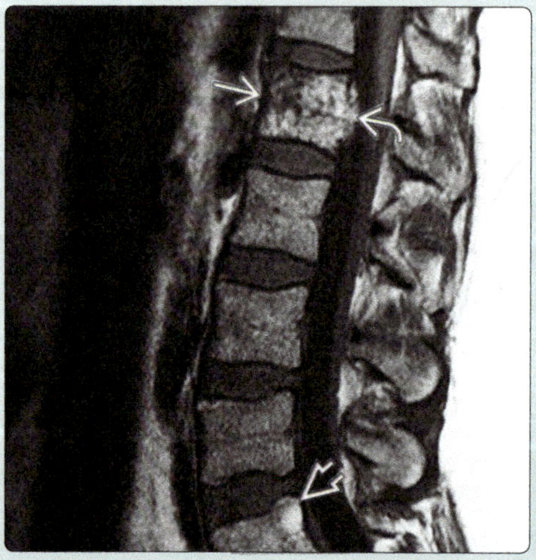

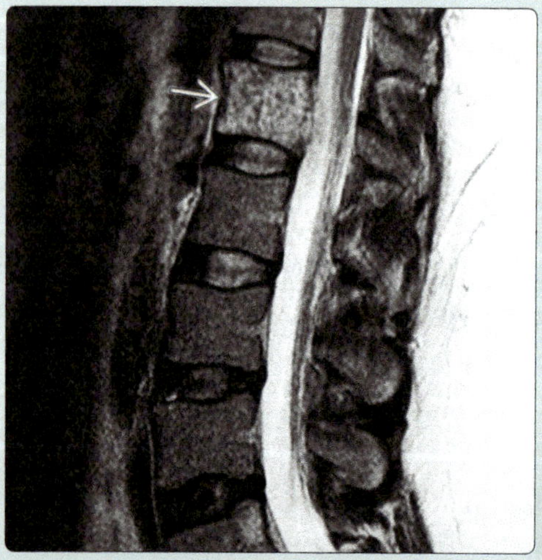

Lymphoma

KEY FACTS

TERMINOLOGY

- Lymphoreticular neoplasms with myriad of specific diseases and cellular differentiation

IMAGING

- Multiple types with variable imaging manifestations
- Epidural lymphoma: Thoracic > lumbar > cervical
  - Enhancing epidural mass ± vertebral involvement
- Osseous lymphoma: Long bones > spine
  - Bone destruction ("ivory" vertebra, rare), vertebra plana
- Lymphomatous leptomeningitis
  - Smooth/nodular pial enhancement
- Intramedullary lymphoma: Cervical > thoracic > lumbar
  - Poorly defined, enhancing mass
- Secondary > primary involvement
- Extradural > intradural > intramedullary
- FDG PET useful for staging, monitoring treatment response, predicting treatment outcomes, and risk stratifying lymphoma patients

PATHOLOGY

- Lymphoma is most common malignancy of epidural space
- Non-Hodgkin lymphoma (NHL) > > Hodgkin disease; 80-90% are B cell
  - CNS lymphoma > 85% NHL (B cell > > > T cell)
- CNS lymphoma may be primary or secondary (hematogenous or direct geographic extension)

CLINICAL ISSUES

- Most common presenting symptom = back pain
- Intramedullary = myelopathy (weakness, numbness)
- Cord compression occurs in up to 5-10% of systemic lymphomas
- Generally poor prognosis for CNS lymphoma
- Markedly sensitive to chemotherapy/XRT
- Depressed humoral and cell-mediated immunity leads to opportunistic infections

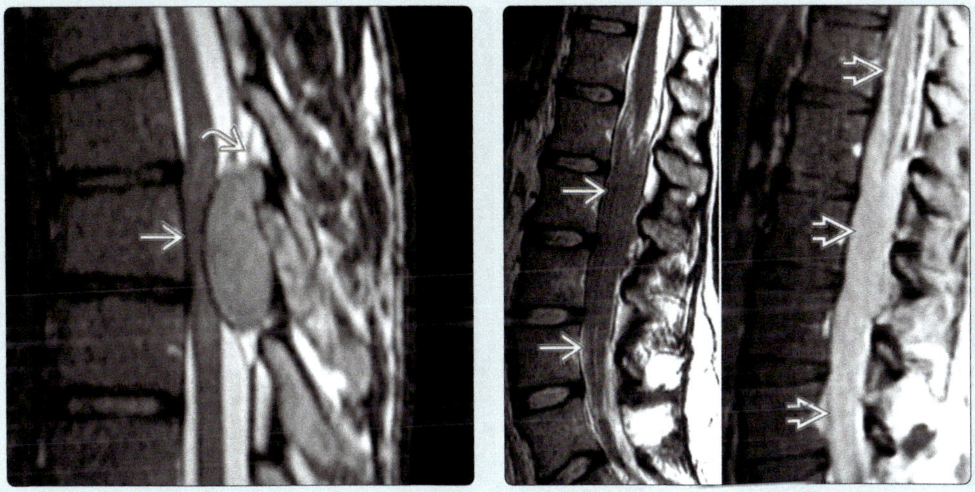

(Left) *Sagittal T2WI MR demonstrates a discrete hypointense mass in the posterior epidural space with a cap of epidural fat. The spinal cord is displaced anteriorly. Biopsy disclosed B-cell lymphoma.* **(Right)** *Sagittal T2WI MR (L) shows amorphous hypointense tumor mass insinuating along the cauda equina. Sagittal T1WI C+ MR (R) reveals enhancing lymphoma within the leptomeninges surrounding the distal conus and involving the nerve roots diffusely.*

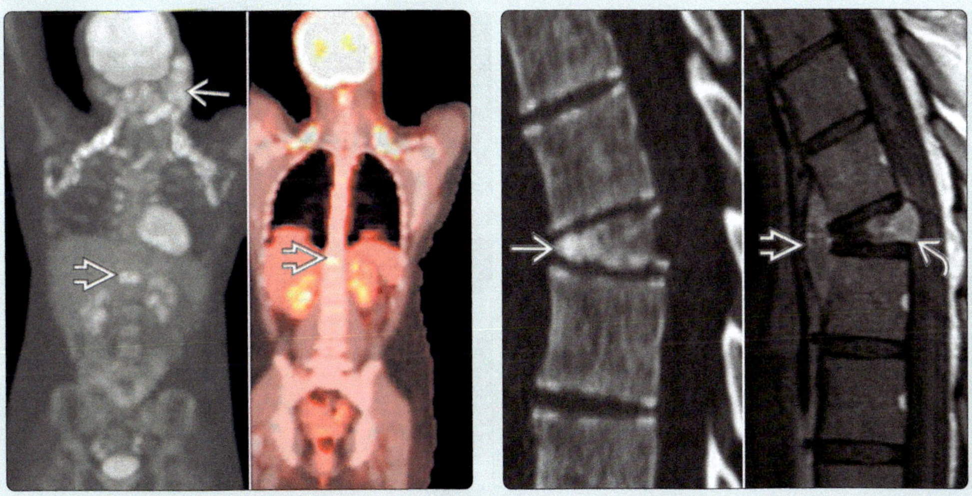

(Left) *Coronal PET (L) shows FDG uptake in the left cervical lymph node mass that was clinically evident. PET/CT fused image (R) shows abnormal activity at T11. This is an example of osseous metastases from cervical Hodgkin lymphoma primary tumor.* **(Right)** *Sagittal CT (L) demonstrates a pathologic compression fracture of a midthoracic vertebral body. Sagittal T1WI C+ MR (R) confirms abnormal marrow enhancement and a ventral paraspinal mass.*

KEY FACTS

TERMINOLOGY

- Acute or chronic myeloid or lymphoid white blood cell neoplasia with spinal involvement as component of systemic disease

IMAGING

- Radiographs/CT
  - Diffuse osteopenia with multiple vertebral fractures ± lytic spine lesions
  - Variable enhancing isodense soft tissue mass with adjacent bone destruction
- MR
  - T1WI: Hypointense marrow and focal tumor masses
  - T2WI: Hyperintense marrow ± focal vertebral mass, cord signal abnormality
  - T1WI C+: Abnormal enhancement of marrow, focal lesion, or leptomeninges

TOP DIFFERENTIAL DIAGNOSES

- Metastases
- Lymphoma
- Ewing sarcoma
- Langerhans cell histiocytosis

CLINICAL ISSUES

- Localized or diffuse bone pain
- Symptomatic patients present with fever, ↑ ESR, hepatosplenomegaly, lymphadenopathy, joint effusions, petechial and retinal hemorrhage, anemia, frequent infections

DIAGNOSTIC CHECKLIST

- Marrow infiltration in child with osteoporosis raises suspicion for leukemia
- Consider leukemia in patient with unexplained compression fractures

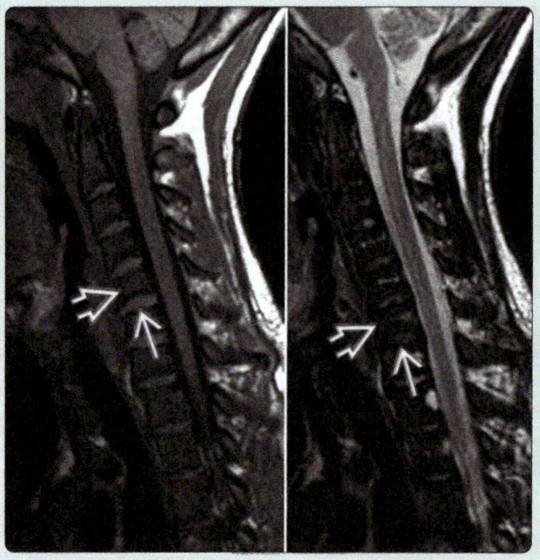

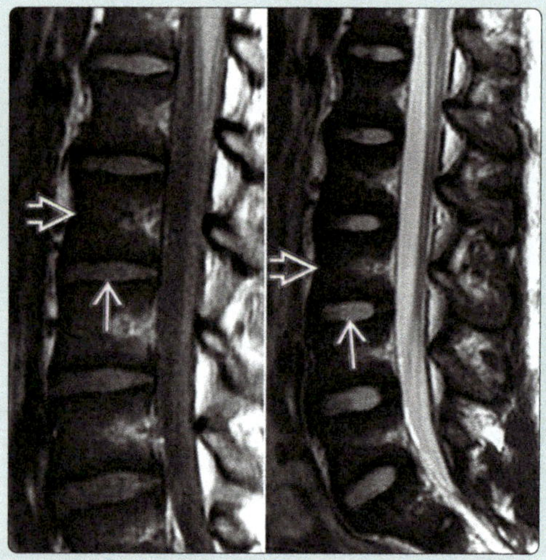

(Left) *Sagittal T1WI MR (L) and T2WI MR (R) of the cervical spine demonstrate diffuse abnormal hypointense signal intensity within the vertebrae ➡. Signal intensity is lower than the adjacent disc spaces ➡.* **(Right)** *Sagittal T1WI MR (L) and T2WI MR (R) of the lumbar spine exhibit diffuse abnormal hypointense signal intensity within the vertebrae ➡ compared with the adjacent disc spaces ➡. Abnormal signal may be a combination of tumor marrow infiltration and hyperplastic marrow secondary to anemia.*

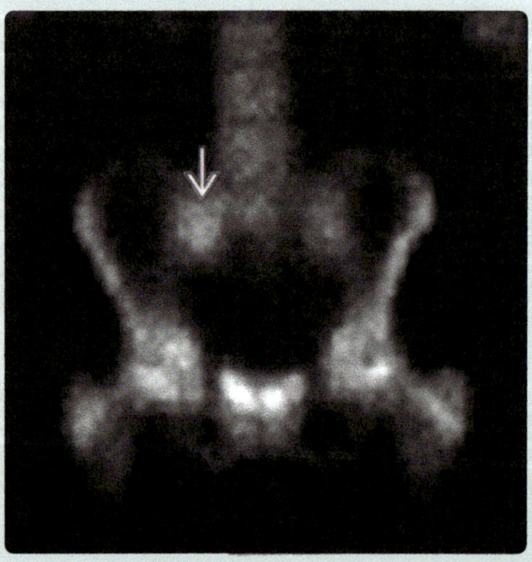

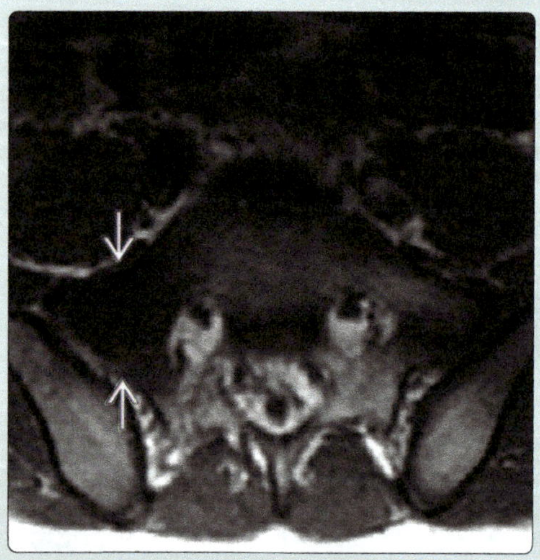

(Left) *Coronal planar bone scan of the pelvis reveals abnormal increased uptake within the right sacral ala ➡ in this case of focal leukemic metastasis to the axial skeleton. Bone scan may underestimate disease extent, especially in absence of significant cortical destruction.* **(Right)** *Axial T1WI MR in the same patient clarifies the right sacral alar metastatic lesion ➡. There is no definite cortical breakthrough.*

KEY FACTS

TERMINOLOGY

- Solitary monoclonal plasma cell tumor of bone or soft tissue
- Diagnosis of solitary bone plasmacytoma (SBP) requires
  - Solitary lesion, biopsy showing plasma cells
  - Negative skeletal survey, negative MR spine, pelvis, proximal femora/humeri
  - Negative clonal cells in marrow aspirate
  - No anemia, hypercalcemia, or renal involvement suggesting systemic myeloma

IMAGING

- Axial skeleton > extremities
  - Thoracic vertebral body most common site
- Radiographs/CT
  - Lytic, multicystic-appearing lesion ± vertical dense striations
  - Pathologic compression fracture common
- T1 hypointense, T2/STIR hyperintense marrow with low signal, curvilinear areas
  - Posterior elements involved in most cases
  - ± associated soft tissue mass (paraspinous or epidural with draped-curtain sign)

PATHOLOGY

- SBP may reflect early (stage I) multiple myeloma
- SBPs considered clinical stage I Durie-Salmon lesions

CLINICAL ISSUES

- Most common symptom = pain due to bone destruction
- Epidural extension may cause compression of cord or nerve root
- Mean age = 55 years (younger than age of patients with multiple myeloma)

DIAGNOSTIC CHECKLIST

- Must exclude 2nd unanticipated lesion (33% of cases)

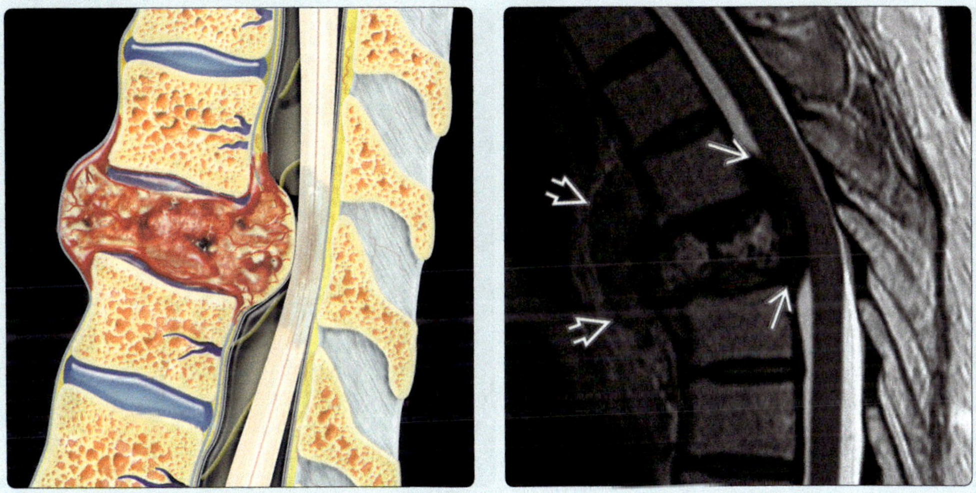

(Left) *Sagittal graphic shows collapse of a thoracic vertebral body due to tumor infiltration. There is retropulsion of the anterior and posterior margins. Posterior retropulsion and tumor mass may result in cord compression.* **(Right)** *Sagittal T2WI MR demonstrates a heterogeneously hyperintense thoracic vertebral body lesion with hypointense ventral epidural ➡ and paravertebral ⇨ soft tissue components producing cord compression.*

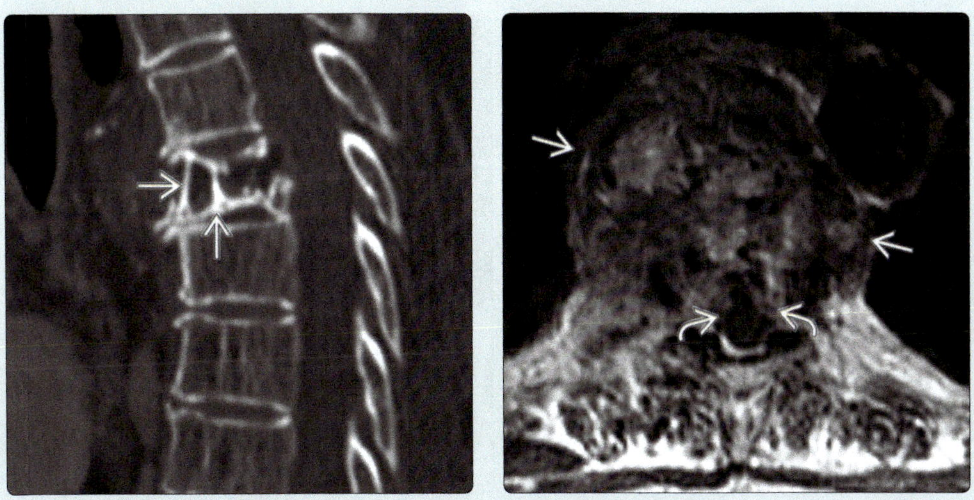

(Left) *Sagittal bone CT exhibits the characteristic appearance of thickened cortical struts ➡, a result of stress phenomenon from the lytic process forcing remaining bone to increase thickness as a compensatory response to weakening bone.* **(Right)** *Axial T1WI C+ MR depicts tumor infiltration of a thoracic vertebral body, with extension into the paravertebral ➡ and epidural ↷ spaces. The latter significantly narrows the canal.*

Multiple Myeloma

KEY FACTS

TERMINOLOGY

- Multifocal malignant proliferation of monoclonal plasma cells within bone marrow

IMAGING

- Skeletal survey is initial diagnostic imaging evaluation
  - Diffuse osteopenia and multiple lytic lesions
- NECT (bone algorithm)
  - Multifocal lytic lesions
  - Vertebral destruction and fractures
- MR patterns
  - Normal
  - Focal marrow involvement
  - Diffuse marrow involvement
  - Variegated pattern (micronodular, "salt and pepper")
- Compression fractures with variable central canal narrowing
- FDG PET
  - Identifies active multiple myeloma; useful in monitoring treatment response
- FSE T2 with fat saturation, STIR, or T1WI C+ with fat suppression increase lesion conspicuity

TOP DIFFERENTIAL DIAGNOSES

- Metastases
- Leukemia/lymphoma
- Osteoporosis

CLINICAL ISSUES

- Bone pain: 75%
- Marrow failure: Anemia, infection
- Renal insufficiency/failure
- Serum protein electrophoresis shows M protein (monoclonal immunoglobulin)
  - Immunofixation electrophoresis more sensitive for small amounts
- Hypercalcemia

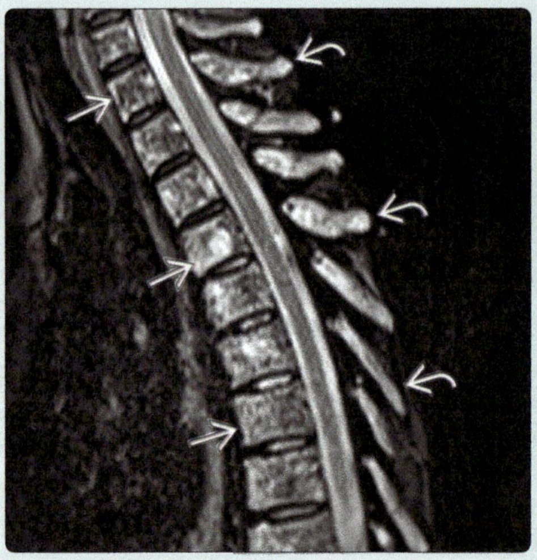
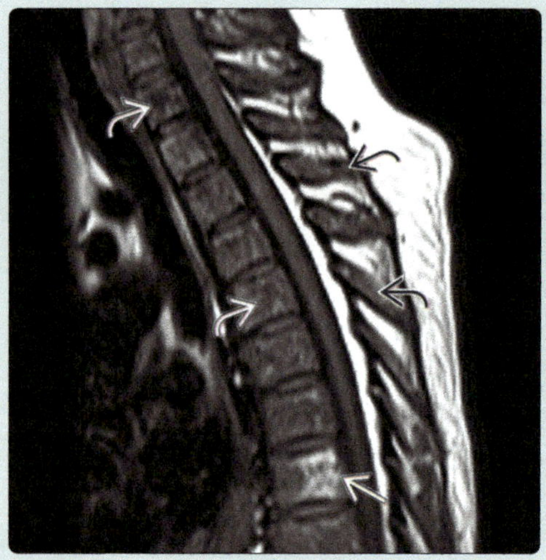

(Left) *Sagittal STIR MR illustrates innumerable hyperintense foci in the cervical and thoracic vertebral bodies → and spinous processes →. Advanced imaging is recommended in those with normal radiographs and monoclonal gammopathy or a solitary plasmacytoma.* **(Right)** *Sagittal T1WI MR demonstrates heterogeneous marrow signal due to fatty replacement by countless hypointense lesions in the vertebral bodies → and the spinous processes →. There is a benign vertebral hemangioma at T8 →.*

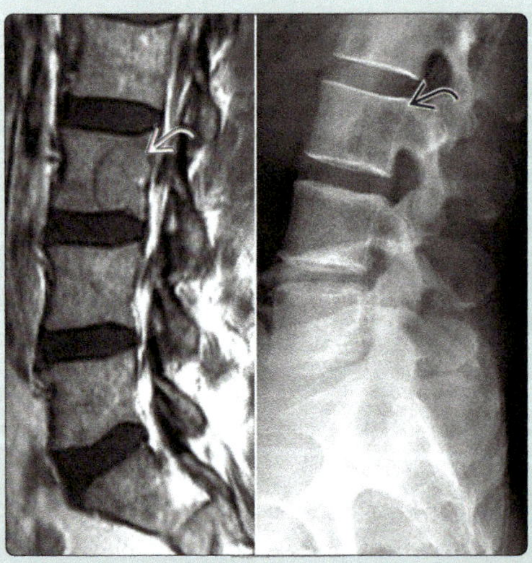
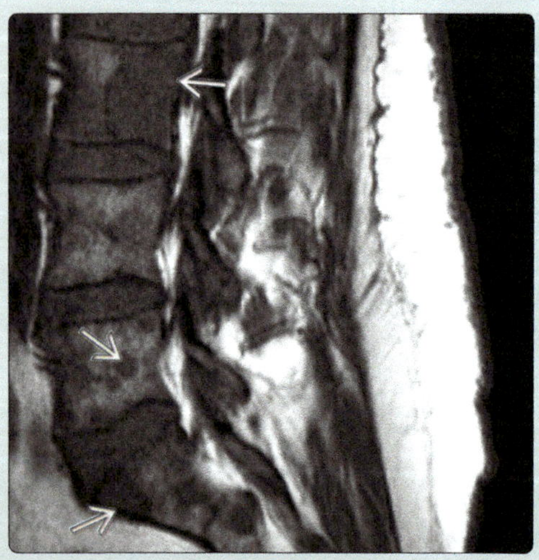

(Left) *Sagittal T2WI MR (L) shows marrow heterogeneity with a hypointense L3 vertebral body lesion →, barely detectable on lateral MR (R) →. Radiographs allow identification of only those lesions with advanced destruction affecting at minimum 30% of trabecular bone.* **(Right)** *Sagittal T1WI MR depicts fatty marrow replacement by several hypointense vertebral body lesions of varying sizes →. Posttreatment T1WI MR shows gradual replacement of infiltrates by red marrow, then by fat.*

KEY FACTS

TERMINOLOGY

- Neurinoma, neurilemmoma (outdated terms)
- Neoplasm of nerve sheath (Schwann cells)

IMAGING

- 70-75% intradural extramedullary
  - Most common intradural extramedullary mass
- 15% completely extradural
- 15% transforaminal, "dumbbell" masses
- Bone remodeling due to large intraspinal or intraforaminal tumor common
- Cystic change common
- Calcifications, hemorrhage are rare
- Uniform, heterogeneous, or peripheral enhancement patterns

TOP DIFFERENTIAL DIAGNOSES

- Neurofibroma
- Perineural root sleeve cyst
- Myxopapillary ependymoma
- Meningioma
- Leptomeningeal carcinomatosis
- Neuroblastic tumor

PATHOLOGY

- WHO grade I
- Neurofibromatosis type 2 (NF2): Loss of tumor suppressor (merlin) on chromosome 22
- Sporadic schwannoma more common than NF2
  - Inactivating mutations of merlin gene in ~ 60%

CLINICAL ISSUES

- Pain, weakness, paresthesias most common clinical findings
- Typically solitary unless part of inherited tumor syndrome

DIAGNOSTIC CHECKLIST

- Schwannoma most likely when solitary enhancing "dumbbell-shaped" spinal lesion present

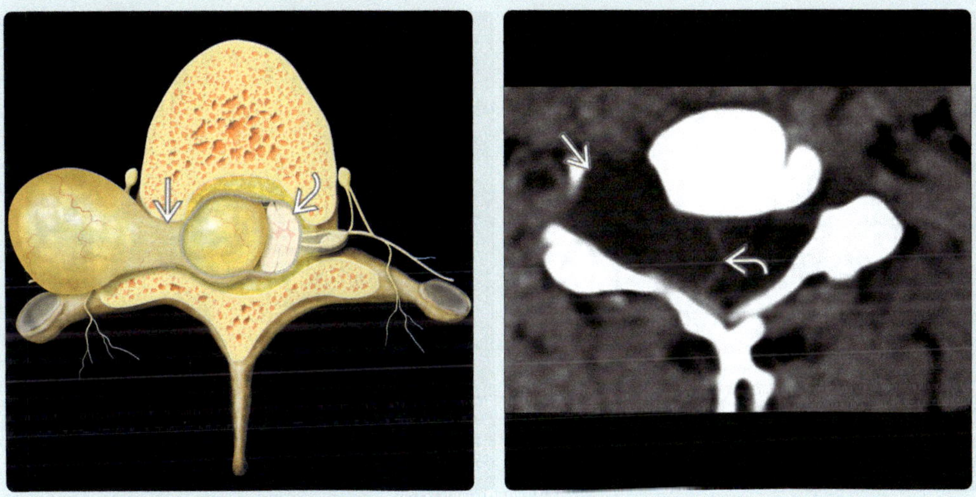

(Left) *Axial graphic portrays a right-sided dumbbell-shaped spinal nerve root schwannoma, enlarging the neural foramen ➡ and compressing the spinal cord ➡. Both intra- and extradural components ("dumbbell") are present.* **(Right)** *Axial CECT shows a hypodense transforaminal mass ➡ enlarging the right neural foramen. The intraspinal component effaces the thecal sac ➡ and causes canal stenosis.*

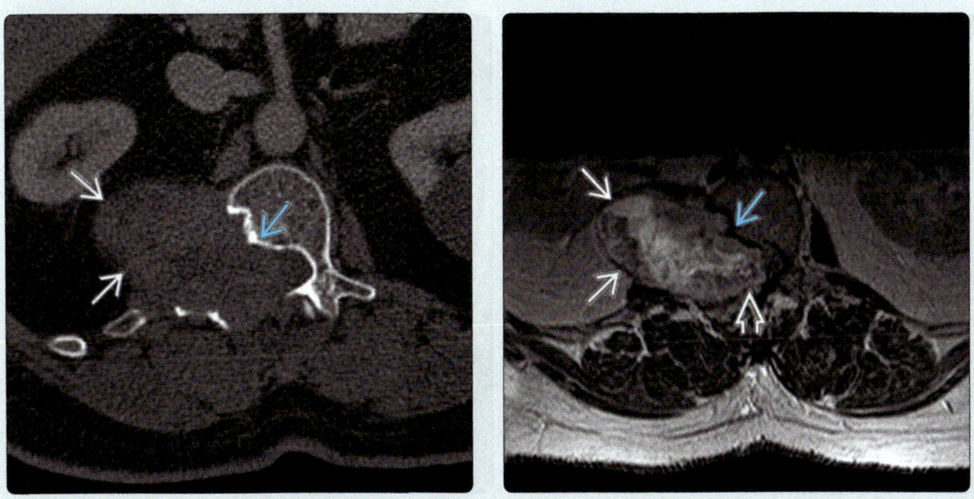

(Left) *Axial NECT demonstrates a large soft tissue mass ➡ enlarging the right L1-2 neural foramen. There is conspicuous scalloping of the vertebral body ⇨. The full intraspinal component is not seen.* **(Right)** *Axial T2WI MR in the same patient reveals heterogeneous mass ➡ signal intensity. Foraminal enlargement and vertebral body scalloping are again seen ⇨. The extradural component within the spinal canal is causing significant canal stenosis ➡.*

KEY FACTS

IMAGING

- Intradural extramedullary mass
- Thoracic (80%) > cervical (16%) > lumbar (4%)
- Typically round or ovoid (en globe)
    - En plaque variety pancaked or flat along dura
- Broad-based dural attachment
- Strong homogeneous enhancement
    - Prominent "dural tail" less common than with intracranial
- Calcification in 1-5%
- No bony remodeling or hyperostosis in spine

TOP DIFFERENTIAL DIAGNOSES

- Schwannoma
- Ependymoma, myxopapillary
- Lymphoma
- Intradural metastases

PATHOLOGY

- Arise from arachnoid cap cells
- > 95% WHO grade I
- Most solitary, sporadic
    - Almost all have 22q12 abnormalities
- Syndromes
    - Multiple lesions with neurofibromatosis 2
        - Intradural extramedullary meningiomas and schwannomas
        - Intramedullary ependymomas
    - Familial clear cell meningioma syndrome
    - Multiple meningiomatosis

CLINICAL ISSUES

- Peak incidence: 5th-6th decade
- > 80% female
- 2nd most common intradural extramedullary tumor
- Sensory and motor deficits (84%)
- Gait disturbances (83%)
- Local pain (47%)

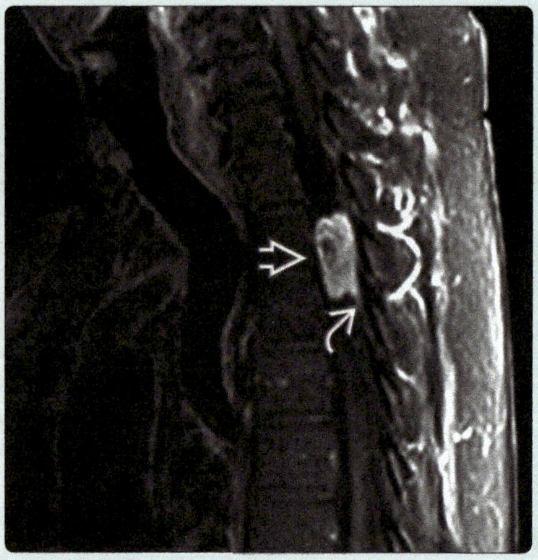
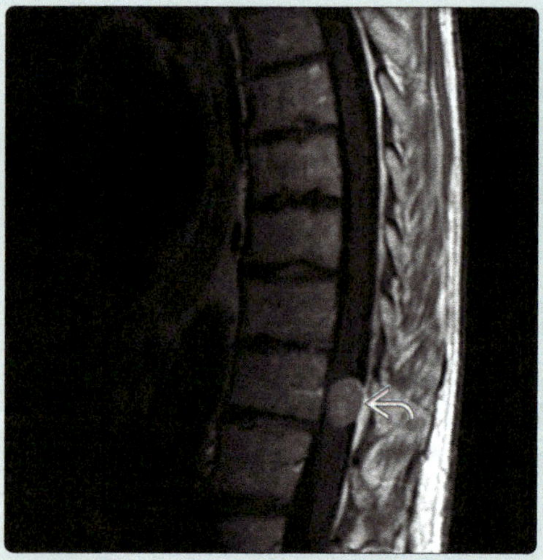

(Left) *Sagittal T1WI C+ FS MR of the upper thoracic spine shows an intensely enhancing intradural mass ➡ with a broad dorsal dural attachment. A small enhancing dural tail ➡ is seen, a finding suggestive of but not exclusive to meningioma.* **(Right)** *Sagittal T1WI C+ MR shows a rounded, circumscribed, intradural extramedullary mass ➡ with homogeneous, intense enhancement positioned dorsal to the thoracic cord. A dural tail is not evident in this case.*

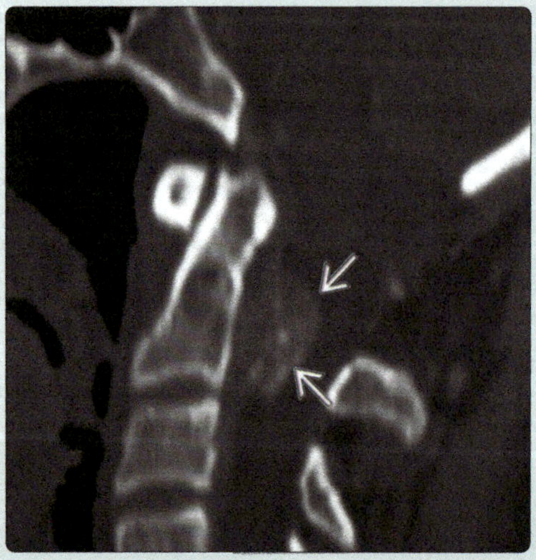
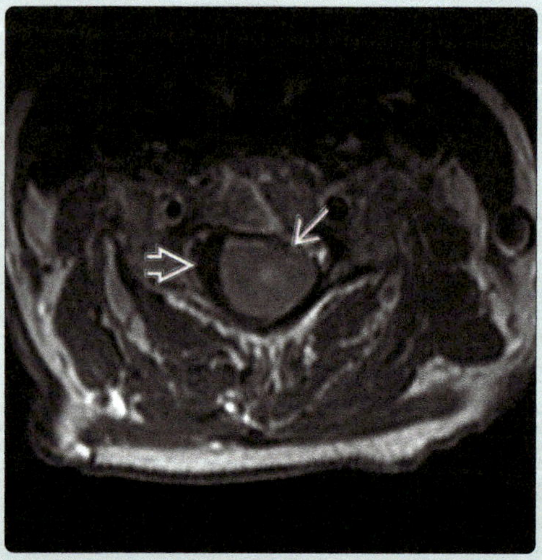

(Left) *Sagittal reconstructed CT shows a sizable, partially calcified meningioma ➡ arising on the ventral margin of the canal at the level of C2. The mass results in significant canal stenosis and cord compression.* **(Right)** *Axial T1 C+ image shows a large cervical meningioma with a ventral, dural-based attachment at the C5-6 level ➡, severely compressing and displacing the cervical cord posteriorly and to the right ➡.*

KEY FACTS

TERMINOLOGY

- Neoplasm containing Schwann cells, fibroblasts, myxoid material, and peripheral nerve fibers

IMAGING

- Locations: Extradural/paraspinal, intradural extramedullary
- Variable involvement of spinal root, neural plexus, peripheral nerve, or end organs
- Size varies from small circumscribed mass to large plexiform neurofibroma (NF) involving multiple body compartments
- Plexiform neurofibroma pathognomonic for neurofibromatosis type 1 (NF1)
- Target sign on T2WI suggestive but not pathognomonic for NF
- PET avidity suggests malignant degeneration

TOP DIFFERENTIAL DIAGNOSES

- Schwannoma
- Meningioma ("dumbbell" with intra-, extraspinal components)
- Perineural root sleeve cyst
- Chronic inflammatory demyelinating polyneuropathy
- Malignant nerve sheath tumors

PATHOLOGY

- Neoplastic Schwann cells + fibroblasts
- Tumor, nerve fascicles intermixed
    - Presence of axons characteristic of NF
- 90% of neurofibromas are sporadic

CLINICAL ISSUES

- Malignant transformation of plexiform NF to MPNST in 10% of NF1 patients

DIAGNOSTIC CHECKLIST

- Rapidly growing NF or atypical pain concerning for malignant transformation to MPNST
- Solitary spinal lesion more likely schwannoma than NF

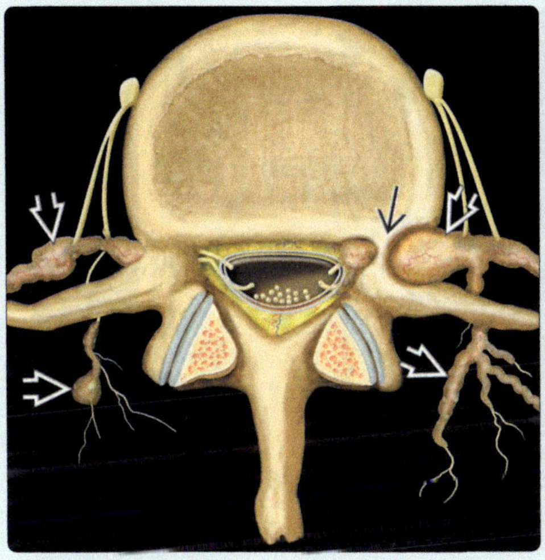

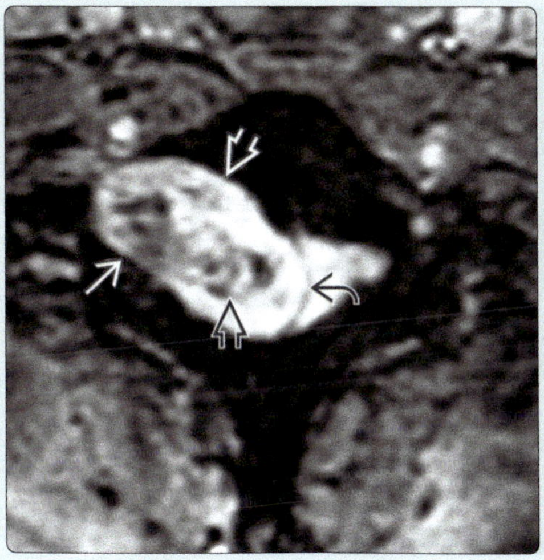

(Left) *Axial graphic portrays bilateral lobulated plexiform neurofibromas in neurofibromatosis 1. There is erosion of the left pedicle by the tumor.* **(Right)** *Axial T2* MR shows a mass widening the right neural foramen and scalloping the adjacent cervical vertebral body. The intraspinal extradural component of the mass causes severe canal stenosis. The mass is predominantly hyperintense with some whorled hypointensity centrally (so-called target sign not specific for neurofibroma).*

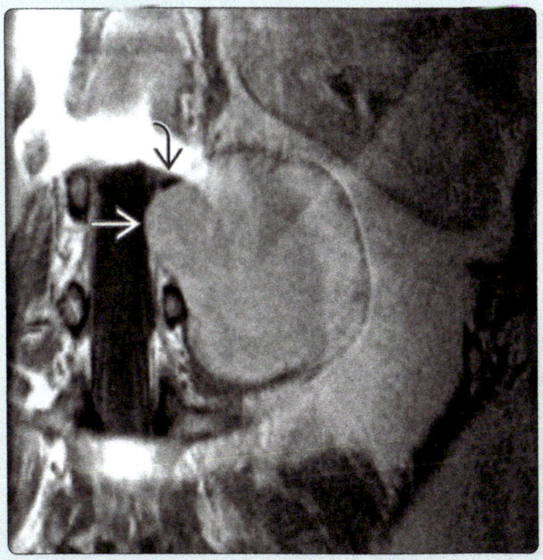

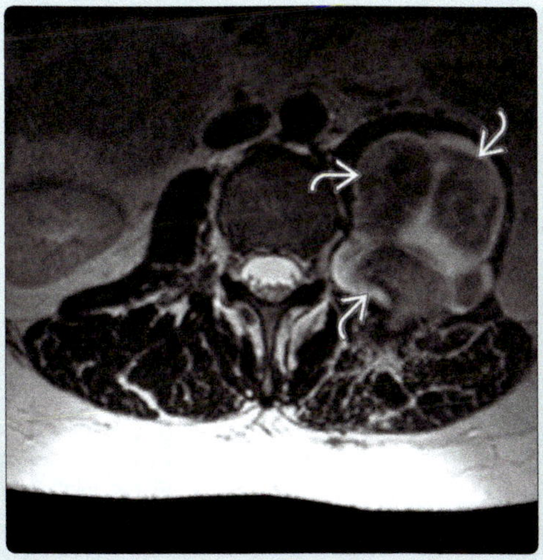

(Left) *Coronal T1WI C+ MR shows an enhancing paraspinal mass on the left at L1-2 extending into the left neural foramen, with minimal impact on the thecal sac. Remodeling causes enlargement of the left L1-2 neural foramen with thinning of the L1 pedicle.* **(Right)** *Axial T2WI in the same patient shows central areas of T2 hypointense signal with peripheral rim of hyperintensity. This target sign is not specific but is seen more commonly with neurofibroma than with schwannoma.*

Metastases, CSF Disseminated

KEY FACTS

TERMINOLOGY

- Spread of malignant tumor through subarachnoid spaces of brain and spinal cord

IMAGING

- Smooth or nodular enhancement along cord, cauda equina
- Located at any point along CSF pathway
- 4 basic patterns
  - Solitary focal mass at bottom of thecal sac or along cord surface
  - Diffuse, thin, sheet-like coating of cord/roots ("carcinomatous meningitis")
  - Rope-like thickening of cauda equina
  - Multifocal discrete nodules along cord/roots

TOP DIFFERENTIAL DIAGNOSES

- Multifocal primary tumor
- Meningitis (pyogenic, granulomatous > chemical)
- Neurosarcoidosis (diffuse or nodular enhancement)
- Recent lumbar puncture
- Thick nerve roots/cauda equina
  - Guillain-Barré
  - Congenital hypertrophic polyradiculoneuropathies
  - Neoplasm (e.g., lymphoma)

PATHOLOGY

- Hematogenous dissemination from solid tumors (1-5%)
- "Drop" metastases from patients with primary CNS tumor (1-2%)
- Leukemia, lymphoma (5-15%)
- Falsely negative CSF cytology in up to 40%

CLINICAL ISSUES

- Typically seen in advanced cancer cases
- Prevalence increasing as cancer patients living longer
- Median patient survival of 3-6 months with treatment

DIAGNOSTIC CHECKLIST

- MR more sensitive than CSF cytology

(Left) *Sagittal T1WI C+ MR shows a mixed nodular and smooth leptomeningeal tumor along the distal cord and conus medullaris due to drop metastases from glioblastoma multiforme.* **(Right)** *Sagittal T2WI shows multiple nodular, low signal intensity, rounded, drop metastases involving roots of the cauda equina, spreading from an intracranial glioblastoma multiforme.*

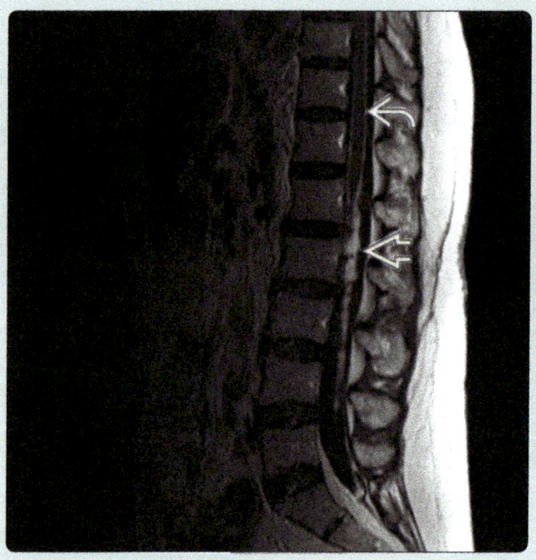

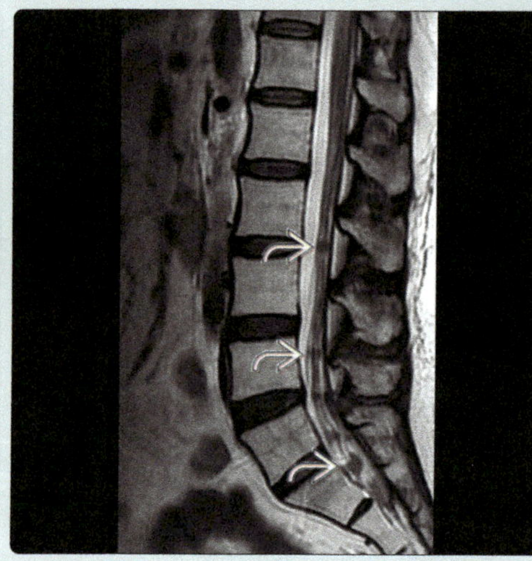

(Left) *Sagittal T1WI C+ MR shows bulky, nodular, drop metastases from a pineal germinoma along the conus and cauda equina.* **(Right)** *Sagittal T1WI C+ MR shows cerebrospinal fluid metastasis from small cell lung carcinoma with a bulky enhancing dural mass compressing the cervicomedullary junction and linear enhancing metastases along the dorsal pial surface of the cord from C7 caudally . An additional enhancing focus is seen in the region of the gracile tubercle .*

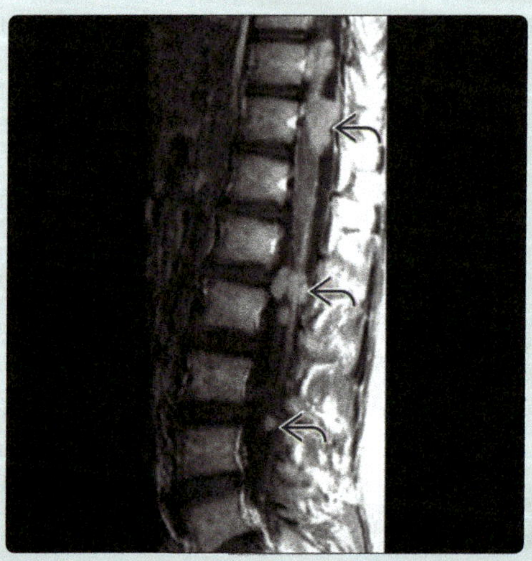

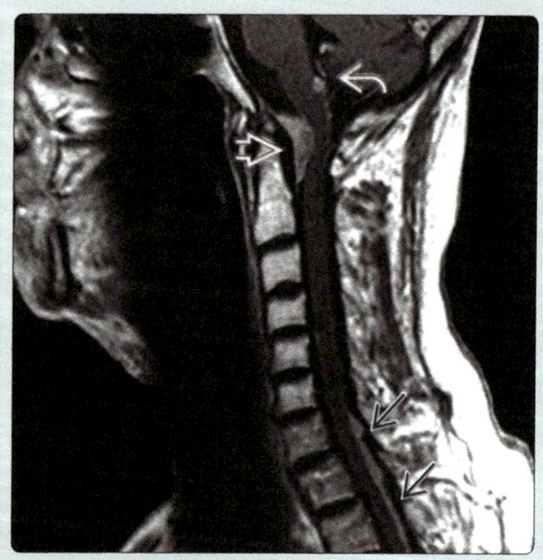

Astrocytoma

KEY FACTS

TERMINOLOGY

- Primary neoplasm of astrocytic origin within spinal cord

IMAGING

- Fusiform expansion of cord with enhancing component of variable morphology
  - Almost always enhances
- Cervical > thoracic
- Usually ≤ 4 segments
  - Occasionally multisegmental, even holocord (more common with pilocytic astrocytoma)
- ± cyst/syrinx (fluid slightly T1 hyperintense to cerebrospinal fluid)
- Hyperintense on proton density and T2WI MR
- Myelopathy should be evaluated with contrast-enhanced MR

TOP DIFFERENTIAL DIAGNOSES

- Ependymoma
- Hemangioblastoma
- Syringohydromyelia
- Autoimmune or inflammatory myelitis

PATHOLOGY

- 80-90% low grade
- 10-15% high grade

CLINICAL ISSUES

- Slow onset of myelopathy
- May cause painful scoliosis
- Most are slow growing
  - Malignant tumors may cause rapid neurologic deterioration
- Most common intramedullary tumor in children and young adults
- Overall, ependymomas > astrocytomas (2:1)

DIAGNOSTIC CHECKLIST

- Myelopathy should be evaluated with MR

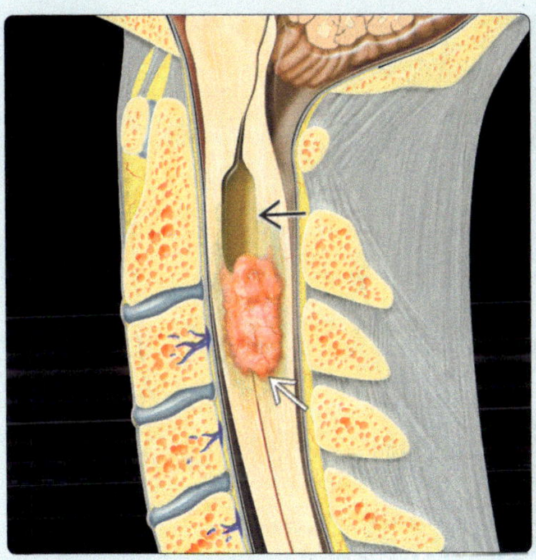
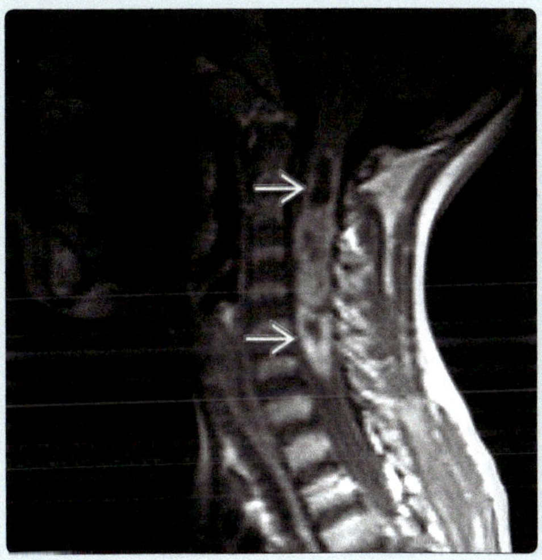

(Left) *Sagittal graphic of cervical spine astrocytoma shows a fusiform solid mass ➡ with a rostral cystic cord component ⇨.* **(Right)** *Sagittal T1WI C+ MR reveals a heterogeneously enhancing cervical cord mass ➡. The tumor subtype and histological grade are the most important prognostic factors. Malignant transformation, although common in recurrent adult low-grade gliomas, is unusual in pediatric low-grade intramedullary spinal cord tumors.*

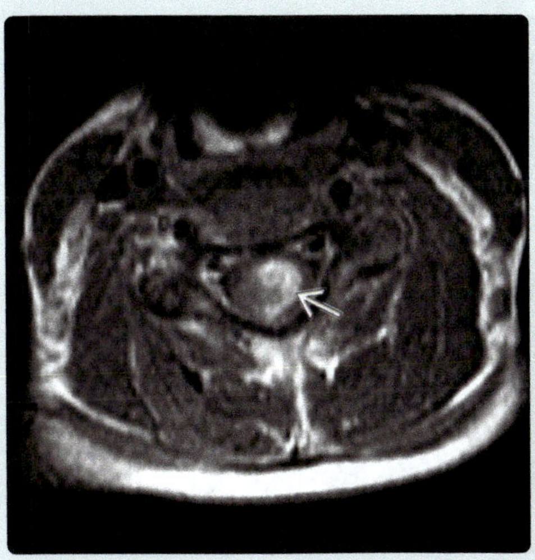
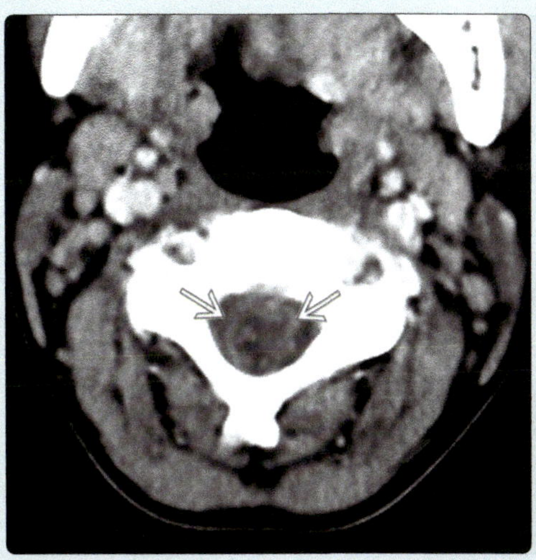

(Left) *Axial T1WI C+ MR depicts an intramedullary enhancing tumor in the cervical cord ➡. Astrocytomas tend to have an eccentric growth pattern and are T2 hyperintense. Up to 1/3 are reportedly nonenhancing but have mass effect and cord expansion.* **(Right)** *Axial CECT illustrates a heterogeneously enhancing mass ➡ within the central spinal canal in this case of cervical spinal cord astrocytoma with holocord edema (not shown).*

Classic Ependymoma

KEY FACTS

TERMINOLOGY

- Neoplasm arising from ependyma lining spinal cord central canal

IMAGING

- Circumscribed, enhancing hemorrhagic cord mass with surrounding edema
- Associated cysts common
- Cervical > thoracic > conus
- T1WI: Isointense or slightly hypointense to spinal cord
- T2WI: Hyperintense relative to spinal cord
- Cap sign: Hemosiderin at cranial or caudal margin
- Most tumors enhance

TOP DIFFERENTIAL DIAGNOSES

- Astrocytoma
- Hemangioblastoma
- Demyelinating disease
- Idiopathic transverse myelitis

PATHOLOGY

- Arises from ependymal cells of central cord canal
    - Most intramedullary
    - Rarely can be intradural extramedullary
- Most WHO grade II
- Rarely WHO grade III
    - Anaplastic ependymoma
- Association with neurofibromatosis type 2

CLINICAL ISSUES

- Most common presentation
    - Neck or back pain
- Other presentations
    - Progressive paraparesis, paresthesias

DIAGNOSTIC CHECKLIST

- Spinal cord neoplasm with associated peripheral hemorrhage suggestive of cellular ependymoma

(Left) *Coronal graphic depicts an intramedullary ependymoma mildly expanding the cervical cord. Cranial and rostral cysts , as well as hemorrhagic products , are associated with this mass.* **(Right)** *Sagittal T1WI C+ MR demonstrates a cervical intramedullary mass with solid and cystic components causing fusiform cord expansion. There are 2 areas of enhancing solid components and rostral cyst extending cephalad into brainstem. The adjacent solid portion shows little enhancement .*

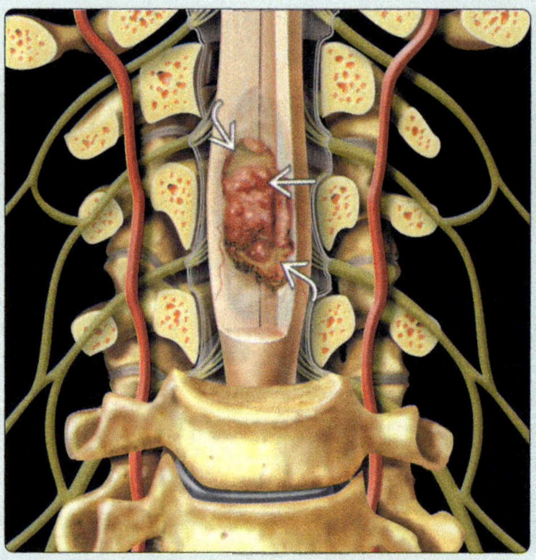

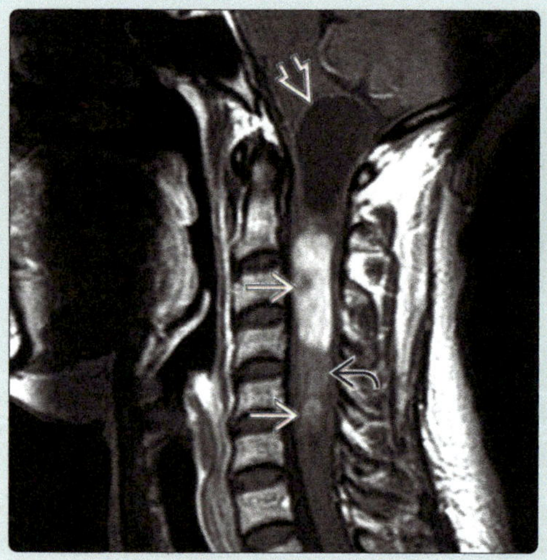

(Left) *Axial T1WI C+ MR reveals an expansile intramedullary ependymoma with robust enhancement pattern.* **(Right)** *Sagittal T2WI MR illustrates the mixed cystic and solid appearance of cervical ependymomas in a patient with neurofibromatosis type 2. In addition, there is a dural-based intradural extramedullary meningioma .*

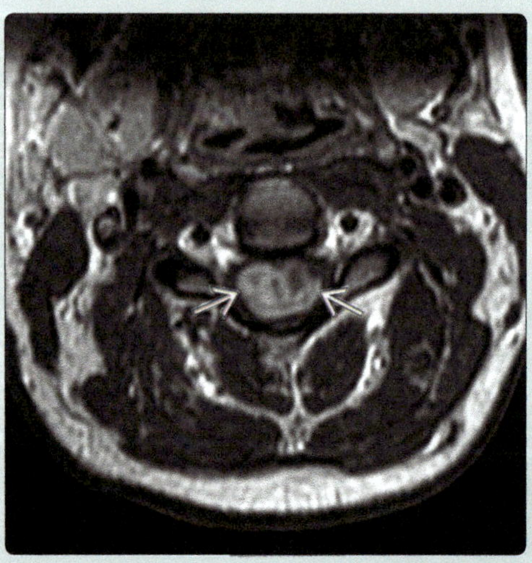

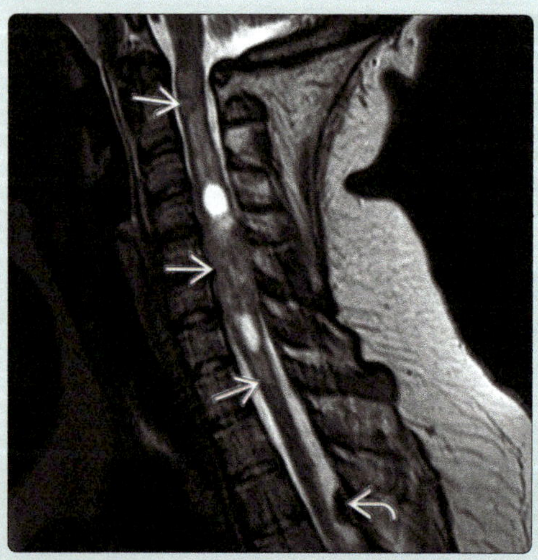

Myxopapillary Ependymoma

KEY FACTS

TERMINOLOGY

- Slow-growing glioma arising from ependymal cells of conus, filum terminale, cauda equina

IMAGING

- Usually spans 2-4 vertebral segments
  - May fill entire lumbosacral thecal sac
- Ovoid, lobular, sausage-shaped
- CT/radiographs
  - ± osseous canal expansion, thinned pedicles, vertebral scalloping
  - May enlarge, extend through neural foramina
- T1WI: Isointense → hyperintense to cord
- T2WI: Almost always hyperintense to cord
  - Hypointensity at tumor margin = hemosiderin
- T1WI C+: Intense enhancement

TOP DIFFERENTIAL DIAGNOSES

- Nerve sheath tumor
- Intradural metastases
- Meningioma
- Paraganglioma

PATHOLOGY

- WHO grade I
- May have local seeding or subarachnoid dissemination
- Subarachnoid hemorrhage

CLINICAL ISSUES

- Symptoms mimic disc herniation
- Back pain most common
- Other issues include paraparesis, radiculopathy, or bladder and bowel dysfunction

DIAGNOSTIC CHECKLIST

- Slow tumor growth may delay diagnosis
- Always image the conus in patients presenting with back pain

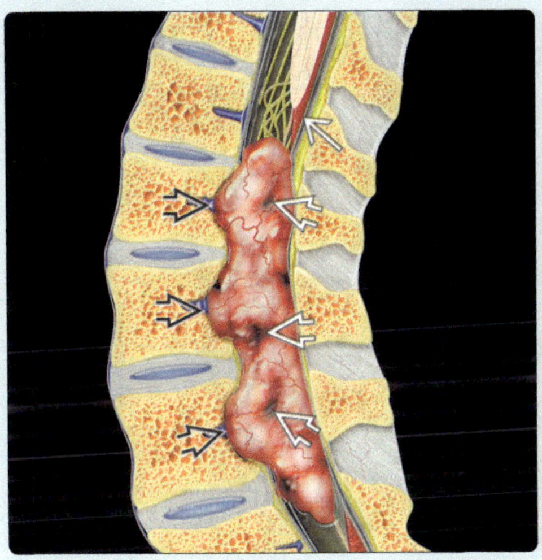

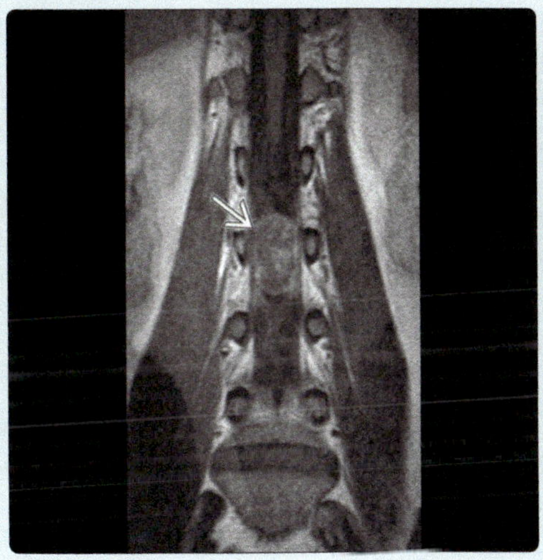

(Left) *Sagittal graphic shows a multilevel cauda equina myxopapillary ependymoma. Mass is vascular, with old intratumoral hemorrhage ➡, acute subarachnoid hemorrhage ➡. Slow tumor growth has enlarged spinal canal and remodeled posterior vertebral cortex ➡.* **(Right)** *Coronal T1WI MR shows a well-delineated, intradural extramedullary mass in lumbar spine ➡. Lesion is predominantly isointense with cord and nerves. Almost 70% of filum terminale masses are ependymomas, mostly myxopapillary type.*

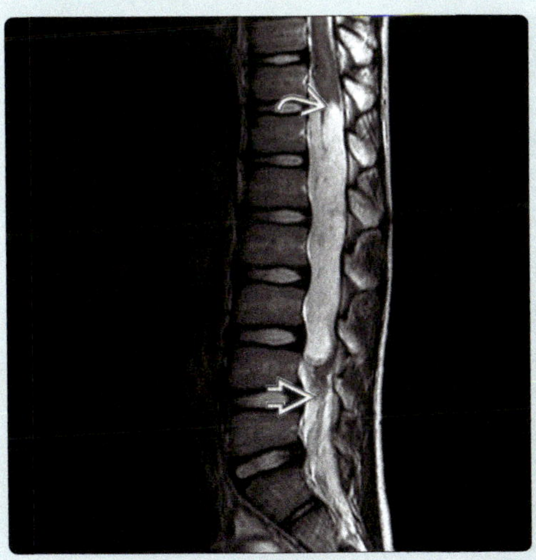

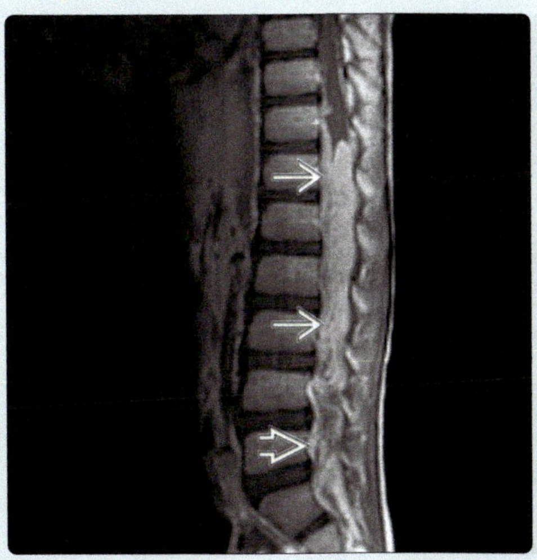

(Left) *Sagittal T2WI MR reveals an extensive intradural tumor distorting the conus ➡ and cauda equina ➡. Myxopapillary ependymomas are unique in their intracellular and perivascular accumulation of proteinaceous mucin, which appears T1/T2 hyperintense.* **(Right)** *Sagittal T1WI C+ MR exhibits avid homogeneous tumor enhancement ➡. Note diffuse intradural tumor seeding ➡. Smaller tumors tend to displace the cauda equina nerve roots, whereas large tumors often compress or encase them.*

Spinal Cord Metastases

KEY FACTS

TERMINOLOGY

- Metastatic lesion from primary carcinoma in another organ (including brain)

IMAGING

- Focal, enhancing cord lesion(s) with extensive edema
- Typically small (< 1.5 cm)
- T1WI: Enlarged cord
- T2WI/PD/STIR: Focal high signal represents diffuse edema
  - Rarely syrinx
- T1WI C+: Focal enhancement
- T2* GRE: Hypointensity due to hemorrhagic components

TOP DIFFERENTIAL DIAGNOSES

- Demyelinating disease
  - Multiple sclerosis
  - Acute disseminated encephalomyelitis
- Primary cord tumor
- Inflammatory granuloma
  - Tuberculosis
  - Sarcoidosis
- Inflammatory myelitis
- Radiation myelopathy

CLINICAL ISSUES

- Brown-Séquard syndrome
- Rapidly progressive flaccid paraparesis
- Sphincter disturbance
  - Urinary and bowel dysfunction with conus involvement predominate
- Intramedullary spinal cord metastatic heralds poor prognosis

DIAGNOSTIC CHECKLIST

- Full craniospinal imaging when focal cord lesion found
- Edema out of proportion to focal small cord lesion suggests metastasis, even if solitary

(Left) *Graphic depicts metastases to the skeleton, epidural space, and cord. The hemorrhagic intramedullary metastasis expands the cord. Rapid onset of symptoms is characteristic for intramedullary spinal cord metastatic (ISCM). Asymmetric dysfunction of the spinal cord mimicking Brown-Séquard has been reported in 30-40% in ISCM but is exceptional in patients with epidural spinal cord compression.* **(Right)** *Sagittal T1WI C+ MR shows an avidly enhancing nonsmall cell metastasis to the conus.*

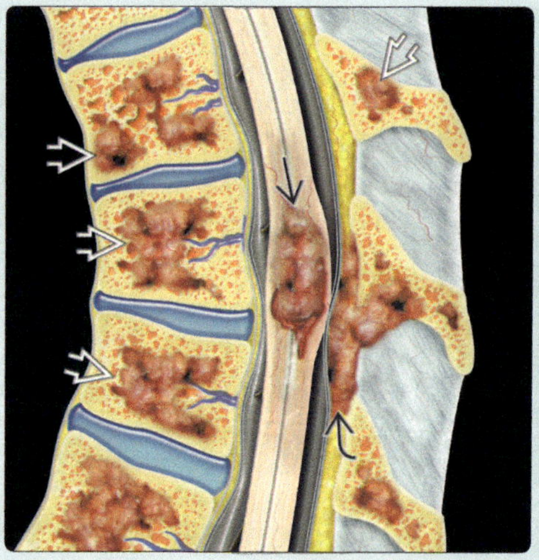

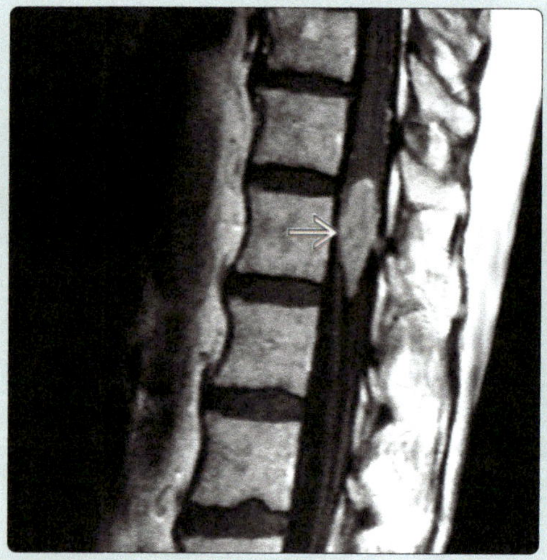

(Left) *Sagittal T2WI MR demonstrates a well-defined intramedullary lesion in the thoracic spinal cord due to angiosarcoma metastases. The lesion has a hyperintense center and hypointense rim. Also note spinal cord edema extending above and below the lesion.* **(Right)** *Sagittal T1WI C+ MR reveals subtle enhancement of the angiosarcoma metastasis. Nonneoplastic lesions, such as radiation myelopathy, demyelinating plaques, and paraneoplastic necrotizing myelopathy, can be difficult to differentiate from ISCM.*

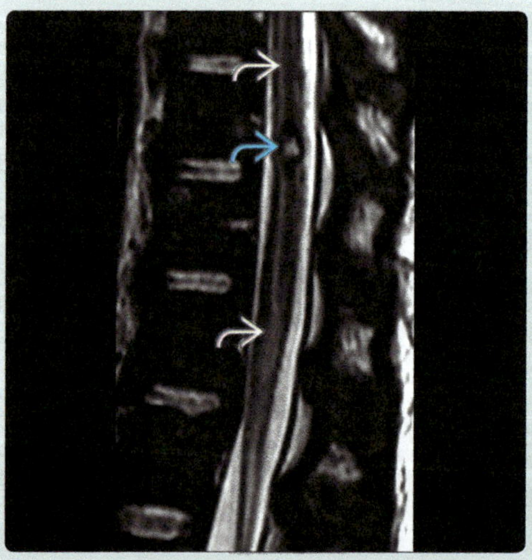

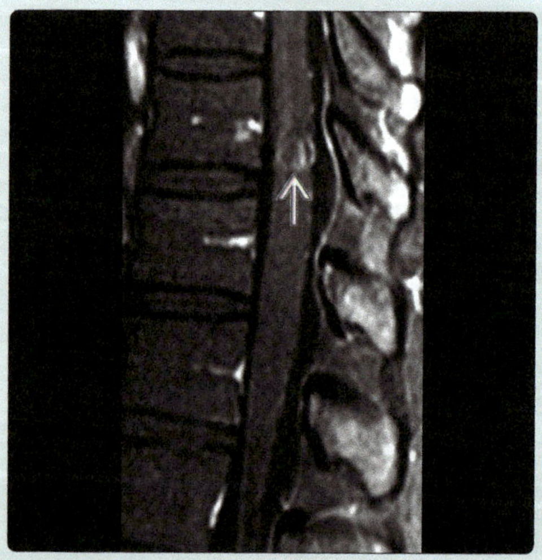

Radiation Myelopathy

KEY FACTS

TERMINOLOGY

- Chronic progressive radiation myelitis
- Delayed radiation myelopathy

IMAGING

- Spindle-shaped cord swelling with irregular, focal rind of enhancement (early)
- Focal cord atrophy (late)
- Clinical signs may reflect longer segment of damage than demonstrated on MR

TOP DIFFERENTIAL DIAGNOSES

- Transverse myelitis
- Multiple sclerosis
- Spinal cord infarct
- Astrocytoma
- Syrinx

PATHOLOGY

- Demyelination, lipid-laden microphages, swollen astrocytes, endothelial damage, necrosis, local Ca++ deposition, hyalinosis of intramedullary vessel walls

CLINICAL ISSUES

- Onset of progressive numbness and weakness ± sphincter dysfunction 1 month → several years after fractionated radiotherapy
- Relentless progression without significant improvement in most cases

DIAGNOSTIC CHECKLIST

- Late focal atrophy at sites of previous enhancement
- Fatty marrow replacement in treatment field provides clue to etiology
- Pathologic cord changes not always visible on MR

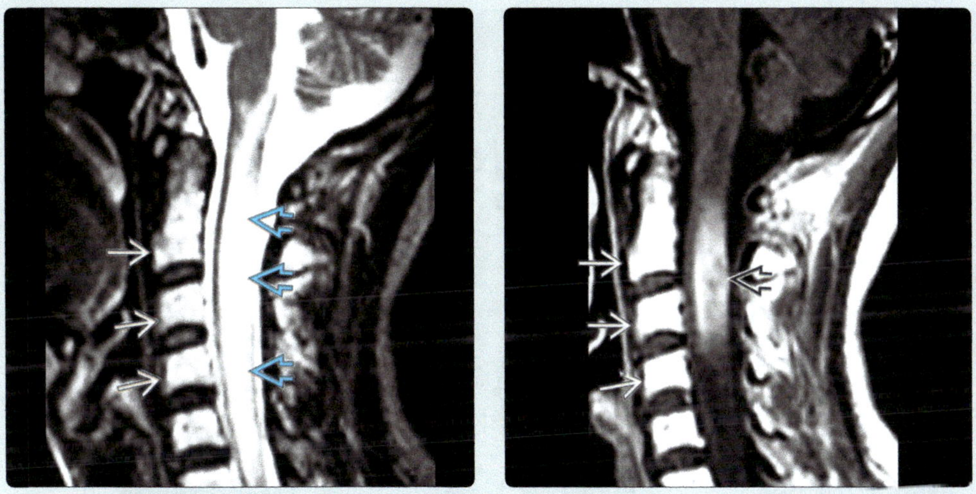

(Left) *Sagittal T2WI MR in a patient following radiation therapy demonstrates abnormal intramedullary T2 hyperintensity ⇨, appearing as bright as the surrounding CSF. High-signal intensity in the vertebral bodies ➡ reflects fatty marrow replacement, characteristic of postradiation changes.* **(Right)** *Sagittal T1WI C+ MR confirms abnormal spinal cord parenchymal enhancement in the area of greatest radiation myelopathic injury ⇨. The fatty replacement of the vertebral marrow is well seen ➡.*

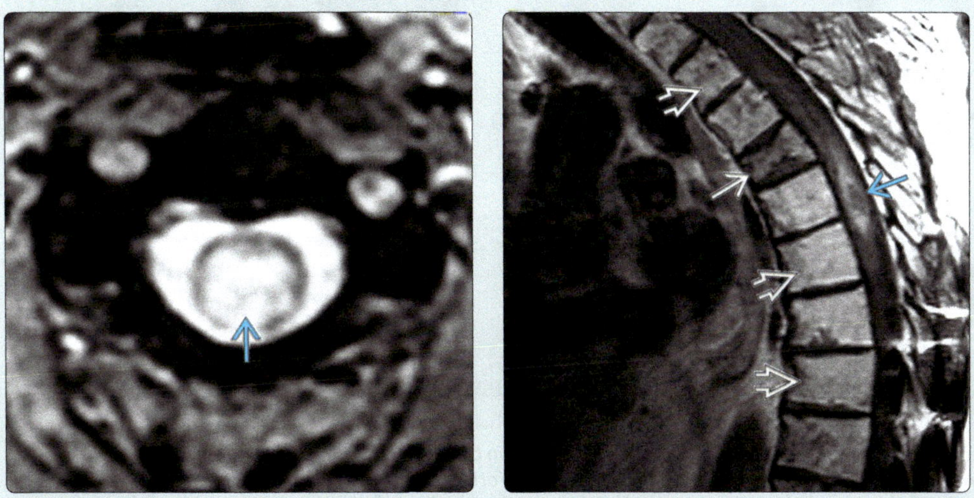

(Left) *Axial T2* GRE MR obtained within the area of greatest cord expansion and cord injury confirms that the majority of abnormal signal → resides within spinal cord central gray matter.* **(Right)** *Sagittal T1WI C+ MR of radiation myelopathy shows spindle-shaped enhancement → in thoracic cord. Fatty marrow replacement ➡ is also conspicuous in this patient following previous radiation therapy for vertebral metastases. A compression fracture ➡ is also seen.*

Postirradiation Vertebral Marrow

KEY FACTS

TERMINOLOGY

- Transformation of cellular vertebral marrow into fatty marrow following therapeutic irradiation

IMAGING

- Sharp demarcation between irradiated and untreated marrow (margins of radiation port)
  - Corresponds to site of irradiation and extent of radiation field
- Marrow signal intensity within radiotherapy portal similar to subcutaneous fat on T1WI
- May demonstrate associated compression fractures

TOP DIFFERENTIAL DIAGNOSES

- Normal fatty marrow
- Vertebral hemangioma

PATHOLOGY

- Marrow changes on MR dependent on radiation dose, fractionation, and time elapsed after treatment
- Complications include osteopenia, osteoporotic compression fracture, osteonecrosis, residual/recurrent metastases, and postradiation myelitis

CLINICAL ISSUES

- Usually asymptomatic
- Development or worsening of pain and neurologic complaints worrisome for radiation necrosis, insufficiency fracture, or tumor recurrence or progression

DIAGNOSTIC CHECKLIST

- Homogeneous fatty marrow sharply delineated from untreated vertebral marrow diagnostic of postirradiation change
- MR is modality of choice for marrow imaging
  - T2WI FS MR or STIR and T1WI C+ FS MR to evaluate for residual or recurrent marrow disease

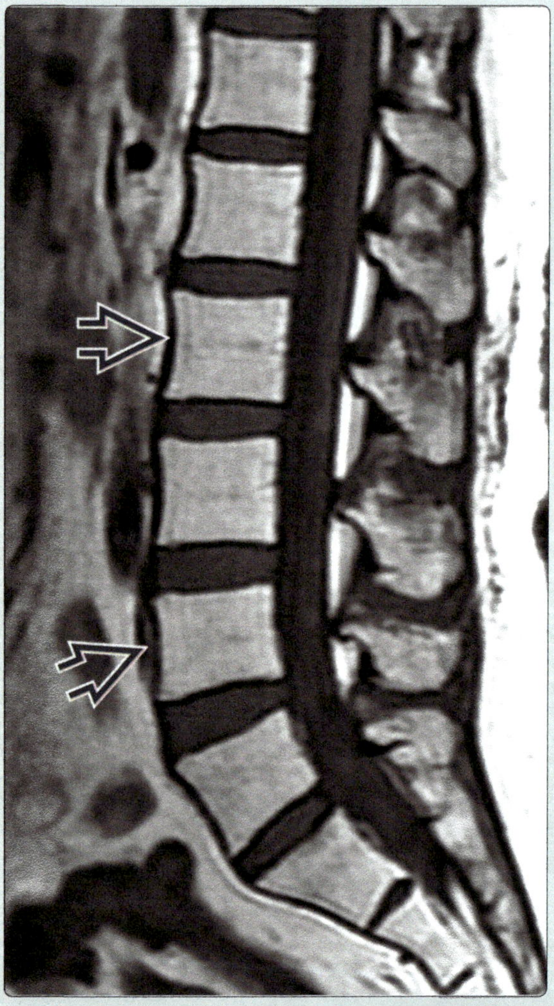

Sagittal T1WI (for metastatic intracranial glioblastoma with "drop metastases") shows typical postradiation "bright" fatty marrow conversion following whole-spine radiation ⇨.

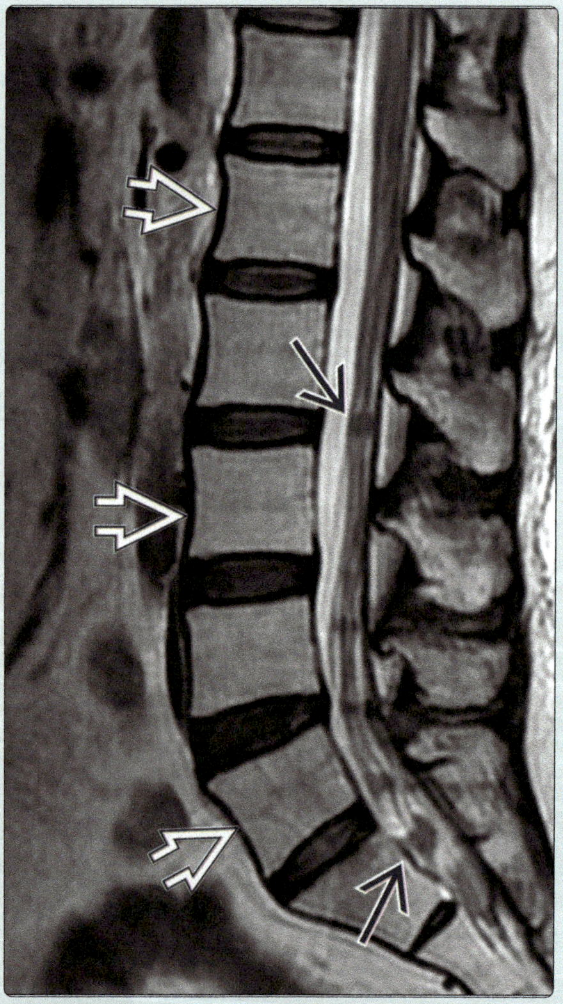

Sagittal T2WI in the same case again demonstrates diffuse postradiation fatty marrow replacement with uniformly "bright" vertebral bodies ⇨. Multiple metastatic nodules can be seen within the cauda equina ➔.

KEY FACTS

TERMINOLOGY

- Uncommon complication following intrathecal chemotherapy
  - Transient or permanent paraplegia
  - Initially described following intrathecal methotrexate (MTX) in pediatric acute lymphoblastic leukemia patients

IMAGING

- Smooth linear enhancement of conus pia, anterior cauda equina nerve roots
- Unenhanced T1W, T2W images normal

TOP DIFFERENTIAL DIAGNOSES

- Guillain-Barré syndrome
- Cerebrospinal fluid (CSF) disseminated metastases
- Postradiation radiculopathy

PATHOLOGY

- Intrathecal MTX, arabinoside (Ara-C) standard prophylaxis, and treatment agents for pediatric CNS leukemia
- MTHFR polymorphism affects folate homeostasis, may modify or predict CNS vulnerability to MTX

CLINICAL ISSUES

- Lower extremity flaccid weakness, most often without sensory deficit
- ↑ CSF protein, mononuclear pleocytosis, CSF immunoglobulin G synthesis
- Most commonly occurs after > 1 intrathecal chemotherapy dose
- Abnormal electrodiagnostic studies correlate with nerve root enhancement
- Most patients are children, but rare reports in adults
- Extent of clinical recovery is variable

DIAGNOSTIC CHECKLIST

- Correlation with clinical information critical to establishing correct diagnosis
- Contrast administration essential to detect cauda equina abnormality

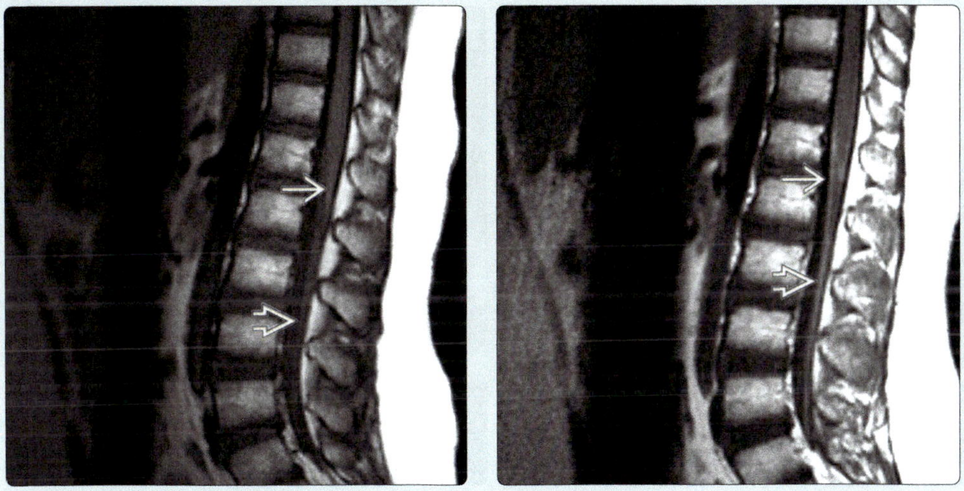

(Left) *Sagittal T1WI MR in a leukemia patient with leg weakness following intrathecal chemotherapy shows normal appearance of the conus ➡ and cauda equina ⮕. The unenhanced images may be normal in patients with anterior lumbar radiculopathy, so contrast should always be given.* **(Right)** *Sagittal T1WI C+ MR in the same patient reveals abnormal smooth, thin, linear enhancement of the ventral conus pia ➡ and cauda equina ⮕. The diagnosis would have been missed without contrast administration.*

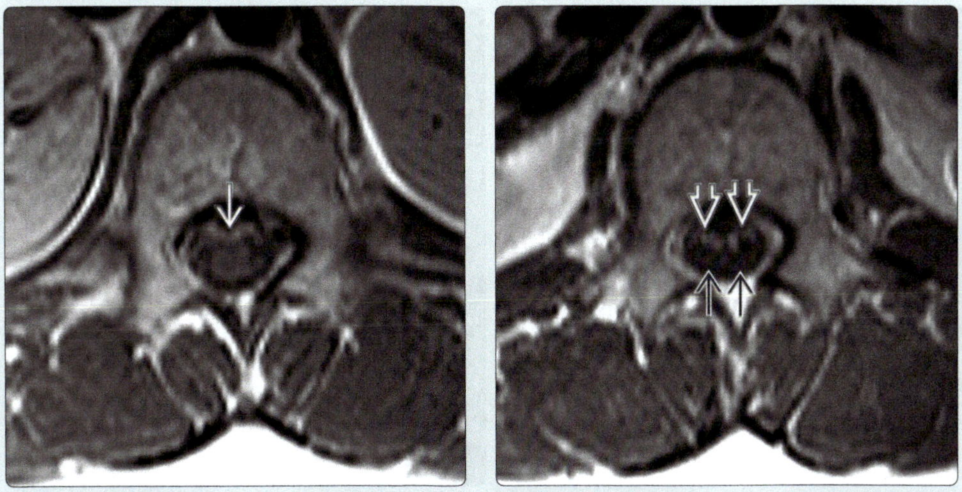

(Left) *Axial T1WI C+ MR through the conus medullaris confirms smooth, thin, linear enhancement of the ventral conus pia and cauda equina ➡.* **(Right)** *At the level of the cauda equina, axial T1WI C+ MR demonstrates characteristic smooth thin linear enhancement of the ventral cauda equina nerve roots ⮕ but not the dorsal cauda equina nerve roots ➡.*

KEY FACTS

TERMINOLOGY

- Cerebrospinal fluid (CSF) flow-related phenomenon due to time of flight (TOF) effects and turbulent flow

IMAGING

- Location: Intrathecal, subarachnoid space
    - Most prominent in cervical and thoracic spine
- Low or high signal intensity
- Ill-defined margins

TOP DIFFERENTIAL DIAGNOSES

- Vascular malformation, type I dural arteriovenous fistula
- Vascular malformation, type IV arteriovenous fistula
- CSF drop metastases

CLINICAL ISSUES

- Time of flight effects
    - Dark CSF signal
    - Positive relationship between CSF velocity and TOF losses
    - Typically occurs in spin-echo or fast spin-echo imaging
- Flow-related enhancement produces bright CSF signal
- Turbulent flow
    - Abnormally dark signal intensity
- Ghosting artifact motion
    - Periodic motion, such as CSF pulsation, cardiac motion, and respiratory motion

DIAGNOSTIC CHECKLIST

- Flow artifacts frequently have bizarre nonanatomic appearance
- Cross-reference other imaging planes and compare with faster imaging sequences (GRE, true FISP) that reduce superimposed flow phenomenon
- Ghosting artifacts in phase-encoding direction often accompany TOF- and FRE-related signal changes, help point out true nature of those changes

(Left) *Sagittal STIR MR shows an ill-defined signal void in the dorsal subarachnoid space of the thoracic spine ➢. This artifact is due to a combination of respiratory and cardiac-related pulsatile cerebrospinal fluid (CSF) flow superimposed on cranially directed bulk CSF flow. There is also contribution from turbulent CSF flow moving from the ventral to dorsal subarachnoid space. This complex CSF motion results in phase incoherence, leading to signal loss.* **(Right)** *Axial T2WI MR confirms the CSF flow artifact ➢.*

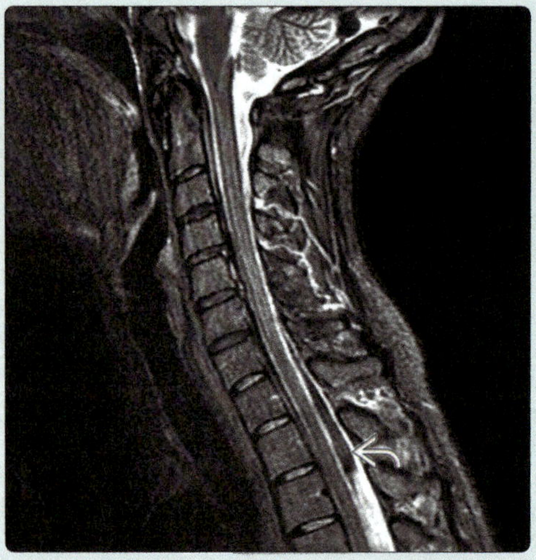

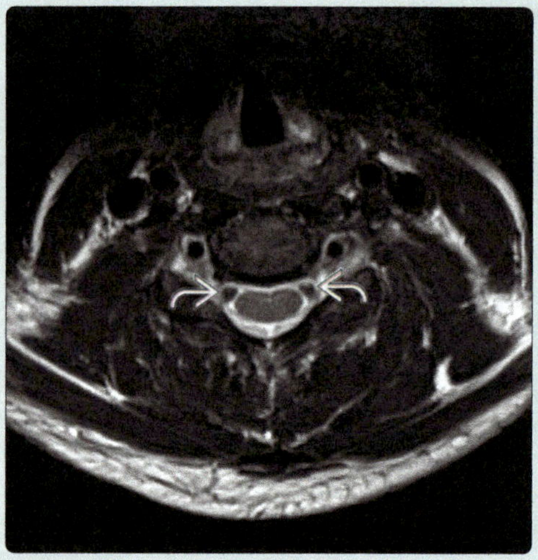

(Left) *Axial T1WI MR depicts isointense CSF flow artifact dorsal to the thoracic cord in the subarachnoid space ➡.* **(Right)** *Sagittal T1WI MR exhibits syringomyelia in the cervical cord ➡. CSF flow dynamics are altered because of the cerebellar tonsillar ectopia ➢. The turbulent flow results in a broader spectrum of proton velocities, which result in more rapid dephasing and signal loss. There is also a positive relationship between CSF velocity and time of flight losses.*

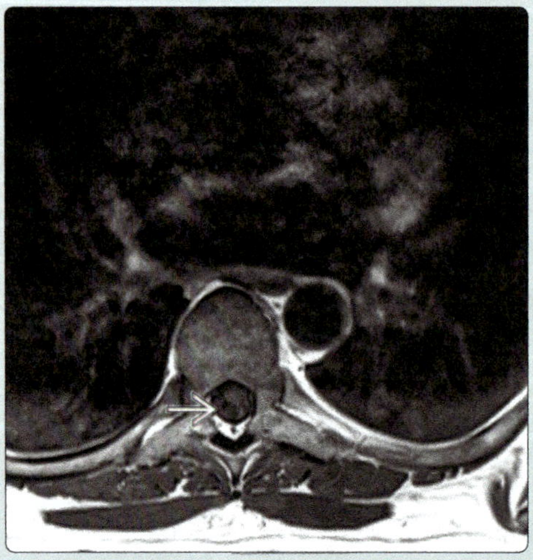

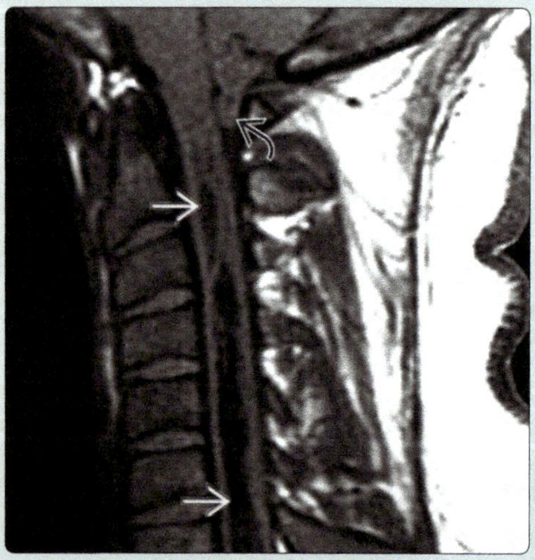

Perineural Root Sleeve Cyst

KEY FACTS

TERMINOLOGY

- Dilatation of arachnoid and dura of spinal posterior nerve root sheath, containing nerve fibers
- a.k.a. Tarlov cyst

IMAGING

- Occur anywhere along spine
  - Most common in lower lumbar spine and sacrum
  - S2 and S3 nerve roots most commonly involved
- Thin-walled cyst mass
  - Contents follow cerebrospinal fluid (CSF) density/signal intensity
  - No enhancement
- ± neural foraminal widening (bone remodeling)

TOP DIFFERENTIAL DIAGNOSES

- Facet synovial cyst
- Nerve sheath tumor
- Spinal nerve root avulsion
- Meningocele

PATHOLOGY

- Nabors classification of spinal meningeal cyst (MC)
  - Type I: Extradural MC without spinal nerve root fibers
    - IA: Extradural MC
    - IB: Occult sacral meningocele (outdated term)
  - Type II: Extradural MC with spinal nerve root fibers
  - Type III: Intradural MC

CLINICAL ISSUES

- Majority asymptomatic: > 80%
- Symptoms may worsen with postural changes, Valsalva maneuvers
- Cyst rupture → spontaneous intracranial hypotension
- Symptoms simulate disc herniation and spinal stenosis

DIAGNOSTIC CHECKLIST

- CSF intensity mass enlarging neural foramen or sacral canal characteristic of perineural root sleeve cyst

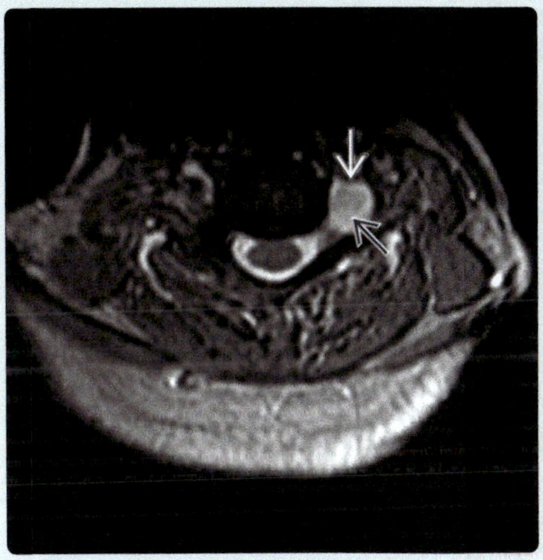

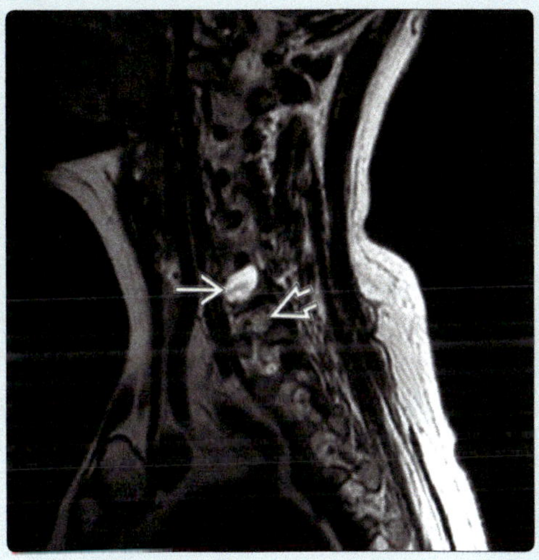

(Left) *Axial T2WI MR demonstrates a focal, well-circumscribed, hyperintense perineural cyst ➡ within the left C6-7 foramen. Subtle linear low signal ⇨ within the cyst represents the exiting nerve within it.* **(Right)** *Sagittal T2WI MR confirms focal expansion of the left C6-7 foramen by a large perineural root sleeve cyst ➡. Note hyperintense cyst signal compared with the normal dorsal root ganglia ➡ within the adjacent level neural foramina.*

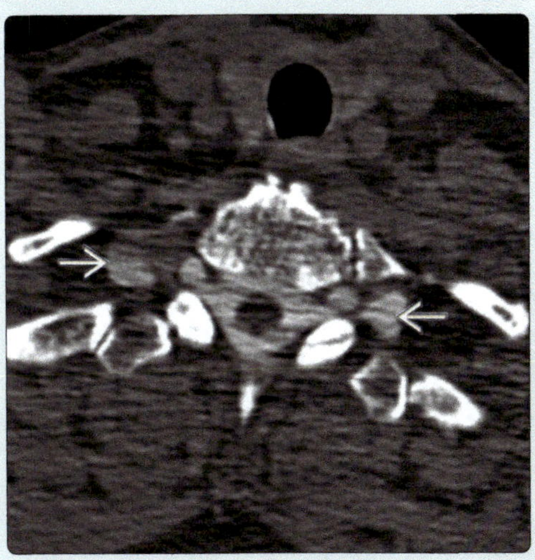

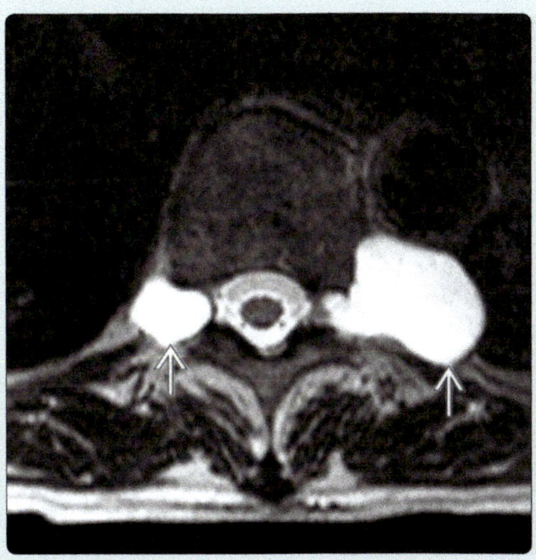

(Left) *Axial CT myelography shows multiloculated bilateral T1 nerve root contrast-filled cysts ➡ confirming contiguity with the contrast-filled dural sac. Only part of the right cyst contains contrast.* **(Right)** *Axial T2WI MR of the thoracic spine demonstrates bilateral, well-circumscribed cerebrospinal fluid intensity perineural cysts ➡ extending through the neural foramina.*

KEY FACTS

TERMINOLOGY

- Excessive accumulation of intraspinal fat causing cord compression and neurologic deficits

IMAGING

- Thoracic spine: 58-61%
    - T6-T8, dorsal to spinal cord
    - Epidural fat ≥ 7 mm thick
- Lumbar spine: 39-42%
    - L4-L5, surrounding thecal sac
- Y-shaped configuration to lumbar thecal sac on axial imaging
- Mass effect on thecal sac and nerve roots
- Follows fat signal intensity on all sequences
    - Fat suppression to confirm adipose tissue, exclude blood products

TOP DIFFERENTIAL DIAGNOSES

- Subacute epidural hematoma
- Spinal angiolipoma
- Epidural metastasis
- Epidural abscess

PATHOLOGY

- Exogenous or endogenous steroids
- General obesity
- Idiopathic

CLINICAL ISSUES

- Gradual progression of symptoms
- Weakness: > 85%
- Back pain, sensory loss, polyradiculopathy, altered reflexes, incontinence, ataxia

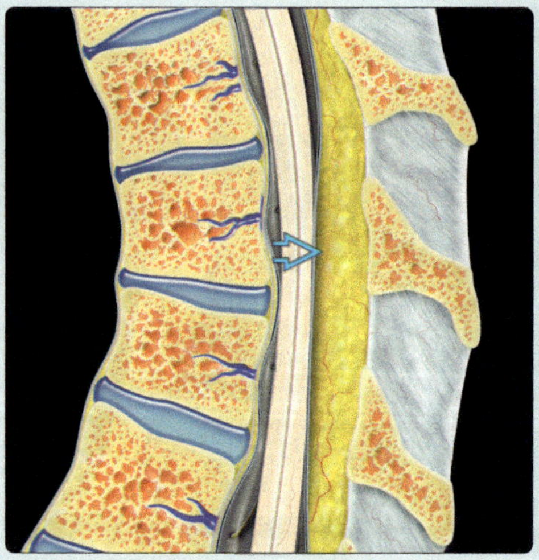
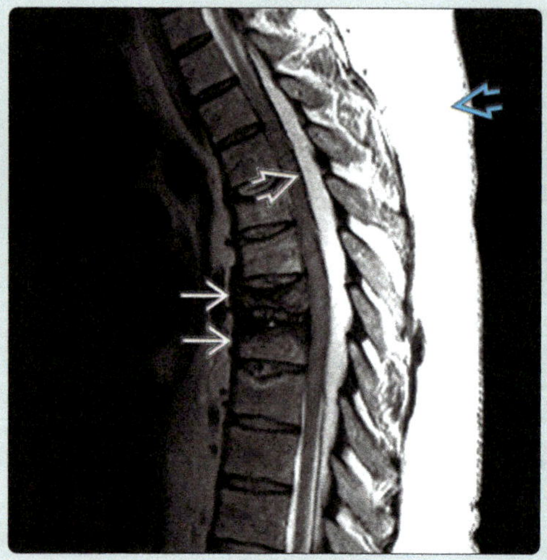

(Left) *Sagittal graphic illustrates confluent abundant epidural fat in dorsal thoracic canal, with effacement of the dorsal thecal sac and mild mass effect on spinal cord, which is displaced ventrally.* **(Right)** *Sagittal T2WI MR of thoracic spine shows smooth and homogeneous dorsal epidural tissue, isointense to subcutaneous fat. Vertebral compression fractures are due to steroid-induced osteoporosis.*

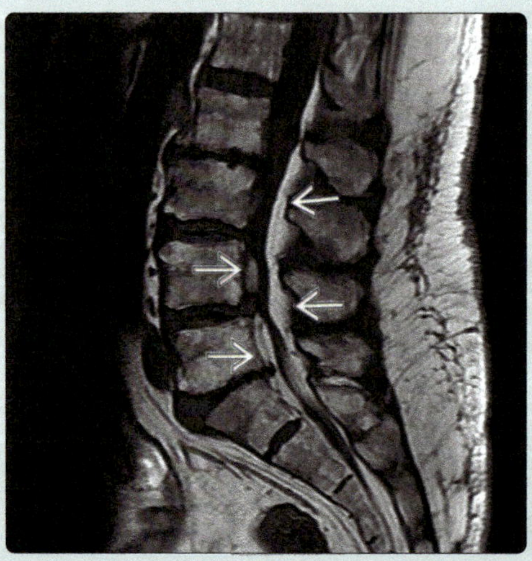
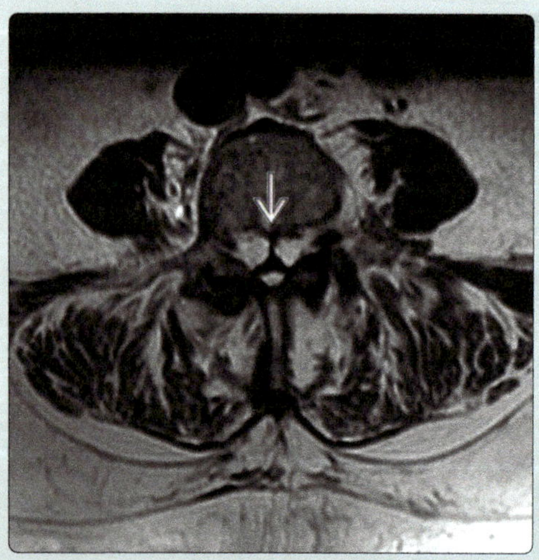

(Left) *Sagittal T1 MR shows abundant epidural fat both dorsal and ventral to the thecal sac. The thecal sac is small in AP diameter due to compression by the fat.* **(Right)** *Axial T1 MR shows marked prominence of the epidural fat in the lumbar canal, which causes the thecal sac to assume a trefoil pattern. The abundant fat in the epidural space allows for good visualization of the normal anatomy of the Hoffman ligament, which connects the posterior longitudinal ligament to the ventral dura.*

KEY FACTS

TERMINOLOGY

- Red marrow: Hematopoietic marrow
- Yellow marrow: Fatty marrow

IMAGING

- Yellow marrow often distributed around central perforating vein
- Yellow marrow adjacent to endplates in degenerative disc disease
- After bone marrow transplantation: Fat centrally located in vertebral body, red marrow at periphery
  - Yellow marrow high T1W signal intensity
  - Red marrow low to intermediate T1W signal intensity
- Signal intensity equal or slightly higher than muscle

TOP DIFFERENTIAL DIAGNOSES

- Leukemia
- Multiple myeloma
- Metastasis
- Myelofibrosis
- Hemangioma

PATHOLOGY

- Normal marrow pattern changes with age
- Primarily erythropoietic marrow in childhood
- Gradually converts to fatty marrow during adulthood
- Fatty marrow 1st seen around central draining vein
- Fatty, erythropoietic marrow often intermixed in marbled pattern
- Converts to predominantly fatty marrow in later adulthood
- Red marrow reconversion occurs with anemia, obesity, high athletic activity, bone marrow transplantation, and erythropoietic stimulating agents

CLINICAL ISSUES

- Asymptomatic

DIAGNOSTIC CHECKLIST

- Marrow fat patterns vary with age, health

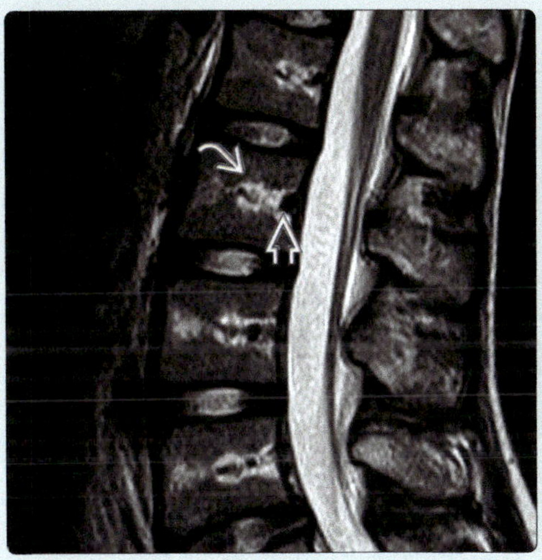

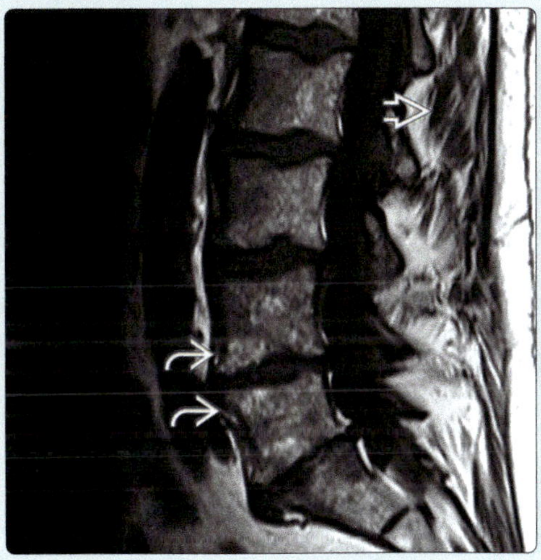

(Left) *Sagittal T2WI MR in a 15-year-old patient shows fat centered on the draining vein at each vertebral level. The remainder of the vertebral body contains red marrow, the usual pattern in young patients.* **(Right)** *Sagittal T1WI MR in a 50-year-old patient shows a polka dot appearance of yellow and red marrow. Fat tends to be centered around the draining veins and adjacent to degenerated discs. Red marrow is of equal or slightly higher signal intensity compared with muscle.*

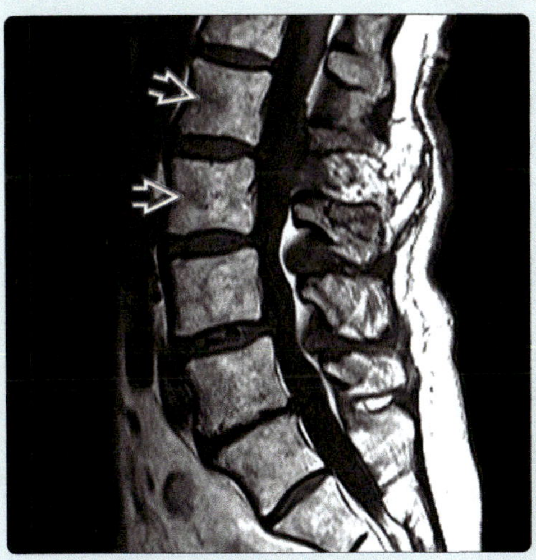

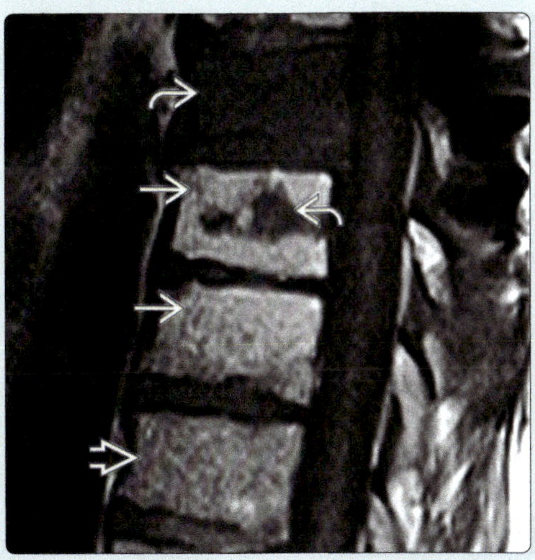

(Left) *Sagittal T1WI MR in an 85-year-old patient shows that marrow is predominantly fatty, but small foci of erythropoietic marrow, appearing as subtle hypointense areas, are still present interspersed throughout. Although red marrow involutes with aging, there is always some red marrow in the spine, unless a patient has been treated with radiation therapy.* **(Right)** *Sagittal T1WI MR shows a difference in signal intensity between normal fatty marrow, irradiated marrow, and tumor infiltration.*

KEY FACTS

TERMINOLOGY

- Idiopathic hypertrophic pachymeningitis
- IgG4-related hypertrophic pachymeningitis
- Multiorgan immune-mediated condition, which mimics multiple malignant, infectious, and inflammatory disorders
  - Chronic progressive diffuse inflammatory fibrosis of dura of brain or spine

IMAGING

- Linear low signal mass involving dura with variable mass effect upon cord
- Low signal linear mass effacing cerebrospinal fluid (CSF) and cord
- Peripheral enhancement related to peripheral zone of active inflammation vs. chronic central fibrosis

TOP DIFFERENTIAL DIAGNOSES

- Meningioma
- Lymphoma
- Tuberculosis
- Sarcoidosis
- Dural metastases
- Venous engorgement (CSF leak)

PATHOLOGY

- Autoreactive IgG4 antibodies observed in IgG4-related disease
  - No evidence they are directly pathogenic
- **Central pathology features**
  - Lymphoplasmacytic infiltration
  - Obliterative phlebitis
  - Storiform fibrosis
  - Mild to moderate tissue eosinophilia

CLINICAL ISSUES

- Spinal presentation as mass with myelopathy or radiculopathy
- Histopathology remains cornerstone of diagnosis

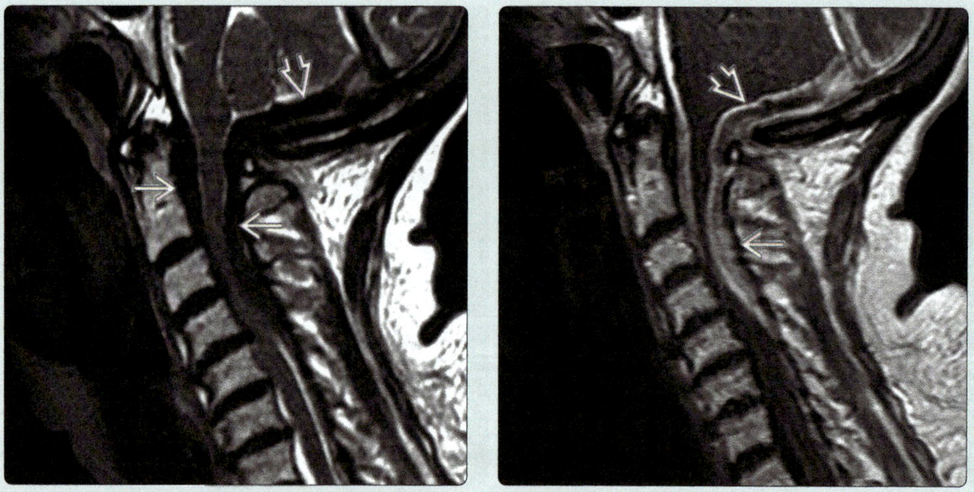

(Left) *Sagittal T2WI MR shows extensive low signal intensity thickening of the dura involving posterior fossa ➡ and upper cervical dura ➡. There is severe cord compression with loss of normal cerebrospinal fluid signal from the C1-C3 level.* **(Right)** *Sagittal T1WI C+ MR in the same patient shows diffuse enhancement of the dural thickening. Note the variable enhancement with areas that homogeneously enhance ➡ and other areas with more peripheral enhancement ➡.*

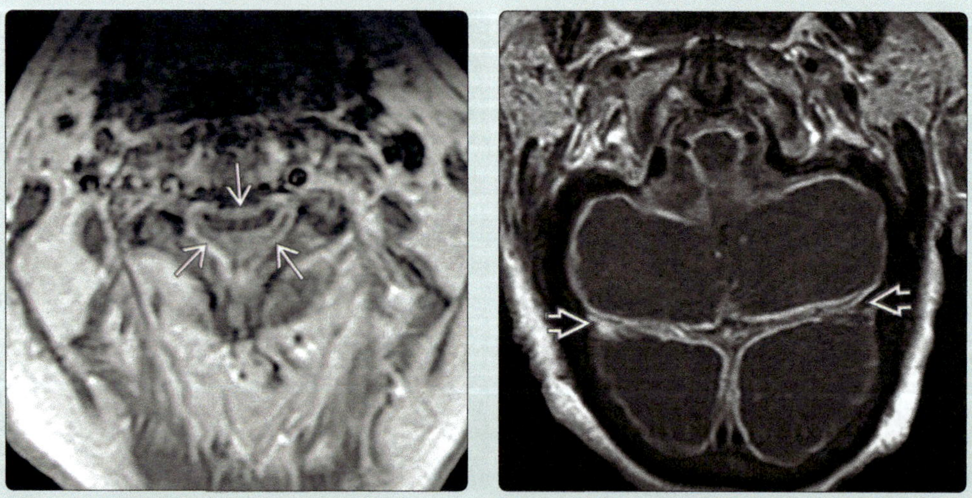

(Left) *Axial T1WI C+ MR shows diffuse enhancement of the markedly thickened dura circumferentially surrounding the cord ➡.* **(Right)** *Axial T1WI C+ MR shows the extension of the diffuse dural enhancement and thickening, including along the tentorium ➡. Note the lack of direct brain parenchymal involvement.*

Terminology

Synonyms: Great anterior radicular artery, arteria radicularis magna = artery of Adamkiewicz radicularis magna = artery of Adamkiewicz

Imaging Anatomy

Vertebral Artery

The vertebral artery is divided into 4 segments. The **1st segment** (V1) of the vertebral artery extends from its origin to the point of entrance into the foramen of the cervical transverse process, which is usually the 6th body. The vertebral artery is usually the most proximal and largest branch off of the subclavian artery. Multiple variations in the anatomic course and origins of the vertebral arteries have been described. The most common variation in vertebral artery origin is in the origination from the proximal subclavian artery. The origin of the left vertebral artery from the aortic arch between the left common carotid artery and left subclavian artery has been described in 2.4-5.8% of cases. When there is an origin of the vertebral artery from the arch, the vertebral artery usually enters the foramen of the transverse process of the 5th cervical vertebrae. With a normal origin of the left vertebral artery from the subclavian artery, the vertebral artery enters the transverse foramen of the 6th cervical vertebrae in nearly 88% of cases. The site of entrance at the level of C4 is seen in 0.5%, C5 in 6.6%, and C7 in 5.4%. Rare examples of origins of the left vertebral artery from the left common carotid artery, or external carotid artery, have been described. Also rare are variations in the origin of the right vertebral artery (< 1%) from the aorta, carotid arteries, or brachiocephalic arteries.

The **2nd segment** (V2) of the vertebral artery extends superiorly through the foramen of the transverse processes in a vertical course until it reaches the transverse process of C2. The **3rd segment** (V3) of the vertebral artery extends from the exit of C2 to its entrance into the spinal canal. After leaving the transverse foramen of C2, it courses laterally and posteriorly to pass through the transverse foramen of C1. The vertebral artery then extends posterior and medially in a horizontal groove on the upper surface of the posterior arch of C1. The vertebral artery turns abruptly as it nears the midline and pierces the posterior atlantooccipital membrane and enters into the vertebral canal. Anomalous connections in this region are uncommon but include the proatlantal intersegmental artery, which can communicate between the internal or external carotid artery and the vertebral artery at this level. Local duplication or fenestration of the V3 segment can occur. The occipital artery also can arise from the V3 segment. A persistent first intersegmental artery can occur where the vertebral artery courses below the C1 arch after exiting the transverse foramen of C2 and enters the spinal canal without passing through the C1 transverse foramen (3-4%). The origin of the posterior inferior cerebellar artery may also be anomalously low between C1 and C2.

The **4th segment** (V4) segment pierces the dura and extends through the foramen magnum, where it lies anterior to the medulla and eventually joins the contralateral vertebral artery to form the basilar artery. Major branches arising off the vertebral artery include multiple muscular branches from the extracranial segments to supply the deep muscles of the neck and meningeal branches. The posterior meningeal branch arises from the vertebral artery above the level of C1, and below the foramen magnum, and supplies the falx cerebelli and the medial portion of the dura of the occipital posterior fossa. Just before joining to form the basilar artery, each of the vertebral arteries give off a branch that will become the anterior spinal artery, which extend downward and medially to join in the midline with a corresponding branch from the other vertebral artery. The posterior spinal arteries can originate from the posterior inferior cerebellar arteries or from the intracranial portion of the vertebral arteries.

Spinal Arteries

The spinal cord circulation is derived from segmental branches off of the vertebral arteries, as well as multiple radicular arteries arising from segmental vessels. These segmental vessels include the descending cervical, deep cervical, intercostal, lumbar, and sacral arteries. The anterior spinal artery arises at the junction of the intradural segment of the vertebral arteries, caudal to the basilar artery. The anterior spinal artery descends in the midline without interruption from the foramen magnum to the filum terminale. The anterior spinal artery supply is reinforced by multiple segmental feeders. The segmental feeders give rise to sulcal, or central branches, which supply the anterior 2/3 of the cord. The anterior 2/3 includes the anterior horns, spinothalamic tracts, and corticospinal tracts. The anterior spinal artery lies in the midline on a ventral aspect of the cord, in the groove of the anterior median fissure. The posterior spinal arteries arise from the posterior rami of the vertebral artery or from the posterior inferior cerebellar artery.

The posterior spinal arteries are a paired longitudinal system of vessels on the dorsal cord medial to the dorsal roots. These form a plexiform and variable network between the 2 dorsal arteries. The posterior spinal artery supplies the posterior 1/3 of the cord, which includes supply to the posterior columns and a variable supply to the corticospinal tracts. Continuation of both the anterior and posterior spinal artery supply is derived from segmental anastomoses. These segmental vessels arise as dorsal rami from vertebral, subclavian, thoracic intercostal, and lumbar intercostal arteries. The dorsal rami enter the canal through the neural foramen and then penetrate the dura and divide into 2 main branches: The dural artery, which supplies the nerve root sleeve and the dura, and the radiculomedullary branch. The radiculomedullary branch then divides into a radicular artery, which penetrates the subarachnoid space to supply the anterior and posterior roots. There is also a variable medullary artery branch, which joins the anterior spinal artery and posterior spinal artery. The radicular arteries arise from the division of the radiculomedullary arteries along the anterior and posterior nerve roots. The anterior radicular artery extends along the anterior surface of the spinal cord, whereas the posterior radicular artery likewise extends along the posterior cord surface.

The multiple fetal segmental vessels will regress with adulthood, leaving 2-14 (average 6) anterior radicular arteries persisting in the adult and 11-16 posterior radicular arteries in the adult. The major cervical radicular feeders to the spinal cord occur between the C5-C7 levels. There are 2-3 anterior cervical cord feeders that measure 400-600 microns in size. There are also 3-4 posterior cervical cord feeders, which are smaller in size, on the order of 150-400 microns. The V3 segment never gives rise to radiculomedullary branches. In the thoracic spine, there are 2-3 anterior thoracic cord feeding segmental vessels. These are usually left-sided and are on the order of 550-1,200 microns in size. Small ventral feeding vessels may also be present on the order of 200 microns. There is an inverse relationship between the number and caliber of ventral radicular vessels. There can occur "pauci-segmental" anatomy with fewer vessels (< 5) with larger caliber or "pluri-segmental" anatomy with more vessels with smaller caliber. The dominant thoracic anterior radicular artery is also called the artery of **Adamkiewicz**. The artery of Adamkiewicz tends to have a left-sided origin (73%) and arises from T9-T12 (62%), with less common origins in the lumbar region (26%) and from T6-T8 (12%). A major segmental feeder may also occur in the upper thoracic spine, often the T5 level. This has been termed the artery of **von Haller**. The number of posterior thoracic cord feeding vessels varies from 9-12, with an average of 8. The posterior thoracic feeding vessels have no right-to-left lateralization. These vessels are on the order of 150-400 microns in size. The lumbosacral and pelvic regions have from 0-1 major feeding vessels to the spinal cord. The anterior spinal artery ends at the conus with communicating branches (rami cruciantes) to the posterior spinal artery. The posterior division of the iliac artery gives rise to the inferior and superior lateral sacral branches, which give rise to the spinal arteries via the anterior sacral foramen. The anterior division of the iliac artery gives rise to the inferior gluteal artery, which supplies the sciatic nerve. The posterior division of the internal iliac artery gives rise to the iliolumbar artery, which supplies the femoral nerve at the iliac wing level.

Spinal Veins

The veins of the spinal cord parallel the spinal arterial pattern. There is a very symmetrical pattern of venous drainage (compared with the highly asymmetrical arterial supply) with minimal anterior-to-posterior, right-to-left segmental variation. There are 2 sets of intrinsic radial draining veins, which drain into the anastomoses on the cord surface. The central group of veins provides for return of the anterior horns and surrounding white matter and drain into the central veins in the anterior median fissure. This forms the anterior median vein. Peripheral dorsal and lateral cord drainage is via small valveless radial vein plexus, which extends to the coronal venous plexus on the cord surface and then drains to the epidural venous plexus of Batson. The epidural plexus consists of anterior and posterior internal vertebral plexus components and connects with the superior and inferior vena cava, azygos and hemiazygos systems, and the intracranial dural sinuses. There are from 30-70 medullary radicular veins. The anterior median vein continues caudally along the filum terminale to the end of the dural sac. The coronal and median veins drain to the medullary veins, which leave the intradural space at the root sleeve and extend into the epidural plexus. Medullary veins have a functional valve-like mechanism at the dural margin, which prevents epidural reflux into the intradural space. There are no intradural valves present.

Embryology

The embryogenesis of the vertebral artery begins at ~ day 32 and is completed by day 40. The vertebral artery is formed from fusion of the longitudinal anastomosis that links cervical intersegmental arteries, which branch off primitive paired dorsal aorta. The intersegmental arteries regress, except for the 7th vessel, which will come to form the proximal portion of the subclavian artery, including the origin of the vertebral artery. As the connections to the primitive dorsal aorta disappear, the vertebral artery takes shape and initially has a more beaded anastomotic appearance and a tortuous course. The basilar artery is formed by fusion of the 2 primitive vertebral arteries.

Spinal cord vessels originate from a capillary network on the ventral lateral surface of the cord connected with segmental aortic branches. Two primitive longitudinal systems are formed. By the end of the 2nd month, the ventrolateral systems transform into longitudinal solitary anterior median anterior spinal artery. The plexus-like pattern remains more prominent on the dorsal surface of the cord. The anterior spinal artery formation is followed by a variable regression of segmental feeding vessels (initially 31) and is completed by the 4th month of gestation. The reduction is most pronounced in the thoracic and lumbar areas. Segmental arteries persist as intercostal and lumbar arteries. In the cervical spine, dorsal intersegmental anastomoses persist as components of the vertebral arteries. The ventral anastomoses persist as the thyrocervical trunk.

Selected References

1. Gailloud P: The artery of von Haller: a constant anterior radiculomedullary artery at the upper thoracic level. Neurosurgery. 73(6):1034-43, 2013
2. Eskander MS et al: Vertebral artery anatomy: a review of two hundred fifty magnetic resonance imaging scans. Spine (Phila Pa 1976). 35(23):2035-40, 2010
3. Becske T et al: The vascular anatomy of the vertebro-spinal axis. Neurosurg Clin N Am. 20(3):259-64, 2009
4. Bell R et al: Neurovascular anatomy: a practical guide. Neurosurg Clin N Am. 20(3):265-78, 2009
5. Debette S et al: Cervical-artery dissections: predisposing factors, diagnosis, and outcome. Lancet Neurol. 8(7):668-78, 2009
6. Goyal MS et al: The diagnosis and management of supraaortic arterial dissections. Curr Opin Neurol. 22(1):80-9, 2009
7. Johnson MH et al: Vascular anatomy: the head, neck, and skull base. Neurosurg Clin N Am. 20(3):239-58, 2009
8. Kim YK et al: Cervical artery dissection: pathology, epidemiology and management. Thromb Res. 123(6):810-21, 2009
9. Tubbs RS et al: Surgical anatomy and quantitation of the branches of the V2 and V3 segments of the vertebral artery. Laboratory investigation. J Neurosurg Spine. 11(1):84-7, 2009
10. Wang S et al: Anomalous vertebral artery in craniovertebral junction with occipitalization of the atlas. Spine (Phila Pa 1976). 34(26):2838-42, 2009
11. Bagheri SC et al: Penetrating neck injuries. Oral Maxillofac Surg Clin North Am. 20(3):393-414, 2008
12. Chen JW: Cervical spine injuries. Oral Maxillofac Surg Clin North Am. 20(3):381-91, 2008
13. Turan TN et al: Treatment of intracranial atherosclerotic stenosis. Rev Neurol Dis. 5(3):117-24, 2008
14. Schmidt WA: Takayasu and temporal arteritis. Front Neurol Neurosci. 21:96-104, 2006
15. Nelson PK et al: Vertebrospinal angiography in the evaluation of vertebral and spinal cord disease. Neuroimaging Clin N Am. 6(3):589-605, 1996

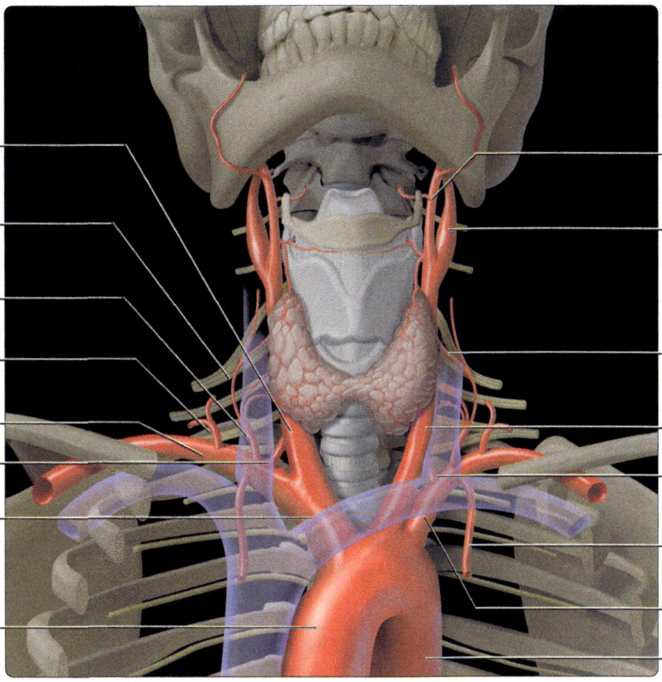

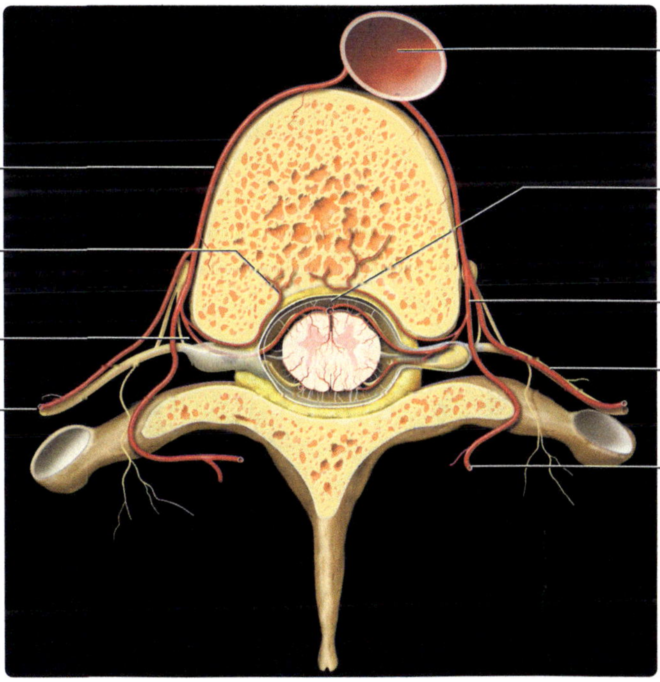

(Top) *AP graphic shows the aortic arch and arterial great vessels in red. The vertebral arteries give rise to the anterior and posterior spinal arteries (ASA and PSA). The ascending cervical arteries, branches of the thyrocervical trunks, give off anterior and posterior segmental medullary arteries that anastomose with the ASA and PSA on the cord surface. Complete spinal angiography includes evaluation of all these vessels.* **(Bottom)** *Axial graphic shows overview of the arterial supply to the vertebral column and its contents, depicted here for the lower thoracic spine. A series of paired segmental arteries (cervical regions arise from the vertebral and thyrocervical arteries, thoracic regions are intercostal arteries, and lumbar regions are lumbar arteries) divide into anterior and posterior branches. The posterior branch gives rise to a muscular branch, a branch to the vertebral body, and the radiculomedullary artery. The radiculomedullary artery enters the vertebral canal via neural foramen.*

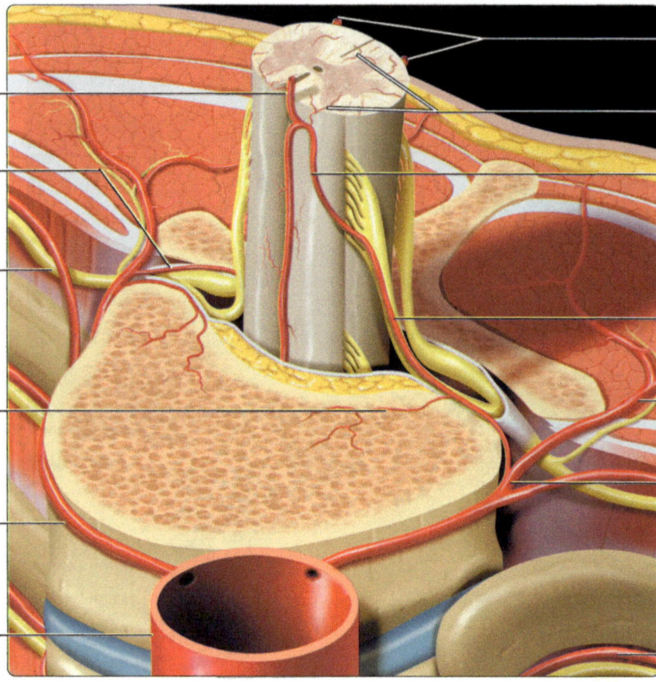

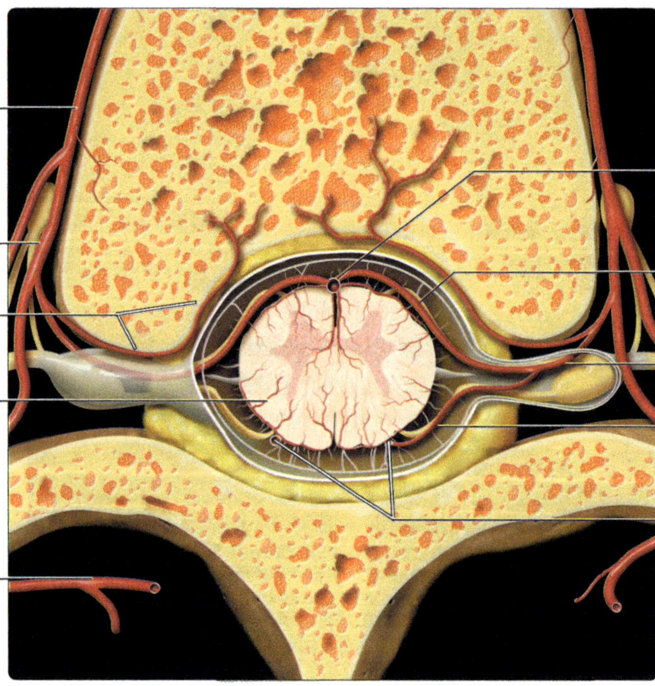

(Top) *Oblique axial graphic rendering of T10 depicts segmental intercostal arteries arising from the lower thoracic aorta. The artery of Adamkiewicz is the dominant segmental feeding vessel to the thoracic cord, supplying the anterior aspect of the cord via the anterior spinal artery. Note its characteristic "hairpin" turn on the cord surface as it first courses superiorly, then turns inferiorly.* **(Bottom)** *Anterior and posterior radiculomedullary arteries anastomose with the ASAs and PSAs. Penetrating medullary arteries in the cord are largely end-arteries with few collaterals. The cord "watershed" zone is at the central gray matter.*

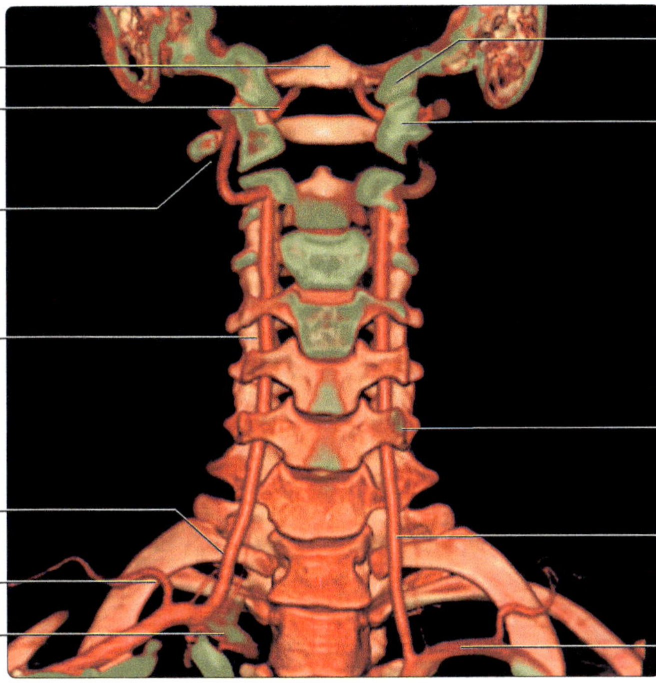

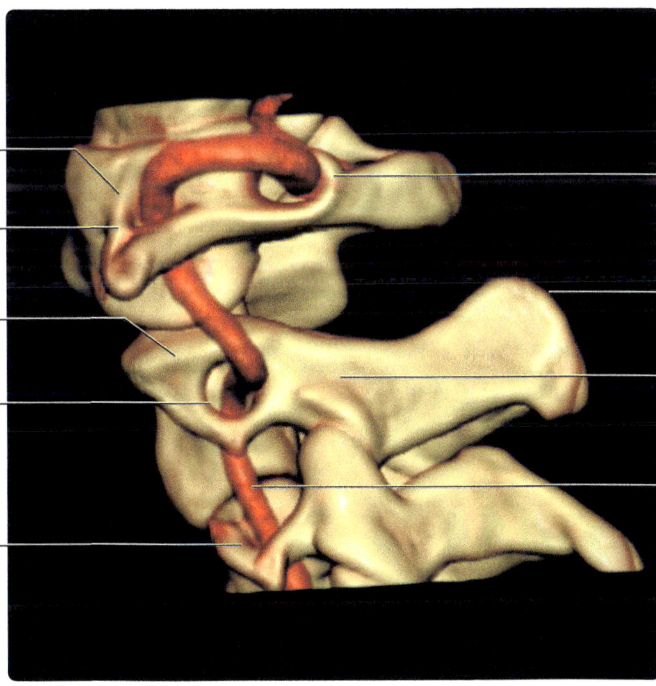

(Top) *AP volume-rendered image of CTA shows the course of the vertebral arteries, entering the transverse foramen and ascending to the foramen magnum. Both vertebral arteries in this patient enter the C6 level, but this can show wide normal variation. Left vertebral arteries arising from the arch enter more cephalad, at C5.* **(Bottom)** *Lateral volume-rendered CTA shows the course of the distal left vertebral artery passing through C1 and horizontally oriented C2 transverse foramen.*

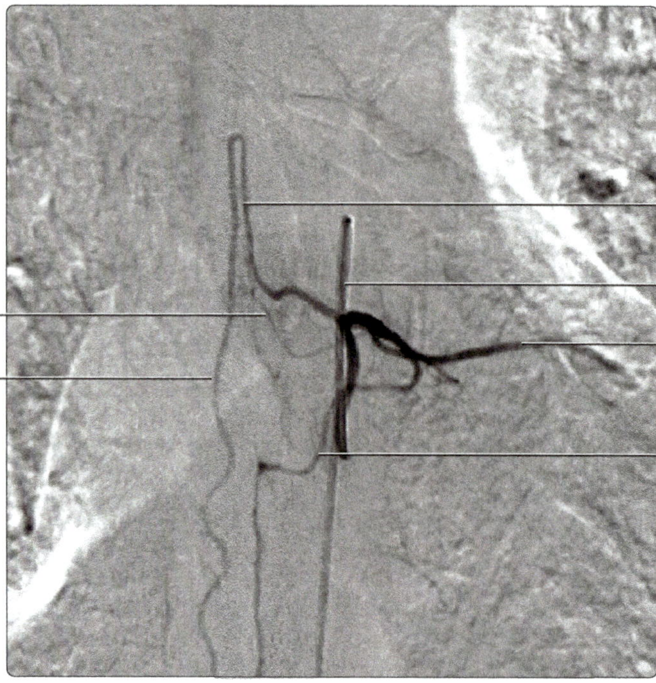

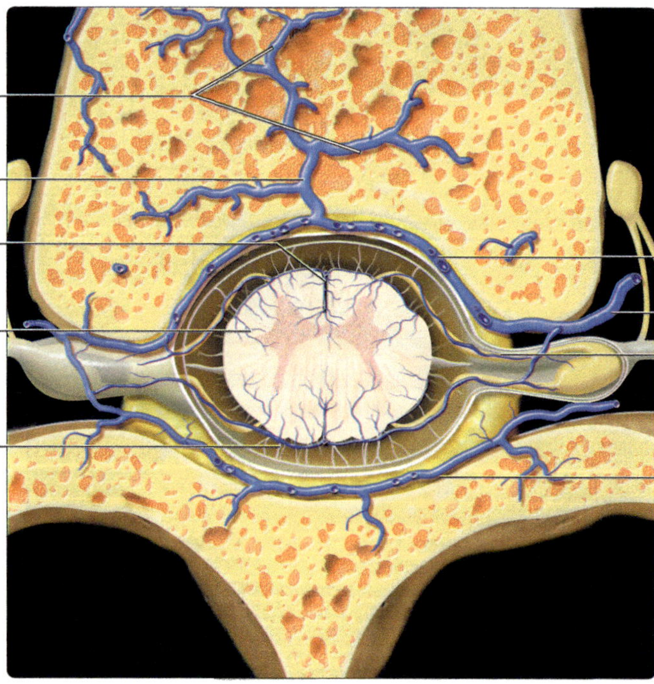

(Top) *AP view of a left T8 intercostal injection gives rise to the characteristic "hairpin" turn of the major segmental feeding vessel to the thoracic cord, the artery of Adamkiewicz. Extending inferiorly from the top of the "hairpin" turn is the ASA, which supplies the anterior 2/3 of the cord.* **(Bottom)** *Magnified graphic of the internal vertebral venous plexus is shown. The radicular veins course along the dorsal and ventral rami, eventually draining into components of the anterior or posterior internal plexus, and subsequently the segmental veins, which will drain into the superior or inferior vena cava.*

Type 1 Vascular Malformation (dAVF)

KEY FACTS

TERMINOLOGY

- Synonyms: Type 1 spinal arteriovenous fistula (AVF), dural AVF, dural fistula
- Definition: Spinal AVF, present within dura, with intradural distended draining veins

IMAGING

- Cord enlarged, T2WI hyperintense, vessel flow voids on cord surface
- Multiple enhancing serpentine veins on cord surface
- Dynamic contrast-enhanced MRA capable of defining dilated intradural veins; very useful to guide catheter angiography
- Spinal catheter arteriography is gold standard for confirming diagnosis/treatment

TOP DIFFERENTIAL DIAGNOSES

- Cerebrospinal fluid pulsatile flow artifact
- Spinal cord tumor
- Spinal cord arteriovenous malformation
- Tortuous "redundant" roots from spinal stenosis

PATHOLOGY

- Venous hypertension from engorgement reduces intramedullary AV pressure gradient, causing reduced tissue perfusion and cord ischemia

CLINICAL ISSUES

- Most common presentation is progressive lower extremity weakness with both upper + lower motor neuron involvement
- Very rarely presents with subarachnoid hemorrhage
- Middle-aged man with progressive lower extremity weakness exacerbated by exercise
- Persistent edema and enhancement of cord can occur even with successful clinical treatment of fistula

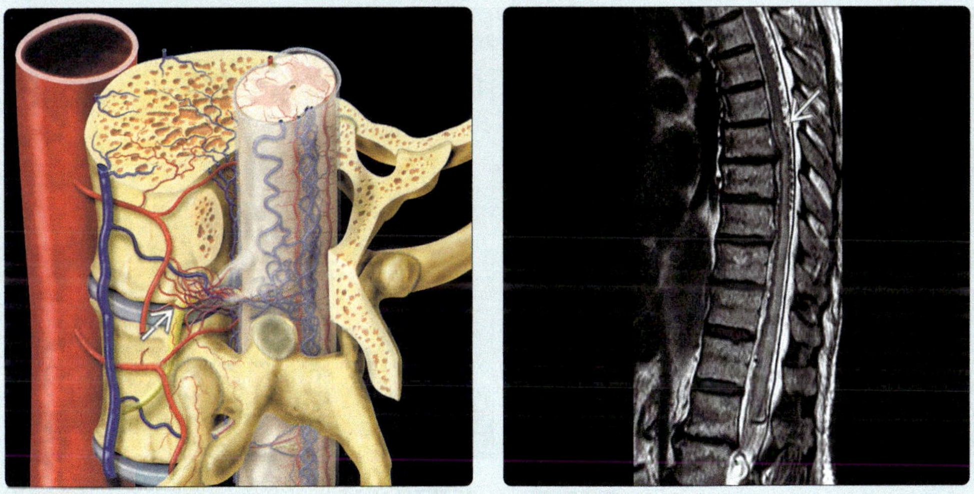

(Left) *Sagittal oblique graphic of the thoracic cord shows site of a type 1 dural fistula at the dural root sleeve level* ➡*, with secondary dilatation of intradural venous plexus due to arteriovenous shunt.* **(Right)** *Sagittal T2WI MR shows central cord T2 hyperintensity (edema) related to venous hypertension from the peripheral fistula shunting, which typically spares the cord periphery. There are multiple serpentine intradural flow voids from the arterialized and distended venous plexus* ➡*.*

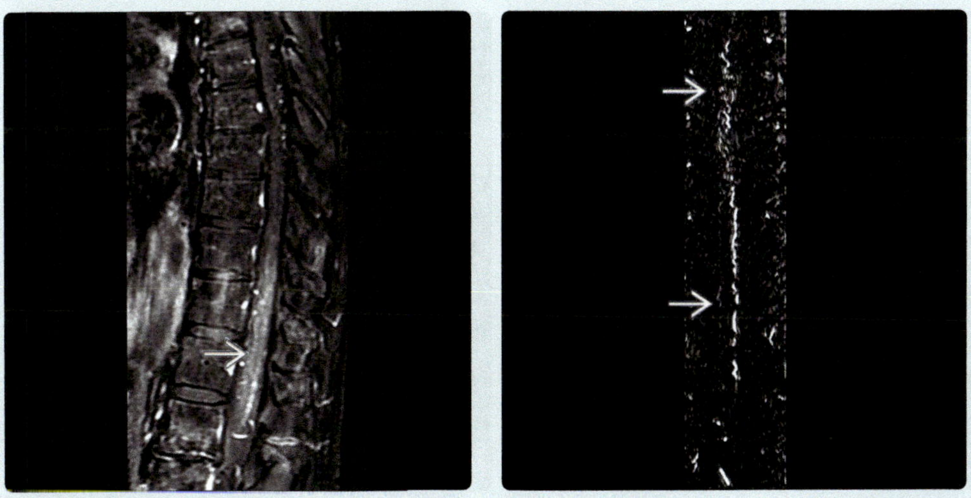

(Left) *Sagittal T1WI C+ FS MR shows ill-defined diffuse enhancement of the distal thoracic cord* ➡ *in this case of type 1 dural fistula. Faint to moderate cord parenchymal enhancement is common with this lesion.* **(Right)** *Coronal reformat of double-dose dynamic enhanced spinal MRA shows the dilated coronal venous plexus throughout the thoracic spine* ➡*.*

Spinal Cord Infarction

KEY FACTS

TERMINOLOGY

- Spinal cord ischemia/infarction
- Secondary to vessel occlusion
  - Anterior spinal artery (ASA); T4-9 most vulnerable
  - Posterior spinal artery (PSA)
- Hypotensive (cord "watershed" zone = central gray matter)

IMAGING

- MR with contrast, + diffusion
- Cord hyperintensity on T2WI; central owl's-eye pattern
  - Central gray matter or entire cross-sectional area
  - Slight cord expansion in acute phase

TOP DIFFERENTIAL DIAGNOSES

- Multiple sclerosis
- Transverse myelitis
- Acute disseminated encephalomyelitis/viral myelitis
- Neuromyelitis optica
- Type I dural fistula
- Spinal cord neoplasm
- Radiation myelopathy

PATHOLOGY

- Most known causes related to aortic pathology
- Other etiologies
  - Systemic hypotension, septicemia, disc embolism
  - Blunt trauma with dissection
  - Iatrogenic (transforaminal steroid injection, selective root block)
- Up to 50% of cases have no known etiology

CLINICAL ISSUES

- ASA: Abrupt-onset weakness, loss of sensation
- PSA: Dorsal column dysfunction (loss of proprioception, vibration)
- Rapid progression; maximum deficit within hours
- Poor prognosis, with permanent disabling sequelae
- Pain is frequent and disabling feature of cord infarct

(Left) *Axial T2WI MR in this case of hypoxic-ischemic encephalopathy (HIE) shows typical "owl's eye" abnormal hyperintensity within the central gray matter from chronic spinal cord infarction.* **(Right)** *Axial T1WI MR in case of severe HIE shows focal low signal within the central cord due to old infarction with myelomalacia.*

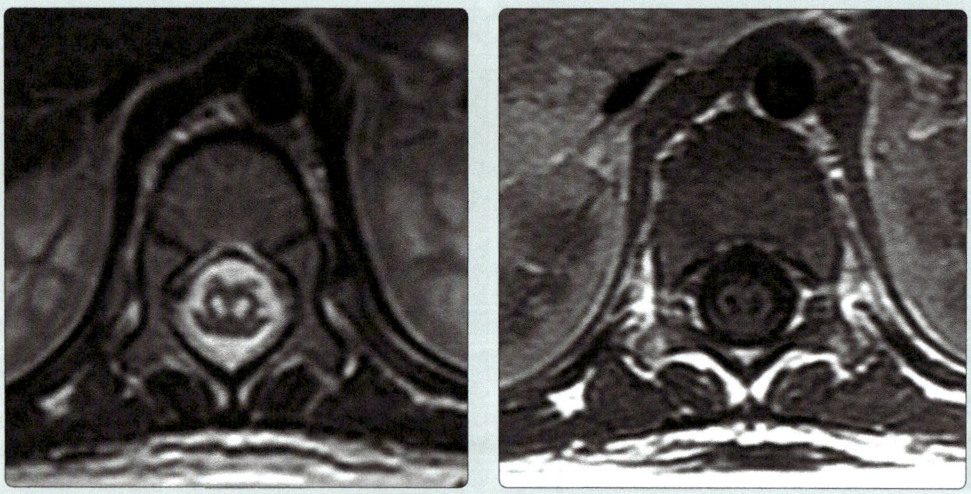

(Left) *Sagittal T2 MR shows slight hyperintensity in the distal thoracic cord ➡ in this patient with acute onset of leg weakness. There is a geographic region of increased signal ➡ in the superior aspect of the thoracic vertebral body due to concomitant cord and vertebral body infarcts.* **(Right)** *Sagittal STIR MR shows the cord hyperintensity involving the mid and dorsal aspect of the thoracic cord ➡, along with the vertebral body infarction ➡. The classic anterior 2/3 of the cord involved is not always present.*

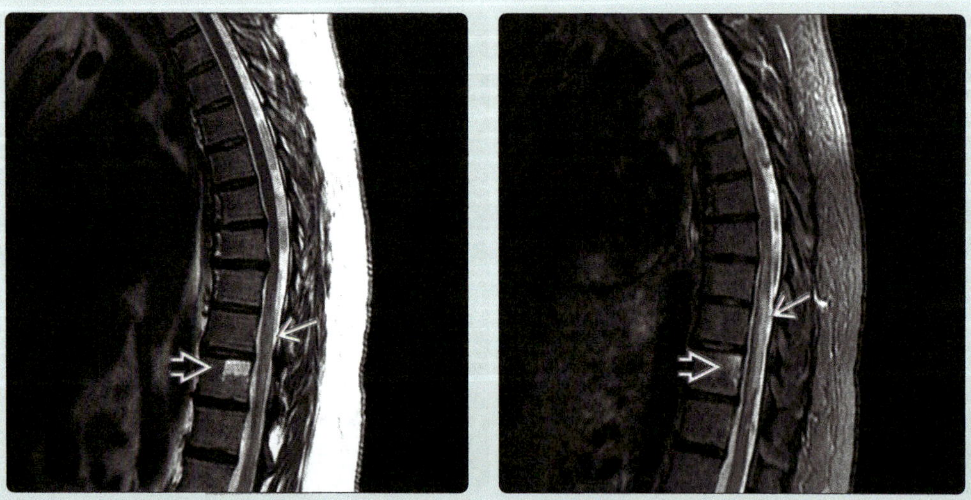

KEY FACTS

TERMINOLOGY

- Skeletal disorder characterized by low bone strength and increased risk of fracture

IMAGING

- Bone scintigraphy and MR are most sensitive to detect osteoporotic spine and sacral insufficiency fractures
- Bone mineral density
  - Standard measure for diagnosis of osteoporosis (OP) and assessment of fracture risk
  - WHO T-score cut-off value for OP: -2.5
- Thinning of cortex on radiographs and CT
- Normal or heterogeneous signal intensity (SI) on T1/T2WI MR
- MR features of **benign** osteoporotic fracture
  - Incomplete replacement of bone marrow, spared normal bone marrow SI of vertebral body
  - Multiple compression fractures
  - Retropulsion of posterior bone fragment
  - Low signal intensity band on T1/T2WI MR

TOP DIFFERENTIAL DIAGNOSES

- Lytic or blastic osseous metastases
- Multiple myeloma
- Hyperparathyroidism

PATHOLOGY

- Risk factors
  - Age
  - Postmenopausal
  - Glucosteroids
- Underlying disease → secondary osteoporosis
- Fragility fracture and insufficiency fracture

CLINICAL ISSUES

- Asymptomatic bone loss
- Affects up to 40% of postmenopausal women
- ↑ Morbidity due to bone fractures

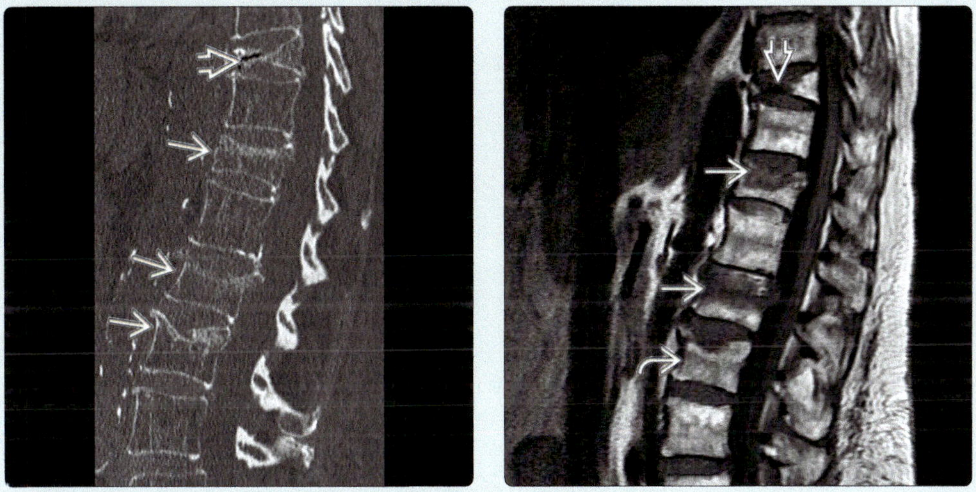

(Left) *Sagittal NECT shows compression fractures ➡ involving multiple levels from L3 inferiorly to T10 superiorly. The T10 anterior wedging compression fracture shows gas within the body ➡, compatible with Kümmel disease (osteonecrosis).* **(Right)** *Sagittal T1 MR in the same patient demonstrates that the L3 fracture is chronic with fatty marrow signal ➡. The L2 and T12 fractures are acute with low signal superior endplates ➡. The gas seen on the CT in the T10 fracture appears black ➡.*

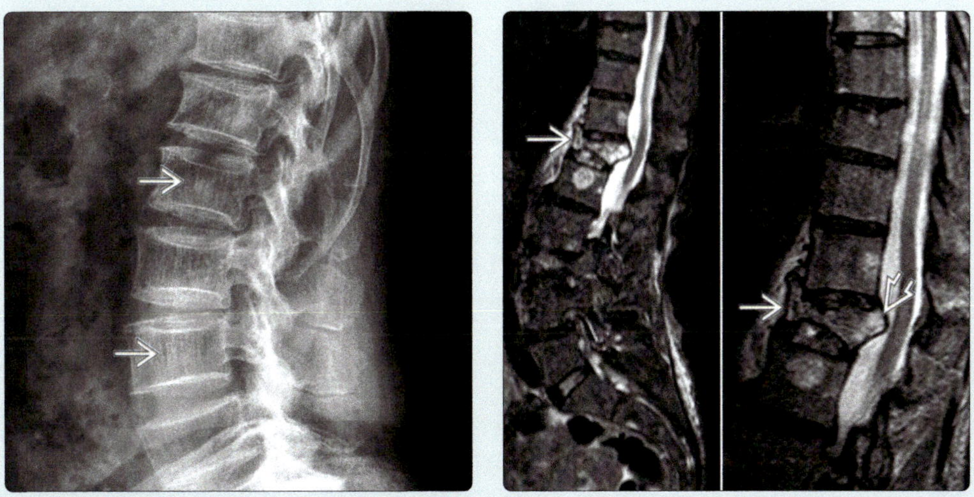

(Left) *Lateral radiograph reveals diffuse osteopenia with thinning of the cortices and accentuated appearance of the bony trabeculae ➡ due to background of demineralized bone.* **(Right)** *Sagittal STIR MR illustrates a benign osteoporotic fracture of the T12 vertebral body ➡ with retropulsion of the posterior cortex ➡. MR findings of metastatic fracture include convex posterior vertebral body border, abnormal signal of pedicle or posterior elements, epidural or paraspinal mass, and other metastases.*

PART II: SPINE
SECTION 6

Peripheral Nerve and Plexi

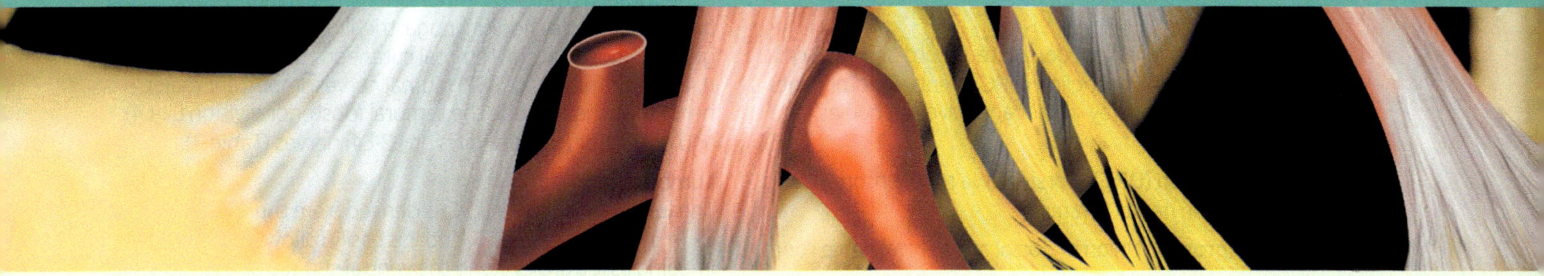

Terminology

Nerve rootlets: Individual neural filaments of dorsal and ventral roots directly exiting from spinal cord

Nerve roots: Composed of multiple individual dorsal or ventral nerve rootlets

Dorsal sensory roots exit from dorsolateral cord and have cell bodies within dorsal root ganglion (DRG). Ventral motor roots arise from anterior cord gray matter and have cell bodies within the cord.

Dorsal root ganglion (DRG): Dorsal nerve root sensory ganglion, resides in neural foramen

Spinal nerve (proper): Union of dorsal and ventral nerve roots

There are 31 nerve pairs (8 cervical, 12 thoracic, 5 lumbar, 5 sacral, and 1 coccygeal). Proper spinal nerve is short in length and bifurcates into ventral and dorsal rami.

Ramus: 1st spinal nerve branch

Larger ventral primary ramus (VPR) supplies ventral musculature and facets. Smaller dorsal primary ramus supplies paraspinal muscles and part of the facet.

Peripheral nerve: Combination of 1 or more rami into single neural conduit

Plexus: Neural network of anastomosing nerves

Imaging Anatomy

Cervical Plexus

The cervical plexus forms from the ventral rami of C1-C4 and variably a C5 minor branch. It has ascending superficial, descending superficial, and deep branches that supply the nuchal muscles, diaphragm, and cutaneous head/neck tissues.

Brachial Plexus

The brachial plexus (BP) forms from the ventral rami of C5-T1 and variably from minor branches of C4 or T2. The BP contributes to several nerves originating above the BP proper, including dorsal scapular nerve, long thoracic nerve, nerves to scalene/longus colli muscles, and a branch to the phrenic nerve. The remaining minor and all major terminal nerve branches arise from the BP proper.

Anatomically, the BP is classically divided sequentially (proximal to distal) into 5 segments: Roots/rami, trunks, divisions, cords, and terminal branches. The roots/rami originate directly from the spinal cord levels C5 to T1. The 3 trunks include the superior or upper (C5-C6), middle (C7), and inferior or lower (C8, T1) trunks. Important minor nerves arising directly from the trunks include the suprascapular nerve and nerve to subclavius muscle. Two divisions are described: Anterior division innervates anterior (flexor) muscles, and posterior division innervates posterior (extensor) muscles. No named minor nerves arise directly from the anterior or posterior divisions. The 3 cords include the lateral cord (anterior divisions of superior, middle trunks) that innervates anterior (flexor) muscles, the medial cord (anterior division of inferior trunk) that innervates anterior (flexor) muscles, and the posterior cord (posterior divisions of all 3 trunks) that innervates posterior (extensor) muscles. The cords branch to form several important named terminal peripheral nerve branches.

Clinically, the BP is divided into 3 discrete segments based on anatomic relationship to the clavicle. These include the supraclavicular (roots, trunks), retroclavicular (divisions), and infraclavicular (cords, terminal branches) plexus.

Lumbar Plexus

The lumbar plexus derives from the L1-L4 ventral rami and a minor branch from T12. Important named minor nerve branches include the iliohypogastric, ilioinguinal, genitofemoral, lateral femoral cutaneous (L2-L3), and superior (L4-S1) and inferior (L5-S2) gluteal nerves. Important major nerve branches include the femoral (posterior division L2-L4) and obturator (anterior division L2-L4) nerves (Table 2).

Lumbosacral Trunk

The lumbosacral trunk (LST) is derived from the ventral rami of L4 (minor branch) and L5, and it is easily followed on axial imaging as it transits along the ventral surface of the sacral ala to join the sacral plexus in the pelvis.

Sacral Plexus

The sacral plexus is composed of the LST, S1-S3 ventral rami, and a minor branch from S4. The sacral rami and LST converge into the upper sacral neural band (LST and S1-S3) that forms the sciatic nerve and the lower sacral neural band (S3-S4) that forms the pudendal nerve.

Coccygeal Plexus

The coccygeal plexus converges from the S5 ventral ramus, Cx1, and a minor branch of S4. The major named branch is the anococcygeal nerve.

Anatomy-Based Imaging Issues

Normal Nerve Findings

Surrounding perineural fat provides excellent visualization of nerves and allows them to be easily distinguished from adjacent soft tissues. The normal peripheral nerve is a round/ovoid shape with well-defined internal fascicular architecture. Normal nerve fascicles are uniform size and shape, and this characteristic fascicular pattern helps distinguish peripheral nerves from other lesions, such as schwannoma or ganglion cyst, which also demonstrate high intrinsic T2 signal intensity.

Intrafascicular signal intensity is determined predominately by endoneurial fluid and axoplasmic water, whereas the interfascicular signal is dominated by fibrofatty connective tissue that is amenable to fat suppression. Therefore, normal nerve fascicles are isointense to adjacent muscle tissue on T1WI and mildly hyperintense relative to muscle interspersed within hypointense fibrofatty connective tissue on fat-saturated T2WI or STIR MR. No abrupt change in nerve caliber or course should be observed in an anatomically normal nerve.

Abnormal Nerve Findings

The acutely abnormal nerve demonstrates 1 or more of the following findings: Segmental nerve enlargement, disruption of nerve anatomic continuity, T2 signal intensity approaching that of regional blood vessels on fat-saturated T2WI or STIR sequences, or disruption or distortion of normal fascicular architecture. Entrapped or scarred nerves may show abrupt change in caliber or course.

The abnormal nerve, therefore, remains isointense on T1WI but becomes increasingly hyperintense to muscle on T2WI. In the setting of injury, it is postulated that increased endoneurial free water content alters the normal signal characteristics of peripheral nerves. The cause of abnormal high signal on T2WI and STIR sequences is not definitively known, but it has been speculated that edema from increased endoneurial fluid due to disordered endoneurial fluid flow or local venous obstruction may explain abnormal T2 hyperintensity. Alterations in axoplasmic flow may also produce increased signal. Axoplasmic flow is impeded by nerve compression, and increased axoplasm proximal and distal to the injury site may produce T2 hyperintensity.

Imaging Pitfalls

It can sometimes be difficult to distinguish peripheral nerve from adjacent vascular structures, particularly if the abnormal nerve displays high T2 signal intensity. Vessels demonstrate internal flow voids, branch at large angles, and show intense contrast enhancement. On the other hand, nerves do not show flow voids, branch at relatively acute angles, enhance minimally, and display a discrete distinctive fascicular architecture on transverse imaging.

Clinical Implications

High-resolution MR technique readily identifies the large major nerves and major plexi and permits visualization of their internal neural anatomy. Conversely, smaller major and essentially all minor peripheral nerves are too small to directly visualize.

Successful peripheral nerve imaging requires a strong working knowledge of normal plexus and nerve anatomy. Additionally, peripheral nerve imaging is time consuming and necessitates constraining the imaging volume to clinically relevant regions rather than general "screening" surveys. It is critical to have all pertinent clinical and electrodiagnostic data available to appropriately constrain imaging volume and help detect subtle abnormalities.

Differential Diagnosis

Normal Nerve/Plexus

The normal nerve/plexus shows normal course, caliber, contour, and internal fascicular architecture. Consider myopathic or other nonneural etiology in symptomatic patients.

Nerve/Plexus Mass

Neural neoplasms are most commonly of neural sheath origin. Consider solitary or plexiform neurofibroma, schwannoma, or malignant peripheral nerve sheath tumor. Less common considerations include neurolymphomatosis and peripheral nerve metastasis.

Trauma

Etiologies include traction (stretch or avulsion), laceration (projectile, fracture fragment, sharp object), or direct compression (hematoma, fracture).

MR is sensitive for the detection and in some cases discrimination of all 3 described peripheral nerve injury levels. **Neuropraxia**, the least severe type of injury, is characterized by focal damage to the myelin sheath without axonal disruption and manifests as identifiable but swollen and hyperintense nerve fascicles. **Axonotmesis** is an intermediate level of crush or traction injury that produces axonal disruption and subsequent wallerian degeneration but leaves the Schwann cells and endoneurium intact. Axonotmesis will display a homogeneously increased signal intensity nerve with loss of fascicular architecture at the injury site. **Neurotmesis**, the most severe form of nerve injury, cannot always be distinguished from axonotmesis in the cases of functional rather than anatomical transaction but may display axonal disruption with discontinuity of some or all of the surrounding connective tissues and subsequent wallerian degeneration in definitive cases.

Entrapment Syndrome

Neural compression occurs at characteristic locations. These injuries are often, but not always, related to poor ergonomics or overuse injuries.

Hereditary Motor and Sensory Neuropathy

Inherited peripheral nerve disorders are characterized by abnormally enlarged peripheral nerves (usually palpable if not deep) and variable clinical neuropathy presentations. Some demonstrate characteristic onion- bulb appearance on micropathology following nerve biopsy, reflecting recurrent episodes of demyelination and remyelination. The most common hereditary motor and sensory neuropathy disorder is Charcot-Marie-Tooth, which has characteristic clinical manifestations and may involve the cauda equina, peripheral nerves, or both.

Infection/Inflammation

Myriad pathological etiologies and clinical manifestations characterize this diverse group of disorders. Important causes include syphilis (tabes dorsalis), leprosy, infectious neuritis (usually viral), and sarcoidosis. Immune-mediated noninfectious disorders include postviral or vaccination (Guillain-Barré syndrome), chronic immune demyelinating polyneuropathy, and idiopathic brachial plexitis (Parsonage-Turner syndrome).

Drug/Toxic Injury

Neural injuries have been linked to vinca alkaloids, therapeutic gold, amiodarone, dapsone, thalidomide, and lead or mercury intoxication.

Vascular Insult

Injury may result from either nerve ischemia related to peripheral vascular disease or vascular trauma or sequelae of vasculitis. The most common vasculitis etiologies are diabetic, Churg-Strauss, polyarteritis nodosa, and Wegener granulomatosis.

Selected References

1. Chhabra A et al: Peripheral nerve injury grading simplified on MR neurography: As referenced to Seddon and Sunderland classifications. Indian J Radiol Imaging. 24(3):217-24, 2014
2. Crush AB et al: Malignant involvement of the peripheral nervous system in patients with cancer: multimodality imaging and pathologic correlation. Radiographics. 34(7):1987-2007, 2014
3. Demehri S et al: Conventional and functional MR imaging of peripheral nerve sheath tumors: initial experience. AJNR Am J Neuroradiol. 35(8):1615-20, 2014
4. Pham M et al: Peripheral nerves and plexus: imaging by MR-neurography and high-resolution ultrasound. Curr Opin Neurol. 27(4):370-9, 2014
5. Sureka J et al: MRI of brachial plexopathies. Clin Radiol. 64(2):208-18, 2009
6. Bowen BC et al: Plexopathy. AJNR Am J Neuroradiol. 29(2):400-2, 2008
7. Hof JJ et al: What's new in MRI of peripheral nerve entrapment? Neurosurg Clin N Am. 19(4):583-95, vi, 2008
8. Kim S et al: Role of magnetic resonance imaging in entrapment and compressive neuropathy–what, where, and how to see the peripheral nerves on the musculoskeletal magnetic resonance image: part 2. Upper extremity. Eur Radiol. 17(2):509-22, 2007
9. Castillo M: Imaging the anatomy of the brachial plexus: review and self-assessment module. AJR Am J Roentgenol. 185(6 Suppl):S196-204, 2005

Brachial Plexus Major Nerves

Nerve	Definition	Motor/Sensory Innervation	Important Branches
Radial nerve	Terminal branch of posterior brachial plexus cord	Innervates extensor muscles of arm and forearm (triceps, brachioradialis, extensor forearm muscles)	Most important branch is posterior interosseous nerve
Median nerve	Terminal branch arises from both lateral and medial brachial plexus cords	Innervates flexor muscles of forearm and thumb as well as 1st and 2nd lumbricals	Most important branch is anterior interosseous nerve
Ulnar nerve	Terminal branch of medial brachial plexus cord	Innervates flexor carpi ulnaris, 3rd and 4th lumbricals, and majority of intrinsic hand muscles	
Musculocutaneous nerve	Terminal branch of lateral brachial plexus cord	Innervates flexor muscles of arm (coracobrachialis, biceps, and brachialis)	
Axillary nerve	Terminal branch of posterior brachial plexus cord	Innervates deltoid and teres minor muscles	

Lumbosacral Plexus Major Nerves

Nerve	Definition	Motor/Sensory Innervation
Obturator nerve	Terminal branch of lumbar plexus (anterior division)	Innervates thigh adductor muscles
Femoral nerve	Terminal branch of lumbar plexus (posterior division)	Innervates iliacus, psoas, and quadriceps muscles
Sciatic nerve	Largest peripheral nerve branch of sacral plexus	Innervates posterior thigh (biceps femoris, semitendinosus, semimembranosus, adductor magnus) and all leg muscles (via tibial and common peroneal nerve)
Common peroneal nerve	Major anterior terminal branch of sciatic nerve	Innervates anterior leg muscles; superficial peroneal nerve innervates peroneus muscles, extensor digitorum brevis; deep peroneal nerve innervates tibialis anterior, extensor digitorum longus, extensor hallucis longus muscles
Tibial nerve	Major posterior branch of sciatic nerve	Innervates posterior leg muscles (gastrocnemius, soleus, tibialis posterior, flexor digitorum longus, flexor hallicus longus)

High-Resolution MR Protocols

MR Pulse Sequence	Technical Parameters	Technical Comments
Coronal T1WI MR	3-4-mm slice thickness, 20-24-cm FOV, no interslice gap	Direct coronal plane, not oblique
Coronal fat-saturated T2WI or STIR MR	3-4-mm slice thickness, 20-24-cm FOV, no interslice gap	Direct coronal plane, not oblique
Direct axial or sagittal oblique T1WI MR	5-7-mm slice thickness, 16-20-cm FOV, no interslice gap	Sagittal oblique plane oriented perpendicular to plexus
Direct axial or sagittal oblique fat-saturated T2WI or STIR MR	5-7-mm slice thickness, 16-20-cm FOV, no interslice gap	Sagittal oblique plane oriented perpendicular to plexus
Coronal and axial fat-saturated T1WI C+ MR (optional)	Same planes as unenhanced imaging sequences	Use if suspected or confirmed mass or infection

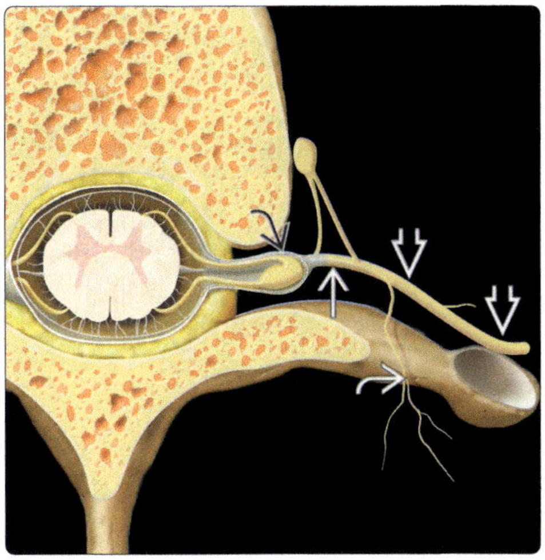

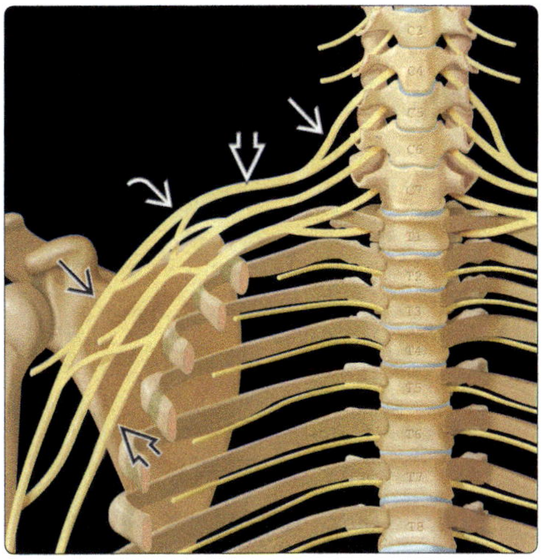

(Left) *Axial graphic shows formation of a spinal nerve from dorsal, ventral rootlets to form the spinal nerve proper. The short spinal nerve bifurcates into large ventral and small dorsal primary rami. The dural sleeve of the nerve root is shown in gray, terminating just past the dorsal root ganglion.* **(Right)** *Graphic shows typical anatomy of the 5 brachial plexus sections from proximal to distal: Roots (technically ventral primary rami) of C5-T1, trunks, divisions, cords, and terminal major branches.*

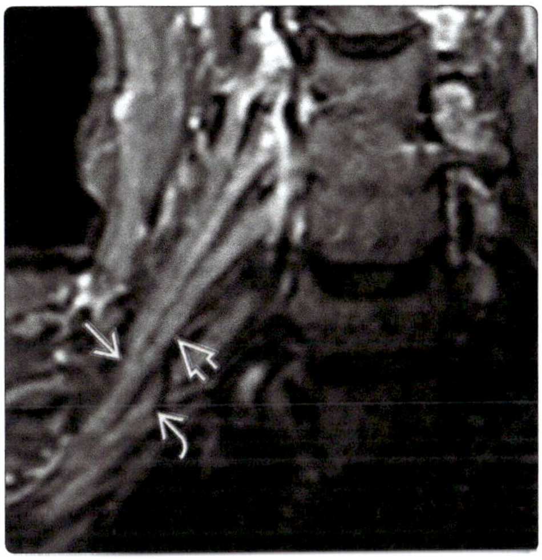

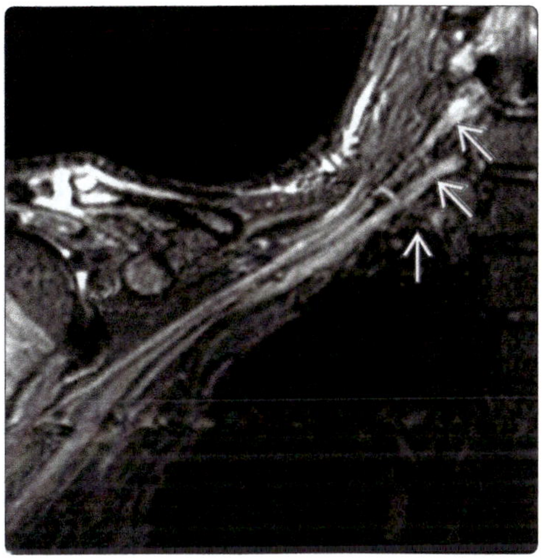

(Left) *Coronal STIR MR of the upper right brachial plexus depicts normal mildly hyperintense brachial plexus roots/rami of C5 to T1. C5 and C6 form the superior (upper) trunk, C7 the middle trunk, and C8 and T1 the inferior (lower) trunk.* **(Right)** *Coronal STIR MR of the lower right brachial plexus demonstrates normal C7, C8, and T1 roots/rami sequentially forming trunks, divisions, and cords. The normal brachial plexus courses retroclavicular into the axilla.*

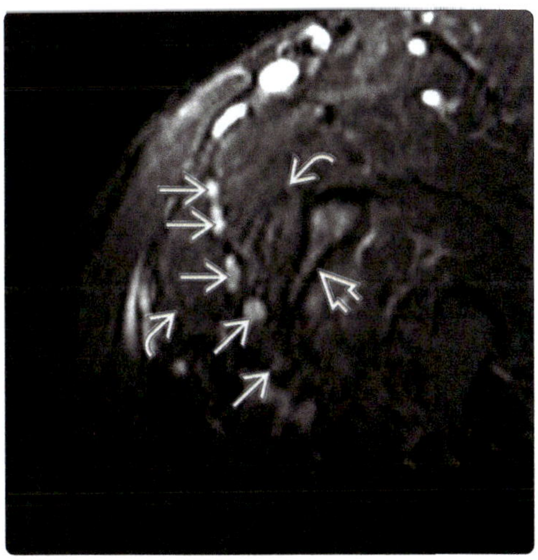

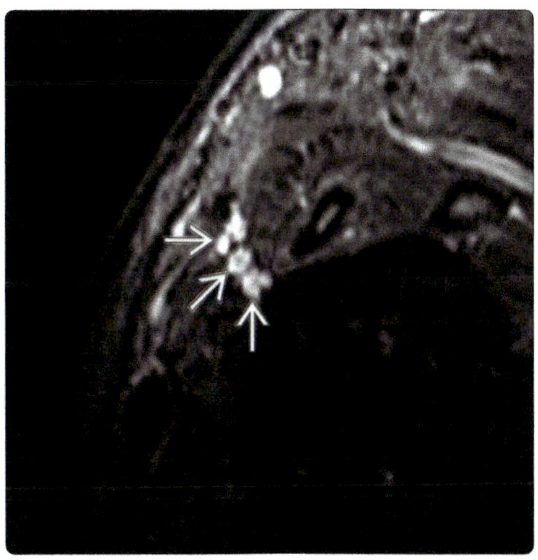

(Left) *Sagittal oblique STIR MR demonstrates the ventral primary rami of C5 through T1 proximal to the trunks. C8 exits above the 1st rib, whereas T1 exits below. The brachial plexus is "sandwiched" between the anterior and middle scalene muscles.* **(Right)** *Sagittal oblique STIR MR distal to the root level shows formation of the upper, middle, and lower trunks arranged in a vertical line between the scalene muscles.*

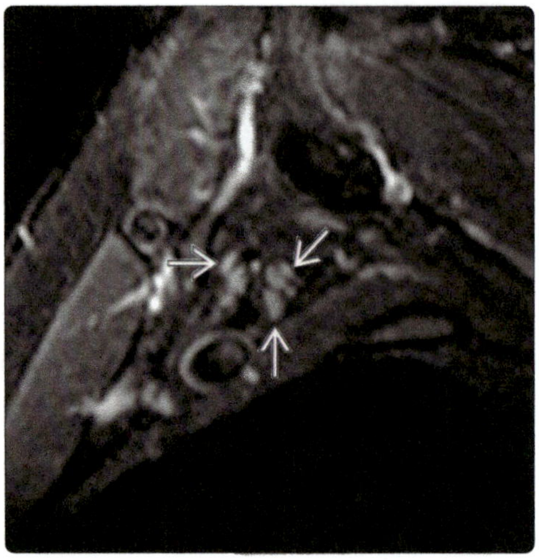

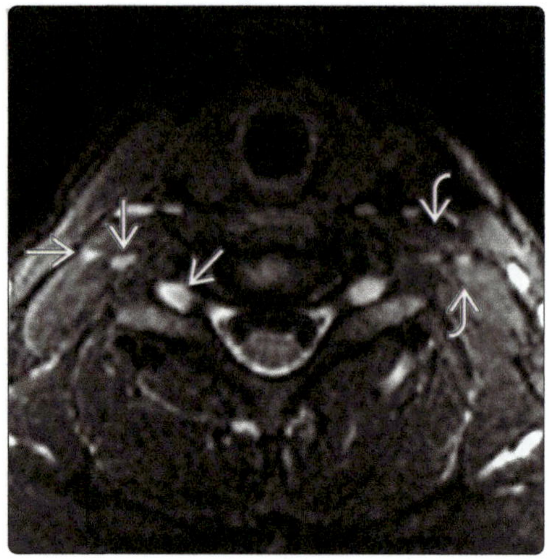

(Left) *Sagittal oblique STIR MR of the right brachial plexus distal to the trunks and divisions demonstrates formation of the 3 cords (lateral, medial, and posterior)* ➡. **(Right)** *Axial STIR MR depicts the C5, C6, and C7 ventral primary rami* ➡ *transiting between the anterior and middle scalene muscles* ➡ *in preparation to form the upper brachial plexus. This image demonstrates the conspicuity of the brachial plexus on routine cervical spine MR studies.*

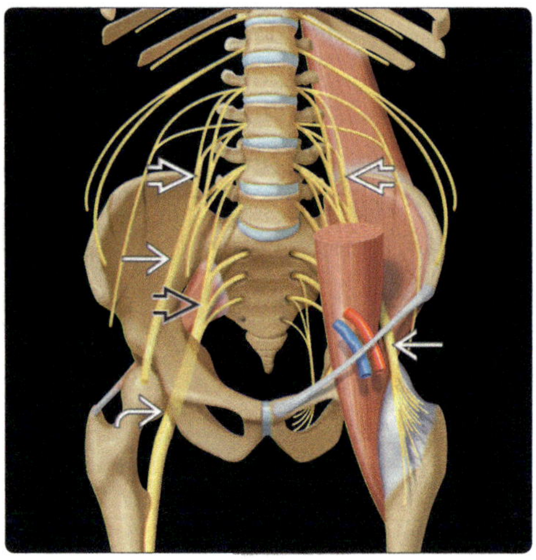

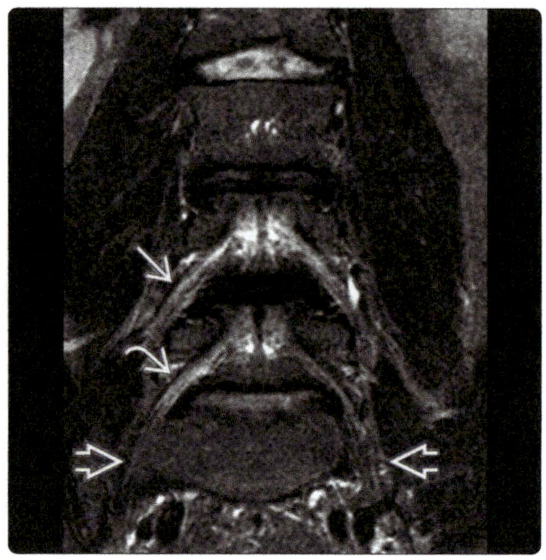

(Left) *Coronal graphic of the lumbosacral plexus demonstrates the lumbar plexus* ➡ *ventral to quadratus lumborum and iliacus muscles and medial to psoas muscle. The femoral nerve* ➡, *the major terminal branch of the lumbar plexus, travels between iliacus and psoas muscles under inguinal ligament. The sciatic nerve* ➡ *is the major output of the lumbosacral plexus* ➡. **(Right)** *Coronal T2WI FS MR shows the L4* ➡ *and L5* ➡ *nerve root forming the lumbosacral trunk* ➡.

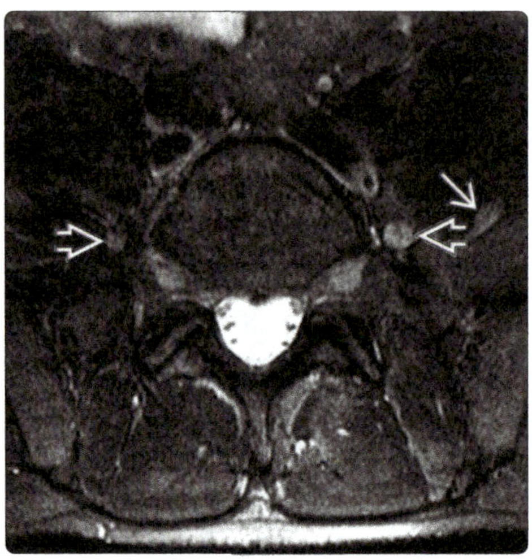

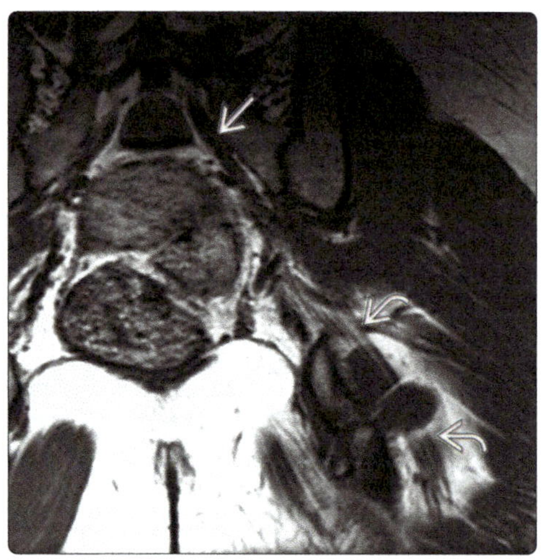

(Left) *Axial T2WI FS MR at the lumbosacral junction demonstrates the bilateral lumbar plexus* ➡ *after the L4 contribution in expected location medial to the psoas muscles. The left femoral nerve* ➡ *has branched off and is tracking within the iliopsoas groove in expected location.* **(Right)** *Coronal T1WI MR through the pelvis demonstrates the normal left S2 nerve* ➡ *transiting its named neural foramen to contribute to sacral plexus and left sciatic nerve* ➡ *as it passes through the sciatic notch.*

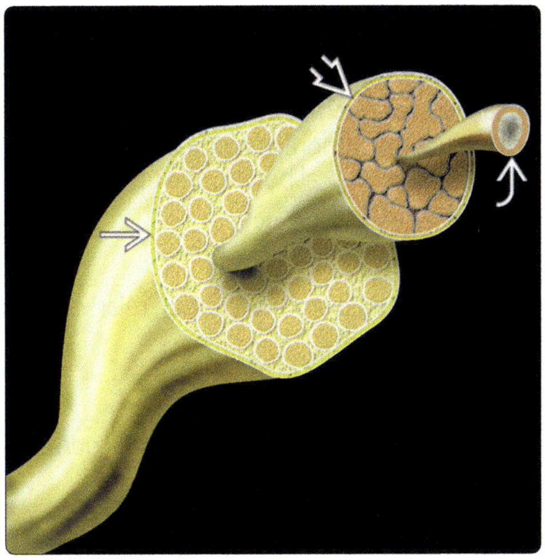

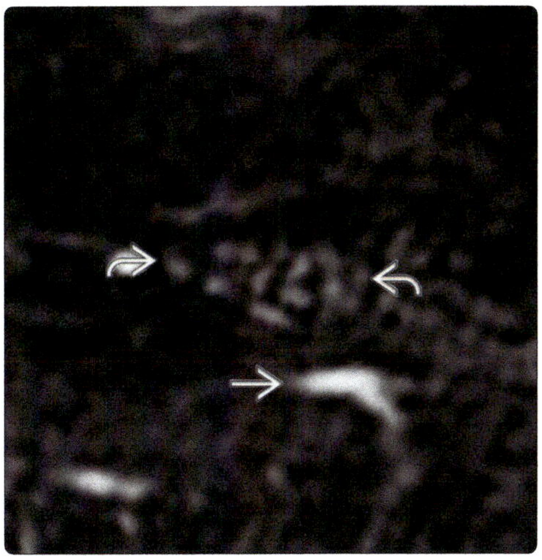

(Left) *3D graphic depicts normal peripheral nerve hierarchical anatomy. The peripheral nerve itself, composed of numerous fascicles, is surrounded by epineurium. Each fascicle is individually enveloped by perineurium. Each fascicle contains many endoneurium-wrapped axons.* **(Right)** *Axial STIR MR of the normal sciatic nerve shows normal peripheral nerve imaging characteristics. The fascicles are mildly hyperintense to muscle but not as bright as regional vessels.*

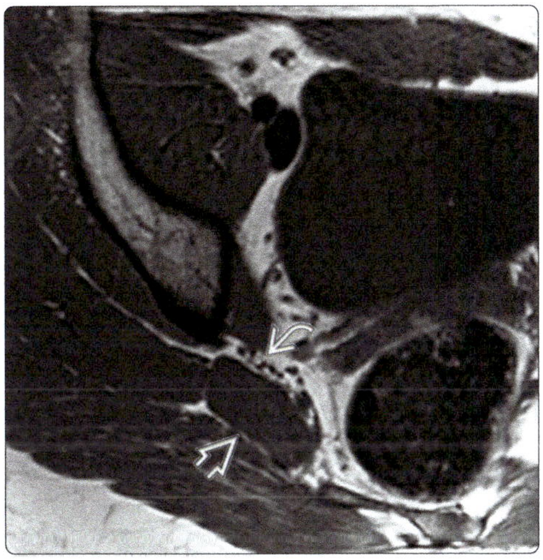

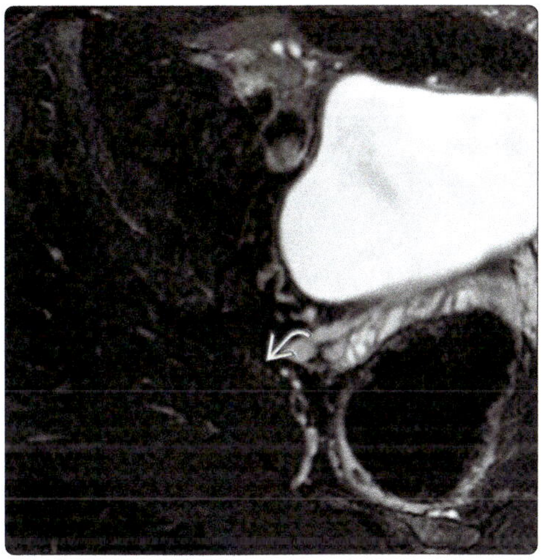

(Left) *Axial oblique T1WI MR shows normal sciatic nerve on the ventral piriformis muscle. Although the nerve (largest single nerve in the body) is enveloped by epineurium, the abundant fibrofatty epineurium gives the impression that individual fascicles are free in pelvic fat.* **(Right)** *Axial oblique T2WI FS MR demonstrates normal sciatic nerve with distinctive mildly hyperintense fascicles separated by interspersed dark (fat-suppressed) fibrofatty connective tissue.*

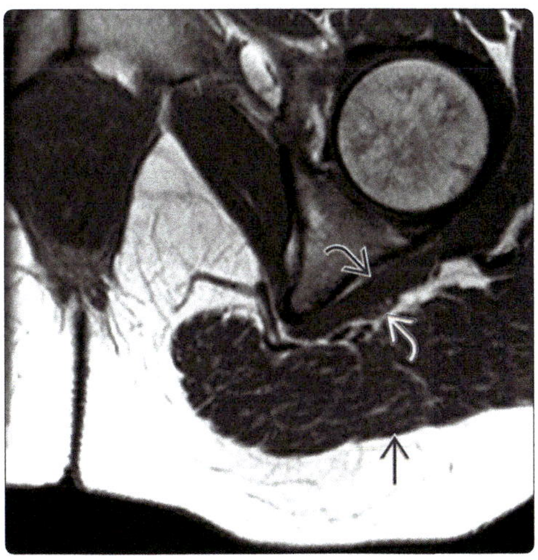

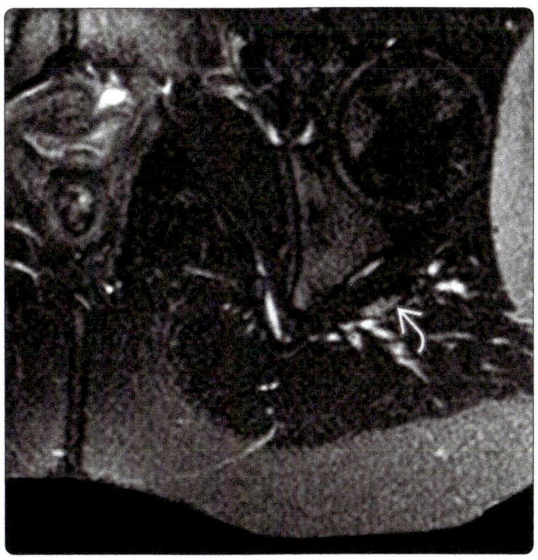

(Left) *Axial T1WI MR of normal sciatic nerve at the obturator internus level is readily identified between the obturator internus and gluteus maximus muscles. Normal sciatic nerve is smaller and flatter at this level than at piriformis level.* **(Right)** *Axial T2WI FS MR shows normal sciatic nerve at level of gluteus maximus and obturator internus. The normal neural fascicular architecture is distinctive and permits nerve discrimination from adjacent veins.*

Superior Sulcus Tumor

KEY FACTS

TERMINOLOGY

- Synonym: Pancoast tumor
- Benign or malignant neoplasm extending to superior thoracic inlet with severe shoulder/arm pain along C8, T1, T2 nerve trunks, Horner syndrome, weakness + atrophy of intrinsic hand muscles (Pancoast syndrome)

IMAGING

- Soft tissue apical lung mass with variable extension into chest wall, adjacent bone destruction, brachial plexus invasion

TOP DIFFERENTIAL DIAGNOSES

- Metastatic disease
- Other thoracic tumors [besides nonsmall cell lung carcinoma (NSCLC)]
- Brachial plexus neural tumors
- Hematologic neoplasms
- Radiation fibrosis
- Vascular (venolymphatic) malformation
- Infection

PATHOLOGY

- Bronchogenic carcinomas may arise from either upper lobe
- Invades parietal pleura, endothoracic fascia, subclavian vessels, brachial plexus, vertebral bodies, and upper ribs
- NSCLC most frequent etiology

CLINICAL ISSUES

- Clinical findings determined by tumor location relative to scalene muscles
- Severe shoulder and arm pain
- Horner syndrome
- Pulmonary symptoms uncommon early in disease course

DIAGNOSTIC CHECKLIST

- Apical lung mass with bone destruction = bronchogenic carcinoma until proven otherwise
- Rare benign tumors or infection may mimic lung carcinoma

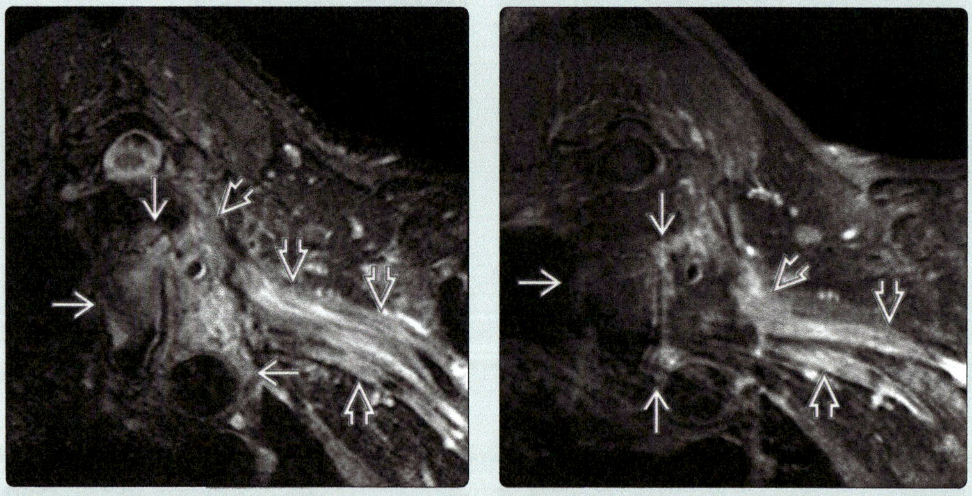

(Left) *Coronal STIR MR [nonsmall cell lung carcinoma (NSCLC), arm pain and weakness] shows extensive architectural distortion of the lung apex by a peripheral lung mass ➡ with extension along the brachial plexus elements ⇨.* **(Right)** *Coronal T1 C+ FS MR (NSCLC, arm pain, and weakness) demonstrates a heterogeneously enhancing apical lung neoplasm ➡ with tumor extension ⇨ along the lower brachial plexus elements.*

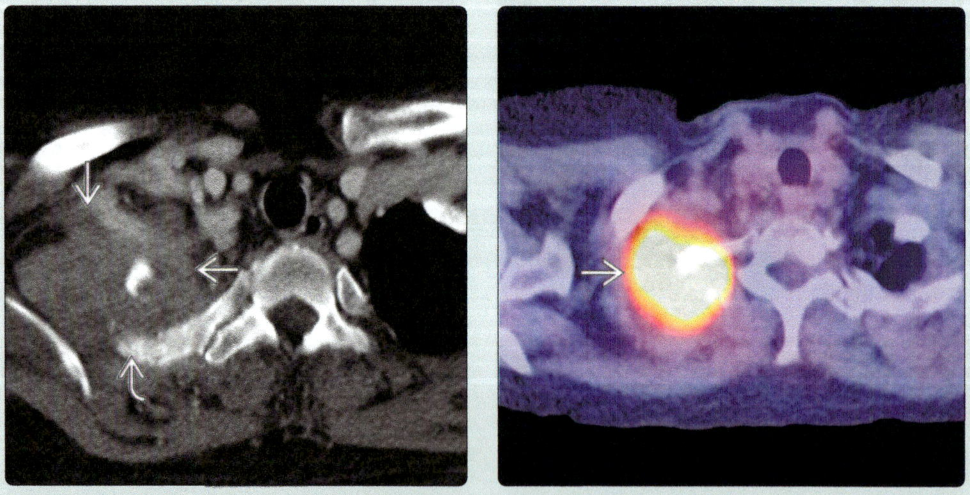

(Left) *Axial CECT demonstrates a soft tissue mass ➡ involving the right upper lobe with extension beyond the chest wall producing destruction of right T1, T2 ribs ↱.* **(Right)** *Axial PET (FDG) CT fusion image reveals marked hypermetabolic radiotracer uptake within the right upper lobe bronchogenic carcinoma ➡.*

KEY FACTS

TERMINOLOGY

- Thoracic outlet syndrome (TOS)
- Neural, venous, &/or arterial compressive syndrome at thoracic outlet (TO)
- Diagnosis made by 1 of 3 methods (by event, affected structure, or compression cause)

IMAGING

- ± cervical rib, elongated C7 transverse process
- ± brachial plexus compression or distortion, scalene muscle inflammation or fibrosis, abnormal vascular flow voids within TO
- Positional occlusion or narrowing of subclavian artery (SCA) with arm hyperabduction, external rotation

TOP DIFFERENTIAL DIAGNOSES

- Primary and secondary plexus tumors
- Radiation plexopathy
- Trauma

PATHOLOGY

- Cervical ribs, abnormal transverse processes, fibrous bands, scalene compression of TO contents
- Neural injury with fibrosis, axonal loss

CLINICAL ISSUES

- "True" neurological TOS: Intermittent arm pain, numbness, and weakness with hyperabduction, external rotation
  - Pain in shoulder, proximal upper extremity → neck
  - Paresthesias, numbness in forearm/hand
- Vascular TOS: Paresthesias secondary to arterial or venous ischemia
  - Obliteration of brachial, radial pulses with arm hyperabduction and elevation

DIAGNOSTIC CHECKLIST

- SCA aneurysm or subclavian vein thrombosis, brachial plexus compression with abnormal T2 hyperintensity at TO strongly suggest TOS

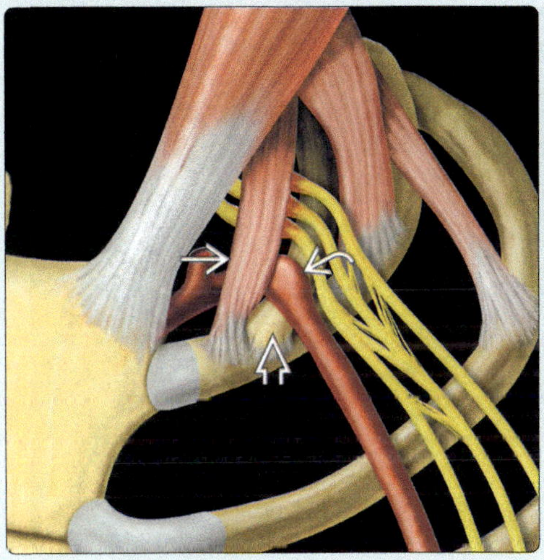

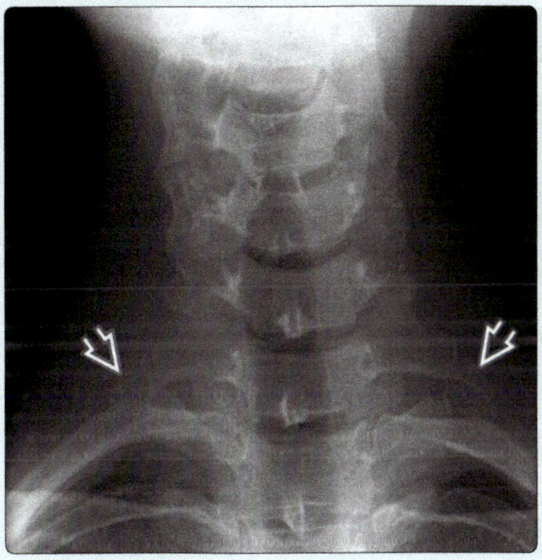

(Left) *Coronal graphic of the thoracic outlet (TO) demonstrates brachial plexus compression and a subclavian artery (SCA) aneurysm arising secondary to the C7 cervical rib and anterior scalene muscle compression.* **(Right)** *Anteroposterior radiograph demonstrates bilateral rudimentary C7 cervical ribs. The right cervical rib articulates with the 1st thoracic rib.*

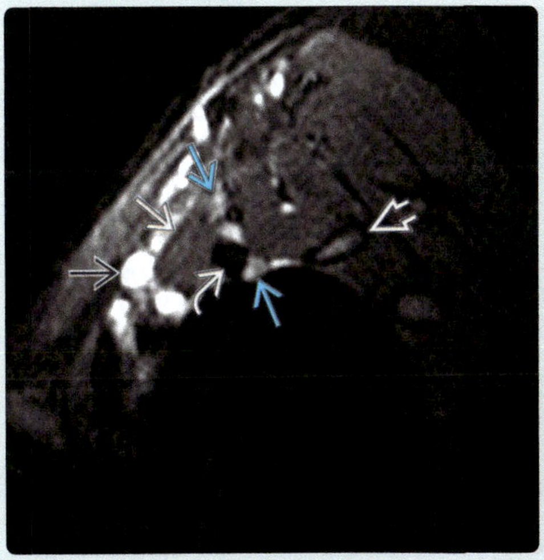

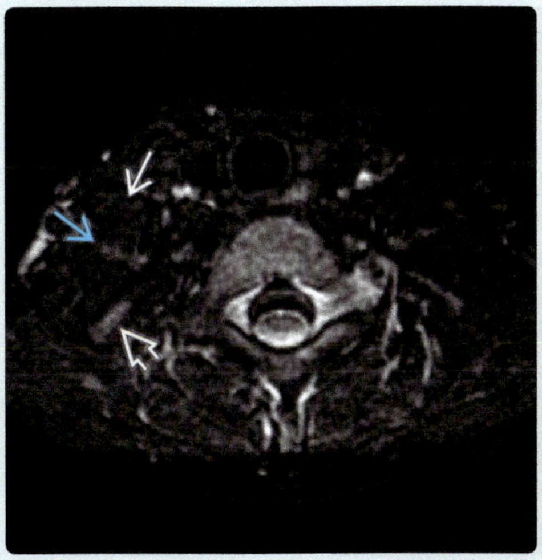

(Left) *Sagittal oblique STIR MR shows normal anatomy of the interscalene triangle: Brachial plexus trunks, anterior and middle scalene muscles, SCA, subclavian vein, and 1st thoracic rib.* **(Right)** *Axial STIR MR demonstrates normal axial thoracic outlet anatomy. The brachial plexus passes between the anterior and middle/posterior scalene muscles and over the 1st thoracic rib.*

Muscle Denervation

KEY FACTS

TERMINOLOGY

- Secondary muscle injury resulting from denervation following nerve injury

IMAGING

- **Acute denervation**
  - Muscle appears normal on T1WI
  - Diffusely increased signal intensity on T2WI, STIR
  - Mild, homogeneous enhancement with gadolinium
- **Chronic denervation**
  - Fatty atrophy evident on T1WI
  - Muscle volume decreased
  - Denervation edema often persists for prolonged period

TOP DIFFERENTIAL DIAGNOSES

- Disuse atrophy
- Muscle trauma
- Muscle inflammation or infection
- Radiation myopathy

PATHOLOGY

- Nerve tumor, infection, autoimmune neuritis, peripheral neuropathy or injury

CLINICAL ISSUES

- Weakness, muscle volume loss in distribution of injured nerve
  - May be painful
- Acute denervation may partially or totally recover depending on nerve injury severity
- Chronic denervation changes permanent

DIAGNOSTIC CHECKLIST

- Distribution of muscle signal abnormalities indicates location of nerve lesion
- Obtain fluid-sensitive sequence that shows muscle of concern in cross section

(Left) *Coronal STIR MR shows denervation edema → of the trapezius, which is innervated by the spinal accessory nerve. This nerve can be traumatized by carrying heavy loads on the shoulder.* **(Right)** *Coronal T1WI C+ FS MR in the same patient shows uniform enhancement → of the affected muscle. Muscle tears, in contrast, had a heterogeneous appearance.*

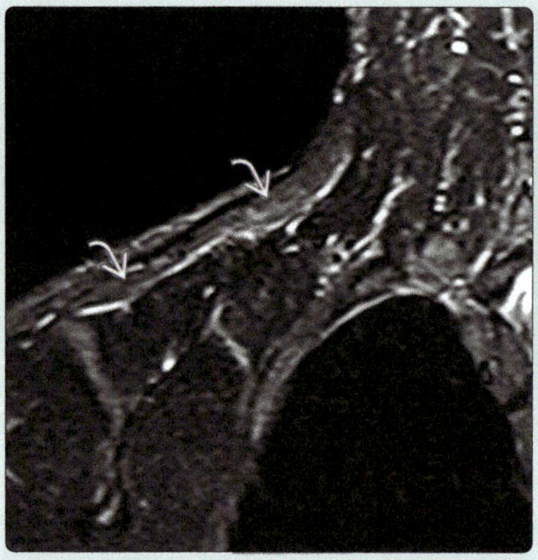

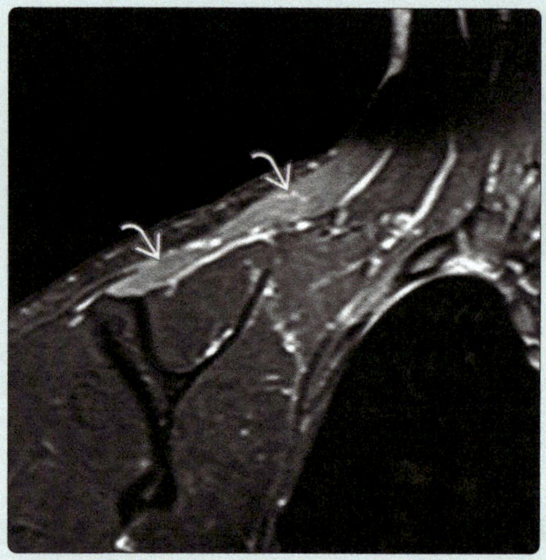

(Left) *Axial T2WI FS MR shows a free muscle flap → to the leg. The muscle shows severe, diffuse edema with a few streaks of fat interspersed. This is an expected finding and should not be confused with infection.* **(Right)** *Coronal T2WI FS MR shows denervation edema → throughout the intrinsic muscles of the foot. Denervation edema due to diabetes primarily involves the feet. It tends to be streakier and less homogeneous than denervation from other causes.*

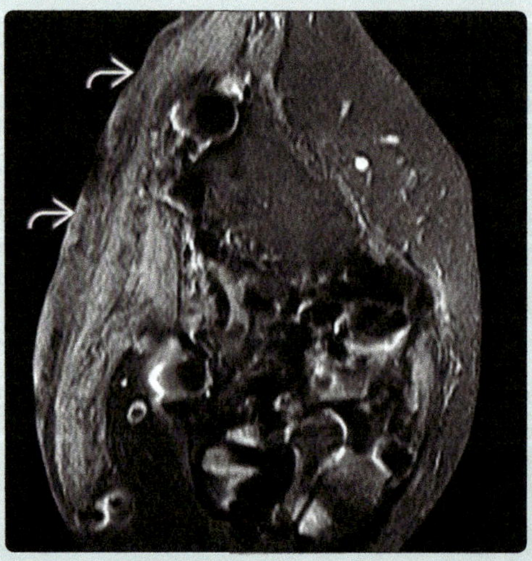

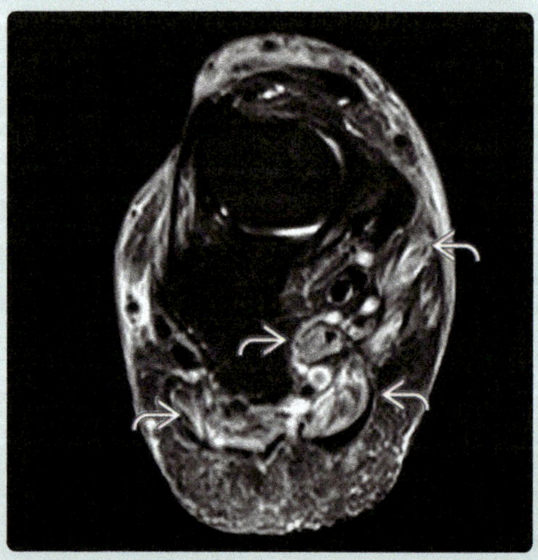

Brachial Plexus Traction Injury

KEY FACTS

TERMINOLOGY

- Synonyms: Brachial plexus stretch injury, brachial plexus avulsion, avulsion pseudomeningocele
- Stretch injury or avulsion of ≥ 1 cervical roots, brachial plexus

IMAGING

- Stretch injury: Enlargement, abnormal edema of neural elements
- Avulsion: Abnormal cerebrospinal fluid signal intensity within empty thecal diverticulum

TOP DIFFERENTIAL DIAGNOSES

- Nerve sheath tumor
- Lateral meningocele
- Nerve root sleeve cyst
- Chronic inflammatory demyelinating polyneuropathy (CIDP); less often acute inflammatory demyelinating polyneuropathy (AIDP)

PATHOLOGY

- Adults: Majority posttraumatic injuries secondary to high-energy force
- Infants: Secondary to excessive traction on plexus during difficult delivery (breech or forceps)

CLINICAL ISSUES

- Complete brachial plexus avulsion produces useless "flail arm"
- Clinical incomplete paralysis possible with complete root avulsion(s) because of redundant muscle innervation from multiple roots
- EMG/NCS helps differentiate traumatic from immune etiologies

DIAGNOSTIC CHECKLIST

- Familiarity with normal brachial plexus anatomy essential for MR interpretation
- Muscle denervation pattern predicts abnormal nerves

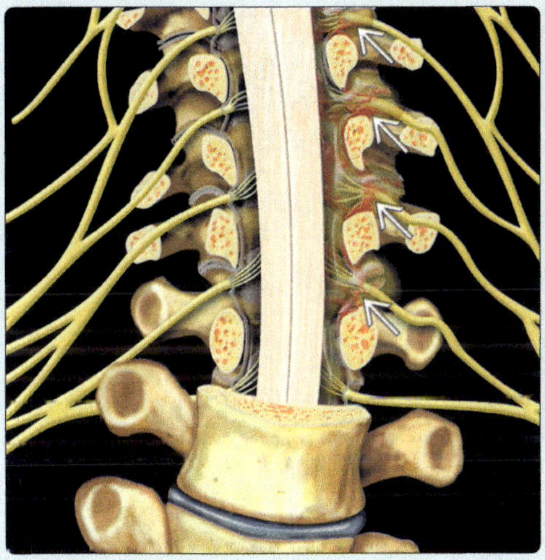

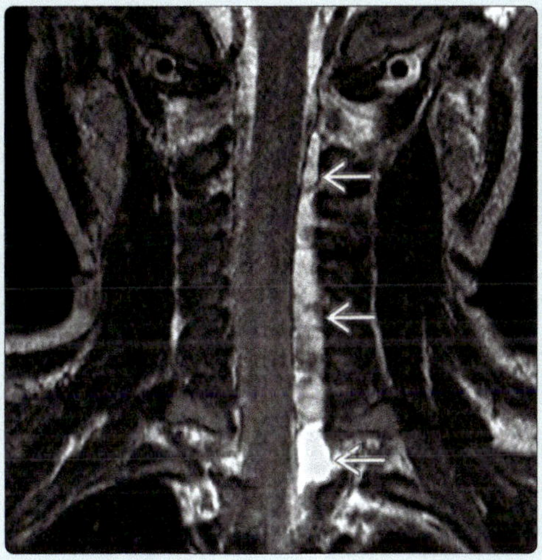

(Left) *Coronal graphic demonstrates posttraumatic avulsion of left C5-C8 nerve roots ➡, producing local hemorrhage at the site of root injury and associated pseudomeningoceles.* **(Right)** *Coronal T2WI MR in a patient with posttraumatic paralyzed "flail arm" demonstrates an extensive extradural cerebrospinal fluid (CSF) signal intensity collection admixed with blood products ➡, representing CSF leakage following avulsion of multiple nerve roots, displacing the spinal cord to the right.*

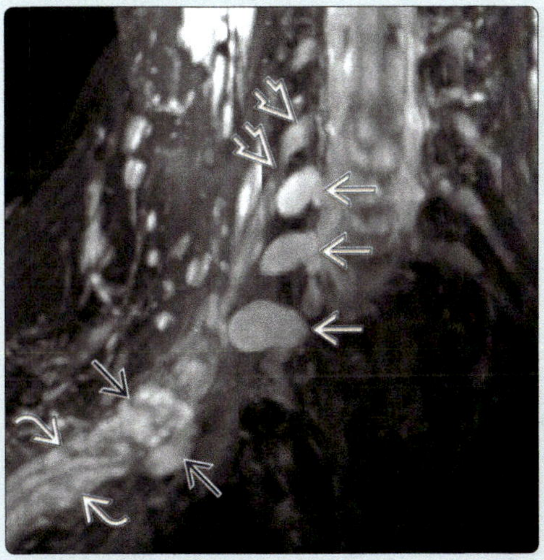

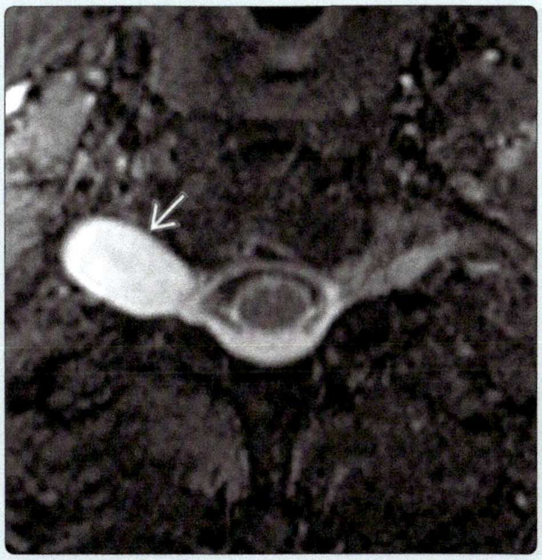

(Left) *Coronal STIR MR in a patient with severe brachial plexus traction injury shows avulsion pseudomeningoceles of right C6, C7, and C8 roots ➡. The C5 root is attenuated with abnormally ↑ signal (incomplete stretch injury) ➡. The avulsed nerve roots have formed a "retraction ball" ➡, with abnormal enlargement and T2 hyperintensity of the distal (denervated) plexus ➡.* **(Right)** *Axial STIR MR confirms the CSF signal and lack of demonstrable neural elements within the right C7 pseudomeningocele ➡.*

Idiopathic Brachial Plexus Neuritis

KEY FACTS

TERMINOLOGY

- Parsonage-Turner syndrome

IMAGING

- Can affect any muscle innervated by brachial plexus
  - Most common: Rotator cuff, deltoid, biceps, triceps
- Denervation edema is earliest finding
  - Diffuse, homogeneous high signal on T2WI, STIR throughout affected muscle
    - Often, muscles innervated by 2 or more different peripheral nerves are affected
  - ± T2/STIR hyperintensity of plexus
- Fatty atrophy occurs in chronic denervation (uncommon)

TOP DIFFERENTIAL DIAGNOSES

- Cervical radiculopathy
- Suprascapular nerve entrapment
- Brachial plexus neoplasm
- Brachial plexus or cervical nerve root avulsion
- Radiation neuritis/myositis
- Quadrilateral space syndrome
- Pancoast tumor
- Muscle injury

PATHOLOGY

- Often idiopathic; can be associated with viral or bacterial infection
- Can also be posttraumatic or postsurgery condition

CLINICAL ISSUES

- Sudden onset of pain, followed by weakness, paresthesias
- M > F
- Most cases resolve in 3 months to 2 years
- Physical therapy to preserve range of motion

DIAGNOSTIC CHECKLIST

- Often an unexpected finding on shoulder MR performed to evaluate weakness, pain

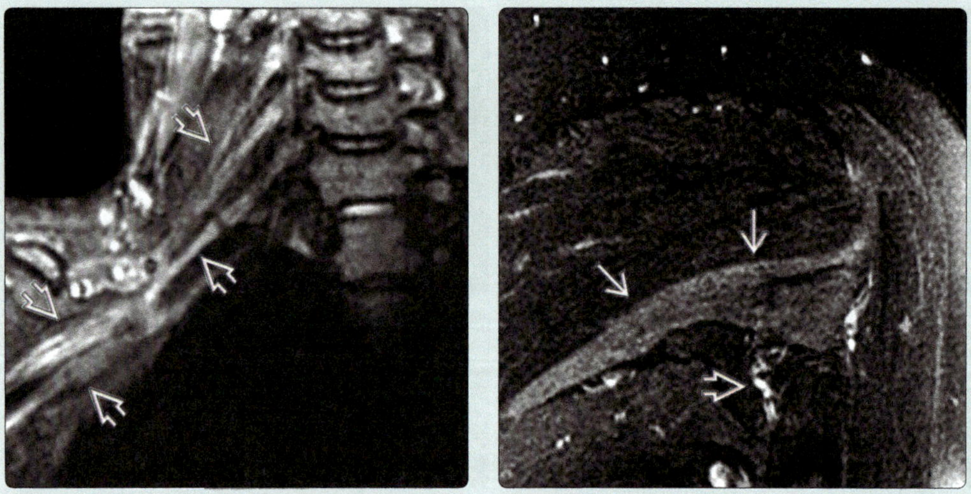

(Left) *Coronal STIR MR shows diffusely increased signal intensity in brachial plexus due to idiopathic brachial neuritis.* **(Right)** *Coronal oblique T2WI MR shows denervation edema of the teres minor due to brachial neuritis. Edema is homogeneous and uniform, and there is no disruption of muscle fibers. Quadrilateral space shows no evidence of mass involving axillary nerve. Whenever denervation edema is seen, a search should be made for nerve mass or extrinsic compression.*

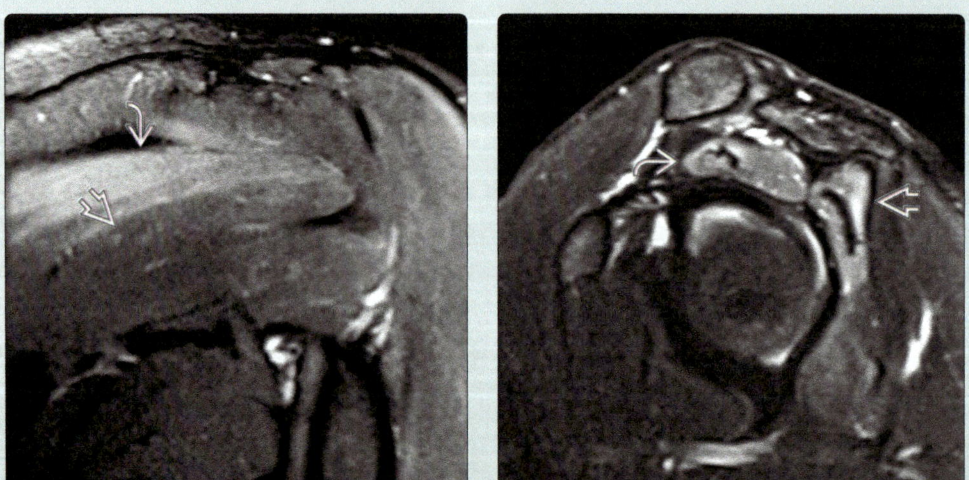

(Left) *Coronal oblique T2WI MR shows diffuse increase in signal intensity throughout superior fibers of infraspinatus muscle. Interestingly, the inferior portion of the muscle is spared. Unusual distributions of denervation edema are common in brachial neuritis.* **(Right)** *Sagittal T2WI MR shows diffusely abnormal signal intensity in the infraspinatus and supraspinatus muscles. Differential diagnosis, in this case, includes suprascapular nerve entrapment.*

KEY FACTS

TERMINOLOGY

- Group of inherited disorders characterized by focal or diffuse peripheral nerve enlargement
- Hereditary motor-sensory neuropathy (HMSN), hypertrophic neuropathy (HN), hereditary sensory neuropathy (HSN), hereditary motor neuropathy (HMN), hereditary sensory and autonomic neuropathy (HSAN), Charcot-Marie-Tooth (CMT) syndrome

IMAGING

- Focal or diffuse fusiform peripheral nerve enlargement
  - Peripheral nerves ± intradural nerve roots
  - ± involvement of cauda equina nerve roots
- Acute &/or chronic muscle denervation changes
- Best imaging tool: High-resolution MR (MR neurography)

TOP DIFFERENTIAL DIAGNOSES

- Guillain-Barré syndrome
- Chronic inflammatory demyelinating polyneuropathy
- Nerve sheath tumor
- Traumatic nerve stretch injury

PATHOLOGY

- Hypertrophic nerve roots, peripheral nerves
- "Onion bulb" formations = nerve thickening caused by repetitive segmental demyelination/regeneration (histologic hallmark of CMT but can occur in others)

CLINICAL ISSUES

- Distal extremity muscle weakness/atrophy (motor > sensory), foot deformities
- Back/lower extremity radicular pain ± myelopathy
- Sensory loss, focal tenderness, dysesthesias

DIAGNOSTIC CHECKLIST

- Consider HMSN when abnormally enlarged peripheral nerves identified on MR
- Genetic consultation recommended for patients with fusiform nerve enlargement on MR

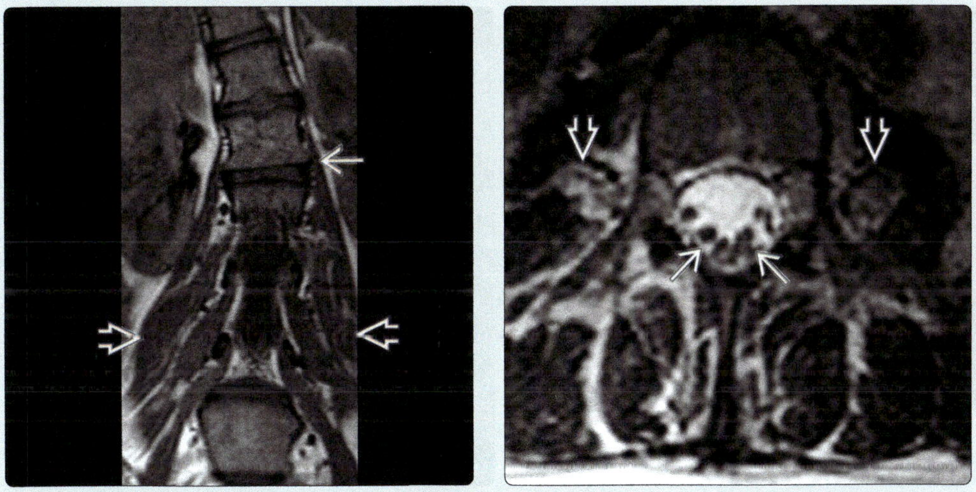

(Left) *Coronal T1WI MR (Charcot-Marie-Tooth, painful scoliosis) demonstrates convex left scoliosis and bilateral abnormal fusiform enlargement of the extradural spinal nerve roots and lumbar plexus.* **(Right)** *Axial T2WI MR (Charcot-Marie-Tooth, painful scoliosis) confirms abnormal enlargement and T2 hyperintensity of the bilateral extradural lumbar nerve roots as well as aberrant enlargement of the intradural cauda equina nerve roots.*

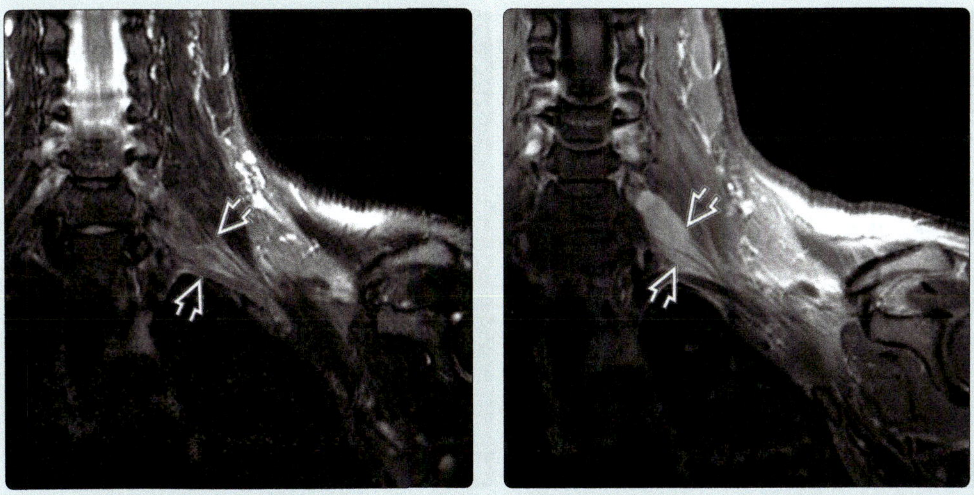

(Left) *Coronal STIR MR (unknown type hypertrophic neuropathy, left arm pain and weakness) demonstrates abnormal fusiform enlargement of the left proximal brachial plexus C7 and C8 roots/rami.* **(Right)** *Coronal T1WI C+ FS MR of the left brachial plexus in the same patient confirms fusiform enlargement and diffuse homogeneous nerve enhancement within the left proximal brachial plexus C7 and C8 roots/rami.*

KEY FACTS

TERMINOLOGY

- Synonyms: Femoral neuropathy, femoral mononeuropathy, femoral nerve (FN) palsy
- FN entrapment or injury secondary to direct trauma, compression, stretch injury, or ischemia

IMAGING

- Nerve enlargement ± loss of internal fascicular architecture, ↑ T2 hyperintensity
- Injury most common in psoas muscle body, iliopsoas groove, or femoral canal

TOP DIFFERENTIAL DIAGNOSES

- Neoplastic femoral nerve infiltration
- Nerve sheath tumor
- Lumbosacral disc syndromes
- Lumbar plexopathy

PATHOLOGY

- Reported causes include self-retaining retractor, thigh tourniquet, traumatic injury, heparin anticoagulation (retroperitoneal hematoma), arterial catheterization complication, obstetrical complication, diabetic neuropathy

CLINICAL ISSUES

- Acute symptom onset, pain/weakness in FN distribution, diminished/absent knee jerk reflex, thigh muscle atrophy
- Severe back/groin pain (retroperitoneal hematoma)
- Recovery is rule over days → months

DIAGNOSTIC CHECKLIST

- Femoral neuropathy is uncommon
- Look carefully for lesion or hematoma in iliopsoas groove or femoral canal

(Left) *Coronal graphic shows the normal course of the femoral nerve ➡ relative to the psoas muscle ➡ and inguinal ligament ➡. The femoral nerve produces multiple peripheral branches to the anterior thigh muscles.* **(Right)** *Coronal STIR MR (femoral neuropathy postsurgical herniorrhaphy) depicts marked enlargement, T2 hyperintensity of the right femoral nerve ➡, with abrupt transition at the right groin. In this case, the femoral nerve was accidentally ligated during herniorrhaphy.*

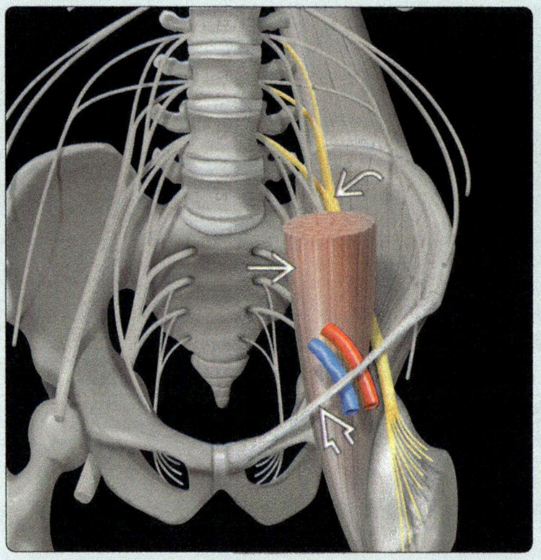

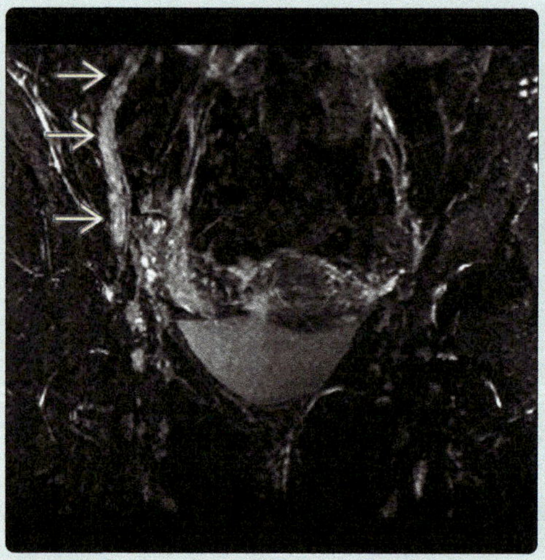

(Left) *Axial STIR MR in the same patient confirms that the right femoral nerve ➡ in the iliopsoas groove is markedly enlarged with discrete T2 hyperintense fascicles (compared to the normal left femoral nerve ➡).* **(Right)** *Axial CECT (severe hemophilia) depicts large left iliacus ➡ and psoas ➡ hematomas. Femoral neuropathy occurs from compression of the adjacent femoral nerve, which runs along the psoas muscle and iliopsoas groove ➡. A normal iliopsoas groove is seen on the right ➡.*

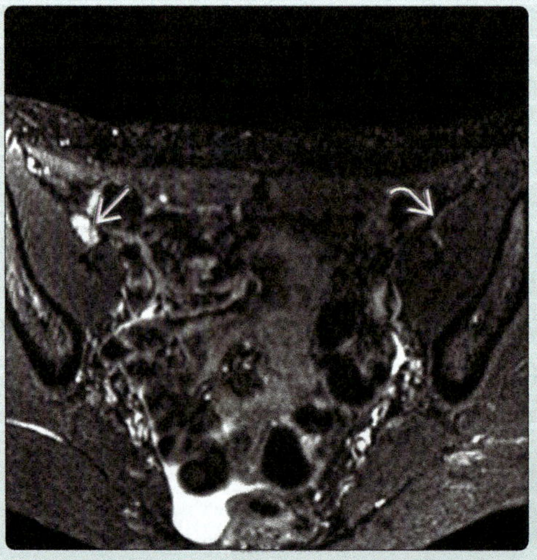

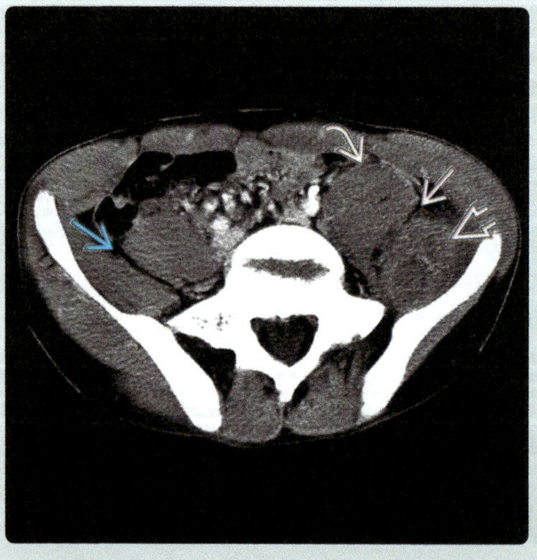

KEY FACTS

TERMINOLOGY

- Synonyms: Ulnar nerve (UN) entrapment, cubital tunnel syndrome
- Partial fixation, compression, or distortion of UN

IMAGING

- UN enlargement ± abnormal T2 hyperintensity, architectural distortion
- Most commonly occurs within cubital tunnel (elbow); uncommon at Guyon tunnel (wrist) or brachial plexus

TOP DIFFERENTIAL DIAGNOSES

- Acute direct nerve trauma
- Idiopathic brachial plexitis (Parsonage-Turner syndrome)
- Nerve sheath tumor
- Enlarged perineural vein
- Medial epicondylitis

PATHOLOGY

- Edematous/indurated UN ± thickened retinaculum, fibrous infiltration, fascicular atrophy/loss
- ± anconeus epitrochlearis, enlarged medial triceps head

CLINICAL ISSUES

- Symptoms range from mild transient paresthesias of 4th and 5th digits → claw hand/digits, intrinsic muscle atrophy
- ± severe elbow/wrist pain radiating proximally or distally

DIAGNOSTIC CHECKLIST

- Focal nerve enlargement, abnormal T2 hyperintensity distal to medial epicondyle
- Search for anatomic abnormalities (enlarged triceps medial head or anconeus muscle, osteophyte, thickened retinaculum)

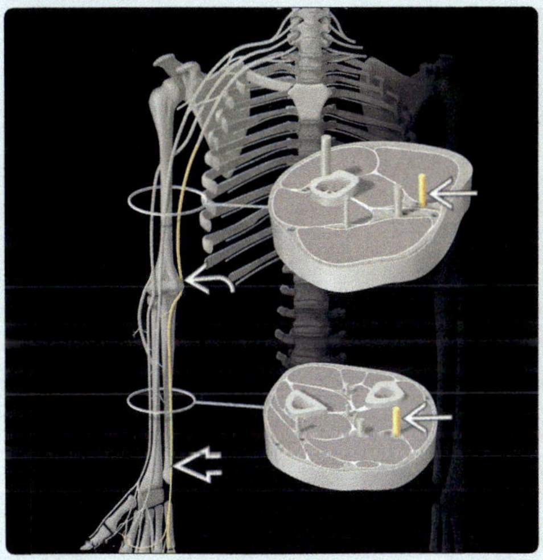

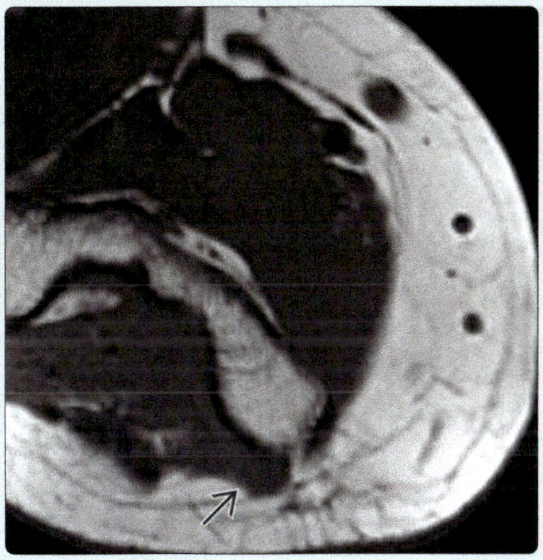

(Left) *Coronal graphic of the right upper extremity demonstrates the normal course of the ulnar nerve → (yellow). Vulnerable locations to injury include the cubital tunnel → at the medial elbow and Guyon canal → at the medial wrist.* **(Right)** *Axial T1WI MR of the right elbow demonstrates mild abnormal enlargement and rounded configuration of the right ulnar nerve → within the cubital tunnel.*

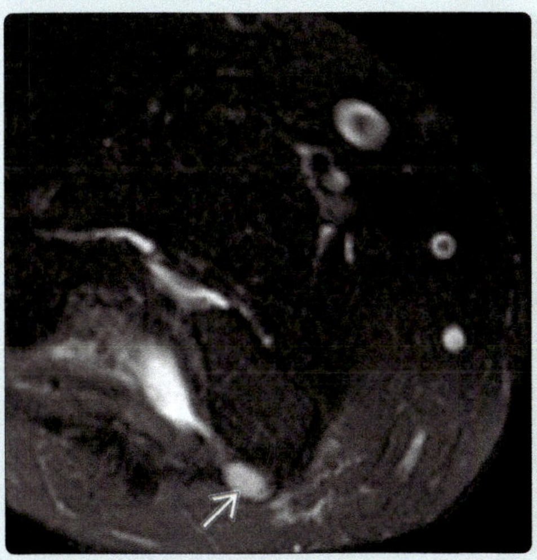

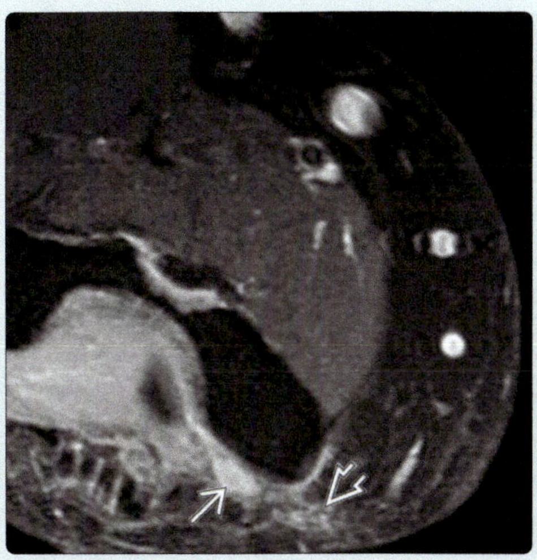

(Left) *Axial T2WI FS MR of the right elbow demonstrates mild enlargement and abnormal T2 hyperintensity of the right ulnar nerve → with complete loss of internal fascicular architecture, indicating an axonotmetic or neurotmetic injury rather than the less severe neuropraxic injury.* **(Right)** *Axial T1WI C+ FS MR of the right elbow confirms diffuse abnormal enhancement of the mildly enlarged right ulnar nerve →. Note also mild edema and inflammation in the adjacent soft tissues →.*

KEY FACTS

TERMINOLOGY

- Suprascapular nerve impingement with muscle denervation

IMAGING

- Suprascapular nerve impingement may occur at either spinoglenoid or suprascapular notch
- Spinoglenoid notch: Between neck and blade of scapula, roofed by spinoglenoid ligament
  - Entrapment affects infraspinatus muscles only
- Suprascapular notch: At superior border of scapula, roofed by superior transverse ligament
  - Entrapment affects both supraspinatus and infraspinatus muscles
- Denervation edema is 1st sign on MR
  - Uniformly increased signal intensity of muscle
- Fatty atrophy occurs later

TOP DIFFERENTIAL DIAGNOSES

- Cervical radiculopathy
- Parsonage-Turner syndrome (brachial neuritis)
- Rotator cuff tear
- Traction neuropathy
- Neural tumor

PATHOLOGY

- Paralabral cyst due to tear of posterosuperior glenoid labrum
- Mass or venous varicosities compressing nerve
- Posttraumatic scar or heterotopic ossification

CLINICAL ISSUES

- Young or middle-aged patients, M > F
- Overhead athletes

DIAGNOSTIC CHECKLIST

- Denervation edema best seen on sagittal fluid-sensitive sequences

(Left) *Coronal graphic shows suprascapular nerve coursing through suprascapular notch ➡, after which it gives rise to motor branch to supraspinatus muscle ➡. Nerve then passes through the spinoglenoid notch ➡ and innervates the infraspinatus muscle ➡.* **(Right)** *Coronal T2WI FS MR shows an elongated, multilocular cyst ➡ extending from a posterosuperior glenoid labral tear ➡ through the spinoglenoid notch. Infraspinatus muscle ➡ shows a mild, homogeneous increase in signal intensity.*

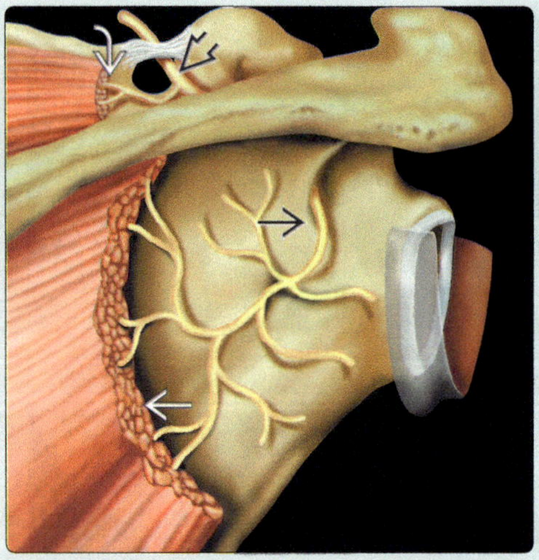

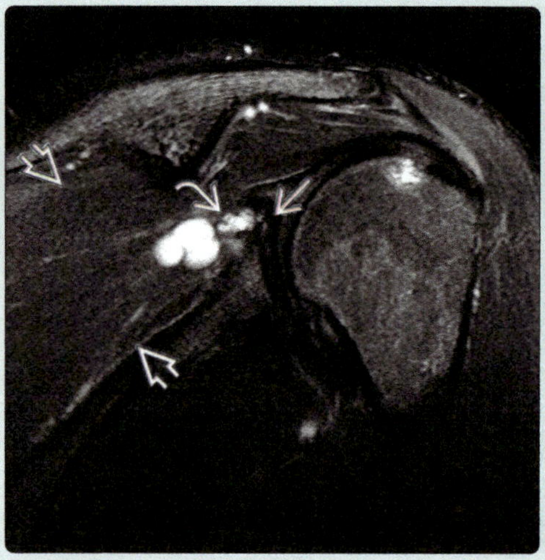

(Left) *Axial PD FSE FS MR in the same patient shows the cyst ➡ at the level of the spinoglenoid notch ➡. Denervation edema is less visible on this sequence than on T2 FS or STIR.* **(Right)** *Sagittal T2WI FS MR in the same patient shows the cyst ➡ at the spinoglenoid notch. The sagittal image most readily shows the abnormal signal intensity of the infraspinatus ➡ relative to the supraspinatus ➡ muscle.*

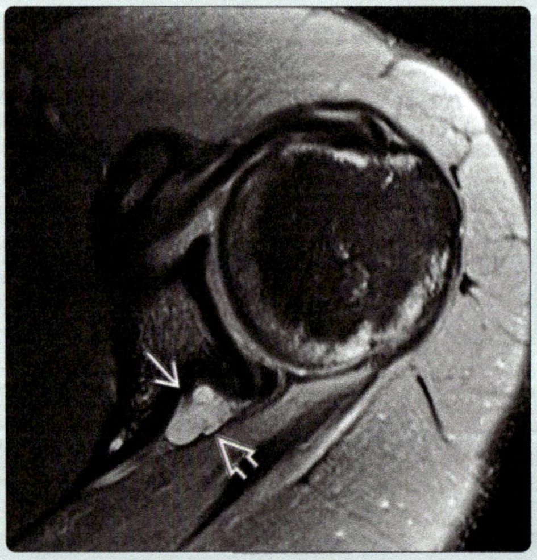

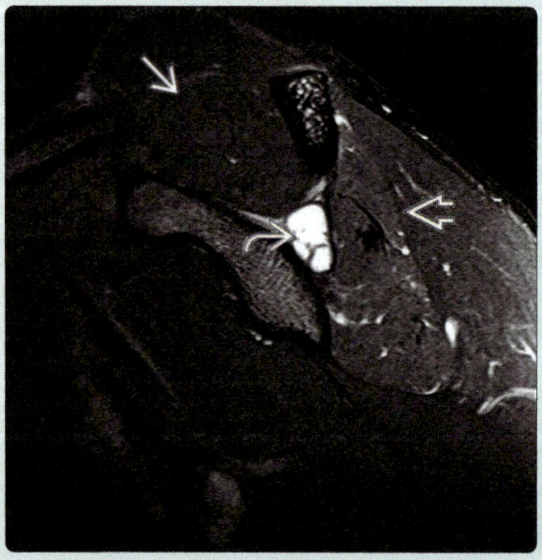

KEY FACTS

TERMINOLOGY

- Pronator syndrome: Nerve entrapment at pronator teres
- Carpal tunnel syndrome: Nerve entrapment at carpal tunnel

IMAGING

- Nerve enlargement distal to region of entrapment
  - Fascicles indistinct
- Perineural enhancement
- ± mass compressing nerve
- Denervation changes in muscles distal to entrapment

TOP DIFFERENTIAL DIAGNOSES

- Cervical radiculopathy
- Tenosynovitis
- Peripheral nerve sheath tumor
- Thoracic outlet syndrome

PATHOLOGY

- Common etiologies
  - Overuse, arthritis, anatomic variants
  - Fractures
- Less common = neoplasm

CLINICAL ISSUES

- Tinel sign: Tingling along course of nerve when nerve tapped at point of entrapment
- IF bilateral look for diabetes, hypothyroid, rheumatoid arthritis

DIAGNOSTIC CHECKLIST

- Diagnosis usually made on EMG, not MR
  - Ultrasound is option
- Imaging diagnosis challenging
  - Nerve normally high signal intensity (in carpal tunnel) on FSE T2WI
  - Nerve normally flattened at level of hook of hamate

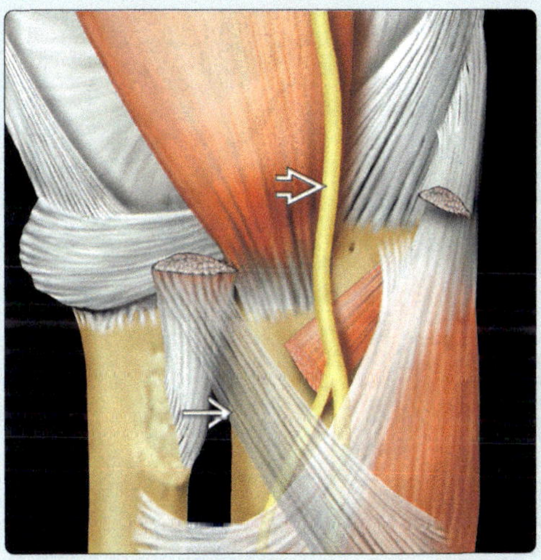

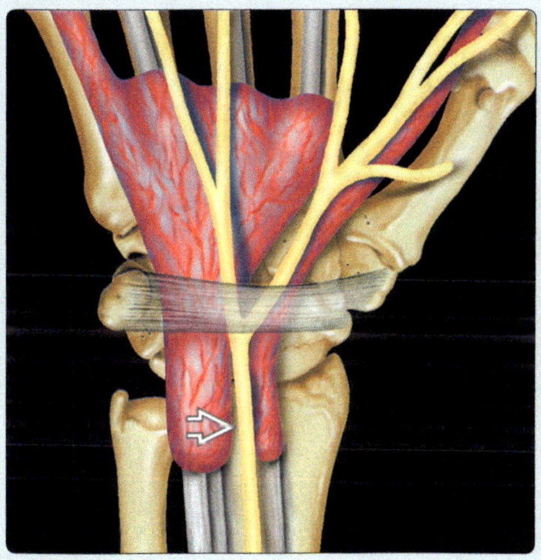

(Left) *Graphic of anterior elbow shows median nerve ➔ passing anterior to brachialis muscle. It extends between the heads of the pronator teres and beneath the biceps aponeurosis ➔. Entrapment of the nerve in this region is rare compared with carpal tunnel syndrome. It usually presents with numbness with repeated pronation/supination of the forearm.* **(Right)** *Coronal graphic of the carpal tunnel shows the median nerve ➔ at the ventral margin of the carpal tunnel, superficial to the flexor tendons.*

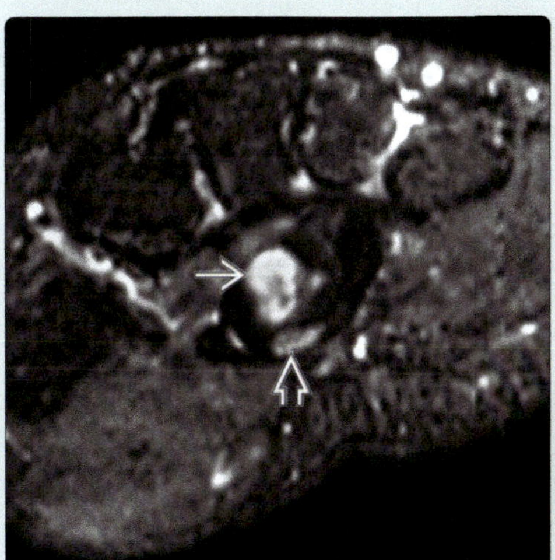

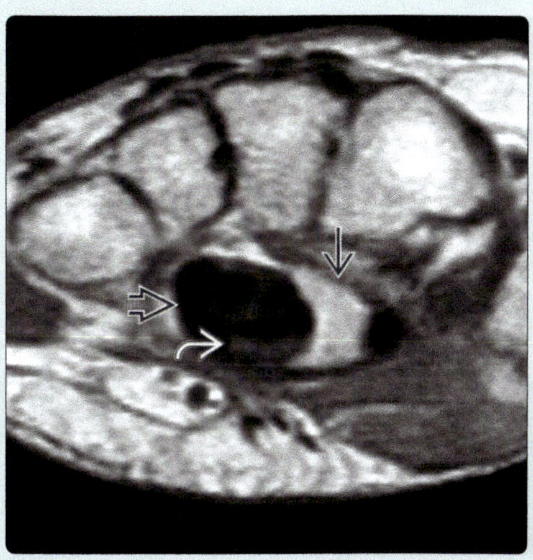

(Left) *Axial T2 FS MR performed at the wrist demonstrates a ganglion cyst ➔ in the carpal tunnel, exerting mass effect on the median nerve ➔.* **(Right)** *Axial T1WI MR reveals a lipoma ➔ within the carpal tunnel. The flexor tendons ➔ are displaced ulnarly, and the median nerve ➔ is compressed.*

KEY FACTS

TERMINOLOGY

- Synonyms: Common peroneal nerve (CPN) palsy, CPN entrapment
- CPN entrapment at fibular head

IMAGING

- CPN swelling, abnormal T2 hyperintensity
    - Fascicular architecture preserved in milder cases (neuropraxic injury)
    - Loss of internal fascicular architecture in more severe cases (axonotmetic, neurotmetic)

TOP DIFFERENTIAL DIAGNOSES

- Ganglion cyst
- Viral neuritis
- Nerve sheath tumor
- Direct acute CPN trauma

PATHOLOGY

- Usual etiology is entrapment or sequelae of continued pressure on CPN at fibular head level
- Edematous/indurated CPN ± thickened "fibular tunnel" at surgery

CLINICAL ISSUES

- Foot drop, sensory abnormality along anterolateral leg
- Prognosis variable; frequently good recovery following conservative management
- Surgical decompression reserved for recalcitrant cases

DIAGNOSTIC CHECKLIST

- Focal CPN enlargement, abnormal T2 hyperintensity at fibular head suggests CPN neuropathy
- MR imaging more sensitive for detecting acute than chronic nerve injuries
- Electrodiagnostics (EMG/NCS) can help localize and detect chronicity

(Left) *Coronal graphic depicts the normal course of the common peroneal neuropathy (CPN). The sciatic nerve ➞ branches into the tibial nerve ➞ (shown behind the femur) and the CPN ➞, which courses around fibular head.* **(Right)** *Axial T1WI MR demonstrates atrophy and fatty infiltration of the right anterolateral compartment muscles ➞ innervated by the CPN. Mild fascicular enlargement within the right CPN ➞ is not as conspicuous on T1WI as it is on T2WI FS MR or STIR MR.*

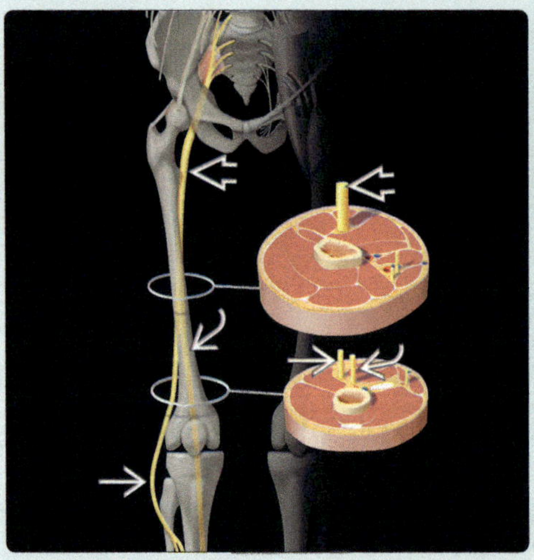

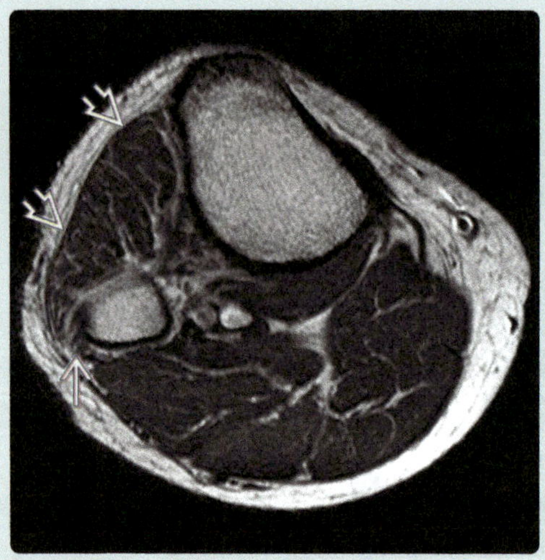

(Left) *Axial T2WI FS MR (same patient) reveals abnormal T2 hyperintensity in some anterolateral compartment muscles ➞, confirming ongoing denervation superimposed on chronic denervation. The right CPN ➞ is mildly enlarged, with swollen, hyperintense fascicles.* **(Right)** *Axial STIR MR confirms abnormal T2 hyperintensity in some anterolateral compartment muscles ➞. The CPN ➞ shows mild enlargement and abnormal signal intensity with preservation of intrinsic fascicular architecture.*

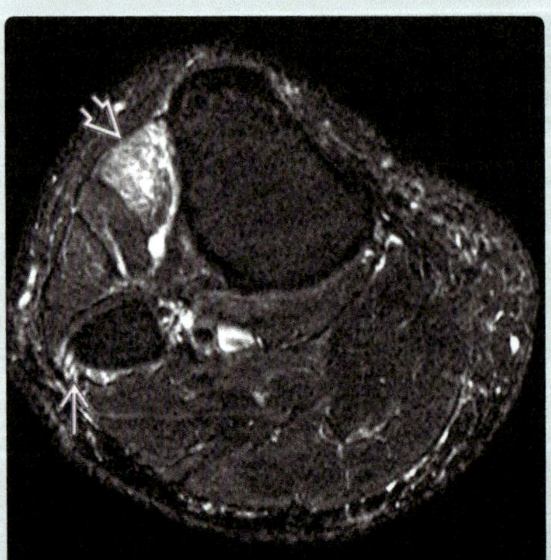

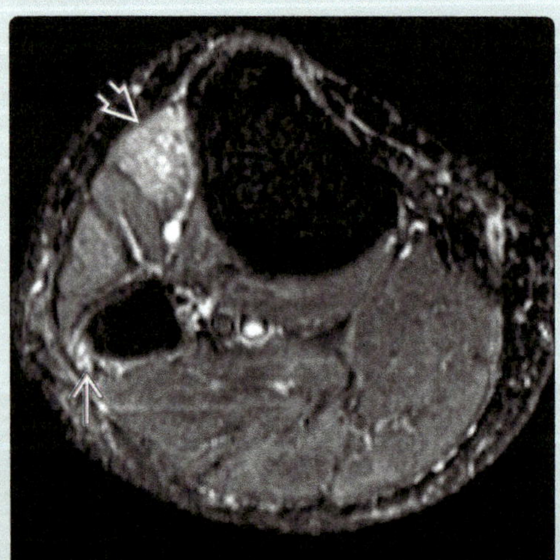

KEY FACTS

TERMINOLOGY

- Tarsal tunnel syndrome

IMAGING

- Denervation of affected plantar intrinsic muscles
    - Uniform high signal intensity on fluid-sensitive sequences
- Mass in tarsal tunnel
    - Ganglion cyst: Follows fluid signal intensity, homogeneous, ± thin rim of enhancement with gadolinium
    - Nerve sheath tumor: Round or ovoid shape, often shows "tail" where it arises from nerve, diffuse enhancement
    - Venous varicosities: Serpentine, enlarged vessels in tarsal tunnel, can be followed beyond tunnel
- Scar: Amorphous material around tibial nerve
- Osseous impingement: Fracture malunion, subtalar coalition

TOP DIFFERENTIAL DIAGNOSES

- Radiculopathy
- Diabetic neuropathy
- Calcaneal stress fracture
- Plantar fasciitis
- Isolated fatty atrophy of plantar muscles

PATHOLOGY

- Up to 50% of cases are idiopathic

CLINICAL ISSUES

- Burning, tingling pain, numbness at plantar aspect of foot

DIAGNOSTIC CHECKLIST

- Fatty atrophy of plantar intrinsic muscles can be incidental finding, increasing with age
- Intramuscular edema is most reliable sign of muscle denervation

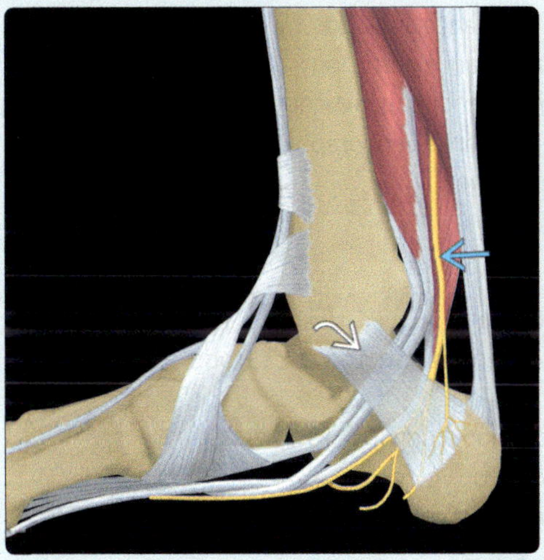
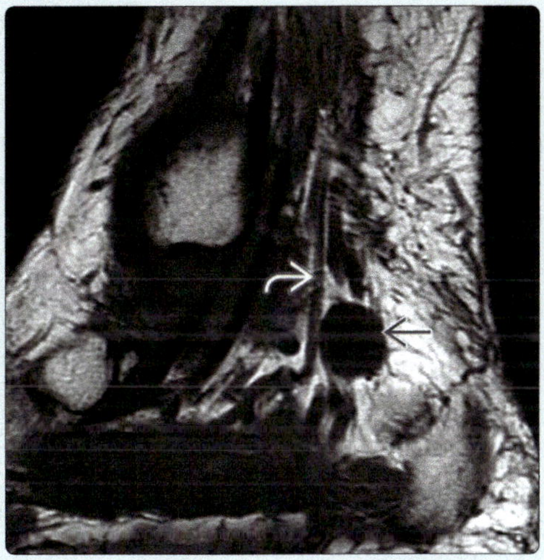

(Left) *Sagittal graphic of the medial side of the ankle shows the tibial nerve → as it courses through the tarsal tunnel, the roof of which is formed by the flexor retinaculum ⇒. The tibial nerve is vulnerable to compression throughout its course from behind the medial malleolus to the midfoot.* **(Right)** *Sagittal T1WI MR shows a lobular ganglion cyst → in the tarsal tunnel adjacent to the posterior tibial vein ↷. The patient presented with tibial neuropathy.*

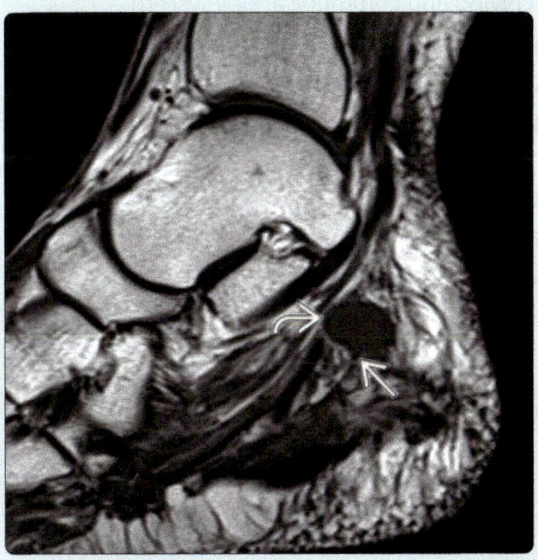
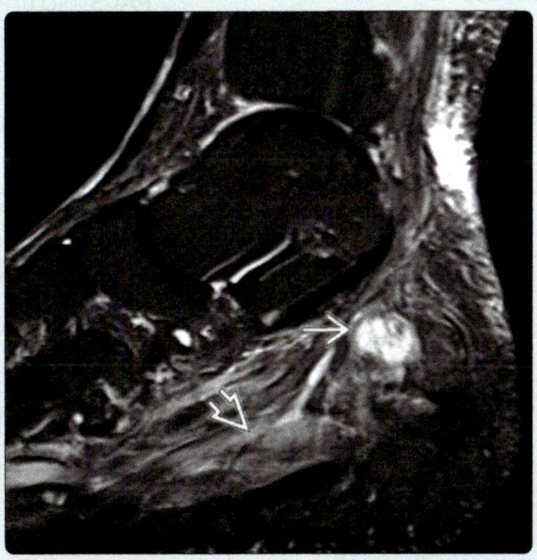

(Left) *Sagittal T1WI MR shows a low signal intensity mass ⇒ in the tarsal tunnel. The mass has a small "tail" ↷, characteristic of nerve sheath tumors. At surgery, this was found to be a malignant peripheral nerve sheath tumor.* **(Right)** *Sagittal STIR MR in the same patient shows that the mass → is heterogeneously high in signal intensity. The degree of heterogeneity is greater than expected for a synovial cyst. There is denervation edema in the abductor hallucis muscle ⇒.*

Radiology Abbreviation Index

A

ADC: apparent diffusion coefficient
AP: anteroposterior
ASL: arterial spin labeling

C

CBF: cerebral blood flow
CBV: cerebral blood volume
CECT: contrast-enhanced computed tomography
Cho: choline
CISS: constructive interference in steady state
Cr: chromium
CT: computed tomography
CTA: computed tomography angiography
CTP: computed tomography perfusion
CTV: computed tomography venography

D

DaT: dopamine transporter
DCE: dynamic contrast-enhanced (MR)
DSA: digital subtraction angiography
DSC: dynamic susceptibility contrast-enhanced (MR perfusion)
DST: dural sinus thrombosis
DTI: diffusion tensor imaging (MR)
DWI: diffusion-weighted imaging (MR)

E

ECD: Tc N,N'-l,2-ethylenediylbis-L-cysteine diethyl ester
EMG: electromyography
F-18 FDG: F-18 fluorodeoxyglucose
FIESTA: fast imaging employing steady-state acquisition
FISP: fast imaging with steady-state precession
FLAIR: fluid-attenuated inversion recovery
fMRI: functional magnetic resonance imaging
FSE T2: T2 fast-spin echo imaging
FS-PGR: focal segmental pulse-generated runoff

G

Glx: glutamic acid
GRE: gradient echo

H

HMPAO: hexamethylpropyleneamine oxime
HU: Hounsfield unit

K

kPS: endothelial transfer coefficient

L

Lac: lactate

M

MDCT: multidetector computed tomography
MIP: maximum intensity projection
MP-RAGE: magnetization-prepared rapid acquisition gradient echo
MR: magnetic resonance
MR T1: magnetic resonance T1
MRA: magnetic resonance angiography
MRP: magnetic resonance perfusion
MRS: magnetic resonance spectroscopy
MRV: magnetic resonance venography
MTT: mean transit time

N

NAA: N-acetylaspartate
NASCET: North American Symptomatic Carotid Endarterectomy Trial
NCS: nerve conduction study
NCV: nerve conduction velocity
NECT: nonenhanced computed tomography

P

PACS: picture archiving and communications system
PC: phase contrast
pCT: positron computed tomography
PD: pulsed Doppler (wave)
PET: positron emission tomography
PiB: Pittsburgh compound B
pMR: proton magnetic resonance
PWI: perfusion-weighted imaging (MR)

R

RF: radiofrequency

S

SPACE: sampling perfection with application optimized contrast with different flip-angle evolutions
SPECT: single photon emission computed tomography
SPGR: spoiled gradient echo
SSP: section sensitivity profile
STIR: short tau inversion recovery
SWI: susceptibility-weighted imaging

T

T1: spin lattice or longitudinal relaxation time (MR scan)
T1 C+: T1 contrast-enhanced (MR)
T1 C+ FS: T1 contrast enhanced with fat suppression
T1WI: T1-weighted imaging
T2: spin-spin or transverse relaxation time
T2*: T2 star, observed or effective T2
T2* GRE: gradient echo T2 star
T2* SWI: T2 star susceptibility-weighted imaging
T2WI: T2-weighted imaging
T2WI FS MR: T2-weighted magnetic resonance imaging with fat suppression
TE: echo time
TOF: time of flight
tPA: tissue plasminogen activator
TR: recovery time
TTP: time to peak

Numbers

11C: carbon-11
123-FP-CIT: [I-123]N-ω-co-fluoropropyl-2β-carbomethoxy-3β-(4-iodophenyl)nortropane
15O: oxygen-15
99mTC: technetium-99m

INDEX

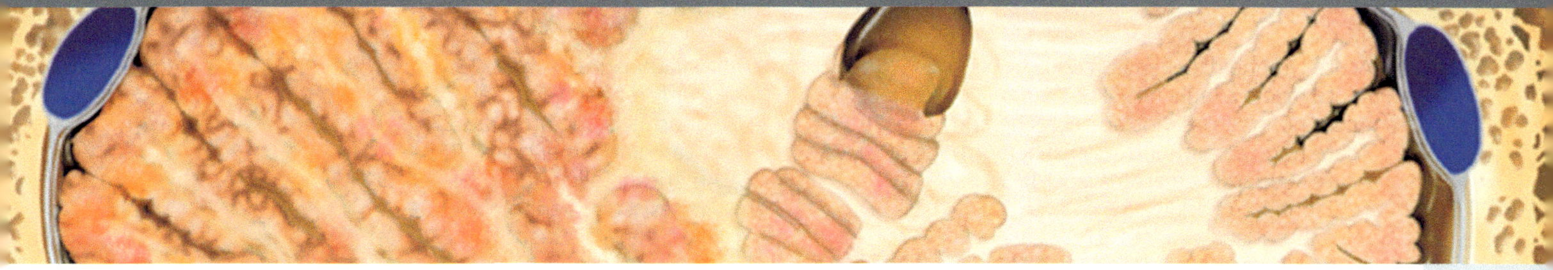

A

INDEX

INDEX

INDEX

B

INDEX

INDEX

INDEX

INDEX

D

INDEX

F

G

INDEX

H

I

J

K

L

INDEX

M

INDEX

INDEX

N

O

P

INDEX

INDEX

INDEX

T

INDEX

U

V

INDEX

W

X

Y

Z

9780323447812